PRACTICAL
PAEDIATRICS

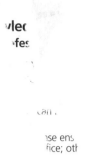

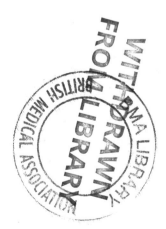

BRITISH MEDICAL ASSOCIATION

0872283

Commissioning Editor: Ellen Green
Development Editor: Lulu Stader
Project Manager: Andrew Palfreyman
Design Direction: Erik Bigland
Illustrator Manager: Bruce Hogarth
Illustrator: Antbits

PRACTICAL PAEDIATRICS

EDITED BY

Professor D. M. Roberton MD FRACP FRCPA
Pro Vice Chancellor, Division of Health Sciences
Dean, Faculty of Medicine
University of Otago
New Zealand

Professor M. South MB BS DCH MD MRCP FRACP FJFICM
Director, Department of General Medicine
Professor & Deputy Head of Paediatrics
University of Melbourne
Australia

SIXTH EDITION

WITHDRAWN FROM LIBRARY
BMA LIBRARY
BRITISH MEDICAL ASSO

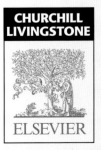

CHURCHILL LIVINGSTONE

ELSEVIER

EDINBURGH LONDON NEW YORK OXFORD PHILADELPHIA ST LOUIS SYDNEY TORONTO 2007

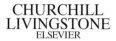

CHURCHILL
LIVINGSTONE
ELSEVIER

An imprint of Elsevier Limited

© 2006, Elsevier Limited.
© Longman Group UK Limited 1986, 1990, 1994. All rights reserved.

The right of Don Roberton and Mike South to be identified as editors of this work has been asserted by them in accordance with the Copyright, Designs and Patents Act 1988.

No part of this publication may be reproduced, stored in a retrieval system, or transmitted in any form or by any means, electronic, mechanical, photocopying, recording or otherwise, without the prior permission of the Publishers. Permissions may be sought directly from Elsevier's Health Sciences Rights Department, 1600 John F. Kennedy Boulevard, Suite 1800, Philadelphia, PA 19103–2899, USA: phone: (+1) 215 239 3804; fax: (+1) 215 239 3805; or, e-mail: *healthpermissions@elsevier.com*. You may also complete your request on-line via the Elsevier homepage (http://www.elsevier.com), by selecting 'Support and contact' and then 'Copyright and Permission'.

First edition 1986
Second edition 1990
Third edition 1994
Fourth edition 1998
Fifth edition 2003
Sixth edition 2007

ISBN: 978 0-443-10280-6

British Library Cataloguing in Publication Data
A catalogue record for this book is available from the British Library

Library of Congress Cataloging in Publication Data
A catalog record for this book is available from the Library of Congress

Notice
Medical knowledge is constantly changing. As new information becomes available, changes in treatment, procedures, equipment and the use of drugs become necessary. The editors, contributors and the publishers have taken care to ensure that the information given in this text is accurate and up to date. However, readers are strongly advised to confirm that the information, especially with regard to drug usage, complies with the latest legislation and standards of practice.

ELSEVIER | your source for books, journals and multimedia in the health sciences
www.elsevierhealth.com

Working together to grow
libraries in developing countries

www.elsevier.com | www.bookaid.org | www.sabre.org

ELSEVIER | BOOK AID International | Sabre Foundation

The publisher's policy is to use **paper manufactured from sustainable forests**

Printed in China

Preface

Welcome to the 6th edition of *Practical Paediatrics*.

Practical Paediatrics was first published in 1986. The initiative for the development of the textbook came from Professor Max Robinson, a member of the Department of Paediatrics of the University of Melbourne, and Max was the foundation editor. The concept was to provide a paediatric text for medical students that would be user friendly, practical in its approach to learning of the needs of children and their families, relevant to curricula in Australia and New Zealand, the Asia–Pacific region and internationally, be up to date in its information, and available at a reasonable price.

Practical Paediatrics has more than met all of these objectives. There has been a new edition approximately every 4 years and we are pleased now to have the opportunity to publish the 6th edition.

It is a source of pride that the textbook has a very wide international following. It is used by medical students, doctors training in paediatrics and other specialty areas in medicine, primary care practitioners, nurses and allied health trainees and practitioners, and many other health professional groups.

Max Robinson has been an editor of all editions up to and including edition 5. Following his retirement from active academic life, he felt that he should also retire from editorial duties for edition 6. However, he retains an active involvement, with coauthorship of one of the chapters of edition 6. We thank Max for his initiative and for all that he has contributed to *Practical Paediatrics*. Its success has been due to his strong contributions, knowledge and authorship.

It was a challenge to find someone to match Max Robinson's enthusiasm and interest. It is a source of great pleasure to Max that Professor Mike South, also of the Department of Paediatrics of the University of Melbourne, agreed to become a coeditor of the 6th edition of *Practical Paediatrics*. Mike is a general paediatrician and a paediatric intensivist, and has a strong and active interest in evidence-based medicine and evidence-based teaching and learning.

The 6th edition of *Practical Paediatrics* continues the approach of the preceding editions. In this edition, all content has been revised, often extensively, and there are new sections such as International Child Health, Obesity in Childhood and Adolescence, and Child and Adolescent Gynaecology.

The layout of the textbook has been changed to incorporate sections on topics as components of larger chapters. In edition 6 we welcome many new authors and, as for previous editions, we thank those who have written for *Practical Paediatrics* in the past.

Reading lists and up-to-date websites that give useful academic and parent and family information have been included as in edition 5. An innovation for this edition, however, is that these, along with the Self Assessment Questions, are now available on a website which is accessible by purchasers of the textbook. This allows easy searching of the reading lists, linkages to the websites, and also linkages to online sections of the textbook itself. There are many new Self Assessment Questions, which have been a popular feature, providing a practical assessment of learning by testing problem-solving skills. The answers to each question are accompanied by a rationale explaining the reasons for the answers.

Many new Clinical Examples have been incorporated to assist the reader place information in context and to aid the learning process. An innovation in edition 6 is the incorporation of highlighted Practical Points in each section to emphasis key issues, and also as an aid to revision.

The 6th edition of *Practical Paediatrics* is the last to have Ellen Green of Elsevier as commissioning editor. She has been a great friend and mentor, and we wish her the very best in her well-earned retirement. As editors, we owe a great deal to our superb development editor, Dr Lulu Stader. She has continually worked with us to manage, edit and improve the content of this edition (from her workplace in the wilds of the beautiful north-west of Scotland) and we are deeply grateful to her for her patience and expertise.

We hope that you will find this edition of *Practical Paediatrics* useful, and that it assists with developing an understanding and interest in the health needs of children, their families and their communities.

Don Roberton   Mike South
Dunedin, New Zealand   Melbourne, Australia

Contributors

Dr George Alex MBBS, MMed, MRCP, FRACP, PhD
Department of Gastroenterology, Royal Children's
  Hospital, Parkville, Victoria, Australia
The child with diarrhoea

Dr Mike Anscombe MBChB, FRACP, DipClinEpi
Department of Paediatric Emergency Medicine,
  Mater Children's Hospital, South Brisbane,
  Queensland, Australia
Child injury

Professor Jennifer Batch
Professor of Paediatrics & Child Health, Royal
  Children's Hospital, Herston, Queensland,
  Australia
Growth and variations of growth

Professor Louise Baur MBBS, BSc(Med), PhD, FRACP
Discipline of Paediatrics & Child Health,
  University of Sydney, The Children's Hospital at
  Westmead, New South Wales, Australia
Obesity in children and adolescents

Professor Spencer Beasley MBChB(Otago),
  MS(Melbourne), FRACS
Chief of Child Health Services, Christchurch
  Hospital, Christchurch, New Zealand
Abdominal pain and vomiting in children
Acute neonatal surgical conditions
Common surgical conditions in children

Professor Bruce Benjamin AO, OBE, FRACS, DLO,
  FAAP, FACS (Hon)
Killara, New South Wales, Australia
*Ear, nose and throat, and head and neck surgery
  problems*

Professor Julie Bines MBBS, FRACP, MD
Department of Gastroenterology and Clinical
  Nutrition, Royal Children's Hospital, Parkville,
  Victoria, Australia
Nutrition

Professor David Brewster AM, BA(Hons), MD, MPH,
  FRACP, PhD
Dean, Fiji School of Medicine, Suva, Fiji Islands
Infections in tropical and developing countries
The child who needs fluid replacement

Dr Justin Brown MBBChir, MA, MRCP, FRACP
Department of Endocrinology & Diabetes, Royal
  Children's Hospital, Parkville, Victoria,
  Australia
Thyroid disorders in childhood

Dr Leo Buchanan
Paediatrician, Lower Hutt Hospital, Wellington,
  New Zealand
Indigenous culture and health

Assistant Professor Fergus Cameron BMedSci, MBBS,
  DipRACOG, FRACP, MD
Department of Endocrinology & Diabetes, Royal
  Children's Hospital, Parkville, Victoria,
  Australia
Thyroid disorders in childhood

Professor Jonathan Carapetis MBBS, BMedSc, FRACP,
  FAFPHM, PhD
Department of Paediatrics, Royal Children's
  Hospital, Parkville, Victoria, Australia
Infections of bone and joints

Associate Professor Anne Chang MBBS, FRACP,
  MPHTH, PhD
Department of Respiratory Medicine, Royal
  Children's Hospital, Herston, Queensland,
  Australia
*An approach to chronic cough and cystic fibrosis in
  children*

Dr Kevin Collins MBBS, FRACP
Senior Paediatric Neurologist, Monash Medical
  Centre, Darling, Victoria, Australia
Cerebral palsy and neuro-degenerative disease

Professor Jennifer Couper MBChB, MD, FRACP
Professor of Paediatrics and Child Health, Women
  & Children's Hospital, Adelaide, South
  Australia, Australia
Childhood diabetes

Dr Peter Cundy MBBS, FRACS
Senior Visiting Orthopaedic Surgeon, Woman's &
  Children's Hospital, North Adelaide, South
  Australia, Australia
*Common paediatric orthopaedic problems and
  fractures*

Professor Brian Darlow MA, MD, FRCP, FRACP, FRCPCH
Department of Paediatrics, Christchurch School of
  Medicine & Health Sciences, Christchurch, New
  Zealand
The newborn infant: stabilization and examination

Professor Geoff Davidson MBBS, MD, FRACP
Director, Centre for Paediatric & Adolescent
  Gastroenterology, Women's & Children's
  Hospital, Adelaide, South Australia, Australia
Gastro-oesophageal reflux and H pylori

Professor Martin Delatycki MBBS, FRACP, PhD
Genetic Health Services Victoria, Royal Children's
  Hospital, Flemington Road, Parkville, Victoria,
  Australia
Genetic counselling

Dr Terry Donald
Women's and Children's Hospital, North Adelaide,
  South Australia, Australia
Child abuse

Associate Professor Trevor Duke MD, FRACP, FJFICM
Centre International Child Health, Royal
  Children's Hospital, Parkville, Victoria,
  Australia
International child health
The child who needs fluid replacement

Dr Daryl Efron MBBS, FRACP, MD
Royal Children's Hospital, Flemington Road,
  Parkville, Victoria, Australia
Failure to thrive

Dr James E Elder MBBS, FRANZCO, FRACS
Melbourne Children's Eye Clinic, Royal Children's
  Hospital, Parkville, Victoria, Australia
Eye disorders in childhood

Dr Jan Fairchild MBBS, FRACP
Paediatric Endocrinologist, Women's and
  Children's Hospital, Adelaide, South Australia,
  Australia
The child of uncertain sex

Dr Peter Flett
Calvary Health Care Tasmania, Hobart, Tasmania,
  Australia
*Large heads, hydrocephalus and neural tube
  defects*

Professor David Forbes MBBS, FRACP
Department of Paediatrics, Princess Margaret
  Hospital for Children, University of Western
  Australia, Perth, Western Australia, Australia
Liver diseases in childhood

Professor Kevin Forsyth MB, ChB, MD, PhD, FRACP,
  FRCPA
Head of Paediatrics & Child Health, Flinders
  University & Medical Centre, South Australia,
  Australia
Electronic learning resources

Dr Mike Gold
Paediatric Allergist, Women's & Children's
  Hospital, North Adelaide, South Australia,
  Australia
The atopic child

Dr Brian Graetz PhD, MPsych(Clin), BA(Hons), DipT
Clinical Psychologist, Women's & Children's
  Hospital, North Adelaide, South Australia,
  Australia
*Common child and adolescent mental health
  problems*

Professor Keith Grimwood ONZM, MD, FRACP
Professor & Head of Department of Paediatrics &
  Child Health, Wellington School of Medicine,
  Wellington, New Zealand
Meningitis and encephalitis

Associate Professor Sonia Grover MBBS, FRANZCOG, MD
Clifton Hill, Melbourne, Victoria, Australia
Child and adolescent gynaecology

Professor Jane Harding FRACP, DPhil
Department of Paediatrics, University of
  Auckland, Auckland, New Zealand
*Low birth weight, prematurity and jaundice in
  infancy*

Dr Simon Harvey MD, FRACP
Department of Neurology, Royal Children's
  Hospital, Parkville, Victoria, Australia
Seizures and epilepsies

Professor Richard Henry MBBS, FRACP, DipClinEpi
Deputy Dean, Faculty of Medicine, University of
  New South Wales, Sydney, Australia
Asthma
Wheezing disorders other than asthma

Dr Harriet Hiscock MB BS, FRACP, MD, GradDip
  Epidemiology & Biostatistics
Centre for Community Child Health, Royal
  Children's Hospital, Parkville, Victoria 3052,
  Australia
Life events of normal children

Dr Neil Hotham B. Pharm
Senior Specialist Drug Information Pharmacist,
  Women's & Children's Hospital, North Adelaide,
  South Australia, Australia
Birth defects, prenatal diagnosis and teratogens

Professor David Isaacs MBBChir, MD, FRACP,
  FRCPCH
Senior Staff Specialist, Paediatric Infectious
  Diseases, Children's Hospital, Westmead, New
  South Wales, Australia
Infectious diseases of childhood

Dr Christine Jeffries-Stokes MBBS, BMedSc, FRACP,
  MPH
Senior Lecturer, Department of Paediatrics,
  University of Western Australia, Kalgoorlie,
  Western Australia, Australia
Indigenous culture and health

Professor Colin Jones MBBS, FRACP, PhD
Director, Department of Nephrology, Royal
  Children's Hospital, Parkville, Victoria,
  Australia
Urinary tract infections and malformations
Bone mineral disorders

Dr Andrew Kennedy MBBS, FRACP
Adolescent Physician Centre for Adolescent Health,
  Royal Children's Hospital, Parkville, Victoria,
  Australia
Care of the adolescent

Professor Nicky Kilpatrick BDS, PhD, FDS, RCPS
Senior Dental Surgeon, Royal Children's Hospital,
  Parkville, Victoria, Australia
Disorders of teeth and the oral cavity

Associate Professor Andrew Kornberg MBBS(Hons),
  Dip TA (ATAA), FRACP
Paediatric Neurologist, Royal Children's Hospital,
  Parkville, Victoria, Australia
Neuromuscular disorders

Professor Peter LeSouëf MBBS, FRACP, MD
School of Paediatrics and Child Health, University
  of West Australia, and Department of
  Paediatrics, Children's Hospital Medical Centre,
  Perth, Western Australia, Australia
*Lower respiratory tract infections and abnormalities
  in childhood*

Dr Jan Liebelt MBBS(Hons), FRACP, MSc
SA Clinical Genetics Service, Women's &
  Children's Hospital, North Adelaide, South
  Australia, Australia
Birth defects, prenatal diagnosis and teratogens

Dr Zoe McCallum MBBS, FRACP
Senior Lecturer, Department of Paediatrics, Royal
  Children's Hospital, Parkville, Victoria, Australia
Nutrition

Dr James McGill MBBS(Hons), FRACP
Department of Metabolic Medicine, Royal
  Children's Hospital, Herston, Queensland,
  Australia
Inborn errors of metabolism

Dr Steven McTaggart MBBS, FRACP, PhD
Child and Adolescent Renal Service, Royal
  Children's Hospital, Herston, Queensland,
  Australia
Glomerular disease, renal failure and hypertension

Dr David Meldrum
Chatswood Assessment Centre, Royal North Shore
  Hospital, Chatswood, New South Wales, Australia
Developmental surveillance

Professor Craig Mellis MBBS, MPH, MD, FRACP
Associate Dean, Clinical School, University of
  Sydney, Sydney, Australia
Acute upper respiratory infections in childhood

Professor Paul Monagle MBBS (Hons) (Monash) M.Sc.
  (Health Research Methodology, McMaster) M.D. (Monash)
  FRACP, FRCPA, FCCP
Director, Department of Clinical Haematology
  Royal Children's Hospital, Melbourne
Chair, Head of Department, Department of
  Pathology the University of Melbourne
Anaemias of childhood

Dr Kevin Murray
Department of Rheumatology, Princess Margaret
  Hospital for Children, Perth, Western Australia,
  Australia
Arthritis and connective tissue disorders

Professor Barry Nurcombe
Director, Child & Adolescent Psychiatry, Royal
  Brisbane Hospital, Queensland, Australia
Major psychiatric disorders

Professor Frank Oberklaid AOM, MD, FRACP, DCH
Director, Centre for Community Child Health,
  Royal Children's Hospital, Parkville, Victoria,
  Australia
Life events of normal children

Associate Professor Mark Oliver
Department of Gastroenterology and Clinical
  Nutrition, Royal Children's Hospital, Parkville,
  Victoria, Australia
The child with diarrhoea

Dr Tracey O'Brien FRACP, MBChB, MHL, BSc
Paediatric and Adolescent Haematologist/Oncologist,
  Head, Cord and Marrow Transplant Program,
  Sydney Children's Hospital, Randwick, New
  South Wales 2031, Australia
Childhood cancers

Dr Mike O'Callaghan MBBS, FRACP MSc
Child Development & Rehabilitation, Mater
  Children's Hospital, South Brisbane,
  Queensland, Australia
Developmental disability

Dr Edward O'Loughlin MBBS, MD, FRACP
Department of Gastroenterology, The Children's
  Hospital, Westmead, New South Wales, Australia
Malabsorption

Dr Rod Phillips MBBS, FRACP, PhD
Paediatric Skin Specialist, Royal Children's
  Hospital, Parkville, Victoria, Australia
Skin lesions in systemic disease

Dr W. Robert Pitt MBBS, FRACP, FACEM
Director, Paediatric Emergency Medicine, Mater
  Children's Hospital, South Brisbane,
  Queensland, Australia
Child injury

Dr Nicola Poplawski MBChB, FRACP, MD
Adelaide, South Australia, Australia
Modern genetics

Dr Jeremy Raftos
Head, Paediatric Emergency Department, Women's
  & Children's Hospital, North Adelaide, South
  Australia, Australia
Causes and assessment

Professor Dinah Reddihough MD, BSc, FRACP, FAFRM
Director, Department of Child Development and
  Rehabilitation, Royal Children's Hospital,
  Parkville, Victoria, Australia
Cerebral palsy and neuro-degenerative disease

Dr Peter Richmond MBBS, MRCP, FRACP
Department of Paediatrics, Princess Margaret
  Hospital for Children, Perth, Western Australia,
  Australia
Immunization

Professor Don Roberton MD (Otago), FRACP, FRCPA
Pro Vice Chancellor, Division of Health Sciences,
  and Dean of Medicine, University of Otago,
  Dunedin, New Zealand
The clinical consultation: history taking & examination
Immunization
Arthritis and connective tissue disorders

Professor Maxwell Robinson AM, MBBS, MD, FRACP
Mt Martha, Victoria, Australia
Infections in tropical and developing countries

Dr Maureen Rogers MBBS, FACD
Emeritus Consultant in Dermatology, Children's
  Hospital Medical Centre, Westmead, New South
  Wales, Australia
Skin disorders in infancy and childhood

Dr Remo Russo MBBS, FRACP, FAFRM (RACP)
Senior Visiting Medical Specialist, Women's &
  Children's Hospital, Adelaide, South Australia,
  Australia
Large heads, hydrocephalus and neural tube defects

Professor Susan Sawyer
Director, Centre for Adolescent Health, Royal
  Children's Hospital, Parkville, Victoria,
  Australia and Professor of Adolescent Health,
  Department of Paediatrics, The University of
  Melbourne, Melbourne, Australia
Care of the adolescent
*An approach to chronic cough and cystic fibrosis in
  children*

Professor Michael Sawyer
Professor in Child and Adolescent Mental Health,
  University of Adelaide, and Head, Research and
  Evaluation Unit, Women's and Children's
  Hospital, Adelaide, South Australia, Australia
Common child and adolescent mental health problems

Dr Ben Saxon MBBS, FRACP, FRCPA
Department of Haematology & Oncology, Women's
  & Children's Hospital, Adelaide, South
  Australia, Australia
Abnormal bleeding and clotting

Professor Jill Sewell MBBS, FRACP
Deputy Director, Centre for Community Child
  Health, Royal Children's Hospital, Parkville,
  Victoria, Australia
Hyperactive and inattentive children

Professor Peter Sly MBBS, FRACP, MDDSc
Head, Division of Clinical Sciences, Institute for
  Child Health Research, Perth, Western
  Australia, Australia
Croup and stridor

Professor Mike South (UK) FRACP, MD, F JFICM
Paediatrician and Specialist in Intensive Care,
  Director, Department of General Medicine,
  Professor & Deputy Head of Paediatrics,
  University of Melbourne, Australia
*The clinical consultation – history taking and
  examination*
Emergency care of the collapsed child

Dr Mike Starr MBBS, FRACP
Paediatrician, Infectious Diseases Physician,
  Consultant in emergency Medicine, Director of
  Paediatric Physician Training, Royal Children's
  Hospital, Parkville, Victoria, Australia
Congenital and perinatal infections

Dr David Starte
Senior Staff Specialist in Developmental
  Paediatrics, Royal North Shore Hospital,
  Chatswood, New South Wales, Australia
Developmental surveillance

Geoffrey Stokes
Wongutha Birni Aboriginal Corporation,
  University of Western Australia, Kalgoorlie,
  Western Australia, Australia
Indigenous culture and health

Dr Andrew Steer MBBS
Clinical and Public Health Research Fellow,
  Medical Coordinator Fiji, Suva, Fiji Islands
Infections of bone and joints

Dr Graeme Suthers PhD, FRACP, FRCPA
SA Clinical Genetics Service, Children's, Youth's and Women's Health Service, North Adelaide, South Australia, Australia
Modern genetics

Professor Barry Taylor
Professor of Paediatrics & Child Health, University of Otago, Dunedin, New Zealand
SIDS and unexpected death in infancy

Professor Rita Teele MD, FRANZCR
Radiologist, Gloucester, Massachusetts, United States of America
Diagnostic imaging in infancy and childhood

Dr Elizabeth Thompson MBBS, MD, FRACP
Clinical Geneticist, SA Clinical Genetics Service, Women's & Children's Hospital, North Adelaide, South Australia, Australia
The dysmorphic child

Associate Professor James Tibballs BMedSci(Hons), MBBS, MEd, MBA, MD, MHlth & MedLaw, FANZCA, FJFICM, FACTM
Intensive Care Physician, Intensive Care Unit, Royal Children's Hospital, Parkville, Victoria, Australia
Principal Fellow, Australian Venom Research Unit, Department of Pharmacology, University of Melbourne, Australia
Poisoning and envenomation

Professor David Tudehope
Director, Neonatology, Mater Mother's Hospital, South Brisbane, Queensland, Australia
Breathing problems arising in the newborn period

Professor Graham Vimpani
Director, Child Adolescent & Family Health Service, Hunter Children's Health Network, Wallsend, New South Wales, Australia
Child health and disease

Associate Professor Neil Wigg MBBS, FRACP, MPolAdmin
Director, Community Child Health Services, Fortitude Valley, Queensland, Australia
The child and the family

Dr Ian Wilkinson MBBS, FRACP
Paediatric Neurologist, John Hunter Hospital, Newcastle, New South Wales, Australia
Children with headaches

Professor James Wilkinson MBChB, FRACP, FRCP, FRCPCH, FACC
Senior Cardiologist, Royal Children's Hospital, Parkville, Victoria, Australia
Assessment of the infant and child with suspected heart disease
Common heart defects and diseases in infancy and childhood

Dr Melanie Wong
Department of Immunology and Infectious Diseases, The Children's Hospital at Westmead, Westmead, New South Wales, Australia
Immunodeficiency and its investigation

Contents

PART 1

CURRENT PAEDIATRICS

Child health and disease 1.1

G. Vimpani

Children and young people (up to the age of 24 years) comprise approximately one-third of the population of Australia.

Some statistics relevant to children and young people in Australia are:

- 19.5% of the Australian population is aged 0–14 years – 38.9% of the indigenous population is aged less than 14 years
- 13.8% of the Australian population is aged 15–24 years – 18.4% of the indigenous population is aged 15–24 years
- 4.5% of Australian children are indigenous
- 86% of Australian children live in south-eastern mainland states
- 5.8% were born overseas – 38% in Asia; 36% have at least one overseas-born parent
- 32% of births are ex-nuptial; nearly 20% of children live in single-parent families
- one in every five children will experience divorce of their parents before their 16th birthday
- 27% of under-2-year-old children participate in formal child care
- just under 12% of children under 14 years live in relative poverty.
- Australia ranks 18th of 26 Organisation for Economic Co-operation and Development (OECD) countries in the proportion of children living in circumstances below 50% of the national median income.

Australia is a highly urbanized nation with a total estimated population in 2004 of 20.1 million, of whom 1.26 million (6.3%) are children aged less than 5 years, 2.72 million (13.6%) are children aged 5–14 years and 2.76 million (13.7%) are young people aged 15–24 years (Table 1.1.1). Following colonization in the 18th century, the proportion of children declined to a low of 24% in 1943 but increased steadily with the baby boom of the 1950s, levelling out at about 30%.

Since then, although the actual number of children aged 0–14 years has increased, the proportion has decreased to a record low of 19.5%. This decline is due mainly to a drop in fertility, from 3.4 children per woman in the baby boom years to the current level of 1.77 children per woman. The projected child population proportion (aged 0–14 years) in the year 2051 is between 12% and 15%, or 2.8–4.8 million.

The majority (86%) of Australian children live in the south-eastern mainland states. 63.5% live in major cities with populations greater than 100 000, with 22% living in inner regional areas, 11% in outer regional areas and less than 5% in remote areas. Children living in rural and remote areas comprise a larger proportion of the total population in those areas.

About 5% of Australia's children were born overseas: 14% of these are from the UK and Ireland, 12% come from other European countries, 38% from Asia and 13% from New Zealand. Reflecting the cosmopolitan nature of Australia today, at least 36% of all Australian children have at least one parent who was born in a country other than Australia. Over 179 000 or about 4.5% of the child population are indigenous and these account for around 39% of all indigenous Australians.

Between 1950 and 2004 the proportion of ex-nuptial births rose from around 5% to 32% – about half of these were to women in de facto relationships. Between 1986 and 2001, the number of one-parent families in Australia increased by 53%. In contrast, the number of couple families with children increased by 3%.

Couple families (two parents or carers, married or de facto) now include 81.3% of children under 15 years, while 18.7% live in one-parent families. Of children living in single-parent families, 70% live with a parent who is separated or divorced, 20% with a parent who never married and 10% with a widowed parent. Of 978 000 children living with only one natural parent in 1997, most (88%) lived with their mother in either a one-parent (68%) or in step- or blended families (20%). Of all divorced couples, 50% involve at least one child – 62% of these children being aged less than 10 years. About one in five children will experience their parents' divorce before their 16th birthday. Children in single-parent families fare less well socially, educationally and physically than children in two-parent families, often because of the accompanying socioeconomic disadvantage these families experience.

The June 2002 Labour Force Survey showed that, in more than half (57%) of all couple families with

Table 1.1.1 Estimated Australian population of children and young people (by age and state), 2004

Age (years)	State/Territory								Australia	% of Australian population
	NSW	Vic	Q'ld	SA	WA	Tas	NT	ACT		
0–4	423 957	305 696	250 870	88 626	123 994	30 153	17 458	20 232	1 262 247	6.27
5–9	441 603	320 104	268 225	96 222	133 517	32 491	16 634	20 984	1 330 019	6.66
10–14	458 573	333 260	280 579	100 902	141 170	34 427	16 308	22 000	1 387 485	6.90
15–19	450 213	329 929	272 420	102 605	142 676	34 166	14 614	23 624	1 370 457	6.82
20–24	454 546	347 189	275 639	101 594	139 171	30 139	15 906	27 982	1 392 312	6.92

children aged less than 15 years, both parents were employed. It was more common for families to have a father employed full-time and a mother employed part-time than for both parents to be employed full-time (34% compared with 19%). Lone parents were less likely to be in the labour force than parents in couple families. Close to one-third of lone fathers (30%) and almost half of lone mothers (47%) were not in the labour force.

Between 1984 and 2002 the proportion of under-2-year-olds in formal (or formal and informal) child care increased from 8% to 41%; for 4-year-olds the proportion in 2002 was 83%. Care was used for less than 10 hours per week for 45%, while 6% used it for more than 45 hours per week. The type of care involved largely depends on the age of the child. 73% of the children under 2 years in formal care are in long-day-care centres, with around 21% in family day care. 39% are involved in informal care from friends and relatives. Only 52% of 4-year-olds are in pre-primary or primary education, the seventh lowest performing country in the OECD.

Poverty is a well-known determinant of population health. The term 'poverty' means different things to different people. There are three different approaches to defining poverty:

- *absolute poverty* – where a family's income does not pay for basic necessities such as shelter and food
- *relative poverty* – where a family's income is low in comparison to the income of other families
- *subjective poverty* – where a poor family is defined as one that believes its income is inadequate for its needs.

Most developed countries, including Australia, adopt the relative approach. UNICEF estimates that one in six children in industrialized countries live in relative poverty. The data on the prevalence of child poverty in Australia since the mid-1990s are confusing. According to UNICEF Australia's rank is behind

many European countries, coming 18th of 23 wealthy countries in 2000, with 14.7% of its children aged under 14 years living in households with incomes lower than 50% of the national median, although Australia performed relatively well in reducing child poverty rates towards the end of the 1990s. However, the OECD estimates that the child poverty rate in Australia (ranked 10th out of 24 countries) was around 12% in 2000. The UNICEF data are consistent with other Australian data (HILDA) showing a recent improvement in poverty rates, with a decline from 16.7% to 14.5% from 2001–2003. However, the overall rate of relative poverty among indigenous children is three times higher than that for non-indigenous children.

Changes in disease patterns

The health status of children has always reflected an interaction between biological susceptibility and their experience of the physical, chemical and psychosocial environment. Greater understanding of the role of gene–environment interactions in child health outcomes is occurring as the result of interdisciplinary research such as that involving the Dunedin, New Zealand longitudinal study cohort, where it has been shown that abused children are much more likely to develop later antisocial behaviour if they carry a particular variant of the monoamine oxidase transporter gene.

Paediatrics has changed dramatically during the last 50 years, as the mortality for all life-threatening conditions: infectious disease in particular has declined substantially (Fig. 1.1.1). Although improved levels of education, housing, hygiene, immunization and antibiotics have not entirely eliminated infectious disease (e.g. the emergence of HIV/AIDS), the morbidity and mortality due to infection, particularly for those aged 14 years and younger, has been reduced markedly in developed societies.

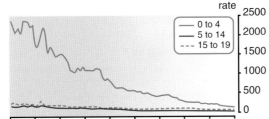

rate

	2500
0 to 4	2000
5 to 14	1500
15 to 19	1000
	500
	0

1907 1917 1927 1937 1947 1957 1967 1977 1987 1997

Rate per 100 000 population.
Source: AIHW Mortality Monitoring System

Fig. 1.1.1 Death due to all causes, by age of child. Source: Australian Institute of Health and Welfare (AIHW) Mortality Monitoring System.

Table 1.1.2 Domains of child health

Health domain	Description
1. Longevity	Projected life expectancy
2. Activity	Functional status, ability/disability
3. Comfort	Symptoms
4. Satisfaction	Satisfaction with own health
5. Disease	Presence and progression of defined disease states
6. Achievement	Social and emotional development
7. Resilience	Ability to resist threats to health

After Starfield B 1987 Journal of Chronic Diseases 40(Suppl 1): 109s–115s.

Examples of the declining incidence of infectious disease are many, but of particular importance is the greatly reduced incidence of tuberculosis; chronic suppuration of chest, bone and ear; rheumatic fever and rheumatic heart disease, and streptococcal infections of all types. It should be noted that the incidence of all infections was falling well before the advent of antibiotic and chemotherapeutic drugs, which, incorrectly, have often been given the major credit for control of infection.

In contrast, some other childhood diseases have shown a rising prevalence, for which the causes are unclear. There has been an increase in the prevalence of asthma symptoms (present in around 20% of children in community surveys) and hospital admissions, with asthma now the leading cause of admission of children to hospital. In addition, new challenges have been posed by the emergence of what have been termed 'problems of developmental health and wellbeing' that are related to extensive changes in social and family life during the past 30 years. Examples are child maltreatment, behaviour and learning problems, youth suicide, obesity and other eating disorders, substance misuse and early onset of criminal behaviour.

Child health

In evaluating disease incidence and the health status of a community, mortality and morbidity figures are used. There has been a centuries old traditional focus on mortality, partly because of compulsory reporting of death in most countries. However, mortality is a very crude index of health and is of limited value in assessing the health status and health needs of a community. A strict disease focus cannot describe the full spectrum of child health. An important difference between child and adolescent health compared with adult health is that the young person is developing rapidly, a process in which genetic and environmental influences are critical. In this transactional process, 'goodness of fit' between young people and their environments is a determinant of good outcomes, including the impact of disease and disorder on functional capacity. The 1946 World Health Organization (WHO) definition defines health as 'a state of complete physical, mental, and social well-being and not merely the absence of disease or infirmity'. A more practical and complete way of thinking about child health involves the seven categories shown in Table 1.1.2.

Describing health therefore requires more than a consideration of morbidity and mortality. It is similarly important to understand risk and protective factors and behaviours that may have positive and negative impacts on health. From a practical point of view, complete paediatric clinical assessment requires a consideration of all of the above domains. This applies equally to the child with leukaemia, cystic fibrosis, acute bacterial meningitis, developmental delay, child maltreatment, behaviour problems or even a child who presents for a well child review.

Mortality

Changing patterns of mortality

Important components of changes in mortality in Australia are:

- increasing life expectancy (77.4 for men, 82.6 for women in 2002) – but for the indigenous population in Australia it is about 20 years less

- improved neonatal mortality associated with better perinatal care. The current neonatal mortality rate (2003) is below 3 per 1000 for the first time
- improved postneonatal mortality associated with the declining rate of sudden unexplained deaths in infancy (SUDi)
- the indigenous infant mortality rate (13.0/1000 live births) is nearly three times higher than the non-indigenous rate (5.0/1000), although the indigenous rate has declined by 3.3% per year. Australia's infant mortality rates are in the mid range for OECD countries
- the indigenous 1–14-year-old mortality rate is 36.9 per 100 000, compared to 16.2 per 100 000 in non-indigenous Australians
- 40% of deaths in 1–14-year-olds are due to unintentional injury, despite a 59% fall since 1979
- cancer accounts for 31% of deaths due to acquired disease
- declining infectious disease mortality has been consolidated by universal immunization programmes
- an 'excess' of deaths of young children (100 per year) occurs in rural and remote areas, 30 of each 100 being non-indigenous
- substantial declines in traffic accident mortality in adolescents (52% males, 21% females since 1961), although the rate of decline has flattened out in the last 5 years
- 40% increase in adolescent male suicide deaths from 1979 until 1997, with a subsequent unexplained fall
- 7.4% of youth deaths in 1998 were related to drug dependence, although the rate has subsequently declined.

The WHO and Australian Bureau of Statistics (ABS) definitions shown in Table 1.1.3 are important in collecting data on mortality. Many countries do not use the WHO definitions, and the ABS alternatives in relevant categories are detailed. Caution should, therefore, always be exercised in comparing published mortality rates internationally.

Life expectancy at birth in Australia increased substantially throughout the course of the 20th century, largely as a result of improved infant and child mortality, and is among the highest in the world. Life expectancy in Australia in 2002 was 77.4 years for males and 82.6 years for females. Regrettably, indigenous children can expect to live about 20 years less than the rest of the Australian population.

Infant mortality rates are important indicators of child health, particularly when analysed as component neonatal and postneonatal rates. Neonatal mortality has always been influenced by pregnancy complications and fetal growth and development, including the presence of congenital anomalies, whereas postneonatal mortality rates are more commonly related to social and environmental conditions. Since the 1920s in Australia, when both these rates were very high, there has been a rapid decline, especially in postneonatal mortality, as social and environmental conditions improved and infectious disease was progressively controlled. With the advent of neonatal intensive care in the late 1960s, the neonatal mortality rate declined even further, to the point where, today, neonatal and postneonatal rates are again at similar, albeit much lower, levels. Despite these improvements in neonatal mortality rates, it is

Table 1.1.3 Definitions of mortality and mortality rates

		WHO		Australian Bureau of Statistics (ABS)	
	Description	Birth weight (g)	Gestation (weeks)	Birth weight (g)	Gestation (weeks)
Stillbirth	Stillborn infant	≥1000	≥28	≥500	≥22
Neonatal death	Death within 7 days of birth (ABS within 28 days)	≥1000	≥28	≥500	≥22
Infant death	Death within 1 year of birth	≥1000		≥500	
Live birth	Any birth that shows signs of life after being born				
Perinatal mortality rate	Stillbirths plus neonatal deaths per 1000 births, live and still				
Infant mortality	Infant deaths per 1000 live births				
Postneonatal mortality rate	Infant deaths between 28 days and 1 year per 1000 live births				

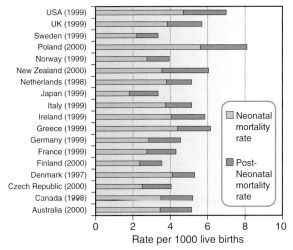

Neonatal & post neonatal mortality

USA (1999)
UK (1999)
Sweden (1999)
Poland (2000)
Norway (1999)
New Zealand (2000)
Netherlands (1998)
Japan (1999)
Italy (1999)
Ireland (1999)
Greece (1999)
Germany (1999)
France (1999)
Finland (2000)
Denmark (1997)
Czech Republic (2000)
Canada (1998)
Australia (2000)

☐ Neonatal mortality rate

☐ Post-Neonatal mortality rate

Rate per 1000 live births

Fig. 1.1.2 Neonatal, postneonatal and infant mortality rates, selected countries, latest year available.

Table 1.1.4 Causes of neonatal deaths in Victoria, Australia, 2004		
Cause of death	No. (terminations)	%
Non-malformations		
Spontaneous preterm	69	
Specific perinatal conditions	17	
Hypoxic peripartum death	14	
Antepartum haemorrhage	9	
No obstetric antecedent	8	
Hypertension	7	
Infection	6	
Fetal growth restriction	4	
Other maternal conditions	3	
Subtotal	*137*	*66*
Malformations		
Chromosomal abnormalities	17 (11)	
Central nervous system abnormalities	11 (6)	
Urinary tract abnormalities	10 (4)	
Multiple abnormalities	9 (5)	
Cardiovascular system abnormalities	8 (4)	
Other	13 (5)	
Subtotal	*70 (35)*	*34*
Total	**207**	**100**

Source: with permission from Consultative Council on Obstetric and Paediatric Mortality and Morbidity, Annual report for 2004.

disconcerting to note that there has been a slight increase in the proportion of low-birth-weight infants (6.8% overall, but 13.5% in indigenous births), and morbidity rates in the smallest surviving infants have increased.

In Australia, indigenous mortality rates are substantially higher at all ages. Although there have been major gains for all Australians in infant and perinatal mortality, from a rate of approximately 100 per 1000 live births at the turn of the 20th century to the 2002 figure of 5.0, the rates are still nearly three times higher for indigenous (13.0) than for non-indigenous Australians. 70% of the 'excess' deaths in rural and remote areas (observed deaths in rural and remote areas compared to what would be expected if city death rates had applied) occur in indigenous children. Injuries, deaths due to undetermined causes and respiratory deaths were the most common causes of 'excess' indigenous deaths in rural areas.

Figure 1.1.2 shows the comparative neonatal, postneonatal, and infant mortality rates for a number of developed countries. A reduction in the indigenous infant mortality rate would significantly improve the Australian figure. An excess of male over female infant deaths is observed worldwide.

Causes of death

Neonatal deaths

Table 1.1.4 shows the major causes of neonatal deaths in Victoria, Australia, in 2004. 60% of these deaths occur on the day of birth, with most being due to extreme prematurity or poor fetal growth, congenital malformations or pregnancy complications. 34%

of neonatal deaths (including late terminations) result from a malformation, although only 24% of these deaths involve a known chromosomal abnormality. Further reductions in the incidence of neural tube defects (NTDs) will occur with use of the now proven preventive effect of periconceptional folate supplementation in mothers of both high-risk (previous NTD-affected conception) and low-risk (no previous NTD-affected conception) infants. The perinatal mortality rate for multiple births is more than double that for singleton births.

There remains major scope for further improvement in neonatal mortality, particularly with the development of an understanding of the determinants of premature labour, intrauterine growth restriction, developmental anomalies and other perinatal conditions. Very little is known about the causes of prematurity, and even less about its prevention. Progress has been hampered by research that has not distinguished between placental insufficiency (leading to intrauterine growth retardation) and preterm labour as causes of low birth weight.

It is not surprising, therefore, that there has been little change in the incidence of low birth weight in recent generations. Indeed, there has been a slight rise in its incidence in the last decade (from 6.3% to 6.8%), which is partly explained by a higher proportion of older mothers giving birth. In 1998 the birth rate in non-indigenous women over 35 years of age exceeded that in those under 19 years for the first time, while the rates in younger indigenous women were similar to those in women aged 30–34 years. Fortunately, however, the perinatal mortality rate is now similar for major birth-weight groups above 1000 g. This has only come about during the last 20 years when newborn intensive care has improved survival for high-risk neonates dramatically. During this time, the reduction in mortality has been greatest for the 1000–2499 g group.

Postneonatal and child deaths

A major contributor to the recent decline in postneonatal mortality (children aged over 1 month and under 1 year) has been the decline in deaths from sudden infant death syndrome (SIDS) (Fig. 1.1.3). SIDS is the commonest cause of sudden unexplained death in infancy (SUDi), for which strict diagnostic criteria must be satisfied. Other causes of SUDi include unintentional overlying and unrecognized homicide. SIDS comprised 24% of postneonatal deaths in Victoria in 2004. However, following a public education campaign during the 1990s that emphasized that babies should be placed on their back or on their side in such a way that they cannot roll on to their stomach, the death rate from SIDS has decreased dramatically. In 2002, the SIDS death rate was 46 deaths per 100 000 live births, compared with 180 in 1982, a fall of 74%, with most of the decline occurring during the early 1990s. Other risk factors have also been identified consistently from epidemio-

logical studies. These include maternal cigarette smoking, lack of breastfeeding, overheating of the baby and a parental history of illicit drug use. This breakthrough with an astonishingly simple intervention seems now to be confirmed, although its precise mechanism is not yet fully explained. However, the rate of SIDS in indigenous infants remains higher than in Caucasians.

Causes of death between 1 and 14 years

More than 98% of children survive from birth to 15 years of age. The mortality rates for children aged 1–14 years declined by 52% between 1983 and 2003. Unintentional injuries, poisoning and violence account for over 40% of deaths, despite a 59% fall since 1979, with rates in boys about 1.6 times higher than in girls. The decline in rates has levelled out in recent years. Motor vehicle accidents (involving occupants, pedestrians and cyclists) account for half the injury deaths, and drowning (domestic pools, bathtubs, dams and drains, rivers and sea, and domestic buckets) for a further one-quarter of the deaths (but one-third of all injury deaths in under-5-year-old children). Swimming pool drownings account for about half of all drownings in those aged under 5 years, a proportion that has shown no significant change since the 1990s. Other causes of unintentional injury deaths were burns, asphyxiation and a number of rarer causes (Table 1.1.5).

The decline in injury mortality has been due to a number of preventive actions, including child resistant packaging of medication (unintentional poisoning deaths are now rare, although hospital admission remains relatively common), traffic and driver control measures (infant and child seat restraints, improved vehicle design, traffic control through speed cameras, random breath testing, local area traffic control, and cyclist helmets), and domestic pool isolation fencing. Added to these measures has been an increase in public awareness of child safety through targeted and mass media education campaigns. As with disease, the challenge to reduce injury morbidity now follows these important gains in saved lives.

Other major causes of death in this age group include malignancy and congenital abnormalities. Of the one-quarter in this age group who die from disease, 60% succumb to cancer despite important advances in long-term survival from surgery (for example, Wilms tumour), chemotherapy and radiotherapy (for example, acute leukaemia and lymphomas).

Another important cause of preventable infectious disease mortality in children is bacterial meningitis. Introduction of universal immunization for *Haemophilus influenzae* (Hib), meningococcal C and pneumococcal infections has resulted in a very

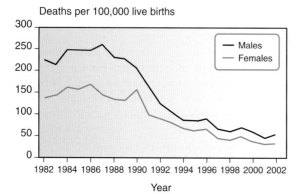

Sudden infant death syndrome rate (infants aged under 1 year).

Deaths per 100,000 live births

Fig. 1.1.3 Sudden infant death syndrome rate (infants aged under 1 year). Estimates based on data from AIHW National Mortality Database.

Table 1.1.5 Causes of postneonatal infant and child deaths in Victoria, Australia, 2004

Cause of death	Postneonatal 1–11 months No.	%	Child 1–14 years No.	%
Determined at birth				
Other conditions	13		3	
Malformation/birth defect	28		25	
Other	2		3	
Subtotal	*43*	*57*	*31*	*30*
Sudden infant death syndrome (SIDS)	*18*	*24*	*–*	*–*
Injury (unintentional)				
Motor vehicle	1		13	
Drowning	–		8	
Asphyxia	1		1	
Other	–		5	
Subtotal	*2*	*3*	*27*	*26*
Acquired disease				
Infection	10		6	
Malignancy	–		29	
Other	–		7	
Subtotal	*10*	*13*	*42*	*40*
Intentional injury	*1*	*1*	*4*	*4*
Undetermined	*1*	*1*	*–*	*–*
Total	**75**		**105**	

Source: with permission from Victorian Council on Paediatric and Maternal Mortality.

significant decrease in invasive disease due to these organisms.

Causes of death between 15 and 19 years

Mortality rates in this age group are about five times higher than in children aged 5–14 years, although substantially lower than rates in the 0–4-year group (Fig. 1.1.1). The principal causes of death in adolescents are injury (50%), particularly traffic-related causes (where alcohol use is an important contributor to mortality), suicide (20%) and cancer (10%). The mortality rate for males is twice that of females in this age group. While death rates for females have declined by 21% since 1961, in males the corresponding decline is 52%, largely as a result of a substantial reduction in traffic-injury mortality, despite an increasing number of vehicles and young drivers and passengers (Table 1.1.6). The disturbing increase in adolescent male suicide that occurred between 1979 and 1998, with the rate increasing by 40%, has begun to fall for reasons that are unclear; in 2002 rates were at their lowest since 1984. The male rate is currently four times higher than the female rate. Drug dependence accounted for 7.4% of youth deaths in 1998 and had risen sharply in recent years, especially among males, but has declined subsequently.

Table 1.1.6 Mortality rates for major causes of deaths in young persons aged 15–19 years, Australia, 1961–1999 and 15–24 years 2003

Cause of death	Deaths per 100 000 15–19 years old					
	1961	1971	1981	1990	1999	2003
Injury (all causes)	57.2	88.2	65.5	49.0	51.3	37.1
Motor vehicle	36.6	63.4	47.3	26.5	24.0	16.7
Drowning	2.2	2.6	1.5	1.0	1.7	–
Suicide	3.8	9.3	6.7	11.5	12.5	10.9
Cancers	6.4	7.6	6.1	4.7	7.2	4.3
Infectious disease	1.6	1.0	0.9	0.9	1.1	–
Drug related					8.8	0.6
All causes	85.9	114.2	85.3	67.0	76.9	53.3

Source: with permission from Australian Bureau of Statistics.

Morbidity

Changing patterns of morbidity

There have been changes in patterns of morbidity also in recent decades:

- the prevalence of asthma in children and young people rose during the 1980s and 1990s (12.3–19.2%) but there has been no further increase since then. Currently, 14–16% of children report asthma as a current problem, with a higher proportion reporting wheeze
- there has been increasing concern about problems of developmental health and wellbeing – 35% of new paediatric consultations are for behaviour problems and 13% for learning problems
- 14% of children have mental health problems – higher rates are associated with low income, coercive parenting, family conflict, blended/single-parent families and children with chronic illness
- 29% and 24%, respectively, of children exposed to coercive and inconsistent parenting styles had mental health morbidity compared with 11% exposed to encouraging styles
- disability affects 7% of 0–14-year-olds, but chronic illness and disability account for 50% of all paediatric consultations
- there has been a rising incidence of cerebral palsy in births under 1500 g (from 10 to 70 per 1000 live births) during the last 25 years
- 10% of all hospital admissions involve children under 15 years.

Information about child health can be obtained from cross-sectional community prevalence surveys or longitudinal cohort studies, health service provider records (e.g. community nurses, school health services, general practitioners, paediatricians and hospitals) and national health insurance data. Growing up in Australia, the National Longitudinal Study of Australian Children funded by the Commonwealth government, is expected to provide important cross-sectional and longitudinal data over the next decade on two cohorts of 5000 under-1-year-old children and 4-year-olds.

Children and adolescents presenting to general practitioners

From an ongoing national survey of general practice statistics, it is known that 15.8% of total general practice encounters in Australia are for children aged 0–14 years, with a further 9.8% for young persons aged 15–24 years. The top reasons for consulting a doctor (including but not limited to general practitioners) in children aged under 15 years were respiratory conditions (upper respiratory infection, including tonsillitis, asthma and acute bronchitis) and immunization. Rates of presentation to GPs for asthma fell by almost one-third in 0–4-year-olds between 1998/99 and 2001/02.

Children and adolescents presenting to specialized paediatric services

In the Australian health care system, children may be referred to a consultant or specialist paediatrician by a general (or primary care) practitioner for consultation on difficult problems, or for management of rare or difficult-to-treat chronic illnesses. Paediatricians work in the community and/or in general hospitals with paediatric facilities (secondary paediatric services) or children's hospitals with extensive subspecialty services (tertiary hospitals). In addition, public and private hospitals provide accident and emergency services for children. The pattern of injuries and acute and chronic illnesses seen in these settings varies according to the mix of private and public paediatric hospitals servicing urban and rural communities. The case mix (pattern of clinical problems) differs for outpatient clinic attendances, emergency department presentations and hospital admissions.

A 12-month survey of the practice profile of paediatricians in the Barwon region of Victoria in 1996/97 found that 10% of the childhood population had consulted a paediatrician practising in the community during this period: 68.9% of consultations concerned medical problems, with central nervous system/disability and the respiratory system each accounting for 16% and gastrointestinal problems a further 14%. Nearly 35% of children seen had behavioural problems, with 76% of these relating to attention deficit/hyperactivity disorder (ADHD), which was the most common diagnosis overall. A further 14.5% of consultations concerned children with epilepsy or another disability, 13% were for children with learning problems and 10% were for asthma. Just over 4% of all consultations involved children with significant social problems. At least 50% of these paediatric medical consultations involved children with a chronic illness.

Attendances at an emergency department provide a further component of the picture of child injury and acute illness. Gastroenteritis, asthma and injuries dominate the mix of clinical conditions treated in this setting. Children 0–4 years with asthma attend emergency departments relatively more often than people of other ages who have asthma.

Around 10% of hospital admissions in Australia are for children under 15 years. The reasons for hospital admission of children vary according to the type of hospital (secondary versus tertiary) and therefore the types of surgical and medical treatments that are provided. The admission case mix is also changing as the pattern of clinical management evolves; for example, the admission rate for asthma in 0–4-year-olds is higher in boys but has declined over the last decade and the average length of stay for asthma has been reduced from 6 days to just over a day during the past 25 years. Minor surgical procedures account for a large proportion of hospital admissions, and asthma is by far the single leading reason for hospital admission in children.

The prevalence of asthma in Australia is one of the highest in the world, with more than 2 million Australians estimated to be affected by the disease. Asthma is more prevalent in young people, with 12.3% of 1–4-year-olds, 19.2% of 5–9-year-olds and 18.7% of 10–14-year-olds reporting asthma as a long-term condition in the 1995 Australian Health Survey. Rates are slightly higher in males in childhood, thereafter higher in females and in indigenous children. In Australia, Queenslanders report a higher prevalence than Tasmanians. Children with asthma report a lower quality of life. Around 40% of children with asthma live with a person who smokes; higher exposure rates occur among socioeconomically disadvantaged children.

Health behaviours

Health status of children and young people is changing as evidenced by health behaviour changes:

- increased immunization uptake has followed establishment of the Australian Childhood Immunisation Register (ACIR) – 90.5% fully immunized at 1 year in 2002, 87.8% at 2 years and 80.6% fully immunized at 6 years
- there has been a plateau in rates of adolescent smoking but with persisting higher rates among girls (32% versus 28%)
- rates of obesity and overweight are rising – 25% of Sydney and Melbourne 7–18-year-olds are overweight.

A number of factors that rely on public participation have a profound impact on child health, and on future good health as an adult. In traditional societies, parenting was a responsibility of the clan, not just the biological parents. The quality of parenting provided in developed countries is now arguably one of the major determinants of public health, being implicated in the high prevalence of academic failure, disruptive behaviour and other mental health problems, intentional and unintentional injuries, substance misuse and juvenile crime.

Other health behaviours may also have benefits or adverse effects; for example, high rates of breastfeeding and immunization, child restraint use in motor vehicles, sun exposure protection using clothing and sun screen creams, healthy nutrition, active lifestyles, pool fences and swimming competence, and bicycle helmets all have a beneficial impact on disease and injury prevention. Harmful behaviours, such as cigarette smoking, may result in the smoker's exposure, or passive exposure of the fetus or infant, to the hundreds of potential carcinogens in cigarette smoke and its other toxic effects on the respiratory and cardiovascular systems. The physician who cares for children has a crucial role in contributing to parent and child awareness of the real opportunities the individual has to make healthy lifestyle decisions that will benefit all members of the family.

Immunization

Immunization is one of the most effective disease prevention tools. Australia has a strong tradition of successful mass immunization through local government, community nurses and general practitioners. Immunization schedules in the various states of Australia are modelled on the National Health and Medical Research Council (NHMRC) recommendations, and the Commonwealth is responsible for providing schedule vaccines free of charge to all Australian children.

The Australian Childhood Immunisation Register, which is managed through the national health insurance scheme (Medicare) was established as part of the National Childhood Immunisation Program begun in 1996. It provides a reminder and recall system direct to parents, and also makes available a mechanism to monitor vaccine uptake within the community. Doctors are paid to notify the ACIR each time they immunize a child. Since the implementation of the register and a range of incentives directed at parents and health-care providers to promote immunization, there has been a progressive increase in the proportion of children immunized from around 65% of 2-year-olds fully vaccinated in 1998 to 90% in 2002 (Table 1.1.7).

Epidemiological evidence suggests that a failure to be immunized is due to a number of factors, including parent apathy linked with lack of awareness of the importance of immunization, its safety and its effectiveness, and health professionals' poor performance in delivering age-appropriate immunization.

Smoking and sun exposure

The massive increase in the incidence of lung cancer in men over the age of 50 years preceding the 1980s and, in more recent years, the rise in women, along with the increase in melanoma in both sexes, stands in stark contrast to the relatively stable incidence of most other cancers. What have these outcomes to do with paediatrics? The answer is that the behaviours associated with an increased risk of these diseases commence in childhood and adolescence.

Table 1.1.7 Proportion of 1-year-old children in Australia who are fully immunized

Data source	DTP (%)	OPV (%)	Hib (%)	All (%)
ABS, April 1995	86.2	86.3	62.3	51.4
ACIR, March 1997	77.4	77.2	77.2	74.9
ACIR, March 2001	91.5	91.4	94.6	91.2
ACIR, March 2002	92.0	91.9	94.5	90.5

ABS April 1995 value for DTP is for pertussis only. Immunization coverage for diphtheria and tetanus at that time was 88.5%. The proportion fully immunized in 1995 (51.4%) includes Hib, which was added to the immunization schedule in April 1993. The proportion fully immunized in 1995, excluding Hib, was 70.8%.
ABS, Australian Bureau of Statistics; ACIR, Australian Immunisation Register; DTP, diphtheria, tetanus and pertussis vaccine; Hib, *Haemophilus influenzae* type b conjugate vaccine; OPV, oral polio vaccine.
Adapted, with permission, from data from ABS, ACIR and the Communicable Diseases Network Australia.

Smoking related disorders

The current patterns of lung cancer incidence and mortality in men (a 2% per year decline) and women (a 1.6% per year increase) probably reflect smoking behaviour patterns 20 years ago. Most smokers commence smoking in adolescence and this behaviour, once established, may be difficult to change. In addition, the number of pack-years of smoke exposure is directly related to the risk of smoking-related cancers, cardiovascular disease and numerous other health problems. The relationship between media exposure to cigarette promotion and the likelihood of young people becoming smokers is strong and well established. With increasing awareness of the profound and irrefutable causal relationship between cigarette smoking and disease, and with new laws restricting the way in which cigarettes may be advertised, the prevalence of adolescent smokers in Australia has finally started to decline during the past 15 years but daily smoking rates are higher in 16–17-year-old girls (14.5%) compared with boys (7.95%).

Furthermore, the recent widespread recognition of the harmful effects of both prenatal and postnatal passive smoke exposure in children (low birth weight and prematurity and all their consequences, respiratory infections, asthma, otitis media, impaired lung growth) has led to rapid changes in public policy, laws and community practices aimed at reducing environmental tobacco smoke exposure, especially for children. The clinician's role is to assist in the education of young parents, to provide access to professional quit programmes and to encourage smokers in the meantime to smoke only outside the family home and wear protective clothing while doing so, and never in the family vehicle or in the company of children.

Melanoma

In the case of melanoma, the incidence rates have increased markedly since 1983, especially for males. Australian melanoma rates are among the highest in the world, with a tenfold difference in incidence between Australia and England and Wales. Melanoma risk is related to ultraviolet radiation exposure and the incidence is higher in individuals with many moles, those with fair, sun-sensitive skin, and those who have intermittent high recreational exposure. It is thought that exposure in childhood may be particularly important. It is therefore disconcerting to note that surveys have found that between 9% and 12% of children and young people in all age groups who have been exposed to the sun have not used sun protection.

Obesity and physical fitness

There has been growing concern about the increasing levels of obesity and lack of physical fitness in children and young people in Australia. In 1985, 4% of boys and 6% of girls were classified, according to their body mass index (BMI, a measure of weight for height) as being overweight. A more recent study (2000) found that about 25% of children aged 7–18 years in Sydney and Melbourne were overweight, practising sedentary lifestyles and consuming a diet high in fat and low in the intake of fruit and vegetables. It is of some concern that around one-third of children under 12 years do not eat any fruit or fruit products and more than one in five do not eat any vegetables or vegetable products. Childhood obesity is now being tackled as part of a national strategy developed by the National Obesity Taskforce.

Disability

In addition to acute problems, modern child health care is very much concerned with the long-term management of a number of disorders associated with physical and intellectual disability. Many of these disorders are determined genetically and until comparatively recently were fatal in early life. Examples include cystic fibrosis, thalassaemia major, spina bifida, phenylketonuria, haemophilia and various malignancies.

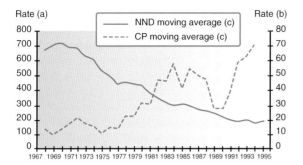

Fig. 1.1.4 Very-low birth weight (less than 1500 g) neonatal death (NND) and cerebral palsy (CP) rates in Western Australia 1987–1996. (a) Neonatal death rate per 1000 live births. (b) Cerebral palsy rates per 1000 live births. (c) 3-year moving averages; note that CP moving average rate for 1994 is derived from 2 years data only. Source: Cerebral Palsy Register, Institute for Child Research, Perth, Australia (unpublished data).

In 2003, the overall prevalence of disability in children 0–14 years was estimated to be about 8%. Approximately 52% of these had a severe or profound restriction in core activities. Older children (5–14 years), especially males, had higher rates of severe disability. The rates have remained relatively constant since 1998. There was a very strong socio-economic gradient in rates of disability with children in families in the lowest income quintile accounting for 32.4% of all those with profound core activity restrictions, compared with only 7.0% of children in the highest income quintile.

An increasingly important cause of disability is very low birth weight (<1000 g). With modern technology, approximately two-thirds of very-low-birth-weight infants will survive, although significant disability will remain in up to 25% of survivors. Indeed, there has been a steady rise in the incidence of cerebral palsy over the past 20 years in infants weighing less than 1500 g at birth (Fig. 1.1.4). Other disabilities include intellectual disability, auditory and visual problems, and epilepsy, alone or in combination. It should be noted, however, that the vast majority of cases of cerebral palsy and of intellectual disability are not related to birth asphyxia or other perinatal events.

Emotional and behavioural problems

The management of emotional and behavioural problems of childhood is an important challenge in a large proportion of paediatric consultations. A national survey of child and adolescent mental health in 1999 found that 14% of children and young people had mental health problems, with higher rates being noted in boys and children living in low income, step/blended and sole-parent families. Although one in five teenagers have mental health problems, most will not seek or receive treatment. Children with chronic illness have a doubled risk of emotional maladjustment and those with chronic physical disorders that affect the brain, notably spina bifida, epilepsy and cerebral palsy, have the highest risk.

Conversely, paediatric disorders that are still poorly understood have frequently been attributed to emotional causes, when there has been good evidence that psychological factors may also be a consequence of the disorder. Maternal mood disorder is common in infancy and in later childhood and is associated with a range of adverse outcomes such as infant cry–fuss behaviour (colic), feeding and sleep problems and cognitive or behavioural problems in older children. Other conditions, such as recurrent abdominal pain, encopresis, enuresis, headache, school refusal and school failure, may be associated with emotional problems in the children themselves but again caution needs to be exercised about the direction of causality. The role of the child's doctor is to recognize that emotional factors may be both a contributor to and a consequence of the child's physical symptoms and there is a duty especially not to diagnose a psychological cause in the absence of overt and specific evidence of psychological dysfunction. Recognizing the emotional as well as the physical consequences of children's diseases is crucial to effective paediatric care.

Social and family factors

It is now recognized that family and social factors significantly modify disease and must be taken into account if total care is to be provided. These factors include family size and financial status, physical characteristics of the home, behaviour and way of life of parents, their education, attitudes, habits and the family's capacity to select and use the various types of care available. Poverty is, in particular, a well established risk factor for a large number of health problems. Often this is compounded in recent migrants, where isolation and acculturation difficulties confer additional stress on young families. Maternal depression in this situation has been shown to be an important accompaniment of child development and adjustment difficulty.

Parenting

The ability of children to self-regulate their behaviour is influenced by the nature of the relationship between children and their caregivers in early life. The risks of disruptive behaviour disorders, such as oppositional defiant disorder and conduct disorder, and later criminality are greatly increased in children where there is insecure attachment between infants and their caregivers in the early years of life and where parental disciplinary styles are coercive or inconsistent. The West Australian Child Health Survey found a substantially increased rate of mental health morbidity in children exposed to these parenting styles (29% and 24% respectively) compared to encouraging styles (11%).

Future directions

There is widespread recognition that social, environmental, family and technological changes during the past 35 years have contributed to the changing pattern of child health mortality and morbidity. There is also increasing awareness that patterns of behaviour, health and wellbeing that are established in fetal life and childhood become to some extent biologically embedded, sometimes through gene–environment interactions, affecting neuroendocrine and neuroimmunological functioning and, as such, have lifelong implications for physical and mental health, coping and competence. The health and wellbeing experience of children is thus increasingly being seen as having wide ramifications for the competence, coping and adaptability of human populations undergoing massive social changes associated with their transformation from industrial to globalized, information based economies. Child health, as it was at the turn of the 20th century but for very different reasons, is once more at centre stage in the grand vision of improving the health and wellbeing of human populations.

Child health in a global context

T. Duke

Introduction

In the last 100 years there have been dramatic reductions in child mortality and general improvements in child health in Western countries. These have resulted from economic development, public health interventions, better nutrition, maternal health, immunization and advances in health technology and curative care. Child mortality rates have fallen from over 100 per 1000 live births in the UK, North America, Australia, New Zealand, Japan, Scandinavian countries and western Europe, at the end of the 19th century, to less than 10 per 1000 live births at the beginning of the 21st century. However, 90% of the world's people, who live in developing countries, have not shared in this prosperity and progress.

The World Health Organization (WHO) estimates that every year more than 10 million children die; 99% of these deaths occur in developing countries. Figure 1.2.1 shows the distribution of child mortality globally; the majority of under-5 deaths being concentrated in sub-Saharan Africa and south Asia. In 2001, 47 countries had child mortality rates higher than 100 per 1000 live births. Ten countries – eight in Sub-Saharan Africa – had mortality rates of more than 200.

Child health inequity

Inequity is unfair distribution, and child health has many layers of inequity. Inequity between regions and countries is brought into sharp focus in the 21st century because of globalization and freedom to travel: countries that are half a day's flying time away from capital cities in Australia, for example, have child mortality rates 10 times higher than that of non-indigenous children in Sydney or Melbourne.

Inequity exists also within countries; for example, in Papua New Guinea in 1999 the median child mortality was 89 per 1000 live births, but some provinces had under-5 mortality rates as low as 49 and others as high as 164 per 1000 live births. Similarly in Cambodia, the child mortality rates in various provinces ranged from 50 to 229 per 1000 live births. Urban child mortality is generally lower than rural mortality, for example: 43 versus 71 per 1000 live births in South Africa. The neonatal mortality rate in remote mountainous area of Vietnam is three times higher than in urban areas. However, regional averages hide further maldistribution: urban slums within cities in many developing countries have rates of child mortality that are much higher than their nation's average.

Income is a major determinant of child mortality risk. In 2003 the average under-5 mortality rate was 123 deaths per 1000 in low-income countries, 39 in lower-middle-income countries and 22 in upper-middle-income countries. In high-income countries the rate was less than 7. Within-country income inequity also has a great effect on child mortality risk. Among the poorest quintiles (the poorest 20%) of the populations of Cambodia and Vietnam child mortality rates are two to three times higher than in the richest quintiles. Equity of income distribution is also an important determinant: countries with low gross domestic product (GDP) but a more even income distribution have much lower rates of mortality than other countries with higher GDP but inequitable income distribution. Maternal education and access to health services are also closely related to child mortality risk.

Disparities exist in the financial, technical and human resources available for child health, globally and within countries, and this is closely related to mortality risk. In 1973 Professor David Morley said of Nigeria: 'Three quarters of our population are rural, yet three quarters of our medical resources are spent in the towns where three quarters of our doctors live; three quarters of the people die from diseases which could be prevented at low cost, and yet three quarters of medical budgets are spent on curative services.' Unfortunately, the same is still true today of most developing countries: the doctor: population ratios of many countries are 20 times higher in cities than in rural areas. Differences in health service access between rural and urban populations manifest in disparities of functional outcomes as well as mortality risk: for example, compared to urban children with epilepsy, children with epilepsy in rural Zimbabwe are less likely to receive treatment (63% rural versus 95% urban), have a greater seizure burden (2.3 versus 1 per month) and are more likely to have problems that impair social and educational attainment.

15

The distribution of global child mortality

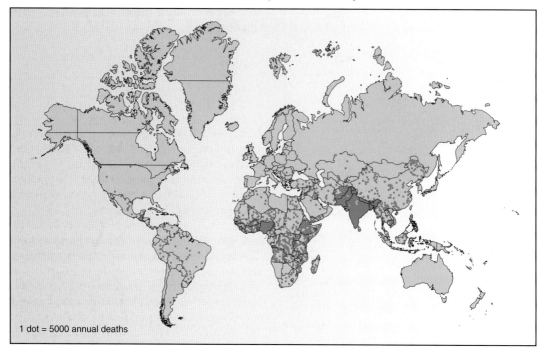

1 dot = 5000 annual deaths

Fig. 1.2.1 The distribution of global child mortality. 1 dot = 5000 annual deaths. Source: Black RE, Morris SS, Bryce J 2003 Where and why are 10 million children dying each year? Lancet 361: 2226–2234.

Human resources in low income countries are being further eroded by the drain of doctors and nurses migrating to richer countries. HIV/AIDS has exacerbated this human resources crisis; to implement effective antiretroviral treatment programmes requires increased numbers of trained health workers. However, the cruel irony is that HIV/AIDS is claiming a major proportion of the young population of doctors and nurses in countries, particularly in Africa, that most need effective prevention and treatment programmes.

Research in child health is also disproportionate to the burden of diseases and inequitably distributed. While $73 is spent on health research per disability-adjusted life-year lost (DALY: an index that combines both mortality and disability) for diseases overall and $8.40 is spent on research into HIV, malaria and tuberculosis, only $0.51 per DALY is spent on research into acute respiratory infection and $0.30 per DALY is spent on diarrhoea. 86% of scientific publications and 97% of patents are held by 16% of the world (the advanced economies), while the remaining 84% publish a mere 14% of the world's scientific papers and hold 3% of the world's patents. Therefore, between countries and for all major diseases, capacities to deal with child health problems are inversely proportional to the magnitude of the problems.

Causes of global child mortality

The major causes of deaths in children under-5 years of age globally are listed in Table 1.2.1. The proportions are region-specific, with skewed distribution in the Africa region. For example, 94% and 89% of the world's malaria and HIV/AIDS deaths occur in Africa.

More than 50% of children who die in developing countries have moderate or severe malnutrition, and malnutrition is implicated in deaths from diarrhoea (61%), malaria (57%), pneumonia (52%) and measles (45%). However, malnutrition is often underreported in national statistics and underrecognized in clinical settings where childhood malnutrition is so common as almost to be the norm. The situation is even more complex than Table 1.2.1 suggests: while children often present with a single condition (e.g. acute respiratory infection), those who are most likely to die will often have experienced several other infections in recent months, have more than one infections currently (e.g. pneumonia and diarrhoea, or pneumonia and malaria) and have malnutrition with micronutrient (such as iron, zinc or vitamin A) deficiency.

Child disability and development

Like mortality, the capacity of countries to prevent and treat child disability is inversely proportional to

Table 1.2.1 The major causes of deaths in children under-5 years of age globally, with estimates for 2000–2003

Cause	No of deaths (000)	% of total annual global deaths
Causes in children 1 month–5 years	**6685**	
Acute respiratory infections	2027	19
Diarrhoeal diseases	1762	17
Malaria	853	8
Measles	395	4
HIV/AIDS	321	3
Injuries	305	3
Others	1022	10
Neonatal causes	**3910**	
Pre-term birth	1083	10
Severe infection	1016	10
Birth asphyxia	894	8
Congenital anomalies	294	3
Neonatal tetanus	257	2
Diarrhoeal diseases	108	1
Other	258	2
Total	**10 595**	**100**

With permission from: World Health Report 2005 – make every mother and child count. Statistical annex, p. 190. http://www.who.int/whr/2005/en/

the burden of the problems. Child disability and developmental problems occur at high rates in poor countries because of the frequency of neurological disease (including perinatal asphyxia, bacterial and tuberculous meningitis, cerebral malaria and neurocysticercosis), the contribution of undernutrition to developmental retardation (maternal malnutrition, low birth weight, iron and iodine deficiency), high rates of trauma and injury, in utero exposure to drugs and alcohol, congenital syphilis and rubella syndromes, and exposure to environmental toxins. Institutionalization of orphans and disabled children in some countries also contributes to severe developmental delay, because of emotional neglect and malnutrition. The lack of primary prevention, screening and rehabilitation services that might mitigate the effect of disabilities on function also worsens the impact of these conditions on individuals and the community.

In some countries community rehabilitation services have improved the lives of many disabled children, iodine and other micronutrient supplementation and fortification programmes are under way, programmes for the primary prevention of injuries are starting and some least developed countries are getting access to vaccines that will prevent meningitis. However, more work in these areas is urgently needed.

Neonatal health

More than one-third of all under-5 deaths occur in the first month of life (Table 1.2.1) and the majority of neonatal deaths occur in the first few days after birth, making the neonatal period the most hazardous time of life. The vast majority of the 3.9 million annual neonatal deaths occur in socioeconomic deprivation in developing countries. Programmes to improve neonatal survival are focusing on supervised clean deliveries, essential care of the newborn (early breastfeeding, skin-to-skin warmth), steroids for preterm labour, antibiotics for premature rupture of membranes, maternal tetanus toxoid to prevent neonatal tetanus, prevention of mother-to-child transmission of HIV and identification of sick neonates requiring referral to hospitals. Recently the WHO has produced guidelines for the management of seriously ill neonates in hospitals in developing countries. Improving neonatal health, particularly the reduction in low birth weight through improved maternal health, may reduce the risk of adult diseases such as hypertension, coronary artery disease and non-insulin-dependent diabetes, which form a large and increasing burden of non-communicable diseases in developing countries. As neonatal mortality falls, however, resources need to be available to deal with the increased morbidity that will occur in survivors. Such morbidities include malnutrition, chronic lung disease and neurological disease among survivors of prematurity.

Adolescent health

The health of young people (defined by WHO as aged 10–24 years) in developing countries has hitherto been a low priority. However, four out of five people between 10 and 24 years of age live in developing countries. Although mortality rates for adolescents in developing countries are much lower than for children under 5 years, the proportion of deaths occurring in adolescents is several times higher in developing countries than in developing countries. However, as pointed out by Goodburn and Ross (see Further reading) it is the future costs of current morbidity and the adoption of unhealthy behaviours by young people that pose the greatest risk and provide the greatest opportunities for prevention. As countries pass through economic transition, as the HIV/AIDS pandemic has developed and with increasing urbanization, the health problems of young people are increasingly on the global agenda.

WHO estimates that half of all HIV infections have occurred in people less than 25 years of age. There is high potential for prevention of many of the major diseases in adults by interventions targeted at adolescents. Indeed, improving the health of young people may be a major key to improving health at all ages: improving adolescent education, delaying reproductive age, improving nutrition and exercise, reducing smoking and drug and alcohol consumption and preventing sexually transmitted infections will have beneficial effects on the young people themselves now and in decades to come, and reduce the burden of disease among newborns and children in future generations.

Children in complex emergencies

Complex emergencies are identified as acute situations in which there is excess mortality (more than one death per 10 000 population per day). They may be due to natural (e.g. flood, tsunami or earthquake) or unnatural (war, famine) disasters, or both. Complex emergencies are dynamic, with variable durations of emergency, recovery, resettlement, rehabilitation and development phases. After the initial disaster, high mortality rates are usually due to diarrhoeal disease, cholera and dysentery, measles, malaria, meningococcal disease, tuberculosis, neonatal causes, trauma, malnutrition and micronutrient deficiency. High rates of mental health problems, including post-traumatic stress disorder, depression and anxiety, also have been reported in many studies of children living in refugee camps or exposed to violence or armed conflict. According to the United Nations High Commissioner for Refugees (UNHCR), as of January 2003 10 million children under 18 years of age were refugees or living in refugee-like situations, such as asylum-seekers, internally displaced persons or returnees, in more than 150 countries in all regions of the world.

Many factors impede the delivery of health care in such situations, including lack of human resources and referral services, security constraints, poor supervision and coordination, and failure of integration with local health services or transition to a sustainable health system. In addition, lack of comprehensive guidelines and approaches, especially for the management of neonatal problems, HIV infection, mental health problems, and child and sexual abuse, limit the impact of health care in these situations.

The effect of poor child health on communities

Childhood disease has major effects on the economy and lives of families, communities and developing nations (see Clinical example). Poor health among children or a family member is a common cause for families sliding into poverty. For affected families, the cycle of poverty, poor nutrition, chronic ill-health and low educational attainment is common.

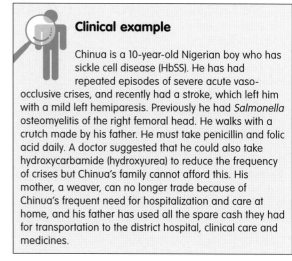

Clinical example

Chinua is a 10-year-old Nigerian boy who has sickle cell disease (HbSS). He has had repeated episodes of severe acute vaso-occlusive crises, and recently had a stroke, which left him with a mild left hemiparesis. Previously he had *Salmonella* osteomyelitis of the right femoral head. He walks with a crutch made by his father. He must take penicillin and folic acid daily. A doctor suggested that he could also take hydroxycarbamide (hydroxyurea) to reduce the frequency of crises but Chinua's family cannot afford this. His mother, a weaver, can no longer trade because of Chinua's frequent need for hospitalization and care at home, and his father has used all the spare cash they had for transportation to the district hospital, clinical care and medicines.

International conventions and child health

There have been several United Nations (UN) conventions designed to improve global child health in the last 30 years. The Declaration of Alma Ata was one of the first to identify primary health as being crucial to child survival, and that improvements in food security, clean water, sanitation, appropriate housing and education were crucial to progress. In 1990 the UN Convention on the Rights of the Child stated that all children have the right to the highest attainable standard of health, and access to care and medicines when they are sick, and held governments responsible for providing comprehensive health services. The mantra of the Declaration of Alma Ata was 'Health for all by the year 2000'. Sadly, for many reasons – the emergence of the HIV/AIDS pandemic, lack of political commitment, inadequate financing, a drastic human resources shortage and inadequate attention to non-health-sector elements – this ambitious aim did not come close to being realized. In 2000 the UN developed the Millennium Development Goals (MDGs), which was signed by all UN member states and set specific goals in eight areas (Table 1.2.2). The fourth MDG calls for a reduction in child mortality. Specifically, MDG-4 states that countries should aim to reduce child mortality by two-thirds of what it was in 1990, by 2015. Some national governments have signed up to a modified target for MDG-4 to reflect what is feasible and realistic. Other MDGs are crucial to child health and development including: to halve the proportion of

Table 1.2.2 The eight Millennium Development Goals and key indicators

1 Eradicate extreme poverty and hunger
Population below $1 a day (%)
Percentage share of income or consumption held by poorest 20%
Prevalence of child malnutrition (% of children under 5)
Population below minimum level of dietary energy consumption (%)

2 Achieve universal primary education
Net primary enrolment ratio (% of relevant age group)
Percentage of cohort reaching grade 5 (%)
Youth literacy rate (% ages 15–24)

3 Promote gender equality
Ratio of girls to boys in primary and secondary education (%)
Ratio of young literate females to males (% ages 15–24)
Share of women employed in the non-agricultural sector (%)
Proportion of seats held by women in national parliament (%)

4 Reduce child mortality
Under 5 mortality rate (per 1000)
Infant mortality rate (per 1000 live births)
Immunization, measles (% of children under 12 months)

5 Improve maternal health
Maternal mortality ratio (modelled estimate, per 100 000 live births)
Births attended by skilled health staff (% of total)

6 Combat HIV/AIDS, malaria and other diseases
Prevalence of HIV, female (% ages 15–24)
Contraceptive prevalence rate (% of women ages 15–49)
Number of children orphaned by HIV/AIDS
Incidence of tuberculosis (per 100 000 people)

7 Ensure environmental sustainability
Forest area (% of total land area)
Nationally protected areas (% of total land area)
GDP per unit of energy use (PPP $ per kg oil equivalent)
CO_2 emissions (metric tons per capita)
Access to an improved water source (% of population)
Access to improved sanitation (% of population)

8 Develop a Global Partnership for Development
Youth unemployment rate (% of total labour force ages 15–24)
Fixed line and mobile telephones (per 1000 people)
Personal computers (per 1000 people)

the population living on less than US$1 per day; to ensure universal primary education; to eliminate gender disparity in all levels of education; to reduce by three-quarters the maternal mortality ratio; to reverse the rising incidence of HIV, malaria and other diseases; to halve the proportion of people

without sustainable access to safe drinking water and sanitation; and targets in development aid, market access, debt relief, employment and information access. Each of these goals has specific targets and indicators that can be used as benchmarks.

Evidence for effective interventions in reducing child mortality

In 2003 *The Lancet* published a series on child survival, outlining the evidence for effectiveness of interventions in reducing child mortality. 23 interventions (15 preventative and eight curative) aimed at the commonest causes of child mortality had high-grade evidence for effectiveness, i.e. large randomized trials, systematic reviews. These interventions were selected for being low-cost and having potential for implementation at near-universal scale in low-income countries. Some interventions protect against deaths from many causes, for example breastfeeding protect against deaths from diarrhoea, pneumonia and neonatal sepsis; insecticide-treated materials (bed-nets, sheets, etc.) protect against deaths from malaria and also reduce deaths from preterm delivery. However, with the exception of breastfeeding (estimated global coverage of 90%) global coverage of known effective interventions for reducing child deaths from common conditions is low.

To promote a comprehensive model of care for the sick child in 1995 WHO developed the Integrated Management of Childhood Illness (IMCI). IMCI is a case management and training strategy that focuses on primary health workers managing the most important causes of childhood illness, including identification and treatment of children with multiple pathologies. Evaluation of IMCI in Bangladesh and Tanzania showed improvements in the quality of case management, and now over 90 countries have adopted the strategy, albeit often in pilot projects with moderate coverage. In recognizing that primary health care will only have an optimal impact on child mortality if there are effective referral services, WHO has produced complimentary guidelines on paediatric care for district or provincial hospitals. These guidelines emphasize that diagnosis and drug treatment are not sufficient for optimal care of the seriously ill child but that triage, supportive care (including fluids, oxygen, nutrition), monitoring, discharge planning and follow-up are essential also. These processes of care were found to be deficient in audits of practice in many developing and transitional countries.

To achieve MDG-4 by 2015, focus will need to be on achieving universal access to health services and on improving equity. Limited resources may need to target interventions towards marginalized populations within low- and middle-income countries. These populations include the poor, refugees and internally displaced persons, families living in remote rural areas and urban slums, disaster areas and war zones, ethnic minorities, indigenous populations, new immigrants, AIDS orphans, child workers, child soldiers and abandoned children. There is also a need for an 'enabling environment' for child health and survival: political commitment, adequate funding, human resources, community awareness and support, improvements in water, sanitation and the environment, and improvements in education and gender equality. The quality of care provided in health facilities and the nature of interactions be-tween health systems, families and communities have major consequences for child health, human rights, poverty alleviation and development.

Table 1.2.3 Principles of global child health
1. Focus on children who have least access to services
2. Support simple, low-cost interventions that can achieve high coverage
3. Improvement in nutrition is vital
4. Support national and local services and institutions, and deliver services where possible through existing local structures
5. Seek out, respect and support local human capacity; it is often greater than you think
6. Local ownership of ideas and strategies is essential for sustainability
7. Support multidisciplinary and multisector collaboration
8. Use a framework that incorporates human-rights and equity
9. Critical evaluation of programs is crucial to the efficient and ethical use of resources
10. Be patient – progress that incorporates these principles may not be fast, but it may be long-lasting

How can child health professionals in developed countries contribute to global child health?

There are many pathways to meaningful contributions to global child health. However, they all require experience, technical expertise, perspective and cultural understanding. These prerequisites can best be gained by an extended time living and working in a developing country. This early experience, and the eventual expression of this work, can be immensely varied: working as a medical officer, nurse, teacher or researcher in a government hospital, university, public health service, mission hospital, research institute, non-government organization working with children, UN organization or collaborative institute for child health. A contribution can be made from virtually any specialty but clinicians familiar with Western models of curative health care need to appreciate the central importance of public health.

Skills in teaching, epidemiology, research and infectious diseases are especially valuable. In the forthcoming decades, increasing numbers of doctors and other health professionals from developed countries will make substantial, ongoing and career-long contributions to global child health, as part of their core work. For others, financial contributions to child health programmes in developing countries may be a preferred option. Whatever the pathways, there are several principles of international health collaboration that should be followed (Table 1.2.3).

The highest priorities for paediatrics in the 21st century are firmly located in the poorest areas of the developing world. Solutions will be largely local, although regional and global support for local initiatives and priorities are essential. Slowly but increasingly this is being recognized by individual health professionals, education institutions, journals and professional societies in developed countries.

Electronic learning resources

K. Forsyth

Medical information resources now are largely electronic. In recent years, most medical publishing companies have provided content that is available through the internet. Many textbooks of medicine are available to purchasers in electronically searchable forms and most medical journals are now provided in electronic form and in print form.

Abstracting and literature search entities rely on recognition of entered keywords to identify resources. When keywords are entered in a search programme using a professional abstracting service, a list of journal references may be provided. Most medical journals have an independent peer-review process that allows confidence in the reliability of the information obtained. Alternatively, a more general search, using an internet search engine, may be used. However, for internet sites available for public search use, we have little indication of the validity or robustness of the information provided, and probably no concept of the authority or integrity of the author. Therefore, in the area of professional information for instruction there are many hazards for the unwary.

Although there are extensive databanks of information available electronically, some of which are of great merit as instructional aids, the process of learning requires that information is taken through a process where it becomes knowledge gained by the learner. Self-directed integrated learning may be assisted using information technology. Information technology can enable learners actively to construct their world of learning and the knowledge that they are gaining. Active learning includes the ability for a learner to represent a construct in multiple modalities. The recognition by Gardner that 'if you only know it one way it's a very fragile knowing' is an articulate way of stating the need for learners to come to an understanding of a concept through a number of different routes. Properly developed educational resource material utilizing information technology enables such construction and the ability to represent concepts in multiple ways.

Increasingly, as computers become more powerful and sophisticated, it is becoming easier to construct 'virtual learning worlds'. In competency-based disciplines such as medicine, creating virtual worlds is, in some situations, more effective and much cheaper than providing concrete experimental learning experiences for students. An example is the management of the fitting child. From informal surveys of final-year medical students, it has been estimated that only 10% of graduating students have witnessed a convulsion. At Flinders University in South Australia, a CD-ROM has been developed that contains videos of all the major seizure types. In addition, there is a virtual emergency room with a 'fitting child' scenario. The student is required to manage this situation. The advantage of this type of learning is apparent from the observation of a medical student that 'it is better for the computer, rather than the coroner, to tell you that you have mismanaged the child'. This type of learning is becoming an important component of curricula in medical schools.

In parallel with these developments, new modes of educational research are needed. Computer-based learning is essentially a new discipline. New tools are required to evaluate the effectiveness of computers as an instructional strategy. Electronic leaning resources are readily available on the internet. In addition, there are many CD or DVD products that deal with specific areas. The better ones provide an interactive approach that enhances the learning experience. One of the real difficulties with internet resources is the highly variable quality of the material: some of it is simply incorrect and some is misleading. In general, government-sponsored websites are of robust quality, as are those hosted by higher education institutions.

Search engines such as Google have revolutionized the utility of the internet. If using a search engine to locate information on a topic, in general it is preferable to select sites that are higher-education- or government-sponsored. Usually this is readily apparent from the web address.

Electronic references have revolutionized research. The ability to find abstracts through either PubMed or other on-line databases such as Medline enhances the researcher's ability to search the literature. There are now software programmes, such as Endnote or Reference Manager, that enable the reference citation to be stored locally and then inserted directly into publications. This aids accuracy and limits time spent on the mechanical process of inserting references.

Paediatric web sites

The following is a list of internet resources that are reliable and that students of paediatrics are likely to find helpful.

Key: A, applications/programs; CE, Windows CE PDA; I, still images; ML, multilingual; P, Palm PDA; Ps, Psion (EPOC) PDA; Q, online quiz; T, text; V, video images.

Core paediatric sites

1. **Medic.Com Paediatric medicine:** http://www.medic8.com/Paediatrics.htm [T, I, V] (UK)
An excellent site with a comprehensive selection of relevant paediatric links including paediatric medicine organisations, journals, databases, online textbooks and educational sites.

2. **General Pediatrics:** http://www.generalpediatrics.com/ [T, I] (USA)
A large site with extensive coverage of paediatric medical conditions and many links to other useful paediatric web pages. Compiled by Dr D. D'Alessandro, University of Iowa College of Medicine.

3. **Harriet Lane Links:** http://derm.med.jhmi.edu/poi/ [T, I] (USA)
The Harriet Lane Links site (formerly Pediatric Points of Interest) provides an edited collection of paediatric resources (6285 links). Maintained and edited by physicians at the Johns Hopkins University, this site attempts to catalogue, review and score existing links to paediatric information on the internet.

4. **COMSEP** http://www.comsep.org/ [T] (USA)
The Council on Medical Student Education in Pediatrics (COMSEP) home page provides a multitude of links to paediatric educational resources, clinical cases sites and paediatric departments. It also provides the common core paediatric curriculum for US medical schools.

5. **PEDIATRIC linx:** http://www.pediatriclinx.com/ [T] (USA)
Regular reviews and updates in the paediatric specialties. Topical articles across the broad spectrum of paediatrics.

6. **BUBL LINK:** http://bubl.ac.uk/link/linkbrowse.cfm?menuid=8230 [T] (UK)
A catelogue of selected and peer reviewed internet resources in medicine, including paediatrics.

7. **Omni:** http://omni.ac.uk/ [T] (UK)
A gateway for reviewed health and education sites in medicine, reviewed weekly. Mostly UK content.

8. **Virtual Children's Hospital:** http://www.vh.org/VCH/ [T] (USA)
This site, maintained by the Children's Hospital of Iowa and the University of Iowa, has an extensive collection of links to useful paediatric sites worldwide. It is the 'virtual hospital' digital library of health information sites.

9. **The Merck Manual:** http://www.merck.com/mrkshared/mmanual/home.jsp [T] (USA)
A full text searchable version of the Merck Manual of Diagnosis and Therapy (17th edn, 2000). A valuable and up to date resource with links to other medical specialties. The Paediatrics section is at http://www.merck.com/mrkshared/mmanual/section19/sec19.jsp

10. **Paediatric Sites For Medical Students:** http://www.health.adelaide.edu.au/paediatrics/medindex.htm [T, I] (Australia)
A collection of links to web based paediatric resources for medical students.

11. **Subspecialty Collection from the American Academy of Pediatrics:** http://www.pediatrics.org/collections/ [T] (USA)
A topic specific archive of specialist paediatric studies published in the journal Pediatrics from January 1997 to the present. Within each category, further links and automated eSearches of Medline have been included to extend exploration of the topic areas.

12. **Martindale's Health Science Guide; Obstetrics, Pediatrics and Gynecology:** http://www.martindalecenter.com/MedicalPed_3_P.html [T, I] (USA)
A wide ranging site covering dictionaries and glossaries, an interactive anatomy browser, interactive patient cases, literature searches and useful links. Developed under the auspices of the University of California Library, USA.

13. **eMedicine Online Medical Textbooks:** http://www.emedicine.com/specialties.htm [T, I] (USA)
A collaborative peer reviewed site containing hundreds of online textbook chapters in many subject areas including paediatrics. A very valuable resource, and the whole site is updated and extended frequently.

14. **Medscape Pediatric Resource Centers:** http://www.medscape.com/pediatricshome?src=pdown pediatrics/pediatrics.html [T] (USA)
Extensive collection of resources for various paediatric diseases including paediatric oncology, group B streptococcal disease, asthma, growth and development and new variant Creutzfeldt–Jakob disease.

15. **Band-Aides and Blackboards:** http://www. lehman.cuny.edu/faculty/jfleitas/bandaides/ [T] (USA)
Stories of paediatric chronic illness written by children and adolescents with these conditions. Although provided primarily as a service for patients, it is a wonderful resource for medical students hoping to gain some understanding of the effect of chronic illness on the lives of young people.

General medical sites with paediatric content or relevance

1. **Medscape:** http://www.medscape.com/ [T, I] (USA)
Medscape contains news, reviews, medline searching, online *Harrisons' Internal Medicine* and links to hundreds of valuable medical sites. The site can be tailored to provide targeted information and automatic weekly update emails for paediatrics or most other specialties. Membership is required but registration is free.
2. **AusDoctors:** http://www.ausdoctors.net/ [T, I] (Australia)
Doctors net UK: http://www.doctors.net.uk [T, I] (UK)
Both these sites provide free online access to the *Textbook of Pediatrics*, 5th edition, by Forfar and Arneil. Registration for both sites is free for medical students and doctors.
3. **Doctors Guide:** http://www.docguide.com/ [T, I, ML] (USA)
A free registration medical site that provides access to online clinical updates and paediatric clinical cases.
4. **PubMed Central:** http://www.pubmedcentral. nih.gov/ [T, I] (USA)
A growing web based archive of journal literature for the life sciences being developed by the National Center for Biotechnology Information (NCBI) at the US National Library of Medicine (NLM). It includes free online access to the British Medical Journal, Arthritis Research, and Critical Care.
5. **Free On-line Medical Journals:** http://www. freemedicaljournals.com/ [T, I] (USA)
Link page to over 1440 free online medical journals.
6. **British Medical Journal:** http://www.bmj.com/ [T, I] (UK)
The 'collected resources' link contains an archive of paediatric papers published in the BMJ.
7. **Student British Medical Journal:** http://www.studentbmj.com/ [T, I] (UK)
Medical news and issues, including paediatric news and articles are presented in a format specifically tailored to medical students.

8. **British National Formulary (BNF) Online:** http://bnf.org/bnf/ [T, I] (UK)
The online BNF is published jointly by the British Medical Association and the Royal Pharmaceutical Society of Great Britain. It is a very concise and accurate drug reference and is updated twice yearly. Registration is required, free for NHS (UK) staff, but not for those from developed countries. There is additionally a Paediatric version of the BNF at http://www.bnfc.nhs.uk/bnfc/
9. **Office of Rare Diseases:** http://rarediseases. info.nih.gov/ [T, I] (USA)
A portal of information to rare diseases.
10. **Genetic and Rare Conditions Site:** http://www. kumc.edu/gec/support/ [T] (USA)
Medical Genetics, University of Kansas Medical Center, with information on genetics of rare diseases.
11. **OMIM™:** http://www3.ncbi.nlm.nih.gov/ omim/ [T] (USA)
Online Mendelian Inheritance in Man (OMIM). A catalog of human genes and genetic disorders. Useful and authoritative site for information on paediatric genetic syndromes.
12. **The CDC Wonder Database:** http://aepo-xdv-www.epo.cdc.gov/ [T] (USA)
This site offers a comprehensive compendium of the official guidelines and recommendations published by the US Centers for Disease Control and Prevention (CDC), with extensive statistics and information on public health matters.
13. **National Cancer Institute's Database:** http://cancernet.nci.nih.gov/ [T] (USA)
The National Cancer Institute's (NCI) comprehensive information database contains screening, prevention, treatment and supportive summaries for health care professionals. The main site links to the NCI's pediatric oncology branch.
Medical Student Resource: http://medicalstudent.com/ providing huge list of educational resources.

Search databases

National Library of Medicine, USA: The National Library of Medicine (NLM) offers '*PubMed*' and '*Internet Grateful Med*', which are two free systems to search MEDLINE: http://www.ncbi.nlm.nih.gov/ entrez/query.fcgi?DB=pubmed [T] (USA)

Free access to Medline is also available from the home pages of Medscape, the British Medical Journal, AusDoctors, Doctor's net UK and from many other medical sites. An online tutorial in the use of PubMed is available at: http://www.nlm.nih. gov/bsd/pubmed_tutorial/m1001.html [T] (USA). Most medical libraries have available searching of medline through on-line databases such as Ovid, including access to full text journals.

Evidence based medicine

The following sites are excellent resources for evidence based medicine reviews:

1. **Cochrane Colloboration:**
   http://www.cochrane.org [T] (UK)
   A core site for EBM information and links to EBM resources on the web.
2. **Evidence based medicine journal:** http://ebm.
   bmjjournals.com/ [T] (USA)
   New research of relevance to health
3. Oxford Centre for Evidence based Medicine.
   http://www.cebm.net/ For learning, doing,
   teaching, including an educational toolbox.
4. New York Evidence based Physicians. http://www.
   ebmny.org/ An evidence based resource centre.

Clinical teaching and clinical cases

1. **The Virtual Pediatric Patient:** http://www.vh.
   org/Providers/Simulations/VirtualPedsPatients/
   PedsVPHome.html [T, I] (USA)
   A useful case based teaching resource for
   common paediatric problems compiled by
   Donna M. D'Alessandro and Tamra E. Takle,
   University of Iowa College of Medicine.
2. **Asthma Management:** Guidelines for the
   Primary Care Physician: http://www.vh.org/
   pediatric/provider/pediatrics/Asthma/Asthma.
   html [T] (USA)
   American guidelines. Dr Miles Weinberger,
   University of Iowa College of Medicine.
3. **Paediatric Critical Care Resource:** http://pedsccm.
   wustl.edu/All-Net/main.html [T, V, I, ML]
   Associated with the picuBook project (http://
   picuBOOK.net) supported by the European
   Commission.
   Excellent peer reviewed articles on a wide
   range of paediatric emergency and critical care
   subjects (European Union).
4. **Correlapaedia** – a Correlative Encyclopedia of
   Pediatric Imaging, Surgery, and Pathology:
   http://www.vh.org/Providers/TeachingFiles/
   CAP/CAPHome.html [T, I, CS, Q]
   Edited by Michael P. D'Alessandro, University
   of Iowa College of Medicine, Steven J.
   Fishman, MD, Harvard Medical School, and
   Deborah E. Schofield, Children's Hospital of
   Los Angeles (USA)
   * 1997 winner of the American Academy of
   Pediatrics *Best of the Pediatric Internet Award*.
5. **COMSEP Clinical Cases**:
   http://www.comsep.org/EducationalResources/
   MultimediaTeaching.htm; A collection of non
   interactive and interactive paediatric clinical
   cases and a self-study online test.

6. **University of Kansas Pediatric Cardiology
   Cases:** http://www.kumc.edu/kumcpeds/
   cardiology/cardiology.html [T, I] (USA)
   Online lectures, images and case studies in
   paediatric cardiology.
7. **OnLine Pediatric Surgery Handbook** for
   Residents and Medical Students: http://home.
   coqui.net/titolugo/handbook.htm [T] (USA)
   A valuable text resource which can be
   downloaded as a PDF file. A branch of the
   parent website **Pediatric Surgery Update:** http://
   home.coqui.net/titolugo/index.htm#psu
   Edited by Doctor Lugo-Vicente, University of
   Puerto Rico School of Medicine, with independent
   teams of international contributors and reviewers.
8. **Pediatric Critical Care Medicine (PedsCCM):**
   http://PedsCCM.wustl.edu/ [T] (USA)
   A peer reviewed, collaborative information site for
   health professionals, this site helps disseminate
   information to promote quality care for critically
   ill and injured infants and children. The site
   also offers free AvantGo updates of the latest
   paediatric critical care evidence based treatment
   available for automatic palm OS download.
9. **American Academy of Pediatrics Policy
   Statements and Clinical Practice Guidelines:**
   http://www.aap.org/policy/pcyhome.cfm [T]
   (USA). An authoritative site with information
   on Policy Statements, Clinical Reports,
   Technical Reports, Clinical Practice guidelines
   and Parent pages.
10. **University of Virginia Pediatric
    Pharmacotherapy**: http://www.healthsystem.
    virginia.edu/internet/pediatrics/pharma-news/
    home.cfm l [T] (USA)
    A monthly brief, referenced, peer reviewed
    online review of new paediatric drugs and drug
    use in the USA.
11. **Great Ormond Street Library Paediatric Resources**:
    http://www.ich.ucl.ac.uk/library/ [T] (UK)
    A collection of paediatric websites particularly
    relevant to practice in the UK.
12. **Medical Connect:** http://www.medconnect.com/
    [T] (USA)
    An online CME/CE centre with weekly
    paediatric cases.
13. **Paediatric ALS:** http://www.mja.com.au/public/
    issues/aug19/arcg/arcg.html [T] (Australia)
    Paediatric advanced life support guidelines from
    the Australian Resuscitation Council Guidelines.
14. **Vanderbilt Pediatric Digital Library:** http://
    www.mc.vanderbilt.edu/vumcdiglib/databases.
    html?diglib=4 [T] (USA)
    The Vanderbilt Medical Center Pediatric
    interactive digital library is an extensive online
    reference for the paediatric specialties.

15. **Pediatric Dermatology:** http://www.edae.gr/
    pediatric.html [T, I] (USA)
    A large list of paediatric dermatology
    resources.
16. **Paediatric Lung and Heart Sounds:** http://www.
    rale.ca/ [T, S] (Canada)
    RALE: Repository of digital lung and heart
    sounds from the University of Manitoba. The
    full program requires payment, a demo is
    downloadable without charge.
23. **OncoLink-Pediatrics:** http://www.oncolink.
    upenn.edu/specialty/ped_onc/ [T, I] (USA)
    A collection of paediatric oncology resources
    with a 'case of the month' and other
    educational material aimed at medical
    students, doctors, parents and sick children.
    Compiled by the haematology and oncology
    specialists at the Children's Hospital of
    Philadelphia, USA.

Anatomy and imaging resources

The following are some sites with good image
resources:

1. **Paediatric Imaging and Radiology Site Collection**
   edited by Dr M. D'Alessandro, University of
   Iowa College of Medicine [T, I] (USA)
   a. **General Pediatric Imaging:**
      http://www.pediatricradiology.com/ [T, I]
   b. **Thoracopedia** – Paediatric respiratory medi-
      cine images: http://www.vh.org/Providers/
      TeachingFiles/TAP/Thoracopedia.html [T, I]
   c. **Paediapaedia** – an encyclopedia of paediatric
      disease with brief text notes, radiological
      images and differential diagnoses: http://www.
      vh.org/Providers/TeachingFiles/PAP/
      PAPHome.html [T, I]
2. **Fetal Echocardiography Homepage:** http://www.
   med.upenn.edu/fetus/ [T, I] (USA)
   An extensive library of still fetal
   echocardiograph images.
3. **Pediatric Imaging and Pathology:** http://www.
   uab.edu/pedradpath/cases.html [T, I] (USA)
   A useful collection of teaching files from the
   Departments of Pediatric Imaging and
   Pathology, Children's Hospital, Alabama.
4. **The Whole Brain Atlas:** http://www.med.
   harvard.edu/AANLIB/home.html [T, I, V]
   (USA)
   An excellent online neuroanatomy resource
   consisting of both still and video images of
   clinical cases with correlated neuroimaging (CT,
   MRI and PET scans). Compiled by Drs K. A.
   Johnson and J. A. Becker of Harvard Medical
   School.

National/International Governmental and paediatric organisations

1. **The Royal Australasian College of Physicians:**
   http://www.racp.edu.au/
2. **American Academy of Pediatrics:** http://www.
   aap.org/
3. **Royal College of Paediatrics and Child Health:**
   http://www.rcpch.ac.uk/
4. **Canadian Paediatric Society:** http://www.cps.ca/
5. **Society for Adolescent Medicine (SAM):** http://
   www.adolescenthealth.org/ [T] (USA)
   A multidisciplinary organisation of professionals
   committed to improving the physical and
   psychosocial health and wellbeing of adolescents.
   The site includes access to online publications
   such as position papers on a range of adolescent
   health related issues and an extensive and
   annotated list of links to web sites of interest.
6. **International Pediatric Chairs Association:** http://
   www.academicpediatrics.org An international
   committee of academic paediatricians.
7. National Health and Medical Research Council:
   http://www.nhmrc.gov.au/
8. WHO: http://www.who.int/en/
9. UNICEF: http://www.unicef.org/

Handheld/PDA resources for paediatrics

The quality and quantity of applications for handheld computers, also known as palmtop computers
or personal digital assistants (PDAs), has improved
significantly in recent years. There are now six major
PDA operating systems (OSs): Palm OS, EPOC,
Windows Mobile Pocket PC, Symbian OS, Black-
berry and Windows Mobile Smartphone. Currently
Palm OS is the most popular PDA OS worldwide; it
is fast, intuitive, memory efficient and requires very
little hardware. The Palm OS is used in Palm, IBM,
Handspring visor, Sony Clio and TRG-pro PDAs.
These PDAs use touch screen handwriting recognition or a screen based keyboard for manual data
entry, but keyboards can be attached. The Palm OS
has by far the largest amount of medically related
software and much of it is regularly updated and
improved.

The Epoc OS is very popular in Europe and is
utilised by the Psion series 3 and series 5 PDAs. The
Psion-Epoc combination is a powerful stand alone
system with excellent integrated software and tech-
nologically advanced hardware. Psions have the
advantage of a large screen and use quality integrated
keyboards for manual data entry. Currently Epoc
medical software is quite limited in scope and quality
compared with that available for the Palm OS system.

The Windows CE OS is also very popular, especially in North America. It is essentially a miniatur-

ised version of Windows, and, like the palm top, usually utilises touch screen handwriting recognition or a screen based keyboard for manual data entry. The newer Windows CE versions are quicker and more memory efficient than previous versions and many Palm OS medical software programs are available in Windows CE format.

1. **The 2000 Guide to Handheld and Palmtop Computing Resources for Health Care Professionals, 2nd edition:** http://themedicalguide. hypermart.net/ [P, Ps, CE, T, A] (Aust)
The essential guide for medical resources for Palm OS, Windows CE, Psion 3/5, and Newton OS handheld computers compiled by Ralph La Tella. Explanatory notes accompany each product and are often accompanied by actual screen shots of the application. It contains an extensive collection of paediatric software (Australia).
2. **Medical Pocket PC:** http://MedicalPocketPC. com/ [CE, T, A] (USA)
Core site for health related resources for the Windows CE platform.
4. **Useful sites containing medical reviews, discussion forum and downloads of freeware, shareware and commercial medical softwares for PDAs** [T, A] (USA)
   - Handango: http://www.handango.com/
   - Palm Gear: http://www.palmgear.com/
   - TuCows PDA: http://pda.tucows.com/index.html
   - Handheldmed.com: http://www.handheldmed. com/
   - Washington University Medical Palm Initiative: http://medicine.wustl.edu/~wumpi/
   - PDAMD: http://www.pdamd.com/vertical/ home.xml
   - Healthy Palm Pilot: http://www. healthypalmpilot.com/
   - Peripheral Brain: http://pbrain.hypermart.net/
   - The Medical Piloteer: http://www. medicalpiloteer.com/
5. **Paediatric pharmacopoeias**
   a. Epocrates: http://www.epocrates.com/ [P, T] (USA)
   The Epocrates package consists of the **qRx 4.0** drug reference guide and the **qID 1.0**, the infectious disease treatment guide for the Palm OS. Adult and paediatric doses, drug interactions and adverse effects are readily assessed. Available free online, where it is revised and peer reviewed monthly.
   b. **Tarascon ePharmacopoeia:** http://www.medscape.com/ [P, T] (USA)

Tarascon ePharmacopoeia is a PDA drug reference guide based on the popular pocket Tarascon drug booklet and similar to Epocrates qRx 4.0. It is available for free download but only within the USA from the medscape site. No equivalent PDA pharmacopoeias comprehensively covering paediatric medications used in the UK, Europe or Australasia are currently available.

6. **The Pediatric Pilot Page:** http://www. keepkidshealthy.com/pedipilot.html [P, T] (USA)
Has links to numerous Palm OS paediatric software sites.
7. **Pediatrics on Hand:** http://www. pediatricsonhand.com/ [P, T] (USA)
Compiled by Dr Stockwell, contains several useful handheld paediatric applications.
8. Handheld hospital patient clinical management applications:
   a. **Palm OS**
   — PatientKeeper: http://www.patientkeeper.com
   — WardWatch: http://www.watch.aust.com/ pilot/wardwatch
   b. **Psion**
   — http://www.psionarchives.com/
   c. **Windows CE**
   — Patient Tracker: http://www.handheldmed. com (Under Software)
9. **Memoware:** http://www.memoware.com/ [P, Ps, CE, T, A] (USA)
Memoware is an extensive repository of PDA documents and applications for the Palm, EPOC and Windows CE operating systems. The medical section has a host of useful paediatric documents such as immunisation regimens, specialised paediatric pharmacopoeias and developmental milestone references. Many of the documents require industry standard PDA document readers of databases such as Doc, SmartDoc, HanDbase, iSolo, Jfile 4, List, TealDoc, TealInfo or WordSmith. These are inexpensive (less than $25) and can be obtained via PDA software sites like Handango, TuCows PDA and Palm Gear (see above). The HanDbase website also has many medically relevant documents available for free download: http:// www.ddhsoftware.com/ [P, Ps, CE, T, A] (USA).

Acknowledgements

The assistance of Dr R. Wilcox, who undertook the initial internet searching and website analyses, is gratefully acknowledged.

PART 2

CLINICAL ASSESSMENT

Clinical consultation: history taking and examination

D. M. Roberton, M. South

History taking and physical examination are essential components of the diagnostic process, and this is especially so in child health. In most presentations, the majority of the information required for a diagnosis comes from the history, with a smaller amount coming from the physical examination. In many cases, no investigations are required. A common paediatric scenario is one in which a difficult diagnosis is able to be made by an experienced clinician who simply takes a thorough history.

Clinical consultations in paediatrics differ from those in adult medicine

The approach to clinical history taking and physical examination of children differs from that used for adults in several respects:

• It is much more common in paediatrics for the history to be given by a third party such as the parent or another caregiver. Be aware that the description of symptoms may be modified by the parent's perceptions or interpretations, and by factors such as anxiety. First-time parents sometimes do not know that what they perceive as a problem is in fact part of the normal range of variation for children
• There are many extra components of the history and examination that are important in children and that require special emphasis according to the age and presenting problem. Examples include details of the pregnancy and birth, feeding history in infancy, immunizations, growth, developmental milestones, behaviour and schooling
• The approach to establishing rapport with the patient and how the examination is conducted will need to be modified according to the age and development of the patient. There are differences in the techniques of physical examination and in expected findings at different ages.

Differences from adult consultation will be emphasized in the sections that follow.

Planning your approach to the consultation

A number of factors will modify the way you should set about the consultation:

• *The age and developmental status of the child.* Your approach will be quite different for a newborn baby, a preschool age child, an older child and an adolescent
• *The urgency and nature of the presenting problem.* In an emergency presentation, urgent treatment will obviously take priority over obtaining a complete history. It is, however, usually appropriate to return to aspects of the history at another time. It is clearly not necessary that a complete past history and developmental assessment be performed if a 4-year-old presents with acute diarrhoea and vomiting; however, it would be essential if the presentation were because of parental concern over the child's speech
• *The possibility of splitting the consultation into more than one session.* This is often appropriate for the assessment of more complex problems. Young children will often become bored, tired, hungry or irritable if a consultation lasts more than about 30 minutes. This can limit their ability to concentrate or cooperate with the assessment.

Clinical example

Louise, a 4-month-old girl, was the first baby in her family. She was taken to the general practitioner by her mother, Mary, who was very anxious because she felt that her baby was constipated, with a bowel action only once every 3 days. Mary was worried that this was because she was not producing enough breast milk to meet Louise's needs. Mary had been advised by a relative to give Louise laxative drops and to switch to bottle feeding.

Careful history taking revealed that Louise was feeding well and was passing a partly formed stool every third day without difficulty. There were no abnormalities on examination. Her growth chart showed that she was gaining weight well and was tracking just above the 50th centile for her age. Mary was shown the chart to reassure her that her baby was thriving. It was explained that Louise's stool frequency was within the normal range for breastfed babies. Mary was encouraged to continue breastfeeding.

Establishing rapport with the child and family

Your success in obtaining valuable information from the history and physical examination will depend partly on your knowledge of what information to seek and greatly on how you go about the task. Establishing a good relationship with the child and family is essential. The parents need to know who you are and to understand the purpose and likely outcome of the consultation. The child needs to feel comfortable in the environment and with you, particularly as you move on to the physical examination. Stranger anxiety, especially in children from about 8 months to 5 years of age, can be a significant obstacle. Experience and understanding help to overcome this.

The physical environment makes a big difference to how children feel. An adult may tolerate undressing in a cold room to be examined but a 2-year-old will probably cry. A bright, colourful room with pictures on the wall and toys on the floor is much more conducive than a 'sterile' clinical environment. A good range of toys, drawing materials, puzzles and other activities for all ages will be helpful.

Introduce yourself to the parents and, for almost all ages, to the child. Explain who you are and your role in the child's care. A common concern from parents of recently hospitalized children or children attending clinics is that they met many doctors and other health professionals, not really knowing who they were or who was 'in charge'.

Ask what name the child likes to be called. Just how much you should talk directly to the child at this stage will vary with the age of the child and with your assessment of how relaxed the child is. Some children respond well to questions and comments about their favourite sports team, school or a toy they have brought with them, while others will be shy and anxious if you address them directly. Learn to read children's responses and adapt accordingly. Young children may initially be very shy and cautious, and become much more confident and interactive later in the consultation.

Children's behaviour will often reflect how their parents are feeling. It is common for parents to feel anxious when attending a medical consultation. If you can form a good relationship with the parents, they will feel more at ease during the consultation and you will also have a better relationship with the child.

Sometimes it is appropriate to reassure the child at the start that nothing unpleasant is going to happen during the consultation (e.g. no blood tests or 'needles'). The child may associate visits to the doctor with memories of past uncomfortable experiences. Never hesitate to explain why you are asking a certain question or why you are performing a particular part of the examination.

Details of appropriate techniques for history taking and physical examination for adolescents are given in Chapter 3.11.

Taking the history

The current problem

Start by asking the parent (and/or child), about the current problem or problems. It is important to find out what they perceive to be wrong, and why they have chosen to seek medical attention at this time. A referral letter from another practitioner may have provided you with some information but it is essential to understand the problem from the parent's and child's perspective.

Questions such as: 'Why have you come to see me?', 'Why have you come to the clinic?' or 'What is worrying you about James?' are good ways to begin. If there is more than one problem, ask the parents to list them. Then approach the problems in order of perceived importance. Leave some space in your written record to add additional problems as they come to light during the history. Let the parent tell the story of the presenting problem/s without interruption. You may need to prompt them to go right back to the onset of the symptoms, as parents sometimes commence their description part way into an illness (e.g. from the time they last saw the family doctor). Questions like 'When was she last completely well?' can be very helpful.

Understanding the sequence and evolution of symptoms can be just as important as listing the symptoms themselves. The pattern of evolution will often reveal the diagnosis (e.g. central abdominal pain, later moving to the right iliac fossa in appendicitis).

When seeking extra detail or clarification, ensure your questions are open (e.g. 'Did he have any vomiting or diarrhoea?') rather than leading (e.g. 'He had no vomiting or diarrhoea?'). Be sure that the parent understands the terminology you use and always avoid medical jargon. Asking if the child has a symptom using a word the parents have never heard of, such as dyspnoea, will nearly always elicit a negative response, whereas an enquiry about breathing difficulties may result in a more accurate answer. Terms that you use every day, such as 'wheezing', may not mean the same thing to the lay person, so try to obtain a clear description. Sometimes it helps to ask parents to mimic the symptoms themselves, such as a cough or type of gait.

Older children can usually provide many of the details themselves. They can be asked if they agree with the description given by the parent or have anything to add.

You will then need to explore the symptoms in more detail (e.g. if the presenting symptom is cough, you will want to learn its character, if it is repetitive, if it occurs under certain circumstances and if it is moist or dry).

You will want to enquire about appropriate epidemiological features such as whether anyone else in the family or other contacts had similar symptoms, or if anyone at home is a smoker.

Clinical example

William, a 5-year-old boy, was brought by his parents for assessment because they noticed that he was tired each day in the late afternoon. He would lie on the sofa for up to an hour and be uninterested in playing during that time. Following this, he would seem to be his normal self.

This had been going on for nearly a year, since he started school. The rest of the history and examination were unremarkable. The parents' concerns seemed out of proportion to what is fairly common behaviour in early school age children. When asked why they had chosen to seek a medical opinion now, they revealed that a child of one of the mother's work colleagues had recently been diagnosed with leukaemia, and tiredness had been one of the features of her illness. The parents' major concern was that William might have the same diagnosis.

Learn to listen carefully and to distinguish comments that represent direct observation (e.g. 'he kept crying and pulling up his legs') from those that represent parental inference (e.g. 'he kept having spasms of tummy pain').

Be as specific as possible when taking the history of the current problems. Summarize your understanding of the symptoms and discuss this with the child and his/her parents once you feel you have a complete picture of the presenting problems and symptoms, to ensure that you have understood the information correctly and also to allow further information to be added if needed.

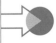

Practical points

- To obtain the trust of a child, you also need to gain the trust of the parent/s
- Do not use abbreviations or medical jargon during discussion with the family (say 'blue' rather than 'cyanosed' and 'breathing difficulty' rather than 'dyspnoea')
- When the family use descriptions such as 'wheezing' or 'croupy', make sure that these words mean the same to them as they do to you

Past history

The initial enquiry about the past history seeks to gain information relevant to the current problem and the age of the child. It is important to ask if the current problem has ever occurred in the past and to ask about past illness that might relate to the current presentation (e.g. a past history of meningitis will be very relevant for a 2-year-old who now presents with a seizure disorder).

For infants, it is important to obtain a history of the mother's pregnancy (her health, nutrition, use of medications, alcohol intake and smoking during the pregnancy, etc.), details of the birth (gestation, problems during labour, breech delivery, use of forceps or caesarean section) and the condition of the infant at birth (including the Apgar score, if known, and the need for any medical interventions such as oxygen therapy). What were the birth weight and other measurements? Ask about the infant's course in the first few weeks, including any illness and details of feeding and weight gain. Parents may have the child health record, which will provide many of these details. Simple questions such as 'Was the mother allowed to hold her baby immediately after birth?', and 'How soon was the baby discharged from hospital after birth?' can probe for problems. In young children, the early feeding history is also important.

Details of the pregnancy, birth and early course of postnatal life are usually of less significance for an older child presenting with an acute illness. They will be important, however, for an older child if the presenting problem is neurological or if there is a concern about developmental progress.

Family and social history

The young child's world is the family and it is very important to obtain an understanding of the family and social contexts of the child's illness and management. Ask about the age and health of the child's parents and siblings. Who else lives in the same household, and who provides most of the child's care? Does the child live in more than one household, as is often the case when parents are separated? Does the child attend day care, kindergarten or school? Is there a family history relevant to the child's presenting problems?

Find out about the family's housing and economic situation. Are the parents employed? Do they receive any financial allowances or community services? Look for factors that might adversely affect the child's health (e.g. smoking by household members), or that may influence management decisions (e.g. if the family live a long way from hospital and don't have a car).

It is usually useful to draw a brief family tree (Fig. 2.1.1).

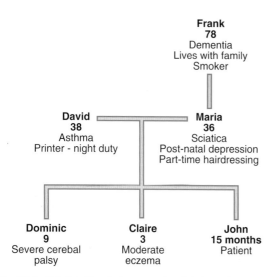

Frank
78
Dementia
Lives with family
Smoker

David
38
Asthma
Printer - night duty

Maria
36
Sciatica
Post-natal depression
Part-time hairdressing

Dominic
9
Severe cerebral
palsy

Claire
3
Moderate
eczema

John
15 months
Patient

Fig. 2.1.1 This brief family tree reveals a lot about the genetic and environmental factors that affect John, who now presents with recurrent cough and wheeze.

Clinical example

Mrs Baker brought her 10-year-old daughter Ruth for assessment. Ruth had previously been an outgoing and active girl but recently had seemed tired and listless, had lost her appetite and often would miss days of school because of headaches and abdominal pain. Mrs Baker was concerned that Ruth had an underlying illness such as glandular fever. Mrs Baker had had glandular fever herself when she was in her teenage years.

As part of the history taking, enquiry was made about the family's current circumstances. Ruth's parents had recently separated, and Ruth, who had been close to her father, saw him only occasionally. Unfortunately, her parents were no longer on speaking terms. On examination, Ruth appeared well although she was rather withdrawn. Blood tests did not suggest any evidence for glandular fever. Ruth's symptoms were due to the changes in her parents' relationship and she was assisted by counselling and support from a child psychologist.

Systems review

A brief check for other symptoms should be undertaken, using the usual organ systems approach. Again, learn to ask your questions in a non-leading way. Questions should be relevant to the current problem and the age of the child, rather than a long list of routine items. Ask about recent travel or potential environmental exposures if they are relevant to the presenting problem.

Growth and development

One of the aspects of childhood that clearly differentiates it from adult life is that children are growing physically and are acquiring new developmental skills. The achievement of a child's full growth and developmental potential is a central component of childhood and it follows that progress in this area requires careful assessment during the clinical consultation.

In infancy, growth is mainly assessed by checking for adequate weight gain, while in older children linear growth and appropriate body weight are both assessed. Where possible, birth measurements and any other previous growth measurement should be plotted on appropriate length/height, weight and head circumference centile charts (Ch. 19.1). This provides two types of information: an estimate of growth achievement in comparison with that expected for the 'normal' population and also growth progression with time in relation to expected genetic potential by observing 'tracking' along centile channels. Measurements are recorded most commonly in the parent-held child health record. Linear growth can also be plotted on growth velocity charts. An appropriate nutritional intake is an obvious and important prerequisite for normal growth: you should find out the usual daily pattern of food intake (breastfeeding in early childhood, type of formula feeds and intake pattern in later childhood) (Ch. 3.3).

You should also ask questions to ascertain whether developmental progress is within normal expectations. This can be done for young children by asking specific 'screening' questions that determine developmental progress at hallmark ages for each of the four major areas of development: gross motor, fine motor/adaptive, language and special senses, and personal–social. This assessment has its greatest importance in the early years of life to enable early detection of developmental difficulties (e.g. hearing impairment, motor difficulties due to cerebral palsy) and allow early intervention.

For older children, ask about progress at kindergarten or school, including parents' assessment as to motor skills and cognitive abilities in comparison with siblings and peers. For school-age children, enquire about special abilities that their child exhibits both in learning and in skills in sports or other activities. Ask children what they enjoy most in their learning activities ('What things are really fun to do?'), and in what activities they see themselves as having special abilities ('What are you really good at?').

More details of developmental assessment can be found in Chapter 2.2.

Behaviour

A brief history of the child's general behaviour is appropriate. Sometimes a perceived behavioural difficulty will be the presenting problem and a more detailed history will be necessary (Chs 4.1, 4.2, 4.3).

Medications

Enquire about current and past medications, including any adverse reactions and suspected drug allergies. Ask specifically about prescription medications and over-the-counter items. Complementary or alternative therapies are now frequently used in children but parents often forget or are reluctant to mention their use.

Immunization status

Full details of past immunizations should always be obtained. Don't just ask 'Is she up to date with immunizations?' or 'Has he had all his needles?' The answer you get will often be 'yes' and may be incorrect. Take time to go through what has been administered and compare this to the recommended schedule. Again, the child health record will be useful if available. Remember that, unless there is a specific contraindication, every clinical consultation should be seen as an opportunity to check immunization status and to offer immunizations that are due or have been missed (Ch. 3.5).

Closing questions

Complete the history taking by providing the parent or child with the opportunity to add extra information that may have been left out and to air their own concerns about causes for the presenting problem. The following closing questions will sometimes bring out very important information:

- Is there anything else that is worrying you?
- Is there anything else I should know or anything I have forgotten to ask you?
- Do you have any ideas of your own about what may be causing your child's symptoms?

Throughout the history taking, you will have the opportunity to observe the child. Remain observant so that you notice symptoms such as coughing or tachypnoea, developmental features of the child's play, and the interaction of the parent and child. This is a part of the physical assessment which is just as important as the more formal physical examination that follows.

Practical points

- Always undertake a brief but accurate assessment of growth and development at any consultation
- Remember to ask about all types of therapy used. Specifically enquire about complementary or alternative medications and other therapies
- Always take the opportunity to check that the child has received all his/her immunizations at the appropriate ages
- The closing questions will often be the ones to bring out the parent's deepest concerns regarding their child's problem. Don't omit this important opportunity, and leave yourself enough time to ask
- Be observant of the child's physical activities and the child/parent interactions during the history taking. These unstructured observations are an important part of the information gathering process

The physical examination

Introduction

The purpose of the physical examination is to provide additional information to aid in the diagnosis, assessment of the response to therapy, clues to comorbidities and important screening data on growth and development.

Young children will not understand why they are being approached and touched by a stranger. Shyness and stranger anxiety may limit their cooperation and some will simply refuse any physical contact. This is particularly the case for children between approximately 9 months and 3 years of age. Obtaining cooperation and a successful examination requires skill, understanding and practice. Don't be surprised or concerned if you are unsuccessful sometimes: this also happens to experienced paediatricians. Try coming back to the examination at a different time or with a different approach. Establishing a good rapport with the parent and child during the introduction and history taking as described above will facilitate the physical examination. The clinical approach to the examination of the adolescent is provided in Chapter 3.11.

Privacy during physical examination is just as important to children as to adults. You need to be friendly and relaxed, with a quiet and calm voice, and use gentle, unhurried physical movements. Undertake the examination by gentle opportunity, and vary the order in which you perform the components of the examination according to the child's cooperation. It is often the case with young children that you are not able to undertake all aspects of the examination at one time because it is tiring or frightening for the child. This means coming back at a later stage to continue.

You need to be prepared to examine the child in the position in which he or she is most relaxed. This might be on the examination couch but for young children is more likely to be on the mother's lap, cuddled over the father's shoulder or even lying on the floor! Undressing a young child completely will often upset him or her, and you should consider what it is necessary to expose according to the clinical situation.

Useful information can be obtained by careful observation from a distance and this is a very important technique for examination of small children. Sometimes it is more important to take a step back than to move forwards!

Clinical example

Ravi, an 18-month-old boy, presented to hospital with a history of cough and noisy breathing. His elder sibling had recently had a cold. Ravi was obviously frightened and upset when placed on the couch for the physical examination. He cried and clung to his mother's blouse when the Emergency Department Resident tried to undress him.

David, the Paediatric Registrar, suggested that Ravi be placed on his mother's lap while he observed him from a short distance. The nurse handed Ravi a brightly coloured toy. He stopped crying and started to examine the toy. David was able to note that Ravi was well grown, did not look seriously unwell and was alert. He was pink in room air, there was a clear nasal discharge and he had an obvious barking cough and mild stridor when resting. David asked that Ravi's mother lift his upper clothing to expose most of his chest. Ravi looked apprehensive but did not cry. David was able to observe good symmetrical chest movements with a respiratory rate of 22 per minute, and there was minimal indrawing of the intercostal soft tissues. David approached with his stethoscope but again Ravi looked as if he was about to cry. David knew that auscultation of the chest would not add much additional useful diagnostic information in this setting and so he desisted.

Ravi was diagnosed as having viral croup of mild to moderate severity.

In situations where you think the child's tolerance of the examination may be limited, ask yourself what are the most important items that you need to examine. It is often useful to do these first rather than adopting the more traditional sequence of examination used in adults and older children. Usually it is best to leave any potentially distressing components until last (e.g. examination of ears and throat).

You will become a skilled examiner of patients of any age if you learn to be a careful observer, and this is particularly so in the case of children. Teach yourself to really listen to what you hear, to look at what you see and to feel what you touch.

Most paediatricians develop their own techniques or 'tricks' for obtaining a child's cooperation with aspects of the examination. Some techniques rely on distraction (e.g. producing a previously unseen toy just prior to auscultation of the precordium). Some may use an incremental approach to obtaining the child's confidence. For example, in an anxious child, one might commence auscultation of the lungs by placing the stethoscope on a less threatening area than the chest, such as the child's thigh, then moving it onto the chest once the child has learned that it is not uncomfortable. Alternatively one might auscultate the father's arm or back first so the child can see that nothing unpleasant is involved. The detail of these techniques is not as important as the principle of learning methods that suit your own style of interacting with children.

As described for taking the history, physical examination of children needs to be adapted according to the presenting problem and the working differential diagnoses as they are formulated during the consultation. It is important to emphasize that successful physical examination of children is not only about ticking boxes in a checklist. Knowing exactly what to examine in any given situation, how to perform the examination techniques in children of differing ages and how to interpret the results are much more important and only come from experience in caring for children. The appendix to this chapter includes a list of the items that are commonly included during the physical examination as a guide only – don't use it as a checklist for every child.

General observation and behaviour

What are your first impressions of the child? Is she happy and relaxed, or does she seem tense and uncomfortable? Is she in pain? Is she of normal appearance or different from what you expect? Is she normally grown or small/large/obese/malnourished? Does she respond normally and in an age-appropriate way to her parents and siblings? How does she respond to you and to the surroundings? Is her understanding and language or other communication age-appropriate? Does she appear to hear and see normally? Is there anything obvious such as noisy breathing, bruising, an abnormality of limb movement, skin rash or abnormal pigmentation? Does she move/crawl/walk/run/climb normally? Are her fine motor movements while playing, drawing or getting undressed and dressed normal?

These initial impressions can be of great importance and provide useful clues for your overall assessment of the nature of the child's health problems and their impact.

Measurements

Except in emergencies, measurement of weight and height and plotting these variables on centile charts should be a routine part of the examination for *all* children. Children are ideally weighed in only light undergarments, and in babies the nappy should be removed. Height should be measured accurately using purpose-made equipment (Ch. 19.1).

Specific examination

It is assumed that the reader already has a good understanding of normal examination technique and expected findings for adult patients. There are many differences in the techniques and expected findings in children and these are emphasized below.

Vital signs

Normal ranges for heart rate, respiratory rate and blood pressure vary with age. Table 2.1.1 gives approximate values for children at rest. Note that blood pressure upper normal values can be different in boys and girls. If hypertension is suspected, consult age- and gender-specific graphs for blood pressure.

Respiratory system

The pattern of respiration in young infants often has a large abdominal component. The chest wall is compliant so that conditions that cause reduced lung compliance or airway obstruction will more readily be manifest by indrawing of the soft tissues of the chest wall, and in more serious disease the rib cage itself may be drawn in during inspiration. The breath sounds in infants are more readily heard because of the thin chest wall and they often sound harsher on auscultation than in older children and adults. These normal differences in auscultation findings are even more pronounced in the upper parts of the right lung, sometimes leading inexperienced examiners to suspect pathology in this area in young children when in fact the breath sounds are normal for this age.

Cardiovascular system

A thorough description of examination of the cardiovascular system is provided in Chapter 15.1. Selection of an appropriate-sized cuff for the age and size of the child is important for accurate measurement of blood pressure.

Abdomen

Compared with older children, the abdomen of a young infant appears protuberant, and the umbilicus may be everted as a normal finding. The liver is normally palpable up to 2 cm below the right costal margin and it is sometimes possible to feel the tip of a normal spleen and the lower pole of the right kidney.

Rectal examination should not be performed routinely. If indicated by the presenting problem, it should be undertaken once only and by the person who will be making management decisions based on the findings (e.g. a surgical registrar in the case of suspected appendicitis).

Genitalia

In infant boys, assessment of the penis and scrotum should be considered part of the normal routine

Table 2.1.1 Some normal ranges for vital signs at different ages in childhood			
Age	Respiratory rate (breaths/min)	Heart rate (beats/min)	Systolic blood pressure (mmHg)
Newborn	40–60	100–160	50–75
1 week to 3 months	30–50	80–160	50–85
3 months to 2 years	20–40	80–140	60–100
2 years to 10 years	14–24	60–100	70–110
>10 years	12–20	50–100	85–120

examination, as unsuspected inguinal herniae, undescended testes and urethral abnormalities may be detected. It is normal for the prepuce to be non-retractile and adherent to the glans up to around 4 years of age.

In girls, examination of the genitalia is usually undertaken only when indicated because of a specific problem. In instances where a genital examination beyond simple external observation is required in a girl this should be done by an appropriate specialist.

Central nervous system

Formal examination of the nervous system is time-consuming and many aspects require cooperation from the patient. In young children, observation of movement and behaviour can provide most of the necessary information, with specific neurological examination being reserved for children where the primary concern is the nervous system. Routine sensory examination is necessary only rarely.

Skin

Examination of the skin is important not only in dermatological problems: congenital skin lesions may give diagnostic clues to other conditions. For example, the characteristic pale patches of tuberous sclerosis may provide the diagnosis in a child who is being assessed for developmental delay and seizures (Ch. 21.2).

Musculoskeletal system

Examination for congenital hip disease should be routine in young infants (Ch. 8.1).

Special senses

From the history and general observation, you should be able to assess that the child can see and hear adequately. Screening examination for hearing and vision must be age-appropriate (Chs 22.1, 22.2) and formal assessment by an audiologist or optometrist may be required.

Development

A brief screen of developmental achievements and progress should be undertaken. Detailed assessment is not routine unless indicated by the clinical problem (Ch. 2.2).

Head and neck

In babies, examine the head size and plot it on the centile chart. Check the head shape, the fontanelles and the sutures (Ch. 11.1). The posterior fontanelle is often closed by 2 months of age and the anterior fontanelle closes between 12 and 24 months of age.

Examine the teeth, if present, for their number, pattern of eruption and the presence of caries or abnormalities (Ch. 22.3). Take this opportunity to remind parents of the importance of good dental care and of regular attendance with a dentist.

Examination of the mouth, throat and ears requires good cooperation or appropriate restraint of the child. Observation of experienced practitioners is the best way to learn these techniques.

Concluding the examination

As for taking the history, it can be helpful to ask the parent or child if there is anything else they would like you to check at this point. Your examination may also have revealed findings that prompt you to return and take further details in the history.

Note taking

It is important that you produce an accurate and clear record of the history and examination findings. This will be needed to help you later and as a record for future staff involved in the child's care. A few items will need to be jotted down briefly as you go along but the rest of the record should be written after the consultation is completed. You will not develop a good rapport with the family if you are constantly gazing at your papers and writing notes.

In younger children, you will have adapted the order of the physical examination to fit the clinical problem and their tolerance of the examination process. Whatever the sequence in which you obtain your information, it is still important to record your findings in a logical and structured format.

The consultation as part of the therapy

Doctors often think of the management of a clinical problem as a chronological sequence commencing with history taking and examination, followed by formulation of a differential diagnosis, appropriate investigations, final diagnosis, treatment, assessment of response and outcome. Most families who have an ill child will not arrive at the consultation with you with that same perspective. They will have come because they perceive that their child has a problem and they will often be anxious that it might turn out to be serious. They will be in a foreign environment and one that may have frightening associations for them. They may not know who exactly you are nor if you are the best person to help them with their child's problem.

You will be in a position to help ease at least some of the family's anxieties long before you have even arrived at a diagnosis. You can achieve this by being friendly, by explaining who you are and by conveying that you are genuinely interested in their concerns and that you value their time and opinions as much as your own. Use language they understand, give them time and opportunities to express their concerns fully, be gentle and caring during your examination, and give a clear explanation of what you think the problem might be and the nature and purpose of any investigations or treatment that you recommend. In this way, you will help to obtain the family's confidence and trust, which in turn will improve their willingness to cooperate with the plan of investigation and treatment that is required.

You will not acquire all these skills overnight but learning them is rewarding and fun, and you will be a much more effective doctor for children and their families at the end of the process.

Practical points

- Skills in history taking and examination cannot be acquired adequately by reading a textbook. Ensure you have lots of practice with children of all ages and in different clinical settings
- Learn to appreciate what constitutes normal growth, development and physical findings on examination. Take every opportunity you can to observe normal children (who might be visiting the hospital or community health centre, in the cafeteria, or even travelling on public transport). Try and guess their ages from your observations (based on size, development and behaviour) and then ask how old they really are
- Adapt the content and techniques of history taking and examination to fit the age of the child and the urgency of the medical problem
- Learn to be flexible in your approach – some patients will need to be examined on the floor, while in a play area, or from a distance

Items that are commonly included in the physical examination

Those items marked (#) are usually included, while others will be noted in selected situations only.

- Height (#)
- Pulse rate (#)

- Weight (#)
- Respiratory rate (#)

- Head circumference
- Blood pressure (#)

General appearance
- Looks well/unwell/sick/very sick (#)
- Alertness (#)
- Distressed/cooperative
- General body build
- Overall development including speech
- Facial appearance/dysmorphism (#)
- Posture, movement
- Interaction with parents (#)

Skin
- Colour/pigmentation/jaundice/cyanosis/pallor (#)
- Bruising/petechiae/rashes/scars
- Turgor
- Visible blood vessels
- Subcutaneous fat

Nails/hair
- Cyanosis/pallor/clubbing
- Haemorrhages
- Distribution and colour of hair

Lymph nodes
- Size/mobility/tenderness of nodes in each group (cervical, occipital, axillary, inguinal, etc.)

Head
- Size/shape/posture
- Fontanelles: presence/shape/tension
- Bruit/percussion

Eyes
- Appearance/blinking/ptosis/nystagmus
- Visual acuity/fields
- Ocular movements/squint
- Lids/discharge
- Fundoscopic appearance
- Light and corneal reflex

Ears
- Position/shape
- Discharge
- Hearing (#)
- Appearance of tympanic membranes

Nose
- Shape/flaring with respiration/discharge/bleeding
- Patency of airway/mucosal appearance/polyps

Mouth/lips/teeth/gums/ palate/pharynx
- Colour of lips, tongue and buccal mucosa
- Presence of exudates/coating/ulcers
- Lip swelling or scaling/fissuring
- Number of teeth and presence of caries
- Breath odour/salivation
- Petechiae/bleeding
- Colour of pharyngeal mucosa
- Size, colour and presence of exudate on tonsils

Chest/lungs
- Shape/symmetry/deformities (including Harrison's sulcus, rickety rosary)
- Expansion of chest and pattern of breathing
- Soft tissue indrawing with respiration
- Pattern and rate of breathing
- Cough/stridor/wheezing
- Percussion note
- Breath sounds/added sounds

Breasts
- Development (Tanner stage)

Heart
- Appearance of precordium: deformity/activity
- Pulse: rate/rhythm/strength/nature
- Blood pressure
- Apex beat/cardiac impulse/thrills
- Percussion of cardiac dullness
- Heart sounds/added sounds
- Features of cardiac failure

Abdomen
- Shape/distension/visible mass/movement with respiration
- Visible veins/peristalsis
- Percussion/ascites
- Tenderness on palpation
- Enlarged organs/palpable mass
- Anus/rectum (avoid examination in children unless specifically indicated)

Genitalia
- Development (Tanner stage)
- Presence of testis in scrotum
- Scrotal swellings/hernia
- Urethral/vaginal discharge
- Evidence of injury

Spine
- Posture/deformity/hair/dimples/tenderness

Limbs
- Deformity/contractures
- Muscle development
- Hip dislocation (Ch. 8)
- Joints: tenderness/swelling/range of movement
- Temperature/colour

Nervous system
- Alertness/responsiveness/general ability
- Abnormal movements/gait/posture
- Tone/power/coordination/symmetry of movement
- Reflexes/primitive reflexes
- Special sensory examination
- Sensation
- Cranial nerves

Developmental assessment
See Chapter 2.2

Developmental surveillance and assessment

D. Starte, D. Meldrum

We continue to develop new skills throughout life but it is during childhood that this process is most dramatic. As with physical growth, the rate of developmental growth is a defining distinction of paediatric medicine. There are major developmental changes in primary and high-school children but it is the first 5 years of life, during which the majority of basic skills are acquired, that is a predominant focus for developmental paediatrics.

Doctors learning about child development often wish to memorize lists of milestones but fail to appreciate the diversity of normal variation. Adults are not expected to have an even distribution of talents themselves, in their families or in their colleagues; yet when we consider children we often assume they will all walk at 12 months, talk in phrases at 2 years and draw faces at 4 years. It is the variability in normal patterns of development that makes the area fascinating and creates complex challenges in screening and diagnosis.

Assessing normal development (developmental surveillance)

Developmental surveillance is a routine part of all paediatric interactions. This requires the doctor to have a working knowledge of normal development in all its forms and to be able to detect variations that may be indicative of significant disorders.

Child development progresses in many areas simultaneously. It is as necessary to know the various developmental systems as it is to know the physical systems. Each will have its component parts and the rate of progress in all of these components may be similar (when delayed, this is described as a global delay) or discrepant (described as specific or selective delay).

The process of determining a child's developmental progress is no different from any other system, and starts with a good history. Parents are often remarkably accurate at recalling recent developmental changes but more distant events may require prior notice so that sources such as relatives and baby books can be reviewed. A simple structured questionnaire filled in before the interview can allow parents to consider the details in the waiting room or at home. Most developmental interactions are best scheduled for a well child visit or review to avoid confusing illness behaviour with developmental delay.

> ### Clinical example
>
> Sinclair, a 3-year-old child of English speaking parents, only had a vocabulary of 20 words. His medical history was normal. The parents were reassured by his normal hearing assessment, as well as by the father's own history of initial poor speech development as a child. However, the preschool staff became concerned about the degree of his language difficulty and whether it was part of a global developmental delay. The words he knew were used singly, were clearly articulated and were used in their appropriate context but, to indicate his needs, he resorted to leading an adult by the hand. No phrases or small sentences were heard. He understood two-step commands and used facial expressions, hand gesturing and eye to eye contact appropriately. At preschool, he was interested in the other children but they often excluded him in play when he couldn't talk properly. He showed examples of imaginative, constructive and cooperative motor play. There were no behavioural concerns and he was an affectionate child.
>
> Assessment with the Griffiths Mental Developmental Scales showed that his abilities tested within the average range for his age, other than a mild delay in speech and language skills. During the assessment, he was cooperative and persevered with the tasks at hand. Sinclair therefore had an isolated expressive language disorder of presumed familial origin, and was referred to a speech pathologist for assessment, therapy and liaison with the preschool teacher to modify his preschool curriculum.

The following are important components when undertaking developmental surveillance:

- adequate time and privacy
- good communication skills
- knowledge of normal developmental ranges
- history of family patterns of behaviour and development
- examination for neurological and syndromic features

Table 2.2.1   Areas of development (input requires sensation; output requires motor control)

Gross motor control	Movement sensation – kinaesthesia, vision and vestibular input Large-muscle coordination produces agility
Vision and fine motor	Vision and visual perception guidance Small-muscle coordination produces dexterity and clear speech
Language and hearing	Hearing and auditory processing distinguish speech sounds Receptive language encodes words and sentences into ideas Expressive language encodes ideas as words and sentences, leading to speech Pragmatic language enables socially interactive conversation
Social and daily living skills	Watching and listening inform imitation Fine and gross motor skills enable imitative actions Feeding, dressing and household tasks lead to self-care Nurturing fosters self-confidence and independence Temperament moderates emotional regulation

- attention to sensory functions, e.g. vision and hearing
- belief in parents' reporting accuracy.

A good history starts with the pregnancy and delivery and progresses through the neonatal, infancy, toddler and preschool years. The areas to consider are covered in Table 2.2.1 and parents should be asked open-ended questions about their child's progress, such as 'Tell me how she is getting around', which would be more likely to elicit revealing answers than 'Is she walking now?' This process is time-consuming and parents need to feel relaxed and unhurried if they are to give their best information. Some of the information may well be sensitive, especially when there are problems, and a private setting without interruptions is important.

The key is to look for areas of development delayed beyond the normal range and not to compare the child with 'normal milestones', which are merely the average age of achievement. Half of the population will not meet median milestones by definition, and their use can worry many parents unnecessarily. It is preferable to use the normal ranges in Table 2.2.2. Many developmental patterns are familial and so are many developmental disorders. Do not accept delay as a normal variation because an uncle did not talk until he was 4 years old, as the uncle may also have had a developmental language disorder or deafness. Other 'causes' such as being a twin, bilingualism or tongue tie should not be accepted, and actual delays need to be excluded by more formal diagnostic assessment. Assuming that the child is significantly delayed because of these causes of minor variation is a common source of late diagnosis and delayed effective intervention.

As each area is reviewed through the different stages of childhood, any apparent delays or unusual features can be clarified with the family. This allows the developmental examination to be targeted. While many children are shy and perhaps fearful, a quiet patient approach will often bring out the showoff in children, especially for tasks about which they are confident. For this reason it is best to start looking at non-verbal areas (blocks, puzzles, drawing, etc.), and having appropriate furniture at the child's height will enable you to get down to the child's eye level. Simple equipment (Table 2.2.3) can be used to elicit a range of skills and the session should remain a play activity. Remember that too much direct eye contact, especially from above, can be threatening, and a relaxed tangential approach across the child may be more successful. Refusal to cooperate is a regular occurrence and it is better to reschedule than to persist and teach the child that your sessions are going to be unpleasant.

The most important conclusion that needs to be drawn from this exercise is to ensure that there are no warning signs of a potential problem (Table 2.2.4). Should doubt exist, it is always better to seek a second opinion and to arrange some simple therapy or intervention than to provide false reassurance. It may make you feel better to reassure, but families who waste months finding help for their child will often feel very angry.

Formal developmental screening

Screening is the process of detecting presymptomatic disorders in order to intervene and change their natural history. Screening uses tests of known

Table 2.2.2 Normal ranges (approximately 25th centile to 90th centile)

Age	Gross motor control	Vision and fine motor	Language and hearing	Social and daily living skills
2–4 months	Head steady in sitting	Follows object through 180°	Squeals with pleasure	Smiles
5–8 months	Sits without support	Passes cube hand to hand	Turns to soft voice Baba/Gaga babble (up to 10 months)	Feeds self biscuit
9–14 months	Stands with support	Neat pincer grasp of raisin	Mama or Dada specifically	Indicates needs by gesture
12–16 months	Walks well alone (up to 21 months)	Stack of two cubes (up to 21 months)	Three words	Drinks from a cup
15–24 months	Walks up steps	Scribbles spontaneously	Points to one body part	Removes garment
21–36 months	Jumps on the spot	Draws vertical line in imitation	Uses plurals and phrases	Puts on clothing Plays tag with other children
3–4½ years	Balances on one foot for 5 s	Copies a ladder Draws a face	Understands cold, tired and hungry Asks 'Wh' questions	Separates from mother

Table 2.2.3 Developmental equipment

Gross motor control	Steps, for walking up and down Tennis ball, for kicking, throwing and catching Tricycle, for riding and pedalling
Vision and fine motor	Raisins, for pincer grasp and self feeding 2.5 cm blocks, for simple stacks, counting and colour matching Simple inset puzzles, for matching and sorting shapes Small crayon/pencil, for scribbling and drawing Paper, for above and folding and cutting
Language and hearing	Doll, for identifying body parts and pretend play Simple picture book, for pointing out items/describing the action Telephone or Dictaphone, for encouraging spontaneous speech
Social and daily living skills	Eyes and ears, for listening to parents and observing interactions Mirror, for watching baby's responses to self Toy cup, plate and cutlery, for demonstrating feeding self or doll

accuracy in healthy or at risk populations to uncover those with the target problem before symptoms arise. Further diagnostic testing can then be performed, before appropriate intervention is carried out. In the developmental context, tests are sometimes used to formalize the surveillance process. Examples are:

• Parent's Evaluation of Developmental Status. 10 simple questions about parent concerns (www.pedstest.com)
• Denver II. American observation schedule of four areas of development (www.denverii.com)
• Australian Developmental Screening Test (ADST). Australian observation schedule (Psych Corp – Australia)

Table 2.2.4 Warning signs to worry about; be concerned if the child is not doing this by the stated age (items marked * are a worry if they are present)

Age (months)[†]	Gross motor control	Vision and fine motor	Language and hearing	Social and daily living skills
3	Complete head lag*	Following with eyes	Searching for sounds with eyes	Smiling
6	Preference for one hand Persistent Moro*	Squint*	Head turn to soft voice	Interest in people
9	Sitting with support	Persistent hand regard*	Ba-ba-ba babble	Awareness of strangers
12	Pulling to stand Standing with support	Pincer grasp	Trying one or two words	Constant mouthing*
18	Walking alone	Constructive play with blocks Casting toys*	Six words Constant dribbling*	Pointing at items Finger feeding
24	Running	Turning book pages	Fifty single words	Interested in other children Helps in dressing
36	Kicking a ball	Drawing lines	2–3 word phrases Echolalia*	Interactive play with peers
48	Pedalling and hopping	Drawing a face	Sentences and 'Wh' questions	Imaginative play Toilet trained by day

† Or at any age if there is parental concern (parents are usually right) or regression in skills.

• Brigance screens. Modern observation schedule (www.curriculumassociates.com)
• Ages and Stages Questionnaires. Structured parent questions for different ages (www.brookes publishing.com).

As developmental delays produce easily detectable symptoms, regular review of the various developmental areas at all doctor visits may well be a more effective method of detection than formal screening procedures at specified intervals. This surveillance is enhanced when combined with parent education about child development.

Diagnosing the problem (developmental assessment)

While this process is broadly a more detailed version of simple surveillance, it is common for doctors with particular experience in the area to be involved in teams with other professionals with specific expertise. These professionals may be:

• social workers or community nurses, who are highly skilled in family support and interactions
• psychologists, skilled in intelligence testing and behavioural interventions
• physiotherapists, with skills in movement and coordination
• speech pathologists, with language and oromotor skills
• occupational therapists (OT), with daily living skills, seating and manual dexterity.

In good teams all members learn from each other and considerable role release can occur. Some specialized teams will need specific expertise from orthoptists, audiologists and orthotists, as well as technical support personnel to help with specific equipment. Clinics specializing in developmental assessment may be located in major hospitals with paediatric services or in community-based health centres.

The history taking, which often includes parental questionnaires, will be very detailed about the nature of the concerns raised as well as the medical, developmental and family history. It is most important to be clear about the family's expectations of the assessment, so that their agenda is covered fully. It may be helpful to arrange a home visit by one of the team initially to break the ice with the family and to see the child in more natural surroundings. Most families are understandably anxious about a formal developmental assessment, as it may lead to bad news. Anything done to reduce the family's apprehension will also be likely to reduce the child's fears and improve the reliability of the assessment as a sample of the child's development. To this end, the venue for the assessment should not be overly clinical and the staff should be understanding and welcoming.

Clinical example

Max was a 3-year-old boy with an unremarkable past medical or family history. However, from the age of 2 years there were concerns about his development, in particular his language and gross motor skills. A previous speech pathology assessment revealed a mild receptive and expressive language delay. Despite progress with speech therapy, a review of his general development was requested because of concerns that he was also stumbling when running. Compared to his sister he was slightly later in sitting (8 months) and walking (15 months) and he initially had difficulties in climbing frames but he still could jump or kick a ball well, and walked up and down stairs one step at a time.

Max was examined using the Griffiths Mental Developmental Scales, which showed age-appropriate puzzle skills, low-average range fine motor and language skills and slightly more delayed gross motor skills. On examination he had a lordotic posture, a waddling gait, only slightly overdeveloped calf muscles, and mild difficulty getting up from a sitting position on the ground. A proximal myopathy was suspected in association with his very mild developmental delay. The initial creatine kinase (CK) was 33 000 units/litre and a dystrophin gene analysis was arranged. Max went on to have a muscle biopsy, which showed the typical changes of Duchenne muscular dystrophy.

Important aspects of the developmental assessment process are:

- multidisciplinary team approach
- colleagues working as equals
- good information gathering before the assessment
- standardized tests of development and intelligence
- standardized behavioural questionnaires
- specific therapist reviews as clinically indicated (physio, OT, speech)
- ample time and privacy to discuss the findings with the family
- written reports to the family with a plan of action
- follow up on any recommendations made.

Information should also be gained from people who know the child, such as teachers, therapists and doctors. This requires consent from the family to approach them but can be very useful if done in advance. The developmental assessment can then be interpreted in the light of the child's wider world. Sufficient time needs to be allocated at the assessment for all the issues to be covered, and this can take several hours. A choice of professionals to see the family can be made based on the concerns expressed and the information gathered. During the assessment, each professional will need some time to work with the child and also to talk with the parents to clarify history details particular to their involvement.

Most teams will attempt some form of formal test of developmental status, often performed by the psychologist, to assess the degree and distribution of any developmental delay or disability. This is not just to gain a score but provides a structured way of reviewing all aspects of cognitive development in an age appropriate framework. In young children, this may be a developmental test such as the Griffiths or Gesell Scales. In older children a standard intelligence test is often used such as the Weschler tests (WPPSI or WISC), the Stanford-Binet or the Differential Ability Scales.

A developmental quotient (DQ or GQ) derived from the former tests includes aspects of self-care and motor development and is a broader concept than intelligence quotient (IQ), which relates more specifically to cognitive capacity. It is usual to talk about a delay in development when the child is young (say under 3 years of age) and the prognosis uncertain. When it seems that the child has a permanent developmental disorder it is better to call it a disability, as many parents assume that any delay will eventually resolve. In addition, specific behavioural questionnaires may be used to assess the severity of symptoms suggestive of autism, attention deficit/hyperactivity disorder (ADHD) or other behavioural disorders such as oppositional defiant disorder or anxiety disorders.

Investigations that may be useful and should be considered in situations of possible developmental delay are:

- formal hearing and vision testing, not screening (see text)
- low average to borderline delay alone: consider variation from family norms.
- mild/moderate delay or above with language delay/dysmorphisms: chromosomes, DNA for fragile X, thyroid function
- boys with above: creatinine kinase
- severe intellectual deficit: lactate/pyruvate, amino and organic acids

43

Clinical example

When Jesse was 2 years 1 month old, he was referred for assessment of his development because of speech and language delays. On the developmental assessment he displayed a mild developmental delay overall, with an age equivalent level of 1 year 5 months. His weaknesses were in the areas of personal–social, language and fine motor skills, which were moderately delayed (1 year age equivalent level). His strength was in gross motor skills, which were normal (2 year 4 month age equivalent level). Speech therapy and occupational therapy were arranged and when he started preschool an individualized educational programme was established for him.

Jesse was reviewed again at the age of 3 years 11 months and still showed an overall mild delay (2 years and 7 months). Gross motor skills remained his personal strength, being within normal limits, and his puzzle-solving skills had improved to a borderline level. However, his weakest areas continued to be language and fine motor skills, which were still moderately delayed. Speech therapy and occupational therapy programmes continued, and a special needs teacher was arranged to provide further educational support at preschool.

At the age of 5 years and 2 months a reassessment was arranged to plan for school placement based on his general learning progress and support needs. He was assessed using the Differential Ability Scales (an IQ test), which demonstrated a general conceptual ability around the 1st percentile (IQ = 63), in the mild deficit range. When considered together with parental, teacher and therapist reports and his two previous developmental assessments, it was clear Jesse had a long-term intellectual disability of mild degree. Mainstream kindergarten placement with integration support was arranged, with possible progression to an appropriate smaller support class at primary school age. Gross motor skills are not a good guide to intellectual development.

- large head, central nervous system or skin signs: computed tomography (CT)/magnetic resonance imaging (MRI); watch for family history of large head
- small head: TORCH titres; mild maternal phenylketonuria; MRI.
- loss of speech skills: sleeping electroencephalogram; neurometabolic tests
- old houses, renovations, pica: blood lead
- syndromic or dysmorphic features: genetics opinion before specific DNA studies.

It should be remembered that investigations in these situations should be offered rather than being insisted on: not all families are as focused on aetiology as medical staff.

The medical examination (Ch. 2.1) will ensure that growth parameters are measured, especially head circumference, and signs of dysmorphism and neu-rocutaneous disorders are sought. The aim is to detect any condition that might be causing the developmental delay, or indeed any general medical problem that may be exacerbating it. While a thorough physical examination is desirable, particular attention needs to be paid to the neurological system, looking for signs of cerebral palsy and other neuromotor disorders (Ch. 17.2).

Some ingenuity may be needed after a long developmental session to engage the child in play again. Indeed much can be learned from observing the developmental testing (preferably through a one-way screen) or working with the physiotherapist or occupational therapist to dovetail the necessary observations. Special attention is often paid to vision and hearing screening at this time, and much has been written about this. However, a note of warning is necessary, as these senses are vital for children's learning. For intervention to be as efficient as possible, these senses need to be acute. It may therefore be more of a service to the child to ensure that he or she is seen by a vision or hearing professional than to perform some rough screening test, especially when the developmental concerns are specific to that sense (i.e. hearing to language or vision to motor skills). Again, false reassurance needs to be avoided at all costs.

Many children coming to developmental teams will already have a diagnosis such as Down syndrome or cerebral palsy, but some conditions are less obvious and need particular vigilance, e.g. velocardiofacial syndrome, fragile X syndrome (Ch. 10.3), the mucopolysaccharide storage disorders, thyroid deficiency or lead excess and, in boys, muscular dystrophy. Investigations or further opinions should be recommended to families as needed, to help exclude any conditions that appear possible. Chromosome analysis or specific DNA tests have the highest positive yield in most developmental presentations. Imaging and EEG testing are less rewarding unless specific signs or symptoms of neurological disorder are present.

Of particular relevance is the referral to a clinical genetics service for the family of a child with any dysmorphic features or a known condition where new information about recurrence or antenatal testing may be available. This is an area of medicine where knowledge is changing with dramatic speed and up-to-date information on diagnosis, prognosis and available testing can be valuable for both the index family and all their relations.

Once all members of the team have had their chance to interact with the child and family, it is time to bring everything together. This fusion of professional opinions should occur before further discussions with the family so that they can be presented as a cohesive view of the child. The feedback session can be scheduled on the same day or later; it is always helpful to have both parents present and any close family supports that they request, e.g. grandparents.

Once the team's view has been clearly stated, it is normal to ask for the family's reaction and to discuss this. This will hopefully lead to discussions covering investigation, aetiology, prognosis, genetic advice and a plan of action. Recommendations can be formulated with the family as to what needs to be done by whom, where and when. This all needs to be recorded carefully and copies given to the family on the day, as much of what is said may be forgotten, especially when the news is shocking. However, the manner in which it is imparted is likely to be remembered for all time and care taken with the time available, privacy and if necessary the use of interpreter services will help optimize a potentially traumatic session.

All parents need copies of all the reports that are generated; further copies can be sent to those professionals involved with the child if the family agree. Follow-up can be arranged to review any investigations or to help establish intervention services. Many parents feel a sense of grief if the child has a serious developmental problem and it may be necessary to provide written material and counselling to help them understand that this is a normal reaction. Failure to resolve the grief reaction can lead to ongoing anger, depression or marital conflict and may delay important remedial action for the child.

> **Practical points**

- Development occurs in many areas, often unevenly. Always check receptive language, expressive language, non-verbal reasoning (puzzles), social interaction/empathy, daily living skills, attention and impulse control
- Listen carefully to parents/carers. An accurate and detailed history will be the best diagnostic guide. Do not reassure unless you are certain of normality. Worried parents are usually right
- Remember to have hearing/vision problems excluded as a cause of possible developmental delay by trained professionals (audiology/optometry), especially when there are language- or fine-motor-based concerns
- Refer for therapy and early intervention early while you observe and review. Do not wait for suspicion to grow into certainty before providing useful help
- Discussion of diagnosis/prognosis requires time, privacy, empathy, honesty, cultural sensitivity and both parents whenever possible. Details of what is said may be forgotten, so detailed written reports are essential (how it is said is always remembered)
- Definite loss of skills when healthy may indicate regression, suggesting serious neurological pathology; this requires urgent assessment
- Developmental diagnosis is not black or white but has many varying shades of grey

Areas of diagnostic dilemma

Developmental disorders are multidimensional in nature. This means that many children do not fit neatly into a diagnostic box; the widely used DSM-IV-TR and ICD-10 classifications cannot be relied on to describe the subtleties of a particular child's developmental profile and difficulties adequately. There may be a range of overlapping problems of varying degree that need to be acknowledged. Having moved from simple categorical classification (boxes) to a linear spectrum model (a line), it is clear that even this is inadequate. One way of viewing the child's diagnosis is as a series of linear spectra, which can be set at various levels rather like a sound mixing board. It is then possible to consider and plan therapy, for example, for a child who has a mild intellectual disability with a lot of attentional and impulse control problems, minor sensory oversensitivities and obsessional features with good gross motor skills. This model allows the intervention plan to be tailored very closely to the child's and family's specific needs. Unfortunately, many bureaucracies that control resource allocation find such a subtle approach too hard and may resort to headline diagnostic labels as an entry ticket to funding support. Also, many families need a clear label to work with, but they also need to understand that any human individual is far more subtle and complex than a single label or even a list of comorbid disorders.

Autism

Since Leo Kanner's original description, the definition of this disorder has expanded considerably (Ch. 4.4). The core diagnosis of autistic disorder has clear criteria involving:

- delayed language and non-verbal communication
- little interest in socialization, with repetitive unimaginative play
- reliance on routines and rituals, repetitive motor mannerisms and unusual sensory sensitivities.

However, there are many children who have some but not all of these features. It is now usual to reserve the diagnosis of Autistic Disorder for children who fulfil the DSM-IV-TR criteria and to use the term 'Autistic Spectrum Disorder' for children who have a basic lack of social empathy or interest in communication, especially with their own peers or siblings. These children will have some of the features of autistic disorder but not all. Indeed, those with more language disorder and less social difficulty may be labelled as having 'semantic–pragmatic language

Clinical example

At 4 years 3 months, Adrian had only three recognizable words. He avoided eye to eye contact, and paid little attention to what was asked of him, preferring to play alone. He made sounds as he wandered around a room, laughing and giggling for no apparent reason, looking at himself in the mirror and often flapping his fingers close to his face. He was quiet, only becoming upset with the sound of a vacuum cleaner or a passing police car siren. He appeared distant, not spontaneously giving or accepting affection. He was toilet trained and could undress completely but needed assistance to get dressed. He could not pedal a tricycle, and had poor ball playing skills and an immature pencil grip with only circular scribbling. At preschool he needed constant direction and encouragement by the staff, and he had not developed any friendships.

Assessment with the Griffiths Mental Developmental Scales indicated a moderate intellectual disability with non verbal skills at around 2–2.5 years, but his verbal skills were found to be further delayed at 12–18 months. His behaviour was consistent with a diagnosis of autistic disorder, as he had a specific impairment in forming social relationships, in communicating and in playing imaginatively, in addition to his developmental disability. Adrian had high support needs and required intensive educational programming and behaviour modification to develop to his optimum potential.

disorder', and those with better language function but poor social interactions, clumsy motor skills and perhaps an unusual speech pattern can be described as having Asperger disorder. This constellation of pervasive developmental disorders is being recog-nized with increasing frequency and may indeed be increasing in actual prevalence (Ch. 4.4).

Attention deficit/hyperactivity disorder

This disorder is very common on its own or with specific areas of developmental weakness, especially language. However, the core deficit of delayed impulse inhibition can occur to an extent in children with intellectual disability or autism. Recognition of this can lead to including additional treatment possibilities in the child's plan of management (Ch. 4.3).

Intellectual disability

By definition, over 2% of the population will have an IQ that is more than 2 SD below the mean or below 70. This is 1 in 50 children, making it by far the most common major disability. The delay occurs fairly evenly in all areas of development, and is described as mild, moderate, severe or profound, depending on the deviation from the mean on testing. It is usual to make the diagnosis from assessment of cognitive function and adaptive function; this latter is the ability of the child to perform everyday tasks in the real world and is sometimes assessed with specific inventories such as the Vineland Adaptive Behaviour Scales. Children with significant discrepancies between their verbal and non-verbal cognitive or reasoning skills are more likely to have a specific learning disability than an intellectual disability and full scale scores should be viewed with caution (Ch. 3.8).

PART 3

SOCIAL AND PREVENTATIVE PAEDIATRICS

The child and the family 3.1

N. Wigg

Virtually all aspects of early human development, from the brain's evolving circuitry to the child's capacity for empathy, are affected by environments and experiences that are encountered in a cumulative fashion, beginning early in the prenatal period and extending throughout the early childhood years.

Shonkoff and Phillips 2000

The concept of health for children is one that involves a broad range of areas. The majority of the health needs for children are met in the context of their family. A healthy child is one who is physically well, whose emotional needs are met and who is socially adjusted. Each of these needs have several parameters, which are discussed below.

The physical needs of the child

- Care and protection from violence
- An adequate diet to provide for nutritional needs
- Protection against heat and cold in early life, and protection against physical dangers, such as fire, electricity, water, poisons and motor vehicles
- Prevention of illness through good living standards, education, health surveillance, immunization and other public health measures.

Children grow and thrive in the context of close and dependable relationships that provide love and nurture, security, responsive interaction and encouragement of exploration. Without at least one such relationship, development is disrupted and the consequences can be severe and long-lasting.

The emotional and social needs of the child

- The opportunity to grow up in a family context with close and dependable relationships with one or more adults (parents)
- Consistent, positive caregiving
- Reasonable limits to be set on the child's behaviour
- Feelings of being worthwhile and concern for the wellbeing of others
- The development of self-help skills and a sense of achievement

- Opportunities for play, recreation and companionship
- Opportunities to learn and explore
- Sensitive responses to emotional needs during illness, particularly in chronic illness
- Recognition of each child's individuality
- Recognition of the basic rights of every child as outlined by the United Nations Declaration of the Rights of the Child.

To meet the physical, social and emotional needs of their children, parents and others in a caring role must fulfil their own needs. These caregiver needs include:

- adequate housing and transport
- freedom from unnecessary economic stress
- freedom from community and domestic violence
- easy access to family support and early childhood services, such as child care, health and education services
- knowledge of how to access community supports and services
- social networks and extended family supports
- an understanding of child development and behaviour.

The growth and development of a child in the family and community context are determined by the interplay of genetic, physical, social and emotional factors and experience. The balance of risk and resilience factors influences a child's developmental pathway.

Risk factors preventing optimal progress might include:

- family conflict and disintegration
- economic disadvantage (low household income)
- parental mental health disorders
- individual child factors, such as low intellectual ability or difficult temperament
- external factors, such as unsafe neighbourhoods, environmental threats, war, etc.

Balanced against these are *resilience* factors, which are protective and promote wellbeing:

- safe, nurturing home environment
- consistent, supportive caregiving
- individual factors, e.g. normal intellectual ability
- sense/experience of success, self-determination and achievement.

The building blocks for intellectual development

There are many components of the family and societal environment that are important in the intellectual development of the child. Some of these are:

- a loving and nurturing caregiving/family environment
- child rearing beliefs and practices that are designed to promote healthy adaptation
- the opportunity to play, learn, explore and communicate
- the growth of self-regulation of physiological systems, emotions, behaviours and social interactions
- positive and consistent human relationships
- access to developmentally appropriate educational settings: children are active participants in their own development and learning
- good physical health.

As a child grows from a newborn infant to an independent young adult, his or her social environment expands and diversifies. A young infant has all its needs met within the immediate family. Contact with other young children is important for the social and emotional development of the preschooler. A young teenager may spend more time with peers than with her or his family. The structure of the family, the style of parenting and the capacity to support the growing child's progressive independence are all important determinants of the health and wellbeing of children.

The Australian family

Australian society, as for many others, is multicultural, with pluralistic values and child rearing practices. Child- and family-centred health care of children and young people should be carried out within the cultural and values framework relevant to the child.

Clinical example

Leeanne was the 4-year-old daughter of professional parents who had migrated from another country in Asia. Her behaviour was demanding, overly active and often aggressive. Her communication skills were delayed. Both parents stated that in their families of origin children were not disciplined until school age and were cared for by the extended family.

Behavioural intervention needed to include these views of parenting.

Traditionally, Australian families have been made up of mother (usually at home), father and two or more children. However, this picture of the 'nuclear' family no longer represents the Australian family.

Many families in Australia do not contain dependent children. The Australian Bureau of Statistics (ABS) reports that, in 2003, for families with dependent children:

- 74% of children aged 0–14 years lived in intact families (where all children lived with both natural parents)
- 19.2% of children lived in one parent families
- of children living in one parent families, 88% lived with the mother and 12% with the father
- over the last 10 years, the proportion of couple families with children has declined while the proportion of one-parent families has increased.

Three demographic trends have altered the structure of Australian families with children:

- the rate of divorce
- the age of marriage and having the first child
- the decision of women not to have children.

During the last 20 years marriage rates have fallen and the age at first marriage and age of first birth have increased dramatically. The median age of first marriage for women is now almost 27 years and the median age of first birth is over 28 years. Consequently, family size is smaller. In contrast, divorce rates rose in the 1970s, stabilized in the 1980s and increased slightly again in the 1990s; however, the rate of divorces involving children declined from 61% in 1986 to 54% in 1997.

There has been an increase in de facto relationships, which have become more socially acceptable in the last 20 years, including those in which children are involved. The proportion of exnuptial births (mothers not married) had risen to 29% in 1998, and at least half of these births were to women in de facto relationships.

Increasingly, women are deciding to remain childless. In the 1990s 27% of women did not have any children. Family size and fertility rate for indigenous women are also falling. During the 1960s indigenous women had a total fertility rate of around six babies per woman, which fell during the 1970s to about three and in the 1990s to 2.4. Indigenous women are often younger at the time of first birth.

Families at work

Workforce participation rates for family members have increased in many developed countries in recent years. However, unemployment is also common, particularly in single-parent families. These changes have the potential for significant effects for children.

• In 2003, in couple families where the youngest child was under the age of 15 years, at least one parent was in employment in 94% of families. Both parents worked in 59% of these couple families
• In lone-mother families where the youngest child was under 15 years of age, nearly 55% of mothers were not employed
• In lone-mother families where the youngest child was aged 0–2 years, only 28% of mothers were employed
• Couple families with children under 15 had an average income 2.8 times that of lone-parent families
• The proportion of all children under 15 years living in families without a parent employed fell from 19% in June 1994 to 17% in June 2004.

For many Australian families with children it is essential financially for both parents to have paid employment. 'Mum at home, and Dad at work' is not the reality for many children. Accessible and affordable child care, family day care or other informal child caring/minding arrangements are needed.

Coincident with these changes in families and communities, the incidence of child abuse (physical, emotional and sexual) is thought to have risen over the last three decades; however, data about the rates of abuse are incomplete and much goes unrecorded.

Clinical example

Casey, age 4, was brought to the emergency department of a busy metropolitan hospital late in the evening, with a temperature of 38°C. Both his parents worked full-time, and Casey had spent his day at the neighbourhood child care centre. After a 2 h wait, Casey was seen and found to have a minor upper respiratory tract infection. He did not need any specific treatment.

His parents had brought him to the hospital as they had not been able to take time off work during the day to seek medical advice for him, and after-hours suburban medical services were not available in their area.

Children of families in distress

Economic disadvantage/poverty

Poor people are more likely to have poor health. There is a gradient of socioeconomic effects on health: the more affluent you are, the more likely you are to experience good health; the poorer you are, the worse your health is likely to be. There is no particular cut-off point for economic advantage above which health is protected.

Low household income is associated with lower purchasing power, material deprivation and reduced ability to participate in everyday community activities.

Low income households tend to occur in neighbourhoods that have fewer communal resources and where the social and physical environments are hazardous. Being poor is also often associated with much greater stress, feelings of lowered self-worth, powerlessness and helplessness. Mental and physical health problems follow.

International standards define poverty as a household income of less than 50% of the median income for that nation or state. In 2005, 12.8% (1 in 8) of Australian children lived in poverty.

Single-parent families are much more likely to live in poverty. The resulting inadequate diet, lack of opportunities and emotional stress may be coupled with the emotional turmoil that children and parents experience in separation and divorce. In general terms, children in one-parent families have poorer mental and physical health than their peers in two-parent families. However, much of this difference can be explained by lower household income and the stress of financial hardship. Fortunately, the majority of children in one-parent families still experience good health.

Low family income may affect the health of the children in many ways, e.g.:

• lower birth weight
• lower rates of breastfeeding
• poor vaccination rates
• poor growth
• higher rates of infectious diseases.

Socially marginalized families/groups

Indigenous Australians (Aboriginal and Torres Strait Islander peoples) have poorer health than other Australians. Indigenous children have poorer nutrition and growth, higher rates of infectious disease, higher injury rates and high rates of infant and child mortality (Ch. 3.2).

The reasons for the persistence of the relatively poor health of indigenous children are complex. Certainly living conditions, fewer educational opportunities and poor access to goods and services all contribute. So do cultural disruption, high levels of poverty, lack of access to culturally acceptable health care, and racism.

Clinical example

Taliah was the third child of a 21-year-old Aboriginal mother. The family lived in a small town in the Northern Territory. Taliah was 6 months old, was growing and developing well, was breastfed and was free of illness. Her older brother and sister had much poorer health. Before her birth Taliah's mother had joined the local 'strong women, strong babies' programme.

Multicultural Australia includes many immigrant groups whose children are at greater health risk. Many families come to Australia to escape persecution and civil disruption in their own countries and they bring with them the legacy of trauma and loss.

The major problems experienced by ethnic minority groups include lack of employment opportunities (and associated low household income), social isolation, unfamiliarity with health care and other social services, and barriers due to communication problems and cultural differences.

Culturally sensitive health care services that include bilingual workers and interpreter services are essential. Doctors and other child health workers should recognize the vast range of child rearing and health care practices of ethnic groups in Australia.

Families affected by mental health problems and drug abuse

Children's early development and health depends on the health and wellbeing of their parents. Postnatal depression is relatively common, affecting about 15% of mothers. Severe postnatal depression impacts on the establishment of infant–mother relationships (known as attachment). Disorders of attachment result in infant health problems, such as sleep problems, failure to thrive, disturbed behaviour such as excessive crying, and subsequent emotional and behavioural problems.

Children who grow up in families where one or both parents have a mental health problem frequently experience inconsistent parenting and disturbed relationships within the family. The scene is set for such children to develop behavioural, emotional and mental health problems.

The Western Australian Child Health Survey identified that 20% of 12–16-year-olds had a significant mental health problem (Zubrick et al 1995). Thus one in five teenage school children will have a mental health problem and most will not seek or receive treatment (Ch. 4.2).

Alcohol is by far the most widely used and abused drug in our society. Drinking alcohol is not only accepted but is expected behaviour in Australia. Approximately two out of three men and one in two women drink alcohol at least once a week. Of those who drink, about 10% of men and 6% of women are in the medium- to high-risk groups. The abuse of alcohol by one or both parents has a profound effect on the family.

Clinical example

Trent, a 9-year-old boy, was noted to be performing poorly at school by his teacher. He was a bright student but had become inattentive and frequently he disrupted other children in the classroom. His writing had deteriorated. When the family was contacted, it was discovered that Trent's father had recently left the family after months of disharmony due to his excessive drinking.

Social worker assistance was obtained and Trent received counselling. Trent is now involved in Scouts and his school performance is improving.

Children of alcohol-dependent parents suffer anxiety and unhappiness and may be exposed to violence and argument. In many cases this leads to the child becoming antisocial, engaging in alcohol/drug use and developing mental health problems such as depression. Alcohol and drug (e.g. heroin) addiction frequently leads to financial stress in a family, together with deterioration in family relationships and parental separation. The consequences on children are severe.

Family violence

16% of Australian couples experience violence in the relationship. For 4% of couples the level of physical violence is such that physical harm is a likely outcome.

Our society tolerates high levels of violence in the media, in sport and in the community generally. However, violence in the family context has a profound effect on children. Violence between parents is frequently associated with violence towards their children.

Children who witness violence as a 'problem solving' technique at home may adopt similar patterns of behaviour, particularly when they themselves become parents.

Services for the child and family

General or primary care practitioners (family doctors) provide the mainstay of health services for children and families. These primary health care services are complemented by a range of government-funded community health and social services. The following are given as examples.

For families with young infants:

- Well-child care in child health centres
- Home visiting programmes for families with additional needs, e.g. Family Care Program, Good Beginnings
- Residential services
- Parent help lines, child health lines (24 h, 7 day telephone advice lines)
- Printed and online information services.

For families with preschoolers:

- Health surveillance, including immunization and health promotion
- Injury prevention and safety promotion
- Health service component to child care and preschool services
- Telephone and other information services
- Health screening prior to school entry – provided by child health nurses
- Developmental assessment clinics and early intervention services

For families with school-age children:

- Support services provided by education departments, e.g. guidance officers, counsellors

- Assessments of children by child health nurses
- Health education
- Community mental health services
- School oral health (dental) services

Family centred care involves:

- partnerships with parents
- services identify and meet parents' goals
- services are delivered in culturally relevant frameworks
- full participation of the parents (and child) in decision making.

The Federal government in Australia provides a number of pensions or benefits administered by Centre Link and the Department of Family and Community Services. These include the family allowance, child care supplements, supporting parents and carer benefits.

State governments and non-government agencies (often church-affiliated) provide many family and community support services.

Similar government-funded services are provided for families in many other countries.

The field of family support services is complex and accessing 'the right service at the right time' is frequently a major problem for families experiencing distress. Family doctors and other child health workers need to know about the child and family services available in their area, and about government benefits for families.

3.2 Indigenous culture and health

G. D. Stokes, C. A. Jeffries-Stokes

Definition

The definition of an Aboriginal or Torres Strait Islander commonly used in Australia requires three criteria be satisfied. It is a person who is of Aboriginal or Torres Strait Islander descent, who identifies as an Aboriginal or Torres Strait Islander and who is recognized as an Aboriginal or Torres Strait Islander within the community in which they live.

Population statistics

The number of Aboriginal and Torres Strait Islander people living in Australia at the time of white settlement will never be accurately known but it was probably at least 300 000 and possibly as many as 1 000 000 people. By the 1920s this number had plummeted to about 60 000 because of the introduction of new diseases, brutal treatment and the effects of rapid social and cultural change. In 2004 almost 500 000 people identified themselves as Aboriginal or Torres Strait Islander, representing 2.5% of the population of Australia.

The age structure of the Aboriginal and Torres Strait Islander population of Australia is markedly different from the rest of the population. High fertility rates and short life expectancy combine to result in a very young population. 40% of the indigenous population is under the age of 15 years compared to 21% of the non-indigenous population, with only 2.5% of the indigenous population over the age of 65 years compared with 12% of the non-indigenous population.

The history of Aboriginal people in Australia

No one knows for sure when Aboriginal people first came to Australia. The Dreamtime stories describe the creation of Aboriginal people, the land, plants and animals as occurring at the same time and Aboriginal people believe that they have always been here in Australia. Scientific evidence suggests that Aboriginal people have been here for at least 50 000 years.

Settlement by non-Aboriginal people in Australia has been relatively recent in historical terms. For example the official British settlement of Western Australia began in Albany in 1826; from here non-Aboriginal people spread out across the state. This took some time. The Goldfields was first explored by non-Aboriginal people just over 100 years ago and in the northern Goldfields white settlement began only about 80 years ago, and in some places as recently as 60 years ago. This represents white settlement of the Goldfields in living memory – there are elderly Aboriginal people who can still recall seeing the first white person who came to their area. This is similar to many areas throughout Australia.

There is ample evidence that the first settlers thought of the Aboriginal people as savages and had very little understanding of Aboriginal culture and way of life. Aboriginal people were shot, poisoned, imprisoned and pushed off their land into camps or reserves on the outskirts of settlements. They had little immunity to the diseases brought by the settlers and hundreds died of infections such as measles, leprosy and influenza. Aboriginal people infected with sexually transmitted diseases or leprosy were arrested and transported to remote isolation camps.

In 1905 in Western Australia the Aborigines Act was passed and remained in force until 1963. This meant that the Chief Protector of Aborigines became the legal guardian of all mixed-race children and Aboriginal people lost all rights of citizenship in their own country. They could not marry, get work, move about, go to school or go to hospital without permission from the Chief Protector. They could not be in town after 6 pm and had to carry a 'Dog

Licence' or identification papers all the time. Their children were forcibly removed and put into missions, where they were deliberately separated them from their families and culture – this is known as the 'stolen generation'. Many were also subject to emotional, physical and sexual abuse. Many never saw their parents again and some still have not been able even to find out who their families are. The missions operated under the 1905 act until 1963 and then continued until the mid 1970s in many areas as, even though the legislation had changed, community attitudes had not.

In 1967 a referendum was conducted and Aboriginal people were finally given equal rights under the law as citizens of Australia. In practice, enormous inequality still exists.

Health status

One area where inequality is most evident is in the health status of indigenous Australians compared to non-indigenous Australians. The life expectancy of indigenous men and women is 20–30 years less than that of their non-indigenous counterparts.

Indigenous Australians suffer higher rates of disease in almost all categories than non-indigenous Australians and are admitted to hospital almost twice as often as non-indigenous Australians. Diseases of the cardiovascular system are the most common cause of death for indigenous adults but multiple pathology is common and diabetes and renal disease are between 10 and 30 times more common than the general population.

The infant mortality rate is between significantly higher for infants of Indigenous parents. In New South Wales the infant mortality for indigenous infants is twice that for the total population but in Western Australia it is four times higher. Indigenous infants are more likely to be of low birth weight (less than 2.5 kg). Aboriginal and Torres Strait Islander children suffer higher rates of upper and lower respiratory tract illness, gastrointestinal illness, renal stones and skin infestation. Many also suffer from diseases more common in third world countries such as rheumatic fever and chronic otitis media. The higher rates of many of these illnesses are probably due to the substandard conditions in which many Aboriginal and Torres Strait Islander people live.

The skin system and family relationships

Many of Australia's Aboriginal people believe that all people in the world belong to a 'skin group'. Most people, however, have long ago lost the tradition of passing on and identifying their skin groups. Aboriginal people all over Australia maintain the skin groups and the customs of relationships defined by the skin groups. Some Aboriginal people have lost contact with their culture and may not know the name of their skin group but they still conduct their relationships within the family and within the wider community according to the customs handed down in their families. These are customs that have their origins in the skin group system.

In the Eastern Goldfields and Central Desert there are four major skin groups, although in some areas these are further subdivided. The names of the skin groups in the Wongutha language of the Eastern Goldfields are Gurrimurra, Boorungu, Panaka and Tjarru.

Each family will have members of all four skin groups. For example if a Gurrimurra man marries a Boorungu woman, their children will be Panaka. A Panaka man marries a Tjarru woman and their children will be Gurrimurra. A child will always be the same skin group as the paternal grandfather.

The four skin groups define all relationships in the Aboriginal community. All members of the same skin groups will be brothers (*goorda*) and sisters (*gaggu*) or grandfather and grandchild (*dhamu*) or grandmother and grandchild (*guburli*). The members of other skin groups will in turn be father, mother, spouse or in-laws. This is regardless of whether any blood relationships exist or not. Marriage is only allowed between people who have the appropriate skin relationship. A member of one skin group can only marry someone from one other strictly defined skin group. Blood relationships are also considered and marriage between people who are closely related by blood, even if their skin groups are compatible, may not be allowed.

The skin groups define how people will relate to each other – grandparents must be treated with respect. Members of the same skin group (brothers and sisters and grandparents) are responsible for each other's social and moral education and conduct. Parents are responsible for the love and nurture of their children. In many areas punishment should not be meted out by the parents – it is the responsibility of the older members of the same skin group. This is particularly important in the medical setting, because the parents alone may not be allowed to make major decisions, give consent for procedures or make a child submit to treatment. In many cases these issues should be dealt with by the grandparents and the whole family needs to be involved.

The skin groups also define important spiritual and ceremonial roles in communities that still practise traditional culture and ceremonies. These are usually secret and not discussed outside the skin group.

Aboriginal people are able to determine the skin groups of a newcomer by recognizing spiritual characteristics and by knowing the newcomer's family and kin relationships. The skin groups have nothing at all to do with physical appearance and do not relate to skin colour.

Non-Aboriginal people also have skin groups. Once they have become familiar to Aboriginal people they will be able to work out their skin groups by observation of the types of relationships that they form with Aboriginal people. Until the skin group of a newcomer is determined it may be very difficult to communicate with Aboriginal people, but once a skin group is recognized that person will be accepted as part of the Aboriginal community and extended family.

A different way of thinking

Australian Aboriginal people do not think of themselves as individuals: they see things from the perspective of the tribe or community. Nothing is owned by an individual: everything, including children, belongs to the group.

Because of this sense of community family, cultural and spiritual responsibilities come before all other responsibilities. Providing for the family today may be much more important than saving for something that may never happen.

Many Aboriginal people do not think of time in the same way as non-Aboriginal people. They rarely keep watches or clocks and things happen when the time is right rather than at the right time.

People are valued not for their achievements but for the people that they are – this is particularly true of strangers and non-Aboriginal people. Titles and academic achievement mean very little. Age, experience and personal qualities are much more important.

Health, illness, and spirituality – an Aboriginal perspective

All aspects of life have a deep spiritual dimension for Aboriginal people. The concepts of health and illness cannot be separated from this and good physical health is not possible without consideration of family, land and spirit.

Many Aboriginal people believe that illness occurs when spiritual health is compromised as a result of wrongdoing or, perhaps, magic. Because of the concept of family and community, illness may strike because of transgressions by another person, usually a family member, and may be seen as a form of payback. Whatever the cause, it may be necessary to take steps to address the spiritual causes of illness before good health can be restored.

Issues surrounding childbirth and gynaecology are seen as strictly women's business and anything to do with the male genitalia, urinary system or body markings is considered to be men's business. This is highly secret for many Aboriginal people and should not even be discussed where a person of the opposite sex might overhear the conversation. Such issues need to be addressed very sensitively and privately.

Death

When an Aboriginal person dies, many believe that their spirit must make the journey to the spirit world. This journey must not be interrupted so the name of the person who has died is not spoken. This is because the spirit may feel that they are being called back to the world of the living and not be able to rest. Even people who have the same or a similar name as the dead person will take another name or use a nickname for a time so there is no confusion for the spirit. Often a special name (*Gunbina* in the Wongutha language) is used by people with the same or a similar name. This usually continues for at least a year, or until after the spring rains that wash the earth and renew it.

Stories about the person who has died will be told and their life will be celebrated, using a special term (*Rubagee* in the Wongutha language) to refer to them, or terms such as 'my brother', 'your father', etc., instead of naming them.

The cause of death needs to be explained and any people who may have contributed to or caused the death need to be identified and appropriate punishment delivered. It is important for any medical staff involved in the care of the person who has died to talk to the family and, if possible, explain the cause of death.

Mourning ('sorry business') is an important part of the ceremonies surrounding death. Many Aboriginal people will feel the need to mourn loudly and even injure themselves as a demonstration of their grief. This may be in part to ensure that the spirit feels suitably appreciated. There is a large public display of grief by the family and the funeral arrangements are usually taken care of by the in-laws to allow the family to grieve properly.

The funeral and burial take place when the family is all assembled and people will often travel great distances to attend. This is very important and is often considered more important than any other responsibilities (including work). Another ceremony is held one year later to complete the burial and mourning.

Approaching Aboriginal people

Many people are unsure of how to approach Aboriginal people and particularly wish to avoid causing offence. This frequently results in missed opportunities for meeting and getting to know Aboriginal people. Here are some simple guidelines to assist in these situations. They are by no means complete and Aboriginal people from different areas will have different customs, but these hints should help to establish relationships so that these differences and customs can be explored.

Eye contact

Most Aboriginal people consider it extremely rude to establish direct eye contact. For some people it will indicate a lack of manners, and for others it is considered highly offensive and a breach of traditional law. It is therefore not usual for Aboriginal people to sit or stand opposite another person. It is better to sit beside or at right angles to the other person so that you both look at the same view rather than at each other.

Introductions

It is usual to introduce yourself by name – Christian name or first name and surname. This helps to establish who you are and who your family is. This also helps in working out your skin group. Names for some groups also have great power and if you know an Aboriginal person's name but they do not know your name they may feel very uncomfortable and in a position of weakness in the relationship. To establish that you are all on an equal footing it is advisable to introduce yourself properly.

Shaking hands

When Aboriginal people meet they usually touch each other, often hugging each other but at least shaking hands. They do not usually expect a non-Aboriginal person to want to touch them so they may not offer their hand to a stranger to shake but you should offer your hand. This establishes that you have no fear of touching them and that you meet as equals. Sometime it may be awkward to shake hands, and in this case a light touch on the shoulder is acceptable and will not cause offence with Aboriginal people of either sex.

Conversation

It is important to give an opportunity for the Aboriginal person to get to know you, to know what you are like and to work out your skin group. It is particularly helpful, if you already know other Aboriginal people, to mention them, as then you may have friends or acquaintances in common. It is also very reassuring for Aboriginal people if you have visited their country – so ask where they are from and mention it if you have visited the area. Equally important is that you show some of your own personality. All Aboriginal people consider themselves related to each other, so they are usually quite informal with each other and although this will depend on the circumstances of the meeting it is usually best to just relax and be yourself.

The right words

The word Aborigine came from the Latin *ab origine* and means 'from the beginning'. It is used to describe the original inhabitants of Australia. This implies that they are a single group but in fact they are many diverse and different groups with different names, languages, traditions and culture, although the groups have strong links with each other. Wherever possible tribal names should be used – Koori, Yamatji, Wongutha, Ngoongar and so on.

When the term Aboriginal is used it is always spelt with a capital A. Prior to 1967 Aboriginal people were classified as part of the native fauna or animals of Australia. After 1967 they were given citizenship in their own country. Therefore a capital 'A' is always used in recognition of their humanity, unlike cats, dogs and other animals who are referred to with lower case. In general, the term 'Aboriginal people' is preferred, rather than 'Aborigines'. Although Aboriginal people may use other terms to refer to themselves, such as Blackfella or Blacks, these terms should not be used by non-Aboriginal people and may cause great offence.

PART 2: MAORI VIEW OF CHILD HEALTH AND ILLNESS

L. Buchanan

Children in the New Zealand population

Children under the age of 15 years currently make up 23% of New Zealand's population. The ethnic breakdown of the more than 830 000 children contains four major groupings:

- European (60%)
- Maori (21%)
- Pacific Islander (8%)
- Asian (7%).

Who is Maori?

Until the 1980s, the official census definition of this question was based on a child having 'half or more' Maori origin. Now, however, census data and common usage define Maori as a person of Maori ancestry who chooses to identify as Maori. It is important to be aware that the unifying term Maori really dates from the time of European occupation of New Zealand. Historically, tribal divisions were quite marked. Informed observers as recently as the 1930s referred to Aotearoa (New Zealand) as a series of islands joined by narrow strips of land!

What are the particular features defining health of Maori

At a national Maori health conference in 1984 the then Minister of Maori Affairs – himself a Maori – suggested that there was no such thing as Maori health but only people health. This question is as alive today as it was then. What, then, are traditionally the particularly strong features of health for Maori (recognizing that elements of the features will be identifiable within many different cultures)? Some of these are:

- the concept that the health of an individual should never been seen in isolation from the extended family, the physical environment and a belief system that saw some things as sacred
- the concept that the healing of an illness could only occur through putting things right with one's spiritual side, one's *whanau* and the environment
- the notion that for health and wellness there was always going to be an interplay between spiritual

matters, thoughts and feelings, the physical functions of the body, the family and the environment.

The Eurocentric notion that there could be a split between functions of the mind and the body would be seen as incomprehensible. Likewise, the idea that the only proper approach in medical practice would hinge around precise scientific principles as epitomized by randomized controlled trials would be seen as alien. In *te ao Maori* (the Maori world) all manner of possible explanatory links between events occurring around the same time or on a certain day would be considered. There would be more empathy in Maoridom with the kind of Hippocratic notion that medicine is primarily an art that might use science for its purposes on occasions. There would be nothing 'schizophrenic' seen in a Maori doctor holding those kind of views while at the same time working with what most would regard as a contemporary mainline scientific approach to humans and health. It would be seen as no different from a brilliant scientist such as Pascal believing firmly in the basic Christian concept that God could become man while continuing with his scientific enquiries.

Mason Durie brilliantly summarized wholeness or wellness for Maori as needing to involve the four walls of a house, each supporting the others. Their four pillars are:

- *taha wairua* (spiritual side)
- *taha hinengaro* (thoughts and feelings)
- *taha tinana* (physical side)
- *taha whanau* (the family).

Measuring all these aspects of health is not easy, with the spiritual side perhaps being the most challenging. Yet *taha wairua* would usually be seen as the most important aspect – the need to acknowledge or have a faith in 'a life force', a God outside yourself. This turning outwards would place the issue of the person being at one with the environment as pivotal.

The special relationship between a person and the environment is reflected in the shared meaning of some key words: *whanau* means birth but it also is the word for the child's more immediate family; *whanua* is the word for the placenta but it is also the word for the land.

The concept of *taha hinengaro* focuses on thoughts and feelings and functions of the brain. Maori might be puzzled by developments only within the last 50 years suggesting that there could be such a thing as psychosomatic medicine. To Maori it is not possible to compartmentalize health into defined areas that have no relationship to other key aspects of the person's life. Again *te reo* (the language) tells the story with the word for intense anger being *pukuriri* – literally fighting within the stomach. Likewise, a word for depression is *manawapouri* – blackness within the heart.

In the realm of *taha tinana* – the physical side – particular importance is placed on the ancient concepts of some things being sacred or *tapu* and requiring a special approach.

A woman who had just had a baby would be an example of a situation needing particular care. The importance of separating off eating facilities or spaces from toileting or washing facilities would be another. The head, breasts and genitalia of the person are seen as special. Breaches of the sacred or *tapu* conventions would traditionally be seen as an important contribution to any sickness or illness coming to an individual.

The significance of the child within Maori culture

The fourth concept of the four walls of health helps place the child – *taha whanau*. Health cannot be considered without regard to the family as a whole. The child is seen as a *taonga* (a special gift) to the *whanau* (family). The child brings a continuation of the inheritance lines (*whakapapa*). The child is seen as the hope for the future. The care and upbringing of the child would be seen as belonging not just to the parents but to the extended family, with grandparents playing a special role. Maori has been described as a culture that puts people before self, so that a young child would be expected to receive considerable *arohatanga* (warmth and love) and *awhinatanga* (help and assistance).

Practical issues in achieving cultural competence in working with the Maori child and family

Cultural competence has become an item of concern on both sides of the Tasman in recent years. The Medical Council of New Zealand has been charged in the Health Practitioners Competence Assurance Act 2003 with setting standards of clinical competence, cultural competence and ethical conduct to be observed by health practitioners. The Council has been struggling with how to define cultural competence. Maori input has been sensitive to the idea that Maori culture might not have a special place in Aotearoa but rather be one culture like a disability culture,

a gay culture, a youth culture, or a rural culture. Maori acknowledge the reality and special contributions of the other ethnic groups within New Zealand – especially sister Pacific Island cultures. Clinical and cultural competence should not be separate and clinical competence is not possible if one is unable to respond adequately and sensitively to the special circumstances, beliefs and backgrounds of a family.

The special status that Maori seek for the culture is firstly tied to the reality of Maori being the original people in Aotearoa ('the land of the long white cloud') and is secondly related to the particular provisions for Maori in the founding document establishing the modern New Zealand nation in 1840.

This Treaty of Waitangi was signed at a time when Maori outnumbered Europeans. There were three clauses to the document, with Maori health concerns being contained in the second and third clauses. The second clause promised Maori protection of their sacred treasures (health has been identified as one of these) and the third clause promised the same rights (taken to include health rights) as their new English brothers and sisters. It is a matter of speculation now how sincere Lord Normanby might have been in the language he suggested should be used in the treaty, when he was contemporaneously dealing with British interests in the opium war in Hong Kong and in diplomatic difficulties with the Russian Court at St Petersburg.

Debate about the special position of Maori in New Zealand has intensified during the last 25 years, with an examination of the status of the Treaty of Waitangi central to the arguments. A degree of acrimony arose from the Maori policies of the two main political parties in the run up to the September 2005 general election in New Zealand. Some Maori thought that the name that Maori had chosen for New Zealand – the land of the long white cloud – had come back to haunt them. In some minds the issue of whether there is or should be any such a thing as Maori health is back on the agenda.

Particular issues and approaches to children and family in the context of the health consultation

Welcoming every member of the supporting family (*whanau*) or just an individual parent needs to be undertaken with courtesy and respect. Some general enquiries about what is happening in the family and where they are from are advisable before taking a formal history of the concerns about the child. Direct eye contact from an older child or some of the *whanau* might not occur at first and should not be interpreted as rudeness or diffidence. If the family are running late or have missed previous appointments, remember that people other than doctors can also have busy lives. Consultants on teaching ward rounds or in multidisciplinary clinic sessions might like to introduce or refer to the others present with them as their supporting *whanau*. If the doctor has some familiarity with Maori greetings and enquiries, this knowledge should first perhaps be used in an exchange with the child rather than the adults present. Maori can feel embarrassed if, from then on, a Maori health professional launches into *te reo* (the language) and they are non-speakers. Ideally some distance and space – especially in the non-urgent outpatient situation – need to be available between the doctor and the *whanau*. This initial encounter for Maori is really like a ritual of engagement.

It is important tactfully to consider what the special significance of a child's symptoms might be to that family. A carefully taken family history is therefore essential. An alertness to the normal Maori view that matters of a psychological nature can cause physical symptoms and that the life of the child has a spiritual and sacred component should not be overlooked.

In terms of assessing various diagnostic possibilities one should be aware that cystic fibrosis and coeliac disease do not seem to occur amongst Maori. This fact is obviously of genetic origin. Anorexia nervosa is exceedingly rare amongst Maori, while marked obesity is all too common. These features could well partly relate to the cultural preference that does not favour slender body shapes as either healthy or desirable. Genetic disposition tendencies have not spared Maori, however, from either attention deficit/hyperactivity disorder or autism. These conditions offer a double challenge to the child's *whanau*:

• The easy participation of a lively, easily distracted 'mind-blind' and possibly somewhat uncoordinated child in codes associated with formal *marae* activities or the action-chanting-singing of *kapahaka* groups is problematic
• The common Western medicine practice of multi-disciplinary assessment is likely to be stressful, given the Maori preference being for the building up a one-to-one relationship with a person whom one learns to trust. Also, the frequent turnover of staff makes the *kanohi* to *kanohi* exchanges with differing people difficult.

Medications that have their effect through alterations of brain function, such as anticonvulsants or psychostimulants, may well be viewed with concern by Maori and the justification for their usage will need to be discussed quietly and carefully with the *whanau*. European concepts of autonomy in decision making by an individual young adolescent are completely out of kilter with traditional Maori views. The *whanau* may well hold quite a different view from what the law allows in regard to informed consent issues relating to issues such as access to contraception or abortion.

When it comes to the clinical examination of the child it should be remembered that the head, the breasts and the genitalia are customarily *tapu* areas, so the usual sensitivities about these parts of the examination should be respected. Scalp vein intravenous access should be avoided.

A doctor should tend towards formality in dress code when working with Maori – especially if a younger person. One needs to remember that the doctor is a kind of Western medicine equivalent of the *tohunga* (person with special training and responsibilities to guard those things sacred and special). Within hospitals, paediatricians should lead the way in ensuring that there are adequate culturally sensitive live-in facilities for *whanau* members supporting a sick child.

Should a Maori child in one's care die, there is a real sense of urgency within the extended family for the child's body to be given over to the family as soon as is feasible. This is partly to facilitate grieving but also to recognize the special spiritual nature of the child and the child's membership of the extended family.

Current social and economic circumstances in which Maori children are being raised

Care needs to be taken in either overcalling or undercalling available population data that measure the social and economic circumstances of a people. One frustration for Maori is that the items that can be measured more readily are external forces that may shape a person's wellbeing (e.g. home ownership, income level, formal educational attainment). Even where apparent or implied deprivation seems to exist, it should be clear that not all people will see themselves as deprived. Seemingly definite solutions to disadvantage such as the significant lowering in recent years of the high Maori unemployment rate may be less clear-cut. What if the employment time or wage is minimal or the work means that the family must move away from their tribal area? The presence or absence of a developed spiritual awareness could either compensate for or compound other perceived deficits in the family circumstances of the child.

The true situation is that modern Maori must live in two worlds. The degree of impingement of the European world on *te ao Maori* (the Maori world) will partly depend on whether they live in an urban or rural setting and the family's involvement in specific Maori activities. One study suggests that nowadays up to 60% of Maori may have limited contact with their culture.

The forces that shape the increased hospitalization or mortality rate of Maori children compared with non-Maori are complex but it is difficult to avoid the notion that measurable socioeconomic disadvantage will only compound the significant loss many Maori suffer of what it means to be Maori.

The organization of health services for Maori

In the 2001 census, only 3% of New Zealand medical practitioners identified themselves as Maori, while the total Maori population was 15%. Even among the doctors identifying themselves as Maori a wide variation exists in their knowledge of *taha Maori* (Maori things). These facts mean that in the short to medium term it is not possible to deliver services by Maori for Maori – which is the preferred option of many Maori. Rather, non-Maori medical practitioners of good will – sensitive to Maori nuances – are going to be needed to support Maori children and their families. Doctors working with children should become familiar with the specific local Maori health initiatives that relate to children. Most public hospitals have a definite Maori liaison service, while *marae*-based or community based Maori health facilities are becoming more common.

The way forward

Back to the future! The first step must be to put the house in order. Durie's idea of the four walls of the house needing to be in harmony cannot be overemphasized. Maori do need to rediscover what it is to be Maori. Strengthening the *whanau* has to be the first step in any 'closing the gaps' policy for *tamariki* (children). The wise use of any monies becoming available to Maori from government compensation for previous forced or doubtful land acquisitions or settlements could help with the reinvigoration of Maori health.

Kia kaha! Kia manawanui! Tihei Mauriora!

3.3 Nutrition

Z. McCallum, J. Bines

Adequate and appropriate nutrition is the keystone of a child's optimal growth and development. Nutrient and energy requirements change markedly during infancy, childhood and adolescence. In the hospitalized child, nutritional requirements may be increased as a result of chronic disease, prematurity or malabsorption. Different mechanisms of enteral feeding or even parenteral feeding may be required.

Many diseases in adult life have their antecedents in childhood nutrition, for example, hypertension, type 2 diabetes, obesity, hyperlipidaemia and some cancers.

Nutritional requirements

Nutrients and dietary guidelines

Nutrients are food components that are required for optimal growth, development and body function. Macronutrients (protein, fat and carbohydrate) are energy sources and are essential for cellular homeostasis. Micronutrients, which include vitamins, minerals and trace elements, are required in much smaller amounts.

Individual nutrient requirements vary with age, size, growth and health status. Recommended dietary intakes (RDIs) are the levels of essential nutrients that are considered adequate to meet the known nutritional needs of healthy people. The RDIs are derived from estimates of requirements for different ages and sex and include a wide safety margin to allow for variation in absorption and metabolism. The RDIs are population standards and do not account for specific individual needs, which vary because of illness, injury or activity. They do, however, exceed the nutrient requirements of most individuals and should only be used as a guide. The Australian RDIs for infants and children are provided in National Health and Medical Research Council (NHMRC) 1992 Recommended dietary intakes for use in Australia. NHMRC, Canberra.

The NHMRC released a document entitled *Dietary Guidelines for Children and Adolescents in Australia* in 2003 (available on line at: http://www.nhmrc.gov.au/publications/_files/n34.pdf). These apply to healthy children from birth to 18 years of age. These,

in combination with the RDIs, assist in the provision of complete nutritional advice.

Dietary Guidelines for Children and Adolescents in Australia (National Health and Medical Research Council 2003)

- Encourage and support breastfeeding
- Children and adolescents need sufficient nutrition foods to grow and develop normally
- Growth should be checked regularly for young children
- Physical activity is important for all children and adolescents
- Enjoy a wide range of nutritious foods
- Children and adolescents should be encouraged to:
  - Eat plenty of cereals, legumes and fruits
  - Eat plenty of cereals (including breads, rice, pasta and noodles), preferably wholegrain
- Include lean meat, fish and poultry and/or alternatives
- Include milks, yoghurts, cheese and/or alternatives
- Reduced fat milks are not suitable for young children under 2 years, because of the high energy needs of young children, but reduced fat varieties should be encouraged for older children and adolescents
- Choose water as a drink
- Alcohol is not recommended for children
- And care should be taken to:
  - Limit saturated fat intake and moderate total fat intake
- Low fat diets are not suitable for infants
- Choose foods low in salt
- Consume only moderate amounts of sugars and foods containing sugars
- Care for your child's food: prepare and store it safely.

Energy

Food is metabolized and provides energy required by the body for growth and synthesis of new tissue, for metabolic processes and for physiological functions and activity.

Fat, carbohydrate and protein provide energy, which is measured in kilojoules (kJ) or kilocalories (kcal: 1 kcal provides 4.182 kJ). Fat provides a concentrated source of energy, contributing 37 kJ/g, approximately twice that provided by an equivalent amount of protein or carbohydrate. Fat contributes 50% of the total energy in breast milk or standard infant formula. The average diet of older children provides 30–40% of total energy from fat, 45–55% from carbohydrate and about 15% from protein. Most of the energy intake in children is used for growth and development. Recommendations for energy intake are difficult to determine, even for individuals of similar age, sex and size, because requirements vary. The NHMRC recommends that for children 5–14 years approximately 30% of energy intake should be fat – with no more than 10% coming from saturated fat.

Nutritional assessment

Nutritional assessment is the process by which the individual is evaluated for normal growth and health, for risk factors contributing to disease and for early detection of nutritional deficiencies and excesses.

Comprehensive nutritional assessment includes:

- dietary assessment
- physical examination, including anthropometry
- laboratory studies.

Dietary assessment

The primary care giver(s) should be asked what the child usually eats in a typical day, in all settings that the child is in – i.e. home, child care, outings. Children derive up to 30% of their energy from snacks, so it is important to include these in the assessment of all food and fluids consumed.

Qualitative methods include a dietary history and food frequency questionnaire. These do not allow for the precise calculation of energy or nutrient intakes but rather determine the pattern, style and types of foods eaten.

Quantitative methods calculate precise energy and nutrient intakes and include a 24-hour food record and a 3-day food record.

If the initial dietary assessment raises concerns, then referral should be made to a dietitian.

Physical examination and anthropometry

Physical examination gives a general impression of nutritional status, including signs of anaemia, jaundice, wasting, oedema, lethargy, muscle weakness and fat stores.

Examination may reveal evidence of specific micronutrient deficiency, including pallor, bruising or bleeding, skin, hair and gum abnormalities, and neurological or ophthalmological disorders. In adolescents, the stage of puberty should be documented.

Anthropometry refers to the measurement of physical dimensions and body composition. Measurement of height/length and weight gives the most useful assessment of overall nutritional status, although normal growth can still occur in marginally malnourished children. Serial measurements of growth add valuable information about the impact and chronicity of nutritional compromise. The following routine measurements are used for the anthropometric component of a nutritional assessment:

- recumbent length before 2 years of age, or height after 2 years of age
- weight for age
- weight for length/height
- head circumference (used until 36 months of age)
- growth velocity
- skinfold thickness (triceps and other sites as indicated)
- midarm circumference

Growth charts for height or length, weight and head circumference are used to monitor growth at different chronological ages (Ch. 19.1). Specific ethnocultural- and even syndrome (Down, Turner)-specific growth charts exist. The percentiles range from 3rd to 97th, with the 50th percentile used as the standard. Intrauterine growth curves have been developed for gestational ages 26–42 weeks using birth weight and length data for infants born at successive weeks of gestation. These charts help to determine the premature infant's size in relation to others born at that gestational age. The growth curves may be used to evaluate the growth of a premature infant provided the measurements are corrected for gestational age. Premature infants should have the weight corrected until the child is 24 months of age, length until the child is 36 months of age and head circumference until the child is 18 months of age.

Patients requiring long-term monitoring of nutritional status should have serial measurements of mid arm circumference and triceps skinfold thickness to assess fat and muscle stores.

Body mass index

Serial body mass index (BMI) is used as a representative measure of body fatness in children (Ch. 3.4). It, however, cannot distinguish between excess weight produced by adiposity, muscularity or oedema. In children with nutritional deficiency, and in the setting of overweight and obesity, it is useful measure of fatness. It is calculated from the formula BMI = weight [kg]/height [m]^2.

Calculated BMI values need to be compared with age- and sex-specific reference standards. In Australia, the recommended BMI charts are the BMI-for-age percentile charts developed in the USA by the Centers for Disease Control (National Center for Health Statistics 2000). These can be downloaded from the CDC website (http://www.cdc.gov/nchs/about/major/nhanes/growthcharts/clinical_charts.htm) and can be used to monitor progress: *Girls*: http://www.cdc.gov/nchs/data/nhanes/growthcharts/set1clinical/cj41l024.pdf; *Boys*: http://www.cdc.gov/nchs/data/nhanes/growthcharts/set1clinical/cj41l023.pdf.

A BMI that is greater than the 85th percentile suggests that the individual is overweight and a BMI greater than the 95th percentile suggests obesity.

Laboratory assessment

Laboratory assessment is used to detect subclinical deficiency states or to confirm a clinical diagnosis. It provides an objective means of assessing nutritional status.

Laboratory assessment is summarized in Table 3.3.1.

Nutrition in utero

Research into the fetal origins of adult health has identified fetal nutrition as being of critical importance. Maternal nutrition is a powerful epigenetic determinant of not only birth size and subsequent growth, but also the future risk of metabolic syndrome (hyperlipidemia, hypertension, coronary artery disease, NIDDM) in adult life. The 'Barker' hypothesis states that adaptations undergone by the starved foetus in utero to become 'thrifty', that is to make maximum use of scarce nutrients, may in the setting of adequate or even abundant nutrition, become counterproductive.

Most in utero malnutrition in Western societies, however, results from placental insufficiency. Periconceptual and antenatal folate supplements are advised as they have been shown to markedly reduce the risk of neural tube defects.

Breastfeeding

Breastfeeding is the best form of nutrition for the growing infant. Australian hospitals are encouraged to adopt the 'ten steps to successful breastfeeding' listed in Table 3.3.2 (http//www.nhmrc.gov.au/publications/_files/n34.pdf).

The weight percentiles and body composition of breastfed infants differ from those who are formula-fed. In general, breastfed infants tend to grow rapidly in the first few months and then grow at a slower rate than current percentiles. This may result in their weight appearing inadequate when plotted on current growth charts, even when they are healthy. In 2006, the WHO Multicentre Growth Reference Study released international growth curves for breastfed infants (available on line at: http://www.foodstandards.gov.au/foodstandardscode/). Current NHMRC recommendations for weight gain in infancy are 150–200 g/week at ages 0–3 months, 100–150 g/week at ages 3–6 months and 70–90 g/week at ages 6–12 months. Preterm breastfed infants require iron supplements from 4–8 weeks of age. Those born at a gestation of less than 32 weeks will usually

Table 3.3.1 Laboratory parameters for assessing nutritional status	
Protein status	Albumin, total protein, pre-albumin, urea, 24 hour urinary nitrogen, carnitine
Fluid and electrolyte and acid–base status	Serum electrolytes, acid-base, urinalysis
Glucose tolerance	Serum glucose, HbA1c
Iron status	Serum iron, serum ferritin, full blood examination
Mineral status	Calcium, magnesium, phosphorus, alkaline phosphatase, bone age, bone density
Vitamin status	Vitamins A, D, E/lipid ratio, C, B$_{12}$, folate, PT/PTT
Trace elements	Zinc, selenium, copper, chromium, manganese
Lipid status	Serum cholesterol, HDL cholesterol, triglycerides, free fatty acids

Table 3.3.2 Ten steps to successful breastfeeding
Every facility providing maternity services and care for newborn infants should: 1. Have a written breastfeeding policy that is routinely communicated to all health care staff 2. Train all health care staff in skills necessary to implement this policy 3. Inform all pregnant women about the benefits and management of breastfeeding 4. Help mothers initiate breastfeeding within half an hour of birth 5. Show mothers how to breastfeed, and how to maintain lactation even if they are separated from their infants 6. Give newborn infants no food or drink other than breast milk, unless medically indicated 7. Practise rooming-in (allow mothers and infants to remain together), 24 hours a day 8. Encourage breastfeeding on demand 9. Give no artificial teats or pacifiers (also called dummies or soothers) to breastfeeding infants 10. Foster the establishment of breastfeeding support groups and refer mothers to them on discharge from hospital or clinic
Source: World Health Organization 1989 Protecting, promoting and supporting breastfeeding: the special role of maternity services, a joint WHO/UICEF statement. WHO, Geneva.

require fortification of breast milk with protein and calories in the preterm period to prevent growth failure. All breastfed infants should receive vitamin K on the first day of life.

Advantages of breastfeeding

Breastfeeding has many benefits for both the infant and the mother. Breast milk is precisely tailored for the infant's needs and contains many factors protective against infection (see Infant formulas, below) and growth factors. The low sodium content of human breast milk is important, given the immaturity of the human infant's renal concentrating mechanisms. Breastfed infants, when compared with formula-fed infants, have improved neurodevelopment and a lower incidence of infections, diabetes, necrotizing enterocolitis and gastroesophageal reflux. Although there is some evidence that breastfeeding may protect against allergic disease in atopic families, the evidence for a population-wide protective effect is inconclusive. Breastfeeding may partially protect women against premenopausal breast cancer, ovarian cancer and osteoporosis. Lactational amenorrhoea may act as a contraceptive adjunct, especially in the developing world.

Breastfeeding initiation and persistence

Approximately 85% of mothers in Australia and other Western countries breastfeed at hospital discharge after delivery. The prevalence of breastfeeding falls to 50% at 3 months and 25–30% at 6 months after delivery. Women of higher socioeconomic and educational status generally breastfeed for longer than the less privileged. Information about the advantages and management of breastfeeding, including where to obtain advice and support, if needed, should be made available to all new mothers.

Reasons given by mothers for stopping breastfeeding include pain and discomfort (e.g. sore nipples, mastitis, thrush); anxiety regarding the adequacy of milk supply, and a return to work.

Common problems with breastfeeding

Problems may exist with both maternal breastfeeding technique and anatomy, as well as with the infant's suck and oropharyngeal anatomy. In addition, insufficient milk supply is often perceived to be a major problem, which may lead to unnecessary cessation of breastfeeding. Most women are physiologically able to produce sufficient milk. Appropriate education, encouragement and support may be all that is needed.

Clinical example

Isabella was born at term following an uneventful pregnancy and delivery. Her mother was very keen to feed her first baby but experienced considerable pain from sore, cracked nipples soon after discharge from hospital. She returned to the hospital to seek advice from a lactation consultant, who noted that Isabella was incorrectly positioned and attached.

Correct positioning and attachment, which is vital for successful breastfeeding, resolved the problem of sore nipples, enabling Isabella's mother to continue to breastfeed without discomfort.

Isabella breastfed on demand, approximately 3-hourly. At 4 weeks of age she started sleeping longer between feeds and suckled less vigorously. Her mother became very anxious and was concerned that her milk supply was inadequate, particularly as it became apparent that Isabella had not gained weight when weighed at a clinic visit. It was evident that the feeding difficulty was the result of infrequent feeding and maternal anxiety. She was encouraged to feed her baby more frequently, including during the night, and to ensure that Isabella drained the first side before offering the second. Her husband was encouraged to bring Isabella to her for feeding during the night. As a result, the milk supply increased and Isabella gained weight appropriately. Timely advice and encouragement and support prevented this mother from ceasing breastfeeding unnecessarily.

Infant formulas and other milks

Health professionals and caregivers are faced with a bewildering array of infant formulas for non-breastfed infants. Health professionals who give advice about formulas should be familiar with the different types and understand when particular formulas should be used. All infant formulas used in Australia are required to be manufactured in accordance with the *Australia New Zealand Food Standard Code*, which specifies the requirements for composition, quality and labelling for infant formulas (Food Standards Australia New Zealand 2006).

While the nutritional composition of infant formulas resembles that of human milk, it is not possible to incorporate the many immunological factors that have been identified in human milk. These include specific immune factors such as IgA, maternal lymphocytes and macrophages, and other non-specific protective factors such as lactoferrin and lysozyme. Additionally, there are many other factors in human milk, including nucleotides, specific long-chain polyunsaturated fatty acids, bile-salt-stimulated lipase, cholesterol, free amino acids, oligosaccharides and growth factors, that cannot be simply added to formulas.

Requirements of formula fed infants

The infant's appetite determines the volume and number of feeds required. Demand feeding for bottlefed infants is appropriate. Term infants require approximately 120–160 ml/kg per day to meet their fluid and nutrient needs during the first 4–6 months of life when milk feeds provide the sole source of nutrition. The number of feeds per day changes as the infant grows, and the number of feeds per day decreases with increased feed volumes.

Establishment of a feeding pattern is often easier for mothers of breastfed infants, as they respond to the infant's demands and do not focus on the volume consumed at each feed. The actual number and volume of feeds taken by bottlefed infants causes considerable anxiety for some parents. Reassurance should be provided that the infant's appetite is the best guide, and as long as the infant gains weight consistently, but not excessively, and is thriving and active, progress is satisfactory.

Composition of standard infant formulas

Standard infant formulas are recommended for healthy term infants who are not breastfed. The nutrient compositions of these standard formulas are very similar, with minor variations in the protein, fat and carbohydrate content (Table 3.3.3).

• *Protein.* All standard infant formulas have cow's milk protein as a basis, which is modified in order to produce a protein composition more like that of human milk. The cow's milk protein is modified through heat treatment processes, with the addition of whey in order to modify the casein:whey ratio so that it is similar to that of human milk. Despite this, the amino acid profiles of infant formulas remain different from those of human milk.

• *Fat.* The fat sources in standard infant formulas are a mixture of vegetable oils with or without butterfat. It is possible to achieve ratios of saturated to unsaturated fatty acids that are similar but not identical to those of human milk. Although the degree of saturation may be similar, the structure of the fats is not the same, resulting in differences in digestion and absorption. The fatty acid composition of human milk also varies with the maternal diet, and can be modified favourably by substituting some of the saturated fats in the diet with appropriate mono- and polyunsaturated fatty acids. Some manufacturers now add long-chain polyunsaturated fatty acids to formulas, as there is evidence that these play an important role in infant development, with advanced visual pathway maturation and a postulated benefit for intelligence. The fat composition in formulas may also promote the formation of soaps in stools, contributing to constipation in some infants.

• *Carbohydrate.* The carbohydrate source in standard infant formulas is lactose.

All formulas are supplemented with vitamins and minerals. These standard infant formulas are suitable for the first 12 months of life and are labelled 'suitable from birth'. The common practice in the community, and with some medical practitioners, of changing from one formula to another because an infant is irritable or unsettled should be strongly discouraged. Changing brands on a frequent basis does not help settle the infant and can lead to mistakes in reconstitution, as scoop size and methods of preparation vary.

Preparation of formula

Having selected an appropriate formula, it is essential that it is prepared correctly and hygienically, using safe water and sterilized utensils and equipment. Formulas should be prepared according to the manufacturer's directions, using the scoop provided to measure the powder carefully. Studies have highlighted significant inaccuracies in measuring the amount of powder for formula reconstitution, and other mistakes in preparation of formula. Health professionals need to ensure that parents understand how to prepare formulas, and should never assume

Table 3.3.3   Breast milk and artificial formulas composition table

	Energy kJ (kcal)/100 ml	Protein source	Fat source	Carbohydrate source	Indication	Concerns
Breast milk	289 (69)	Protein source is whole protein	Short-, medium- and long-chain fats	Lactose	The preferred infant feed	HIV infection in mother
Breast milk fortified with FM85 (5%) and Polyjoule (4.2%)	432 (103)	Protein source is whole protein	Short-, medium- and long-chain fats	Lactose	Pre-term infant	
Preterm formula, e.g. S26 LBW LCPs	340 (81)	Whey : casein 60 : 40	Coconut, oleic, palm, soy. LCPs, MCT2.5%	Lactose	Pre-term infant	Does not contain immunoglobulins, and other non-specific protective and growth and factors
Term formula – cow's-milk based, e.g. S26, Nan1	273 (65)	Whey : casein 60 : 40	Oleo, coconut, soy, oleic, palm, canola, corn	Lactose	If breast milk not available	Does not contain immunoglobulins, and other non-specific protective and growth factors
Soy formula, e.g. Infasoy	274 (65)	Soy isolate	Oleo, coconut, soy, oleic	Corn syrup solids, sucrose	Soy formulas should be used in galactosaemic infants and for infants of vegetarian families reluctant to use cow's milk	Does not contain immunoglobulins, and other non-specific protective and growth factors Soy formulas are commonly and usually inappropriately used for suspected cow's milk protein intolerance, lactose intolerance, colic and in an attempt to prevent allergies. Up to 50% of children with cow's milk protein intolerance will also be allergic to soy protein, and it is preferable for these children to be given a formula with hydrolysed protein. Soy formula is not required for lactose intolerance as there is no need to eliminate milk protein. The presence of phytates in soy formulas may inhibit absorption of minerals, particularly calcium. Soy formulas have a higher aluminium content than other formulas. This places preterm infants or infants with poor renal function at risk of toxicity, especially renal osteodystrophy

Table 3.3.3 Breast milk and artificial formulas composition table—cont'd

	Energy kJ (kcal)/100 ml	Protein source	Fat source	Carbohydrate source	Indication	Concerns
Lactose-modified formulas, e.g. De-Lact	286 (69)	Casein dominant	Vegetable oil	Maltodextrin, glucose, galactose	Low-lactose or lactose-free formulas are the feeds of choice for formula-fed infants with true lactose intolerance	In older children with lactose intolerance, enzymatic drops containing lactase may be used with cow's milk
Hydrolysed formulas (peptide), e.g. Pepti-Junior	280 (67)	Whey hydrolysate. The protein in these formulas is partially hydrolysed to peptides and free amino acids	Vegetable oil, MCT (50%)	Corn syrup solids	Semi-elemental formulas are designed to meet the needs of infants who are intolerant of intact protein, who maldigest protein and fat, or who have problems with severe diarrhoea, food intolerance or allergy	These formulas are expensive and should only be used with medical guidance
Extensively hydrolysed (amino acid) formulas, e.g. Neocate	298 (71)	Amino acids (elemental)	Safflower, soy, coconut	Dried glucose syrup	Infants with multiple food allergies or an abnormal gut may require elemental formula in which the protein has been totally hydrolysed to amino acids	These formulas are expensive and should only be used with medical guidance. Taste bitter

that they can readily follow the instructions. Parents can be tempted to use less formula powder to save money, resulting in an underfed infant, or to over-feed by adding extra powder in an attempt to achieve more rapid growth. Both diluting and concentrating formula can lead to serious electrolyte disturbance in the infant and should be discouraged.

Breastfed babies do not require other fluids, even in hot weather, if they are fed frequently. Formula-fed infants may be offered small amounts of cooled, boiled water between feeds during very hot weather.

Other milks

Cow's milk should be introduced for infants over 12 months. The fat in milk is an important source of energy, fat-soluble vitamins and fatty acids for young children.

Cow's milk has a low iron content and higher levels of protein, sodium, potassium, phosphorus and calcium than human milk or formula. It also has a higher renal solute load and lacks vitamin C and essential fatty acids. Low-fat (2%) cow's milk can be given to children over 2 years of age. Skim milk (no fat) is not recommended unless there is a specific medical condition, such as hypercholesterolaemia. Soy milk should not be used for children under 2 years of age. Calcium-supplemented brands should be chosen if used for older children.

Clinical example

Thao brought her 13-month-old child, Madison, to the doctor for review of her cold. She reported that Madison constantly had a cold and was always tired but she had attributed this to the fact that she was still little and had recently started child care. Madison's height and weight were both on the 50th centile. The GP noticed that she was pale, however, and asked about her diet. Thao replied that Madison was a 'fussy eater' but loved her milk. On further questioning the GP discovered that she had commenced cow's milk at 9 months of age and was currently consuming 800 ml per day. Iron studies and a blood count revealed iron-deficiency anaemia. Thao was advised to reduce Madison's milk intake to less than 500 ml/d and offer a diet rich in meat and leafy green vegetables. It was explained that the cow's milk was 'filling Madison up' but was not providing her with iron and the other vitamins essential for her growth. Madison was commenced on an iron supplement. Thao was advised to delay the introduction of cow's milk until after 12 months of age in future children.

Goat's milk is not recommended for infant feeding. It has a similar macronutrient composition to cow's milk but there are micronutrient deficiencies. If parents insist on goat's milk, a goat's milk infant formula fully supplemented with vitamins and minerals should be used because goat's milk is markedly deficient in folate and other vitamins. If fresh goat's milk is used, it must be pasteurized or boiled and supplemented with folic acid and vitamins B_{12}, B_6, A and C. A child with a true cow's milk protein intolerance will almost certainly be intolerant to goat's milk protein. Goat's milk is also unlikely to reduce atopy.

Nutrition in the well child in the community

Timing of introduction of solids

Breast milk or an appropriate formula will be sufficient to meet the needs of the healthy, growing infant until 4–6 months of age. At this time solid foods can be introduced safely, supplementing the milk intake, which remains the major source of nutrition until about 12 months of age.

By 4–6 months of age infants have lost the tongue thrust or extrusion reflex, have head control, and are able to sit without support, allowing them to manipulate solid foods. The digestive system has also matured, with pancreatic amylase levels sufficient for digestion of starches. Most infants at this age are showing an interest in the world around them and are receptive to trying new foods. Healthy full-term infants are born with iron stores that are sufficient for the first 4–6 months of life, after which these become depleted and milk feeds need to be supplemented with other dietary sources of iron, particularly haem-derived iron.

Introduction of solids before 4 months of age can displace breast milk or formula, but the solids do not necessarily supply sufficient energy and nutrients for the rapidly growing infant. Solids can also result in decreased breast milk supply, as a result of reduced frequency and intensity of sucking. Early solids may also possibly result in food allergy. Delaying the introduction of solids until later during the second 6 months of life may compromise growth and nutritional status, as breast milk alone is insufficient after 6 months to supply energy and micronutrient needs.

The first foods

The introduction of a variety of foods is often referred to as the 'educational diet' as it begins the child's lifetime experience of food. The first foods to be introduced should be soft and smooth, although the infant quickly learns to manage foods of different textures, with the 'chewing reflex' using the gums developing around 7–9 months. Iron-fortified infant cereals are usually introduced first, as these can be mixed to the desired consistency with breast milk or formula. Fruit and vegetables are introduced gradually. Sources of haem iron such as meat and poultry are recommended at about 7 months of age. Custard, yoghurt and cheese can also be introduced. Egg yolk is suitable from this time, but it is advisable to leave egg white until around 12 months of age, because ovalbumin is one of the commoner causes of allergic reaction in infants. Most infants will be eating a variety of modified family meals by 12 months of age.

Feeding the toddler

Between 1 and 3 years of age, growth and appetite slow markedly. The child displays independent thought and action. Young children have limited control over their food choices and rely on caregivers to provide a variety of foods. Caregivers should understand the normal behaviour and eating patterns of toddlers – such as the fact that a child may require eight separate offers of a new food before it is eaten! Unrealistic expectations may create feeding problems. Threats, scolding, bribery and use of food as a reward are likely to create rather than resolve problems. Food fads are relatively common at this age, and may develop for no apparent reason or following illness or a traumatic event. Such fads disappear as quickly as they start and are only rarely a danger to health.

Some children may persistently choose only one food (such as custard) or may avoid foods of certain textures (lumps). If a very limited diet is consumed, a dietitian should be consulted in order to assess the adequacy of energy and nutrient intake. Speech pathologists can assist with oral stimulation and the introduction of different tastes and textures.

Bottle feeding should be avoided beyond 18 months of age. Excessive milk intake may result in iron deficiency. Infants should not be settled in bed with a bottle, as this can cause nursing bottle caries (Ch. 22.3).

Excessive intake of milk or fruit juice may reduce appetite and, as a result, may limit the variety of food intake. Excessive fruit juice consumption, particularly apple and pear juice, can result in toddler diarrhoea due to saturation of the facilitated diffusion of fructose. It can also result in poor growth. Fruit juice is high in sugar and does not contain the vitamins and fibre that are in fresh fruit. It should not replace the consumption of water as the best drink for children.

Practical points

- Nutrition in childhood, starting from in utero, is a key determinant of a child's growth, development and is a future adult health status
- Nutritional assessment requires a dietary history, physical exam and blood tests
- Breastfeeding has many benefits over infant formula for both mother and infant
- A range of infant formulas are available and have differing protein sources and indications
- Solids may be introduced after 6 months
- 'Fussy' toddler eating is a normal developmental phenomenon and threats, scolding, bribery and use of food as a reward are likely to create rather than resolve problems
- Water is the best non-milk drink for children (not juice or other sugar sweetened drinks)
- Low-fat milk is appropriate for children over the age of 2 years

Specific nutritional concerns during childhood

Low-fat diets during childhood

The NHMRC currently advises against the use of low-fat diets, specifically reduced fat milk, for young children (<2 years).

Vegetarian diets

The lower energy and higher fibre content of vegetarian diets can limit children's total energy intake, as they may not consume sufficient volume to meet their needs.

Children on well planned semi-vegetarian, lacto or lacto ovo vegetarian diets are adequately nourished if appropriate attention is given to selection of suitable iron sources, and sufficient vitamin C is consumed to maximize iron absorption. Vegan diets place children at risk of iron deficiency anaemia. Children on vegan diets require calcium-fortified soy milk to ensure adequate calcium intake. The risks of vegetarian diets for adolescents, particularly vegans, are significant, because of the rapid growth that occurs during puberty. Sufficient energy and an adequate intake of iron, calcium, zinc and, if vegan, vitamin B_{12} must be ensured.

Providing that the mother is consuming an adequate vegetarian diet, infants can be successfully breastfed. Strictly vegan mothers who are not receiving vitamin B_{12} place their child at considerable risk of profound neurological impairment. Vegetarian mothers who formula-feed often prefer not to use formulas based on cow's milk. An appropriately fortified infant soy formula may be used. Solid introduction should commence in the usual way, between 4 and 6 months of age, but particular attention needs to be given to iron, if haem-iron-containing foods are being avoided. Infants placed on vegan diets are most at risk of nutritional deficiencies. Children who develop iron deficiency anaemia may be at risk of a persistent small neurocognitive impairment, even with iron repletion. Breastfed infants whose mothers are exposed to little direct sunlight (including cultures where women are veiled), may require vitamin D supplements to prevent rickets.

Hypoallergenic diets

There is a role for elimination diets in children with documented multiple food allergy. However, food restriction in children places them at risk of macro and micronutrient deficiency. This highlights the importance of communication with the treating doctor and or dietitian to ensure that the diet is nutritionally sound.

Nutrition issues in adolescence

Common features of teenage eating include skipping meals, consumption of a limited variety of foods, frequent consumption of high-fat, high-sugar, low-nutrient foods, a lack of fibre and fad dieting. Fast food consumption may contribute to the increasing prevalence of adult obesity in Western society, particularly when combined with a sedentary lifestyle (Ch. 3.4). Poor and sometimes inappropriate body image may account for the fad diets that are quite common among teenage girls and boys. Girls in particular will often modify their diets to avoid food that they see as high in fat and energy, such as meat or milk, which may result in an entire food group being omitted from their diet. The avoidance of milk and milk products during the time of peak accumulation of bone mass and calcium accretion may play a role in osteoporosis later in life. Limiting sources of iron, such as red meat, can lead to iron deficiency. Appropriate nutrition education and role modelling needs to be provided both at home and in the school setting.

Overnutrition

The startling rise in the prevalence of obesity amongst Australian children over the last three decades indicates that the aetiology is not purely genetic. Australia is now the second 'fattest' nation on earth. Clearly there are complex genetic and environmental factors at play. These are discussed fully in Chapter 3.4. It is important to note that overweight children may still be at risk of micronutrient malnutrition such as iron and calcium deficiency. A poor-quality diet rich in excess calories may lack adequate micronutrients.

Undernutrition

Malnutrition

Malnutrition is the leading cause of childhood morbidity and mortality worldwide. The root causes of malnutrition vary between the industrial and the developing world. Currently ample food is produced to feed the world's population but social and political forces, such as war, lack of transport infrastructure and degradation of arable land, conspire to keep food from the most needy.

A malnourished child has a weight-for-length (or height) less than 70% or less than −3 SD of the normalized reference figure (World Health Organization 2005 Management of the child with a serious infection or severe malnutrition. WHO, Geneva. Available on line at: http://www.who.int/child-adolescent-health/publications/referral_care/Referral_Care_en.pdf). Children below 60% of weight-for age may be stunted, and not severely wasted.

Generalized reduction of food intake or starvation results in protein–energy malnutrition. The ultimate result of protein calorie malnutrition is marasmus (from the Greek 'to waste away'). Children who have a proportionately greater deprivation of protein than energy may develop kwashiorkor (from the Ghanaian 'deprived child'). These children are malnourished and oedematous. Children with kwashiorkor have a typical appearance consisting of a protuberant belly, muscle wasting, dependent oedema, flaking skin with depigmentation ('flaky paint' dermatitis), glossitis and angular cheilitis. These children often have other vitamin deficiencies, especially deficiencies of B vitamins such as thiamine, leading to beriberi, and niacin, leading to pellagra. Vitamin A deficiency can result in blindness and may significantly worsen mortality from diarrhoea and measles. Long-term consequences include insulin-dependent diabetes mellitus secondary to tropical pancreatitis, and also a significant reduction in IQ and school performance.

If malnutrition has occurred relatively acutely, height and weight discrepancies may result. If malnutrition has been severe and protracted, stunting may occur and often future growth is compromised, even after adequate energy provision.

Malnutrition in the developing world

Malnutrition is endemic in the developing world. Children often receive insufficient energy. Malnutrition and kwashiorkor frequently date from the cessation of breastfeeding and the arrival of a new infant. In some parts of the developing world, high-quality protein, particularly meat, poultry and fish, is in short supply. The cessation of breastfeeding also predisposes the child to respiratory and diarrhoeal disease. The increased metabolic demands of infection may result in further nutritional deficits. Both humoral and cell-mediated immunity may be compromised and this may result in further infection. Immunization may not be freely available and sanitation may be rudimentary. Water is frequently contaminated. Infection with human immunodeficiency virus (HIV) is a major contributor to malnutrition, particularly in Africa. All these factors combine to contribute to the synergistic spiral of malnutrition and disease.

Malnutrition in the developed world

Poverty plays a role in malnutrition in the developed world. However, other factors such as ignorance, food faddism and psychopathology also contribute. Some factors, such as societal concern about obesity, which may engender concern quite inappropriately in children, are seldom seen in the developing world.

In Australia marasmus rarely develops in a malnourished child, usually because of intervention from social agencies or because medical intervention occurs. Kwashiorkor is virtually never seen, even in the indigenous population, where protein–energy malnutrition often occurs. Both food intake and increased metabolic demands secondary to infectious disease burden contribute to protein–energy malnutrition.

A 1995 study estimated a 20% minimum prevalence of malnutrition (wasting or stunting) in Aboriginal children under 2 years of age living in the Darwin rural region. A prospective study conducted between 1997 and 2000 of Aboriginal paediatric admissions in Darwin, with a mean age of 16 months, found that 41% were underweight (after rehydration), 32% were microcephalic, 26% were wasted and 17% were stunted. These figures are not dissimilar to those seen in studies of indigenous Northern Territory children in the 1960s. Apart from substantially increasing the risk of infant mortality, long-term somatic growth and neurocognitive function may be compromised by the microcephaly often accompanying malnutrition.

Malnourished children may also have specific vitamin and trace element deficiencies. These should be assessed and corrected. By far the most common deficiencies in developed societies are in iron and folate. Rickets is seen in the breastfed children of dark-skinned women who wear religious veiling, limiting sun exposure. In deprivation situations children also may suffer from scurvy. The patterns of vitamin and trace element deficiencies in the developing world are quite different.

Eating disorders: anorexia nervosa and bulimia

The diagnostic criteria for these disorders are discussed in Chapter 4.4. These conditions are common, with prevalence rates for anorexia nervosa alone of 0.5–1.0% being reported in Australia and New Zealand. They contribute disproportionately to hospital costs and bed stay statistics.

Therapy consists principally of nutritional rehabilitation and emotional support (Ch. 4.4). However, care is needed during refeeding, as described below.

Clinical example

Mohammed, aged 18 months, was brought to hospital by his parents when they noticed he was still not walking. Lower limb X-rays revealed his bones were osteopenic and had the appearance of rickets. Fatima reported that her son had been born at term and that she was still breastfeeding him. She would have to stop soon as she had just discovered that she was pregnant with her fifth child. The family was Muslim and ate a varied diet. Fatima had always thought her son was a healthy boy. Blood tests revealed a very low calcium and vitamin D. X-ray of Mohammed's ribs and wrist revealed rachitic changes.

Fatima's blood had a normal serum calcium but low vitamin D.

A newborn's vitamin D status is heavily dependent upon maternal status. Fatima was of Somali origin and, being both dark-skinned and adherent to the Muslim practice of veiling the body and face (thus limiting exposure to sunlight), had developed vitamin D deficiency. This led to her breast milk being low in vitamin D. Both mother and son were treated with calcium and vitamin D supplements and encouraged to spend some time exposing their skin to sunlight. Fatima was closely monitored throughout her subsequent pregnancy to ensure adequate calcium intake.

Nutrition in the hospitalized child

Acute and chronic protein energy malnutrition is common in children admitted to a tertiary hospital, occurring in over 50% of infants 3–12 months of age (Fig. 3.3.1). Malnutrition and obesity in hospitalized patients is associated with increased infectious and non-infectious complications, mortality, costs and length of stay.

Factors affecting a hospitalised child's nutritional status

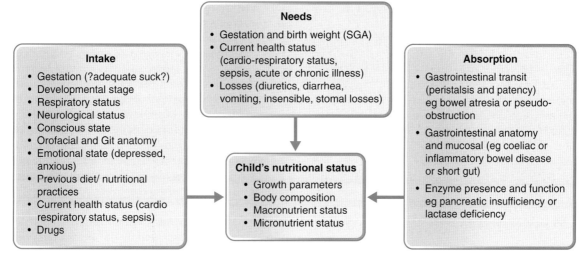

Fig. 3.3.1   Factors affecting a hospitalized child's nutritional status. GIT, gastrointestinal tract; SGA, small for gestational age.

Nutritional assessment of patients at admission and during the period of hospitalization provides the basis for the identification and treatment of nutrition deficits. Indicators for early nutritional intervention include:

- height-for-age and weight-for-age % or z scores more than 2 SD below the mean for age
- height-for-age <95% expected
- weight-for-height <90% expected or >120% expected
- height velocities <5 cm/year after 2 years of age.

In contrast to prolonged fasting, that responds to simple protein–energy repletion, the nutritional management of a patient with metabolic stress due to critical illness requires consideration of glucose metabolism, and specific micronutrient and energy requirements. Energy requirements during critical illness are usually reduced but will increase during the rehabilitation phase. The total energy expenditure (TEE) is the sum of:

$$\text{TEE} = \text{BMR} + E_{activity} + E_{growth} + E_{losses} +$$
$$\text{Thermic effect of feeding } (\sim 10\%).$$

Basal metabolic rate (BMR) is the largest component of TEE and can be estimated in children using predictive equations (Table 3.3.4). BMR is increased by clinical conditions including fever, major surgery, cardiac failure, sepsis and burns.

Routes of feeding

Acute illnesses such as gastroenteritis and respiratory infections usually result in inadequate intake to meet increased metabolic needs. This usually results in transient weight loss only. Children may require supplemental hydration, receiving fluids either by nasogastric tube or the intravenous route. Children with chronic illness, however, may require long-term assistance with nutrition. This may be in the form of supplemental feeding either through a nasogastric tube or a gastrostomy tube. The latter form of feeding is especially useful in chronic illness or neurological compromise, such as cystic fibrosis or cerebral palsy and in children with chronic illness for whom re-establishment of oral feeding has not been possible.

Some children are unable to feed enterally and require parenteral (intravenous nutrition). These include extremely premature or ill neonates, children recovering from intestinal surgery and children with intestinal failure (short gut).

Table 3.3.4   Schofield equation for calculating basal metabolic rate (BMR) in children

Age	Sex	BMR (kcal/day)
0–3 years	Male	0.167W + 1517.4H – 617.6
	Female	16.252W + 1023.2H – 413.5
3–10 years	Male	19.59W + 130.3H + 414.9
	Female	16.969W + 161.8H + 371.2
10–18 years	Male	16.25W + 137.2H + 515.5
	Female	8.365W + 465H + 200
H, length/height (in m); W, body weight (in kg).		

Prematurity

Premature infants have increased nutritional metabolic demands due to a rapid growth phase, tissue development, stresses of illness, poor temperature control and the particularly increased demands of small for gestational age (SGA) infants. These factors, combined with immature organ function, poor nutrient stores and altered feeding patterns mean that the majority of premature infants will require a combination of parenteral and/or specialized enteral nutrition. The former provides the recommended fluid and electrolyte requirements until the latter is tolerated at sufficient volumes for growth and development.

Short bowel syndrome

Short bowel syndrome (SBS) is the clinical syndrome of severe malabsorption and maldigestion that occurs after a major surgical resection or a congenital shortening of the intestine. In a full-term neonate the small intestine is about 250 ± 40 cm at birth. Short bowel syndrome occurs when the small bowel remnant is less than 30% of normal length, equivalent to less than 75 cm. Some patients with SBS require long-term parenteral nutrition to provide the nutrition, fluid and electrolytes necessary to sustain life. Failure to wean from parenteral nutrition in children with SBS is associated with less than 30 cm jejunoileum, lack of enterocolic continuity, residual disease of the intestine and lack of early feeding tolerance.

Chronic illness (with intact gut)

Monitoring of nutritional status should be an integral component of the care of children with chronic illness. Malnutrition and growth failure is common in children with cerebral palsy due to abnormalities in feeding skills, oromotor incoordination, gastroesophageal reflux, constipation and behavioural problems. Nutritional deficits place these patients at increased risk of pressure sores, skeletal abnormalities and infection. Enteral nutrition provided by a nasogastric or gastrostomy tube has been associated with improvement in energy levels, behaviour and mobility. Patients with renal disease, liver disease and cystic fibrosis are at risk of developing specific micronutrient abnormalities in addition to protein–energy malnutrition.

Parenteral nutrition

Infants and children who are unable to feed enterally require intravenous nutrition using lipid and nutrient solutions. These are delivered either by a peripheral intravenous line (maximum dextose concentration of 10%) or via a central venous line (maximum dextose concentration of 30%). The nutrient solution is comprised of amino acids (both essential and non-essential), glucose, electrolytes, minerals, vitamins, trace elements and water, and may contain heparin. The main source of non-protein calories is D-glucose (dextrose). The lipid emulsion is a concentrated source of calories with low osmolarity. Patients receiving parenteral nutrition (PN) require daily weighing, urinalysis and fluid balance. Baseline and frequent subsequent blood tests are required to monitor for electrolyte imbalance, glucose metabolism and to tailor the parenteral nutrition accordingly.

Parenteral nutrition (in addition to the underlying illness) can be complicated by life-threatening electrolyte imbalance, hypoglycaemia, hyperglycaemia, line sepsis thrombosin and extravasation of the nutrient into the tissues resulting in a parenteral nutrition 'burn'. Most infants and children are on parenteral nutrition for short periods of time during acute illness or recovery from surgery. However, children with intestinal failure may require total parenteral nutrition (TPN) life-long. In addition to the acute complications, these children are at risk of vitamin and micronutrient deficiency, growth failure, parenteral nutrition liver disease and vascular access complications.

Refeeding syndrome

Refeeding syndrome is the term used for the metabolic complications that may occur when aggressive nutritional therapy is used to treat the severely malnourished patient. In particular, the delivery of intravenous or enteral carbohydrate loads may precipitate these potentially fatal electrolyte disturbances. The potential metabolic disturbances that may occur include hypokalemia, hypophosphataemia, hypomagnesaemia and hyponatremia. Potential side effects of these electrolyte and mineral disturbances include: cardiac failure, respiratory compromise, seizures, myocardial infarction and arrhythmias.

Under most circumstances of prolonged starvation or significant weight loss, renourishment should commence slowly with small increases in nutrition delivered once electrolyte and mineral disturbances have been corrected. For example, commence feeding at basal energy requirements, increasing to full requirements over 7–10 days. Patients most at risk during refeeding include those with anorexia nervosa, weight loss more than 10–20% body weight, pro-

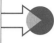

Practical points

- The consumption of excess calories, combined with an increasingly sedentary lifestyle has resulted in a dramatic increase in the prevalence of obesity in Australian children and adults
- Malnutrition is the leading cause of childhood morbidity and mortality worldwide
- Malnutrition continues in our own indigenous population, with up to 20% of hospitalized Aboriginal children in Australia's Northern Territory estimated to be malnourished
- The most common micronutrient deficiencies in developed societies are in iron and folate. Rickets is seen in the breastfed children of dark-skinned women who wear religious veiling, limiting sun exposure
- Hospitalized children are at particular risk of malnutrition and require careful nutritional assessment of needs, losses, intake and absorption
- Nutrition is safer when given enterally. Parenteral nutrition should only be used when enteral nutrition is contraindicated or unsuccessful
- Refeeding syndrome describes the metabolic complications that occur when aggressive nutritional therapy is used to treat the severely malnourished patient
- The delivery of intravenous or enteral carbohydrate loads may precipitate potentially fatal electrolyte disturbances and therefore requires close monitoring

longed fasting or a minimal intake of longer than 7–10 days.

Monitoring refeeding is essential and includes daily/regular monitoring of glucose, electrolytes, urea, creatinine, phosphate, magnesium and fluid balance until stable. Supplementation of potassium, phosphate and magnesium may be required during the initial feeding period guided by blood levels.

3.4 Obesity in children and adolescents

L. A. Baur

Childhood obesity is one of the most serious public health problems facing the developed and, increasingly, the developing world. The prevalence of obesity is increasing in children of all ages and obese children and adolescents may suffer from a host of co-morbidities. Some of these are immediately apparent, while others act as warning signs of future disease.

Obesity is a chronic disorder of energy imbalance that arises as a consequence of a complex interaction between genetic, social, behavioural and environmental factors. While primary prevention may ultimately be the most effective strategy in curbing the epidemic, treatment of those children who are currently obese is needed to improve both their immediate and longer term health outcomes.

The definition of overweight and obesity in childhood and adolescence

Body mass index – a measure of total body fatness

Body mass index (BMI), calculated by dividing weight in kilograms by height in metres squared, is a simple measure of body fatness. Body mass index varies dramatically with age and sex during childhood and adolescence: it rises in the first year, falls during preschool years and then rises once more in adolescence. The point at which BMI starts to increase again, between 4 and 7 years of age, is termed the point of 'adiposity rebound' (Figs 3.4.1, 3.4.2).

Until recently, no standard definitions of overweight and obesity existed for children and adolescents. The International Obesity Task Force (IOTF) has developed a table of age- and sex-specific BMI cutoff points that can be used in epidemiological research to classify overweight and obesity and to allow international comparisons. The IOTF definition is, however, not designed for general clinical use.

Several countries have developed their own BMI-for-age growth charts, and these can be used clinically in order to chart an individual's BMI and to monitor changes over time. An example, from the US Centers for Disease Control and Prevention, is shown in Figures 3.4.1 and 3.4.2. Until further research helps establish the relation between BMI-for-age cutoff points and health outcomes in childhood and adolescence, the decision as to which specific centile lines denote overweight and obesity in clinical settings ultimately remains arbitrary.

Waist circumference – a measure of fat distribution

In children and young people, just as in adults, waist circumference is correlated with abdominal fat, as well as with cardiovascular risk factors. While waist circumference charts are available for some individual countries, there are no internationally accepted criteria for high- or low-risk waist circumference in this age group. Of course, as with BMI-for-age charts, nationally developed waist-circumference-for-age charts can be used to monitor the clinical progress of an individual patient.

Racial and ethnic variations in definition

Racial and ethnic variations exist in the biological response to excess adiposity. Among adults, Asians generally have a higher percentage of body fat for a given BMI, and an associated increased health risk at lower BMI values compared with Europeans. In contrast, Pacific populations generally have a lower percentage of body fat and a decreased health risk at the same BMI levels. These differences are also likely within the child and adolescent age group and ultimately require the development of ethnic- or race-specific definitions or criteria for obesity. There are additional implications for the primary prevention and management of overweight among racial and ethnic groups.

Body mass index-for-age percentiles: Girls, 2 to 20 years

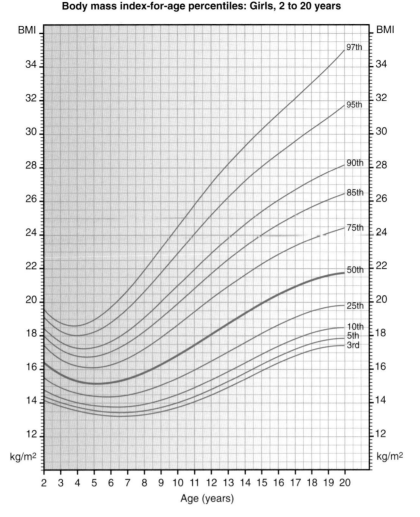

Fig. 3.4.1 Body mass index for age chart for girls aged 2–20 years. Source: US Centers for Disease Control; developed by the National Center for Health Statistics in collaboration with the National Center for Chronic Disease Prevention and Health Promotion (2000).

The prevalence of overweight and obesity among children and adolescents

International prevalence rates and secular trends

The worldwide prevalence of overweight (including obesity) in children and young people aged 5–17 years is approximately 10%, with that of obesity alone being 2–3%. However, certain regions and countries have particularly high rates of paediatric obesity. For example, more than 30% of children and adolescents in the Americas, and approximately 20% of those in Europe, are overweight or obese, with much lower prevalence rates being seen in sub-Saharan Africa and Asia. In 1995–1997 in Australia, the prevalence of overweight and obesity in children and adolescents varied between 19% and 23%; more recent nationally representative prevalence data are awaited. In 2002 in New Zealand, 31% of children and adolescents were overweight or obese, with higher rates being found in Pacific and Maori children.

Of most concern are data showing the rapid change in obesity prevalence in many countries in several continents. This is the case even for China, with its relatively low overall obesity prevalence compared with some Westernized countries (although the caveats about the definition of obesity in Asian populations mentioned above should be noted). A related finding is that not only is the prevalence of obesity increasing in several countries but overweight children are heavier than in the past. Such findings have very significant implications for future population health strategies.

Body mass index-for-age percentiles: Boys, 2 to 20 years

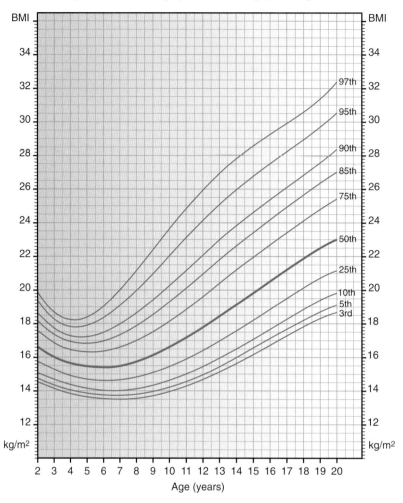

Fig. 3.4.2   Body mass index for age chart for boys aged 2–20 years. Source: US Centers for Disease Control; developed by the National Center for Health Statistics in collaboration with the National Center for Chronic Disease Prevention and Health Promotion (2000).

Obesity-associated complications

The potential complications of obesity among children and adolescents may be immediate (i.e. affecting the obese child or young person), or may not manifest until the medium to long term. These complications may affect many body systems, as outlined in Table 3.4.1.

Complications during childhood and adolescence

Psychosocial complications

The most common consequences of obesity in childhood and adolescence are those related to psychosocial dysfunction and social isolation. In pre-adolescent children, physical appearance and athletic competence self-esteem are lower than in their normal-weight peers, but global self-esteem appears to be preserved. In adolescent girls, excess weight is significantly related to body dissatisfaction, drive for thinness and bulimia. Cross-sectional studies of teenagers consistently show an inverse relationship between weight and both global self-esteem and body esteem. Adolescence is a period when there is marked self-awareness of body shape and physical appearance and so it is not surprising that the pervasive negative social messages associated with obesity in many communities may have an impact at this stage.

Recent studies of health-related quality of life in children and adolescents show differences between obese and non-obese children. Severely obese

Clinical example

Trudy presented to her GP with a respiratory tract infection. Her mother commented incidentally that Trudy was concerned about her weight and was being teased at school. Indeed, she had left her previous school because of bullying and now it appeared to be starting afresh in the new school.

Trudy was the only child, with a good relationship with her parents and some peers. She was in good general health, apart from the weight gain. Several family members were obese (mother and three grandparents), her paternal grandfather had type 2 diabetes and her maternal grandfather had hypercholesterolemia and ischaemic heart disease. Trudy was leading a sedentary lifestyle: she enjoyed playing music, sewing, reading and talking on the phone. Trudy was driven to and from school each day and watched 3 hours of television per day. Her dietary intake included skipping breakfast, full-cream milk, 'something nice' for morning and afternoon tea, buying food at the milk-bar in the afternoon, a daily intake of 500 ml of soft drink and free access to biscuits at home.

On examination, Trudy's height was 161.5 cm (<75th centile), weight 74.3 kg (>97th centile), BMI 28.4 kg/m^2 (>95th centile for age; adult overweight range) and waist circumference 89 cm (adult female 'at significant risk of metabolic complications' range). She was in mid puberty and had abdominal and upper thigh striae. Her blood pressure was 120/80. A fasting blood test showed a normal glucose (4.6 mmol/l; normal range 3.5–5.5), mild hyperinsulinaemia (115 pmol/l) and a lipid profile characteristic of central obesity: total cholesterol 5.3 mmol/l (normal range 2.6–5.5), HDL cholesterol 0.8 mmol/l (normal >0.9), triglycerides 1.9 mmol/l (normal range 0.6–1.7).

To manage Trudy's weight problems, her GP arranged to see Trudy and her mother, separately and together, initially every 3 weeks and then less frequently. Two visits to a local dietitian were also arranged; more frequent follow-up could not be organized. Trudy was encouraged to set her own goals for food and activity changes; these goals were revisited at the consultations. She was helped to look at ways in which eating cues could be recognized and modified. The family was supported to make changes to their eating patterns and the use of the television in the home.

In time, Trudy's mother lost some weight as a result of altered cooking practices and being more active. Water was offered at the evening meal instead of soft drink, less healthy snacks were no longer stored in the cupboards and the family started eating more vegetables and had smaller meat and rice/potato portions at the evening meal. Trudy ate something for breakfast each morning and started walking to and from school. She started tennis lessons and found an interest in tap dancing.

Ten months later, Trudy's weight was 69.3 kg, her height was 163.0 cm, her BMI was 26.1 kg/m^2 and her waist circumference was 81 cm. She reported being more fit and said she was greatly enjoying school and was no longer being bullied. A repeat fasting blood test showed an improved lipid profile (total cholesterol 4.8 mmol/l, HDL cholesterol 1.0 mmol/l, triglycerides 1.4 mmol/l) and a decreased insulin concentration (85 pmol/l), consistent with a reduction in central obesity.

patients in a clinical setting report significantly reduced health-related quality of life compared with healthy children: their quality of life scores are similar to those of children diagnosed with cancer. In randomly sampled populations, the physical and social domains of health-related quality of life for obese children are lower than for non-overweight children, although less significantly reduced than seen in a clinical sample.

Orthopaedic complications

Slipped capital femoral epiphyses occur much more commonly in obese young people, and obese patients have an earlier onset of slippage than non-obese patients. Blount disease (tibia vara) is a deformity of the medial portion of the proximal tibial metaphysis that arises as a result of increased, and possibly unconventional, weightbearing on cartilaginous bone, with subsequent compensatory overgrowth and bowing of the tibia. Young people who are overweight or obese have low bone area and bone mass relative to their body weight, making them more prone to fractures than lean individuals.

More minor orthopaedic abnormalities associated with obesity include knock knee (genu valgum), a decreased recovery from soft tissue ankle injuries and flat, wide feet with increased static and dynamic plantar pressures. These conditions may seem relatively trivial in health terms but could have a significant impact on a child's ability to fully participate in activities.

Hepatobiliary complications

Obese children and adolescents may experience a range of gastrointestinal and hepatobiliary disorders, the most significant being non-alcoholic fatty liver disease (NAFLD). This is an umbrella term that includes steatosis as well as steatohepatitis. It typically presents as an asymptomatic elevation of transaminases. The degree of steatosis is associated with the severity of obesity, a central fat distribution, hypertriglyceridaemia, insulin resistance and the presence of raised transaminases, with a raised alanine aminotransaminase being most specific for steatosis. Liver fibrosis and even evolving cirrhosis have been identified in liver biopsy findings of paediatric patients with NAFLD.

Several clinical audits from paediatric surgical units have demonstrated an association between cholesterol cholelithiasis and obesity in children and adolescents. Gastro-oesophageal reflux appears more prevalent in obese individuals, possibly secondary to increased intra abdominal pressure.

Table 3.4.1 Potential obesity associated complications among children and adolescents

System	Health problems
Psychosocial	Social isolation and discrimination, decreased self esteem, learning difficulties, body image disorder, bulimia *Medium and long term:* Poorer social and economic 'success', bulimia
Respiratory	Obstructive sleep apnoea, asthma, poor exercise tolerance
Orthopaedic	Back pain, slipped femoral capital epiphyses, tibia vara, ankle sprains, flat feet
Hepatobiliary	Non-alcoholic fatty liver disease, gallstones
Reproductive	Polycystic ovary syndrome, menstrual abnormalities
Cardiovascular	Hypertension, adverse lipid profile (low HDL cholesterol, high triglycerides, high LDL cholesterol) *Medium and long term:* Increased risk of hypertension and adverse lipid profile in adulthood, increased risk of coronary artery disease in adulthood, left ventricular hypertrophy
Endocrine	Hyperinsulinaemia, insulin resistance, impaired glucose tolerance, impaired fasting glucose, type 2 diabetes mellitus *Medium and long term:* Increased risk of type 2 diabetes mellitus and metabolic syndrome in adulthood
Neurological	Benign intracranial hypertension
Skin	Acanthosis nigricans, striae, intertrigo

Neurological complications

Idiopathic raised intracranial pressure (pseudotumour cerebri) is a rare but potentially very serious complication of obesity. The role obesity plays in the pathogenesis of the disorder is unknown.

Asthma and sleep-disordered breathing

Respiratory outcomes can be poor in obese children. Asthma appears to be more prevalent in obese than non-obese children. When compared with lean children with asthma, overweight and obese children use more anti-asthma medications, have more wheezing episodes and experience more unscheduled visits to hospital. Obese children also have a lower exercise tolerance than their lean peers, possibly compounding their obesity.

Potentially more serious is the complication of obstructive sleep apnoea. The prevalence of obstructive sleep apnoea in cohort studies of obese children varies, depending upon the definitions of obstructive sleep apnoea and of obesity, with rates of 13–26% being reported. Obstructive sleep apnoea is associated with severity of obesity, insulin resistance and dyslipidaemia among children and adolescents. Profound hypoventilation and even sudden death have been reported in severe cases of sleep apnoea associated with obesity.

Risk factors for cardiovascular disease

Risk factors for cardiovascular disease are one of the most common problems facing the obese young person. In the Bogalusa Heart Study, from the USA, 60% of overweight 5–10-year-olds had one cardiovascular risk factor, such as hypertension, high low-density lipoprotein (LDL) cholesterol or high triglycerides, while over 20% had two or more risk factors. Overall, when compared with their lean peers, overweight children were 2.4 times more likely to have elevated total cholesterol and diastolic blood pressure, and 4.5 times more likely to have elevated systolic blood pressure. A central fat distribution is particularly associated with the clustering of cardiovascular risk factors.

Endocrine complications

Overweight children are much more likely to have elevated fasting insulin concentrations (indicative of insulin resistance) than their lean peers. Impaired glucose tolerance and impaired fasting glucose have been documented in obese children and adolescents in a range of studies.

Originally extremely rare among children and adolescents, the incidence of type 2 diabetes mellitus is now increasing and is inextricably linked to the prevalence of obesity among young people. In the late 1970s and early 1980s, the first reports of type 2 diabetes in native American and Canadian First Nation young people were published, with subsequent reports in the 1990s being particularly of other minority groups in the USA. There are now affected children and young people in a wide range of countries. Youth with type 2 diabetes are generally in the adolescent age group, are obese, have acanthosis nigricans (see below) characteristic of insulin resistance, have a family history of type 2 diabetes and are female.

The metabolic syndrome, a term describing a cluster of highly prevalent disorders in Western countries that appear to be linked to insulin resistance and central obesity, was initially identified among adults. Among adolescents in the USA, the overall prevalence of the metabolic syndrome is approximately 10%. However, among overweight adolescents, the metabolic syndrome affects almost one-third of individuals. Any further increases in the prevalence of obesity are likely to be accompanied by increases in the significant morbidity associated with this disorder.

Reproductive system complications

Menstrual abnormalities occur more frequently in obese girls, including the early onset of puberty and menarche, as well as menstrual irregularities and polycystic ovary disease. There is a strong association between abdominal fat, increased levels of the androgenic hormones, hirsutism, insulin resistance and polycystic ovaries, which grouped together is termed polycystic ovary syndrome.

Skin complications

Obese children suffer from overheating because their fat tissue acts as insulation, resulting in profuse sweating with any physical activity. Thrush occurs more commonly in obese subjects, especially in such moist, overheated areas as skin folds or the groin. Striae can also occur, particularly on the abdomen and thighs.

Acanthosis nigricans is a relatively common dermatological feature of insulin-resistant states such as obesity. It is characterized by thickened areas of hyper pigmentation, with later development of hypertrophy and sometimes papillomatosis. The skin lesions typically occur in intertriginous regions such as the base of the neck, axillae, groin, antecubital and popliteal fossae and umbilicus. The condition is more frequently seen in darker-skinned ethnic groups.

Adult complications arising from child and adolescent obesity

Obesity in adulthood

The most significant health risk faced by obese young people is that they are at risk of becoming obese adults and therefore are at increased risk of cardiovascular disease, diabetes and some cancers. Tracking of obesity from childhood and adolescence through to adulthood is more likely with a family history of parental obesity, the presence of obesity in late childhood or adolescence or with increased severity of obesity.

Long-term cardiovascular complications

Obesity in childhood and adolescence is associated with an increased risk of heart disease in adulthood. Non-invasive assessments of vascular structure show that carotid intima media thickness in adult life is associated with a variety of child or adolescent cardiovascular risk factors, especially obesity. Long-term (55–57 years) follow-up studies of cohorts in the USA and the UK have shown that both all-cause mortality and cardiovascular mortality is associated with higher childhood BMI. Study participants who, as young people, were above the 75th centile for BMI were twice as likely to die from ischaemic heart disease than those who had a BMI between the 25th and 75th centiles.

Long-term endocrine and metabolic complications

Individuals who are overweight as children have an increased risk of endocrine and metabolic complications as adults. Childhood BMI predicts the development of diabetes in adulthood. Results from the Bogalusa Heart Study show that childhood obesity is the strongest predictor of the development, in adult life, of the cluster of risk factors that characterize the metabolic syndrome: those children who were in the top quartile of BMI were 11 times more likely to develop the metabolic syndrome as adults than their lean peers.

Long-term psychosocial complications

Being overweight in adolescence may also be associated with later social and economic problems. Obese adolescent females and young women are more likely, as adults, to have lower family incomes, higher rates of poverty and lower rates of marriage than women with other forms of chronic physical disability who are not overweight. This finding suggests that discrimination plays a role in adverse outcomes. However, obesity limited to childhood does not appear to be associated with adverse socioeconomic, educational, social and psychological outcomes in adulthood.

Aetiology of obesity

Obesity is a complex condition with interactions between genetic, metabolic, behavioural and environmental factors all contributing to its development.

Physiological basis of obesity

Obesity is a chronic disorder affecting energy imbalance. This means that there is a perturbation in the balance between energy intake and energy expenditure. This balance is influenced by a complex set of physiological pathways, for which the hypothalamus acts as the central regulator of energy homeostasis and energy intake. The resultant energy regulation system is very protective against weight loss, which has been the dominant physiological threat to the individual until the past couple of decades in most Westernized societies. However, the system is not protective against weight gain.

Genetic associations of obesity

The heritability of obesity

There is a strong familial association with obesity, with numerous studies indicating that a major part of this association is via a shared genetic predisposition. Twin, family and adoption studies suggest an overall heritability of BMI and body composition of 25–50%.

Genes associated with common obesity

Recent studies have shown that at least 135 different candidate genes are associated with obesity-related phenotypes. Not surprisingly, the range of actions, or presumed actions, of the many gene products of candidate genes is extremely varied, reflecting the numerous physiological pathways influencing total body energy balance and fat distribution. Thus, genes influencing appetite and satiety signals, fat cell signalling, adrenal action, resting metabolic rate, diet-induced thermogenesis, nutrient partitioning, peripheral insulin action, deposition of visceral fat and obesity-related comorbidities are all the subject of active investigation.

Monogenic forms of obesity

Mutations in several genes that encode proteins with probable roles in central appetite regulation have been described. Single gene mutations in at least 10 different genes have been reported, involving 173 individuals with obesity. Most of the mutations are associated with severe early-onset obesity and have a recessive form of inheritance, with the exception of mutations in the melanocortin 4 receptor gene, which has an autosomal dominant mode of inheritance.

Syndromic forms of obesity

Many rare syndromes that are caused by discrete genetic defects or chromosomal abnormalities have obesity as one of a constellation of physical and development abnormalities. The most frequent of these syndromes is Prader–Willi syndrome, characterized by diminished fetal activity, obesity, muscular hypotonia, mental retardation, short stature, hypogonadotropic hypogonadism and small hands and feet, as well as a number of other features.

Environmental and behavioural associations of obesity

Genetic factors make a major contribution to an individual's susceptibility to the development of obesity. However, unless the 'correct' environmental conditions exist, an individual's genetic predisposition for obesity may not be fully expressed, a situation that was presumably the norm in most countries prior to the last decades of the 20th century. The increased prevalence of obesity in recent decades in genetically stable populations highlights the central role of recent important environmental trends in the development of the obesity epidemic.

Television viewing

The association between television viewing and obesity in childhood and adolescence has been demonstrated in both cross-sectional and longitudinal studies, although there are no clear data linking obesity with the viewing of interactive video games, computers or other 'small screen' time. Several possible mechanisms for the association between television viewing and obesity include:

- increased exposure to food marketing
- increased snacking of energy-dense foods and drinks while watching television
- displacement of time spent in more physical activities
- reinforcement of sedentary behaviour
- reduction in basal metabolic rate while watching television
- television viewing is a proxy for a generally obesogenic lifestyle, reflecting parenting style and limit-setting around food choices and recreational choices.

Physical activity and sedentary behaviour

In cross-sectional studies, lower physical activity levels and sedentary behaviours have been shown to be associated with a higher prevalence of obesity in children. Prospective studies in childhood suggest that physical activity has a protective effect on the development of excess weight gain in childhood. Major changes in urban and transport planning and the broader physical activity environment may have contributed to a reduction in physical activity and an associated increase in obesity through the following:

- loss of public recreation space
- increased high-rise housing
- increased motorized transport
- decreased access to public transport
- increased use of passive forms of entertainment, e.g. television, computers
- perceptions of lack of safety in local neighbourhoods.

Dietary intake and eating patterns

The increased prevalence of obesity in recent decades has resulted, in part, from changes in dietary intake. Factors that are likely to have contributed to this include:

- an increased consumption of energy-dense, micronutrient-poor foods
- a high intake of sugar-sweetened drinks, and possibly fruit juices
- intense marketing of energy-dense foods and fast food outlets
- increased fast food restaurant meal frequency
- early feeding styles: parental feeding restriction is associated with increased child eating and weight status.

Breastfeeding has a small but protective effect against obesity. Additional protective factors include high dietary fibre content and school environments that support healthy food choices for children. The relative contributions of dietary fat (versus energy) intake, glycaemic index, portion sizes and specific eating patterns to the development of obesity remain unclear, although all may play an important role.

Socioeconomic conditions

The prevalence of being overweight is high among the poorer children in developed countries and the richer children in developing countries. Potential contributors to obesity in urbanized developing countries include increased availability of cheap energy dense foods and widespread access to tele-

Table 3.4.2	Medical conditions associated with obesity
Endocrine	Hypothyroidism, hypercortisolism, growth hormone deficiency or resistance
Central nervous system damage	Hypothalamic–pituitary damage due to surgery, trauma or cranial irradiation
Post-malignancy	Acute lymphoblastic leukaemia
Side effects of drug therapy	Glucocorticoids, some anti-epileptics (e.g. sodium valproate), some antipsychotics (e.g. risperidone, olanzapine), insulin

vision which favours a more sedentary, indoor lifestyle.

Medical conditions associated with obesity

Obesity may occur secondary to a range of medical conditions, some of which are outlined in Table 3.4.2.

Other factors associated with obesity

Other factors that are associated with obesity are:

- growth patterns that are associated with an increased risk of subsequent obesity, which include an earlier adiposity rebound and rapid catch-up growth in the first 2 years
- parental obesity, which more than doubles the risk of adult obesity among both obese and non-obese children aged less than 10 years. Having two obese parents increases the risk of mid childhood obesity by more than 10 times when compared with children neither of whose parents is obese
- parental (especially maternal) dietary disinhibition, which is associated with development of excess weight gain in the child.

The management of child and adolescent obesity

Clinical assessment

Clinical history

The clinical history should be conducted sensitively. The features that should be covered in a clinical history are outlined in Table 3.4.3.

Table 3.4.3 History to be sought as part of the clinical assessment of the obese patient	
General history	Pregnancy details, including maternal gestational diabetes Early medical history Ethnicity
Weight history	History of obesity including onset and duration of obesity Pubertal history (including menstrual history if relevant) Impact of obesity on the life of the patient and his/her family Reasons for seeking clinical help
Complications history	Psychological effects of obesity, including teasing and bullying Presence of sleep apnoea/disturbed sleep Asthma Specific symptoms such as knee/hip pain Menstrual history (girls) Exercise tolerance
Family history of obesity and disorders associated with insulin resistance	Relative weights or BMIs of family members Family history of obesity, type 2 diabetes, cardiovascular and cerebrovascular disease, fatty liver disease and obstructive sleep apnoea
Lifestyle history	Physical activity, including transport to/from school, participation in organized sports or other activities, access to recreation space or equipment for games, availability of friends or family for games or play Sedentary activities, including TV, video games, computer use, other passive entertainment time, mobile phone use Dietary history, including meal patterns, fast food intake and snacks, soft drink intake

Anthropometry

BMI and waist circumference are most useful when measured serially and when used to monitor change over time:

- BMI is calculated as weight/height^2 and then plotted on a BMI-for-age chart (Fig. 3.4.1)
- waist circumference is measured at the midpoint between the lower edge of the ribs and the iliac crest, approximately at the level of the umbilicus, although in severely obese patients with a fatty apron this measurement can be difficult to ascertain.

Physical examination

Features to be sought on physical examination include:

- hypertension (ensure that the blood pressure cuff width is adequate)
- skin findings, e.g. acanthosis nigricans, striae, intertrigo, skin chafing, hirsutism
- adenotonsillar hypertrophy
- clinical signs of asthma
- hepatomegaly (fatty liver), right upper quadrant tenderness (gall stones)
- an abnormal gait due to joint or other musculoskeletal problems; clinical signs of hip, knee or ankle problems; bowing of the tibiae.

Findings on physical examination that may indicate other causes for obesity (e.g. hypothyroidism, hypercortisolism or Prader–Willi syndrome) and that call for further assessment include short stature, dysmorphic features, violaceous striae, intellectual disability and visual or neurological defects indicative of a central nervous system lesion.

Laboratory investigations

For overweight and mildly obese children, laboratory investigations are generally not necessary. However, if a child or adolescent is very obese (especially if centrally obese), has a family history of disorders associated with insulin resistance, or history and examination findings that suggest the presence of complications of obesity or other risk factors, then the following biochemical screening for dyslipidaemia, insulin resistance, glucose intolerance and liver abnormalities is recommended:

- fasting lipid profile (total cholesterol, LDL cholesterol, HDL cholesterol, triglycerides
- fasting glucose
- liver function tests (specifically alanine aminotransaminase)
- consider fasting insulin
- consider oral glucose tolerance test.

Further assessment of liver function (e.g. liver ultrasound, exclusion of other causes of liver dysfunction) may be required. More detailed endocrinological assessment may be needed if there is short stature, hirsutism or menstrual irregularities. If obstructive sleep apnoea is suspected, referral for polysomnography is warranted.

Defining treatment outcomes

The goals of therapy should initially be clarified with the parents or young person as appropriate. Markers of a successful outcome of therapy may include:

- resolution of medical complications
- improvement in self esteem and psychosocial functioning
- an increase in the level of fitness or aerobic capacity
- improvement in family functioning
- changes in weight status: slowing of weight gain, or weight maintenance (especially in prepubertal children); in some, weight loss
- a decrease in waist circumference ('waist loss') is a useful indicator of reduction in abdominal obesity.

Education of the family and, where appropriate, the young person, about the nature of obesity, including the realization that it is a chronic disorder of energy balance, is also important, as the need for long-term changes in behaviour will then be more readily apparent. Helping the family or young person identify small, achievable goals is important. Examples may include aiming initially for one extra walk per week, or reducing television viewing by 1 hour per day every few weeks.

Broad principles of management

The broad principles of management include:

- clarification of treatment outcomes
- family involvement
- a developmentally appropriate approach
- long-term behaviour change
- long-term dietary change
- increased physical activity
- decreased sedentary behaviour.

Conventional treatment approaches

Family focus

Long-term maintenance of weight loss (i.e. 2–10 years) is achieved when the intervention is family-based. Families influence food and activity habits, and thus it is not surprising that effective therapy of obesity must take this into account. Altered food patterns within the whole family, as well as support of the child and parental reinforcement of a healthy lifestyle, are important factors in successful outcomes.

A developmentally appropriate approach – pre-adolescent children

Treatment of pre-adolescent obesity with the parents as the exclusive agents of lifestyle change is superior, in terms of long-term weight and psychosocial outcomes, to a child-centred approach. Thus, when dealing with the obese pre-adolescent child, sessions involving the parent or parents alone, without the child being present, are likely to be the most effective.

Adolescent-focussed interventions

With adolescents, consider having separate sessions for the young person and parent(s). Short-term weight management success is associated with a range of interventions, all involving intense support for behavioural change, i.e. increased physical activity, phone- and mail-based behavioural interventions initiated in primary care settings, pharmacological therapy and a low-glycaemic-load diet.

Behaviour modification

There are a range of potential behavioural modification strategies that can be used in the management of childhood obesity, including:

- monitoring behaviour
- setting goals
- rewarding successful changes in behaviour
- controlling the environment.

The nature of each of these strategies will vary depending upon the age and developmental status of the patient.

Dietary management

Involvement of the entire family in making the change to a sustainable and healthy food intake is vital. The focus should be on behaviour change, healthier food choices and a reduction in the consumption of energy-dense, micronutrient-poor foods and high sugar drinks. Avoidance of severe dietary restriction may be important in both helping the development of the child's capacity to self-regulate dietary intake and avoiding the subsequent development of disordered eating.

Clinical example

Anna, aged 2 years and 2 months, at a consultation for an intercurrent illness, had her height and weight assessed by her GP. Her height was 92 cm (97th centile for age) and she was noted to be obese, with weight 19.8 kg (>97th centile for age) and BMI 23.4 kg/m² (>>95th centile for age).

Anna's birth weight was 3.7 kg. Review of her growth records showed that her weight had tracked along the 90th centile for the first 6 months, and that from 12 months of age her weight had steadily veered above the 97th centile. In the past 14 months, Anna had been eating the same foods as her parents and two older siblings. This included two or three 'fast food' meals per week, several 'treat' snacks per day (e.g. biscuits or a packet of crisps) and a regular soft-drink intake. When outside, Anna tended to sit and play in the sandpit rather than actively play. There were three televisions in the household and Anna was estimated to watch 3–4 hours of television per day. Both of Anna's parents were mildly obese and her siblings were also overweight.

The GP sensitively raised the issue of Anna's excess weight gain with Anna's mother and encouraged a whole-family approach to lifestyle change. Support for change was given by the GP, and the mother also attended a children's healthy nutrition group programme offered in the local community health centre. Changes that occurred during the next 6 months included offering the children water instead of soft drink, a reduction in serve sizes at the evening meal and provision of healthy snack choices. The parents instituted some rules about television viewing, limiting it to less than 90 minutes per day. The children, including Anna, were encouraged to play outside more often. The sandpit was covered and Anna spent more time in active play.

Six months later, Anna's weight remained unchanged and her height was now 97 cm (97th centile for age). The resultant BMI was 21.0 kg/m², which was still above the 95th centile but showed a marked 2.4 unit decrease over the time period.

Dietary interventions should follow national nutrition guidelines and should have an emphasis on the items listed in Table 3.4.4.

Physical activity and sedentary behaviour

Participation of obese children in a lifestyle programme (e.g. walking, running, cycling or swimming, based on the family's preference) leads to greater long-term reductions in overweight than a programme of isocaloric programmed aerobic exercise. Targeting decreased sedentary behaviour may be as effective as targeting increased physical activity in terms of medium-term weight and fitness outcomes.

Recommendations regarding physical activity and sedentary behaviour are listed in Table 3.4.4.

Settings for treatment

Time-efficient interventions such as group sessions, holiday camps or mail- and phone-based behavioural interventions may do at least as well as individual sessions in the management of child and adolescent obesity.

Non-conventional approaches to therapy

As yet, there is little information to guide the use of more aggressive treatment approaches such as very-low-calorie diets, drug therapy or bariatric surgery in the treatment of severe paediatric obesity. Such therapies should occur in the context of a behav-

Clinical example

Peter, a 15-year-old Australian boy of Lebanese ethnic origin, with a strong family history of central obesity, type 2 diabetes, premature heart disease and hypertension, had significant central obesity (weight 102.8 kg, BMI 39.3 kg/m², waist circumference 115 cm). He had a very sedentary lifestyle and a large intake of soft drink and 'fast food' meals. Peter was aware that he was 'not able to keep up with his mates' but was otherwise unconcerned about his large size. He had a wide circle of friends. Findings on physical examination included hypertension (blood pressure 130/85 with a wide cuff; >95th centile for age, sex and height) and marked acanthosis nigricans at the base of his neck and in his axillae and groin flexures, indicative of insulin resistance.

Fasting blood tests showed normoglycaemia (4.8 mmol/L), hyperinsulinaemia (280 pmol/L), low HDL cholesterol (0.8 mmol/L), hypertriglyceridaemia (2.2 mmol/L) and a mildly raised alanine transaminase (60 U/L; normal range 10–50). An oral glucose tolerance test excluded glucose intolerance and diabetes. Liver ultrasound was consistent with diffuse fatty infiltration (in keeping with non-alcoholic fatty liver disease). Thus, Peter had several features of the metabolic syndrome: hyperinsulinaemia, dyslipidaemia, central obesity, hypertension, acanthosis nigricans and fatty liver disease.

Peter was encouraged to limit his television viewing and he also took out a gym membership, although he found it difficult to attend regularly. A dietitian provided counselling about dietary change and provided initial frequent review, but again Peter was unable to sustain the lifestyle change, largely because of lack of motivation for change. Weight gain continued. Orlistat was prescribed, but Peter found the side effects (bloating, steatorrhoea, abdominal pain) unacceptable and thus discontinued therapy. After review by a paediatric endocrinologist, Peter was commenced on the insulin-sensitizing agent metformin. There was some initial weight loss on this therapy (2.0 kg in the first month of therapy) but he was relatively non-adherent to therapy after the first couple of months.

Table 3.4.4 Interventions for changes in dietary intake and physical activity and sedentary behaviour

Dietary interventions	Modified eating patterns, e.g. regular meals, eating together as a family, avoiding eating while watching the television
	Parents modelling healthy food choices
	Food choices that are lower in energy and fat and have a lower glycaemic index
	Increased vegetable and fruit intake
	Healthier snack food options
	Decreased portion sizes
	Reduction in soft drink, cordial and fruit juice intake
	Water as the main beverage
Physical activity and sedentary behaviour	Focus on increasing incidental activity, e.g. playing with friends or family, walking to the local shops, helping with housework
	Look at active transport options, e.g. walking, cycling, using public transport
	Choose organized activities that the child enjoys
	Improve access to recreation spaces and play equipment (e.g. balls, Frisbees, skipping ropes)
	Limit time spent watching television, or using the computer, play stations or other such 'small screens', to less than 2 hours per day
	Consider alternatives to motorized transport
	Parents should be role models of a physically active lifestyle

ioural weight management programme and should be restricted to specialist centres with expertise in managing severe obesity.

Existing national guidelines on management of overweight and obesity in children provide little guidance on the use of pharmacological therapy, reflecting the paucity of clinical studies. It would appear that the pancreatic lipase inhibitor orlistat and the serotonin- and noradrenaline (norepinephrine)-reuptake inhibitor sibutramine can be used in obese young people with complications who have failed conventional management. Such therapy should be given in the context of a behavioural management programme, with specialist supervision, and only when there is a reasonable expectation of benefit over risk.

Primary prevention of child and adolescent obesity

Because child and adolescent obesity is so common in many countries and has such pervasive consequences, it is important that not just the overweight and obese are targeted with treatment interventions, but that effective primary prevention strategies are also identified and put in place. Interventions simply focussing on educating individuals and communities about behaviour change have had limited or no success in modifying the prevalence of obesity. This is because the broader environment in many communities does not readily support healthy food choices for physically active lifestyles.

Many predisposing factors (physical, economic and sociocultural) contribute to obesity in individuals, and these can operate at both a microenvironmental level (i.e. the settings where individuals live, eat, play or go to school) as well as at a macroenvironmental level (i.e. the broader sectors that ultimately influence dietary intake and physical activity, which are beyond the ability of an individual to influence). Microenvironments relevant to obesity include homes, schools, community groups (e.g. clubs, churches), food retailers (e.g. supermarkets), food service outlets, recreation facilities and local neighbourhoods (e.g. cycle paths, street safety). Macroenvironments relevant to obesity include food production and importing, food manufacturing and

Practical points

- Obesity is a chronic disorder of energy imbalance. The focus should be upon both sides of the energy balance equation: energy in and energy out
- Measure BMI and plot the result on a BMI for age chart. Measure and record waist circumference
- In prepubertal children, weight maintenance or reduction in the rate of weight gain are appropriate goals of therapy
- For younger children, focus upon the parents as agents of change. Adolescents will require a different, developmentally sensitive approach
- Long-term behavioural change is required, involving an increase in incidental physical activity, a reduction in sedentary behaviour and a sustainable change to a lower energy intake

importing, food marketing (e.g. fast food advertising), the sports and leisure industry (e.g. instructor training programmes), urban and rural development (e.g. town planning, local government) and the transport system (e.g. public transport systems).

Considering this, a range of opportunities exist for prevention strategies in a given community or country. These might include:

- development of town planning policies that promote active transport or public transport in contrast to motorized transport
- regulation of the nature and amount of food marketing directed at children
- provision of high-quality recreation areas

- regulation of the types of food and drink provided in school canteens
- improvement in public transport
- subsidies on fruit and vegetables
- provision of safe cycle paths and safe street lighting in local neighbourhoods
- provision of economic incentives for the production and distribution of vegetables and fruit
- support for walk-to-school programmes.

Such interventions will require intersectoral and intergovernmental cooperation, supported by adequate resourcing and significant community ownership.

Immunization 3.5

P. C. Richmond, D. M. Roberton

Immunization provides protection against specific infectious diseases and is one of the greatest achievements of medical science and public health. It is the right of every child to be protected against vaccine-preventable diseases; parents, caregivers and health professionals need to ensure that immunization is available to all children.

Protection against subsequent infection after surviving the initial challenge has been recognized for many centuries for some infections. The use of material from smallpox lesions for vaccination was practised in early dynasties in China. Edward Jenner has been credited with the recognition that vaccination with cowpox virus could protect against challenge with smallpox. Smallpox was declared eradicated worldwide in 1979.

Diphtheria immunization began in Australia in the 1920s and immunization campaigns against pertussis (whooping cough) were initiated in the 1940s. Triple antigen vaccine (DTP: diphtheria, tetanus and pertussis) was used in Australia from 1953. Endemic poliomyelitis began to decline after the introduction of immunization in the early 1950s and has now been eradicated in the developed world. It is likely that poliomyelitis will be the second vaccine-preventable disease to be eradicated worldwide. Measles immunization has been available in Australia for more than 30 years.

Immunization remains one of the most important public health priorities in developed and developing countries. In the developing world, many millions of childhood deaths occur each year from vaccine-preventable diseases such as tetanus and measles because of lack of access to vaccines and vaccine provider services. Thus immunization and its promotion remains one of the major activities of the World Health Organization, with the aim of achieving universal immunization for children.

Principles of immunization

Immunization may be passive or active.

Passive immunity

Passive immunity refers to the acquisition of pre-formed antibody. The fetus receives maternal IgG antibodies during the later weeks of pregnancy, and breastfeeding supplies IgA antibody at the mucosal surfaces of the gastrointestinal tract.

Passive immunization as a means of disease prevention is used in the form of:

- normal human immunoglobulin for protection against measles and hepatitis A
- specific high-titre preparations against cytomegalovirus (CMV), varicella, tetanus, rabies, hepatitis B and diphtheria
- humanized monoclonal antibody against respiratory syncytial virus (RSV) infection.

Passively acquired immunoglobulin has a relatively short half-life and does not lead to active immunity.

Active immunization

Active immunization involves administering antigen so that an immune response develops that is similar to that occurring after naturally acquired infection. This immune response should be one that entails the development of lifelong immunological memory and lifelong prevention from the disease that results from infection with that infecting agent.

Active immunization to prevent infection or the effects of infection may be performed using:

- whole organisms (live or killed)
- purified components of organisms (subunit vaccines, polysaccharide vaccines)
- modified products of the infecting organisms (toxoid vaccines)
- manufactured components of organisms (recombinant vaccines).

Requirements of vaccines

Ideally, a vaccine should:

- give complete protection from the disease caused by the infection
- give lifelong protection
- cause no adverse effects
- need to be given once only
- be able to be given in combination with other vaccines

- be able to be administered easily and without discomfort
- be stable under a wide range of storage conditions
- have a long storage life
- be easy and cheap to manufacture.

Principles of vaccine selection

Diseases and the vaccine types used for prevention of these diseases are listed in Table 3.5.1. The immunization strategies used for these diseases have been developed to take account of the following factors:

- *The nature of the disease process.* For example, toxoid vaccines are used to prevent diseases in which exotoxins are responsible for the disease such as diphtheria and tetanus.
- *The route of infection.* For example, oral rotavirus vaccines have been developed to provide protective mucosal immune responses to rotaviruses, which are a major cause of severe gastrointestinal tract infections in infants.
- *Variability of the organisms causing disease.* For example, influenza vaccines need modification regularly to provide protection from prevalent circulating strains; polio vaccines (oral and inactivated) contain

the three strains of the poliovirus that cause disease, and pneumococcal polysaccharide vaccine contains polysaccharide from the 23 most common strains that cause disease out of more than 80 strains of pneumococcus.

- *The nature of the immune response.* For example, *Haemophilus influenzae* type b (Hib) vaccines, meningococcal C vaccine and pneumococcal vaccines are much more effective in children under the age of 2 years when given as polysaccharide–protein conjugate vaccines rather than purified polysaccharide vaccines because of the poor immune response to polysaccharides at this age. Another example is measles immunization, which is not undertaken until the age of 9–12 months in most countries because passively acquired maternal antibody remains in sufficiently high concentration to neutralize the administered live attenuated vaccine virus strain in the infant prior to this age.
- *The age at which children are most susceptible to infection.* Indigenous infants in Australia are recommended to receive a Hib vaccine (PRP-OMP) that provides better protection after the first dose at 2 months of age because of the early onset of invasive Hib disease in that population; Meningococcal C conjugate vaccines are given as a single dose at 12 months of age, as meningococcal C disease is rare before that age in Australia, whereas a vaccine for

Table 3.5.1 Vaccine types for schedule vaccines and other commonly available vaccines	
Disease	Vaccine type
Schedule vaccines	
Hepatitis B	Recombinant subunit vaccine
Diphtheria	Toxoid (formaldehyde treated toxin)
Tetanus	Toxoid (formaldehyde treated toxin)
Pertussis	Acellular vaccine containing two to five purified or recombinant antigens from *Bordetella pertussis* (killed whale-cell pertussis is still used in some countries)
Haemophilus influenzae type b (Hib)	Polysaccharide protein conjugates (PRP-OMP, PRP-T)
Poliomyelitis	IPV: inactivated poliovirus vaccine (types 1, 2 and 3)
Measles	Attenuated live virus (freeze dried)
Mumps	Attenuated live virus (freeze dried)
Rubella	Attenuated live virus (freeze dried)
Varicella	Attenuated live virus (freeze dried)
Pneumococcal infections	Conjugate vaccine containing seven serotypes
Meningococcal C disease	Meningococcal C conjugate vaccine
Other commonly used vaccines	
Hepatitis A	Inactivated hepatitis A strain
Bacillus Calmette–Guérin (BCG)	Live attenuated bacteria
Influenza	Subunit vaccine derived from inactivated virus
Pneumococcal infections	Polysaccharide vaccine containing 23 pneumococcal polysaccharides (not conjugated)
Meningococcal infections	Quadrivalent vaccine containing A, C, W135 and Y polysaccharides (not conjugated)

meningococcal B disease (currently being trialled in New Zealand) needs to be given in early infancy as the incidence is highest under 12 months of age.

• *The effects of infection on the host.* For example, rubella immunization is provided for all children at age 1 year and again at preschool age to provide long-lasting immunity for girls before their child-bearing years, and to decrease the circulation of rubella in the community, and therefore the risk of exposure of pregnant women to rubella. These strategies have resulted in a dramatic decrease in fetal rubella infection and the associated malformations that occur in early pregnancy (congenital rubella embryopathy).

• *The ability to optimize immunization coverage for the at-risk population.* A targeted strategy of hepatitis B vaccination in newborns of mothers who are hepatitis B carriers to prevent perinatal transmission was ineffective in immunizing the at risk infants, so universal newborn hepatitis B immunization has been implemented in Australia.

Immunization schedule for routine childhood immunization

The immunization schedule recommended in Australia by the National Health and Medical Research Council (NHMRC) is presented in Table 3.5.2. There are differences in the schedule in individual states/territories in Australia because of the contract prices for supply of different types of combination vaccines and variations in the epidemiology of some diseases (such as Hib disease).The immunization schedule has changed significantly in recent years with the availability of new vaccines and is likely to change frequently in the future, so it is important to keep up to date.

Vaccines are provided to registered immunization providers and are generally free of charge. Immunization providers are general practitioners, local authority immunization services, some hospital services (particularly in children's hospitals) and some maternal and child health agencies. All immunization providers must be familiar with:

• the immunization schedule
• vaccine storage and handling requirements
• requirements for informed consent for vaccine administration
• adverse effects of immunization
• potential contraindications to immunization.

These details are provided in Australia at approximately 2-yearly intervals by the NHMRC Immunization Technical Advisory Group as *The Australian Immunisation Handbook*, which is made available to

Table 3.5.2   The NHMRC Standard Immunization Schedule for immunization for Australian children

Age	Vaccine	Route	Milestone
Birth	HBV	i.m.	
2 months*	DTPa	i.m.	
	Hib	i.m.	
	IPV	i.m.	
	HBV	i.m.	
	PCV	i.m.	
4 months*	DTPa	i.m.	
	Hib	i.m.	
	IPV	i.m.	
	HBV	i.m.	
	PCV	i.m.	
6 months*	DTPa	i.m.	
	IPV	i.m.	
	Hib* }	i.m.	
	HBV* }	i.m.	
	PCV	i.m.	Milestone 1
12 months	MMR	s.c.	
	Hib	i.m.	
	MCC	i.m.	Milestone 2
18 months	Varicella	s.c.	
4 years	DTPa	i.m.	
	OPV	oral	
	MMR	s.c.	
10–13 years†	Varicella	s.c.	
	HBV 1	i.m.	
1 month later	HBV 2	i.m.	
5 months later	HBV 3	i.m.	
Prior to leaving school (15–19 years)	dTap	i.m.	
50 years	Td (ADT)	i.m.	

* The availability of different combination vaccines has led to differences in the schedule in the various states. A hexavalent DTPa–HBV–IPV/Hib combination vaccine is being used in New South Wales, Victoria and Western Australia. In other states DTaP–IPV combination vaccines are used with a Hib–HBV combination vaccine.
† This course of HBV is only for those children born before 1 May 2000, who did not receive HBV in infancy as it was not part of the routine schedule for infants at that time. This part of the immunization schedule will only continue until 2010, when the HBV-immunized 2000 birth cohort will have reached the age of 10 years.
DTPa, infant formulation acellular diphtheria, tetanus and pertussis vaccine; dTpa, reduced antigen formulation diphtheria–tetanus–acellular pertussis vaccine for adolescents and adults; HBV, recombinant hepatitis B vaccine; Hib, *Haemophilus influenzae* b conjugate vaccine (PRP–OMP – this particular Hib conjugate vaccine is used because it gives high-level antibody responses after the 2- and 4-month immunizations and therefore gives improved protection in early infancy in comparison with other conjugate Hib vaccines); i.m., intramuscular; IPV, inactivated poliovirus vaccine; MCC, meningococcal C conjugate vaccine; MMR, measles, mumps and rubella vaccine; PCV, pneumococcal conjugate vaccine; s.c., subcutaneous.

all immunization providers and to other health care providers who have a role in immunization services, and is also available as an up to date electronic version on the internet (http://immunise.health.gov.au/handbook.htm).

Administration of vaccines

Storage of vaccines

Most vaccines need to be stored in a temperature range between 2°C and 8°C. Maintenance of the cold chain is required from the time of manufacture until the time of administration. Vaccine storage temperature conditions must be monitored continuously, using thermometers capable of recording maximum and minimum temperatures. Generally, freezing of vaccines is more deleterious to vaccine efficacy than short periods of time above the recommended temperature range.

Consent for immunization

Parents or guardians must be given adequate information that will allow them to make an informed decision about immunization for their child. The information given should include:

- the benefits and risks of immunization
- the common side effects of the various vaccines.

This information preferably should be available in written form, and is provided in a form suitable for parents and guardians in *The Australian Immunisation Handbook*. Valid consent is necessary prior to each immunization episode.

Preimmunization questionnaire

In some circumstances, the risk of adverse reactions to immunization is increased in the presence of some conditions. A standardized questionnaire should be used routinely prior to each immunization episode. The questionnaire should enquire whether the child:

- has had any previous severe reactions to any vaccine
- has any condition that may lower immunity (e.g. treatment with systemic steroids – >1 mg/kg prednisolone per day for >4 weeks – chemotherapy, pre-existing immune deficiency disorder or disorder affecting immunity, such as leukaemia)
- lives with someone with lowered immunity
- might be pregnant (for girls of childbearing age)
- has had a vaccine containing live viruses within the last month
- has any severe allergies (although this is not a contraindication to scheduled immunization)
- has received a blood transfusion or immunoglobulin preparation in the last 3 months
- identifies as being an Aboriginal or Torres Strait Islander person (to ensure that they receive any additional immunizations required).

Children should be assessed to ensure that they are well enough to have vaccine administered: immunization should be deferred only rarely but may be delayed temporarily if there is a temperature over 38.5°C, if the child has diarrhoea or vomiting (for oral vaccines only) or if he or she is obviously unwell for other reasons.

Sites of vaccine administration

Intramuscular vaccine administration in infants under the age of 1 year should be at the junction of the upper and middle one thirds of the anterolateral thigh. If three separate intramuscular vaccines are being given, two vaccines are given in one thigh at least 2.5 cm apart and the other vaccine in the other thigh. In children over the age of 1 year, intramuscular vaccines are given into the mid-deltoid region of the upper arm. Vaccines should *not* be given in the buttocks because of possible suboptimal immune response or sciatic nerve damage.

Adverse effects of immunization

Immunization promotes a protective immune response. As part of this there is often some evidence of minor inflammation in association with parenterally administered vaccines. The most common side effects in the past in Australia were with whole-cell pertussis vaccines: local swelling, crying, irritability and fever. These occur very much less frequently with the acellular pertussis vaccines (DTPa) although large local reactions may occur, especially in older children. Vaccines containing Hib cause minor local swelling and erythema in about one in 20 infants. Measles immunization may be followed by a mild and transient measles-like illness, with fever and a brief rash, about 7–10 days after immunization. All these side effects are generally transient, require no specific treatment and do not preclude further vaccination.

Rarely, there may be major events in association with immunization procedures. Anaphylaxis is very rare (fewer than 1 in 100 000 immunizations) but every immunization provider must have the appropriate equipment and training for dealing with anaphylaxis. The most important components of management of anaphylaxis are maintenance of the airway and the administration of adrenaline (epinephrine).

Convulsions are sometimes seen in association with immunization procedures. Simple febrile convulsions may occur in conjunction with febrile responses to DTP or measles immunizations in children predisposed to febrile convulsions; however, these are not contraindications to further immunization. Immunization is not associated with sudden or unexpected infant death syndrome (SIDS). Several studies, including a recent well controlled study in New Zealand, have shown that the relative risk for SIDS is decreased in immunized children.

Disorders that are not contraindications to immunization

Immunization is not contraindicated in children:

- with minor upper respiratory tract illness (colds, cough, sore throat) or low-grade fever at the time immunization is due
- using inhaled steroid medications for control of asthma or topical steroids for dermatitis
- with atopic disorders
- receiving antibiotics
- with controlled epilepsy, a history of febrile convulsions, a family history of epilepsy or stable neurological disorders

Clinical example

Joshua, aged 6 months, was brought to the community health centre by his 18-year-old mother to see a doctor for advice about a rash on his cheeks, behind his ears and over his upper trunk. The rash was due to infantile eczema. On questioning, it was found that he had not yet received any of his childhood immunizations. His mother said that this was because he always seemed to have a runny nose when due for immunization and she had been concerned that immunization might make his rash worse.

She was reassured that immunization was not contraindicated in the presence of rhinitis or eczema and that immunization was important in infancy. Advice on the management of eczema was given. Joshua received his first DTPa, Hib, hepatitis B, IPV (poliovirus vaccine) and pneumococcal immunizations that day from the health centre's immunization clinic. The immunizations were recorded in his health record and in the Childhood Immunization Register, and appointments were made for further DTPa, Hib, hepatitis B, IPV and pneumococcal immunizations at ages 8 and 10 months. He achieved his second immunization 'milestone' by receiving MMR, meningococcal C vaccine and HBV on his first birthday.

- who have been premature or who are growing poorly.

Children who have documented allergic reactions to eggs can be immunized, as egg proteins are not found in vaccines in the routine childhood immunization schedule, including measles, mumps and rubella (MMR) vaccine. However, advice should be given about immunization with influenza and yellow fever vaccines, which are not recommended for egg-allergic children because of the increased amount of egg protein in these vaccines.

Specific immunization considerations

Prematurity

Premature infants should receive their immunizations at the appropriate age after birth, regardless of their gestational age. For example, an infant born 8 weeks prematurely should commence the immunization schedule at the age of 2 months, even though the gestational age would only be 'at term' if not born prematurely.

Because of a slight risk of reversion of the live virus vaccine strains if passaged repeatedly within

Clinical example

Jake was born at 26 weeks gestation after his mother unexpectedly went into premature labour. He had significant respiratory distress in the first 3 weeks after birth, requiring surfactant, and he was ventilated for 2 weeks. He then needed supplementary oxygen for 4 weeks. He needed parenteral nutrition for the first 4 weeks of life, then nasogastric tube feeding for 4 weeks before he was able to suck and be fed expressed milk from a bottle.

The day he was born, he received his first dose of hepatitis B vaccine as part of the routine schedule of vaccines. At 8 weeks after birth, when he was still equivalent to 34 weeks gestation, he received pneumococcal conjugate vaccine (PCV), DTPa vaccine, Hib and IPV and his second dose of hepatitis B vaccine as part of the routine immunization schedule. The DTPa, IPV, hepatitis B and IPV vaccine were given as a single combination vaccine, DTPa-HBV-IPV/Hib, into his lateral thigh, and the PCV vaccine was given at the same time into the other thigh. His equivalent gestation when he was discharged was 38 weeks. At the time of discharge, arrangements were made for Jake to have his 4-month schedule immunizations DTPa-HBV-IPV/Hib and PCV 4 weeks after discharge, when he was 4 months old and again at 6 months of age. This was followed by meningococcal C, MMR and Hib on his first birthday.

neonatal units, attenuated live poliovirus vaccine (OPV) was not recommended in Australia until the time of discharge from hospital for premature infants, or inactivated poliovirus vaccine (IPV)-containing vaccines were used. The recent introduction of universal IPV immunization in Australia means that preterm infants can be immunized for poliomyelitis with the usual schedule vaccines at the age-appropriate time even if they continue to require inpatient care.

For some vaccines such as hepatitis B and Hib, extremely premature infants (<29 weeks gestation) may require additional doses to ensure protection.

Missed or delayed immunizations

If a child has not received immunization at the appropriate ages, 'catch-up' immunization schedules are used. The immunization schedule does not have to be recommenced nor are additional doses of vaccine needed. Schedules for catch-up immuniza-

tion for DTP, hepatitis B virus (HBV) and Hib immunization are available in *The Australian Immunisation Handbook*.

Live virus vaccines

Live virus vaccines such as MMR and varicella can be given on the same day if necessary, for example for catch-up immunization; however, if different live virus vaccines cannot be given on the same day they should be given at least 4 weeks apart.

Comparison of effects of diseases and vaccines

The benefits of immunization greatly outweigh the risks of any adverse events associated with administration of vaccines used in the childhood immunization schedule. Table 3.5.3 lists some comparisons for vaccine-preventable diseases and effects that may be

Table 3.5.3 Benefits and side effects of childhood immunizations		
Infection	Effects of infection	Side effects of immunization
Hepatitis B	Persistent carrier state common after infection Long-term risk of chronic hepatitis and primary liver cancer	Minor fever in 2–3%, local inflammation in 5–15%
Diphtheria	Toxin causes nerve and heart damage Mortality 1 in 15	DTPa may cause minor local reactions such as swelling, redness and discomfort in approximately 15% of recipients
Tetanus	Toxin causes nerve and muscle changes resulting in paralysis, convulsions Mortality 1 in 10	As under diphtheria, above
Pertussis	Whooping cough Mortality and morbidity highest in infants Mortality 1 in 200 if infected in first 6 months of life	As under diphtheria, above
Poliomyelitis	Febrile illness, followed by paralysis in many Mortality 1 in 20 hospitalized patients Permanent paralysis in many	Paralysis related to vaccine strain virus in 1 in 2.5–5 million recipients or close contacts
Haemophilus influenzae b	Systemic infections such as meningitis, epiglottitis, bone and joint infections Meningitis mortality 1 in 20, long-lasting morbidity 1 in 4	Discomfort or local inflammation in 5%. Fever in 2%
Measles, mumps and rubella	Measles encephalitis in 1 in 1000–2000 Mumps encephalitis in 1 in 200 Congenital rubella syndrome if infected in first trimester of pregnancy	Minor fever, local inflammation in up to 10% 1 in 1 million may develop measles vaccine strain encephalitis; 1 in 3 million may develop mumps vaccine strain encephalitis
Source: Modified from *The Australian Immunisation Handbook*, NHMRC, 2003.		

associated with the corresponding vaccines. A more complete listing is available in *The Australian Immunisation Handbook*.

Recording of immunization administration

Accurate recording of vaccine administration is essential. This must include:

- the vaccine administered
- the vaccine batch number and any other appropriate identifying information
- identification of the immunization service provider
- the date at which the next immunization is due.

This information should be recorded in a parent-held Child Health Record and in the records of the immunization service provider. It should also be entered in nationwide immunization databases. The Australian Childhood Immunization Register (ACIR) was commenced in January 1996 for this purpose and a similar register is used in New Zealand. The register is used for providing a reminder system to inform parents and caregivers when the next immunization is due for their child. Within Australia, uptake of immunization is encouraged by using financial incentives within the family allowance funding programme for immunization completed according to the 'immunization milestones', and by payment of immunization providers for high rates of immunization and for notification to the ACIR.

Other vaccines

Other vaccines are available that are not part of the routine childhood immunization schedule.

Bacillus Calmette–Guérin

Immunization with bacillus Calmette–Guérin (BCG) is no longer provided for all children in Australia nor in many other countries where the overall prevalence of tuberculosis is low. However, it may be recommended for:

- neonates in Aboriginal and Torres Strait Islander communities in regions of high incidence
- neonates or young children in households containing immigrants from countries of high incidence, e.g. south-east Asian and Indian subcontinent countries
- children who are going to live in countries of high tuberculosis prevalence.

Hepatitis A vaccine

Hepatitis A vaccine normally is given as a two-dose schedule for travellers to endemic areas, and has recently been recommended for Aboriginal and Torres Strait Islander children at 18 months of age in northern parts of Australia because of the incidence in that population of hepatitis A with significant morbidity.

Pneumococcal polysaccharide vaccine

In addition to infants, pneumococcal immunization also is important in older children at high risk of pneumococcal disease, such as those with nephrotic syndrome asplenia or sickle cell disease. Adults over the age of 65 years should receive pneumococcal vaccine (over 50 years for Aboriginal and Torres Strait Islander people).

Meningococcal quadrivalent ACW$_{135}$Y polysaccharide vaccine

This is used for the control of outbreaks of meningococcal disease, in those with complement deficiency disorders and in those with asplenia or splenic dysfunction, and is required for pilgrims attending the Hajj as well as being recommended for travellers to sub-Saharan Africa and other countries where these strains are common. Protection following this vaccine is short-term, so boosters are required after 3–5 years.

Influenza vaccine

Annual immunization with influenza vaccine is recommended for:

- children and adults receiving immunosuppressive therapy, for example chronic steroid use and with malignancy, and those with human immunodeficiency virus (HIV)
- children with over 6 months with chronic heart conditions, including cyanotic congenital heart disease
- children with chronic suppurative lung diseases, including cystic fibrosis
- children over 6 months of age with chronic illnesses requiring regular medical follow-up (diabetes mellitus, chronic renal failure, chronic metabolic disorders, haemoglobinopathies)
- adults over 65 years of age
- contacts of high-risk patients, particularly household members.

Clinical example

Holly was brought in by her mother to her GP at 18 months of age to discuss her varicella immunization. Her parents were confused as they had heard that she was better off getting chickenpox as an infection because it gave longer-lasting immunity and giving the vaccine at this age would put her at risk of more severe disease as an adult. Also they were concerned that, if she had the vaccine, she would be at risk of giving the disease to her brother Tom (4 years of age) who was undergoing chemotherapy for acute lymphoblastic leukaemia and had not had chickenpox or been vaccinated.

Her GP advised Holly's parents that varicella vaccine provided good long-term protection against varicella infections and any breakthrough infections (1–2% per year) were mild. In contrast, while chickenpox infection is generally self-limiting, there are risks of severe varicella infection or secondary bacterial infection, which results in 1 in 200 children being hospitalized. The GP also advised that vaccinating Holly was the best way of protecting her brother, as vaccinated healthy children do not pass on the infection and this will decrease the risk of her brother being exposed to a potentially dangerous infection.

Immunization in special circumstances

Travel

Advice for specific vaccines to protect against infection while travelling in other countries depends on the nature of the endemic infections in those countries. Information can be obtained in Australia from the Commonwealth Department of Health and Aging, or from the World Health Organization. It is important for all children travelling to be up to date for all their routine childhood immunizations, as these infections are prevalent in many countries, and for parents to be aware of simple hygiene and protective measures for preventing infection.

HIV infection

Infected or potentially infected infants and children should receive the standard immunization schedule, including MMR vaccine, and it is recommended that IPV be given in place of OPV in countries where OPV is still part of the usual schedule.. Pneumococcal conjugate vaccine is recommended for HIV-infected infants and pneumococcal polysaccharide vaccine for older children and adults. Varicella vaccine can be given to HIV-infected individuals who are asymptomatic or mildly affected with a normal CD4 count. Annual influenza vaccination is also recommended.

BCG should not be given to children with HIV because of risk of disseminated disease.

Bone marrow transplantation

Following allogenic and autologous stem cell transplantation, pre-existing immunity to vaccine preventable diseases is completely or partially lost and reimmunization is necessary. All routine childhood immunizations should be included, although the timing and number of doses required will vary between units and the degree of the patient's immune reconstitution.

Asplenia

Children with asplenia (congenital; after splenectomy, e.g. for hereditary spherocytosis or trauma) or splenic dysfunction (e.g. in sickle cell disease) should receive pneumococcal vaccine (conjugate vaccine if less than 5 years of age and polysaccharide vaccine for older children) and meningococcal C conjugate vaccine followed by quadrivalent meningococcal polysaccharide vaccine. Hib vaccine should be given if it has not been received in infancy.

Primary immunodeficiency disorders

Live viral vaccines and BCG should not be used in children with primary immunodeficiency disorders.

Passive immunization

Passive immunization entails the use of normal human immunoglobulin preparations or hyperimmune (high-titre) immunoglobulin. Passive immunization may be used in children in the circumstances described below.

Normal human immunoglobulin

- Immunoglobulin replacement in primary or acquired immunodeficiency disorders
- Measles prophylaxis
- Hepatitis A exposure

High titre immunoglobulin

- Cytomegalovirus infection or prophylaxis in immunocompromised individuals
- Varicella prophylaxis (zoster immune globulin)
- Tetanus or tetanus-prone wounds
- Rabies exposure
- Hepatitis B exposure, including babies born to hepatitis B carrier mothers

- Diphtheria antitoxin (horse-serum-derived)
- RSV prophylaxis in very-high-risk ex-premature infants with severe ongoing cardiac or pulmonary disease

Future vaccines and vaccine development

Potential changes to immunization strategies for children in the near future in Australia and many other countries include:

- live attenuated intranasal vaccines against influenza
- human papilloma virus vaccines in adolescent girls for the prevention of cervical cancer
- availability of efficacious and safe rotavirus vaccines for infants
- new combination vaccines such as MMR–varicella.

Other developments in immunization during the next 5–10 years are likely to lead to the availability of serotype-independent pneumococcal and meningococcal vaccines. There is a great need for vaccines against malaria and other parasitic diseases causing widespread morbidity globally, and for vaccines with greater efficacy against tuberculosis. Public health strategies will have as their primary focus procedures and community campaigns to ensure the highest possible uptake, in both developing and developed countries, of the highly effective vaccines already available.

Child injury

W. R. Pitt, M. Anscombe

The impact of child injury

In Australia, injuries are the leading cause of death and the second most common cause for admission to hospital in children between the ages of 1 to 14 years. In 2002/03 approximately 66 000 children were hospitalized and 276 died as a result of injury. Most such injuries are preventable. The science of injury prevention is well developed but is not widely applied. Doctors need to be well informed and to be community leaders in this field.

Prioritizing injury control strategies

As health resources are limited, injury prevention programmes must target the most severe injuries, those injuries that affect the most vulnerable members of society and those most amenable to prevention. Figures 3.6.1 and 3.6.2 show the major causes of mortality and reason for hospital admission for children injured in 2002/03. Hospital admission is only one indicator of morbidity. Children can be left with life-long scarring from burns and a significant number of near-drowning survivors are left with some degree of permanent neurological dysfunction. The federal government's National Injury Prevention Plan Priorities for 2004 and beyond identify children as a major priority for injury prevention.

Principles of child injury control

The agent–host–environment model forms the foundation of injury prevention. The *agent* of injury may be any active form of energy that damages body tissues, e.g. the kinetic energy resulting from rapid deceleration, or chemical reaction interrupting the body's ongoing metabolic processes, e.g. hypoxia that damages cells, tissues and blood vessels. The *host* is the injured individual described not only by age and sex but crucially by a child's developmental level.

Cognitive factors influence a child's capacity to recognize and avoid hazards. Toddlers are a particular at-risk group as they explore the home environment, with a physical capability to access hazards they lack the judgement to avoid. Adolescents are prone to risk taking, are vulnerable to peer-group pressure, experiment with alcohol and drugs and are often resistant to education campaigns.

Physical factors that can expose a child to injury include small size (less visible to motorists), large head-to-body ratio (increased risk of head injuries) and narrow airways (risk of foreign body aspiration).

The developmental vulnerability of the child enhances the importance of the *environment* in the injury equation both directly and indirectly. The psychosocial environment has particular importance for children because significant stresses within the family, such as moving to another house or a parent in hospital, may create an environment in which a child is more likely to be injured. However, it is the hazardous physical environment – from motor vehicles to scalding hot tap water – that poses a direct threat to the young child, who lacks the perceptual skills and organized defences of the older child and adult.

The agent–host–environment model has a temporal dimension. Prevention strategies can target pre-event, event and post-event phases. Primary prevention involves measures that prevent an injury event from occurring, secondary prevention minimizes the extent of physical damage incurred by the host during an injury event, and tertiary prevention focuses on optimal treatment after the injury event.

Socioeconomic factors

The risk of child injury is higher in families with a single parent, young maternal age at birth, poor housing, large family size and parental drug or alcohol abuse. Injury and death from injury is strongly associated with poverty. These socioeconomic factors have a profound impact on the capacity of the caregiver to adequately supervise and provide a safe environment for their children.

During the period 2001–2003, the injury mortality rate for indigenous children was nearly three times that of other Australian children.

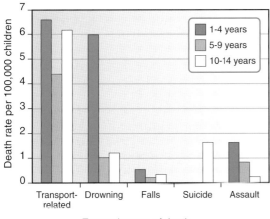

Injury death rate for children aged 1-14 years, 2001-2003 (rate per 100,000 children).

Fig. 3.6.1 Injury death rate for children aged 1–14 years, 2001–2003 (rate per 100 000 children). Source: AIHW National Mortality Database.

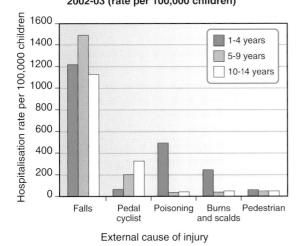

Hospitalisation rates for children aged 1-14 years for specific external causes of injuries, 2002-03 (rate per 100,000 children)

Fig. 3.6.2 Hospitalization rates for children aged 1–14 years by specific external cause of injury, 2002–2003 (rate per 100 000 children). Source: AIHW National Mortality Database.

Perceptions of preventability

The single greatest impediment to progress in injury prevention is the notion that injuries are random chance occurrences that cannot be predicted or prevented. The use of the term 'accident' implies an element of unpredictability. However, the reality is that injuries are no more likely than diseases to occur by chance. The unscientific term 'accident', with its connotations of chance and fate, deflects attention from rational investigation and intervention and must be replaced by descriptions of injuries that reflect the distinct epidemiology of every category and subcategory.

Strategies for prevention

Strategies for prevention should primarily be aimed at removing hazards from the child's environment. Examples include child-resistant packaging for medicines, pool fencing, placing plastic plugs in power sockets, reducing hot water temperatures or installing a smoke alarm.

Education and supervision are less effective but important elements of a targeted injury control program. Informing parents about a hazard provides the opportunity to protect the child from or supervise the child near the hazard. However, encouraging the supervision of children is not a scientific or measurable prevention method.

Supervision means different things to different people in different situations at different ages. For toddlers crossing the road, supervision means physical contact with someone old enough to protect the toddler. In the context of toddler near-drowning, it means keeping the child in direct line of sight. In order to prevent these deaths, direct line of sight supervision is the minimum level of supervision that might make a difference. In reality, for most parents adequate supervision means knowing approximately where a child is in relation to non-lethal home hazards. Higher levels of supervision are only realistically sustainable for brief periods, which will vary from parent to parent.

Successful intervention at the community level can only be achieved if the community recognizes and owns the problem. A sustainable prevention strategy must be socially and politically acceptable. Because prevention often involves some limitation of pre-injury choices, the community must be convinced of the need to act. The collection and dissemination of local injury statistics can help a community to understand the problem. Community engagement and Safe Community programmes are an important part of this process. However, community change will often require some level of enforcement through political and legislative processes.

The doctor's role in injury prevention

Every doctor who provides health care to children or parents of children has the opportunity to reduce the injury disease burden. They should take opportunities for anticipatory guidance about injury prevention issues. Specialists who deal with injured children have the necessary experience, influence and credibility to take a leading role in advocating for injury prevention. A successful child injury advocate is a life-long agent of change who pleads, defends, vindicates or espouses their cause to change the individual or community's perception of injury.

Injuries in the home

Over half of all child injury occurs at home. More than half of these injuries occur in preschool children as this age-group spends most of their time in the home. Younger children are injured most commonly in the living room, bedroom or kitchen whereas older children are more frequently injured in the yard.

The most common cause of injury death in the home is drowning, mainly in swimming pools, followed by asphyxia, driveway runovers, poisoning and crush injury.

Contact with a hard or sharp object after falling is the most common mechanism of home injury. There are different reasons for falling at different ages. Infants are more likely to be injured after falling from a bed or a change table, or while in a baby walker. Toddlers, with their new-found mobility, fall while walking or running. Older children are more likely to injure themselves by falling off bikes or trampolines or out of trees. Skateboards, roller skates and roller blades appear amongst the top ten injury factors in 10–14 year olds. Infants are more likely than older age-groups to sustain head injuries from their falls. Older children present more frequently with limb fractures, sprains and strains, or open wounds.

The next most common reason for presentation due to injury in the home for the under-5 year olds is poisoning. Burns from hot liquids or objects are another common mechanism of injury in the very young. Older children are more likely to be injured by being struck by or colliding with an object. Eye injuries from projectiles are of particular concern because of the risk of blindness.

Injuries at school

After the home, school is the most frequent location for injury amongst school-age children. As with home injury, falls are the most common cause of injury. Fractures, sprains and strains are the most common injuries sustained. Play equipment such as the horizontal ladder is the most common injury factor in primary school children.

Sport is the most frequent activity resulting in injury in high school children, with football codes responsible for nearly two-thirds of the injuries. Injuries due to aggressive behaviour, particularly in males, has been cited as a significant cause of injury in schools, with nearly one-quarter of injuries being attributed to intentional acts.

Some specific illustrative examples of child injury

Low-speed run-overs

A typical low-speed run-over involves a toddler reversed over by a close relative driving a vehicle with limited rearward vision in their own driveway in the late afternoon. Low-speed run-overs are the third biggest cause of injury death in Australian toddlers and account for half the pedestrian death in this age-group. Very young children are difficult for the reversing motorist to see and can move surprisingly quickly.

Opportunities for prevention

Opportunities for prevention may include increasing the public awareness of the driveway as a hazardous environment for young children, better housing design to ensure separation of a child's play area from the driveway and installing reversing cameras on vehicles.

 Clinical example

Ryan, aged 2 years, is the youngest in a family of three children. On a Saturday morning, Ryan's father was getting ready to take Brett, his older son, to football, and his mother was at the same time hurrying her daughter as she was late for her violin lesson. The family had recently bought a large four-wheel-drive vehicle. In the rush and confusion, Ryan wandered out of the open front door and began to explore around the driveway. Unaware of Ryan's presence, his father got into the car and began to back it down the driveway, at the same time yelling quite loudly to his older son to 'get a move on'. Just then, Brett emerged from the front door and screamed for his father to stop. From his vantage point he could see that his father was about to back the car over Ryan.

Four-wheel-drive vehicles are usually higher than conventional cars, and this makes it very difficult to see behind the vehicle. Note that the near-injury also occurred at a time of family distraction and high levels of activity.

Automatic dishwasher detergent ingestion

Poisoning is one of the most common reasons for paediatric injury presentation to an Emergency Department (ED). In the 1970s, child-resistant packaging dramatically reduced poisoning due to prescription medications. Non-medicinal poisonings now account for two-thirds of poisonings in children under 5 years. In the case of automatic dishwasher detergent ingestion, the typical case is a toddler ingesting dishwasher detergent powder either as slurry from the dishwasher detergent compartment or from the container. Caustic burns sustained can cause life-threatening swelling in the early stages of injury and long-term scarring in survivors, necessitating multiple surgical procedures.

Opportunities for prevention and advocacy

The reason child-resistant packaging was so successful as a prevention strategy was that it combined a simple, inexpensive design solution to remove a hazard from a child's environment with legislative support. It has proved more difficult to prevent non-medicinal poisoning. In 1987, in an attempt to reduce alkali burns, legislation was introduced that required strongly alkaline automatic dishwasher detergents in gel or liquid form to be packaged in a child-resistant container with a label cautioning the consumer to keep the product out of reach of children. Almost 20 years later, it is the powder formulations which cause by far the most caustic injury. A working group including doctors and personnel from injury surveillance, toxicology, child safety and product safety organizations is collaborating to advocate for a change in legislation that will include powder formulations.

Asphyxia

Sleep-related deaths occur predominantly in those children under 1 year. Strangulation by a rope, cord, or strap is the most common cause of asphyxial death in the 1–4 year age-group. Foreign body aspiration is the next most common cause of asphyxia. While food is the most frequent cause choking in young children, non-food items such as toys and coins are more likely to have fatal consequences.

Opportunities for prevention

Young children should not be fed small, round, firm or pliable foods that may lodge in the airway. Dangerous foods include chunks of meat or raw carrot, nuts, grapes, hard sweets, bubble gum and popcorn. Small objects such as coins, batteries and parts of toys or games should be kept out of reach. Strings and cords on infant toys, clothing and bedding should be avoided and blind and curtain cords should be kept out of reach. Labels that indicate that toys are unsuitable for children under 3 years should be heeded.

Scalds

Scalds are the most common cause of hospital admission due to thermal injury. A child's thin epidermis is more likely to be damaged than that of an adult. Toddlers are the group most vulnerable to scalds. Scalds may occur in hot baths, tipping over pots or kettles containing boiling water or pulling hot drinks down from a table. In addition to the suffering due to the initial burn there are the risks in deeper burns of long-term cosmetic and functional impairment due to scarring.

Opportunities for prevention

Opportunities for prevention include installation of fitted stove guards, using the back elements for preference or turning pot handles rearward, using place mats instead of tablecloths, and lowering of hot water temperature to 50°C. Referral of children with serious scald injuries to specialized paediatric burns units has a role in minimizing the extent and impact of the injury.

Drowning in domestic swimming pools

Drowning is the most common cause of death in toddlers aged 1–4 years. Half of these occur in domestic swimming pools. The majority of children are on the property with permission and most children were thought to be safe within the house at the time of immersion. Most drowning occurs in unfenced pools or pools with a defective gate, allowing the toddler unintended access to the pool area.

Opportunities for prevention

Death rates due to drowning in domestic swimming pools halved in Queensland after the introduction of mandatory pool fencing in the early 1990s. The benefit is sustained through ongoing education programmes and compliance checks. Early basic life support may save children who have been submerged for only short periods of time.

Crush injuries

Injuries associated with doors are the fifth most common reason for Emergency Department attendance in children aged 1–4 years. These finger-jam injuries may result in a permanent injury, including amputation. Deaths occur when heavy objects such as televisions, bird-baths, trampolines or shelving fall and crush young children.

Opportunities for prevention

The use of door protection devices can reduce the incidence of finger jam injuries. Heavy objects with the potential to topple can be secured, for example tethering a television to the wall.

Falls from playground equipment

Items of playground equipment most associated with injuries from falls are the trampoline at home and the horizontal ladder at a playground. The most represented age-group is 5–9 year olds. One-third of the injuries requiring admission due to falls are forearm fractures.

Opportunities for prevention

It is a important to design and permit play equipment that provides children of different developmental levels with a sufficient physical challenge for enjoyment and skill development without putting them at risk of significant injury. Limiting heights of playground equipment to 1.5 m and the provision of safe fall zones reduces fractures without reducing the fun. New Australian standards minimize the risk of entrapment of body parts.

Clinical example

Louise, aged 6 years, was playing in the school playground with her new friend Melissa. Louise had been reluctant to start school and had tended to stay in the background at playtime. Now, after a whole year at school, she was much more confident and with the arrival of Melissa at the school she really enjoyed playtime. They climbed all over the climbing towers and went down the slippery dip. Then Louise began to make her way across the 'monkey bars'. This equipment is like a horizontal ladder, often 1.5 m or more off the ground. Not having acquired sufficient skill, she fell after two rungs, sustaining a greenstick fracture of her radius. Although the surface of the playground had been covered with tanbark, which should have provided a soft fall, this had been scattered by the many children playing there, and the soft surface had not been maintained.

Many believe that monkey bars are unsuitable play equipment for young children, who do not have sufficient skill to negotiate them safely. Height of play equipment off the ground remains an issue. Maintenance of a soft surface is very important.

Bicycle injuries

Bicycles are the most common consumer product associated with child injury in Australia. 75% of all ED presentations with bicycle-related injuries are children under 15 years. Twice as many males as females are injured. The most common age-group is 10–14 year olds, making up almost 40% of the cases. The most common injuries leading to ED presentation in the child cyclist are limb fractures and open wounds. Most fatalities are due to head injuries and involve a collision with a motor vehicle.

Opportunities for prevention

The Cochrane Review of bicycle helmet effectiveness found that helmets provide a 63–88% reduction in the risk of head and brain injury in all ages of cyclist. Bicycle paths have the potential to reduce serious injury in cyclists but only if these paths are unidirectional and completely separated from other traffic (vehicular and pedestrian).

Suicide

There has been an increase in admission rates for attempted suicide in recent years for children 10–14 years. Suicide is the most common cause of death, after transport-related causes, in older children. Death rates due to suicide in 2002/03 were similar for boys and girls and hanging is a frequent method in this age group.

Opportunities for prevention

It is important to consider stressors and risk factors for suicide in the assessment of any school-age child. Children who have recently attempted suicide need a support network and appropriate therapy. The factors involved are often complex and multifactorial and it is important to work directly with the child and their environment to minimize the risk of a repeat attempt. Publicity can encourage copycat suicide.

Summary

Child injury control is important. Injury is the leading cause of death and is a major reason for hospital admission and long-term disability in this age group. It is known that almost all these injuries are preventable. Concern about injury and action to enhance its control need to operate at several levels

Practical points

- Injury is the leading cause of death in children over 1 year in developed countries
- Injuries are not 'accidents' but predictable, preventable events
- Cognitive and physical factors contribute to the developmental vulnerability of the child to injury
- Environmental modification is more effective at preventing injury than education and supervision
- Falls are the leading cause of injury in children of all ages
- In toddlers, drowning is the leading cause of death and poisoning the most common cause of admission to hospital
- Bicycles are the most common consumer product associated with injury in children
- Suicide is the leading cause of death in children 10–14 years

in the community. Injury prevention must be seen to be relevant to everyone and to be of concern to the individual family, local government, schools and the broader community. Doctors in all branches of the profession have a key role in the community in identifying hazards and providing leadership for change.

Acknowledgement

The authors thank the staff of the Queensland Injury Surveillance Unit and the Queensland Safe Communities Support Centre for their assistance.

3.7 Failure to thrive

D. Efron

Satisfactory growth is a key marker of good health in infancy and early childhood, and so the failure of a child to grow as expected is naturally a cause for concern for parents and health professionals. Failure to thrive (FTT) can result from a broad range of organic and environmental factors, with a combination of influences usually operating. The family often feel confused, worried and guilty, so evaluation needs to be conducted sensitively.

Definition

Failure to thrive can be defined using various criteria. The term is generally applied to infants, although on occasion it is used in children up to 2–3 years of age. Concern is often raised when an infant's weight is below the third centile, that is, more than approximately 2 SD below the population mean. However, this occurs normally in 3% of infants, most of whom are healthy but who are genetically destined to be small. Of more interest is the growth trajectory with time. The criterion of weight crossing two major centile lines with time is more clinically meaningful, and a useful standard by which to decide when to describe an infant as having FTT, and to evaluate accordingly.

Growth patterns

When a child is failing to thrive weight gain is affected first, however, if the problem persists, length also may be affected. If length is affected disproportionately, then the possibility of a skeletal dysplasia syndrome or endocrinopathy should be considered. Head circumference is only affected when failure to thrive is severe.

Irrespective of birth weight, full-term infants tend to assume their genetically determined growth pattern some time in mid to late infancy. This often results in babies who were born large 'crossing down' to reach their predestined track on the growth chart. Measures should be plotted against age corrected for prematurity until approximately 2 years of corrected age.

It is often possible to identify a critical point or period at which a child's growth began to falter. This may enable recognition of an important factor that has adversely influenced growth, such as the introduction of a food to which the child is intolerant, intercurrent infection or change in environmental circumstances causing family stress.

Causes

In developed countries, failing to thrive usually relates to an inadequate intake in the context of psychosocial difficulties. Parental mental illness, substance abuse, poverty, family violence or intellectual disability may result in limited parental capacity or other priorities competing with adequate care of the child. The relationship between mother and infant is often disturbed. Maternal depression is very common in these situations. This may have been present from the postnatal period or may develop as a consequence of feeding difficulties and associated FTT.

In some cases, parents hold alternative belief systems, which influence their care of their child. These may include unconventional diets and feeding practices, opposition to immunization and mistrust of mainstream health care providers. These cases can be extremely challenging and require great skill to maintain a therapeutic relationship with the family.

Chronic or recurrent illness in any system can result in impaired growth (Table 3.7.1). Mechanisms of growth failure include reduced intake (poor appetite/fatigue), increased losses (e.g. vomiting, diarrhoea) and in some cases increased calorie utilization (e.g. chronic infection, cardiac failure). Malnourished infants are vulnerable to infection and these infections may further compromise their nutritional state.

There are often multiple contributing causes for failing to thrive. For example, an infant may have an underlying syndromic diagnosis that is associated with growth restriction but also results in recurrent infections, gastro-oesophageal reflux and irritability with poor feeding behaviour. Psychosocial problems may also be present in the family of a child with organic illness.

Table 3.7.1 Organic causes of failure to thrive

System	Examples
Craniofacial	Cleft palate Pierre Robin syndrome
Neurological	Cerebral palsy with pseudobulbar palsy Spinal muscular atrophy Embryopathy, e.g. in utero infection, fetal alcohol syndrome
Genetic	Chromosomal abnormality, e.g. trisomy 18 Dysmorphic syndrome, e.g. Smith–Lemli–Opitz syndrome
Gastrointestinal	Severe gastro-oesophageal reflux Malabsorption, e.g. giardiasis, coeliac disease, cystic fibrosis Chronic liver disease
Renal	Recurrent/persistent urinary tract infection Chronic renal failure Renal tubular acidosis
Respiratory	Chronic lung disease, e.g. bronchopulmonary dysplasia, cystic fibrosis Chronic upper airway obstruction
Metabolic	Inborn errors of metabolism, e.g. amino acidopathies, mitochondrial disorders
Cardiac	Chronic congestive cardiac failure
Endocrine	Hypothyroidism Adrenal insufficiency
Immunological	Severe atopic disease Food protein allergy Severe combined immunodeficiency
Infectious	Human immunodeficiency virus Tuberculosis

Assessment

The initial step in the evaluation of a child who is failing to thrive is to chart the growth pattern to determine whether it is a cause for concern. Birth measures should be plotted against gestation, and then serial weight, length and head circumference should be plotted on percentile charts through to the present time. Where available, it is preferable to use a chart constructed from a population of the child's particular ethnic group or syndrome, e.g. Down syndrome. Mid-parental height gives an indication of the child's genetic growth potential. The point at which growth began to falter may provide a clue as to the cause, e.g. after the introduction of wheat products in coeliac disease.

A careful evaluation of dietary intake is necessary in the assessment of a child with FTT. A detailed history of feeding patterns is required, including frequency, duration and quality of breastfeeds or total daily volume of formula. If the infant is breastfed, the mother's milk supply should be assessed. In formula-fed babies, check to ensure that the feeds are being made up using the correct concentration of powder to water. It is important to know both the range and quantity of solids being consumed. A 3-day feed diary can be helpful in quantifying the nutritional intake. This history can be difficult to obtain reliably when there is psychosocial disadvantage or neglect.

A detailed systems review is necessary to identify any organic illness that might be contributing to the growth failure, either as the primary cause or as an exacerbating factor. Particular inquiry needs to be made about vomiting, diarrhoea, respiratory symptoms, lethargy and irritability.

Failing to thrive is commonly associated with developmental delay. Infants with FTT often fall

105

Clinical example

James, aged 9 months, was referred by his maternal and child health nurse with concerns about his weight crossing the major centiles. He was born at 38 weeks with a birth weight of 3.6 kg (90th centile) and his current weight was 7.9 kg, which was just above the 10th centile. He had generally been a healthy infant, apart from some upper respiratory tract infections (URTI) and had had a nocturnal cough for 3 weeks since his most recent URTI. He was still breastfed. Solids were introduced at 6 months and he was taking small amounts of rice cereal, vegetables and fruits, as well as some meat and chicken. Examination was normal. He was an alert, interactive infant and responded well to his mother.

His mother was 154 cm tall (3–10th centile) and his father was 170 cm tall (10th centile).

His parents were reassured that James appeared to be a very healthy infant and that he seemed to have settled into his genetically determined growth pattern. Arrangements were made to see him again in 2–3 weeks to ensure that the cough had settled, or, if not, for a chest X-ray to be performed. The review would also allow the opportunity to ensure that he continued to gain weight, with further review to confirm weight gain along the 10th centile as expected.

Clinical example

Taylah, aged 11 months, was brought for assessment by her mother, who was concerned that she 'wouldn't eat'. Her mother also said that Taylah would not sleep during the day, whinged too much and was often 'so worked up she would make herself vomit'. She said that she was finding it extremely difficult to look after Taylah on her own. She reported that Taylah had diarrhoea at times, as well as a constant runny nose. She was bottlefed but lately had not been enjoying her milk. She had little interest in solids.

Taylah's birth weight was 2.3 kg at 36 weeks (10th centile). Her mother did not have the Child Health Record and reported that she did not like the local maternal and child health nurse. Her mother did not interact with Taylah, who was sitting in the pram during the consultation. At one point, when Taylah cried, her mother said: 'See! This is what she's like all the time!' Taylah's mother appeared pale, thin, and anxious. She appeared defensive and angry when asked some questions about her support system.

On examination, Taylah appeared scrawny, pale and miserable. Her clothes were soiled, her nappy was wet and she had an extensive nappy rash, as well as facial and scalp dermatitis. Her hair was sparse, particularly over the occiput, which was flat. Her weight was 6.6 kg (below the 3rd centile, corrected for prematurity). Her length was 68 cm (10th centile), and her head circumference was 43 cm (2–50th centile). Physical examination was otherwise negative. She was unstable when placed in a sitting position. It was not possible to elicit a smile from her. Her urine was negative on a dipstick test.

Taylah was referred to a paediatrician, who admitted her to the regional hospital. Taylah spent a week in hospital, where she fed well and gained 300 g within a few days. The hospital arranged a mental health assessment for Taylah's mother. Her mother was diagnosed with chronic depression and anxiety, and a follow-up appointment was arranged for soon after Taylah's discharge. The enhanced home visiting maternal and child health service was engaged for home-based support, along with close paediatric follow-up.

behind in their gross motor development. Poor muscle bulk and tone results in immature truncal and neck posture and generalized weakness. Commonly the infant's emotional development is also delayed. Malnourished and deprived infants may demonstrate apathy, anxiety, irritability and poorly regulated behavioural states. Some underfed infants become depressed and withdraw from social contact with primary caregivers. Important signs include gaze aversion, lack of a responsive smile and lack of interest in social overture or reciprocal play activities. On the other hand, poor feeding may result from neurodevelopmental impairment, with irritability, oromotor dysfunction and an abnormal swallowing mechanism.

A good social history is critical as part of the assessment. The family's social circumstances may be a central factor in the cause of the growth failure and may also influence therapeutic effectiveness.

A thorough physical examination is required in infants with FTT. The child's general appearance is important. Note whether the child appears small but well (i.e. good colour, alert, active) or malnourished and unwell (i.e. pale, miserable, lethargic).

A poor state of hygiene such as unclean skin and clothes, as well as a marked flattening of the occiput with hair loss, raise the possibility of neglect. The quality of the child's interaction with the examiner,

and more importantly with the mother, should be noted. Irritability, withdrawn behaviour or an anxious appearance are important signs. Observe how the parents respond to the child's distress or signs of hunger such as the rooting reflex, or biting his or her own fist in hunger.

Gross indicators of nutritional state include fat stores, particularly around the buttocks and thighs, and muscle bulk. The severely malnourished infant has prominent ribs, thin limbs and a bony face. Signs of micronutrient deficiency include pallor, rashes and sparse hair. Dysmorphic features raise the possibility of a genetic syndrome. Each system needs to be examined carefully for signs of malformation or disease. Candidiasis raises the possibility of an immune deficiency, although this is more likely to be secondary to malnutrition than the primary cause.

A developmental assessment should be completed as part of the examination. Direct observation of the child's feeding is important to enable better understanding of the feeding behaviour, e.g. intensity of demanding/interest in food, parent's feeding technique, coordination and vigour of suck and swallow, acceptance or rejection of bottle/spoon.

Investigation

If there are no specific signs or symptoms, a diagnosis of organic disease is uncommon. Investigations undertaken to identify a hidden cause for FTT have a low yield. It is appropriate, however, to check electrolytes, creatinine, full blood examination, ferritin and urine microscopy and culture. Other investigations may be indicated if there are specific findings on history or examination. These might include inflammatory markers, thyroid function tests, sweat test, karyotype, immune function tests, stool microscopy, coeliac disease serology, urine organic acid profile and brain imaging.

Management

The management of FTT depends on the severity, whether the child appears healthy or unwell, and psychosocial factors. Establishment and maintenance of rapport and trust with the family is an essential element of successful treatment. Clearly, any identified organic causes need specific therapy.

Mild FTT in an otherwise well child can be managed initially with dietary advice and close monitoring. Catch-up growth requires increased caloric intake. If the infant is breastfed then supplementation after breastfeeds, with either expressed breast milk or formula by bottle, may be necessary. For formula-fed infants, an increased caloric intake can be achieved by increasing the concentration of formula by 25%, or adding a spoonful of glucose polymer powder to bottles. Depending on the age of the infant, the introduction of solids or adding extra calories to solids (using formula milk, butter, cream or margarine) may be indicated.

Admission to hospital is often necessary for children with severe FTT, those who are unwell, where the parents are very anxious, or where there is concern about the quality of the care of the child. A thorough evaluation of the feeding behaviour and routines, mother–infant interaction and the emotional status of both mother and infant can be achieved over several days. A multidisciplinary team approach is optimal in the assessment and management of these children. This includes a dietitian to assess nutritional intake, a speech pathologist to assess feeding and a social worker to assess psychosocial stressors and the family's support system.

In some cases a mental health assessment of mother and/or infant is required. Contact should be made, with parental permission, with professionals in the community who have been involved with the family. This may include a lactation consultant, maternal and child health nurse, general practitioner and/or psychiatrist. Child protection services may need to be involved if there are concerns regarding the child's care.

Satisfactory growth with feeding in hospital (or out-of-home care) suggests that the failure to thrive is psychosocial. In some cases, refeeding may be required using a nasogastric tube. This must be done carefully to avoid complications such as vomiting, diarrhoea and electrolyte disturbance (Ch. 3.3).

The desired feeding pattern for care at home needs to be established first in hospital. On discharge a clear, written feeding plan is essential. Professional supports in the community need to be engaged to continue monitoring and support. Frequent medical review is necessary initially. Children who have suffered severe FTT in infancy/early childhood are at risk of long-term growth, developmental and behavioural problems and so should be followed up by a paediatrician into the school years.

Practical points

- Failure to thrive is commonly due to a combination of factors, with psychosocial issues often prominent
- Chronic illness in any system can result in failure to thrive
- Investigations are unlikely to reveal a cause that was not apparent from a thorough history and examination
- A multidisciplinary approach is necessary, with input from paediatricians, maternal and child health nurses, dieticians, speech pathologists and sometimes mental health professionals
- Admission to hospital is required in severe malnutrition, unwell infants, or where there are concerns about the child's care at home
- Infants who have had a period of failure to thrive are at risk of long-term problems with growth and development

3.8 Developmental disability

M. O'Callaghan

Definition

Disability describes lack of skill in important areas of development that affect age-appropriate functions and participation of the child in the activities of daily life.

A developmental disability may arise prenatally, or during childhood. Approximately 3–5% of children have a moderate to severe disability and up to 20% a mild disability. Many of these disorders are more common in males. The disability may be associated with a specific medical diagnosis or may occur in the absence of an identified cause or medical diagnosis and be descriptive of problems affecting movement, cognitive and sensory functions or behaviour. A child may have multiple disabilities.

Commonly included low and higher prevalence disorders are shown in Table 3.8.1. Although the lower prevalence disorders are usually more severe, all these conditions may have a substantial impact on the quality of life for the child and family.

The World Health Organization International Classification of Function (ICF) for disability and health describes not only how a condition affects body structures and function but also its influence on how a person may perform their personal, family and social roles, together with personal and environmental factors that affect this. Legislative frameworks, recognition of rights, opportunities for education and work, access and community attitudes all influence the ultimate quality of life. The biopsychosocial approach, with emphasis on the child as a person and on their overall function, together with a strong developmental and family perspective, provides a necessary framework for care of children with developmental disability.

A number of low prevalence severe disabilities including hearing and visual impairment, cerebral palsy, spina bifida and autism are covered in other sections of this book. The focus of this section includes general issues of management for all children with a developmental disability; the child with intellectual impairment and selected syndromes associated with this; and children with high prevalence but less severe disorders.

General issues of management

Developmental disabilities are chronic disorders, and this perspective is also required for management, in addition to the interventions that are specific for individual disorders. Four important general aspects of management are:

• *Family-centred care.* This includes an ongoing partnership with families, advocacy, the provision of information regarding the disorder, support groups, access to treatment and respite services, and to sources of financial support. When initially discussing the diagnosis with families, the consultation should include the presence if possible of both parents, sufficient uninterrupted time, a realistic and balanced acknowledgement of potential problems and strengths, and the opportunity for follow-up discussion. Long-term care of the person with severe developmental disability is likely to be stressful to parents, siblings and marriages, with major transitions such as commencing or finishing school and adolescence often being challenging periods
• *One child.* The focus is not only on the management of the medical disorder but also the child's longer-term growth, health, development, emotional wellbeing and independence. Associated behavioural difficulties may be of equal or greater concern to the family than medical aspects of the disability
• *Prevention.* Knowledge of the genetic implications or natural history of a disorder, or common issues arising in the family management of children with a disability may allow prevention of some problems in the future and early identification of others.
• *A plan.* As interventions are frequently multidisciplinary and may involve more than one service, they should be coordinated, have an outcome focus and should involve families in defining realistic short- and longer-term gaols. Interventions should begin early with programmes that occur, where possible, in the child's own community. An important goal is to strive as far as possible to normalize the experiences of the child.

The medical role in the management of a developmental disability is important. It includes initial

Table 3.8.1	Developmental disabilities
Low prevalence	
Cerebral palsy	
Moderate–severe intellectual impairment	
Autism	
Spina bifida	
Severe sensory impairment	
Higher prevalence	
Developmental delay	
Mild intellectual impairment	
Speech and language	
Developmental coordination disorder	
Learning difficulty	
Attention deficit/hyperactivity disorder	
Mild autistic spectrum disorder	

diagnosis, management of the medical disorder, accessing services and meeting normal and specialist health and developmental needs of the child. Management is often facilitated by seeking to understand the 'predicament' of the child and family, i.e. how they may feel and think and experience the situation. There is a need also for an evidence-based medicine approach in discussing traditional and alternative interventions. Increasingly, such evidence is becoming available. The role requires acceptance of cultural and ethnic differences, realistic hope, advocacy and helping families to maintain their overall wellbeing. The medical role is also limited, as the needs of a child and family can often only be met by a range of professionals.

Clinical example

Angie was aged 6 years and had a mild intellectual impairment of unknown aetiology. Her behaviour had always been difficult and had recently become more difficult. She also had a diagnosis of attention deficit/hyperactivity disorder in association with aggression that was only partially responsive to stimulant medication. Reviewing the situation using a biopsychosocial approach, her doctor realized that her behaviour had become worse when her father started working away from home, as a result of which Angie's mother, who always assumed the majority of Angie's care, had to cease her studies. Her mother described feeling socially isolated and depressed.
Angie was in an integrated classroom with a modified programme, although she was acutely sensitive to her lack of academic success compared to her peers. Medication was still required, although this further understanding allowed additional interventions that markedly improved Angie's aggressive outbursts and adjustment.

Intellectual impairment

Terminology

Words used to describe children with lower intellectual abilities may be offensive to the children and their families. It is important not only to use language that describes the child with a particular disorder but also to use currently accepted terminology. Medical terms such as mental retardation (DSM-IV), intellectual impairment and general learning difficulty are often used synonymously, although these terms all focus on important deficits in the child and do not describe competencies of individual children.

Definition

Mental retardation, the term used in DSM-IV, is defined as significantly subaverage intellectual functioning accompanied by limited adaptive function and with onset before 18 years. Adaptive function describes activities of daily living and social competence. Tests of general intellectual function, such as the Stanford–Binet and Weschler Intelligence Scales, have a distribution that is approximately normal, with a mean intellectual quotient (IQ score) of 100 and a standard deviation of 15. The individual's score is, however, an estimate, as performance is affected by a range of child, tester and environmental factors.

Mild intellectual impairment is diagnosed in children with an IQ score between 70 and 55–50 who also have impaired adaptive function. Though the normal curve distribution suggests that 2–3% of children will be in this category, studies generally report a lower prevalence and an association with social disadvantage or family history of similar difficulties. The children may present with speech or behavioural difficulty, or may be identified with developmental concerns in early childhood education centres or with learning difficulty in the early school years. Physical and neurological examinations are usually normal.

Moderate intellectual impairment requires an IQ of 35–50 for diagnosis, with more severely or profoundly affected children having an IQ score below this. Only approximately 0.3% of children have an IQ score lower than 50. These children often have a dysmorphic appearance, a recognized syndrome or other known aetiology for their intellectual disability. Presentation may be by recognition at birth, or with global developmental delay during early childhood. More severely affected children may also have other physical and sensory disorders with many having multiple disabilities.

Medical examination

A standard medical and family history and physical and neurological examination are important. Development is assessed from milestones, current abilities on history from the parent, and testing as required. An identifiable aetiology is more likely if there are:

- minor physical anomalies present, e.g. simian crease or low-set ears
- disturbances of growth, e.g. micro- or macrocephaly, extremes of stature or weight
- abnormal skin lesions, e.g. multiple depigmented or pigmented naevi
- malformations or abnormal findings in several organ systems
- behaviour that in conjunction with other findings suggests a particular disorder
- family history of a similar disorder.

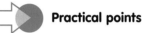

Practical points

Examination of the child with suspected developmental disability

Informal observation
- Appearance
- Behaviour (eye contact, attention, activity level and anxiety)
- Play (symbolic, imaginative or repetitive)
- Movement (skills, symmetry and quality)

Formal observation
- Developmental assessment (strengths and weaknesses)
- Minor physical anomalies
- Vision and hearing
- Physical and central nervous system examinations
- Growth (plot percentiles)
- Behaviour observations from interaction with child

Differential diagnosis

The differential diagnosis of intellectual impairment includes children:

- who have been severely deprived or abused
- with a progressive neurodegenerative disorder or unrecognized epilepsy
- with severe sensory or specific developmental disorders
- where the child's apparent lack of skills is due to cultural differences, mental health disorders or ill health
- infants with severe movement difficulties.

There are many prenatal, perinatal and postnatal aetiologies for intellectual impairment and multiple associated syndromes. A cause is not always able to be identified especially in children with less severe impairment. A child with intellectual impairment may have other associated specific developmental delays such as speech, behaviour problems, health difficulties or additional disabilities. This section describes a limited number of causes of intellectual impairment as examples. Although an approximate stereotype of disorders is described, the expression of the disorder varies and each child requires individual assessment.

Investigations

Investigations and their indications are shown in Table 3.8.2.

Practical points

Assessment goals for the child with developmental disability
- Developmental diagnosis
- Aetiological diagnosis
- Presence of associated disorders (co-morbidity)
- The psychosocial context (predicament)

Fragile X syndrome

X-linked intellectual impairment may explain the male predominance among children with intellectual impairment. It exists in both syndromic and non syndromic forms (Ch. 10.3).

Fragile X syndrome is the commonest form of X-linked intellectual impairment and is the most common inherited cause, with population estimates in males of approximately 1:4000. The condition arises because of an expanded CGG triplicate repeat sequence at Xq27.3 that interferes with the production of fragile mental retardation protein (FMRI). A repeat sequence of less than 55 is normal, while a sequence of more than 200 copies results in loss of function of the gene. Individuals with 60–200 repeats are usually normal, although they may have learning or mild intellectual difficulties. Clinical testing should include DNA studies for the trinucleotide repeats, rather than being restricted to fragile site identification on chromosomes cultured in folate-deficient medium.

The condition predominately affects males as they have a single X chromosome. Girls are less commonly affected and the expression of the disorder may be less marked. Genetic counselling is complex as expansion of the repeat sequence only occurs in female carriers in pregnancy, though the extent of this is not predictable. Males with this disorder will have normal sons though their daughters will be carriers.

Table 3.8.2　Investigations and indications for mental retardation

Test	Indication
Chromosomes	Children with dysmorphic appearance, multiple anomalies or moderate-severe intellectual impairment
Fragile X	Consider in all children with intellectual impairment, especially male children, those with a family history of X-linked intellectual impairment or children with other clinical features of the syndrome
Microdeletion	Specific rare clinical syndromes, usually requested by specialist or geneticist
Thyroid function	Short stature, constipation, dry skin or hair, goitre or no neonatal screen
CPK	If muscle weakness or prominent calves are present. Duchenne dystrophy is associated with developmental disorders
Metabolic screen	Hypoglycaemia, acidosis, altered consciousness level, unusual odour or multiple body systems affected
Ca, PO_4	Short fourth metacarpal, short stature in pseudohypoparathyroidism
Electroencephalogram	If clinical seizures or history of sleep related seizures
Computed tomography or magnetic resonance imaging	If abnormal neurological signs, possible regression or moderate-severe intellectual impairment of unknown cause
Lead	Exposure history, at-risk environment

Table 3.8.3　Clinical features of fragile X syndrome

Appearance
Prominent jaw
Long, narrow face
Large ears
Joint hypermobility
Testicular enlargement in adolescence

Development
Moderate mental retardation
Reduced coordination
Risk of epilepsy

Behaviour
Attention deficit/hyperactivity disorder
Social shyness
Autistic spectrum disorder features

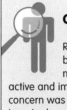

Clinical example

Raymond was 4 years old and his mother had become concerned that his development was mildly delayed for his age and that he was active and impulsive. On questioning, her particular concern was that Raymond might be intellectually impaired, as were her own brother and maternal uncle. Physical and neurological examinations were normal. Genetic testing indicated that Raymond had fragile X and that his mother was a carrier for this disorder. Genetic counselling and formal assessment were provided.

Affected individuals may look normal, especially when younger. Typical physical characteristics and comorbidities are shown in Table 3.8.3. Recurrent otitis media, strabismus or refractive errors in vision, and seizures may also occur. The intellectual impairment is usually of a moderate degree. DNA testing for fragile X syndrome should be considered in all children with intellectual impairment, and especially in males; if there is a family history of intellectual impairment or the child's appearance or behaviour is characteristic of fragile X syndrome.

Down syndrome

Down syndrome or trisomy 21 (Ch. 10.3) is the commonest genetic cause for moderate intellectual impairment, with an overall incidence of approximately 1:800 births. Risk varies, however, increasing especially with maternal age. Screening programmes in pregnancy may involve first- and second-trimester serum markers such as low alpha-fetoprotein levels, high human chorionic gonadotrophin levels, low oestriols in blood, and ultrasound findings including nuchal thickening or characteristic malformations (Ch. 10.1). Chromosomal studies indicate a full trisomy 21 secondary to non-disjunction in 95% of affected children, with translocation or more rarely mosaicism in the remainder.

At birth the diagnosis is usually made from the overall dysmorphic appearance of the infant and clinical findings (Table 3.8.4). Confirmation by chromosomal analysis is always necessary. Children with Down syndrome have an increased risk of malformations with congenital heart disease being present in 30–50% of children. A spectrum of cardiac lesions may be found, although abnormalities of the atrioventricular canal or ventricular septal defect are most common. Gastrointestinal malformations that may be found include duodenal atresia, imperforate anus and Hirschsprung disease.

Intellectual impairment is generally moderate in degree in children with Down syndrome, with a high risk of Alzheimer disease from 40 years of age onwards. The majority of children do not exhibit marked behaviour difficulty, although there is an increased prevalence of oppositional and autistic disorders. Health surveillance recommendations are shown in Table 3.8.4.

Prader–Willi syndrome

This is a rare disorder (1 : 25 000 live births per annum) due to loss of paternal expressed genes at 15q11–13. In 75% of cases, a paternal deletion is present, while in 20% of children two maternal copies of the gene are present. This is described as uniparental disomy (Ch. 10.2), with Prader–Willi syndrome arising because of normal inactivation of the maternal genes by imprinting. A small number of children with Prader–Willi syndrome have other rare genetic causes involving this region. Prader–Willi syndrome illustrates the complex nature of developmental disabilities, the burden on families especially when behaviour difficulty is marked, and the need for multidisciplinary services.

Children with Prader–Willi syndrome have a characteristic appearance and clinical expression involving health, growth, development, learning and behaviour, with the latter often being the greatest burden for families. Initial severe neonatal hypotonia, often with a need for nasogastric feeds, is followed by the development of excessive appetite, lack of satiety and risk of obesity from 3–5 years. During this period, marked behaviour difficulties emerge, including food seeking, oppositional and obsessive compulsive behaviour. Difficulties with concentration and socialization are often also evident. Skin picking may be a particular problem. The risk of psychosis as an adult is increased. Gross motor skills are initially markedly delayed in association with the hypotonia. Affected children are usually mildly intellectually impaired and experience learning difficulties. Endocrine problems secondary to hypothalamic dysfunction affect growth, and the risk of type

2 diabetes is increased in association with obesity. Sleep disorders with central and obstructive apnoea are common and the risk of scoliosis is increased.

Angelman syndrome is a similarly complex, although different, neurodevelopmental disorder arising from loss of maternal expressed genes in the same chromosomal region. The children are ataxic, lack speech and have severe intellectual impairment and a characteristic appearance. They tend to be very happy children and have an interest in water.

Table 3.8.4 Down syndrome: clinical features and surveillance

Neonatal clinical features
Hypotonia
Brachycephaly
Eyes slanted, epicanthic folds, Brushfield spots
Tongue appears large
Ears poorly formed and small
Hands broad, simian crease
Gap between first and second toes

Health surveillance

Issue	Comment
Growth	Use Down syndrome growth charts Initial feeding difficulties common Avoid obesity
Thyroid	Yearly thyroid tests*
Coeliac disease	Consider testing if symptoms, or screen at 3–4 years
Neck	X-ray atlantoaxial joint if symptoms of neck pain or central nervous system signs in legs
Leukaemia	No routine screen, although increased risk of leukaemia or neonatal leukaemoid reaction
Hearing	Initial screen and repeat as indicated for chronic otitis media
Sleep	Risk of obstructive sleep apnoea
Vision	Refractive errors, strabismus
Development	Early intervention/educational plan Specific therapy if needed Behaviour/adjustment
Family	Genetic counselling, knowledge of condition, support, groups, respite, financial benefits

* Under review.

Microdeletion syndromes

Velo-cardio-facial syndrome arises from a chromosomal microdeletion at 22q11.2. There is a wide spectrum of clinical findings including cardiac anomalies, commonly involving the conotruncal region, thymus-associated immune deficiencies, developmental problems of speech, often in association with nasal escape from a cleft of the soft palate, intellectual and learning difficulties, behaviour difficulties and risk of later schizophrenia.

Smith–Magenis syndrome arises from a chromosomal deletion at 17p11.2. It similarly has a wide spectrum of findings, although it is associated with severe behavioural difficulty, particularly involving sleep and aggression to self or others.

Environmental causes

Teratogens in pregnancy include intrauterine infection and significant alcohol intake. Fetal alcohol syndrome is of concern as a cause of developmental delay and in more severely affected children is associated with microcephaly, growth retardation, characteristic facies and later intellectual, learning and behaviour problems. Brain damage from causes such as infection or trauma and severe emotional deprivation can all lead to intellectual impairment. Severe neonatal encephalopathy only rarely leads to isolated intellectual impairment and is usually associated with the presence of other disabilities, especially cerebral palsy. The interaction of both nature and nurture are important in influencing the development and health of children.

High-prevalence disorders

Developmental delay

Children show a broad range of skill at any age. Separating normal variation from mild delays is difficult and is also influenced by the extent of parental concern, the past medical history of the child and family history, including the development of siblings and parents. A developmental disability results in a clinical meaningful degree of functional impairment. The pace of development may vary in individual children and predictors from early childhood have limited accuracy unless development is substantially delayed or disordered, or is associated with a condition of known poor prognosis. Delays may affect all or most areas of development or may be restricted to specific aspects such as speech or coordination. Because ill health, motor or sensory impairment, or family adversity may all affect performance in young children, the term 'global developmental delay' is often used initially even if intellectual impairment is suspected. The term may also be applied where two or more aspects of development are affected. Parents need, however, to understand that 'global developmental delay' does not imply either that their child will necessarily 'catch up' or that the extent of the delay in months is fixed. The ratio between developmental and chronological age, sometimes termed the developmental quotient, is more stable, while the actual gap in months may increase with age.

Clinical example

At 2 years, John's parents were concerned that he was not speaking. He was able to jump and run, and responded to his name and 'no', although he knew no body parts and had just begun to attempt to stack blocks and use a pencil. From the Denver Test, his skills, apart from age appropriate gross motor skills, were approximately those of a 12-month-old child. Referral for further assessments and investigation confirmed that John had a global developmental delay and possible intellectual impairment. When John was seen at age 4 years, his skills developmentally were at approximately a 2-year level. He had continued to gain skills in accordance with his developmental quotient of approximately 50, although his delay in development has increased from 12 to 24 months.

Speech and language impairment

Disorders of communication may affect voice, fluency, articulation of words, grammar, comprehension, the pragmatics of language and non-verbal communication. The term 'pragmatics' describes the social use and understanding of communication. Because of the number of areas of speech and language that are potentially affected and the continuous nature of the distribution of these skills, defining what constitutes a meaningful delay to parents or child health professions is imprecise. Nevertheless, in speech a child would be expected to be using two-word combinations by 2 years, to use sentences by 3 years and to be mostly intelligible to strangers by $3^1/_2$–4 years (Ch. 2.2). The doctor has a responsibility to consider the differential diagnosis and common causes of speech and language delays (Table 3.8.5). For any child with speech or language impairment a formal hearing test is mandatory. Children with global developmental delay or intellectual impairment will present not only with problems of speech and comprehension but also with impaired non-verbal abilities with block construction, puzzles or drawing and deficits in self-care and social skills. Children with associated autism will manifest the behavioural features of that disorder.

Table 3.8.5 Differential diagnosis of speech and language disorders

Hearing impairment
Intellectual impairment
Autism
Environmental deprivation
Anatomical, e.g. palate abnormality
Bulbar or pseudobulbar palsy
Seizures (Landau–Kleffner syndrome)
Developmental speech and language disorder

Clinical example

Mary presented at age 3 years with speech delay. She recited jingles but did not use words to communicate. The doctor assessing her was unable to gain her attention or make eye contact with her. Her parents stated that they experienced similar difficulties with Mary and that she spent her time in isolated repetitive play lining up toys, rather than imaginative play. She wasn't interested in other children and became distressed if they attempted to join her play. A diagnosis of autism was later confirmed.

Where other causes for speech and language delay are excluded or unlikely, the term 'developmental speech and language disorder' is used. Twin studies indicate a strong genetic role in aetiology. Comorbid behaviour disorders, especially difficulties with attention, are common. More moderate or severe delays are often followed by later learning or cognitive difficulties.

Interventions include not only assistance provided by a speech pathologist but also recognition of the importance of play group and early educational programmes with other children. These are settings that are likely to promote speech and language development and social competence.

Developmental coordination disorder

Other terms used to describe the lack of motor skills in these children include dyspraxia or clumsiness. Developmental coordination disorder is a diagnosis made when other neurological and muscle diseases have been excluded, usually on the basis of history and examination. Although uncommon, it is important to consider mild forms of cerebral palsy, cerebellar disorders including progressive spinocerebellar disorders or tumour, and neuromuscular conditions in the differential diagnosis. There is an association with learning difficulty and with behavioural disorders, including attention deficit/hyperactivity disorder and Asperger syndrome (Ch. 4.3).

Learning difficulty

The largest group of children likely to experience learning difficulty is the approximately 14% of children who are slow learners, with intellectual abilities in the borderline range of 70–85 IQ points. Generally, all subject areas are affected.

Specific learning disorders occur in particular subject areas where there is an unexpected discrepancy between intellectual ability and the level of academic attainment in that subject. These disorders were assumed to have a specific neurological basis. The DSM-IV describes specific learning difficulties in reading, maths and writing. The medical term dyslexia describes a specific language-based reading disorder, usually with problems in mastering phonetics. Dyscalculia is a medical term describing difficulties with calculation and mathematics. Behavioural problems are common in children with learning difficulty (particularly attention deficit/hyperactivity disorder), anxiety and loss of self-esteem. As in all developmental disorders, learning and behaviour may also be affected by family stress and ill health in the child.

Although physical and neurological examination are generally normal, important aspects of the medical role in the child with learning difficulty are to ensure that the child is in good health, with normal hearing and vision, that there are no associated comorbidities and that other family and environmental factors are not adversely affecting opportunities for learning. It is also important to advocate for educational assessment and support within the school, to seek specialist consultation when indicated and to help the child and family understand the nature of the child's difficulty.

Child abuse 3.9

T. Donald

Child abuse – development of current concepts

Child abuse is physical or psychological harm caused by the behaviour of parents or carers (in these situations the harm results from acts of commission).

Harm from neglect occurs when a child has not received adequate care from parents or carers (e.g. lack of nutrition, hygiene, health and housing). In these situations the harm results from acts of omission.

The reasons that parents or carers harm their children are complex and are still not fully understood. Between 50% and 70% of parents who abuse their children suffered the same fate when they were children. Common to all families in which abuse occurs is significant psychosocial adversity such as poor education, poverty, young parental age, single parenthood, mental ill health, intellectual disability, substance abuse and intrafamilial violence.

In any family where child abuse has occurred, various combinations of adverse psychosocial factors will be present but the same patterns and levels of adversity are found in non-abusive families. Identification of psychosocial adversity in families as early as possible and the introduction of programmes for its management is a useful strategy in the prevention of child abuse.

That children are harmed or even killed by their parents has been known at various levels in society for centuries. However, the sanctity and privacy of the family and the relative lack of government involvement in social issues precluded any intervention on behalf of children until the late 19th century and the first half of the 20th century.

The neglect of children by their parents or carers first received attention from governments in Australia in the early 1920s. Laws were introduced in various Australian states that led to the creation of state child welfare departments and authorised state child welfare officers to intervene through Children's Courts when it was evident that children were being seriously neglected by their carers. This usually led to children being removed from their parents. They were made state wards and placed in state institutions.

Child welfare legislation, however, did not allow state intervention when a child was harmed in ways other than through neglect. Even when it was known and established that a child had been physically assaulted by a parent, and irrespective of the seriousness of the injuries, intervention by the state welfare authority could not occur unless neglect was also apparent. When children were seriously physically assaulted or killed, the police could intervene but only through common law legal provisions. Police action was not possible in less serious assault that occurred within the 'sanctity of the family'.

Concerns related to child abuse (specifically the physical abuse of infants and young children, which was referred to as the battered baby syndrome) were first raised as an issue in the 1960s in the USA by Dr Henry Kempe. Child abuse became an active professional concern and was considered to be a health, welfare and education sector responsibility between the early 1960s (in the USA) and the mid 1970s (in some Australian states).

Australian reports of physical abuse were published in 1966 by Birrell and Birrell, and of neglect causing growth disturbance by Bialestock. Subsequently, during the next 10–20 years most Western governments introduced specific child protection legislation and management approaches.

The feminist movement in the 1960s and 1970s drew attention not only to the sexual assault of women but also to the sexual abuse of children (i.e. the harming of children through various forms of sexual contact or sexual involvement by their parents, carers or non-family-members).

Physical, sexual and psychological abuse – a general overview

Physical abuse is defined as injury that has been inflicted by a caregiver. It includes injury sustained during physical discipline. An inflicted injury is a manifestation of physical abuse whether or not the caregiver intended to injure the child.

Since physical abuse was first recognized it has been known that it not only causes physical injury, which may have permanent residual effects, but also significant and often serious psychological harm. Psychological harm causes, for example, problems in children's personality development and their ability to self-regulate their behaviour and to interact socially.

Psychological abuse can occur in its own right, apart from its association with physical and sexual abuse. As a separate category of abuse it results from parental behaviour that specifically harms the child psychologically, e.g. parents who constantly belittle, terrorize or a scapegoat their children.

It has now been well established that severe, unresolved psychological trauma in young children has significant effects on their developing brains. The consequences are manifest in behaviour and developmental problems in preschool children, learning problems in older children and antisocial and criminal behaviour in adolescents.

Psychological abuse is defined as a repeated pattern of caregiver behaviour or extreme incidents that convey to their children that they are worthless, flawed, unloved, unwanted, endangered or of value only in meeting another's needs (American Professional Society on the Abuse of Children 1995).

Sexual abuse is defined as the involvement of dependent, developmentally immature children and adolescents in sexual activities that they do not fully comprehend, to which they are unable to give informed consent or that violate social taboos or family roles (Kempe 1978). When non-family-members are responsible for sexual molestation they are almost invariably known to the child and usually to the child's family.

Rarely is sexual abuse physically harmful to children. However, the behaviour may have serious psychological consequences for the child. Sexual molestation is particularly harmful when it occurs on multiple occasions and over a period of time, when it is associated with physical injury, when the child is threatened with physical harm if s/he does not comply with the behaviour, when the child is bribed, coerced or threatened into keeping the behaviour secret, and when family members become aware of the sexual abuse but choose to disbelieve the child and 'turn a blind eye'.

Child protection legislation and the concept of mandatory reporting

Child protection legislation began to be introduced by Western governments primarily because of pressure from medical professionals dealing with victims of the battered baby syndrome. It was introduced in

the USA in the late 1960s and in the Australian states beginning in the late 1970s through to the mid-1980s. Initially the legislation only covered situations of physical abuse or serious neglect. Subsequently, sexual and psychological abuse was also addressed.

Child protection legislation asserts the right of children to be free of harm from abuse or neglect caused by their parents or carers. Most child protection legislation states that the safety of children in their family environment is of paramount importance and must always be considered above the rights or opinions of the parents or carers.

Child protection legislation:

- defines, from a legal perspective, the various forms of abuse and neglect. The definitions vary from state to state
- authorises state statutory welfare authorities to receive notifications of suspected child abuse or neglect from professionals or members of the public
- requires that welfare authorities investigate notifications that they consider indicate possible child abuse or neglect and, when abuse has been confirmed, decide on the most appropriate form of intervention to ensure the future safety and wellbeing of the abused child
- allows courts to:
  - order an investigation when parents or carers are not cooperating with statutory authorities
  - obtain information concerning parents and require that they are assessed and that assessment reports are provided to the court
  - grant various types of order, when a successful application has been made by a statutory welfare agency, that remove the authority of a parent over a child, replacing parental authority with state authority (known as state guardianship).

A web link to the various Australian states' child protection legislation is http://www.aifs.gov.au/nch/issues/issues22.pdf.

When child protection legislation was introduced in the USA, Canada and Australia it contained the requirement for mandatory reporting. Each state in the USA and each of the Canadian provinces has the mandatory reporting requirement. Each Australian state and territory has some level of legislation requiring the compulsory reporting to the state or territory statutory agency of a suspicion of harm due to child abuse or neglect. The breadth of professionals mandated to report varies widely across the states and territories in Australia. For example, in Western Australia the reporting of all children less than 14 years of age with sexually acquired sexually transmitted infections and the reporting of children 14 and 15 years of age with a sexually transmitted infection acquired through abuse is mandated. On the other hand, in the Northern Territory anyone who has reason to believe that a child may be abused or neglected must report this to the appropriate authority.

There is no mandatory reporting requirement in the UK or in New Zealand.

Mandatory reporting refers to the legal requirement placed on specified individuals to notify the designated statutory authority (usually the statutory welfare authority) when the individual has reasonable grounds to suspect that a child has been harmed by abuse or neglect. The precise requirement varies from legislature to legislature.

The list of specified individuals also varies between legislatures but medical practitioners are always specified as mandated notifiers. In addition to medical practitioners, most legislatures include professionals whose work bring them into contact with children, e.g. nurses, psychologists, social workers, child-care professionals and teachers.

Mandatory reporting was introduced when child abuse was considered to be manifest primarily as physical abuse. It was reasoned that physically abused children would usually be brought to medical attention and the abuse would be suspected by the doctor. Mandatory reporting would then allow the doctor to make a notification to the appropriate statutory authority and not be in breach of the professional requirement of patient confidentiality. Also, if a doctor suspected abuse then the legal requirement for notification did not require the doctor to specifically challenge the responsibility of the parents in relation to the suspicion.

Most child protection legislation requires that the anonymity of notifiers is maintained and provides protection for notifiers against legal action that might be initiated by parents or carers.

The value of mandatory reporting in the management of suspected child abuse is still debated. Those regions in which it is not present argue against its introduction. No region that has mandatory reporting has withdrawn it.

A useful summary of the issues related to the mandatory reporting of child abuse was published by the Australian Institute of Family Studies in 2005. The web reference is: www.aifs.gov.au/nch/sheets/rs3.html.

Prevalence of child abuse in Australia

During the past decade the Australian Institute of Health and Welfare has collated prevalence data from the states and territories. During the last 6 years the number of child protection notifications, which is equivalent to the number of suspected cases of child abuse or neglect in Australia, has increased from 107 134 in 1999/2000 to 252 831 in 2004/05. From 2003/04 to 2004/05, the number of notifications increased in all states. Some of this increase reflected changes in child protection policies and practices in the various states but it also reflected increased public awareness of child abuse. The number of substantiations in most states also has increased during the last 6 years, the most notable being Tasmania and the Australian Capital Territory. Again, this increase is affected by changes in policies and practices in the various jurisdictions. It is also an indication of a better awareness of child protection concerns in the wider community and more willingness to report problems to state and territory child protection services.

In all states and territories a large proportion of investigations were not substantiated, i.e. there was no reasonable cause to believe that the child was being, or was likely to be, abused, neglected or otherwise harmed. For example, 62% of finalized investigations in New South Wales and South Australia, 54% in Western Australia and 26% in Queensland were not substantiated.

Generally, physical abuse and neglect are the types most often substantiated (25–30% of notifications of physical abuse or neglect are substantiated). The presence of these forms of harm is obvious, because of the presence of either injury, poor growth or lack of hygiene.

Sexual abuse is less often substantiated (10–25%). Sexual abuse is more difficult to substantiate because its confirmation depends not on the presence of physical signs but on a reliable allegation being made by or on behalf of a child or a person witnessing sexually abusive acts.

Accurate national data on death due to child abuse is not available in Australia. Child death review committees are now spread across Australia and New Zealand and this information will be more readily available in the future. Generally, death from abuse or neglect is not common. Serious physical assault resulting in intracranial or intra-abdominal injury is the usual cause. The most vulnerable age group is those less than 2 years of age, with most deaths occurring in infants less than 12 months of age. Deaths due to upper airway obstruction from suffocation mainly occur in infants less than 6 months of age. In Australia the present estimates of the incidence of child abuse range between 10 and 20 cases per 1000 live births.

Child protection – broadening the concept of child abuse

The concept of the 'continuum of child protection' has developed to incorporate the prevention, early intervention, recognition and management of children who might be or have been harmed through abuse or neglect.

Clinical example

Christine was a previously well 6-week infant brought to hospital by her parents after she had 'coughed up' some bright red blood. On examination, she had a torn frenulum of her upper lip, a small bruise over the left temporal region and three old bruises around her right eye. Her parents did not know how these injuries had occurred. A diagnosis of suspected child abuse resulted in Christine's admission to hospital, where a bone scan revealed 'hot spots' in the midshaft of the left tibia, at the left knee and right chest. Subsequent X-rays were performed (Figs 3.9.1 and 3.9.2).

The clinical features of torn frenulum, bruising of different ages without adequate explanation and unexplained fractures confirmed the diagnosis of child abuse. Protective Services were involved and following investigation and a Children's Court hearing, Christine was placed in the care of her grandmother under a Supervision Order.

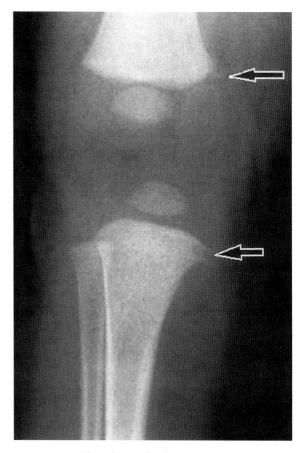

Fig. 3.9.1 See Clinical Example, Christine: epiphyseal fractures of femur and tibia.

The implementation of child protection policies is primarily the responsibility of government agencies, both statutory and non-statutory. Non-government agencies also have a significant role in prevention and early intervention. This role is manifest primarily through family based support and parenting programmes.

Statutory agencies are established through legislation. They have a central role when it is suspected or believed that a child has been abused or neglected. Such children have usually been notified to the statutory agency. Statutory agencies have the responsibility and authority to assess children suspected of having been abused or neglected. They are also able to intervene in the most appropriate way on behalf of abused or neglected children to protect them from further harm and to ensure that the physical and psychological effects of the harm are properly treated.

The two statutory agencies involved in child protection matters are departments for community welfare and the police (whose primary role and responsibility relates to the criminal aspects of child abuse and neglect).

The continuum of child protection

The 'continuum of child protection' stretches from those situations where it is considered that children may be harmed through those children who have been abused or neglected to those children who have died as a result of abuse or neglect.

It is important to identify those children who may be harmed and their families as early as possible in their lives. Identification of such families can then facilitate the provision of services to assist them in their parenting, thus reducing the likelihood that the children will be abused or neglected.

There is no reliable way of predicting which children will become victims of abuse or neglect. However, retrospective study of families in whom children have been abused or neglected reveals the presence of clusters of 'risk factors'. These include (for example) substance abuse, domestic violence, significant parental mental ill health or intellectual disability, poor educational levels, young maternal age and poverty. Premature and complicated birth is

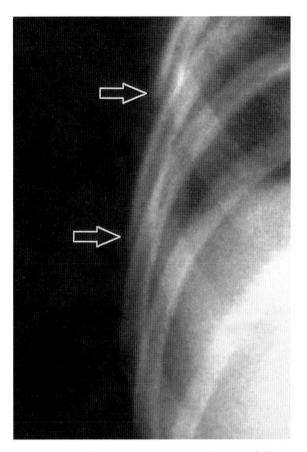

Fig. 3.9.2 See Clinical Example, Christine: fractures of ribs at sites indicated by arrows.

also over-represented in abused or neglected children, as well as poor development of the primary attachment relationship between infant and carer (usually the mother). This is manifest in infants as disturbances in feeding, sleeping and self-regulation and in their mothers as a limited capacity to anticipate and meet the needs of their infant above their own and a restriction in the mother's ability to reflect on the possible effects of adverse circumstances such as violence, anger or threatening behaviour on their infant.

Another 'risk factor' found in families where abuse or neglect has occurred is a history of a parent having suffered abuse in their own childhood. Such a parental history does not reliably predict which individuals will become abusive as parents, as only roughly half of parents abused in childhood go on to harm their own children. The 'risk factors' (psychosocial adversities) that are over-represented in families in whom abuse or neglect has occurred are also seen in families whose children have not been harmed.

The 'continuum of child protection' links together families who are experiencing adversity (which implies there is a potential for abuse to occur) with those in which abuse or neglect has been established. Therefore, even though there is no predictable causal relationship between the presence of adversity and the occurrence of abuse or neglect, the population of families suffering significant adversity will contain the majority of children who will experience abuse or neglect. As a result, child protection from the health professional's perspective begins with the identification of family adversity in pregnancy or early childhood and then the provision of services to assist in the eradication of the adversity or the minimizing of its effects. Such services are generally community-based programmes provided to families with young children with the aim of lessening their social isolation, strengthening the interpersonal relationships of the parents, assisting the parents' understanding of the developmental demands of young children and providing practical home-based parenting advice.

While there is evidence to support the efficacy of such preventative programmes in families where adversity is present but abuse has not occurred, there is no definitive evidence available to indicate that similar programmes reduce the recurrence of incidents of abuse or neglect once they have occurred. Hence to maximize successful intervention it is critical to identify and address adversity in families before children are harmed. Surveying women early in their pregnancy or soon after they have given birth is the most useful means of identifying adversity.

Doctors and nurses are in an ideal position to recognize adversity in families. It is important for them to discuss with the family their concerns about the effects of adversity on their parenting and to facilitate a referral to local community-based early intervention programmes. The aim of reducing adversity is to improve family functioning, particularly relationships within the family and the parenting capacity of the carers. By reducing adversity, the chance of the children of the family being abused or neglected is also significantly reduced. A delay in the provision of services to families experiencing adversity may predispose the child to abuse or neglect.

The recognition by health professionals of adversity and providing assistance with its resolution assists professional engagement with the family. This maximizes ongoing professional involvement with the family if the children are subsequently abused or neglected and state statutory agencies become involved. Continued involvement of health professionals in such families is important because once children enter the child protection system they and their families often become isolated from previous health care providers.

Child protection systems – the interagency child protection process

This refers to the systems and services contained within them that are specifically responsible for child protection at either a state or country level.

The provision of services to children anywhere on the child protection continuum (as described above) occurs through the cooperation and collaboration of different agencies, within both the government and non-government sectors. No single professional or agency can adequately provide fully comprehensive services across the whole continuum.

The principles of interagency practice in relation to the management of suspected child abuse or neglect

The important principles are:

- the development and implementation of inter-agency policies, procedures and guidelines, particularly in relation to such issues as roles, responsibilities, referral practices, time frames for assessments
- the development of an interagency process for the exchange of information in relation to children who are suspected of having been abused – for each professional group this means ensuring that it is legally appropriate to pass on information that has originated from their professional dealings with a client or patient
- the development of systems and processes that encourage joint decision making in relation to the outcomes and interpretations of assessments, the types of intervention and the provision of treatment to abused children.

Health, community services and the police each have specific roles and responsibilities in managing suspected child abuse or neglect. These roles, in summary, include the following.

Health

- Identification of adversity in families and active involvement in its resolution
- Recognition of children in whom abuse/neglect may have occurred
- Ensuring that the child's situation is properly assessed
- Fulfilment of local legal requirements (if any) related to the reporting of suspected abuse to the appropriate statutory agency
- Discussing with community services and the police (according to agreed interagency practices) the ongoing role of the health agency in the management of suspected or substantiated child abuse/neglect
- Maintenance of an ongoing professional relationship with families after abuse has been suspected, irrespective of whether or not investigation by community services and the police is occurring
- Provision of specialist services to children suspected of having been abused/neglected when requested by community services and the police. These services include forensic medical and psychosocial assessment and treatment. They are provided through designated specialist facilities, which are usually based in or connected with tertiary health facilities, e.g. children's hospitals. The forensic medical role includes, for example, deciding whether or not an injury has been inflicted, whether there are any physical findings that would support an allegation of sexual molestation, whether an infant's poor growth is due to a disease process or adverse psychosocial circumstances
- Provision of ongoing therapeutic input to the child and family members after it has been established that abuse or neglect has occurred.

Community services

- Investigation of notifications/reports of suspected child abuse/neglect
- Coordination with health units and police (according to agreed interagency practices and their re-spective roles in the management of suspected or substantiated child abuse/neglect)
- Facilitation of the assessment of children in whom abuse/neglect is suspected
- Establishment of the level of danger/safety of children who have been abused or neglected
- Seeking of court child protection orders in those abused/neglected children who remain in unsafe circumstances
- Optimal placement of children removed from their families because of abuse/neglect
- Ensuring that adequate therapy is provided to children in whom abuse/neglect has been substantiated.

Police

- Investigation of the criminal aspects of child abuse/neglect
- Discussion with community services and health units (according to agreed interagency practices) the police role in the ongoing management of suspected or substantiated child abuse/neglect
- The prosecution, when appropriate, of those who have abused, molested or neglected a child.

Clinical management of suspected child abuse and neglect

The clinical management of suspected child abuse and neglect includes:

- recognition of the child who may have been abused or neglected
- initiation of the interagency process for the assessment of the suspicion
- establishment of the ongoing management needs of the child when abuse or neglect is confirmed
- the health professional's ongoing responsibility to the child in whom abuse or neglect is suspected and their family.

Recognition by health professionals of children who may have been abused or neglected

Whenever a health professional becomes suspicious that a child may have been abused or neglected s/he should make a report to the local statutory child protection agency, whether or not there are local mandatory reporting requirements. Such reports will bring to light any previous similar concerns in the family or involving current family members, ensure that a properly coordinated response occurs and facilitate the optimal assessment and investigation of the suspicions.

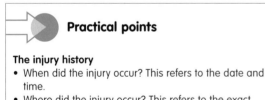

Practical points

The injury history
- When did the injury occur? This refers to the date and time.
- Where did the injury occur? This refers to the exact location.
- What actually went wrong? This refers to the detail of what caused the injury.
- Was the incident actually witnessed and if so by whom?
- On review of the history, has the child had any previous injuries?
- What is the developmental level of the child, particularly in relation to their gross motor abilities (sitting/crawling/walking/running/climbing)?

The suspicion that a child may have been abused or neglected arises in one or more of three ways.

1. An allegation is made on behalf of a child to a professional by another person

These allegations are most often made by one parent against another (from whom they are estranged) or by a family member against a parent. They are often in the context of Family Court proceedings relating to the residency and visitation arrangement of the child.

The role of the doctor in such situations is to:

- facilitate a notification of suspected child abuse to the appropriate statutory authority
- establish what, if any, clinical findings are present that support or refute the allegations – e.g. a suspicion may have arisen that a child has been sexually interfered with solely on the basis of dysuria; if a urinary tract infection is confirmed the suspicion may be resolved
- ensure that any other medical problems the child has are established and understood in relation to the allegations of abuse, e.g. Henoch–Schönlein purpura and the appearance of 'bruising'.

The doctor should never discount the allegations on the basis of a lack of supportive physical findings. All suspicions should be reported and be assessed optimally through the interagency process.

When allegations relate to sexual abuse it is only necessary for the doctor to conduct a superficial genital examination to check for external genital inflammation, discharge or bleeding. The definitive examination must be undertaken by an experienced paediatric forensic physician and will occur as part of the forensic medical assessment, which will be initiated by the interagency process.

When there are physical findings present that may support the allegations they must be carefully and thoroughly documented. For example, superficial or genital injury must be recorded photographically. Normally, this is the responsibility of a paediatric forensic physician and is part of the forensic medical assessment.

2. An allegation is made directly to a professional by a child or young person

This may occur as part of a clinical presentation related to the allegation or may arise during an apparently unrelated consultation, for example, in the process of assessing a child for behaviour disturbance an allegation of physical abuse or emotionally harmful parenting may be made.

When allegations arise in this way they must always be notified to the appropriate statutory agency. When the complainant is an older child or adolescent it is critical that they are informed of the doctor's obligation to notify. Also they must be assisted to deal with the issues that subsequently arise, particularly whether or not they are safe to return home when they have made the allegations against their parent.

The role of the doctor in these situations is to establish if there are any clinical findings that support or refute the allegations.

3. The suspicion arises out of a clinical assessment undertaken for other reasons

Concerns may arise in the context of a consultation and be related to:

- non-specific presentations
- presentations that of themselves should raise suspicions
- the injury history.

Non-specific presentations
These include:

- sexualized behaviour in young children.
- aggressive and violent behaviour in preschool and primary school children.
- adolescents who are self-harming or manifesting serious and repetitive risk-taking behaviour.

None of these behaviours is specifically indicative of abuse having occurred. However, in each case careful consideration must be given to the possibility. Such children and adolescents should be engaged in a counselling process and the opportunity should be provided to them to discuss situations of harm that they may have experienced. When a child or adolescent subsequently makes an allegation or the professional involved believes that abuse has occurred, then reporting to the statutory authority is necessary and a more comprehensive assessment will commence.

Presentations that of themselves should raise suspicions
These include:

- injury in infancy and early childhood that is either unexplained (e.g. a skull fracture with no history of blunt trauma) or inadequately explained (e.g. a spiral fracture of the femur in a 6-month-old occurring when she was having her nappy changed).

The younger the child is when presented with injury the lower should be the threshold for suspecting that the injury may have been inflicted. It is rare for infants who are not independently mobile to sustain any significant injury. Adequate independent mobility is rare before 14 months of age.

Patterns of injury in mobile infants reflect incidents of self-harm and are therefore manifest as injury over bony prominences of the forehead, chin, knees and shins. Facial bruising over soft areas and bruising over muscle masses (thighs, calves, upper arms), the anterior trunk or abdomen are all rare in young children, the more so in those not mobile. When bruising occurs in any of these sites in infancy, inflicted injury should be suspected.

Fractures in normal infants are rare and the forces necessary for their production are only able to be self-generated when young children are able to run and climb or when another person, usually an adult, is involved (e.g. young infants may sustain skull fractures from being dropped from the carrying height of a parent).

The torsional forces necessary to produce a spiral fracture in either the femur or tibia are only able to be self-imposed by young children who are able to run and climb.

Scalds are the commonest heat injury in infants and young children. Most often the scalds involve the child pulling down cups of hot drinks or containers of hot liquids on to themselves. Sometimes these incidents of self-injury are indicative of poor parental supervision or neglect.

Immersion scalds occur when a child is immersed in hot liquid or the liquid surrounding a child becomes hot. The circumstances surrounding immersion scalds require careful and thorough evaluation. Often there is a suspicion that the scald may have been inflicted or occurred through parental neglect. When such suspicions arise they should be reported to the statutory agency.

The sequence of events leading to any serious injury in infancy should be easily ascertainable by speaking with the infant's carers. Serious injuries include head injury, abdominal injury, chest injury or widespread multiple injuries.

When no adequate history is available, a report of the suspicious nature of the injury(ies) should be made to the statutory welfare agency. Subsequently, a comprehensive forensic medical assessment will ensure that the best informed opinion is able to be formulated in relation to whether or not the injuries were inflicted.

The threshold for suspicion of abuse in such infants, particularly when head injury is the presenting problem, must be low. Head injury in infancy may be manifest as blunt trauma to the cranium with or without intracranial haemorrhage or may present solely as intracranial haemorrhage without any obvious external signs of injury. Such head injury is most likely to be a manifestation of intracranial acceleration/deceleration injury, which may occur from such harmful behaviours as violent shaking, which is often associated with severe blunt trauma as well.

A systematic, structured approach to the taking of an 'injury history' assists in evaluating the adequacy of the provided history and therefore in deciding whether the injury should be considered suspicious.

- injuries where the mechanism is apparent and indicates that the injury has been inflicted (e.g. a patterned bruise to the face indicating a slap mark or punch)
- infections that are normally considered to be transmitted by sexual contact (e.g. gonorrhoea, syphilis, human immunodeficiency virus (HIV))
- genital infections that may be transmitted by sexual contact (e.g. herpes simplex, human papilloma virus)
- infants with unexplained poor growth who gain weight quickly in an environment where their intake is normal and controlled, e.g. in hospital or out-of-home care.

Clinical example

Ruth presented at the age of 13 years because of physical and behavioural problems. For the past 6 months she had been listless and uninterested in school and had broken off several friendships at school. During the last month she had complained of recurrent abdominal pain, urinary frequency and dysuria. On physical examination she was withdrawn, with some tenderness over the suprapubic region. Her pubertal status was Tanner stage 4 for breast and pubic hair development. She denied sexual activity.

Microscopy of Ruth's urine revealed numerous white cells and there was a mixed growth on culture. Because of problems in obtaining an appropriate urine sample for further culture and because of the lower abdominal pain and tenderness she was referred for a gynaecological opinion. Pelvic examination was performed in the presence of a chaperone. There was pain in the region of the cervix and there was a purulent vaginal discharge, culture of which resulted in a mixed growth of Gram-positive and Gram-negative cocci and bacilli. Specific antigen for *Chlamydia trachomatis* was detected by enzyme immunoassay.

When told of the diagnosis of a sexually transmitted vaginitis and a pelvic infection, Ruth admitted sexual intercourse. After further discussion she tearfully told of sexual abuse by her stepfather during the previous 6 months. Notification was made to the Child Protection Services and the police charged the stepfather. A care order from the court prevented any further contact between Ruth and her stepfather. Sexual abuse had been the cause of her altered mood and behaviour, as well as causing the recurrent abdominal pain.

Each of these presentations should be reported to the appropriate statutory agency. Interagency discussions will then lead to a comprehensive forensic medical and psychosocial assessment being undertaken. A forensic psychosocial assessment in this context involves the interviewing of children who are sufficiently developmentally advanced.

The injury history
It is not always clear to doctors who first see an injury whether or not it is adequately explained.

As a general rule the parents of children less than 3 years old will either be aware of how their child was injured (because they were witness to the incident) or will clearly state that they lost visual contact with their child for a period of time and heard but did not see the incident of trauma that caused the injury. There will be readily available quantities of useful detail to help the doctor decide whether to be suspicious of how the injury occurred.

The following is a useful protocol to follow when assessing injury in a child.

- When did the injury occur? This refers to the date and time
- Where did the injury occur? This refers to the exact location
- What actually went wrong? This refers to the detail of what caused the injury
- Was the incident actually witnessed and if so by whom?

The parents may have witnessed the incident themselves. However, parents who claim that the incident 'must have happened when . . .' are not providing useful witness information but merely speculating as to the cause of the incident. Such a speculation is not an explanation.

An injury history must always address the developmental capabilities of the child, particularly in relation to gross motor skills. The pattern of injury observed in young children changes dramatically once they are able to move around independently.

Initiation of the interagency process for the assessment of the suspicion

Once a suspicion arises that a child may have suffered abuse or neglect, the interagency process, which introduces the statutory welfare agency and the police, is begun by making a child protection report according to local child protection notification procedures.

At this time the primary concern of the doctor should be the immediate safety and protection of the child. The doctor must decide whether or not to inform the child's parents of the suspicion and will be guided in this decision by factors such as his/her previous relationship with the parents and their behaviour at the time of the presentation of the child.

With infants and young children in whom physical abuse or neglect is suspected the issue of safety, in the first instance, is often best addressed by admission to hospital. This allows the optimal assessment and management of the suspicious injury, the child and the family. Early discussions must occur between the managing team in the hospital, the statutory welfare agency and the police to clarify roles and responsibilities and to ensure the ongoing safety of the child during the assessment and investigation process. The statutory agency workers will explain to the parents the 'child protection process' and the immediate plans for the investigation. They will seek the parents' cooperation for the child to remain in hospital. It there is resistance from the parents to the management plan, the statutory workers may consider applying to court for a child protection order to enable the process to continue.

A range of professionals who are experienced in child protection work will be involved at this time; however, the primary task is to establish whether or not the suspicion of abuse or neglect is sustainable. This is primarily a medical responsibility.

Establishing the ongoing management needs of the child when abuse or neglect is confirmed

The confirmation process incorporates the outcome of the assessment related to the suspicions of abuse or neglect as well as the investigation undertaken by the statutory agency and the police.

The primary ongoing issue once abuse has been confirmed is the child's safety and whether or not there is an ongoing need for protection from the abusive carer. If safety cannot be assured then the statutory workers will consider legal intervention to enable the child to be placed out of home in a safe and nurturing environment.

Children who have been physically injured may have ongoing medical needs. Their ongoing medical management should be coordinated through the statutory worker allocated to the child.

As part of the assessment process the infant or child will have been evaluated for the manifestations of psychological trauma secondary to the harm they have experienced. Addressing these psychological effects of abuse must occur as part of a comprehensive therapeutic programme that should begin as soon as possible after abuse has been confirmed and should involve the carers (whether they are the parents or the providers of out-of-home care).

The health professional's ongoing responsibility to the child in whom abuse or neglect is suspected

Families that have been involved in the child protection system often become isolated from health systems because of their concerns that they will be 'targeted' as abusers in the future.

If a family has previously been well engaged with a particular health professional then ongoing care should be attempted and should begin if possible during the investigation by the child protection system.

Ongoing care may be difficult if the particular professional has made the report of suspected abuse. However, if the carers were informed of why the notification needed to be made at the time, continuing care may be possible.

When children who have been harmed do not receive ongoing therapeutic input then the health professional should establish whether or not this was intended and rectify any omission.

Once children have been placed in 'out-of-home care' their ongoing health needs must be systematically identified and addressed. Many health units give service priority to these children, who are generally under state guardianship.

Forensic assessment of children in whom abuse or neglect is suspected

Once a suspicion of abuse or neglect has been reported to the appropriate statutory authority, a formal forensic assessment should occur. There are two components to an optimal forensic assessment:

- the forensic medical assessment
- the forensic psychosocial assessment.

The forensic medical assessment establishes the extent of injury in a child and whether or not the injury is considered to have been inflicted. When sexual abuse is suspected a forensic medical assessment will establish whether or not there is any sign of genital injury or other condition (e.g. a sexually acquired infection) that could support the suspicion.

Practical points

The five steps of a forensic medical assessment
1. Determining the extent of obvious injury
2. Establishing the biomechanics or mechanism of each injury
3. Ascertaining the history provided for the injury(ies)
4. Assessing the relevance of additional information – site visit evaluation, witness statements
5. Formulating an objective opinion based on the identified injuries

The forensic opinion must be based solely on the result of the medical evaluation.

The forensic psychosocial assessment involves the formal interviewing of a child (when developmentally possible and appropriate) to establish the child's account of events as well as the evaluation of the child's psychological state in relation to the suspicions or allegations. The forensic psychosocial assessment is most important in children in whom there are suspicions of sexual abuse because rarely is there supportive physical evidence or first-hand witnesses to the abuse. If the forensic medical assessment of children in whom there is a suspicion of sexual abuse is conducted first, and is normal, the forensic interview should still proceed because the majority of children who have been sexually abused have no demonstrable physical abnormality.

The opinion that is formulated at the completion of the forensic medical assessment is important to the statutory welfare agency and the police and may influence the ongoing investigation. The outcome of a forensic medical assessment may be that physical evidence was found to support the suspicion or allegation of abuse. It may conclude that an injury was or was not inflicted.

Doctors who are not trained and experienced in forensic paediatric medicine should not undertake forensic medical assessments. A forensic medical assessment is not an extension of a standard paediatric medical assessment. The aim of a standard paediatric medical assessment is to formulate a diagnosis optimal for medical management and health, whereas the aim of a forensic paediatric medical assessment is to formulate a diagnosis optimal for legal purposes. Forensic physicians must also ensure that general health concerns of the children they assess are identified and managed.

What follows is an outline of the principles followed when forensic medical assessments are undertaken.

Forensic medical assessments provide information that may be used as evidence in the investigation of the statutory welfare agency or the police. They must follow specific principles of forensic practice because of the potential for court involvement (children, family or criminal jurisdictions). The standard of a forensic assessment must be adequate for the criminal jurisdiction.

The most important forensic principle that must be followed is the 'chain of evidence'. The chain of evidence is a legal concept which requires that the origin and history of any clinically gathered material that may be presented as evidence in a court must be clearly demonstrated to have followed an unbroken chain from its source to the court.

In the conduct of a forensic medical assessment the 'chain of evidence' relates specifically to:

- the documentation (by clinical description and photography) of the physical findings related to the suspicion of abuse or neglect
- the accurate recording of the explanation offered (when available) to account for the physical findings.

The standard non-forensic medical history and examination is not adequate for forensic purposes.

There are five steps in a forensic medical assessment:

1. *Determining the extent of obvious injury.*

2. *Establishing the biomechanics or mechanism of each injury.* This means the types of 'force' involved (tensile or impact, torsional, bending, thermal and combinations) or how the injury was caused (an incision is caused by a sharp object, e.g. a knife).

3. *Ascertaining the history provided for the injury(ies).* The explanation(s) must account for the appearance and biomechanics of the suspicious injury in the context of the child's developmental capacity (e.g. if an injury is reported to have occurred by an infant rolling off a flat surface of table height then the infant must be observed to establish that rolling is possible).

4. *Assessing the relevance of additional information* – site visit evaluation, witness statements. Site visit evaluation is undertaken, usually in conjunction with the police, to document features of the site where the injury is said to have occurred, e.g. the height of a table, the temperature of hot water from the bath tap, the composition of the surface on to which a child is reported to have fallen. Witness statements are only taken by the police. Their content may assist in establishing a time frame for when an injury occurred (e.g. the time a neighbour heard an infant scream, or whether a facial bruise was present when the child visited the neighbour the day before the suspicion was reported.

5. *Formulating an objective opinion based on the identified injuries.* The forensic opinion must be based solely on the result of the medical evaluation. Factors such as the known level of violence in the child's family and a previous history of physical abuse are critical in the management decisions that will be taken by statutory welfare agencies and the police but such factors cannot influence the forensic opinion. When they do, the forensic opinion is subjective and of no value in the legal context.

Figure 3.9.3 illustrates the possible outcomes after a 'suspicion' is assessed.

If the conclusion of the forensic medical assessment resolves the suspicion (e.g. the dropping of a 2-month-old from the carrying height of a parent adequately explained the skull fracture), no further investigations are necessary. If the conclusion is

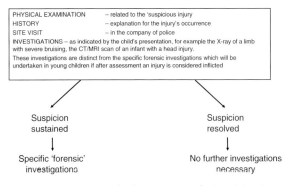

PHYSICAL EXAMINATION — related to the 'suspicious injury
HISTORY — explanation for the injury's occurrence
SITE VISIT — in the company of police
INVESTIGATIONS – as indicated by the child's presentation, for example the X-ray of a limb with severe bruising, the CT/MRI scan of an infant with a head injury.
These investigations are distinct from the specific forensic investigations which will be undertaken in young children if after assessment an injury is considered inflicted

Suspicion sustained → Specific 'forensic' investigations

Suspicion resolved → No further investigations necessary

Fig. 3.9.3 Forensic medical assessment of a 'suspicious' injury.

unclear but there is a possibility that the injury was inflicted, then specific 'forensic investigations' should be undertaken. These are explained further below.

When the forensic medical assessment establishes that the injury remains suspicious and has or may have been inflicted, further investigations should be undertaken. In infants and young children covert injury will frequently be present (most often bony trauma or intraabdominal organ injury) that was not obvious on external examination at presentation.

Such injuries are detected by undertaking specific forensic investigations. These investigations are not generally 'medically' indicated, i.e. they are not undertaken in response to the child's clinical condition. Specifically, they are undertaken to identify covert injuries.

Additional tests will confirm the child's status in regard to clotting and other potential disorders that may have forensic implications.

The specific forensic investigations vary, primarily according to the age of the child. They include:

• imaging studies (skeletal survey, radionucleotide bone scanning, intracranial imaging), which should be undertaken in infants less than 18 months of age and considered in children up to 3 years of age
• adequate X-rays to attempt the ageing of fractures
• laboratory studies, in particular 'organ enzymes' (liver enzymes, pancreatic enzymes)
• bleeding/clotting studies, including the measurement of the coagulation factors, platelet numbers and function
• toxicology studies to analyse for the presence of drugs and poisons.

On completion of the forensic medical assessment the extent of both overt (the presenting suspicious injury) and covert (those injuries revealed by the forensic assessment) will have been documented, an opinion formulated and a report provided to the statutory agency and the police. The police will decide on any criminal proceedings and the statutory welfare agency on whether legal intervention is necessary to ensure the child's safety.

Treatment of any physical and psychological harm will have been organized and should have begun soon after the abuse was confirmed. As stated previously, health professionals who have been previously involved with families in whom abuse has been confirmed should make an effort to continue the association. In these situations families are helped by the support, explanation of the child protection processes and advocacy that a health worker is able to provide.

Needs of health professionals involved with child protection

There is the potential for any clinician who deals with children or families at some time in their practice to have to consider child abuse or neglect as a possible diagnosis.

When the concern of possible abuse or neglect is first raised by the doctor, parents generally challenge the suggestion and frequently become threatening or aggressive. If the doctor is clear with the parents that they are not being accused but, nonetheless, the injury is suspicious and a report needs to be made to the child protection services, they may be reassured and remain engaged. As previously stated, being open and honest with parents is always the best policy, unless it is apparent that such an approach could be dangerous.

It is not good professional practice to offer to make deals with parents when abuse is suspected (e.g. 'if you tell me what happened then I can help sort out this problem quickly').

As a general principle of good practice, health professionals should have in place a support system that enables them to debrief difficult interactions with patients. Such a system should be used when child protection issues arise.

Because the clinical decision as to whether or not a particular situation should raise a suspicion of abuse or neglect is often difficult, clinicians who are non-specialist in the child protection area should establish links with colleagues who can provide support and counsel whenever thorny situations arise.

Sudden infant death syndrome and sudden unexpected death during sleep in infancy

B. J. Taylor

Until 1991, the following was true of sudden infant death syndrome (SIDS):

> When theories compete in profusion
> Then the experts conclude, in confusion,
> There'll be flaws in all laws
> Of this unexplained cause
> Till the problem is solved by exclusion.
>
> Lady Limerick, 1976

In the last 15 years it has become clear that the majority of deaths previously labelled as SIDS, and now more accurately called sudden unexpected death in infancy (SUDI), were related to the intersection of a vulnerable infant, at a particular vulnerable age, with an unsafe environment. Research up to now has defined many 'unsafe' environments and the underlying reasons. More recently, and in the future, there needs to be a focus on childcare practices that are protective in high-risk situations and on how to get current knowledge adopted, again especially in high-risk situations.

Definitions

Infant (0–1 year) mortality has declined consistently during the last 70 years and New Zealand data are used to illustrate this (Fig. 3.10.1).

The majority of this decline has been through falls in neonatal (0–1 month) mortality; postneonatal (1–12 month) mortality declined at a much slower rate until the early 1990s, when most countries, led by New Zealand and the Netherlands, introduced focused public health campaigns to change infant care practice. All areas that have introduced these changes have had dramatic decreases in postneonatal mortality rates. In both Australia and New Zealand, as well as the UK and USA, between 40% and 60% of deaths in the postneonatal period are unexpected and usually occur outside the hospital in the infant's own home.

In 1970, Beckwith defined the sudden infant death syndrome as 'The sudden death of an infant or young child which is unexpected by history, and in which a full postmortem examination fails to demonstrate an adequate cause of death'. There has been an important addition to this definition: namely, an on-site investigation of the death is just as important as the postmortem in making the diagnosis. This definition remains widely accepted and for most purposes is synonymous with the terms 'cot death' (NZ and UK) and 'crib death' (USA), although these terms should not be used, because many of the deaths occur outside the 'cot'.

In 1979, the World Health Organization (WHO) assigned International Classification of Diseases (ICD) code 798.0 to SIDS. It is important to note that any other condition noted on the death certificate takes priority over SIDS in the coding rules, such that if the pathologist believes the death is due to SIDS and puts this as the first diagnosis, but as a secondary diagnosis puts down 'pneumonitis', then the latter takes precedence and national statistics will not include this case as SIDS. Thus, comparing SIDS rates between countries is very difficult and it is generally better to compare total mortality rates within a tightly specified age group. More recently, many mortality review processes are using the label SUDI, as there are many differences still between different areas in the level of death scene investigation and paediatric pathology expertise, as well as access to expensive genetic testing in cases of sudden infant death, making identification of exact SIDS rates very difficult.

There are three characteristic postmortem findings in most babies who are labelled as having SIDS. These are:

- multiple intrathoracic pleural, pericardial and thymic petechiae (found in 80–90% of SIDS and thought to suggest the occurrence of obstructive apnoea before death)
- congested heavy lungs with marked pulmonary oedema (present in any asphyxial death)
- liquid blood in the heart (cause totally unknown).

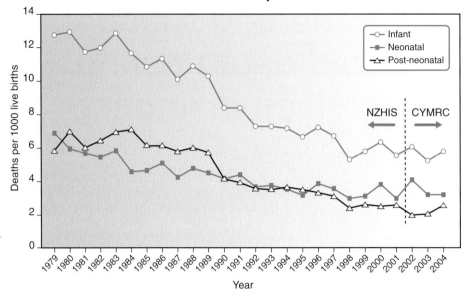

New Zealand Infant mortality 1979 to 2004.

Fig. 3.10.1 New Zealand infant mortality 1979–2004. Information prior to 2002 from NZ Health Information Service and subsequently from the NZ Child and Youth Mortality Review Committee.

Historically, until early in the 20th century, SIDS would have been labelled as 'overlaying' (as in Solomon's judgement – 1 Kings 3: 16–22). Subsequent labelling has included the terms below, and many others since:

- 1890s: 'capillary bronchitis or suffocating catarrh of children'
- 1900–1945: 'status thymico-lymphaticus' (pressure on trachea, lungs and great vessels by an enlarged thymus)
- 1940s: 'accidental mechanical suffocation'
- 1950s: 'fulminating respiratory infection'.

Incidence and geographical variation

There are many difficulties in making any comparisons between countries, as there are important differences in labelling and in postmortem rates. Of some use is the comparison of postneonatal mortality rates or 1–5-month mortality rates. Comparison of deaths from congenital defects suggests no major differences between countries but there are major differences in postneonatal death rates because of differences in the numbers of deaths labelled as SIDS. Because of specific campaigns in different countries, there have been some dramatic changes in SIDS and postneonatal mortality. Thus, until the early 1990s, the highest rates of SIDS were found in

New Zealand and Tasmania (≈4 per 1000 live births), an intermediate incidence in Australia, the USA and the UK (≈2 per 1000) and low rates in Scandinavia (≈1.2 per 1000), Singapore, Hong Kong and Japan (≈0.5 per 1000). Most Pacific Island communities have low rates.

Since 1989, major campaigns promoting:

- supine sleeping
- avoidance of smoking in pregnancy
- breastfeeding
- avoidance of overheating

have been associated with at least a 50% decline in the number of SIDS deaths. Further analysis suggests that this is almost entirely due to change in infant sleep position, with no significant changes in smoking behaviour or other factors. Thus, in the UK SIDS rates are down to less than 0.5 per 1000, and in New Zealand have fallen to less than 2 per 1000.

In most countries with significant minority indigenous populations, their rates of SIDS are higher than in other ethnic groups. In New Zealand, the rates for Maori infants remain approximately three times the non-Maori rate and there have not been the same decreases in SIDS deaths that have been seen in other groups, with some evidence that the rates may even have risen. It has been suggested that this may be specifically because of the specific combination of high rates of maternal smoking and all-night 'bedsharing' between infants and adults, where there

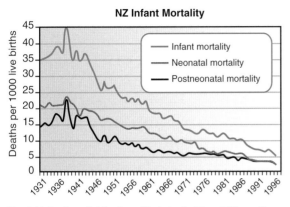

Fig. 3.10.2 Age distribution of 'cot deaths' (n = 343), southern New Zealand, 1979–1984.

is a known interaction increasing dramatically the risk of sudden unexpected death.

Demography

For babies who die of SIDS, the distribution of the age of death is typical (Fig. 3.10.2) and is replicated in almost every study of SIDS from all countries. This is one of the main epidemiological facts that all theories of SIDS must take into account or explain.

Until the change in sleep position, there was a marked seasonal variation, with a winter excess in most countries. With most babies now sleeping on their backs there is now only a minor increase in the number of SIDS in winter. There is an over-representation of infants who die in those born to young mothers (aged <20 years), mothers who are smokers and those in lower socioeconomic groups.

Aetiology of sudden death in infancy

Because SIDS is a diagnosis of exclusion (no obvious cause at postmortem examination or on investigation of the site of death), the investigating team must think of the known causes of sudden and unexpected death in infancy before allocating the label SIDS. The medical causes that must be considered are the following.

• *Cardiac.* Cardiac arrhythmias can cause sudden death, and the most obvious of these is a genetic disorder called the prolonged QT syndrome. Thus, a family history of sudden death, deafness and/or epilepsy may be relevant and could lead to other family members having an electrocardiogram (ECG) or 24-hour Holter monitoring in order to make this diagnosis. Genetic studies are possible on a child who has died but this is still not a routine procedure.

• *Metabolic.* A small percentage (<1% in the UK) of babies dying of SIDS probably die as a result of medium-chain acetyl co-enzyme A deficiency (MCAD). MCAD should be suspected if the baby was starved before death or if there was any unusual smell about the baby. The cause of death in these babies is hypoglycaemia, as they are unable to use medium-chain fatty acids for energy. At postmortem, the clue may be extreme fat droplet deposition in the liver.

• *Homicide.* This must always be kept in mind, especially in the situation where there have been other siblings who have apparently died of SIDS. In general, it is thought that around 10% of SIDS cases may in fact be homicide. There is a helpful statement about these issues from the American Academy of Pediatrics.

• *Infection.* Sudden and overwhelming infection is a possible cause of sudden death. Pneumococcal or meningococcal septicaemia or meningitis are often of particularly sudden onset but it should usually be possible to detect them at postmortem examination.

• *Seizure causing apnoea.* This is theoretically possible but impossible to be sure about without a clear history. There are no pathological markers of this in infancy.

Usually it is not possible to make a clear diagnosis of a medical condition, and the death is then labelled as SIDS. Our current understanding of SIDS is based to a large degree on the interaction of three factors, as illustrated in Figure 3.10.3.

The vulnerable baby

Many studies have reported an association with low birth weight and the presence of other factors that suggest the baby is not as responsive as others, either generally or in the hours before death. There is some evidence that 40–50% of SIDS victims demonstrate poor weight gain prior to death but this is not a very helpful predictor as approximately 35% of control infants will show similar growth patterns.

Necropsy data have shown that more SIDS babies (but not the majority) than controls (which are hard to find) have some evidence of chronic hypoxia, acute hypoxia (elevated hypoxanthine levels in the vitreous humour), small scars in the respiratory centre of the brain stem and increased fetal haemoglobin levels and alterations in brain-stem kainate receptors and serotonergic networks. Microbiological studies have suggested the presence of toxin-producing staphylococcal species more often in the

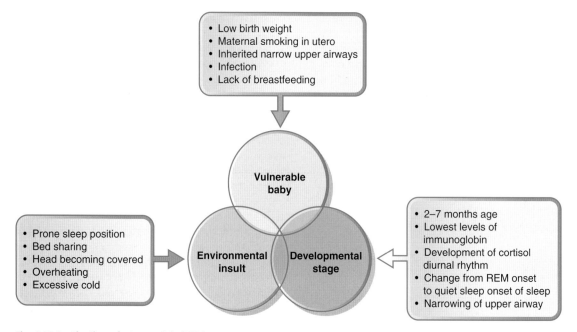

Fig. 3.10.3   The three-factor model of SIDS.

nasopharynx or stools and it has been shown that the presence of nicotine increases the toxicity of these staphylococcal toxins manyfold. Finally, it has been suggested recently that babies that have died of SIDS may have a genetically determined different cytokine response to infection.

The environment

The main contribution of epidemiology to solving some of the mysteries of SIDS started with the description of large differences in the incidence of SIDS between different countries; these were confirmed by similar large differences in postneonatal mortality rates. This strongly suggested that some environmental variables were influencing SIDS and led to many case-control studies of infant care practices that identified prone and side sleeping as increasing the risk of SIDS. The risk of dying when placed to sleep prone compared to supine is approximately five times higher in countries where babies tend to sleep on soft surfaces, and somewhat lower in countries where babies sleep on very firm surfaces.

There is now convincing evidence that side sleeping is also dangerous, but mainly because it increases the risk of the baby turning to the prone position while asleep. It is also most dangerous the first time the baby turns or is put to sleep prone.

Other environmental factors that may contribute appear to be the baby being either too hot or too cold, being found with the head covered by bedding,

or sharing the sleeping surface with adults who are smokers. The interaction of bed sharing and maternal smoking is particularly important. Bed sharing with non-smokers minimally increases the risk of SIDS, while the combination is associated with a very high risk (odds ratio of 4.55). This interaction perhaps explains the high rate of SIDS in indigenous peoples, where the bed sharing/maternal smoking combination is particularly common.

More recently, there has been increasing evidence that having the head completely covered is a particularly dangerous risk factor. Practices parents can initiate to avoid this risk appear to be the avoidance of blankets and sheets, using a sleeping bag arrangement instead. Recent European case-control data suggest a decreased risk with the use of a sleeping bag. Some recommend placing babies to sleep with their feet at the base of the cot so that they are unable to move further under the bedding, but this is unproven and babies can still move sideways under the bedding.

Finally, there is some evidence to suggest that babies that are excessively insulated, are in excessively hot rooms or are underinsulated in cold rooms have a higher risk of SIDS. Because of the many different thermal environments in which a baby may sleep, it is hard to recommend any particular room temperature. Instead, it is wise to recommend that mothers check the temperature of their babies' hands and feet and compare this with the core temperature. The hands and feet should be slightly cooler than core (by about 2°C). If they are cold, either more insulation (bedding or clothing) or a warmer room is needed. If the peripheries are the same temperature as core, the room is either too hot or less bedding and clothing are needed. Obviously, infection could interfere with this assessment and parents should be told not to increase the amount of clothing or bedding of a baby with an infection.

Some environmental factors appear to be protective. These are:

- the use of a dummy (pacifier) during sleep. The American Academy of Pediatrics, somewhat controversially, recently advised the use of a pacifier during sleep in infants from birth if formula-fed and from 1 month of age in breastfed infants. There is good epidemiological evidence that pacifier use is strongly protective (even when not used in the last sleep before death) and, more importantly, one study suggests that pacifier use is especially protective in 'high-risk' situations such as maternal smoking and bedshar-ing. There remains real concern, however, that this may decrease breastfeeding duration and have other unforeseen consequences. Currently, in high-risk situations where the baby is formula-fed, pacifier use is unlikely to do significant harm
- the sharing of the sleeping room (but not the bed) with adults (but not children)
- breastfeeding, although this factor is more controversial.

There is now also convincing evidence that immunization in infancy decreases the risk of SIDS.

Multiple hypotheses and SIDS

There is a long list of popular and not so popular theories as to the cause of SIDS. These range from the 'ammonia theory' (where the increased risk in male babies is attributed to the fact that they are more likely to pass urine closer to the face), to other theories which have had many millions of dollars spent on research disproving them (e.g. the central apnoea theory). Current theories with considerable evidence backing them are the following.

- *Obstructive apnoea.* The relative dimensions of the upper airway appear to be a strongly inherited feature. It appears that babies' upper airway dimensions actually get smaller during the first 6 weeks of life, and this supports the idea that infants are at more risk of significant obstruction at 6 weeks of age than in the first few weeks of life. At the clinical level it is important to remember this if a baby is seen in the newborn period with signs of upper airway obstruction or significant indrawing. Remember that if these features are seen awake they could be much worse when asleep and overnight oximetry may be needed to document this. It appears that this is one aspect that makes a child 'vulnerable'.

- *Decreased arousal responses.* It is now clear that many babies encounter various environmental insults that require them to wake from sleep and attract their caregiver's attention. Many of these stresses appear to be respiratory in nature; in particular, babies, especially those who put their faces into bedding, need to able to move the face away, or increase ventilation dramatically, or finally rouse and cry for help. The causes of poor arousal are being sought but already it is clear from physiological studies that babies do not rouse so well to a variety of stimuli when sleeping in the prone position. It is thought that maternal smoking in pregnancy may specifically affect the baby's ability to rouse from pure hypoxia and it is clear that some sedatives decrease the ability to rouse. More controversial and not really proved in human infants are the effects of overtiredness, hyperthermia or hypothermia, and certain stages of viral infection.

- *Abnormal immunological responses in the lung.*

- *Prolonged QT syndrome.* The evidence supporting this theory was recently boosted considerably by the publication of a large prospective study of ECGs in the first few days of life in many thousands of Italian babies. This suggested that, in their population, many babies who subsequently died of SIDS had a prolonged neonatal QT. As the risk of death in the prolonged QT syndrome can be decreased by the use of beta-blockers, this study must be taken seriously. However, there have been many criticisms of the study and most authorities do not believe that the evidence is strong enough for screening of the newborn population. In practice, an ECG should, however, be done where siblings are born to families who have a strong family history of SIDS and in infants presenting with apparent life-threatening events (ALTEs).

Parent support after an unexpected infant death

Following the unexpected death of a baby, parents feel a profound sense of loss, guilt and depression. This may be complicated if a babysitter, relative or sibling was looking after the child at the time that the death occurred. For young parents, this is often their first experience of a death in the family. Because of the need for an on-site investigation, parents should meet either the paediatrician or the pathologist involved and this places some significant obligations on these practitioners. Initially, a somewhat abbreviated medical history is taken and this needs to be followed up with further meetings and history taking once a postmortem has been carried out. Some parents value support at this early stage from someone who has been through the same trauma, but many do not appreciate this until later. Initially, simply offering such contact is sufficient. If parents wish this support, it can usually be organized with the local SIDS parent support organization.

During the first few days, parents need to be given the result of the postmortem examination and very practical advice on where their baby is, what happens next and who they can turn to for help. They also need to be given some understanding of the syndrome. This is very important in helping them to understand what has happened and to come to terms with the reality of their baby's death.

Although this is a distressing time, and decisions will be difficult to make, both the parents and other family members should be encouraged to be involved in making decisions; 'taking over' by professionals is equally disabling. When the baby is certified dead at home, parents should be consulted about when the baby leaves the house to go to the mortuary.

Over the next few weeks and months, parents will hear, read and experience a whole range of reactions and theories from others, which may often compound their guilt, anger and distress. Unexpected infant deaths have a profound effect on relationships. Some couples will share the experience and become closer but, more commonly, the stress shows up differences that may be hard for individuals to reconcile.

Every parent will experience the process of grieving in his or her own different way. Some will re-experience the past; others will protect themselves from the pain by denial. With time, most parents come to terms with their baby's death; some continue searching for answers for themselves, while others turn to helping others. The time of the anniversary of either the birth or the death often rekindles some of the emotions.

The effects on other children, grandparents and the extended family need to be considered, and advice offered on how best to involve other children in the family in the process of grieving. Siblings need to be told clearly that the death was not because of anything they did or thought, as the 'magical' thinking of younger children can leave them feeling responsible for the death.

Practical points

Checklist for dealing with the sudden death of a baby

- Read and take a copy of *Information for Parents* (available from local SIDS associations)
- Sympathetically interview the parents about their baby's past health
- Examine the baby and confirm death
- Record the history and examination, including recent consultations, family illness and any physical signs
- Clothe and wrap the baby, and take him/her to the parents to see and hold as long as they desire
- Explain what you think is the cause of death
- Explain to the parents that the police and coroner have a duty to investigate all sudden and unexpected deaths and that they will have to make a statement to the police, who may want to examine the baby's room and bedding
- Offer support. Often very practical advice about the postmortem examination, funeral arrangements, cremations, registration of death and other details will be needed during the next few days. It is important that this information is given in written form because parents of children in this age group often have no experience of making funeral arrangements
- Check care needs of dependent relatives and other children
- Inform the on-call paediatrician at the local hospital
- Ask whether the parents would like to see a chaplain or minister, or have their baby blessed
- If the mother is breastfeeding, offer advice on suppression of lactation and expression of milk
- Inform the coroner of the death
- Discuss the clinical story with the on-call coroner's pathologist, who may want some early tissue samples taken
- Suggest that the parents might like to photograph the baby and/or take a lock of hair
- Leave an *Information for Parents* leaflet and local support contact telephone number
- Explain that a paediatrician will contact them in the next few days with the preliminary results of the postmortem
- Inform the Child Health Department, primary care practice and others involved to cancel clinical, surveillance and immunization appointments

Eventually, many parents think of having more children. At this time, preventable factors and support after the birth should be discussed. If it is done before this time, it may compound the guilt they are feeling.

Care of the adolescent 3.11

S. Sawyer, A. Kennedy

What is adolescence?

Adolescence describes the developmental stage between childhood and adulthood. The World Health Organization defines the ages of an adolescent as 10–19 years old, and defines youth as 15–24 years old. We commonly combine these definitions (10–24 years) and use the encompassing term 'young people'.

The onset of puberty has long been accepted as the starting point of adolescence, while key social transitions such as completion of education, financial independence, marriage and children have historically marked the end of adolescence. These endpoints formerly occurred within the few years from the late teens to the early twenties. As young people now commonly participate longer in education and are marrying and having children later, the end of adolescence has become less distinct.

Another approach to the description of adolescence has been provided by Ingersoll, who described this stage of life as:

> A period of personal development during which a young person must establish a sense of individual identity and feelings of self-worth which include an alteration of his or her body image, adaptation to more mature intellectual abilities, adjustments to society's demands for behavioural maturity, internalizing a personal value system, and preparing for adult roles.
>
> Ingersoll 1989

Adolescent health surveys show that the majority of adolescents rate their own health, including their mental health, as good. Many adolescents describe the period of adolescence as enjoyable and exciting, and as a time of satisfaction with the achievement of many milestones such as first relationships, completing school, first job and learning to drive a vehicle. In contrast, adolescence was historically described by adults as a period of turmoil. Certainly, it is a time of increased health risk, for healthy young people as well as for those with chronic illness, and there are a significant number of young people for whom adolescence is not 'smooth sailing'. Furthermore, while many health indicators in younger children and older adults have improved, there is a wide range of public health indicators in young people that have remained static or have declined.

While in many parts of the world, specialist children's hospitals still effectively 'end' at 14 years of age, in that they do not care for young people older than this. Most tertiary children's hospitals in Australasia now embrace adolescence as an important developmental period within the discipline of paediatrics (which is increasingly referred to as 'Child and Adolescent Health'). Young people up to the age of 18 years are now commonly managed in tertiary children's hospitals in Australia and New Zealand, in both inpatient and outpatient settings. While many parts of the world also recognize the subspecialty of adolescent health, all doctors must learn the knowledge, attitudes and skills to manage young people's health concerns, regardless of their likely future roles.

Adolescent development

Just as monitoring infant and child development is an important part of child health, attention to adolescent development is equally central to the provision of quality health care to young people. Maturation in physical, sexual, social, emotional, ethical and spiritual development is the hallmark of adolescence. Each of these components has significant implications for young people and their health. As seen later in this chapter, an adolescent in the early 21st century is exposed to more opportunities than ever before but also faces many health risks.

In order to facilitate monitoring, it can be useful to think about three domains of adolescent development, namely *physical*, *cognitive* and *psychosocial* development. The most important aspect of physical development is the timing of the onset of the adolescent growth spurt and the associated changes of puberty, which mark the acquisition of reproductive capacity. In response to these hormonal changes, the prepubertal unisex silhouette becomes characterized by a larger, muscular male physique and a more rounded female shape. The onset of the pubertal growth spurt is, on average, 1 year younger in girls than boys, but lasts longer in boys (Fig. 3.11.1).

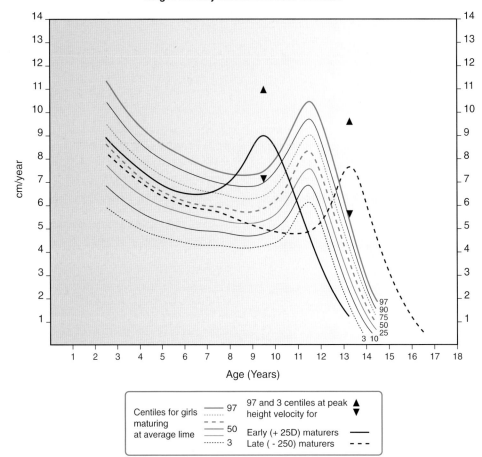

Height velocity centile chart for females.

Fig. 3.11.1   Height velocity centile chart for females.

Neurocognitive maturation is responsible for an increased capacity for abstract thinking, the capacity to think about thoughts. These neurobiological changes are associated with increasing reasoning, executive and planning functions, such as the increasing ability to delay immediate gratification for perceived future benefits. Given how much of health management relates to future health outcomes, understanding young people's cognitive maturation is an important element of the monitoring of adolescent development and of working with young people clinically. Clinical strategies that might influence self-management behaviours in adults who are motivated by future health goals will not be influential in adolescents, who are more motivated by events in the 'here and now'. Neurocognitive maturation is now believed to continue into the early 20s.

Psychosocial development is characterized by aspects of personal individuation, such as the development of a coherent sense of self and an understanding of individual versus family responsibilities, coming to terms with one's physical self, understanding one's sexuality and being able to provide for oneself financially.

While there is close association between the different domains of development, adolescent development is characterized by being uneven and complex: like earlier child development, it is influenced by the environment, is mediated by relationships and is triggered by social participation. Chronic illness can affect each of these domains but the effects are inconsistent. For example, while chronic illness may delay the physical changes of the adolescent growth spurt and of puberty, earlier exposure to challenging life decisions or to friends dying can result in premature consideration of the more spiritual elements of life.

The increasing cultural diversity of Australia and New Zealand results in many young people having parents who were born overseas, who may hold different views of what adolescence is or should be about. Adolescents in these families can sometimes struggle with the discrepancy between the different expectations of their Australian peers and their family about the general aspects of role and identity, as well as specific elements of what is acceptable behaviour at given ages.

Adolescence is commonly divided into three stages of early, mid and late adolescence that highlight these intersecting developmental domains.

Early adolescence is characterized by the physical changes of puberty. It can be a time of increased physical activity and may also be a time where mood changes are noticed by the family. The developmental tasks associated with this period are about establishing a realistic body image and also becoming aware of oneself as a sexual being with a sexual orientation.

Mid-adolescence is characterized by increasing independence, commonly with more time spent with peers outside the home. Education is more demanding of young people's maturing cognitive skills. The developmental tasks of this stage include a stronger sense of oneself as an individual and a greater focus on personal and social values.

Late adolescence is characterized by a greater focus on vocational goals, the transition between school and work, and a greater enjoyment of intimacy, including sexual intimacy. The developmental tasks are to establish adult roles and responsibilities, including longer-term relationships and less reliance on a peer group.

Dramatic social changes in the developed world have resulted in young people being generally healthier, wealthier and better educated than previous generations. More young people now complete 12 years of school than previously, with more continuing on with some form of tertiary study. Social roles have widened for females as well as males. In Australia, the mean age of marriage is older than in previous generations, as is the age that women have their first child, which recently exceeded 30 years. In the 1950s most people had left school, got a job, got married and had children by their early twenties. Many contemporary young people achieve these milestones much later – if at all.

However, there are still many aspects of adolescence that have not changed over the centuries:

> Our youth love luxury. They have bad manners and contempt for authority. They show disrespect for their elders and love idle chatter in place of exercise. Children are now tyrants not the servants of the household. They contradict their parents, chatter before company, gobble up their food and tyrannize their teachers. . . .

Socrates, 450 BC

Practical points

Teenagers, adolescents, youth and young people
- Most teenagers are healthy and happy
- Like younger children, adolescents continue to develop physically, emotionally and cognitively. All consultations with young people should involve an assessment of adolescent development
- As children mature through adolescence, they are exposed to greater health risks from involvement in behaviours with significant health consequences, such as drugs and alcohol and sexual intercourse
- The burden of illness in youth differs from younger children and from adults, being disproportionately affected by mental health problems, the consequences of drug and alcohol use, accidents and self-harm, and complications of sexual activity
- Healthy adolescent development results from complex interactions between risk and protective factors within the individual, family, peers, school and community
- Chronic illness in adolescence is a risk factor for poor health and social outcomes

Risk and protective factors

Learning by doing and maturing by experimenting is a normal part of adolescence (such as learning to drive a car, getting one's first job, experiencing sexual intimacy). Some behaviour, however, can have harmful consequences, and adolescence marks a time of change in relationship to certain risk behaviours and mental health states. While learning about the harmful effects of alcohol by drinking some alcohol is considered normal in Australia, binge drinking is associated with more harmful effects, such as later regretted sexual activity, alcohol dependence in early adult life and deaths from road traffic accidents.

Similarly, while sexual experimentation is considered to be a prelude to healthy sexual relationships in adult life, unsafe sexual activity can result in unplanned pregnancy or sexually transmitted infections.

Generally, the earlier the onset of these 'risk behaviours', the greater the risks or poor health outcomes. For example, while 80% of adult smokers start smoking in adolescence, the onset of smoking at an early age marks a greater risk for continuing smoking as an adult. Similarly, while approximately half of Australian 16-year-olds have had sexual intercourse, people who are first sexually active at a younger age are at increased risk of unsafe sexual activity.

Young people with one identified health risk behaviour are more likely to have other 'comorbid'

Clinical example

Jennifer, a 15-year-old girl, was taken to her general practitioner by her mother because she had been moody and tearful for the last few weeks. She had also been missing school regularly and often complained of an 'upset stomach' in the mornings. On direct questioning, Jennifer offered very little information about the nature of her symptoms or possible causes. The doctor then asked Jennifer's mother to leave the room for a short time, after having explained confidentiality and its limitations. After the assurance of confidentiality and in taking a psychosocial history, Jennifer revealed that she had unprotected sex about 5 weeks ago, had not had a period since, and was worried that she might be pregnant. She had been too fearful to tell her parents, stating 'they would kill me!'

A pregnancy test revealed that she was indeed pregnant. The doctor had a brief discussion about available options and offered to help Jennifer tell her mother, to briefly discuss the various options with her mother and to arrange for them to come back for a more detailed visit. Jennifer agreed with this plan. While her mother was very surprised and upset, these discussions were able to take place, as well as discussion about the importance of future contraception. The doctor also asked about Jennifer's partner, because of child protection concerns. Her partner was her 16-year-old boyfriend.

Jennifer and her mother left the surgery relieved that it was 'out in the open' and having been made aware of the various supports and available services. At a later appointment Jennifer said she would never have been able to say anything at the time without seeing the doctor alone. As they go out the door Jennifer turned to her mother, saying, 'What are we going to tell Dad?'

behaviours. Thus, a young person who is depressed is more likely to smoke tobacco, engage in unsafe sexual activity and have disordered eating.

While the phenomenon of 'extended adolescence' is not of itself problematic, the previous milestones of marriage and children commonly marked the 'maturing out' of risk behaviours. The changing social experiences of contemporary young people result in many continuing to engage in risk-taking behaviours over a longer period of time, with important health consequences.

There are common risk factors that predict earlier engagement in a range of health risk behaviours and social outcomes. These include factors within the individual, family, peer and community domains. For example, living in a family where a parent smokes increases the risk that a young person will start smoking.

There are important additive or synergistic associations between risk factors.

For example, being in a peer group where most of your friends smoke greatly increases the risk of smoking. This risk is even greater if a young person is depressed. Lack of family connectedness or support, lack of engagement with friends, bullying at school and poor academic performance are risk factors in adolescence for a wide range of poor health and social outcomes, such as substance use, poor mental health, early school leaving and antisocial behaviours. Chronic illness in adolescence is always considered a risk factor.

While identifying risk-taking behaviours and their consequences is an important part of any adolescent health assessment, there are also protective factors that are important to identify. These are factors that can ameliorate risk factors or increase the likelihood of positive health and social outcomes. Important protective factors are an intact and well functioning family, connectedness with school, community and peers, and participation in enjoyable extracurricular events such as sport or creative activities.

Put simply, the more protective factors in a young person's life, the more likely they are to make healthier choices in adolescence. While many family factors cannot be changed or 'treated', efforts to alter the school environment can be especially powerful.

Burden of illness in adolescence

The burden of illness in young people differs greatly from that of infants, who are disproportionately affected by congenital disorders, and younger children, in whom acute infectious disease is still a major cause of morbidity.

The burden of illness in adolescence is similarly very different from adulthood, where chronic diseases, including ischaemic heart disease and cancers, predominate. While 15–20% of young people experience some form of special health-care need, the causes of ill health are more commonly psychosocial than biological in adolescence and tend to reflect unhealthy patterns of risk behaviours. The leading cause of mortality and morbidity in the adolescent age group is from accidents and injuries (unintentional and self-inflicted), mental health problems and behavioural problems such as substance abuse. Other prominent health issues are unplanned pregnancy and sexually transmitted infections.

Accidents and injuries

Two-thirds of all deaths between 12 and 24 years of age are due to accidents and self-inflicted injuries, most commonly due to motor vehicle accidents.

Mental health

Mental health and behavioural disorders make up more than 50% of the total burden of illness in adolescents. It is estimated that up to 20% of young people have a mental health problem at some time.

Substance use

Some 15% of Australians aged 14–19 years are daily smokers and an even higher proportion of 20–29-year-olds smoke tobacco. 38% of 14–24 year olds report marijuana use in the previous 12 months. About 70% of 16 year olds drink alcohol.

Sexual health

Chlamydia trachomatis is the main sexually transmitted infection that affects young people, with a threefold increase in notifications in both men and women in the past decade. There has also been a significant rise in hepatitis C infection in young people. While unplanned pregnancy rates have declined, unplanned teenage conception rates remain high.

Nutrition

There has been a twofold increase in overweight children and adolescents and a threefold increase in obese adolescents in the past decade (Ch. 3.4). Rates of physical activity are declining and associated disorders such as type 2 diabetes are on the rise in younger patients.

There are many sociocultural factors that affect the health of some groups of young people more than others. Some examples of these are:

- the death rate for Aboriginal and Torres Strait Islander youth is nearly three times higher than for non-indigenous youth in Australia
- the death rate for young males is three times that for females, but females have three times higher levels of depressive illness
- there is a higher death rate from injury and suicide in young males who live in rural communities
- higher levels of depression and suicide are reported in gay and lesbian young people
- young people from lower socioeconomic backgrounds are hospitalized more often than their more advantaged peers.

Summary

In summary, many adolescent health problems are a consequence of health risk behaviours and developmental challenges. Health problems in adolescents don't occur in isolation, and one identified health problem raises the likelihood that there will be other health and social problems. Many health risk behaviours are established in adolescence and continue into adult life, where they contribute to the adult burden of illness. Early identification and intervention of these behaviours is a desired outcome of any contact by adolescents with the health care system.

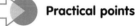 **Practical points**

Engaging young people in clinical consultations
- Introduce yourself to the young person and then the parent
- Explain confidentiality, including limitations, to all adolescents and families
- Be relaxed and non-judgemental
- Avoid jargon or slang but use simple language that the young person will understand
- See the young person alone for part of each consultation
- Psychosocial screening should start with less sensitive questions before proceeding to more personal questions
- Be sensitive and respectful during physical examinations

Medicolegal context

Historically, children were legally viewed as property items of their parents. The law now recognizes the growing maturity of adolescents and their capacity to make independent choices and judgements on matters affecting their future, including their rights to autonomy and privacy in health care, even when they are not legally mature (i.e. under the age of 18 years in Australia). This legal view is consistent with the medical evidence. Studies demonstrate that concerns about confidentiality are a major barrier to young people accessing health services. Once young people have accessed health care services, they are also more willing to disclose important information about health risk behaviours, seek health care and return for follow-up when they understand a service is confidential. Thus, attention to confidentiality should be as much a cornerstone of clinical relationships between doctors and adolescents as it is in adult health care. Nearly one in 10 adolescents report not visiting their health care provider in the past year – despite wanting to do so – because of the fear that their parents would find out.

In young people aged less than 18 years old, judgement about whether to maintain confidentiality in consultations with younger adolescents is linked with assessment of maturity. In deciding whether a person is competent or mature enough to consent to medical treatment, a doctor must decide if the young person is able to understand the nature of the problem, the nature and side effects of any proposed treatment, and other treatment options.

The doctor can accept consent provided that the treatment is in the young person's best interests and the treatment is not complex or likely to have serious consequences. For more complex or contentious procedures, doctors must balance several factors in making a decision, including the age, maturity and characteristics of the adolescent, the gravity of the presenting illness and treatment, and family issues. It is important to remember that all doctors have a legal and ethical duty of confidentiality to competent young people. This duty should only be breached in serious situations such as risk of self-harm or suicide, or in cases of suspected abuse, as well as some other exceptions discussed below. Doctors should become familiar with the specific laws on this issue in the state or region where they practise. In all Australian states and territories, anyone over the age of 15 years can have their own Medicare card and a doctor may bulk-bill a consultation without advising the parents.

Chronic illness

Children with special health care needs have been defined as those who 'have or are at increased risk for a chronic physical, developmental, behavioural or emotional condition requiring health and related services of a type beyond those required by children generally'. According to this definition, 15–20% of children and adolescents have a significant, ongoing health-care need.

There is a greater prevalence of young people with chronic illness in our community, because of improved survival rates from various paediatric illnesses that, as recently as 20 years ago, were associated with extremely poor prognoses. Examples include childhood leukaemias and other cancers, congenital heart disease and cystic fibrosis. Improved medical technologies result in the survival of more young people with complex and severe health-care needs who are reliant on advanced technology and multifaceted health care systems. In addition to improved survival, most developed countries have experienced a true increase in the incidence of certain conditions, such as asthma, diabetes, obesity, mental disorders and leukaemia.

It is important to remember that young people with chronic illness are first and foremost adolescents. Thus, while it might be assumed that adolescents with chronic illness would not add to their health risk profile by engaging in health risk behaviours, there is no evidence that this is the case. Instead, there is some evidence that young people with chronic illness might be even more likely to participate in health risk behaviours.

Importantly, many young people with chronic illness have a greater attributable risk from these behaviours. For example, in addition to the universal health risks of smoking, smoking in young people with asthma, cystic fibrosis or diabetes mellitus can be readily conceptualized as being 'more risky' in terms of their underlying health condition. Another example is the greater attributable risk from alcohol use in young people with diabetes mellitus or epilepsy.

Adolescent development is not a simple linear journey but is a dynamic process that is experienced differently by each individual. Thus, chronic illness can affect adolescents in diverse and complex ways. Physical growth and pubertal development can be delayed, although pubertal development can also commence earlier (precocious puberty) in other conditions (e.g. spina bifida). In addition to these universal elements of adolescent growth and development, adolescence is a time where various physical changes commonly become more significant (e.g. scars from previous surgery such as cleft lip repair or infant bowel obstruction, long-standing clubbing or scoliosis) as cognitive maturation brings greater capacity for both the imagination of an ideal body as well as critical comparison with one's peers. This sense of physical inadequacy can be associated with complex adjustment problems in terms of body image, self-esteem, bullying, peer relationships and mental disorder.

Some adolescents with chronic illness may be less well developed socially because of extended hospital admissions over many years with reduced opportunity for normal peer relationships. More specifically, certain chronic illnesses or disabilities can be associated with reduced cognitive or intellectual functioning. As a result, these young people may be relatively more reliant on their parents. Regardless of the explanation, poor peer relationships and fragile educational engagement can reduce educational achievement and limit career opportunities and future socioeconomic status.

Clinical example

Karen, a 19-year-old woman with cystic fibrosis, was soon to be transferred to a specialist adult cystic fibrosis centre for ongoing care. However, during the last few admissions, concerns had been raised about her mental state as well as the fact that she had twice discharged herself early against medical advice. The adolescent team was informed that her usual treating team felt her mood was 'pretty flat'.

In taking a detailed psychosocial history, the adolescent team identified that Karen had discharged herself against advice as she had a part-time job and an active social life. These were more important to her than her health, as another few days 'never made any difference'. It emerged that Karen had told no-one outside of her immediate family of her illness, including her current boyfriend. Her workplace was also unaware she had cystic fibrosis or had been admitted to hospital. Until recently, she had not required hospitalization for some years. She had hidden the recent admissions by keeping in touch with friends by mobile phone. She finally revealed that the main reason for keeping her illness secret was that a previous boyfriend had broken up with her when she had told him about her cystic fibrosis.

Her depressed mood was confirmed and was thought in most part to be due to the stress of living a 'double life'. While, at least superficially, she denied the severity of her respiratory status, it was considered that the implications of her lung disease (there had recently been discussions about the role of lung transplantation) were likely to have contributed to her depressed mood. She was very poorly adherent with physiotherapy and regular clinic review but had better adherence with antibiotics.

As a result of these and other discussions, Karen was supported in revealing her illness to some close friends and work colleagues, who were relieved there was an explanation for her significant coughing and supportive of her taking time off for treatment. There was further frank discussion about the severity of her illness, and she felt gradually more able to discuss aspects of day-to-day care, including adherence with treatment and transfer to the adult clinic, as well as the possible need for transplantation. Her lung function stabilized.

Practical points

Self management in adolescents with chronic illness
- As young people mature, they should be encouraged to take on more responsibility for managing their health, with less reliance on their parents for day-to-day care
- Seeing young people alone for at least part of the consultation will help build young people's confidence and skills in communication with doctors and health professionals
- Normalize the challenges of adherence in adolescents
- Rather than focusing on problems, work with the young person to develop practical solutions
- Short-term adolescent-focussed goals are more likely to motivate self-care than longer-term health-orientated goals
- Development of self-management skills is an important part of young people's transition towards adult health care

Little is known about what age adolescents begin to take more responsibility for different elements of self-care (such as taking medications, making appointments or seeking care when unwell). Further, it is not known what affect disease severity or intellectual capacity has on these practices. In practical terms, health professionals should encourage parents to support the emerging capacity for self-care in their children as they mature through adolescence. Health professionals can do this by educating the family about adolescent development. For example, many parents can become frustrated when their teenager no longer simply 'does what they are told' in relationship to adherence with requests by parents and doctors to 'take their medicine'. Informing parents of the developmental appropriateness of this behaviour and of ways of making it more likely that young people will adhere to treatment regimens is an important educational role for health professionals. Promoting greater self-management in young people with chronic illness is a specific part of the broader 'package' of working with young people that includes understanding adolescent development, health risk screening, appreciation of the value of confidential health care and understanding the transition to adult health care. This can be summarized as the provision of developmentally appropriate health care to adolescents.

Adherence with treatment

The terms 'adherence' and 'compliance' are often used interchangeably, but there are subtle distinctions between them.

Chronic illness in adolescents can also affect wider family functioning, including sibling experiences and parent marital relationships. Attention to the wider family and its functioning is an important part of looking after adolescents with chronic illness and disability.

Towards self-management

Adolescents with chronic illness are naturally interested and are able to take on a greater role in looking after themselves as they mature, although the skills for self-care do not magically develop but must be practised by young people and supported by their parents and health professionals.

Compliance is defined as the extent to which a patient is obedient and follows the instructions and prescriptions of health professionals. In contrast, adherence is defined as a more active, voluntary and collaborative involvement of the patient in a mutually acceptable course of behaviour aimed at producing a therapeutic or preventive outcome.

Most clinicians who work with young people know that to be authoritarian and prescriptive does not work well; most adolescents, like adults, wish to be included in the decision-making process regarding treatment options. The term adherence better reflects this preferred style of communication with young people. The main practical implication of using the term 'adherence' denotes that adherence behaviours are not exclusively the responsibility of patients but are a reflection of the doctor–patient relationship and the support that young people receive from their families.

Adolescents are commonly conceptualized (and judged) as being 'non-compliant'. Like adults, many adolescents struggle to achieve sufficient adherence with treatment. However, there is little evidence that adherence in adolescents is worse than in adults. Indeed, it is worth remembering that many studies show that adherence to treatment in adults with chronic illness is as low as 50%.

Strategies to improve adherence in adolescents need to take into account the challenge of adolescent development and the ways in which parents can both support and hinder adherence behaviours. Young people are less influenced than adults by the concept of health as a general life goal, or by specific longer-term health risks. For example, while adults with diabetes may be concerned about long-term complications, young people are generally more influenced by things in the 'here and now'. For adolescents, rather than threats to long-term health, development of routines and a focus on short-term goals are more likely to be influential.

In discussions with adolescents, do not assume that adolescents are fully adherent. Rather, use language that reflects the reality that poor adherence is common (labelling someone as 'non-compliant' is generally unhelpful). Likewise, instead of viewing poor adherence as the patient being irresponsible or uncooperative, understand that poor adherence can reflect different priorities, a busy life and the difficulty we all have in forming new routines.

Ask questions of adolescents that explore adherence behaviours in detail. For example, asking 'Which dose do you find hardest to remember, the morning or the evening dose?' can readily lead to greater discussion about the medication itself, and about routines that they have or do not have around different medication dosed. This can then lead to the young person finding their own solutions.

Seeing the young person alone for part of the consultation and listening to the concerns of both parents and young people can be helpful in facilitating better communication around adherence behaviours and other elements of self-management. Parents are very helpful in describing the reality of adherence behaviours but are less helpful in exploring solutions. Engaging young people as well as their parents is the challenge. Many young people feel that their parents constantly 'nag' them about their medication. Notwithstanding that the young person might need parent support with their medication, many young people report that parent 'nagging' makes them less likely to want to take their medication responsibly! Negotiating a short period of 'no nagging', especially when combined with strategies to promote the development of treatment routines, can be helpful. Following such approaches, some young people understand how much they need their parents to assist them, while some parents realize that their teenagers can actually manage quite well!

Improved knowledge about the importance of medication does not, of itself, generally lead to behaviour change. Rather, exploration of practical strategies is more likely to be effective. For example, comparison of treatment routines will commonly help teenagers appreciate that they are adherent with that part of their treatment that they have routines for and less adherent when they don't have routines. Solution-focused work to develop routines is a natural intervention following this insight, especially if it can be linked to short-term goals. Praising any practical change at follow-up visits is also strongly encouraged. Attention to adherence should be part of every consultation with teenagers.

Transition to adult health care

An important component of self-management for those young people who will continue to require specialist health care as they mature is that their care is transferred from a paediatric to an adult health care setting. Managing young adults in an adult setting promotes their ongoing development and independence whereas retaining their care in a paediatric setting is likely to have the opposite effect.

In relation to the provision of health care to adolescents with chronic health problems, transition is defined as 'the purposeful, planned movement of young people with chronic physical and medical conditions from child-centred to adult oriented health care systems'. Thus, the *physical transfer* of care from one setting to another is part of a broader *process of transition* to adult health care.

Clinical example

Paul was a 14-year-old boy with attention deficit/hyperactivity disorder (ADHD) who had been treated with stimulant medication for many years. His mother was concerned because he had recently stopped taking his medication and his school marks were deteriorating quite rapidly. She said that Paul was impossible to talk to about it, as he just shouted at her when she tried to broach the subject. Paul somewhat reluctantly admitted that the medication helped his concentration but he didn't care about educational success so he didn't feel there was much point in taking it.

Paul was referred to an adolescent specialist, who saw him alone. The specialist identified that Paul was being teased and bullied at school, particularly about his ADHD, which had contributed to him stopping taking the lunchtime dose at school. He also hated the way his mother nagged him in the morning to take his tablets as though he were a 'stupid little kid'. Paul revealed that his mood was very low and that during the last few months he had occasionally wished he was dead. He had no active suicidal plan. After a discussion with Paul and his mother, he was changed to a long-acting form of the medication that only had to be taken in the morning. Discussions were held about how Paul could take greater responsibility for remembering to take the medication, which included a conversation about medication routines and reminder charts.

After a few months of regular follow-up, Paul's mood and school performance gradually improved. Initially he was still a bit forgetful about taking the medication but, with the help of his mother, he developed a morning bathroom routine that included his medication. His mother no longer 'nagged' him but instead 'checked in now and then' to monitor the situation. Paul and his mother were communicating much better about this and other issues.

There are many barriers to transition to adult health care, with a significant proportion being *attitudinal*. The young person may fear the unknown and be reluctant to leave the security of a system and a group of health professionals that they have come to know and trust. Parents likewise may be concerned that they will be 'shut out' of the decision-making process in the adult setting. This fear may be more acute if parents have continued to be very actively involved in medical consultations without the young person starting to take on greater responsibility.

Some paediatricians (and parents) fear that the young person will receive less optimal care in the adult setting, and they too have trouble 'letting go', especially if they have looked after the young person for many years. Some adult physicians may fear taking on 'paediatric' patients, as they may be uncomfortable communicating with patients in this age group.

Other barriers are more *structural*, such as the lack of specific expertise (e.g. congenital heart disease, metabolic disorders, intellectual disability) or the lack of multidisciplinary services within the adult health care setting. Funding may perversely reduce the desire to transfer care (e.g. if elements of health care such as total parenteral nutrition or dressings are funded within the paediatric but not the adult setting). Lack of established communication channels between facilities and health care providers may be another barrier to transferring care.

There is no single model or ideal transition model to follow. Rather, a set of principles has been developed that promotes timely transfer to adult settings. Preparation is a very important component of planning, which should start well before the planned physical move. Each individual should have a health professional in the paediatric setting who has the primary responsibility for developing a transition plan. The family doctor or primary health care provider is an important link for continuity for the patient and family and should be actively involved.

While it has been argued that transfer to adult settings should not occur until the young person has the skills to function in an adult service, it can be equally argued that young people may only develop the required skills once they experience a more challenging environment. If possible the transfer should occur when the adolescent's health is in a relatively stable phase.

There is no correct age for transfer, and different approaches have developed in different countries. In Australasia, most children's hospitals plan to transfer young people to the adult setting once they have completed their secondary education, commonly in their 18th or 19th year.

The clinical approach

Meeting the patient

Many younger adolescents, especially those with chronic illness, will only have consulted doctors together with their parents and may therefore not expect anything else. Doctors can actively promote engagement with medical consultations by reinforcing that the young person, not the parent, is the patient. The doctor should introduce themselves to the young person first, then ask them to introduce the accompanying adult. This immediately signals to the young person that they have some control in the consultation. First impressions matter.

Confidentiality

Following introductions, an important step is to explain the confidential nature of health consultations, as it cannot be assumed that young people understand or expect this. We encourage a confidentiality statement to be made when parents are also in the room – as they also need to know. A brief discussion of the limits of confidentiality is also encouraged (the main limitations are risk of suicide or self-harm, risk of homicide or harm to others and any disclosure of abuse). With practice, this only takes a minute or so:

> 'What we talk about is confidential, which means I won't discuss it with anyone else without your permission. There are three exceptions to this, which are if I am worried that you are at risk of harming yourself, at risk of harming others or are being abused and are not safe. If these things come up we will deal with them together. I will involve you in any decisions that need to be made around who we need to talk to.'

Negotiating for time alone

An important component of self-management is that young people are able to participate fully in medical consultations, rather than having to rely on their parents. Seeing doctors alone for at least part of the consultation is a mechanism by which, over time, young people can develop the confidence to speak for themselves. When framed this way, most parents appreciate the opportunity for young people to spend time with the doctor, value the opportunity for the son or daughter to discuss sensitive issues with the doctor, and understand the importance of confidentiality. It is important, however, not to undermine the role of parents and to make sure that they are actively included. This is commonly done by inviting them back at the end of the consultation to discuss the diagnosis and management, having negotiated previously with the young person whether anything needs to be kept confidential.

This is generally not difficult for new consultations. However, it can be harder where a family doctor or paediatrician has seen a child together with the parent for many years. There is no set age to start seeing young people alone for at least part of the consultation. However, it is generally appropriate to offer some time alone from about the age of 13–14 years. Initially, the young person may be seen alone for only a short time. Gradually, however, more time will be spent with the young person alone and less time with the parents and young person together as young people develop the skills that enable them to be more independent within consultations.

Psychosocial screening (HEADSS)

Health risk screening is an important component of the clinical care of all adolescents. One approach to health risk screening has become known by its mnemonic, HEADSS, an approach that was first described in the US in the early 1980s While it provides a framework for health risk screening, it is perhaps better described as a method of engaging adolescents in the medical consultation, identifying both risk and protective factors, providing opportunities for anticipatory counselling and identifying short-term goals that be can used in promoting adherence with treatment.

H – Home
E – Education/Employment, Exercise and Eating
A – Activities (peer-related)
D – Drug use
S – Sexual health and Sexuality
S – Suicide, Self-harm and Safety

The original HEADSS approach (questions about Home, Education, Activities, Drugs and Alcohol, Sexuality, and Suicide and depression) has been recently updated and extended. In addition to the previous focus, the newer HEEADSSS is a prompt to question about Home, Education, Eating and exercise, Activity, Drugs and alcohol, Sexuality, Suicide and depression, and Safety from violence and abuse.

The HEADSS screen is a mnemonic to help the clinician to remember the key aspects of the psychosocial history that are important when seeing young people. It facilitates a holistic approach in which the doctor can engage the young person in discussing a range of behaviours and mental health states that have significant health implications. This approach to taking a psychosocial history extends the consultation beyond treatment of the presenting complaint to a greater focus on more preventative and health-promotional aspects of common behaviours.

This approach to health risk screening should be explained to the young person, as it may be confusing to be asked about personal behaviours such as drug use when seeing a doctor for asthma. One approach is to say:

> 'When doctors do check-ups with older people they measure physical things like blood pressure. Younger people are more likely to be physically healthy, but their health can be affected by different behaviours, which I'm now going to ask you about. This is something we do with all young people.'

There is no need for the HEADSS topics to be discussed in any particular order, although generally clinicians prefer to start with less sensitive questions and proceed to more personal topics. For this reason, many clinicians actually start with questions about education, as questions about home can be challenging when young people have complex family arrangements. At times, it will not be possible to complete a full HEADSS assessment at the first consultation. It is however important to ensure that the issues are discussed at a later date.

Most doctors discuss the presenting complaint first and then move on to the HEADSS screen. It is often useful to remind young people about confidentiality again at this stage and to also let them know that they don't have to answer questions if they feel uncomfortable.

It is important to remember to ask about and discuss protective as well as risk factors. The use of open-ended questions is encouraged to more actively engage young people beyond simple 'yes or no' responses. One of the main reasons for the success of the HEADSS approach is that, when used sensitively, it empowers adolescents to discuss their health seriously with a professional. It also provides opportunities for questions that would not usually be asked of doctors. Discussions such as this are uncommonly initiated by young people, but the majority participate willingly when given the opportunity and the confidentiality. This approach gives the doctor an important opportunity to frame what is going well with young people, to identify areas of concern, to engage in anticipatory counselling and to develop a plan of action.

In consultations with young people, doctors are urged to be respectful, unhurried and non-judgemental. It is not a good idea to try to use current slang or to be 'chummy' with adolescents. Young people, like all patients, are more concerned that their doctors are professional and skilled rather than that they are 'cool' or a friend.

Physical examination

Adolescence is a time of increased sensitivity about one's body and appearance in general. Therefore, even a 'routine' physical examination may be a confronting prospect for a young person. It should therefore be conducted in a professional, respectful and sensitive manner.

This must obviously be balanced with the need for a thorough clinical examination and, in all cases, measurements of height, weight and pubertal assessment are recommended. Ensure that the patient will not be exposed if someone else enters the room by using curtains or screens. Avoid unnecessary exposure of the body. When a particular area must be examined, the judicious use of clothing and sheets is recommended to keep other areas covered. A screening test of pubertal assessment can be made by self-report using the standard pictures of Tanner staging on growth charts and confirmed clinically if there are concerns.

While not a legal requirement, the use of chaperones for a physical examination is increasingly recommended, especially when male doctors are examining female adolescents, in order to make the patient feel more comfortable and reduce allegations of misconduct.

Some further details of the HEADSS assessments are given below.

> ### Practical points
>
> **A summary of psychosocial screening (HEADSS)**
> - **Home**
>   - where do you live?
>   - who lives with you?
>   - who are you closest to at home?
>   - is there anyone at home you can talk about personal issues with?
> - **Education and Employment**
>   - do you go to school? What year are you in?
>   - what are your grades like?
>   - have you changed schools recently?
>   - do you have many friends at school?
>   - do you have any problems with bullying at school?
>   - do you work?
>   - how many hours a week?
> - **Eating**
>   - has your weight changed recently?
>   - have you dieted in the last 12 months?
>   - how much exercise do you do per week?
> - **Activities**
>   - what do you and your friends do for fun?
>   - do you play sport?
>   - are you in any clubs or groups?
>   - what are your hobbies?
> - **Drugs**
>   - do you smoke cigarettes?
>   - do you drink alcohol?
>   - do you use any other drugs?
>   (If yes to any of the above then need to quantify)
> - **Sexuality**
>   - do you have a partner currently? OR Are you in a relationship currently?
>   - have you been sexually active?
>   - have you been pressured into sex?
>   - what do you understand by the term 'safe sex'?
> - **Suicide and depression**
>   - how would you describe your mood lately? (Can ask for score out of 10)
>   - are you ever sad/tearful for no reason?
>   - do you have any trouble sleeping?
>   - have you lost interest in things you used to enjoy?
>   - have you ever felt like hurting yourself?
>   - have you had any suicidal thoughts?
>   - have you ever had a suicide plan?
>   - have you previously attempted suicide?
>
> *Continued*

> **Practical points—cont'd**

- **Safety**
  - have you ever been seriously injured?
  - do you ever drive with people who have been drinking or taking drugs?
  - is there any violence at home?
  - have you ever been physically or sexually abused?
  - does your eating ever seem out of control?

See also Goldenring 2004.

H – Home

It is important to find out where and with whom young people live, and to explore which relationships are most supportive. Do not assume that all young people live within a nuclear family. Consider asking a question like, 'Who lives at home with you?' or, 'Where do you live?' to start. This is also the time to ask about the medical history of family members, as well as parent employment, ages of parents and siblings and other demographic information. Depending on their circumstances, some adolescents find talking about their family quite difficult; experienced clinicians commonly commence a psychosocial history with questions about education.

E – Education and Employment, Exercise and Eating

Most adolescents attend school, so initial questions such as 'Do you go to school?' and 'What school do you go to?' are useful. If asked 'Do you like school?' or 'What year are you in?' the young person can respond with a simple yes or no, which limits further discussion. Questions about what they like best or least about school can be more informative. As well as asking about academic achievement, young people should be specifically asked about their experiences of bullying. If the young person has left school, focus questions about employment or further education.

In recognition of increasing rates of overweight and disordered eating, the recent revision of HEADSS adds screening about levels of exercise and physical activity, as well as diet.

A – Activities

Questions about activities are a good opportunity to focus on peer relationships. Ask about aspirations, hobbies and clubs, as well as about how they entertain themselves away from family or school. Remember to ask about part-time work as this may not come up when talking about school. Questions about future life and career goals are a useful approach to exploring cognitive maturation.

D – Drug use

In questioning about drug use it is important to normalize experimentation with drugs without condoning drug use. Reference to the third person can be a helpful technique, such as, 'Some young people your age try drugs. What have been the experiences in your group of friends? And what about you?' Most clinicians start by asking about cigarettes and alcohol, as these are the two drugs most commonly used by young people, but remember to enquire about the full range of drugs. A brief reminder of confidentiality and a reiteration that your interest is health-related sometimes puts nervous teenagers at ease when moving to these questions. Without being judgemental, it is reasonable to comment supportively on healthy choices that the young person may describe.

S – Sexual Activity and Sexuality

Questions about what sexuality education the young person has received at school can be a helpful starting point for this sensitive topic. Other approaches include normalizing statements, such as, 'Many young people your age are starting to develop more meaningful relationships. Are you in a relationship at the moment?' Some young people report that they would simply prefer to be asked directly about issues like sexual activity and safe sex (contraceptive and condom use). A degree of judgement is always required. Remember not to assume that all relationships will be heterosexual.

S – Suicide, Self-harm and Safety

By this stage, rapport should be well established and questions that screen for anxiety, depression and suicidality usually proceed calmly and easily. One way of introducing this discussion is to ask the person to score their average mood out of 10 and to comment on the variation from this number in both directions.

It is important to ask directly about suicidal ideation and plans, and to act promptly if the person is actively suicidal. Contrary to claims that discussing such issues 'puts ideas into their heads', talking about suicide does not increase suicidal behaviour in young people who are not suicidal but can be protective in those who have been thinking of it but have not discussed it with anyone.

Questions about safety from abuse of any sort, particularly sexual abuse or violence, should be asked. Even if no disclosure is made, it is suggested that the young person be informed that sharing this information with others is important and that you would always be available to talk to them about this and any other issues they would like to raise in the future.

Many health practitioners are uncomfortable and even fearful when working with adolescents. Using this approach will guarantee an easier and more enjoyable experience for both the young person and the doctor. Working with young people is highly enjoyable, often very rewarding and at times great fun.

3.12 Paediatric and adolescent gynaecology

S. Grover

Development of the genital tract occurs between the 7th and 12th weeks of gestation. The gonads arise from the gonadal ridge and their formation is quite separate from that of the urogenital tract. Therefore congenital malformations or variations do not usually affect both the gonads and the urogenital structures.

At birth, under the influence of maternal hormones, the genital tract is well oestrogenized.

During childhood the reproductive tract is relatively quiescent, although small follicles on the ovaries may be an incidental normal finding and may be detected for example at the time of a pelvic scan performed for investigation of the urinary tract. Occasionally, this background ovarian activity can be more prominent, with idiopathic isolated follicle activity and with an isolated vaginal bleed that resolves spontaneously.

The uterus and upper vagina is formed by fusion of the Müllerian ducts. As this occurs in close proximity to the development of the urinary tract, it is not surprising that when anomalies are present in one system they may also be found in the other. Incomplete fusion of the Müllerian ducts can result in a uterine septum. More extensive incomplete fusion can cause a bicornuate uterus or uterine didelphys (with two uterine horns, two cervices and even two vaginas). These variations are relatively common and do not cause problems in paediatric or adolescent gynaecology.

Obstructed and rudimentary uterine horns can also occur – often in association with renal tract anomalies. Clarifying the presence or absence of a uterus and vagina or defining uterine shape can be extremely difficult after maternal oestrogen effects have declined within the initial months of postnatal life. There is little indication for extensive investigation in this age group, as interventions would be left for puberty.

Other genital tract anomalies can be seen in association with endocrine and congenital anomalies. Although surgical correction to reproductive tract anomalies may be part of the correction of these anomalies, e.g. for girls with congenital adrenal hyperplasia, bladder extrophy or cloacal anomalies, further follow-up and possible intervention from the genital tract perspective is not usually required until

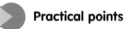

Practical points

- Vaginal examination is inappropriate in paediatric patients. An ultrasound or examination under anaesthesia (depending on the clinical problem) will provide the required information
- For adolescent patients, vaginal examination is infrequently undertaken unless they are sexually active and have given consent for this examination
- Transabdominal ultrasound will almost always provide the necessary information in the adolescent population.

the onset of puberty, when referral to a gynaecologist with experience with these anomalies may be appropriate.

Gynaecological problems in neonates

The decline of maternal oestrogens within a week or two of birth may result in a small vaginal bleed in neonates.

In the neonate with an imperforate hymen, a bulging hymen may be noted, representing a hydrocolpos. Surgical incision of the hymen allows drainage and resolution.

Common gynaecological problems for prepubescent girls

Labial fusion or labial adhesions

Labial adhesions or labial fusion are a relatively common finding in childhood. Labial adhesions are often first noted by the maternal and child health nurse, are not present at birth but may develop within a few months. The onset correlates with the decline in maternal oestrogen effects on the skin of the newborn and infant and the adhesions are thought to occur secondary to skin irritation.

As persistent labial adhesions are not seen in adolescent girls it can be safely presumed that the natural history of labial adhesions is spontaneous resolution. In the past, some have advocated the use of lateral traction and surgical division, or alternatively the use of topical oestrogen cream. Both these approaches are associated with a high relapse rate. Lateral traction can also be distressing for the young girl. As labial adhesions rarely cause any significant symptoms apart from occasional dribbling post-micturition, no intervention is necessary and parents should be reassured.

Clinical example

A 3-year-old girl was noted by the maternal and child health nurse to have an 'abnormal perineum', with no vaginal opening visible. The possibility of an absent vagina was raised, and the mother was advised to take her daughter to the doctor.

On examination of the perineum, the urethral and vaginal openings could not be visualized, as the labia appeared to be joined in the midline. Close examination revealed a fine midline stripe and the general practitioner was able to reassure the parents that the diagnosis was labial adhesions, which would resolve spontaneously. Her parents requested further reassurance that the vagina was actually present, as they had been reading about vaginal agenesis on the internet. Further reassurance was given that vaginal agenesis is a rare problem – and that investigations by any imaging technology in this age group to identify a vagina were unreliable. Instead arrangements are made to review the girl when she was older.

Review 3 years later revealed that the adhesions had almost completely resolved, and the urethral and vaginal opening with hymenal edge were now visible.

Vulvovaginitis

Vulvovaginitis occurs in the context of low oestrogens, with thin, atrophic vaginal and vulval skin. Hence it is seen in girls from early childhood through to the establishment of puberty, when the onset of oestrogen production causes thickening of this skin. The natural flora in the vagina of young girls is mixed bowel flora, similar to the distal bowel. Candida is not found in the non-oestrogenized young girl. Overgrowth of the bowel flora in the vagina is thought to irritate the atrophic skin, causing a discharge which then irritates the vulval skin. The affected skin is primarily the contact surfaces between the labia.

Vulvovaginitis can present with symptoms of:

• offensive vaginal discharge
• skin irritation
• burning with micturition.

The typical history is that the symptoms are intermittent. A specific infectious agent is not identified in most cases. The possibility of sexual abuse sometimes needs to be considered in a child with vulvovaginitis (Ch. 3.9).

Swabs are rarely required, except when there is a profuse discharge or there is skin erythema extending beyond the contact surfaces of the labia majora. In these cases a single organism may be responsible for the problems and specific antibiotics may be required.

Management includes the application of a simple barrier cream (such as zinc–castor oil or Vaseline) and bathing. The addition of vinegar (half a cup to a shallow bath) is often advocated. Parents need reassurance that the natural history is intermittent recurrence until puberty. In the presence of this skin irritation it is advisable to avoid other potential irritants such as bubble baths and soaps. Faecal soiling as a consequence of poor toileting habits may also be an issue. When the skin irritation extends beyond the contact surfaces of the labia, additional irritants such as prolonged periods in wet bathers may have an aetiological role.

A vaginal foreign body needs to be considered in the presence of a persistent vaginal discharge, particularly if the discharge is blood-stained. Vaginal foreign bodies are most often found to be a small amount of toilet tissue, although occasionally there may be beads and other small objects that can be seen on ultrasound.

Occasionally, small foreign bodies can be flushed from the lower vagina using a syringe and saline, but usually a general anaesthetic to enable a careful examination is required.

If itch is a significant component of the symptoms, pin worms need to be excluded. Alternatively, if there is evidence of a generalized eczema then superimposed eczema may occur on the irritated skin of the vulvovaginitis. The approach to management is the same as for vulvovaginitis, with the addition of topical steroids to settle the eczematous component.

Lichen sclerosis, with whitened skin changes and superficial splitting of skin, and atrophic changes in the anterior and posterior fourchette and between the labia minora and labia majora, is also a cause of vulval itch. This may occur secondary to the skin irritation of vulvovaginitis but can also be due to a relatively uncommon autoimmune skin problem. In the presence of vulvovaginitis symptoms and findings, the management of lichen sclerosis is as for vulvovaginitis, with the addition of topical steroid cream. A more potent steroid may be required for a short duration. Diprosone and Advantan are often best tolerated, with others having irritant components in the cream or ointment base.

Vaginal bleeding in childhood can occur in association with a foreign body. Alternatively it can be seen as a result of the ovarian activity of precocious puberty (Ch. 19.1). Rhabdosarcomas (sarcoma botryoides) is a rare childhood lower genital tract malignancy that presents as either sultana like polyps at the vaginal introitus or persistent vaginal bleeding.

Adolescent gynaecology

Overview of puberty, adolescence and the menstrual cycle

The age of onset of menarche has gradually declined during the last 150 years but now appears stable at about 12.5 years. It is influenced by living standards, although genetic factors have some impact when environmental factors are optimal. Although the commonest sign marking commencement of puberty is breast bud development followed by pubic and axillary hair, variations to this can occur (Ch. 19.1).

Breast development may be asymmetric initially and may be mistaken for a 'breast lump'. Body changes associated with puberty and hence body image can provoke concerns in some adolescent girls. In general, the time from commencement of breast development to the onset of first menses should be no longer than 4 years. The absence of menses by the age of 16 years is an indication of the likely need for further investigation.

During puberty, maturation of the reproductive tract, development of secondary sexual characteristics and an increase in bone density occurs. The latter continues up until about 20–25 years of age. Persistent low levels of oestrogen during adolescence may therefore have significant long-term consequences on bone density.

With the onset of ovarian activity, multiple follicles can often be seen on ultrasound. The identification of up to 15–20 follicles is a normal finding. With each cycle, six to 10 follicles in each ovary are recruited from their resting state as primordial follicles. When ovaries are functioning in a mature cyclic pattern, these follicles will each reach several millimetres in diameter before one becomes a leading follicle and increases to a size of up to 3–4 cm at the time of ovulation. On ultrasound this will appear as a simple 'cyst', which can be expected to resolve and disappear during the subsequent 2–6 weeks. It is important to reassure young women that this cyst is normal and demonstrates that the reproductive system is functioning normally.

Ovulation can be associated with some pain (Mittelschmerz or mid-cycle pain). Occasionally, haemorrhage into an ovulation cyst can occur, giving rise to a more complex appearance of the cyst on ultrasound (haemorrhagic corpus luteum). Knowledge of the timing of onset of this pain can be helpful in establishing this diagnosis.

During the first 2–3 years of menstruation it is common for the menstrual cycle to be irregular because of anovulation.

Consultation with young teenage girls needs to be undertaken with careful consideration for their developmental and cognitive stage, recognizing that consultation *without* a parent may be essential to explore relevant issues (Ch. 3.11). Establishing with the parent(s) at the beginning of a consultation that consultation without the parent is part of the standard care of adolescents is important. Raising the issue of confidentiality of the medical consultation with adolescents increases the likelihood of disclosure of health concerns.

Adolescent health risk behaviours need to be identified, as they can impact on reproductive health. Eating disorders may be responsible for menstrual problems (amenorrhoea and infrequent menses), smoking may influence choice of medications, sexual activity raises concerns regarding the need for contraception and risk of sexually transmitted infection, and drug and alcohol intake significantly impacts on the chances of risky, unsafe sexual activity.

Delayed onset of menses – primary amenorrhoea

The onset of periods usually correlates with exposure to oestrogens over some months, during which time breast development, pubic hair and axillary hair growth have occurred. Assessment of the time of onset of breast development and onset of pubic and axillary hair is useful to assess if progression through puberty has been normal. It is important to establish the general health of the young woman as well as the activities in which she participates.

If the young woman has no secondary sexual characteristics then the investigations are guided by the potential causes of delayed puberty (Ch. 19.1).

Assessment of the presence and extent of hair growth can give valuable clues to the diagnosis. Excess hair can be familial and may be related to ethnic origin or due to hormonal causes, with polycystic ovarian syndrome being the commonest. Late-onset congenital adrenal hyperplasia and other endocrine causes such as androgen-secreting tumours, mixed gonadal dysgenesis and 5-α-reductase deficiency are all relatively uncommon.

Scant pubic and axillary hair in the presence of good breast development is seen in complete androgen insensitivity syndrome.

The presence of normal secondary sexual characteristics should lead to clinical questions regarding abdominal pain. If menstruation has been occurring but an obstruction exists, then cryptomenorrhoea can result in cyclic abdominal pain. Clinical examination for a pelvic/abdominal mass should be performed. The commonest cause is an imperforate hymen, which can be confirmed simply by viewing the perineum while applying gentle pressure to the abdominal mass. Pelvic ultrasound can assist in confirming the presence of cryptomenorrhoea and in clarifying the level of the obstruction.

Uterovaginal agenesis is absence of the vagina and uterus. Ovarian function will be normal, as will all secondary sexual characteristics. The creation of a vagina is most often achieved with the use of dilators (and sexual activity). In the absence of a uterus, carrying a pregnancy is clearly impossible, although surrogacy can now be offered, as ovarian function is normal.

Clinical example

At the age of 16 years, Tanya was brought to see her general practitioner because of delay in the onset of menses. She began breast development at the age of 12 years. She was a state champion gymnast and trained intensively 7 days a week. She was of slight build. Examination revealed normal breast development at Tanner stage 3, and pubic hair at Tanner stage 3.

The provisional diagnosis was hypothalamic hypogonadism secondary to the level of physical activity. Follicle stimulating hormone (FSH), luteinizing hormone (LH) and oestrogen concentrations were found to be low. Thyroid stimulating hormone (TSH) and prolactin concentrations were normal. Pelvic ultrasound demonstrated a small normal uterus.

Tanya was reassured that there was no significant underlying problem and that her relatively low weight combined with her exercise level was the cause for the delay.

Irregular periods

The pattern of the periods can be quite irregular during the first few years after the onset of menarche. This can be attributed to an immature hypothalamic–pituitary–ovarian axis. Unless the irregularity is the cause of significant problems, simple reassurance is all that is required. Multiple follicles may be seen on ultrasound, although this is a normal finding in over 20% of young women. Unless there is evidence of hyperandrogenism (i.e. acne or hirsutism) the term 'polycystic ovary syndrome' should not be used.

Polycystic ovary syndrome

This is a syndrome usually associated with insulin resistance and skin changes of acanthosis nigricans as well as hyperandrogenism (excess hair and acne). Many but not all young women with this condition will be obese. The investigation findings can demonstrate an elevated follicle stimulating hormone (FSH) to luteinizing hormone (LH) ratio, ultrasound may show 20–30 follicles with increased ovarian stromal density; and fasting glucose and insulin measurements may show elevated glucose concentrations in relation to the insulin values.

Management consists of improving the diet and increasing the amount of exercise. Additional approaches such as hormonal treatment to regulate irregular and heavy periods and cyproterone acetate or spironolactone to reduce hair growth may be added in some individuals.

Heavy periods

Care needs to be taken when taking a history of menses as what is 'normal' or 'heavy' may vary with different individuals and in different families. Changing super pads (or tampons) that are soaked as frequently as 2-hourly is probably a reasonably heavy period. The presence of anaemia (in the absence of other dietary or gastrointestinal problems) is supportive evidence. Having flooding or 'disasters' regularly is a further symptom. The presence of clots is usually not significant unless the clots are large (>4–6 cm). Small clots are normal and simply mean that there is adequate time between blood leaving the endometrial surface and reaching the perineum to allow coagulation to occur.

Heavy menses in teenagers can be the result of anovulatory bleeding. Additionally, the possibility of a bleeding disorder needs to be considered, with reports suggesting that 10–15% of girls with menorrhagia (in a population without known bleeding disorders, and without predisposing factors such as chemotherapy or warfarin usage) may have an underlying bleeding disorder such as von Willebrand disease or platelet dysfunction.

Further information regarding a family history of heavy periods, postoperative bleeding and easy bruising increases the likelihood of a bleeding problem, but these features are not present in all individuals who are found to have a bleeding disorder. To investigate a young girl with menorrhagia the tests set out in Table 3.12.1 are recommended.

The management of the young girl with heavy menses is with the use of non-steroidal anti inflammatory drugs. These reduce menstrual loss by 30%. Where the loss is heavier and there is concern about a potential bleeding disorder it would be wise to avoid non-steroidal agents in the first instance and instead use tranexamic acid (500 mg, two tablets q.i.d. p.r.n.) on days of heavy bleeding. Additionally, the use of progestogens in anovulatory bleeding may be helpful in stopping the acute bleed. Provera 10 mg b.d. to t.d.s., or norethisterone acetate (NEA) 5–10 mg b.d. to t.d.s. but up to 2-hourly, can be used and then tapered during the next week. It needs to be remembered that complete withdrawal of progestogens is likely to be associated with a withdrawal bleed, so continuation of progestogens for a total of 3 weeks is advised. Ongoing use of cyclic progestogens at a lower dose (Provera 10 mg daily, or NEA 5 mg daily, for 21 d with a 7 d break to allow a withdrawal bleed), or alternatively the oral contraceptive pill can be used as a follow-up for the next 3–6 months.

In the acute context of very heavy bleeding (metrostaxis), resuscitation including blood transfusion may be required. High dose oestrogen may be necessary (estradiol valerate 2–4 mg 6-hourly), combined with tranexamic acid. This can be followed by the oral contraceptive pill commencing 48 hours later.

Table 3.12.1 Useful investigations in menorrhagia

- Full blood examination, iron studies
- Prothrombin time, activated partial thromboplastin time
- Von Willebrand antigen/factor VIII studies
- Platelet aggregometry or platelet function assays

Secondary amenorrhoea

Periods can stop for a range of reasons other than pregnancy – from central (hypothalamic) causes to pituitary and ovarian abnormalities. A careful history will correctly identify several of these underlying causes for secondary amenorrhoea.

Useful investigations for secondary amenorrhoea are presented in Table 3.12.2.

Hypothalamic causes

In a slim young woman, having established a good rapport while using HEADSS as a screening tool (Ch. 3.11) to explore the young woman's physical activities and self perception, the young woman who is taking a great deal of exercise or the teenager with the eating disorder should be identified. Weight loss associated with other medical conditions can also be responsible for central causes of amenorrhoea.

Pituitary causes

Pituitary problems related to prolactinoma or related to thyroid disease can cause secondary amenorrhoea.

Polycystic ovary syndrome

Weight gain and associated insulin resistance and evidence of acne or hirsutism make up the syndrome of polycystic ovary syndrome, which can be responsible for amenorrhoea or oligomenorrhoea (see above).

Ovarian causes

Ovarian failure can be due to gonadal dysgenesis (most commonly Turners syndrome (Ch. 10.3)) or premature ovarian failure.

Table 3.12.2 Investigation of secondary amenorrhoea

Cause of amenorrhoea		Investigation result
Central (hypothalamic)		Low FSH, low LH, normal TSH, low oestrogen, normal prolactin
Pituitary	Thyroid disease	Abnormal TSH
	Prolactinoma	Elevated prolactin (needs to be elevated on more than one occasion)
Ovarian: ovarian/gonadal failure		FSH and LH very high, oestrogen low
Pregnancy:		elevated βHCG

FSH, follicle stimulating hormone; HCG, human chorionic gonadotrophin; LH, luteinizing hormone; TSH, thyroid stimulating hormone.

Pregnancy

The sexually active teenager is at risk of secondary amenorrhoea related to pregnancy.

Pelvic pain

Dysmenorrhoea

Primary or prostaglandin-induced dysmenorrhoea is usually not present during the first menses but may begin within a few periods. It may occur in ovulatory and anovulatory cycles.

It usually consists of a symptom cluster of cramping lower abdominal pain and low back pain. Bowel symptoms varying between constipation and diarrhoea are common, with nausea, vomiting and headaches also occurring frequently. Dizziness, fainting, paleness, lethargy and generalized aches can be part of the same symptom cluster and may precede the onset of bleeding by a few days or may occur on the first or second day of bleeding. These symptoms are usually absent by the final days of bleeding. Symptoms may be exacerbated at times of stress.

These symptoms are generally attributed to prostaglandins, which play a role in coordinating the onset of menstruation. Management consists of general approaches such as exercise, and the use of non-steroidal anti inflammatory drugs optimally commenced prior to onset of symptoms.

Retrograde menstruation occurs in almost all women. This is menstrual flow upwards through the fallopian tubes and into the peritoneal cavity. The presence of free fluid in the peritoneal cavity causes a variable amount of pain. It can cause pain with defaecation and micturition as well as pain on movement. Reducing the menstrual loss by the use of non-steroidal medications or tranexamic acid will usually reduce the amount of retrograde loss and hence will reduce pain.

Endometriosis

Endometriosis is the presence of ectopic endometrium in the peritoneal cavity. As endometrial cells are present in the retrograde menses it is likely that most endometriosis can be attributed to this origin. Endometriosis can vary in severity from a few small spots to extensive endometriosis with adhesions and cyst formation (endometriomas). It is now generally agreed that mild endometriosis is a physiological finding. Endometriosis can be found in adolescents. Care needs to be taken to exclude or adequately manage other causes of period and pelvic pain, and to ensure that menstrual loss is reduced, as heavy and/or frequent periods are known to be a risk factor for endometriosis. Consideration of other factors that may be contributing to the symptoms also needs to be given (careful screening using HEADSS is valuable).

A pelvic ultrasound should be done prior to considering a diagnostic laparoscopy if symptoms are not controlled by other interventions.

Atypical dysmenorrhoea

Dysmenorrhoea that progressively worsens through menstruation and lasting beyond the end of bleeding is atypical and an obstructive Müllerian anomaly needs to be considered. Pelvic ultrasound can often be more helpful in diagnosis than laparoscopy. Assessment for an absent kidney can also give useful supporting evidence for the likelihood of a Müllerian anomaly.

Ovarian cysts

Ovarian cysts can be physiological (see above), occurring in the context of normal ovarian activity, or they can be pathological. Benign dermoid cysts are the most common non-physiological cysts, although even these are relatively uncommon in the paediatric and adolescent setting. Many ovarian cysts are asymptomatic even when they are very large and may be found incidentally at the time of other tests. They may cause vague lower abdominal pain or may present more acutely if torsion of the ovary occurs.

Ovarian torsion

This can be a difficult diagnosis because of the relatively non-specific nature of the symptoms. Failure to consider this diagnosis and late identification of this problem can lead to loss of an ovary.

Ovarian torsion is more common in childhood and adolescence than in adulthood. The abdominal pain is often colicky in nature, with associated nausea and dizziness. As the ovarian cyst may not be palpable, it is essential to consider the diagnosis if there is significant and persistent localized tenderness. A pelvic ultrasound demonstrating an enlarged ovary corresponding to the side of maximal tenderness is supportive evidence. Exploration with laparoscopy may the only way to clarify the diagnosis and is necessary if the ovary is to be preserved.

In the postmenarchal adolescent a history of regular menses with onset of pain occurring approximately midcycle may be adequate to diagnose midcycle pain, or mittelschmerz. However, consideration of the diagnosis of torsion needs to be made if there is significant tenderness. As normal ovaries do not usually undergo torsion, ultrasound may be helpful to identify the enlarged ovary.

Pelvic inflammatory disease

Sexual activity (or a gynaecological surgical procedure) enabling pathogens to access the upper genital tract is the prerequisite for the development of pelvic inflammatory disease (PID).

The commonest pathogen causing PID is chlamydia. Tubal disease and damage as a consequence of PID is a significant cause of infertility, and early diagnosis and adequate treatment is important. For the young woman who is sexually active and is febrile with significant pelvic tenderness, intravenous antibiotics should be used to cover the possibility of polymicrobial infection. The antibiotics chosen should cover chlamydia, *Neisseria gonorrhoea* and other anaerobic and aerobic organisms.

Screening for chlamydia in sexually active young woman under the age of 25 years has been advocated because of reported rates of silent infection in up to 15% of young women. Treatment with a single dose of azithromycin ensures good compliance and is effective. Identification of young women with silent carriage should lead to contact tracing of partners. Follow-up should be offered, and further discussion regarding contraception and safe sex is essential.

Contraception

Discussing and providing contraceptives to teenagers requires careful consultation. The need for contraception will often not be raised by teenagers but if part of the consultation has occurred without parents and has utilized a careful assessment of social activities and relationships, the young woman who is sexually active should be readily identified.

Ideally, involvement of an adult in the decision-making process regarding contraception is preferred but the younger teenager who demonstrates a clear understanding of the risks and benefits can be provided with contraception. Careful documentation and assessment of the competency of the teenager in demonstrating their understanding is essential (a House of Lords ruling in 1984 on this issue has given rise to the expression 'Gillick competence' for this assessment).

Ensuring that the teenager is aware of the need for condoms for 'safe sex' to reduce her risk of acquiring a sexually transmitted infection, as well as informing her of the need for cervical Papanicolaou smears commencing 2 years after the onset of sexual activity, should also be undertaken.

Options for contraception

Emergency contraception

This form of contraception is now usually provided as a single-dose progestogen, and is used as soon as possible after unprotected intercourse. The success of this contraception method correlates with the time interval since unprotected intercourse. It is important to do a pregnancy test prior to use.

Oral contraceptive pill

Although there are a wide variety of oral contraceptive pills available, for simplicity being familiar with two or three variations is all that is required. A standard monophasic pill (which allows the possibility of altering the time of the withdrawal bleeds and allows the option of skipping menses for several months at a time) using ethinyl estradiol and levonorgestrel is a good first-line contraceptive pill. If acne is a major concern then an oral contraceptive pill containing cyproterone acetate can be valuable. Pills with a higher oestrogen content (using ethinyl estradiol 50 µg) are essential for a young woman using anticonvulsant medications where liver enzymes are induced and metabolism of the oral contraceptive pill is accelerated.

Progesterone-only pills

These pills contain low-dose progesterone only and require greater reliability in use, with the pills needing to be taken at the same time every day (±1 h) This is usually difficult for teenagers to manage in their daily routine and hence is usually not considered a good or reliable choice for contraception for this age group.

Injectable – depot medroxy progesterone acetate (Depo-Provera)

This is a very reliable contraceptive and is usually administered every 3 months as an intramuscular injection. Measurement of beta-human chorionic gonadotrophin (βHCG) must be carried out if an injection is overdue, as ongoing amenorrhoea may be due to a pregnancy rather than to effective menstrual suppression.

Etonogestrel

This is a subcutaneous hormone released from a filament inserted into the upper arm, which provides contraception for 3 years. It is a very reliable form of contraception but causes irregular bleeding in 20–30% of women, resulting in requests for removal.

Progesterone-releasing intrauterine device (IUD)

This is also very reliable as a contraceptive, although it is generally not advised for the younger population because of the risk of multiple partners and hence the risk of pelvic inflammatory disease. It is effective for 5 years and causes a 98% reduction in menstrual loss. It has an important place in some specific adolescent populations.

Intrauterine device – copper IUD

These are effective for 5 years, and are very reliable. They generally are not used in the younger population because of the risk of multiple partners and hence pelvic inflammatory disease.

Teen pregnancy

Teenagers often present late with their unplanned pregnancy. If the presentation is early in pregnancy the opportunity to explore choices with respect to the pregnancy needs to be offered. Young women who are part of a positive educational environment with career plans are more likely to decide to terminate a pregnancy.

For teenagers who are pregnant, antenatal care in a young women's clinic offers the opportunity to address their specific needs using a multidisciplinary team. Careful assessment is required to identify their housing and financial support requirements. Dietitian involvement is valuable to ensure that eating disorders or poor nutrition secondary to lifestyle and poverty do not impact on the health of the young woman and the fetus.

Alcohol, smoking and illicit drug taking need to be explored, with links made to appropriate services. Screening for sexually transmitted infections needs to be offered to all pregnant young women as there is evidence that the asymptomatic carriage rate and prevalence in the under-25-year-old age group is significant. Exploration of possible past physical or sexual abuse should be undertaken.

It should not be presumed that any of the preceding issues will be spontaneously volunteered. A positive rapport is essential to gain the confidence of the young woman. Linking the pregnant young woman to educational resources and opportunities may be required, as limited education is a significant factor in lifelong poverty.

Pregnancy in teenagers generally is not associated with additional risks, although gastroschisis occurs more frequently in the babies of teenage mother.

Parenting as a teenager poses real challenges because of the conflicts between adolescent and parenting tasks. The developmental tasks of adolescence include seeking independence, risk taking, being part of a peer group and participating in peer activities. As a parent, provision of a stable environment with responsible and committed time to the care of a baby is clearly in contrast to adolescent tasks.

Intellectual disability – menstrual and contraceptive management

With the onset of puberty, parents and carers of young women with an intellectual disability often become acutely concerned by the further challenges that this sexual development may pose. Although concerns regarding the capacity of the young woman to cope with menstruation itself are often the reason for presentation, underlying worries about the need for contraception, risk of pregnancy and sexual abuse are usually present also.

It is impossible to predict exactly when menstruation will begin. Likewise it is impossible to know what problems, if any, the young woman will experience. As for other young women without disabilities, there is a range of options available to assist in the management of menstrual difficulties, and these need to be used in response to the specific problems and issues for the individual.

Identification of associated medical problems will assist in management decisions. All young women with chronic illness have an increased risk of vitamin D deficiency and the subsequent potential negative impact on bone density. The young woman with

Practical points

- In the presence of a problem that has an impact on the long-term reproductive health of the young woman, care and sensitivity with respect to the impact of this diagnosis on her self-esteem is critical
- Careful use of appropriate language, open discussion and disclosure, psychological support, and the opportunity to become involved in a support group are all considered important components in care

Table 3.12.3   Menstrual and contraceptive management in the young woman with intellectual disability

Management	Clinical effects	Additional comments
Non-steroidal anti-inflammatory drugs	Reduce menstrual pain Reduce menstrual loss	No contraceptive effect
Tranexamic acid	Reduces menstrual loss	No contraceptive effect
Cyclic progestogens	May reduce menstrual pain Regulate bleeding pattern May reduce menstrual loss	No contraceptive effect
Oral contraceptive pill	Reduce menstrual pain Reduce menstrual loss	Contraceptive
Continuous oral contraceptive pill	May eliminate menses May reduce cyclic epilepsy	Contraceptive
Depot medroxy progesterone acetate (Depo-Provera)	May eliminate menses May reduce cyclic epilepsy May have a negative effect on bone density and require replacement oestrogen	Contraceptive
Etonogestrel	May reduce menstrual bleeding but significant risk of irregular bleeding	Contraceptive
Levonorgestrel IUD	Significantly reduces menstrual loss (often achieves amenorrhoea)	Contraceptive
Tubal ligation	No impact on menstrual symptoms	Contraceptive In Australia requires Family Court of Australia approval for those less than 18 years of age
Hysterectomy	Eliminates menses and menstrual pain	Contraceptive In Australia, requires Family Court of Australia approval for those less than 18 years of age
Endometrial ablation	Reduces menstrual loss (may achieve amenorrhoea)	Not contraceptive In Australia, requires Family Court of Australia approval for those less than 18 years of age

reduced mobility has additional risks for osteoporosis. In young women already at risk of negative bone influences, any technique that lowers oestrogens, such as the use of depot medroxy progesterone acetate, should be avoided or only used if replacement oestrogen is also provided. For the young woman with unstable epilepsy, seizures may occur cyclically and achieving a stable hormonal state may be helpful in reducing frequency of seizures.

Menstrual and contraceptive management in the young woman with intellectual disability is summarized in Table 3.12.3.

PART 4

BEHAVIOUR AND MENTAL HEALTH NEEDS IN CHILDHOOD

Life events of normal children

H. Hiscock, F. Oberklaid

Child development, from conception through to adolescence and on to adulthood, proceeds in ways that generally are predictable. Children achieve developmental milestones at certain ages (Ch. 2.2) and these anticipated milestones provide an important yardstick against which to assess the individual child's development. A departure from these predictable developmental milestones, usually in the form of delay or unusual and unexpected behaviours, provides the first sign that development is not proceeding normally.

The development of infants and young children is greatly dependent on their interaction with the environment. In the early years it is the parents, most often the mother, who shape the infant's environment. Research in recent years has served to re-emphasize the importance of the caretaking environment on the developing brain. The sort of environment that a young child is exposed to has a major impact on functioning later in life.

A key requirement for optimal child development is secure attachment to a trusted caregiver, usually the mother, with consistent affection and caring in the first few years. A child's and subsequently an adult's emotional health are significantly influenced by these early relationships between the young child and his or her caretakers.

Assessment of the development of behaviour of a child is therefore never undertaken in isolation: the environmental context is a critical part of the assessment. The child's behaviour and development are always the result of a complex series of transactions between the child and the environment and assessment always considers both.

Risk and resilience

There are well-documented risk factors that make the child vulnerable to a less than optimal outcome. Similarly, there are protective factors that increase the resilience of the child and increase the likelihood of a good outcome. Some of the risk and protective factors can be:

- biological (prematurity, chronic health problems)
- temperamental (difficult versus easy temperament)
- parental (level of education, genetics); familial (family cohesion); socioeconomic (level of income, poverty)
- community (type of neighbourhood, facilities).

Appropriate caretaking by the parents provides some of the most important protective factors in promoting optimal development. Recent research suggests that this caretaking environment actually influences the structure of the brain, with the development of neural pathways that are determined largely by environmental inputs.

Risk and protective factors are not inevitable in individual children, operate differently at different ages, and tend to be cumulative, so that combinations of risk or protective factors are more powerful than individual factors.

Developmental stages

In the course of the child's development there are certain periods that can be viewed as important transition points. Each of these transitions is associated with predictable developmental events and behaviours, stresses and potential problems. The negotiation of each of these transitions is an important milestone that allows the child and the family to proceed to the next level of development. Stresses and problems encountered during these transitions may result in the child progressing down developmental pathways that lead to later problems.

A number of important transitions are considered below. Risk factors and professional interventions that may be of assistance are outlined.

Birth

The goal is to produce a healthy, full-term infant, together with a healthy mother who can cope with the inevitable stresses and change in lifestyle that come with a newborn baby.

Risk factors include maternal physical and mental illness, substance abuse, smoking, adolescence/single pregnancy and poverty. Infant risk factors include genetic defects, birth trauma and prematurity.

Professional interventions. Regular antenatal care enables early detection and intervention for many maternal and fetal complications. During labour the presence of a supportive partner or trusted friend has been shown to decrease time in labour and reduce complications. Early mother–baby contact facilitates breastfeeding and sets the stage for a positive mother–infant relationship. While in hospital it is important to establish linkages with postnatal services such as maternal and child health nurses, general practitioners, home visiting and other community services.

Home with the new baby

This is often a challenging time for the family. Parents and family aim to establish a routine incorporating the needs and demands of the new infant. Parents bring to this transaction their own beliefs and experiences, with varying levels of confidence and competence and skills at handling stress, uncertainty and fatigue. Parents begin to understand their baby's visual, motor and verbal cues and respond appropriately. This is the beginning of a reciprocal relationship or 'dance'. This relationship shapes the baby's brain, especially during the first 3 years of life. If things do not go smoothly, and the mother perceives the infant as difficult and demanding, the long-term mother–child relationship can be compromised, setting the stage for possible future parenting and behaviour difficulties.

Establishing appropriate feeding patterns, preferably breastfeeding as this has many advantages, is another crucial task.

Risk factors include an unwanted child, prenatal complications, problems with bonding and attachment, maternal depression, social isolation, few or no identified supports and a stressful family situation.

Professional intervention. Providing support to parents through what is inevitably a stressful time, even in well functioning families, is essential. Assisting parents with realistic expectations and understanding of their baby's developmental needs and linking them up with a network of family and professional supports are crucial interventions. Sometimes there are early clues as to serious dysfunction, such as maternal depression or major difficulties in the mother–child relationship, so that more intensive intervention may be required.

Early infancy (first 6 months)

All parents need to learn how to manage the following inevitable issues:

• *Crying.* All infants cry. This is now understood to be a normal part of development. However, some infants are difficult to console and their crying causes major stress for their parents. About 10% of infants cry for more than 3 hours per day, 3 or more days per week for 3 or more weeks. These infants are often labelled 'colicky'. Underlying medical causes for crying are uncommon (<5%) and include cow's milk protein allergy, lactose intolerance and possibly gastro-oesophageal reflux. Most crying abates by age 3–4 months, and crying persisting after this raises the possibility of organic illness or concerns in the mother–baby relationship.

• *Feeding.* Most mothers want to breastfeed their infant but not all mothers find breastfeeding easy. Problems with incorrect attachment to the breast are common and may lead to difficult and painful breastfeeding and ultimately to early weaning.

• *Sleeping issues.* Most infants establish a sleep pattern after 3 months of age, although they may not begin to sleep through the night until 6 months. Common parental complaints include difficulties settling their infant and frequent night waking.

Clinical example

A mother presented with her 7-week-old baby boy. She said he was crying 2–3 hours a day and appeared hungry. She was breastfeeding her baby every 1½ hours and said she had no milk so she wanted to wean to formula. Her baby vomited a small amount after most feeds and her general practitioner had prescribed a medication for reflux. After a careful examination to exclude a physical cause of the crying, it was explained to her that all babies cry, and that crying reaches a peak around 6–7 weeks of age and then decreases by age 3–4 months. She was encouraged to keep breastfeeding and to space the feeds to every 2–3 hours so that her baby had a good feed and was not snack feeding. Tiredness signs in babies were discussed, and strategies for settling her baby when he was tired were explained. She was asked to keep a feed/cry diary and to stop the reflux medication. Two weeks later, her baby was crying less and was settling to sleep better. He was feeding every 3 hours and seemed content.

If issues of crying, feeding and sleeping are not addressed, parents may become tired, frustrated, inconsistent and even potentially abusive. A secure attachment may not form between the infant and caregiver, and infants may miss out on the consistent and affectionate caretaking environment that has been shown to have such a major impact on brain development and function throughout childhood and beyond.

Another important task is the introduction of solids, with many mothers beginning to think about weaning towards the end of this period (Ch. 3.3).

Risk factors include postnatal depression, parental conflict, inappropriate maternal expectations, and stress and fatigue. Infant risk factors include difficult temperament, excessive crying and irritability, sleep problems and difficulty feeding.

Professional intervention. Providing support and appropriate information so that parents have realistic expectations and adequate coping strategies is important. Parenting needs to be consistent and caring, and a 'goodness of fit' needs to be established between parenting style and infant needs and behaviours. Medication and frequent formula changes are usually inappropriate for sleeping and crying problems. Rather, parents need reassurance that their infant is healthy and does not have any underlying medical condition. They should aim to settle their infant with a consistent approach that enables the infant fall to asleep on his or her own rather than being held, rocked or fed to sleep. Mothers experiencing problems with breastfeeding should be managed by someone experienced in the area, such as a community nurse or a lactation consultant.

Late infancy (6–12 months)

This is a time of rapidly emerging cognitive, developmental and social competencies in the infant. S/he is interested in the environment and will very often initiate interaction with caregivers, wanting to play and to be stimulated in appropriate ways. Paradoxically, during this time period the first signs of stranger anxiety and separation protest become evident. The infant becomes anxious around strangers and is no longer willing to be picked up by an unfamiliar person. The infant also may begin to become distressed when the parent is out of sight, e.g. at bed time or if left in the care of a babysitter or in childcare.

During this time, food issues become increasingly important, with most mothers completing weaning during this time and moving towards a varied diet with regular meals.

Risk factors include maternal and family stress, inappropriate responses to increasing infant needs for stimulation and social interaction, difficulty changing from breast/bottlefeeding to an educational diet, sleep difficulties and irritability.

Professional intervention. Continued support for parents, provision of accurate information about developmental and other needs of their rapidly developing infant, and ensuring that there is a 'goodness of fit' between the infant and his or her parents are essential. Parents should realize that much of their infant's behaviour is exploratory and that the infant is not being deliberately naughty. Sleep problems can be managed with behavioural interventions such as

'controlled crying', where parents leave their infant for increasing periods of time to enable them to fall asleep on their own. Good eating habits can be established with regular mealtimes of a short duration (typically 20 minutes or less) and encouraging the older infant to finger feed. Parents should offer a variety of foods, understanding that their infant may try a food many times before finally accepting it.

Toddler period (1–3 years)

This is a very major transition time, as the child moves from being an infant, who still is almost totally dependent, to being an active, curious toddler with an increasingly complex set of developmental competencies, including language. One of the normal developmental tasks in this age group is to develop autonomy, and this often challenges the parents as the toddler is oppositional, stubborn, seems always to be testing boundaries and likes to get his or her own way. Temper tantrums are common when the child is frustrated at being unable to master a task, or restrictions are placed on his or her autonomy by parents saying 'no'. Sleep problems and problems around mealtime also are very common. They are more common in children with a difficult temperament and are made worse by inconsistent parenting.

Most children will begin, and some will complete, toilet training during this time period and this sometimes becomes a symbol of the struggle between the parents and the child regarding the child's autonomy. Signs of developmental delay, including language problems, also become evident during this time period.

Risk factors include difficult temperament, difficult behaviours (tantrums, overactivity, eating and sleeping problems, difficulty with socialization) and developmental delay. Family factors include inconsistent parenting, lack of warm and appropriate parenting, inappropriate responses, poor social support and family stress.

Professional intervention. Parents need to know what is normal and how to effectively manage common problems. For example, when a child has a temper tantrum, parents should:

- stay calm
- walk away
- ignore the behaviour until the tantrum stops
- praise the child when appropriate behaviour begins again.

Most tantrum behaviour will escalate initially and then will decline with this approach. For more aggressive behaviour, 'time out' may be used. This involves placing a child in a quiet room or corner for a maximum of 1 minute per year of age whenever the undesired behaviour occurs. The child is allowed out from the 'time out' place when s/he is quiet. This is effective in children over 18 months of age and its use should be limited initially to only the two or three most problematic behaviours.

Preschool period (3–5 years)

During this period, there continues to be a rapid explosion in language, cognitive ability and social skills. While the young child may have been left in childcare or in other child-minding situations, the child now begins to participate in a more structured learning environment. This is an enriching experience in which the child's natural curiosity is stimulated by systematic input from trained preschool teachers and by exposure to other children of the same age. Language continues to develop rapidly, as does the child's cognitive ability.

At the end of this period the child makes the very important and symbolic transition to school, so issues of school readiness become apparent. To undertake a successful transition to school, children need to master a range of motor, cognitive and social skills. They need to:

- be toilet trained
- be able to use a pencil
- be able to focus and maintain attention on a task
- have sufficient language skills
- be able to understand instructions and to make their needs understood
- have the social skills that enable them to interact with peers and with adults
- have the developmental competencies to function in a much more structured learning environment.

The rate of maturation during the preschool period may be uneven and is certainly not linear. The child who appears 'immature' at the age of 4 years, for example, may mature rapidly during the following 6 months. Generally, girls are more mature than boys when they start school.

Risk factors in children include language or other developmental delay, poor social skills, difficulty focusing attention, separation difficulties from parents, and behaviour problems (especially aggression). Family risk factors include low maternal educational levels, bilingual background, poverty and being a single parent.

Professional intervention. Parents of preschool children often seek professional help for concerns about language or developmental delay, behaviour problems, delayed toilet training, or questions about school readiness. Assessment at this age needs to be cautious because of the variability in maturation

rates. Providing parents with information about realistic expectations in this age group and teaching them basic skills in behaviour modification is often very helpful. Many problems are minor and are often transient, and simple, short-term interventions are often effective. However, in some children there are emerging signs of more serious problems, including developmental delay, communication problems, attention difficulties and more serious behaviour problems. These children may require vision and hearing testing, a speech assessment and, where an autism spectrum disorder is suspected, a multidisciplinary assessment.

Most children are toilet trained by 4 years of age. A delay in training may be due to a global developmental delay or may reflect a toddler's 'battle' with parents as the toddler tries to establish autonomy. A programme of regular toileting together with frequent praise and rewards (e.g. stickers) will often achieve continence.

A number of tests assess school readiness but none is sufficient in isolation. The decision to send a child to school should be made by the parents, with input from those involved with the child, especially the preschool and primary teachers.

School years (over 5 years)

School is an important formative experience for all children. Children who have difficulty functioning at school, because of learning difficulties, attention or behaviour problems or social difficulties, will almost always experience their impact beyond school. The child's experience at school can be either a protective or a risk factor for adjustment in childhood and for functioning later in life. Children who struggle academically or socially have been shown to be at major risk in adolescence and later life for poor outcomes, including delinquency, unemployment and depression.

The early years of school are particularly important. Children who have difficulty reading from the outset and who are not established readers by the end of grade 2 are likely to continue to have problems throughout their school career.

Risk factors include chronic health problems, vision and hearing deficits, problems with concentration and subtle developmental weaknesses in the areas of motor function, visuomotor integration, temporal sequential organization (problems remembering the order of information) and language. Risk factors in the family include low parental education, low expectations of school achievement, parenting difficulties and other family dysfunction. Other risk factors include a poor match between the child's temperament and preferred style of learning and classroom placement or teacher expectations and teaching style.

Professional intervention. It is important to identify school learning and behavioural difficulties as soon as possible so that appropriate interventions can be put in place. The longer this is delayed, the greater the chance of a poor outcome. Assessment should involve close evaluation of biological, developmental, behavioural and environmental factors that may be contributing to problems. Hearing and vision should be assessed. Often in this age group a multidisciplinary evaluation that includes a special educational assessment is the most appropriate. Where possible, a child should be referred to an educational psychologist for formal cognitive testing, including tests of intelligence. A detailed and comprehensive assessment will often point to the need for specific developmental and educational interventions that address the individual needs of the child. These may include remedial classes at school and/or tutoring outside school.

Clinical example

A mother presented with her 8-year-old son Ed. His teachers had complained that he was 'mucking around' in class and was disruptive. He had problems with spelling and writing. His father had had similar problems at school and left in year 10. His mother said that Ed was fine at home and tended to play computer games or ride his bike. He was noted to be quiet during the consultation and he said he had few friends at school. His vision and hearing were assessed and they were normal. A neurodevelopmental assessment was performed, which revealed weaknesses in auditory sequencing and language processing. The school psychologist performed a cognitive assessment, which revealed that Ed had normal intelligence but a specific learning difficulty involving reading, writing and spelling. This was discussed with his teachers, who arranged remedial teaching and more computer time for Ed's class work.

Adolescence

Adolescence is a time of immense change (Ch. 3.11). The young person needs to adjust to physical and emotional change, acquire an appropriate gender role, join peer groups, become emotionally independent of parents and other adults and prepare for career and relationships in life. While most adolescents negotiate this period successfully, up to one in five will experience significant physical or emotional problems. Adolescents often experiment with drugs, alcohol and cigarettes, and nicotine addiction usually begins in adolescence.

Risk factors include chronic health problems, learning disability, social isolation, parental physical or mental illness and family dysfunction.

Professional intervention. Health professionals need to address the concerns of the young person as well as the parents. Clarifying the professional obligation of confidentiality at the start of a consultation will reassure and facilitate rapport. In addition to addressing specific problems, screening questionnaires that encompass home, school, recreation, drug use, sexual activity and suicide/depression issues enable a full picture of the adolescent to emerge (Ch. 3.11). Parents need to know what is normal during adolescence and be given effective strategies for both communicating with their adolescent and managing common problems.

Practical points

- Organic causes of infant crying are uncommon but should be suspected if there is associated atopic disease, poor weight gain, frequent (i.e. >3 times per day) vomiting, or blood/mucus in the infant's bowel actions
- In toddlers, low-priority misbehaviours (e.g. tantrums, whining) are best managed by ignoring or distraction
- High-priority misbehaviours (e.g. hitting, kicking) are best managed by asking the child to stop and, if they do not, by putting them in 'time out'
- A child with school-based behaviour or learning problems needs a multidisciplinary assessment, including vision and hearing testing and, where possible, cognitive testing by an educational psychologist
- Up to one in five adolescents will experience significant physical or emotional problems. Screening questionnaires that encompass home, school, recreational drug use, sexuality and suicide/depression issues can help to detect these problems

Common problems presenting in the preschool and school environment

Preschool

Hitting and biting are common in the preschool setting. Occasional biting is usually experimental. Repeated hitting or biting may occur when a child is frustrated, is stressed or feels powerless. The key to management is identifying the cause of the frustration or stress (e.g. not wanting to share a toy) then removing, redirecting or distracting the child away from the cause. Parents should respond promptly and calmly, telling their child not to hit or bite when they remove the child from the situation.

Tantrums are very common (see Toddler section above). Where possible they should be ignored, as any form of attention tends to increase their frequency.

Language delay affects around 10% of preschool children (Ch. 2.2). Causes include simple language delay (expressive and/or receptive), deafness, autism spectrum disorder, global developmental delay and social–emotional deprivation. Referral for a speech therapy assessment is recommended if a child uses fewer than 20 words at 2 years of age, or does not understand simple instructions without gesture, or has no two-word combinations at $2^1/_2$ years. Any child with a language delay needs to be referred for audiology testing to exclude hearing problems.

School

Attention difficulties manifest in many ways, including:

- poor concentration
- 'daydreaming'
- quiet withdrawal
- disruptive behaviour.

Causes include attention deficit/hyperactivity disorder (ADHD), learning difficulties, intellectual disability, language delay, absence seizures, hearing and vision problems and depression/anxiety. Each of these can affect a child's learning. Treatment depends on the underlying cause and health professionals need to liaise with the child's teacher to ensure that the teacher understands the child's difficulties and how they may affect learning (Ch. 4.3).

Learning difficulties occur when a child of normal intellect performs at least 1 SD below their potential ability in one or more areas of reading, spelling, writing or mathematics. Learning difficulties affect 10–15% of school children. Early recognition, diagnosis and remedial teaching are vital to ensure that the child does not lose confidence and become angry, depressed or frustrated. Children with learning difficulties should also have their vision (Ch. 22.2) and hearing (Ch. 22.1) assessed and any problems treated so that their ability to learn in the classroom is optimized. Children with learning difficulties will not, in all likelihood, grow out of their problems, so reassurances that the child will improve with maturity are usually ill founded and inappropriate.

Bullying is the deliberate desire to hurt someone with words or actions. Children who are bullied may refuse to go to school, be very tense and unhappy after school, or show other signs of unhappiness such as difficulty sleeping. Children who bully may be physically punished at home and are more likely to grow up to hit their own partners and children. Managing bullying involves the whole school, with increased awareness, teaching students about conflict resolution and assertiveness training, peer counselling and improved adult supervision.

Common child and adolescent mental health problems

M. Sawyer, B. Graetz

Child and adolescent mental health problems are common in the community. They have a significant impact on the lives of children and parents, and also impose a substantial financial burden on families and communities. In Australia, the National Survey of Mental Health and Wellbeing estimated that 14% of children and adolescents experience significant mental health problems (Table 4.2.1). Adolescents with mental health problems frequently exhibit a range of other health risk behaviours, including smoking, drinking and drug abuse (Ch. 3.11). They also report much higher rates of suicidal ideation and behaviour than other adolescents in the community. Only a minority of children and adolescents with mental health problems receive professional help.

This chapter describes common mental health problems experienced by children (for brevity, the term 'children' will be used to refer to children and adolescents). It also describes practical steps that can be taken to help children, parents and families. The chapter is divided into three components. The first describes the features of common mental health problems, the second describes general approaches to the assessment and management of these problems, and the third provides information about some specific problems experienced by children.

Features of mental health problems

Two approaches are used to describe childhood mental health problems. One approach views childhood problems as lying on a continuum from those with very few problems to those with a large number of problems. Children identified as having a very large number of problems are considered to fall in the 'clinical range' of the continuum and to be in need of help. Typically, problems are divided into two broad groups called externalizing problems and internalizing problems.

The former includes problems such as overactivity, aggressive or antisocial behaviour. The latter includes problems such as anxiety, depression or shyness. Questionnaires completed by children, parents and teachers are used to identify those children in need of help. When a continuum approach is used it is possible to compare the number of problems reported for an individual child with the number typically reported for others of the same age and sex in the community. It is also possible to assess the effectiveness of treatment by evaluating whether there is a reduction in the number of children's problems.

The second approach divides childhood mental health problems into a range of different mental disorders. Each mental disorder consists of a different group of symptoms. There are two main classification systems that identify these symptom groups. One is the International Classification of Diseases developed by the World Health Organization (ICD-10), and the other is the *Diagnostic and Statistical Manual* developed by the American Psychiatric Association (DSM-IV; Table 4.2.2). This categorical approach is used widely in mental health services to describe children's problems. A common feature of both of these approaches is their focus on observable features of children's problems rather than on the presumed aetiology of these problems. This has encouraged a broad investigation of the aetiology of children's problems during the last three decades.

Features of internalizing problems

Many children experience anxiety or sadness. However, when these problems are severe or persist over time, they may indicate the presence of a mental disorder and the need for professional help. In particular, children with high levels of internalizing problems should be assessed for the presence of depressive disorders or anxiety disorders.

Children with depressive disorders feel sad, lack interest in activities they previously enjoyed, criticize themselves and are pessimistic or hopeless about the future. DSM-IV identifies two types of depressive disorder. *Major depressive disorder* consists of acute episodes of depressed mood, loss of interest and pleasure in activities, appetite and sleeping disturbance, low energy, low self-esteem, poor concentration and feelings of hopelessness. Children with *dysthymic disorder* experience similar problems but

Table 4.2.1 Prevalence of mental health problems among children and adolescents aged 4 to 17 years in Australia

Child behaviour checklist scale	Prevalence (%)*
General areas	
Total problems	14.1
All externalizing problems	12.9
All internalizing problems	12.8
Specific areas	
Somatic complaints	7.3
Delinquent behaviour	7.1
Attention problems	6.1
Aggressive behaviour	5.2
Social problems	4.6
Withdrawn	4.3
Anxious/depression	3.5
Thought problems	3.1

Problem areas are not mutually exclusive, and thus 'Total problems' does not equal the sum of externalizing and internalizing problems.
* Percentage of children scoring in the clinical range on the Child Behaviour Checklist Scales in the Child and Adolescent Component of the Australian National Survey of Mental Health and Well-being (Sawyer et al, 2000).

Table 4.2.2 Important DSM-IV disorders among children and adolescents

DSM-IV category	Specific disorders
Disruptive behaviour disorders	Attention deficit/hyperactivity disorder Conduct disorder
Mood disorders	Major depressive disorder Dysthymic disorder Bipolar disorder
Anxiety disorders	Separation anxiety disorder Social phobia Obsessive-compulsive disorder Post-traumatic stress disorder
Learning disorders	Reading disorders Written expression disorders
Pervasive developmental disorders	Autistic spectrum disorders
Elimination disorders	Enuresis Encopresis

their symptoms are less severe. The main feature of dysthymic disorder is the persistence of symptoms over a very long period of time. Children with both disorders may think that life is not worth living and they may contemplate suicide. It is essential that all children with depressive disorders be carefully evaluated for suicidal risk (Ch. 4.4).

While fear and anxiety are common to the human condition, some children experience anxiety that is well beyond that which occurs during normal development. These children suffer personal distress and their anxiety interferes with their daily functioning. Children with anxiety disorders exhibit physiological symptoms (e.g. tremors, sweating and palpitations), maladaptive behaviours (e.g. avoidance of feared situations) and maladaptive thinking (e.g. 'I cannot talk in front of the class because people will think I'm stupid').

DSM-IV identifies a number of different types of anxiety disorder. One of the most common among children is *separation anxiety disorder*, which is defined as excessive and developmentally inappropriate anxiety regarding separation from home or from major attachment figures. Separation anxiety disorder is a common cause of persistent school refusal.

Obsessive compulsive disorder is characterized by obsessions (persistent thoughts, impulses or images that are intrusive and distressing) and compulsions (repetitive behaviours or mental acts employed to reduce anxiety or distress). This disorder causes considerable distress for children and parents. It is important for medical practitioners to be familiar with the typical symptoms of this disorder as effective interventions are available to provide help. These include both psychotropic medications and behavioural treatments. *Social phobia*, which typically begins during the teenage years, comprises fear of social or performance situations in which embarrassment can occur. This condition can adversely affect the development of social skills and can also hinder academic progress at school. Adolescents with this disorder may be reluctant to attend professional services because of their insecurity and fear of social embarrassment.

Features of externalizing problems

Externalizing problems refer to problems such as temper tantrums, aggressive behaviour, stealing and truancy. Boys are more frequently identified as having externalizing problems than girls. Problems in this area, particularly those involving aggressive behaviour, can persist over long periods of time. For example, infants with a difficult temperament may exhibit oppositional and defiant behaviour as preschoolers and may subsequently develop behavioural disorders during later primary school or high school.

Two common mental disorders in this area are *conduct disorder* and *attention deficit/hyperactivity disorder (ADHD)*. The typical behaviour of those with conduct disorder includes bullying, frequent physical fights, deliberate destruction of other people's property, breaking into houses or cars, staying out late at night despite parental prohibitions, running away from home and frequent truancy from school.

Attention deficit/hyperactivity disorder is defined as a persistent pattern of inattentive behaviour and/or hyperactivity–impulsivity that is more frequent and severe than is typically observed in individuals of the same age. Children with inattentive behaviour problems make careless mistakes with schoolwork, find it hard to persist with tasks and are distracted easily. Those with problems in the area of hyperactivity/impulsivity often fidget and talk excessively, interrupt others and are described as constantly being 'on the go' (Ch. 4.3).

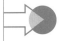

Practical points

Assessment of mental health problems
- Careful assessment is essential before initiating any treatment programme for mental health problems
- Assessment requires knowledge and understanding of children's presenting problems, developmental history, family and social environment
- Information must be obtained from multiple informants (children, parents and teachers)
- Aetiological factors can be divided into predisposing, precipitating, perpetuating or protective factors

Assessment and management of mental health problems

Assessment

A careful assessment of children's problems is an essential prerequisite to effective treatment. This should include information about the child's current problems, a developmental history, and relevant information about the child's family and social environment. It is important to develop a clear understanding of the nature of a child's presenting problems and the factors that have given rise to these problems. One way of organizing these factors is shown below:

- predisposing factors
- precipitating factors
- perpetuating factors
- protecting factors.

In each area, consideration should be given to the possible influence of biological, psychological and social factors.

Information about children's problems should be obtained from children, parents and teachers. Children are the key source of information about their internal state, including their experience of subjective feelings such as anxiety and depression. Parents can provide information about more readily observed behaviour such as sibling conflict or school refusal. Parents are also an important source of information about the early development of children and the chronicity and severity of current problems. Teachers are the best source of information about children's academic progress and they can provide important information about the quality of children's peer relationships. The assessment and treatment of ADHD relies heavily on reports from teachers.

Clinical example

Peter, a 12-year-old boy, lived with his single mother. Peter's mother had a history of depression and his father had been treated for alcohol abuse. Peter's mother sought advice about how to manage his defiant and aggressive behaviour. She said that from the time he was born, she had struggled to cope with Peter's difficult temperament and behaviour. This problem had greatly worsened since she divorced Peter's father last year. Since the divorce Peter had had little recent contact with his father and he was suspended from school on one occasion after damaging property in the school science centre. Peter's teacher described him as being easily distracted and impulsive during the last year. Despite these problems, Peter had continued to maintain satisfactory academic progress and his teacher believed that Peter's intelligence was above average.

The following factors were important in this problem:

- Predisposing factor: family history of psychiatric disorder
- Precipitating factor: divorce of parents
- Perpetuating factor: rejection by father
- Protecting factor: child's intelligence.

Management

The management of childhood mental disorders is complex. Many disorders persist over long periods of time (e.g. ADHD) or tend to recur (e.g. major depressive disorder). In the light of this, the development of long-term management plans is often necessary. The development of such plans requires consideration of several key issues.

Firstly, it is important to recognize that specific interventions are now available for many disorders.

It is important to be familiar with these interventions and to avoid 'one size fits all' methods of counselling. Secondly, the management of children's problems often involves the use of a combination of biological (for example, psychotropic medications), psychological (for example, behaviour modification programmes) and social interventions (for example, school based programmes). Finally, the management of children's problems requires the cooperation of children, parents and teachers. Medical practitioners responsible for the treatment of children with mental disorders must involve all of these groups in the care of children.

A range of psychological interventions is available to help those with mental disorders. These include:

- individual psychotherapy, which focuses on helping children
- family therapy, which focuses on relationships between all family members
- behaviour modification, which focuses on the antecedents and consequences of children's behaviour
- cognitive therapy, which focuses on maladaptive thinking styles.

Recent reviews have drawn attention to the importance of correctly implementing these interventions. It appears that a failure to do this may explain why their effectiveness, when delivered in clinic settings, is less than that achieved in the university or research environments where they were developed.

A wide range of medications are used to treat children with mental disorders. However, an ongoing concern is that, while many of these medications have the potential to provide help, evidence of their efficacy is largely based on studies of adults. With the exception of psychostimulant medications used to treat ADHD, there is a paucity of evidence to guide clinicians in the appropriate use of medications for the treatment of childhood mental disorders.

There has been particular concern in this area in relation to the use of antidepressant medications. Several national authorities have advised medical practitioners to be particularly cautious when using these medications to treat depressive disorders experienced by children and adolescents. When psychotropic medications are used to help children, very clear treatment goals should be identified, along with careful monitoring of effectiveness and adverse effects. Pharmacological treatment should always be used as part of a broader management plan developed in conjunction with children and parents. Only one psychotropic medication should be prescribed at a time to manage a child with a mental disorder. After an appropriate trial, if one medication is ineffective an alternative may be selected. Only after consultation with a child psychiatrist or paediatrician experienced in paediatric psychopharmacology should multiple psychotropic medications be used concurrently to treat a child with a mental disorder.

> ## Practical points
>
> **Treatment of mental health problems**
> - Treatment plans need to be individualized
> - It is important to obtain cooperation from children, parents and teachers
> - Psychological interventions should generally be employed before the use of medication
> - In general, only medical practitioners with specialist knowledge should initiate treatment of child and adolescent mental health disorders with psychotropic medications.

Problems of infancy

Infant mental health is a rapidly developing field. Debates about nature versus nurture have been abandoned in favour of interactional models that link the styles of parenting to an infant's physical health, developmental maturity and evolving personality. This is set in a cultural and extended family context. Attachment theory describes the relationships thus produced between infant and parent. There is increasing evidence that these interactional styles, already measurable by 12 months of age, predict children's interactional patterns later in life.

Recent work has shown that early experiences have a measurable effect on infant's brains. It is believed that tract and synapse development is significantly conditioned by the style of parenting. An infant's brain has the potential to develop and mature, and this potential can best be achieved by parenting that is attuned to the needs of the infant. Thus, appropriate parenting in which love and limits are evident, along with a focus on helping with developmental stages, is likely to promote tract development.

It is known that a wide range of parent and infant issues can interfere with optimal parenting. These include postnatal depression and anxiety, troubled marital relationships and compromised role models of parenting and prematurity. Physical or emotional abuse has particular and long-lasting consequences. There are a growing number of interventions being developed to address these problems in the early years. There is also a growing body of knowledge about the benefits of early (e.g. antenatal) identification of parent risk factors and the potential for health promotion and early intervention at this early stage of an infant's development.

Special issues

Suicidal ideation and behaviour

All suicide attempts should be treated seriously. Although suicidal ideation and behaviour are very rare before the age of 12 years, they become more frequent during adolescence (Ch. 3.11). Approximately 2% of school children attempt suicide, and attempts are often associated with serious mental health problems. Completed suicide is less common. Completed suicide occurs more frequently among boys (2–3/10 000 adolescents per year), who tend to choose more lethal methods than girls. The Child and Adolescent Component of the Australian National Survey of Mental Health and Wellbeing found that adolescents with more emotional and behavioural problems reported substantially more suicidal ideation and behaviour (Fig. 4.2.1).

Suicidal ideation and behaviour is often associated with symptoms of a depressive disorder along with a history of abuse of alcohol or other drugs. Many young people who attempt suicide live in families where there is a high level of interpersonal conflict and where parents have a history of mental disorder or drug and alcohol abuse. As well as a history of chronic adversity, many young people report an immediate precipitant to their suicide attempt. This may involve an argument over parental or school discipline, or a difficulty in a relationship with a friend.

All children who report thoughts of suicide or who attempt suicide should be assessed carefully. This should include assessment of the mental state of the child and the seriousness of the suicidal attempt. Characteristics that suggest that a suicide attempt was serious include:

- family history of suicide attempts
- previous history of suicide attempts
- presence of a mental disorder (e.g. major depressive disorder)
- evidence of premeditation and planning
- an expectation by the young person that the attempt would result in death
- a suicide attempt made while alone or isolated
- precautions taken to make discovery unlikely during or after the suicide attempt.

During the period of time that a young person remains at high risk for suicide, it is important that they be in a safe environment where their behaviour can be monitored. During this time their mental status should be assessed and help provided to address personal or family problems. In some circumstances, such as when a young person has a serious mental disorder or where they have no secure place of residence, it is necessary to arrange hospital admission.

It is important to provide appropriate treatment for depressive disorders experienced by young people who make suicide attempts. This should include the use of specific counselling techniques such as cognitive behaviour therapy and, where appropriate, the use of antidepressant medication. Every effort should be made to reduce the impact of ongoing stressors, such as family conflict, that may precipitate further suicide attempts. When appropriate treatment methods are employed, a high rate of recovery can be achieved. However, major depressive disorder often recurs and it is important that young people and their parents are advised of this continuing risk of further episodes and the symptoms that may signal the onset of a recurrence.

Attention deficit/hyperactivity disorder

Attention deficit/hyperactivity disorder is one of the most common mental disorders experienced by children. The core symptoms of the disorder are inattentiveness, impulsivity and hyperactivity. It is important to recognize that this behaviour may not be evident in the structured office environment of a medical practice. In light of this, it is essential to obtain reports from parents and teachers about the child's home and school behaviour. Many children with ADHD meet the criteria for other mental disorders such as anxiety or conduct disorders, and experience learning difficulties, family conflicts, peer relationship problems and low self-esteem. During assessment it is important to determine the extent to

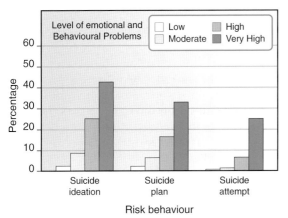

Suicidal Ideation and Suicidal Behaviour

Fig. 4.2.1 Suicide ideation and suicidal behaviour

which these associated disorders and difficulties are comorbid or the source of the child's ADHD symptoms.

The management of ADHD requires the use of a range of different interventions including:

- medication
- parent training
- classroom behaviour management
- remedial education
- family support.

It is important to explain the basis of the child's behaviour to children, parents and teachers. Stimulant medication is an effective treatment for children with this condition. However, to achieve the maximum effect, careful titration of medication dosage is necessary using reports from parents and teachers to identify the effectiveness of different dosage regimens.

Even when a good effect is achieved, however, the child's inattentiveness and impulsivity may be more problematic than that of other children. For this reason, parents will need ongoing help with effective management strategies. It is also important to ensure that children receive appropriate remedial education when a learning problem is identified. One of the disappointing findings from studies that have evaluated the effectiveness of stimulant medication in the longer term is evidence that the academic progress of many children with ADHD continues to lag behind that of their peers.

School refusal due to anxiety problems

A small number of children exhibit high levels of distress when they first commence school, and this may be associated with temper tantrums, excessive fearfulness and complaints of somatic symptoms (e.g. stomach aches or headaches) for which no biological cause can be identified. In some children, this pattern persists and it may give rise to a situation where children do not attend school for long periods of time. School refusal adversely affects these children in two ways. First, the children are at greatly increased risk of receiving an inadequate education. Secondly, they miss out on important socializing experiences. As a result, they may enter later life lacking important social skills. For these reasons, school refusal is a very serious problem that requires urgent and effective management. Often, it will be necessary to provide help to children and parents over long periods of time.

Among younger children who refuse to attend school there may be a history of separation anxiety disorder. Children with this disorder have a history of anxiety when separated from their primary caregiver, may insist on sleeping in their parents' bedroom at night, and may refuse to stay overnight with friends. In primary school, the children will describe their fear of separation from parents, describe worrying about their parents at school and may be excessively anxious if their parents are late to collect them from school. They may also express fear of punishment from teachers or concern about bullying by peers.

Adolescents who refuse to attend school may be suffering from social phobia. Adolescents with this condition experience marked fear of social or performance situations. As a result, they are reluctant to attend school where they have to mix socially with peers and demonstrate adequate academic progress.

Assessment should be initially broad-based and aimed at understanding the cause of children's problems. A developmental history should be obtained with a particular focus on symptoms of anxiety. Information should be obtained about the child's environment both at home and at school. This should include information about family functioning, the classroom and school environment, and peer relationships. It is essential that contact be made with children's teachers to obtain information about these latter issues. Information should also be obtained about the severity, duration and pervasiveness of school non-attendance, noting possible antecedents of the problem and consequences that may be responsible for maintaining the behaviour.

There are a number of specific approaches that can be used to help children with school refusal due to anxiety problems. Implementing these requires the combined efforts of children, parents and teachers. Children need help to better manage their anxiety. This should include the use of techniques such as:

- relaxation training
- systematic desensitization
- cognitive restructuring
- shaping and contingency management.

Parents need to be taught how they can manage children's temper tantrums and how to help children who report somatic complaints. In two-parent families, it is important that both parents participate in treatment programmes. In situations of chronic school refusal, assessing the significance of children's somatic complaints can be helped by close liaison with a general practitioner who can quickly assess a child and advise parents whether the presence of a physical illness precludes school attendance. This support can reduce the pressure on parents who must decide whether or not to allow their child to miss further schooling. Where there is no evidence of a physical illness, every effort should be made to ensure that children return to school at the earliest possible opportunity. Teachers can play a vital role supporting the child's return to school after an absence and helping to reduce anxiety at school due to bullying or performance pressure.

Enuresis and encopresis

Nocturnal enuresis

While most children have achieved bladder control by the age of 5 years, a significant number continue to have problems with nocturnal enuresis. This is embarrassing for children and is a burden for their parents.

In the absence of physical causes, such as a urinary tract infection, nocturnal enuresis is generally not a serious problem. Indeed, it may simply reflect normal variation in the development of bladder control where there is a familial tendency to later maturation of bladder control. Discussing this familial pattern with parents may help them better understand the nature of their child's problem. Exposure to stressful events may also induce children with previously good bladder control to recommence bed wetting.

For younger children, management consists of reassurance and the establishment of a convenient pattern of hygienic care of bed and clothing. Simple procedures such as fluid restriction at night or getting children to empty their bladder when the parents are ready to retire may help. Incentive systems can be put in place to assist children's motivation to remain dry. One method is to reward children for achieving a given number of consecutive dry nights, with the number of nights gradually extended over time.

For more persistent cases of bed wetting, an enuresis alarm has been shown to be an effective treatment in the majority of cases. The alarm consists of a detector mat placed on a child's mattress. The mat is connected to an alarm and when the child begins to urinate during sleep, a circuit is completed and the alarm sounds. The procedure (often called a 'bell and pad') uses simple conditioning rules to train children to achieve better bladder control. Many children's hospitals or chemists have such devices available for hire. However, it is important to ensure that both the mat and alarm function properly, or they will not condition children to achieve better bladder control. Children who are not easily awoken by the alarm will initially require parental assistance to finish voiding in the toilet. This is important in ensuring that the conditioning treatment achieves success.

In recent years, desmopressin has been used as a short-term treatment for children with nocturnal enuresis. It is administered orally or as a nasal spray and acts to decrease urine production at night. Studies report varying success rates but relapse is high and side effects such as headache and abdominal pain have been noted. Tricyclic antidepressants such as imipramine should no longer be used to treat bed wetting because of high relapse rates, the possibility of adverse cardiac side effects and the risks of severe morbidity or even mortality if taken in significant overdose.

Encopresis

Encopresis affects between 2% and 8% of primary school children. It is more common among boys and a high proportion of children with encopresis have concomitant constipation. The problem is distressing for children and may be associated with parent child conflict. Several types of encopresis have been described:

- constipation with overflow
- failed toilet training
- toilet phobia
- stress-induced loss of control
- provocative soiling.

Considerable overlap may occur between these different types of encopresis. However, the descriptions provide a general indication of the types of issue that must be considered when assessing children with encopresis. Before treatment is commenced, it is important to identify the causes of the child's encopresis. This should include a physical examination to identify whether a child has constipation.

There are three elements to the treatment of encopresis. Firstly, it is important to treat constipation when this is present. This generally can be achieved through the use of laxatives or microenemas. Less commonly, it will be necessary to employ a bowel washout. Secondly, it is important to ensure that the diet contains adequate fibre to reduce the likelihood of future constipation. Finally, it is important to establish a routine of regular toilet use. Establishing a new pattern of regular toilet use can be difficult with children. There may be a history of conflict between parents and children about toilet use. Children may also be unclear about the linkage between irregular toilet use and encopresis, particularly if previous interventions have focused largely on punishing children who soil their clothes. Children may also be upset or embarrassed by their problem and may refuse to participate in treatment programmes.

It is important to ensure that children understand why they are experiencing constipation and soiling. A simple schematic diagram showing the key features of the gastrointestinal system can be used to help children understand the nature of their problem. Children need to understand that constipation occurs when there is a build up of faeces because of a failure to empty the bowel regularly. Once they understand this, it is easier to work with them to plan a programme of regular toilet use.

Small rewards given after each use of the toilet can be helpful with young children. In children with toilet phobia, rewards may be given initially for simply sitting on the toilet for a few minutes and then progress to rewards provided when the child empties their bowel in the toilet. To achieve maximum effect, rewards need to be given immediately after children use the toilet, they need to be inexpensive (because of the need to reward each use of the toilet) and they must be given consistently when the child uses the toilet. Jointly identifying appropriate rewards can be used to build a therapeutic alliance with children and encourage their cooperation with the treatment programme. Seeking children's active involvement in treatment planning can also be used to reduce the conflict between children and their parents, with the latter taking on a more supportive and advisory role.

Hyperactive and inattentive children

4.3

J. Sewell

Hyperactive and inattentive behaviours are common in children, ranging in a continuum from normal behaviours, especially in young children, to developmentally inappropriate behaviours that impair daily activities at home and at school.

Developmentally inappropriate levels of hyperactivity and inattention may be the result of many factors, both intrinsic and environmental.

These risk factors (Table 4.3.1) must all be considered in the assessment of children with difficult behaviour, especially when considering the diagnosis of attention deficit/hyperactivity disorder (ADHD).

Definition of attention deficit/ hyperactivity disorder

Attention deficit/hyperactivity disorder is considered to be a developmental disorder of self regulation, characterized by inattention and hyperactivity/ impulsivity. The underlying neurobiological pathway involves the frontal–striatal–cerebellar networks, with deficits occurring in executive functioning, particularly response inhibition, vigilance, working memory and planning.

The diagnosis of ADHD is made using DSM-IV criteria. It is a descriptive diagnosis without implying cause, as it is not a discrete entity and has multiple causes. There must be developmentally inappropriate symptoms of inattention (Table 4.3.2) and/or hyperactivity/impulsivity (Table 4.3.3) with onset before 7 years of age, impairing social, academic or occupational functioning across multiple settings, and these symptoms are not a result of pervasive developmental disorder, psychosis or severe emotional disorders. Subtypes include mainly inattentive, mainly hyperactive or combined.

ADHD is common. The prevalence in the school-age population generally is considered to be 3–5%. Boys are affected more commonly, particularly with hyperactivity. There is a higher incidence in disrupted families and in those with low incomes, again particularly with hyperactivity. There is a strong genetic factor, with about 30% of siblings, 25% of parents and 80% of identical twins affected. Molecular genetic studies have focused on chromosomes

Clinical example

Sammy, aged 6 years, was in his second year of school. His teacher complained that he never sat still, did not complete tasks, talked too much, interrupted and was well behind with reading.

His mother recalled that he had been 'on the go' since about 2 years of age, always preferred playing outdoors rather than settling to games inside, never seemed to remember instructions or the house rules, and acted without thinking about the consequences. He hated homework and 'often forgot' to bring home his school reader.

Sammy's problems are consistent with a diagnosis of ADHD and learning difficulties. Stimulant medication and consistent structure at home and at school helped his behavioural symptoms but he also required educational assessment and specific reading support in the classroom.

that regulate dopamine, the neurotransmitter most associated with learning, motivation, goals and movement, and noradrenaline (norepinephrine), involved in maintaining alertness and attention, particularly with novel stimuli. Two candidate genes, the dopamine transporter and dopamine receptor genes, are reported to be associated with ADHD.

Many children with ADHD have associated neurodevelopmental or mental health problems (comorbidities) (Table 4.3.4). Because of overlapping features, separation into these diagnostic categories is complex; however, it is helpful in completing a descriptive assessment and recommending specific management programmes.

Assessment

The assessment of children for ADHD with its multiple risk factors and comorbidities requires skilled interpretation of information from the child, family and teachers. Relevant factors include:

- medical
- developmental
- family history
- family and social environment

Table 4.3.1   Risk factors for hyperactivity and inattention

- Difficult temperament
- Poor parenting skills
- Family dysfunction
- Child abuse, particularly deprivation
- Developmental delay
- Language disorders
- Learning difficulties
- Anxiety/mood disorders
- Sleep disorders
- Medical conditions, e.g.
  - very low birth weight or small for gestational age
  - fetal alcohol syndrome
  - prenatal exposure to smoking and stress
  - lead poisoning
  - acquired brain syndrome (head injury)
  - chromosomal abnormalities, e.g. fragile X
  - food intolerance (rare)

Table 4.3.2   DSM-IV: Symptoms of inattention

- Poor attention to detail, careless mistakes
- Difficulty sustaining attention
- Seems not to listen
- Seems not to follow through
- Difficulty with organization
- Avoids tasks requiring sustained attention
- Loses things
- Easily distracted
- Forgetful

Table 4.3.3   DSM-IV: Symptoms of hyperactivity/impulsivity

- Fidgets
- Often leaves seat
- Runs, climbs excessively
- Difficulty playing quietly
- 'On the go'
- Talks excessively
- Blurts out answers
- Difficulty awaiting turn
- Interrupts others

Table 4.3.4   Comorbidities with attention deficit/hyperactivity disorder

- Learning difficulties (10–30%)
- Language disorder (30–50%)
- Oppositional defiant disorder (30–50%)
- Conduct disorder (16–20%)
- Anxiety, mood disorders
- Developmental coordination disorder
- Tics, Tourette syndrome

- the school setting
- academic progress
- socialization skills.

General family functioning, behavioural patterns over time, antecedents and consequences of behaviours, and family and school management of behaviours must be understood. Standardized behavioural rating scales completed by parents, teachers and adolescents help to put the behaviours into a normal community context. Thorough physical examination helps to exclude the rare associated medical conditions. Neurodevelopmental assessment provides information on motor skills and auditory and visual processing. Many children require formal assessment of auditory, cognitive, language and educational function. Neuroimaging, quantitative electroencephalograms and psychophysiological tests (e.g. of continuous performance) are research tools only at this stage and are not yet ready for use in clinical diagnosis.

The diagnosis of ADHD can only be made against a thorough understanding of normal patterns of development and behaviour. This is particularly important when considering the diagnosis in a preschool aged child, with wide variations expected in normal behaviour, development and temperament, and vulnerability to adverse family and social circumstances.

Clinical example

Byron, aged 3½ years, was extremely active, aggressive and oppositional, and had a mild language delay. Recently, his mother had separated from Byron's father and begun a new relationship. The family had moved several times and had been involved with a number of family support agencies. His mother wanted Byron to go on stimulant medication like his older half brother.

Byron was diagnosed with oppositional defiant disorder and language delay, in the context of a dysfunctional but committed family. He could also have been diagnosed with ADHD on DSM-IV criteria, but such a diagnosis at this age might be misleading and could shift focus away from the critical issue of effective family support.

Management

ADHD is a chronic condition requiring long-term management based on partnership with the child, the family and the child's teachers from year to year. Counselling on the nature, causes, risk factors and course of ADHD, setting realistic expectations in the light of such understanding, and making accommodations at home and at school will help the child maintain confidence and self-esteem.

Multimodal management includes:

- stimulant medication
- parental behaviour management
- classroom behaviour management
- management of comorbidities, e.g.
  - special education support for learning difficulties
  - treatment of anxiety, depression
- family support, parent support groups.

Stimulant medication

Stimulant medications, which increase dopamine levels in the brain (methylphenidate and dexamphetamine), are the most effective treatment for ADHD and improve target symptoms in about 75% of children with the condition. Improved concentration and decreased hyperactivity, impulsivity and distractibility lead to enhanced task completion, academic progress and social interaction sustained over time.

These medications are safe and have a low profile of adverse effects that either subside spontaneously within the first 2–3 weeks of treatment or can be managed by altering the dose or timing of medication. Insomnia, appetite suppression and headache can be troublesome in some children. There is some evidence that height growth may be suppressed initially, particularly with higher doses, and therefore growth must be monitored carefully.

Long-acting preparations of methylphenidate are now available, enabling morning-only dosage. Atomexetine, a noradrenergic reuptake inhibitor, is now approved for use with ADHD.

There is considerable community concern that too many children are taking stimulants and other psychotropic drugs, with overdiagnosis and medicalization of social problems. There is community concern also about a perceived risk of psychological dependence on drugs instead of developing self-responsibility. The reality is that ADHD is a developmental disorder with significant long-term risk factors in educational, social and vocational outcomes, and only 2% of school-age children in Australia have been prescribed stimulant medication, despite the prevalence of ADHD of at least 3–5%. There is very good scientific evidence for the long-term safety of these drugs. There is also clear evidence that effective treatment with stimulants of adolescents with ADHD protects against substance abuse.

Medication treatment is only one of the treatment modalities for ADHD. It is also critically important for health professionals to advocate community services and family support for children who are at risk for adverse developmental, behavioural and social outcomes, whether or not they have ADHD.

Clinical example

Julie, aged 13 years, was in year 8 at school. Although she had coped academically in primary school, she was having difficulty with organizing herself, working through assignments and getting homework completed on time. Her written work was messy, she was distracted easily and she daydreamed in the classroom. She was worried that she would not do well enough at school to go to university.

Julie's assessment indicated long-term problems with attention, distractibility and impulsivity. She commenced stimulant medication for her ADHD and developed better organization, task completion and interest in work, and neater handwriting. She began to feel that she was much closer to reaching her academic potential.

Behaviour management

Behaviour management programmes use a structured setting to promote behavioural control, reinforcing appropriate behaviours and reducing negative behaviours with specific strategies. Emphasis should be on antecedent support and control, rather than on consequences, i.e. anticipation of the difficulties and plan/teach to avoid (Table 4.3.5).

In the classroom, additional techniques include seating the child close to the teacher, breaking tasks down into small units, frequent exercise breaks (preferably productive and responsible, e.g. taking a message to the office), structured teaching materials adapted to the child's needs, and unrelenting positive encouragement.

Behavioural therapies are particularly important when conditions such as persistent oppositional behaviour and parent–child discord coexist with ADHD.

Alternative/complementary therapies

A small number of children react to synthetic food colours with severe irritability and restlessness. These children, who are very few in number, are helped by dietary restriction. There is no evidence that a sugar

Table 4.3.5 Behavioural strategies
To reinforce: 'catch 'em being good'; use verbal praise and concrete rewards
• Teach listening skills
• Teach problem solving skills, i.e. 'game plan'
To reduce: ignore unwanted behaviours
• 'Act, don't speak', i.e. clear discipline with minimal reprimands and discussion
• Logical consequences

free diet, megavitamins, sensory integration training or neurofeedback are of therapeutic benefit.

Outcome

Hyperactivity tends to diminish in adolescence, although physical restlessness may continue. Inattention, impulsivity and distractibility can continue into adulthood, although self-understanding and self-regulation improve with developmental, cognitive and emotional maturation. Comorbidities, such as learning difficulties, subtle language disorders and conduct disorders, and associated risk factors, such as family dysfunction and poor educational opportunity, can contribute to adverse outcomes, including poor school retention, a limited vocational outlook and risk-taking behaviours in adolescence and early adulthood.

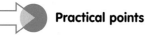

Practical points

- Not all children with hyperactivity and inattention have ADHD
- Genetic and environmental influences contribute to the diagnosis
- Assessment is complex – consider risk factors and comorbidities
- Stimulant medication is safe and effective
- Long-term behavioural, family and educational support is required
- Adverse outcomes in adolescence and early adulthood are common, particularly in association with reading difficulty and aggressive behaviour

Prevention

Externalizing behaviour problems such as hyperactivity, oppositional defiance and aggression are very common in young children, some of whom will go on to a diagnosis of ADHD in the future. Group parenting programmes can help established externalizing behaviour problems by improving nurturing and responsiveness and diminishing harsh discipline. Evidence is now building regarding prevention of externalizing behaviour problems by using effective parenting programmes that start in infancy, raising the possibility of universal prevention in primary care settings.

From the above, it is clear that there are many reasons why children have hyperactive and inattentive behaviours. These behaviours must be interpreted with an understanding of normal development and behaviour, and how these interact with family and community function. When such behaviours are excessive and pervasive, a diagnosis of ADHD may be made, paying attention to causes, risk factors and comorbidities.

Treatment of ADHD is multimodal, with stimulant medications being safe and most effective, but adjunctive behavioural management and family support are essential. Understanding and adjustment in the school setting, with appropriate educational support, are paramount for the child's long-term psychological health.

Universal prevention and targeted early intervention of externalizing behaviour problems may help more children to start school with better self-regulation and capacity to learn, both academically and socially.

Major psychiatric disorders 4.4

B. Nurcombe

The major psychiatric disorders are characterized by relatively specific symptomatology and severe impairment of social, educational and recreational functioning. The primary care physician's role in the management of these disorders is to recognize them as early as possible, assess the patient for risk of harm, refer the family for psychiatric evaluation, collaborate in shared care treatment and ensure that the patient's general health is maintained.

The following symptoms should alert the primary physician to the possibility of a serious psychiatric disorder:

- Infancy and early childhood:
  - failure to thrive without physical cause
  - rumination (i.e. regurgitation, chewing and spillage of gastric contents)
  - delay in spoken language
  - failure to respond normally to parental physical contact or voice
  - stereotyped, repetitive movements (e.g. hand flapping)
- Middle childhood:
  - severe, persistent oppositional behaviour, aggressiveness or impulsive temper
  - persistent stealing
  - developmentally inappropriate sexual behaviour
  - persistent fire setting
  - cruelty to animals
  - truancy
  - unexplained absences from school
  - persistent unexplained physical symptoms (e.g. abdominal or limb pain)
  - severe, persistent separation anxiety (e.g. on leaving home to go to school)
  - failure to speak outside the home
  - obsessions and compulsions
  - persistent depressive or irritable mood
  - deterioration in school performance
  - failure to make friends, solitary interests
- Adolescence:
  - unexplained loss of weight, uncontrolled dieting
  - secretive bingeing and vomiting
  - deterioration in school performance

- social withdrawal and cessation of sporting/recreational activities
- disorganized thought processes, hallucinations, delusions
- persistent or recurrent depressive mood
- suicidal ideation or attempted suicide
- panic attacks
- excessive risk taking, running away from home, sexual promiscuity
- recent gravitation toward 'bad companions'
- unexplained school absences/truancy
- frequent fighting/explosive rage
- persistent unexplained physical symptoms.

The following components of this chapter describe some of the major psychiatric disorders that may occur at various ages in childhood and adolescence.

Practical points

The role of the primary care physician
- Recognize as early as possible the signs of a major psychiatric disorder
- Exclude as quickly as possible non-psychiatric causes of the symptoms
- Refer as soon as possible to psychiatric consultant
- Explain the nature of the problem and the reason for referral to the patient and family
- Collaborate with the psychiatrist in the shared extended care of the patient
- Support the patient and family in adhering to the treatment plan
- Maintain the patient's general health

Infancy and early childhood

Reactive attachment disorders

This group of disorders is associated with deficiency in the infant's capacity to elicit care, or impairment in the caregiver's emotional responsiveness, or a combination of both. Typically, the infant fails to initiate or to respond appropriately to social interaction, exhibiting social withdrawal, inhibition, avoidance or heedlessness and a superficial, undiscriminating sociability.

Often, as a result of depression, psychosis, personality disorder or severe psychosocial stress, the parent has failed to attend to the infant's basic needs for affection, contact comfort and stimulation, or there have been so many changes of caregiver that the infant has not been able to develop a stable attachment. In severe reactive attachment disorder, the infant's physical development (height, weight, head circumference) slows or stops, a condition known as non-organic failure to thrive. Attachment disorder should be distinguished from pervasive developmental disorder, intellectual retardation and developmental language disorder. Non-organic failure to thrive should be differentiated from physical causes of failure to thrive (Ch. 3.7).

Psychosocial dwarfism is usually encountered in children from 18 months to 7 years of age. It is associated with physical and intellectual growth failure, reversible neuroendocrine dysfunction and bizarre eating patterns (e.g. polyphagia, food hoarding). Typically, after hospitalization, the child gains weight dramatically only to stall after returning home. The prognosis for intellectual and social development is poor unless adequate surrogate care is provided or the primary caregiver's parental capacity can be addressed.

Rumination involves the persistent, repeated regurgitation, chewing and spilling of gastric contents, not due to a gastrointestinal or other medical condition. In infants it is associated with emotional neglect. In older, intellectually retarded children it used to be encountered in circumstances of gross institutional neglect. Rumination may be so severe as to lead to inanition and death. In infants, the treatment is to provide consistent contact comfort, with holding, rocking, eye contact and soothing vocalizations. In older children, behavioural treatment is required.

Pervasive developmental disorders

This group of conditions is characterized by delay and deviance in intellectual, communicative and social development, together with stereotyped behaviour and circumscribed interests.

Autistic disorder occurs in about 1 in 1000 children, with a male to female ratio of 3 : 1. The features of autistic disorder are provided in Table 4.4.1. The incidence of all *autistic spectrum disorders* may be as much as 3–6/1000 children. In a minority of autistic children, usually the most severely retarded, a physical cause can be diagnosed (e.g. congenital rubella, fragile X syndrome, herpes encephalitis, neurofibromatosis, phenylketonuria, tuberose sclerosis). For other autistic children there is evidence for a genetic causation, probably involving several genes; however, the precise method of genetic transmission is unclear.

The child suspected of autistic disorder should be assessed as follows:

- physical examination
- dental examination
- assessment of hearing and vision
- psychological testing for cognitive level and pattern of intellectual abilities
- speech and language assessment
- laboratory testing and chromosomal examination to exclude known physical causes of the autistic syndrome
- electroencephalography.

Autistic disorder should be differentiated from:

- developmental language disorder
- intellectual retardation
- sensory impairment (e.g. deafness)
- selective mutism (see below)
- severe psychosocial deprivation
- childhood schizophrenia
- other types of pervasive developmental disorder (see below).

> **Practical points**

Reactive attachment disorder
- Caused by defect in infant's capacity to elicit parental care and/or by failure of the parent to provide adequate or consistent care
- Reflected in the infant's failure to initiate or respond to social contact
- Can lead to stunting of physical or intellectual growth
- Must be differentiated from organic failure to thrive
- Treatment involves the provision of adequate surrogate parental care while the mother/child unit is treated

---

Table 4.4.1   Clinical features of autistic disorder

- Marked impairment of eye-to-eye gaze and communicative gestures
- Failure to develop peer relationships
- Lack of socioemotional reciprocity
- Impaired capacity for joint attention
- Incapacity for make-believe play
- Failure to imitate others
- Delay of language development
- Unusual use of language (e.g. for self-enchantment rather than communication)
- Stereotyped, restricted interests and rituals
- Motor mannerisms (e.g. finger flicking or hand flapping).

Although many parents become concerned that their child is abnormal by the time s/he is 6–12 months of age, autistic disorder is often not diagnosed until much later in childhood. This is regrettable because the earlier the diagnosis, the sooner effective treatment can be provided. In a minority of cases, the child is described as developing normally at first, only to regress into an autistic state when 2 or 3 years old.

Clinical example

Jerry, aged 4 years, had been referred by his mother because his preschool teacher was concerned about his poor language and lack of interest in other children. His mother said that Jerry had always been 'different'. He did not seek or give affection. He did not play properly with his toys but preferred to line them up or watch them falling, one by one, off a table. If anyone interrupted this game, he would scream. He was fascinated by light switches and electric fans, and liked to parrot television commercials. Jerry avoided looking at people by averting his gaze to one side. He did not respond to the doctor's questions. At one point, he suddenly became upset and began to run around the office on tiptoes, flicking his fingertips. He was referred to a developmental paediatrician for a full diagnostic workup.

The best predictors of outcome are IQ and the presence of functional speech at 5 years of age. Epilepsy occurs in about 20%, usually in adolescence. Treatment is multidisciplinary and involves habit training, social reinforcement, the alleviation of avoidant, stereotyped behaviour and the promotion of communicative development. There is evidence that early intervention, commencing in the second or third year of life, can be effective in promoting language and social development. Pharmacotherapy has a limited role, and is of use mainly in children who exhibit severe hyperactivity, aggressiveness or self-harm.

Parents are not usually concerned about children with *Asperger disorder* until the child is 2–4 years old. By middle childhood, the child exhibits the following characteristics:

- impairment of non-verbal communication (e.g. impaired eye contact, lack of facial expression and gesture, and monotonous vocal intonation but intact language development otherwise)
- average intelligence or above
- lack of interest in peer relationships
- lack of social reciprocity, shared enjoyment and humour

- circumscribed interests (e.g. computer games) and inflexible routines
- mannerisms (e.g. hand flapping) and motor clumsiness.

It is unclear whether Asperger disorder is a variant of, or different from, autistic disorder and whether it is distinct from non-verbal language disability, semantic pragmatic processing disorder and schizoid personality disorder. Because of uncertainty about the boundaries of this condition, its prevalence is unclear, perhaps 1–2/10 000, with a 9:1 ratio in favour of males. By adolescence, many children with this condition become frustrated by their lack of friends and the teasing or social rejection to which they are prone. Treatment involves social–cognitive language programming in the educational mainstream. As adults, people with Asperger disorder are more effective in jobs that make few social demands.

Middle childhood

Disruptive behaviour disorder

Oppositional defiant disorder and *attention deficit disorder* are described in Chapters 4.2 and 4.3. *Conduct disorder* refers to a group of children characterized by some or all of the features listed in Table 4.4.2.

Conduct disorder can emerge first in adolescence but the more serious kinds of conduct disorder evolve in middle childhood from earlier oppositional defiant behaviour. A recent study has found a prevalence of 3% in Australian children and adolescents, with a male to female ratio of about 3:1. Conduct disorder is commonly associated with other problems, particularly attention deficit disorder (Ch. 4.3), alcohol and substance use disorder, mood disorder, post-traumatic stress disorder and learning disorder.

The genetic background of conduct disorder is unclear, but twin and adoption studies suggest that there is an inherited component. Other risk factors

Table 4.4.2 Features of conduct disorder

- Persistently aggressive behaviour (bullying, intimidation, frequent fighting, cruelty, coercive sexual behaviour, use of a weapon)
- Destructiveness (fire setting, vandalism)
- Deceitfulness (breaking and entering, stealing, lying, trickery)
- Rule violation (truancy, staying out late at night, running away from home, refusal to accept rules at home or school).

form a cumulative, sequential developmental cascade, as follows:

- maternal smoking during pregnancy
- difficult infant temperament
- early parental neglect with disruption of infant attachment
- callousness and an impaired capacity for empathy with others
- coercive, inconsistent parental discipline
- exposure to parental antisocial behaviour, domestic violence or substance abuse
- coaching by parents who promote violent behaviour
- exposure to physical or sexual abuse
- growing up in a marginalized, socially disadvantaged environment
- minority group status
- relatively impaired verbal intelligence
- learning problems
- the mindset that other people will be hostile, rejecting or unfair to one
- gravitation toward like-minded antiauthoritarian companions
- truancy
- early initiation into smoking, sexual activity and alcohol or drug taking.

If conduct problems do not first appear until adolescence, and few of the above risk factors are operative, the individual will probably not go on to become antisocial as an adult. When behaviour problems begin at an early age and many of the cumulative risk factors apply, it is more likely that the individual will become an adult criminal.

Children with conduct problems are usually referred for evaluation during late childhood or adolescence. It would be preferable if this serious disorder could be detected and treated earlier. The combination of early educational intervention with parenting programmes (e.g. triple-P) designed to alter coercive child rearing holds promise.

Until the last 10 years, no intervention programmes had been found to be effective for older children. Recently, multisystemic therapy involving goal-directed strategic/behavioural family therapy aimed at promoting effective parenting, along with individual counselling and environmental intervention, has produced good results. The placement of offenders in therapeutic foster homes has also shown promise. In foster home programmes, the house parents are trained to be firm and consistent in their discipline and to ensure that the adolescent does not mix with antisocial peers. It is ineffective to treat children who have conduct disorder in community or institutional groups composed of like-minded peers.

Anxiety disorders

Separation anxiety disorder is described in Chapter 4.2. *Generalized anxiety disorder* is characterized by persistent, excessive worrying about life events (e.g. school performance, clothes, dating) accompanied by physical symptoms (e.g. abdominal pains, headaches, fatigue, diarrhoea, urinary frequency). Children with this disorder are likely to have been behaviourally inhibited as preschoolers and to have a parent with anxiety disorder. Generalized anxiety disorder overlaps with *social phobia*, in which the child is particularly fearful of performance situations that incur the scrutiny of others (e.g. reading in front of the class, going to the toilet away from home, athletic competition).

Panic disorder involves repeated attacks of sudden, disabling anxiety, often without any apparent precipitant, associated with the physiological concomitants of anxiety (e.g. hyperventilation, racing heart, cold sweaty hands, choking sensations, dizziness, fainting, fear of dying). The onset of panic disorder is most often in mid-adolescence; it is rare in middle childhood. *Selective mutism* is probably a variant of social phobia. In this condition, the child, more often a girl, fails to speak in social situations outside the home or to strangers. The average age of onset is 2–5 years. In about 30% of cases there has been a premorbid speech or language problem. Selective mutism should be differentiated from deafness, intellectual disability, developmental language disorder, aphonia and the inability of a migrant child to understand English.

Anxiety disorders frequently coincide with attention deficit disorder and depressive disorder. Anxiety disorders are often familial, but without specificity as to type. Whereas behavioural inhibition (which may precede anxiety disorder) has a genetic component, parental anxiety (especially separation or social anxiety) is highly contagious. Treatment, therefore, must involve the parents.

Obsessive compulsive disorder has the features listed in Table 4.4.3.

Obsessive compulsive disorder has a 6-month prevalence of 0.5–1%. The onset is usually between 6 and 11 years, with bimodal peaks. The male to female ratio is probably equal, although males predominate in the younger age group. Neuroimaging, neuropsychological and genetic studies support the concept that the disorder is neuropsychiatric in nature and possibly related to a single major gene superimposed on multiple genes of minor effect. A subgroup of patients may have sustained an autoimmune reaction between caudate nucleus neurones and antibodies to beta-haemolytic streptococci. Obsessive compulsive disorder should be distinguished from:

Table 4.4.3	Features of obsessive compulsive disorder

- Recurrent, distressing thoughts about such matters as germs, contamination or harming the self or others, or preoccupation with excessive moralization or religiosity (obsessions)
- Recurrent distressing rituals involving excessive washing, repeating, checking, touching, counting or ordering (compulsions)
- These thoughts or actions are regarded by the patient as abnormal and are resisted, but the patient is forced to continue to think thus, or to continue the actions
- Symptom exacerbation in times of stress (e.g. starting at a new school)
- Impairment of functioning (e.g. completing chores, getting ready for bed, finishing schoolwork, relating to other family members)

Table 4.4.4	Symptoms of major depressive disorder

- Persistent depressed or irritable mood
- Feelings of worthlessness and hopelessness
- Suicidal ideation
- Loss of pleasure in activities that were formerly enjoyed
- Social withdrawal and cessation of sporting and recreational activities
- Insomnia or hypersomnia
- Loss or gain of weight
- Loss of concentration and deterioration in school performance
- Lack of energy, ready fatigue.

- transient benign habits and rituals such as 'not stepping on the crack' (no impairment)
- the worries associated with generalized anxiety disorder (in which the worries are about daily events)
- Tourette disorder (associated with tics)
- Pervasive developmental disorder (in which the rituals are not distressing and there is marked social impairment).

Obsessive compulsive disorder is commonly comorbid with other anxiety disorders, mood disorder, tic disorder and disruptive behaviour disorders. Obsessive compulsive disorder often persists into adulthood.

Clinical example

Barbara's mother reported that she was worried because Barbara, aged 10 years, had begun to behave in an odd manner. She would touch doorknobs again and again, and spent ages getting to bed because she had to arrange her teddy bears just so around her pillows and at the foot of the bed. She had reluctantly admitted to her mother that she arranged the teddy bears in that way in order to ward off aliens who might abduct her at night. She would wriggle her toes and clench her jaw in a special way but did not know why she did so. When she tried to resist wriggling her toes, she became very anxious and had to give in and do it. Barbara was referred to a psychiatrist, who confirmed that Barbara had obsessive compulsive disorder. She was started on sertraline and referred to a clinical psychologist for behaviour therapy.

Anxiolytic drugs (e.g. benzodiazepines) should be avoided in the treatment of anxiety disorders because there is no evidence that they are effective, and they have addictive and sedative potential. The most effective treatment is a combination of relaxation training, systematic desensitization and cognitive behaviour therapy. Since parental anxiety is commonly associated with childhood anxiety disorder, family therapy is always indicated.

In obsessive compulsive disorder, cognitive behaviour therapy involving exposure to anxiety provoking situations, systematic desensitization and the prevention of compulsive responses to anxiety-provoking stimuli has been found to be effective. Behavioural treatment is the treatment of choice in this disorder, although clomipramine (a tricyclic antidepressant) and serotonin-specific reuptake inhibitors are effective and well tolerated. Family therapy is aimed at educating the family and disentangling the parents from the child's rituals.

Adolescence

Major depressive disorder

Although there is no doubt that children can feel sad, it is not clear that they can develop a true major depressive disorder. There is better evidence for the validity of this diagnosis in adolescence. The characteristic symptoms of major depressive disorder are listed in Table 4.4.4.

Depressive symptoms are commonly associated with anxiety, conduct problems, post-traumatic symptomatology, eating disorder, learning disability, substance abuse and school refusal. A recent Australian population survey found the 6-month prevalence of depression to be 3% in childhood and adolescence. Typically, there is an increased prevalence of depression in the families of depressed children. However, the genetic background of the disorder is still unclear, as is the nature of the interaction between genetic propensity and the adverse life events that often precede depressive episodes.

The clinician should be alerted to the possibility of depression whenever school performance inexplicably drops or there is a change in mood, control of temper, social involvement or sleep patterns. Information is needed from both parent and child with regard to the clinical features of the case and the psychosocial stressors that have affected and are affecting the patient. In less serious cases, individual and family counselling can be effective. In more serious cases, the child should be assessed for risk of suicide (Ch. 4.2) and, if appropriate, admitted to hospital.

Treatment should be individualized and goal directed. Cognitive behavioural therapy, psychodynamic therapy, interpersonal psychotherapy and family therapy may be required separately, or in various combinations. There is no evidence that tricyclic or heterocyclic antidepressant drugs are effective in child/adolescent major depression. Furthermore, they can have serious side effects and may be lethal in suicide attempts. There is evidence for the efficacy of serotonin specific reuptake inhibitors, but there has been recent concern about a connection between this kind of medication and suicidal ideation. Although most depressed adolescents recover from depression within a year, many relapse, and the risk of subsequent episodes continues into adulthood.

Bipolar disorder

There is controversy over the validity of the diagnosis of bipolar disorder in childhood, and its prevalence. It is not clear whether some cases of apparent attention deficit hyperactivity disorder are really suffering from a form of mania, or whether attention deficit/hyperactivity disorder can be a precursor of bipolar disorder. It is clear, on the other hand, that bipolar disorder is underdiagnosed in adolescence and that it is often confused with schizophrenia at that time.

In bipolar I disorder, the patient has experienced at least one manic or mixed manic–depressive episode. In bipolar II disorder, the patient has experienced at least one episode of both major depression and hypomania, but no manic or mixed episodes. Mania is characterized by the following symptoms:

- abnormally elevated or irritable mood persisting for at least 1 week
- grandiose thinking
- pressured speech, racing thoughts and distractibility
- increased activity and recklessness
- marked deterioration in functioning at school, with peers and at home.

Hypomania is characterized by similar but less intense symptoms and less functional deterioration. In a mixed episode, manic and major depressive symptoms coincide. Adolescents with mania often have hallucinations, paranoid ideas and marked lability of mood, causing the aforementioned diagnostic confusion with schizophrenia. The risk of suicide is increased in bipolar disorder, especially during depressive phases.

Bipolar disorder is familial but the mode of genetic transmission has not been elucidated. Bipolar disorder should be differentiated from schizophrenia, major depression with agitation, post-traumatic stress disorder, disruptive behaviour disorder and disorder of mood or delirium secondary to a medical condition (e.g. hyperthyroidism, porphyria) or intoxication with illicit or prescribed drugs (e.g. amphetamines, phencyclidine). The treatment of bipolar disorder is primarily pharmacological. The drug of choice is lithium, the blood levels and side effects of which must be monitored closely. Valproate and carbamazepine may be preferred if the patient's family is chaotic or unreliable. The relapse rate may be reduced if the patient remains on lithium throughout

---

Clinical example

Bill, aged 14 years, was referred by his mother because the school had become concerned about his surliness, rebelliousness and tendency to submit class assignments with macabre content. His mother said that Bill would do nothing to help her at home and that he spent most of his time in his bedroom listening to 'heavy metal' rock music. Bill's father had left her and the four children several years before to live in a distant city and start a new family. Bill presented as a slim adolescent, dressed all in black, with close-cropped hair and a nose ring. After initially sparring verbally, he admitted that he hated his life. He said that he slept poorly and was too tired to concentrate in school. He had recently begun to smoke marijuana. He had no friends he could rely on except, maybe, 'potheads'. He reported that he thought often about committing suicide, probably by jumping from a bridge. A mood disorder was diagnosed and Bill was referred for psychiatric evaluation.

Practical points

Depressive disorder

- Presents in adolescence with physical symptoms, irritability, social withdrawal, deterioration in school performance
- Have a high index of suspicion for this disorder because of the potential for suicide
- Usually associated with environmental stress (e.g. parental divorce, abuse) or loss
- Refer early if condition severe or if patient is suicidal
- Psychotherapy is effective for mild/moderate depression
- Specific serotonin receptor inhibitor medication should be used only in moderate/severe cases

adolescence. Recently, atypical neuroleptics such as risperidone have been used, with promising results.

Schizophrenia

Although schizophrenia can occur in preadolescence, it is rare at that time. It is predominantly a disorder of late adolescence and early adulthood. Schizophrenia is a neurodevelopmental disease, foreshadowed, in many cases, by delayed developmental milestones and impaired development of language and cognition. Common prodromal symptoms are:

- social isolation or withdrawal
- deterioration in functioning at home, at school, and in grooming and personal hygiene
- lack of energy
- hypersomnia
- inappropriate or dulled affect
- unexplained panic
- disorganized, vague conversation with poverty of content
- odd, overvalued beliefs (e.g. of telepathy), rituals or magical thinking
- unusual perceptual experiences (e.g. that the body or face is changing, feelings of unreality, fear of losing control).

The following symptoms are typical after the onset of schizophrenia:

- hallucinations (most commonly auditory)
- delusions (e.g. of persecution, thought insertion, thought loss)
- thought disorder with disorganized or incoherent conversation
- disorganized behaviour (e.g. posturing, catatonic stiffness, agitation)
- flattening of affect, poverty of speech, anergia.

Schizophrenia is a familial disorder with a complex mode of genetic transmission and variable expressivity, operating according to a multifactorial threshold or mixed model of transmission. Schizophrenia should be differentiated from:

- mood disorder (especially bipolar I disorder)
- psychosis due to medical disease (e.g. epilepsy, brain tumour, porphyria, acquired immune deficiency syndrome (AIDS)) or substance abuse (e.g. stimulants, cocaine, hallucinogens, phencyclidine)
- other psychoses (complex post-traumatic stress disorder with dissociative hallucinations, schizophreniform disorder).

Acute schizophrenia conveys a risk of suicide or self endangerment. Acute cases should be hospitalized for diagnosis and stabilization. Patients are usually treated initially with a rapidly acting neuroleptic such as haloperidol. Most patients do not respond to medication until 2–4 weeks have elapsed. The newer ('atypical') antipsychotic drugs (such as clozapine, risperidone, olanzapine and quetiapine) are associated with relatively few side effects other than weight gain, sedation and, in some cases, sexual dysfunction. Psychoeducation for parents is essential in order to foster compliance and independent living skills, and to counteract the high levels of emotional expression between family members that increase the likelihood of relapse. Liaison with the school is necessary. A poor prognosis is associated with early or insidious onset, low socioeconomic status, family history of schizophrenia, absence of precipitating stress and severe negative symptoms.

Clinical example

Annabelle, aged 15 years, had always been an emotionally fragile child who tended to have intense, dependent relationships with her peers. However, recently she had become withdrawn and self absorbed, telling her mother that she wanted to drop out of school and pursue religious studies. At interview, she was fearful and apparently distracted. She asked whether the interview was being videotaped. After some time she revealed that she had been 'chosen' to do something very important in the world. She had become aware of this as a result of a revelation, one day recently, when the earth shone and she 'knew' her destiny. Her conversation meandered and was often difficult to follow. Several times during the interview she stopped talking and smiled to herself. Physical examination was normal. Annabelle was referred to a psychiatrist who confirmed the diagnosis of schizophrenia, admitted Annabelle to hospital and commenced antipsychotic medication. After Annabelle's discharge, her medication was monitored by her family doctor, and appointments were made for her to see the psychiatrist every 6 weeks.

Post-traumatic stress disorder

Post-traumatic stress disorder occurs in response to the personal experience of overwhelming, terrifying, potentially lethal stress directed toward the child or someone with whom the child has a close attachment. In childhood and adolescence, the commonest kinds of threat causing post-traumatic stress disorder are motor vehicle accidents, burn injury, natural or man-made disasters, animal attack, criminal assault, observation of parental homicide or suicide, and war.

A particularly pathogenic stress or threat involves repeated exposure to coercive intrafamilial physical or sexual abuse when the child is unable to disclose or escape the abuse and when, after disclosure, the non-abusive caregiver fails to provide adequate support. The clinical features of post-traumatic stress disorder in childhood are very similar to those in adulthood:

- persistent intrusive imagery concerning the traumatic event
- repetitious play representing the event
- generalized nightmares and trauma nightmares
- the conviction that one is destined for an early death and that there were omens before the trauma
- avoidance of things, people or situations that remind one of the event
- persistent autonomic arousal with an exaggerated startle response.

When post-traumatic stress disorder is caused by repeated physical or sexual abuse, dissociative symptoms are likely to be manifested, e.g.:

- amnesia for all or part of the event or events
- vagueness, daydreaming and the sense of being estranged from others
- trance-like states
- audiovisual hallucinations that represent fragmentary memories of the abuse
- bodily symptoms (such as pseudoseizures or pelvic pain) that represent somatic memories of the abuse.

Post-traumatic stress disorder is likely to be comorbid with, or to be succeeded by:

- mood disorder
- anxiety disorder
- hyperactivity
- alcohol/drug use
- dissociative and somatoform disorders
- intermittent explosive disorder
- borderline personality disorder.

Recent clinical research suggests that children under the age at which sequential, narrative, autobiographical memory can be encoded and recounted (i.e. below 3 years of age) can also manifest a form of post-traumatic stress disorder. The outcome of acute stress is affected adversely if the child is separated from parents, if the parents die, if the parents develop psychiatric symptoms (especially post-traumatic stress disorder) or if there is a contagion of symptoms between children.

After civilian catastrophes, family reunification and assistance with shelter and physical needs take precedence. Group debriefing of affected children has been recommended, but its efficacy is uncertain. Only those children who continue to manifest symptoms after 1 month should be referred for individual treatment. In post-traumatic stress disorder associ-ated with child maltreatment, cognitive behaviour therapy and family therapy have proved helpful. If medication is required, serotonin-specific reuptake inhibitors such as sertraline may be useful in alleviating hyperarousal.

Somatoform disorders

This group of disorders is characterized by physical symptoms that suggest an underlying physical disease but for which either no such basis can be found, or the symptoms are disproportionate in intensity or duration to a known physical disorder. *Somatization disorder* and *hypochondriasis* involve the conviction that physical symptoms have a physical cause and the tendency to present repeatedly for medical care even though no physical cause can be found. The commonest presentations are abdominal pain, headaches or fatigue and muscle weakness. This kind of problem is generally associated with other family psychopathology such as parental anxiety, depression or somatization, and may be based on the parent's conviction that the child has a physical disease such as chronic fatigue syndrome. It is frequently encountered in sexually abused children.

In *conversion disorder* the dramatic symptoms suggest a physical disease but no such disease can be found and the symptoms are distributed or displayed in accordance with a naive view of bodily functioning (e.g. glove and stocking anaesthesia). The commonest conversion symptoms are paralysis, paresis, seizures, anaesthesia, paraesthesia, vomiting, aphonia, headaches, blindness and deafness. Conversion disorder typically follows or accompanies a severe psychosocial stress such as sexual abuse, bereavement or family conflict.

The prevalence of somatoform disorders is probably high. They are closely related to the emotional climate of the family and to parental psychopathology. The primary physician should investigate thoroughly to rule out organic pathology, avoiding interminable testing lest the symptoms become chronic and irreversible. Psychiatric consultation should be sought as early as possible. In conversion disorder, once the hidden stressor is disclosed, symptoms usually dissipate with suggestive therapy such as graduated exercises. In somatization syndromes, the family can be helped to interpret the symptoms as signs of stress and to manage stress, for example with relaxation exercises.

Eating disorders

Anorexia nervosa is characterized by:

- an intense fear of becoming fat or losing control of eating

- a relentless pursuit of thinness
- secretive food refusal, dieting and exercise causing marked loss of weight (below 85% of weight expected)
- the perception of being overweight despite extreme thinness
- amenorrhoea.

Bulimia nervosa is characterized by:

- binge eating with a sense of loss of control
- self-induced vomiting
- the use of dieting, laxatives, diuretics, enemas and exercise to control or reverse weight gain.

Both eating disorders are much more common in girls than in boys; ballet dancers, gymnasts and fashion models are particularly at risk. The prevalence of these conditions has increased greatly during the last 30 years, possibly because of the publicity given in the media to tall, slim fashion models. In the 15–25-year-old group, bulimia is more common than anorexia nervosa. The onset of anorexia occurs in two peaks: early and late adolescence. Bulimia usually begins in late adolescence and may be a sequel of earlier anorexia nervosa.

The adolescent who develops anorexia nervosa is likely to have been a compliant, conscientious child who had an enmeshed relationship with her mother. Secretive dieting and exercise often begin after a minor precipitant, such as being told that one is overweight. The child hides the amount of weight loss from her parents. Menses cease. The child becomes moody, irritable and withdrawn. Eventually, the physical signs of starvation appear:

- emaciated facies and body
- fine body hair growth
- dry hair
- cold hands
- slow pulse
- low blood pressure.

The child resists medical help and is unable to appreciate how emaciated she has become.

The adolescent with bulimia nervosa has dramatic weight fluctuations and develops swollen salivary glands, abraded knuckles and dental caries. Eventually, as a result of chronic metabolic alkalosis, kidney function may be compromised.

Eating disorders are best conceptualized as the product of family psychopathology expressed as eating disorder in one family member. Excessive dieting may represent the pursuit of an idealized body image and self-control by a child who perceives herself as helpless to direct her own life. The retching of the bulimic adolescent reflects the self-loathing and self-harm associated with chronic depression and guilt.

Eating disorders must be differentiated from other disorders that can cause weight loss, e.g. malabsorption disorders, chronic infection, occult malignancy, substance abuse, chronic depression, paranoid schizophrenia and psychogenic vomiting.

Hospitalization and paediatric/psychiatric collaboration are required if the patient is metabolically unstable, as evidenced by dehydration, inanition, electrolyte imbalance, bradycardia and low blood pressure, if she resists treatment or if outpatient treatment has failed. Nasogastric feeding is required in extreme cases. The patient is not discharged from hospital until a reasonable target weight is attained. Treatment plans should be individualized and goal-directed. Anorectic patients respond best to a combination of family therapy and psychodynamic psychotherapy. Bulimic patients, who are usually older, generally respond best to cognitive behaviour therapy. Long-term follow-up studies have revealed that about 50% of anorectics recover, 25% have chronic anorexia nervosa and 25% have other psychiatric disorders. There is a significant mortality. Recovery is uncommon after 12 years of anorexia nervosa. The outcome of bulimia nervosa has not been studied.

> ### Practical points
>
> **Eating disorder**
> - Adolescents with eating disorders are skilled in their ability to conceal loss of weight and failure to eat
> - Exclude other causes of weight loss as soon as possible
> - Hospitalize if the child is metabolically unstable (electrolytes, heart rate, blood pressure, dehydration)
> - Otherwise, the child should be treated as an outpatient with family and individual psychotherapy
> - The older the patient, the worse the prognosis

PART 5

PAEDIATRIC EMERGENCIES

Paediatric emergencies: causes and assessment 5.1

J. Raftos

There are many causes of collapse leading to the need for emergency medical intervention in the child. Table 5.1.1 lists some of the causes of common paediatric emergencies.

The following information outlines the requirements for early assessment and reassessment in paediatric emergencies. Details of the emergency care of the collapsed child are provided in the subsequent chapter.

In approaching the critically ill child, the diagnosis is of secondary importance to:

- *primary assessment*, which is a structured activity, and
- *timely resuscitation procedures.*

The *primary assessment*, sometimes also known as the primary survey, follows progression through the following A, B, C, D, E steps:

- **A**irway
- **B**reathing
- **C**irculation
- **D**isability (deficiency of cerebral function), with attention to
- **E**xposure.

This structured approach is based on the knowledge that the brain requires a continual supply of its two main metabolites: oxygen and glucose. An airway problem, by depriving the brain of its oxygen supply, will rapidly lead to death and therefore must be corrected first. A breathing problem preventing oxygen moving into the lung and carbon dioxide out of the lung is the next priority. A circulatory problem preventing the oxygen being carried to the brain is next, and so on.

The resuscitation measures required and management of the collapsed child are described in detail in Chapter 5.2.

The primary assessment

Airway

The child and infant airways, compared with those of the adult, present particular anatomical and physiological differences that increase their susceptibility to compromise. Infants are obligate nose-breathers. Infants and small children have smaller airways and a smaller mandible, a proportionately larger tongue and more floppy epiglottis and soft palate. The narrowest portion of their airway is below the cords at the level of the cricoid ring, in contrast to adults, where the narrowest portion is at the level of the vocal cords. The trachea is short and soft and hyperextension or flexion of the neck may cause obstruction.

Ensuring that the patient has a patent airway is of the highest priority. In evaluating the airway a look, listen and feel approach is used.

Movement of the chest wall and the abdomen should be carefully looked for. The degree to which intercostal and other accessory muscles are being used to overcome obstruction should be noted. Paradoxical movement of the abdomen may be noted if there is upper airway obstruction.

Listening over the mouth and nose for air movement should follow. Particular note should be made of inspiratory stridor, which is a sign of tracheal, laryngeal or other upper airway obstruction. In severe obstruction, expiratory sounds may also be heard but inspiratory noises will still predominate. A stethoscope should be used to listen over the trachea and in the axillae for air movement.

Finally the examiner, by placing his or her face close to the child's mouth, may feel evidence of air movement.

Breathing

In childhood, conditions that result in respiratory compromise are the most common reason for emergency intervention and are the major cause of a poor outcome.

As with the airway, there are important differences between the child and the adult. Children have a higher metabolic requirement. They have more immature musculature, with easy fatigability of the diaphragm, which is the major muscle of respiration. The chest wall is more compliant and the ribs are more horizontal, decreasing the efficiency of the bellows effect.

The airways in the child are proportionately smaller and therefore produce an increased resis-

Table 5.1.1   Causes of paediatric emergencies

Airway	Breathing	Circulation	Disability	Exposure
Croup	Asthma	Congenital heart disease	Seizure	Hypothermia
Epiglottitis	Bronchiolitis	Duct dependent lesions:	Meningitis	Hyperthermia
Laryngeal foreign body	Pneumonia	Critical aortic stenosis	Encephalitis	Inflicted injury
Bacterial tracheitis	Foreign body	Hypoplastic left heart	Head injury	
Trauma	Congestive heart failure	Coarctation	Raised intracranial	
Angioneurotic oedema	Neuromuscular diseases	Dysrhythmias:	pressure	
Retropharyngeal	Trauma:	Bradycardia	Hypoglycaemia	
abscess	Pneumothorax	Tachycardia	Metabolic disorder	
	Haemothorax	Supraventricular	Poisoning	
	Lung contusion	Ventricular	Envenomation	
	Flail chest	Torsade de pointes		
	Near drowning	Fibrillation		
	Smoke inhalation	Pulseless electrical activity		
	Metabolic acidosis:	Shock:		
	Diabetic ketoacidosis	Cardiogenic		
	Poisoning	Cardiomyopathy		
	Salicylates	Heart failure		
	Methanol	Myocardial contusion		
		Hypovolaemic		
		Haemorrhage		
		Vomiting/diarrhoea		
		Burns		
		Distributive		
		Septicaemia		
		Anaphylaxis		
		Spinal cord injury		
		Obstructive		
		Cardiac tamponade		
		Hypertension		
		Dissociative		

tance to air flow, especially when traumatized or inflamed. Resistance across an airway is inversely proportional to the fourth power of the radius:

$$R = 1/r^4.$$

Thus, halving the radius increases the resistance very significantly.

Having established patency of the airway, evaluation for the presence and adequacy of breathing should follow. It is helpful to divide this into three aspects:

- effort of breathing
- efficacy of breathing
- effects of respiratory inadequacy on other organs.

Effort of breathing

Respiratory rate is age-dependent (Table 5.1.2). Tachypnoea is an early response to respiratory failure. Increased depth of respiration may occur later as respiratory failure progresses. However, it should be noted that tachypnoea does not always have a respiratory cause and may occur in response, for example, to metabolic acidosis. As the intercostal muscles and diaphragm increase their contraction, intercostal and subcostal recession develop. In the infant, sternal retraction may also occur.

The ribs are horizontal in young children. This reduces the 'bellows' effect that the intercostal muscles give to the adult. In the child the sternomastoid muscles must be recruited to further raise the ribs to increase ventilation.

In infants and small children, flaring of the alae nasi may be seen. It must be remembered that, in this age group, 50% of airway resistance occurs in the upper airway and flaring is an attempt to reduce this resistance. This is a late sign and is indicative of severe respiratory distress.

The effort of breathing is diminished in three clinical circumstances. These must be recognized, as urgent intervention may be required. Firstly, exhaustion may develop as a result of the increased respira-

Table 5.1.2 Vital signs by age			
Age (years)	Respiratory rate (breaths/min)	Heart rate (beats/min)	Systolic blood pressure (mmHg)
<1	30–40	110–160	70–90
1–2	25–35	100–150	80–95
2–5	25–30	95–140	80–100
5–12	20–25	80–120	90–110
>12	15–20	60–100	100–120

tory demands. The younger child is even more prone to this due to more immature musculature. Secondly, respiration requires an intact central respiratory drive centre. Conditions such as trauma, meningitis and poisoning may depress this centre. Thirdly, neuromuscular conditions that cause paralysis, such as muscular dystrophy and Guillain–Barré syndrome, may result in respiratory failure without increased effort.

Symmetrical movement of the chest should be confirmed. In the younger child the diaphragm is the main muscle of respiration; therefore, one should also look for movement of the upper abdomen.

Inspiratory and expiratory noises should be noted. Wheezing is heard with lower airway narrowing, as in asthma, often with a prolonged expiratory phase. Crepitations may be heard with pneumonia and heart failure.

Efficacy of breathing

Auscultation of both sides of the chest will confirm air movement. Beware the silent chest! Oximetry is useful for providing a measure of arterial oxygen saturation (S_aO_2), which reflects the efficacy of breathing; however, oximetry may be difficult to obtain in the cold or shocked child because of poor perfusion, and is less accurate when the S_aO_2 is less than 70%.

Effects of respiratory inadequacy on other organs

The impact of hypoxia on the cardiovascular system is to cause tachycardia, but preterminally it may cause bradycardia.

Cyanosis is also a preterminal sign. Hypoxia may also cause peripheral shutdown and pallor secondary to sympathetic stimulation. The effect of hypoxia on the brain is to cause initial agitation and irritability in infants, followed by increasing loss of consciousness.

Clinical example

A 1-week-old infant presented after a 3-day illness, cyanosed and with marked tachypnoea. He was severely ill.

In this situation, rapid systematic assessment and resuscitation measures must go hand in hand. The airway and breathing must be assessed first. This infant was breathing fast and was cyanosed. Points that have to be considered urgently are: is there intercostal, sternal or subcostal recession, or use of accessory muscles indicating increased effort of breathing? Are there inspiratory or expiratory noises? Is grunting or flaring of the alae nasi present? Efficacy of breathing needs to be assessed by assessing the degree of chest expansion, breath sounds and oximetry. The effect of respiratory inadequacy can be seen in an increased heart rate, change in skin colour and mental status.

He was found to have a marked increase in effort of breathing, flaring of the alae nasi, bilateral crepitations and tachycardia. In addition to the cyanosis, he was drowsy.

Assessment of the cardiovascular system showed normal pulse volume, capillary return and blood pressure. A search for evidence of heart failure revealed no gallop or heart murmur, no liver enlargement and the presence of femoral pulses.

With high flow oxygen his colour improved, as did his mental status. A diagnosis of severe bronchiolitis was made.

To complete the assessment he was found to have no rash, his initial temperature was 35°C, and with appropriate warming his temperature rapidly reached 36°C.

Circulation

Cardiac output is the product of stroke volume and heart rate. The normal heart rate decreases with age (Table 5.1.2). Infants have a small, relatively fixed cardiac stroke volume; thus they must increase their heart rate to respond to increased demand.

Infants have a relatively larger intravascular volume (85 ml/kg) that decreases with age to 60 ml/kg in the teenager. The normal ranges for blood pressure increase with age (Table 5.1.2 and Ch. 18.2). This is due to the fact that systemic vascular resistance increases as the child gets older.

Assessment of circulation

An increase in heart rate is the earliest response to any reduction in intravascular volume. As shock progresses, bradycardia may develop as a preterminal sign. It is important to assess pulse volume both peripherally and centrally. Weak central pulses indicate severe shock. Capillary refill can be a sensitive indicator of vascular status. To assess this, light pressure should be applied to the skin over the sternum for 5 seconds. In the normal individual, capillary return of blood, seen as a slight flush of the pallid area where pressure was applied, will occur in less than 3 seconds. Caution should be used in interpreting this sign in the child who has been exposed to a cold environment.

In the shocked child, hypotension is a late preterminal sign.

Effects of circulatory inadequacy on other organs

Circulatory inadequacy leads to poor tissue perfusion, which in turn leads to metabolic acidosis. Tachypnoea occurs to compensate for this.

Initial sympathetic stimulation may cause agitation, but later poor cerebral perfusion causes increasing drowsiness and coma in the preterminal phase.

Prerenal failure develops with hypovolaemia and hypotension, with reduction of urine output. Normal urine output is greater than 1 ml/kg/h in the child and greater than 2 ml/kg/h in the infant.

Signs of cardiac failure

The signs of cardiac failure should be sought. Raised jugular venous pulse height is important in the older child but may be difficult to determine in the younger child because of the relatively short, often chubby neck. Listen for a gallop rhythm and for lung crepitations. Palpation of the abdomen may reveal an enlarged liver.

Disability

The assessment of neurological function as part of the primary assessment has three main aims:

- to rapidly determine the level of consciousness
- to find localizing intracranial lesions
- to determine whether there is raised intracranial pressure.

It must be remembered that respiratory and cardiovascular failure can cause decreased consciousness and must be dealt with first.

Conscious level

Conscious level can be rapidly assessed using the AVPU method:

- *A* Alert
- *V* responds to Voice
- *P* responds to Pain
- *U* Unresponsive.

The child who is unresponsive or who only responds to pain has a Glasgow Coma Scale (GCS) score of 8 or less. The GCS has no place in the primary survey but it is a useful tool for monitoring changes in neurological status after initial stabilization (Table 5.1.3).

Posture and tone

Hypotonia may be seen in the seriously ill child no matter what the underlying diagnosis. Hypertonia and posturing should be observed, if present, and any asymmetry noted. Decorticate posturing is evidenced by flexed upper limbs and extended lower limbs, whereas in decerebrate posturing both the upper and lower limbs are extended. These are both preterminal signs and must be acted on immediately.

Pupil size and reactivity

Examination of the pupils can give valuable information. It is important to determine whether there is dilatation, non-reactivity or inequality. Most importantly, unequal pupils may indicate tentorial herniation or a rapidly expanding lesion on one side of the brain. Small, reactive pupils may indicate a metabolic disorder or medullary lesion.

> **Practical points**
>
> - In the collapsed child, a careful and orderly primary assessment and timely resuscitation measures are of more importance than the diagnosis
> - Children differ from adults physiologically and anatomically
> - Conditions affecting respiration are a common pathway to collapse in the child
> - Cyanosis and hypotension are preterminal signs
> - Decerebrate and decorticate posturing are preterminal signs

Table 5.1.3 Glasgow Coma Scale and Children's Coma Scale

Glasgow Coma Scale (4–15 years)		Child's Glasgow Coma Scale (<4 years)	
Response Eye opening	Score	Response Eye opening	Score
Spontaneously	4	Spontaneously	4
To verbal stimuli	3	To verbal stimuli	3
To pain	2	To pain	2
No response to pain	1	No response to pain	1
Best motor response		Best motor response	
Obeys verbal command	6	Spontaneous or obeys verbal command	6
Localizes to pain	5	Localizes to pain or withdraws to touch	5
Withdraws from pain	4	Withdraws from pain	4
Abnormal flexion to pain (decorticate)	3	Abnormal flexion to pain (decorticate)	3
Abnormal extension to pain (decerebrate)	2	Abnormal extension to pain (decerebrate)	2
No response to pain	1	No response to pain	1
Best verbal response		Best verbal response	
Orientated and converses	5	Alert; babbles, coos, words to usual ability	5
Disorientated and converses	4	Less than usual words, spontaneous irritable cry	4
Inappropriate words	3	Cries only to pain	3
Incomprehensible sounds	2	Moans to pain	2
No response to pain	1	No response to pain	1

Table 5.1.4 Putting it all together: the primary assessment

Airway – Assess patency

Look for	Listen for	Feel for
Movement of the chest wall Intercostal and accessory muscle use	Air movement Abnormal sounds – stridor	Air movement

Circulation – Assess adequacy of breathing

Effort of breathing	Effectiveness of breathing	Effects of inadequate respiration
Recession Respiratory rate Inspiration or expiration noises Grunting Accessory muscle use Flare of the alae nasi	Breath sounds Chest expansion Abdominal excursion	Heart rate Skin colour Mental status

Circulation – Assess adequacy of circulation

Cardiovascular status	Effects of circulatory inadequacy on other organs	Signs of cardiac failure
Heart rate Pulse volume Capillary refill Blood pressure	Raised jugular venous pulse height 　(not in infancy) Respiratory rate and character Skin appearance and temperature Mental status Urinary output	Gallop rhythm Crepitations in lungs Enlarged liver

Table 5.1.4 Putting it all together: the primary assessment—cont'd
Disability – Assess neurological function A rapid measure of level of consciousness should be recorded – AVPU Note the child's posture and tone – especially any lateralizing features Check pupils for size, equality and reactivity Note the presence of convulsive movements
Exposure Take the child's core temperature Look for a rash or injury
Reassessment Should be performed regularly, especially if there is deterioration

Respiratory patterns in neurological failure

Raised intracranial pressure can lead to a number of abnormal breathing patterns, ranging from hyperventilation to apnoea.

Circulatory changes in neurological failure

Hypertension, bradycardia and hypoventilation form the Cushing triad. These are late signs of raised intracranial pressure and must be acted on immediately. Hypotension is a preterminal event.

Exposure

Infants and small children have a proportionately greater surface area and therefore lose heat more rapidly than older children and adults. Infants are also less able to respond to hypothermia. Early measurement of core temperature is therefore important, and appropriate warming during resuscitation should be maintained.

Fever may indicate infection.

It is important to fully expose the child for the primary assessment, as valuable clues such as rashes in meningococcal disease or bruises in inflicted injury may be missed.

The child may respond with fear or embarrassment to exposure and therefore it must be undertaken sensitively.

Reassessment

Frequent reassessment should be undertaken, especially if there is any deterioration during the resuscitation. A search for a definitive diagnosis should now be completed.

Putting it all together

Table 5.1.4 summarizes the components of the primary assessment in table format.

Emergency care of the collapsed child

M. South

The term 'collapse' is used here to describe a state in which a child's neurological and/or cardiorespiratory function is acutely and severely impaired.

Diagnosis

Collapse may occur because of a primary neurological process; when there is loss or reduction of oxygen supply to the brain; or when metabolic disturbance or toxins affect brain function. Collapse may be the result of many different disease processes, some examples of which are shown in Table 5.2.1. A more thorough differential diagnosis and approach to assessment of the collapsed child are presented in Chapter 5.1.

Sometimes the cause of collapse is immediately obvious, as in head injury or drowning, but sometimes it may be a diagnostic problem initially, e.g. sepsis or drug ingestion. In this latter setting, resuscitation will usually have to take priority over obtaining a complete history, examination and investigation. With sufficient personnel available, diagnostic and resuscitative procedures may progress in parallel. One important investigation to consider early when the cause of collapse is unknown is a blood glucose estimation.

Resuscitation

If you might find yourself responsible for the immediate care of a collapsed child, you should be familiar with at least the procedures used in basic life support. The general principles might be the same as used in the resuscitation of adults but specific techniques are required in children.

The primary aim is to restore an adequate supply of oxygenated blood to the brain – to prevent secondary brain damage. The resuscitation procedures required will vary, depending on the degree of physiological impairment, from simple ones, such as application of an oxygen facemask or administration of a bolus of intravenous fluid, through basic cardiopulmonary resuscitation to advanced life support measures including endotracheal intubation, mechanical ventilation and the use of vasoactive drugs.

Resuscitation techniques for newborn infants are discussed in detail in Chapter 11.1.

Life support

The environment is important: make sure you are in a safe situation – you will be of no value to the collapsed child if you, the rescuer, become a second victim (e.g. at a road accident scene). Get someone to summon sufficient extra help.

Quickly evaluate the degree of collapse:
- assess the child's response to verbal or physical arousal (e.g. gentle shaking)
- assess the circulation: look for pallor, cold limbs, weak or absent pulses, poor capillary refill (press on the fingers and see how quickly the colour returns) and tachycardia (don't rely on the blood pressure: in young children this may be initially maintained even in the presence of significant hypovolaemia)
- assess oxygenation (is the face or tongue blue?).

Clinical example

David, a 2¹/₂ year old boy, was found collapsed in the bedroom while visiting his grandmother's house. He was taken immediately to a local hospital where he was noted to be floppy and poorly responsive to voice or physical stimulation. He had an adequate airway, his breathing was a little shallow and slow, and he was slightly dusky in colour. His limbs were pink and felt warm, and he had strong pulses.

David was placed on his side and oxygen was administered by facemask: his colour improved immediately. He was afebrile, with normal blood glucose on bedside testing, and no other physical abnormalities were found.

A careful history showed that he had been very well all day. He had been playing unobserved in his grandmother's house for about an hour before he was found. His grandmother kept some sedative drugs (nitrazepam) in the bedside cabinet and a telephone call back to the house revealed that the tablet bottle was lying open on the bedroom floor.

David continued to receive oxygen and close observation and his clinical condition improved steadily over the next 12 hours. He was discharged home well the following day.

Table 5.2.1 Some causes of collapse in children

Category	Diagnosis
Primary neurological process	Meningitis Head injury Encephalitis Seizures
Failure of oxygen supply to brain	Acute asphyxia (e.g. drowning, birth asphyxia) Respiratory causes (e.g. severe asthma, croup) Cardiac causes (e.g. arrhythmias, myocarditis) Hypovolaemia (e.g. dehydration, haemorrhage) Sepsis Anaphylaxis
Metabolic disturbance or toxins	Hypoglycaemia Hyponatraemia Drug or other toxic ingestion Envenomation Bacterial toxins

In obviously more advanced states of collapse, do not waste time on assessment but commence cardiopulmonary resuscitation immediately. The term ABC is a useful reminder of not only the manoeuvres required (Airway, Breathing, Circulation) but also the correct sequence in which to apply them.

Clinical example

Jodie, a 6-year-old girl, was a rear seat passenger when her family's car was involved in an accident while travelling at around 60 km/h. She was not wearing a seat belt.

On arrival at hospital, she was awake but agitated with multiple superficial abrasions to her face, trunk and limbs. Within 20 minutes her state of consciousness deteriorated, she developed increasing tachycardia and her blood pressure had fallen.

Jodie was intubated to protect her airway; during the procedure careful attention was paid to prevent excessive movement of her cervical spine. The doctor had already inserted a large-bore cannula into a vein in her antecubital fossa, and through this she was given 40 ml/kg of saline. She was re-examined for possible sites of hidden bleeding, including the abdomen and limbs (especially fractured femur). Her abdomen was noted to be distended and she underwent computed tomography (CT), which showed small lacerations of the liver and spleen. CT of her brain, performed at the same time, was normal. Jodie was managed with supportive care, including mechanical ventilation and blood transfusion. Surgical exploration of the abdomen to control bleeding was considered but not performed as she stabilized with medical treatment. She was discharged from the Intensive Care Unit 4 days later.

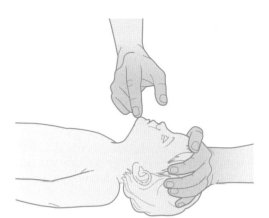

Fig. 5.2.1 Optimal head and neck position for airway protection in an infant. Do not overextend the neck. This head and neck position may be used with the child on its side or lying on its back.

Airway

If conscious, the child will usually adopt the best posture to maintain his or her own airway: don't force the child to lie down.

An unconscious child should be placed on the side: this improves the size of the airway (gravity pulls the jaw and tongue forward), allows saliva and other secretions to drain from the mouth and reduces the risk of aspiration of gastric contents should they be regurgitated. Moving the child in this way may be harmful if there is a possibility of cervical spine injury (e.g. following road trauma); in this case, work to obtain an optimal airway in the existing position without excessive rotation, flexion or extension of the neck.

Assess the adequacy of the airway by observing the degree of chest movement and by listening and feeling for breath at the mouth (place your ear close to the child's mouth).

Sometimes the airway may be further improved by extending the neck to the neutral, or slightly extended, position, and supporting the jaw in a forward position (Fig. 5.2.1). This may be done by placing your fingers behind the angle of the mandible and applying gentle forward pressure. If secretions, gastric contents or food might be obstructing the airway suck them out, preferably with a wide-bore rigid sucker. If the airway is still not optimal then an oropharyngeal airway device may be tried. It must be of the correct size, and appropriately inserted. If too large, it may increase airway obstruction and induce laryngospasm; it may also stimulate vomiting if the patient is partially conscious. The best size may be approximated by laying the airway beside the face: select a size that reaches from the front teeth to the angle of the mandible.

If it is not possible to secure an adequate airway by these means then endotracheal intubation will be required (see below).

Breathing

Once you are sure that the airway is patent, assess the adequacy of breathing: look at the rise and fall of the chest and the rate of breathing. If strong breathing movements are present but they appear obstructed (with poor chest expansion and indrawing of the soft tissues) then recheck the airway. If breathing remains inadequate or you are uncertain, commence artificial respiration. Do not delay, as ongoing hypoxaemia and hypercarbia are dangerous to a child whose brain is likely to be already compromised by the primary problem.

Artificial respiration may be given to assist existing breathing efforts, or as the sole source of gas exchange. If you are assisting the patient's existing but inadequate breathing efforts, you should attempt to synchronize artificial breaths with any taken by the patient. Additional breaths may also be required.

Respiratory support may take various forms: expired-air breathing, bag and facemask breathing; or endotracheal intubation and mechanical ventilation by machine or bag. The choice will depend on the state of the child, the availability of equipment and your experience. If inexperienced with endotracheal intubation, do not attempt this unless it is not possible to provide adequate respiration by other means (this is unusual in children). Appropriate sizes of endotracheal tube are given in Table 5.2.2.

In children less than 1 year of age, expired air resuscitation should be administered with the rescuer's mouth covering the entire mouth and nose of the infant, in older children, mouth to mouth respiration is used, as for adults.

Facemask and bag resuscitation may be performed with a variety of systems. Those with self-inflating bags are easiest to use.

Ideally, any collapsed child should receive high concentrations of inspired oxygen. This may be by simple facemask or through the circuit of the resuscitating bag. It is important to recognize that with most self-inflating bag systems, a flow of oxygen is only supplied to the patient when the bag is squeezed. An alternative delivery system with a simple facemask is more appropriate for administering oxygen to a spontaneously breathing patient. Choose a facemask that provides a good seal around the child's mouth and nose.

Assess their effectiveness of delivered breaths by watching the chest move. Ensure the administered breaths are of sufficient volume, but try not to blow excessively hard as this can lead to gastric distension.

Table 5.2.2 Resuscitation card

Age	Weight kg	Min sys BP mmHg	HR bpm	RR bpm	Adrenaline 1:10 000 mls	Adrenaline 1:1000 mls	ETT int. diameter mm	ETT lip/nose cm	DC shock 2/4 J/kg J	Fluid bolus 20 ml/kg mls
Term	3.5	50	100–170	40–60	0.4	–	3.0/3.5	8.5/10.5	14/07	70
3 months	6	50	100–170	30–50	0.6	–	3.5	9.5/11	24/12	120
6 months	8	60	100–170	30–50	0.8	–	4.0	13/10	16/32	160
1 year	10	65	100–170	30–40	1.0	0.1	4.0	14/11	20/40	200
2 years	13	65	100–160	20–30	1.5	0.15	4.5	15/12	26/52	260
4 years	15	70	80–130	20	1.5	0.15	5.0	14/17	30/60	300
6 years	20	75	70–115	16	2.0	0.2	5.5	15/19	40/80	400
8 years	25	80	70–110	16	2.5	0.25	6.0	16/20	50/100	500
10 years	30	85	60–105	16	3.0	0.3	6.5	17/21	60/120	600
12 years	40	90	60–100	16	4.0	0.4	7.0	18/22	80/160	800
14 years	50	90	60–100	16	5.0	0.5	7.5	19/23	100/200	1000
17+ years	70	90	60–100	16	10	0.5	7.5/8.0	19/23	150/300	1000

Adrenaline 1:1000, volume of 1:1000 adrenaline (epinephrine) to give a dose of 10 µg/kg; adrenaline 1:10 000, volume of 1:10 000 adrenaline (epinephrine) to give a dose of 10 µg/kg; bpm, beats or breaths per minute; ETT int. diameter, endotracheal tube size (internal diameter); ETT lip/nose, depth of endotracheal tube for fixation at lip (oral tubes) or nose (nasal tubes) – always verify that tube is in mid-trachea by clinical examination and X-ray; DC 2/4, DC shock energy in joules for 2 J/kg and 4 J/kg – use same values for both monophasic and biphasic defibrillators (exact settings may have to be modified according to those available on the specific defibrillator); fluid bolus (saline), volume of saline for 20 ml/kg; HR, heart rate normal range; min sys BP, minimum acceptable systolic blood pressure; RR, respiratory rate normal range; term, term newborn infant.

If there is no adequate chest movement, try re-establishing the airway as described above. Move on to manage the circulation, but quickly return to artificial breathing unless adequate spontaneous respiration has commenced.

Circulation

The circulation is inadequate if:

- no central pulses (e.g. carotid or femoral) are palpable
- the heart rate is less than 60 in a collapsed child, or
- the pulses are weak, with other signs of poor tissue perfusion (pallor, coldness, poor capillary refill).

Cardiac compression is indicated for a child with no pulses, weak pulses, bradycardia, or if there is any uncertainty. If in doubt, commence compressions – you will be unlikely to do any harm.

The optimal technique for chest compression varies with age:

- *Infant.* Encircle the chest with the hands, with the thumbs over the lower sternum (Fig. 5.2.2). This technique is not very suitable for solo rescuers as it is time consuming to re-establish the position after administering a breath; in this situation compress the chest with two fingers of one hand over the lower sternum
- *Small child.* Use the heel of one hand, centred one fingerbreadth above the xiphisternum
- *Larger child.* Use the heels of both hands (one atop the other), centred two fingerbreadths above the xiphisternum.

For children of all sizes, the chest should be compressed around 100 times/minute, depressing the anterior chest wall about one-third of the anteroposterior diameter.

Any child who requires chest compressions will also require artificial respiratory support; the con-

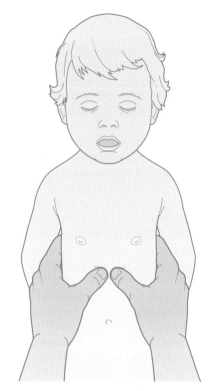

Fig. 5.2.2 In an infant, the chest may be effectively compressed by encircling the chest with your hands, with the thumbs over the lower sternum. This technique is not very suitable for solo rescuers as it is time-consuming to re-establish the position after administering a breath; in this situation, compress the chest with two fingers of one hand over the lower sternum.

verse is usually true also. Chest compression and artificial respiration should be given at a ratio of approximately 15:2, with resumption of chest compressions towards the end of the child's expiration. Once the child has an endotracheal tube in place, chest compressions should not be interrupted during the delivery of each breath.

Fluid administration

Hypovolaemia is commonly an important factor in a collapsed child. Rapid infusion of a fluid bolus should be tried in any patient with signs of an inadequate circulation. Again, if in doubt go ahead and give some fluid: you are unlikely to do any harm and you can assess the effects on the patient's circulation. Initial boluses of 10–20 ml/kg are appropriate; these may be repeated as necessary. Normal saline is usually used, but colloid solutions such as 5% albumin may also be used. Avoid hypotonic fluids, such as dextrose solutions with low concentrations of sodium.

Vascular access

A collapsed child will need vascular access for the administration of fluids and drugs.

Clinical example

Marco, a 2-year-old boy, was found at the bottom of his uncle's unfenced swimming pool during a family barbecue. No one knew how long he had been missing. When the ambulance arrived, his father was giving CPR and Marco was floppy and unresponsive, with no spontaneous respiration or palpable pulses. The ECG monitor showed asystole. He was intubated by a paramedic and an intraosseous needle was inserted. He received continuing CPR and multiple doses of intraosseous adrenaline (epinephrine) during transfer to hospital. Despite 30 minutes of further resuscitation efforts in hospital, he remained in asystole. It was clear that the prognosis for survival was hopeless and resuscitation was discontinued.

Cannulation of a peripheral vein will provide adequate initial access. Try to place a large cannula if possible; or more than one cannula, particularly if you suspect that the collapse is related to haemorrhage.

Cannulation of a peripheral vein can be very difficult in a collapsed child; do not waste time trying for more than a few minutes. Central venous catheterization is an option but can be very difficult in this setting, even for experienced operators; it also takes a significant amount of time. A better alternative is the insertion of an intraosseous needle, whereby a needle is inserted into the bone marrow (which is a vascular space that cannot collapse because of the surrounding bone cortex). This technique is simple, quick and provides access for the administration of fluids and drugs that will reach the central circulation as quickly as if administered into a peripheral vein.

Commercially available intraosseous needles that include a stylet and handle are most commonly used, but a wide-bore lumbar puncture needle is a satisfactory alternative. With the stylet in place, insert the needle through the skin, perpendicular to the surface of the bone in all directions. Local anaesthesia is not required unless the patient is conscious. Twist the needle back and forth along its long axis while firmly pushing it into the bone. Do not rock it from side to side. A 'give' is usually felt as the needle tip enters the marrow cavity. Once you feel this, or once the needle has been inserted a centimetre or two into the bone, remove the stylet and aspirate the needle with a small syringe. Aspiration of dark, blood-like fluid confirms you are in the correct spot. Commercially available needles usually come with a plastic fixation device. If using a lumbar puncture needle, you can fashion a suitable fixation from plaster of Paris. The aim is for the needle to be well supported, to prevent it being dislodged and to prevent sideways movement and enlargement of the entry hole in the bone. Administration of fluid may require pressure on the infusion bag or the use of a syringe and three-way tap.

Appropriate sites for intraosseous needle insertion include:

- the distal tibia (the medial aspect where the shaft of the tibia meets the malleolus; Fig. 5.2.3)
- the proximal tibia, about one-third of the way down from the knee to the ankle (on the flat part of the anteromedial aspect of the tibial shaft)
- the anterior iliac crest.

The tibia is most suitable for children under 5 years of age.

Putting it all together

The basic life support approach to a collapsed child and the advanced management of established paediatric arrest are summarized in Figures 5.2.4 and 5.2.5.

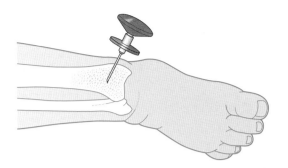

Fig. 5.2.3 Insertion of a needle into the bone marrow at the distal end of the tibia. The black handle facilitates the twisting motion and application of steady pressure as the needle is inserted. The handle, along with the attached stylet, is removed once the needle is in place.

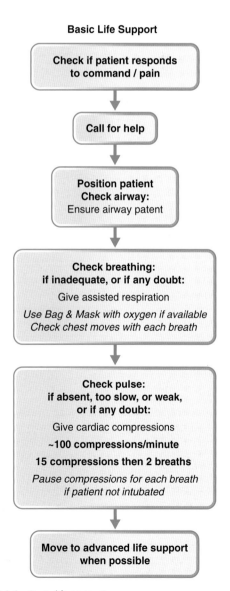

Basic Life Support

Check if patient responds to command / pain

↓

Call for help

↓

Position patient
Check airway:
Ensure airway patent

↓

Check breathing:
if inadequate, or if any doubt:
Give assisted respiration
Use Bag & Mask with oxygen if available
Check chest moves with each breath

↓

Check pulse:
if absent, too slow, or weak,
or if any doubt:
Give cardiac compressions
~100 compressions/minute
15 compressions then 2 breaths
Pause compressions for each breath
if patient not intubated

↓

Move to advanced life support
when possible

Fig. 5.2.4 Basic life support

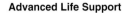

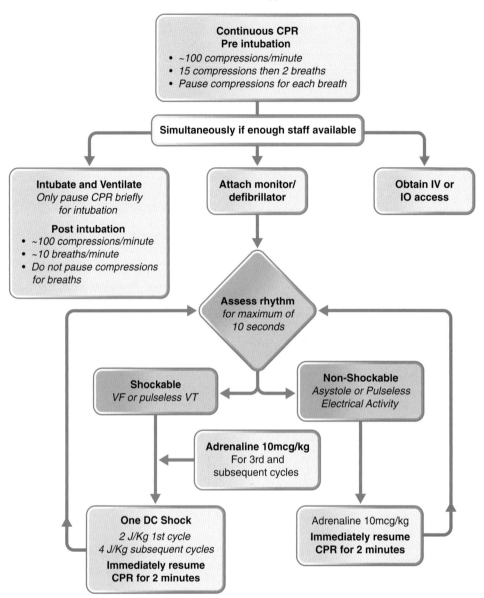

Fig. 5.2.5A Advanced life support. CPR, cardiopulmonry resuscitation; DC, direct current; IO, intraosseous; IV, intravenous; VF, ventribular fibrillation; VT, ventricular tachycardia.

It is important that life support measures are applied *continuously*. They should only be interrupted very briefly to assess response, heart rhythm, etc. They should not be terminated until stability has been clearly achieved or the decision to abandon further attempts has been made definitively.

Ongoing resuscitation

If the child has persistently poor circulation despite the presence of sinus rhythm, and after 40–60 ml/kg of intravenous fluid have been given, look for causes of hidden bleeding (especially abdomen, chest and fractured femur); also consider the use of an inotropic infusion such as dobutamine (10 μg/kg/min – put 15 mg/kg of the drug into 50 ml of saline and run at 2 ml/h).

If the child is successfully resuscitated, careful ongoing monitoring will be required. It is a mistake to terminate intubation and mechanical ventilation too soon. Ensuing brain swelling may lead to a secondary deterioration.

It is important to know when to stop if resuscitation efforts are producing no effect. Except in cases

Advanced Life Support - Notes

Double check:
- ETT position
- Oxygen supply
- Function of self-inflating bag
- ECG leads in contact
- Defibrillator paddles in contact
- IV or IO access is secure

Cardiac Compression is tiring
- Monitor technique
- Change operators every few minutes if possible

Do not waste time when cardiac compressions might be given.
- Commence CPR immediately.
- If in doubt about circulation - give CPR.
- No prolonged attempts at intubation without CPR.
- During resuscitation cycles, do not check for pulse unless ECG shows an organised rhythm.
- Do not check rhythm immediately after DC shock - give CPR for 2 mins then check.

Correct treatable causes
- Hypoxaemia
- Hypovolaemia
- Hypo/hyperthermia
- Hypo/hyperkalaemia
- Tamponade
- Tension pneumothorax
- Toxins/poisons/drugs
- Thrombosis

Other drugs to consider

Atropine
for persistent asystole / bradycardia (20mcg/kg)
(min 100mcg, max 600mcg)

Amiodarone
If VF or pulseless VT persists after 3-4 DC shocks.
(5mg/kg, max 300mg) by bolus injection if patient unstable, or over 40 mins if stable.
Flush IV well after.

Lignocaine
same indications as Amiodarone. (1 mg/kg)
(0.1 ml/kg of 1%)
Amiodarone is the preferred agent, use lignocaine only if unavailable. Never give lignocaine after Amiodarone.

Magnesium Sulphate
For hypomagnesaemia
or for polymorphic VT (torsade de pointes)
50% solution: 0.05-0.1 ml/kg
(0.1-0.2mmol/kg) (max 2g) by intravascular infusion over 5 mins.

Sodium bicarbonate, calcium,
and doses of adrenaline >1 0mcg/kg/dose have no place in routine resuscitation.

Other issues

Blood gas analysis
Arterial (and to some extent venous) blood gas analysis can help determine degree of hypoxaemia, adequacy of ventilation, degree of acidosis, and presence of electrolyte abnormalities such as hyopmagnesaemia. It is not a priority in initial resuscitation attempts, and obtaining a sample should not distract from other resuscitation manoevres.

Fig. 5.2.5B Advanced life support – notes. CPR, cardiopulmonry resuscitation; DC, direct current; ECG, electrocardiograph; ETT, endotracheal tube; IO, intraosseous; IV, intravenous; VF, ventribular fibrillation; VT, ventricular tachycardia.

of extreme hypothermia, as occur in drowning in near freezing water, persisting cardiac arrest after 20–30 minutes of good resuscitation is an indication of a hopeless prognosis. When hypoxia or hypovolaemia have resulted in cardiac arrest with asystole, particularly in an out-of-hospital setting, the prognosis for recovery or survival is very poor.

Temperature control following resuscitation is an area of controversy. Traditional teaching was to maintain normal body temperature using blankets and overhead heaters. There is now animal research, and some human studies, that suggest improved neurological outcome after cardiac arrest, or head trauma, if body temperature is quickly lowered to around 32–33°C for a period of 48–72 hours following

Practical points

- Learn the basics of paediatric life support before you need them – you won't have time to consult a textbook in an emergency
- Do not waste time assessing the adequacy of breathing and circulation in a collapsed child. Assessment can be misleading and time-consuming
- If the circulation or breathing are inadequate or you are uncertain, administer cardiac compressions and artificial respiration
- Never hesitate to give a trial of an intravenous fluid bolus to a collapsed child
- Learn the technique of intraosseous needle placement – this simple technique can be life-saving
- Call for extra assistance early

the insult. More research is needed before firm conclusions can be drawn regarding the use of therapeutic hypothermia in resuscitation of children.

Appendix

Resuscitation guide A

Table 5.2.2 provides a summary of acceptable physiological parameters for children according to age, along with endotracheal tube sizes, DC shocks and doses of adrenaline (epinephrine) used in resuscitation. This table can be photocopied (or downloaded and printed from the internet at http://www.rch.org. au/clinicalguide/forms/resusCard.cfm). If folded horizontally at the centre, it can be laminated and punched to attach conveniently to a hospital ID badge, so making it readily available for reference in the clinical setting.

Resuscitation guide B

Another useful aid to resuscitation can be downloaded from the internet at http://www.rch.org.au/clinicalguide/cpg.cfm?doc_id=5137. It will run as a utility with any recent internet browser. It produces a table of appropriate drug doses, DC shocks and endotracheal tube sizes according to the age and weight of the patient.

Poisoning and envenomation

J. Tibballs

Poisoning and envenomation are two important areas of emergency care that should be familiar to any health practitioner involved with acute care of children and young people.

Poisoning

Poisoning is a common health problem among children. In children's hospitals it is responsible for numerous attendances to emergency departments: over 3500 children aged 0–4 years are admitted annually to Australian hospitals as a result of poisoning incidents. Worldwide, poisoning is the third most common cause of death among young children. A great deal of effort is expended upon a problem that is largely preventable. A Poisons Information Centre serving a population of 5 million receives approximately 40 000–50 000 telephone inquiries per annum; two-thirds concern actual poisoning and, of those, 60–70% concern children aged 4 years and younger.

Epidemiology

The nature of poisoning varies for different age groups in children. Although poisoning in childhood is usually unintentional, the possibility of deliberate poisoning in the younger child as part of child abuse should not be forgotten. Pharmaceutical substances are involved in 70% of poisonings. In hospitals, errors in drug administration are frequent causes of poisoning.

Newborns

Poisoning is almost always iatrogenic in this age group. For example, newborns are at risk at delivery, when they may be given ergometrine instead of vitamin K, causing severe hypertension, convulsions and coagulopathy. In intensive care units, the frequent use of potent cardiovascular drugs, chloramphenicol, gentamicin, barbiturates, phenytoin, theophylline, digoxin, furosemide and opiates predispose the infant to poisoning.

It is not acceptable to perform noxious procedures without analgesia and sedation, and it is commendable that opiates are used in the newborn, but great care should be taken to ensure that overdose does not cause cardiorespiratory failure. Repeated doses or infusions of opiates should be confined to newborns who are mechanically ventilated, and, wherever possible, local or regional anaesthesia should be employed for surgical procedures. Local anaesthetic agents or opiates administered to the mother during labour may poison the newborn.

Care should be exercised with the use of topical antiseptics. Mercurochrome, commonly applied to the umbilical stump, may cause mercury poisoning if used in excess. Hexachlorophene should not be used as a regular bathing solution because it is readily absorbed percutaneously, causing neurotoxicity. If used in excess, iodinated compounds may cause hypothyroidism. Occasionally, mistakes in the preparation of artificial foods may cause serum electrolyte disorders and dehydration.

Age 1–5 years

Poisoning occurs most frequently in this age group. Most instances are said to be accidental, in which the young child discovers a drug or a household cleaning or chemical agent. The majority of serious poisonings occur with prescribed drugs or with over-the-counter drugs. Parents are often unaware that drugs must be stored safely and they underestimate the capabilities of young children who, at this age, become increasingly mobile and curious. They eat substances that are not palatable to adults, and tablets and capsules that resemble lollies (sweets).

The incidence and severity of accidental poisoning from drugs has been reduced markedly by the use of blister packs and bottles with child-resistant lids. Poisoning in the home often occurs between 10 am and noon and between 6 pm and 8 pm when the child is active or hungry and when supervision has lapsed because the parent is involved in other household activities.

Age 6–12 years

Poisoning is relatively uncommon in this age group but it may be truly accidental, such as drinking a poison from a bottle that has been labelled wrongly, or when toxic agents have been stored inappropriately. A common example is storage of potentially toxic liquids in soft-drink containers in garden sheds. Although uncommon, self-poisoning in this age group may occur as drug abuse or manipulative behaviour.

Age 13–17 years

Emotionally disturbed adolescents and young adults may poison themselves deliberately, usually by ingestion, to manipulate their environment, or they may harbour a genuine suicidal intent. They may seek the thrill of drug abuse by inhalation or injection, sometimes as group behaviour. The peak incidence of teenage poisoning is at 14–16 years of age. Repeated episodes occur more frequently among girls but boys' suicide attempts tend to be more successful.

Management

The immediate aim in the management of poisoning, whether serious or not, is to attend to the effects of the poison on the patient. Later, attention should be given to the circumstances with the aim of preventing a recurrence. There are innumerable poisons. All medicines and many household substances are poisonous if taken in sufficient quantity. Upon presentation, the action to be taken, if any, will be determined by the substance involved, its amount, the interval between ingestion and presentation, and the effect of the poison. The following principles of management may be applied universally.

Support vital functions

It is imperative to maintain and support vital functions if these are depressed. Many poisons are excreted adequately or metabolized by the body if the vital functions are maintained. If the patient is unconscious, the airway, the depth and frequency of breathing and the circulation should be examined for adequacy. Chapter 5.2 provides a full discussion on the management of deficiencies of the airway, breathing and circulation.

Establish the diagnosis

It is important to establish:

- what poisons are involved
- in what quantity
- when exposure occurred.

Often the diagnosis of poisoning is self-evident, but at times the diagnosis is not obvious. When a poison has been identified, it should never be assumed that other poisons could not be involved. The symptoms and signs of poisoning are diverse but dangerous drugs threaten vital functions. Seriously poisoned patients present commonly with:

- unconsciousness
- cardiorespiratory failure
- convulsions.

If any of these are present and the cause is otherwise not known, poisoning should be high on the list of differential diagnoses. A meticulous physical examination and history provides invaluable help in diagnosis and treatment. Laboratory investigations may be necessary to establish a diagnosis, determine the amount of poison in the body and help determine specific treatment for certain poisons.

Prevent absorption

Some poisons contaminate the skin, conjunctivae and mucous membranes and other poisons are inhaled as gases. Surface contamination requires copious irrigation with water, while inhalational poisoning may require oxygen therapy and mechanical ventilation. The great majority of poisons are ingested, for which the options for therapy include induced emesis, oral or gastric administration of activated charcoal, gastric lavage and whole bowel irrigation. If the poison has been absorbed already and has reached the vascular compartment, invasive techniques such as:

- plasmafiltration
- haemofiltration
- charcoal haemoperfusion
- haemodialysis
- peritoneal dialysis
- exchange transfusion

may be required.

The poison, its amount and the seriousness of its effects determine the treatment of the poisoned patient. These must be weighed against the hazards of removal. Unconscious or drowsy patients or patients who cannot protect their own airway should not undergo induced emesis or gastric lavage or be given activated charcoal or colonic washout solutions. The consequences of aspirating gastric contents during vomiting or regurgitation in a less than fully conscious state far outweigh the dangers of many untreated poisons, as the mortality from severe pneumonitis is approximately 50%. However, it is appropriate to remove a wide variety of ingested poisons with either:

- activated charcoal
- whole bowel irrigation
- gastric lavage, or
- a combination of these techniques.

Circumstances of presentation and ingestion dictate the choice of technique.

Induced emesis, using ipecacuanha, was a commonly applied form of therapy but has now been largely abandoned because of limited effectiveness, the development of more effective techniques (e.g. activated charcoal) and risk of aspiration of gastric contents.

Activated charcoal is probably the most appropriate therapy in the emergency or casualty department, although whole bowel irrigation may be preferable for some agents. Gastric lavage should be reserved for a recent (within 1 hour) serious life-threatening ingestion in a conscious patient or for serious poisoning in a less than fully conscious patient who has airway protection. The circumstances for the employment of each technique are summarized in Figure 5.3.1.

Activated charcoal

Activated charcoal is itself not absorbable but it adsorbs many different poisons in the gastrointestinal tract and thus prevents absorption of poison into the circulation. However, activated charcoal does not adsorb some poisons, including some elemental metals, some pesticides, ferrous sulphate, ethanol,

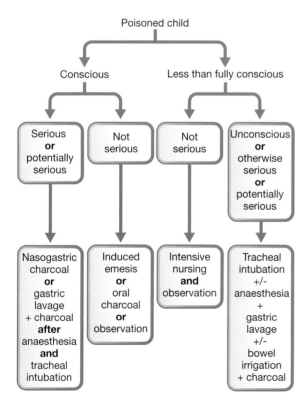

corrosives and petrochemicals. There are many different preparations of activated charcoal, some with sorbitol as a laxative, but with these excessive diarrhoea and hypernatraemic dehydration may result.

To be effective, activated charcoal should be administered within 1 hour of ingestion by mouth or by a nasogastric tube in a fully conscious patient, or by gastric tube in a less than fully conscious patient after the airway has been secured with an endotracheal tube. Children may be more likely to drink it if it is cooled and offered in an opaque paper cup with a lid and a black straw. The dose of activated charcoal is 10 times the ingested poison by weight or 1–2 g/kg of the child's body weight followed by 0.25 g/kg 4–6-hourly. An alternative dosage regimen is 0.25 g/kg hourly for 12–24 hours. Continued or repeated doses of activated charcoal are useful if the poison is in a sustained-release preparation or if the charcoal is known to increase the total body clearance of the poison by interruption of its enterohepatic circulation or by leaching it from the circulation of the gastrointestinal mucosa. It should not be administered if gastrointestinal ileus is present as this may cause regurgitation. Aspiration of activated charcoal may have a fatal outcome.

Activated charcoal is often administered, probably unnecessarily, with a laxative, notably magnesium sulphate, to prevent constipation. If magnesium sulphate is used, care should be taken to avoid hypermagnesaemia, a potential risk with repeated doses. Activated charcoal does not adsorb ipecacuanha and thus there is nothing to be gained by administering it to the patient whose induced emesis is excessive.

Gastric lavage

Gastric lavage was a commonly applied form of therapy but has now been largely abandoned. It is an invasive procedure and is justified only for significant recent poisoning when other techniques are contraindicated or are unreliable. It may also be indicated when the poison delays gastric emptying or forms concretions in the stomach. To be effective, however, it must be performed well and care must be taken to prevent complications. It should never be performed in a less than fully conscious patient unless the airway is protected by prior endotracheal intubation. Loss of consciousness due to poisoning may be associated with cardiorespiratory failure. Endotracheal intubation in this situation should be performed only by those experienced in the techniques of rapid intubation and resuscitation.

Gastric lavage should not be performed after the ingestion of a corrosive substance because additional damage to the oesophagus (perforation, mediastinitis) and stomach (perforation) may occur. It is also unwise to perform gastric lavage after ingestion of

Fig. 5.3.1 Management of poisoning. Modified from Tibballs J 2003 Poisoning and envenomation. In: Smart J, Nolan T (eds) Royal Children's Hospital Paediatric Handbook. Blackwell Science, Carlton.

petrochemicals or hydrocarbons as these substances have a very low surface tension and cause severe pneumonitis, even after minor contamination of the oropharynx, which may occur after the passage of the lavage tube renders the gastro-oesophageal sphincter incompetent. The risk of causing or exacerbating chemical pneumonitis exceeds the benefit of poison removal, despite the depression of central nervous system function that may follow. Such patients recover if vital functions are preserved.

Gastric lavage is a potentially traumatic procedure, particularly to the oropharynx, even when indicated. Occasionally the oesophagus and stomach have been perforated. It is psychologically as well as physically traumatic. For physical safety, the child must be restrained: this is best achieved by wrapping the child in a sheet with the arms pinned by the side. The child must be held in a lateral head down position. For gastric lavage to be performed well, safely and atraumatically in a small child, it should be preceded by induction of general anaesthesia with endotracheal intubation.

Whole bowel irrigation
This is an effective technique to limit absorption of a poison. It is the preferred technique when the poison has passed beyond the pylorus and therefore cannot be removed by induced emesis or gastric lavage and when the substance is a drug or substance not adsorbed by activated charcoal. In the latter category are foreign bodies such as miniature disc batteries. Slow-release drug preparations may also be removed with this technique.

The agent used is a mixture of polyethylene glycol and electrolytes that flushes out the contents of the bowel without disturbing the serum volume, osmolality or electrolytes. It is administered via nasogastric tube at a rate of 30 ml/kg/h for 4–8 hours until the rectal effluent is clear. It should not be administered to a less than fully conscious patient or when gastrointestinal ileus is present. Concomitant administration of activated charcoal is counterproductive.

Removal from the circulation
If the poison reaches the circulation, an invasive extracorporeal technique may be necessary to achieve removal. Usual techniques include forced diuresis, haemodialysis, plasmapheresis and charcoal haemoperfusion. These techniques are usually reserved for recognized circumstances when there is deterioration of vital functions despite maximal therapy (mechanical ventilation, inotropic/vasopressor therapy and artificial renal therapy) or the lack or failure of an adequate excretory or metabolic pathway (renal, hepatic) to eliminate the poison. For these techniques to be effective, however, the poison must have a relatively small volume of distribution.

Peritoneal dialysis is not an efficient technique to remove poisons from the blood. Occasionally, the small size of a patient and the properties of a poison permit its removal by exchange blood transfusion.

Administer an antidote

Only relatively few poisons have antidotes but knowledge and use of these can be life-saving. The appropriate dose of each is determined by the amount of poison and its effects. A list of common important antidotes is given in Table 5.3.1 (see also Further Reading).

Recognition of poisons

There are literally thousands of poisons and no one person can be expected to be familiar with them all. However, it is vital to recognize that any substance that has effects, or side effects, on the central nervous system, cardiovascular system and respiratory system is a potential serious poison. It is prudent to be familiar with serious poisons that are ingested commonly (Table 5.3.2) and those that have delayed actions, such as colchicine, paracetamol and paraquat. The content of unfamiliar proprietary preparations should be sought, as effects may not be obvious from common usage. For example, the antidiarrhoeal drug Lomotil contains atropine and the opiate diphenoxylate, which may cause respiratory depression. Swallowed disc or 'button batteries' that impact in the gastrointestinal tract may cause ulceration into surrounding structures (trachea, aorta), whether by release of corrosive chemicals or by electrical activity, and may cause mercury poisoning when corroded by gastric acid.

It is important to have access to a Poisons Information Centre by telephone, fax or e-mail. These centres maintain a vast store of up-to-date information and are usually accessible on a 24-hour basis. While Poison Information Centres provide an invaluable service, the management of the poisoned patient is the responsibility of the treating physician.

Clinical example

Simon, a 15-month-old toddler, was noted by his mother to be irritable, drooling saliva and have inflamed lips after tasting the residue of the powder in their automatic dishwasher door. On examination, oropharyngeal ulceration was observed. An intravenous cannula was inserted for fluid and nutrition therapy and an endoscopy of the upper gastrointestinal tract was performed. Significant burns to the mid-oesophagus were discovered; these healed with stricture formation, necessitating repeated dilatation with bougies.

Table 5.3.1 Antidotes to some serious poisons

Poison	Antidotes	Comments
Amphetamines	Esmolol i.v. 500 µg/kg over 1 min, then 25–200 µg/kg/min	Treatment for tachyarrhythmia
	Labetalol i.v. 0.15–0.3 mg/kg or phentolamine i.v. 0.05–0.1 mg/kg every 10 min	Treatment for hypertension
Benzodiazepines	Flumazenil i.v. 3–10 µg/kg, repeat 1 min, then 3–10 µg/kg/h	Specific receptor antagonist. Beware convulsions
Beta blockers	Glucagon i.v. 140 µg/kg, then 0.2–1 µg/kg/min	Stimulates non catecholamine cAMP, preferred antidote
	Isoprenaline i.v. 0.05–3 mg/kg/min	
	Noradrenaline (norepinephrine) i.v. 0.05– 1 µg/kg/min	Beware hypotension
Calcium channel blocker	Calcium chloride i.v. 10%, 0.2 ml/kg	
Carbon monoxide	Oxygen 100%	Decreases carboxyhaemoglobin. May need hyperbaric oxygen
Cyanide	Dicobaltedetate i.v. 7.5 µg/kg (max 300 mg) over 1 min, then 300 mg at 5 min	Give 50 mL 50% glucose after each dose
	Sodium nitrite 3% i.v. 0.33 ml/kg over 4 min, then sodium thiosulphate 25% i.v. 1.65 ml/kg (max 50 ml) at 3–5 min	Nitrites form methaemoglobin–cyanide complex. Beware excess methaemoglobin >20%.
		Thiosulphate forms non-toxic thiocyanate from methaemoglobin–cyanide
Digoxin	Magnesium sulphate i.v. 25–50 mg/kg (0.1–0.2 mmol/kg)	
	Digoxin Fab i.v: acute – 10 vials per 25 tablets (0.25 mg each), 10 vials per 5 mg elixir; steady state – vials = serum digoxin (ng/ml) × BW(kg)/100	
Ergotamine	Sodium nitroprusside infusion 0.5–5.0 µg/kg/min	Treats vasoconstriction. Monitor BP continuously
	Heparin i.v. 100 units/kg then 10– 30 units/kg/h	Monitor partial thromboplastin time
Heparin	Protamine 1 mg/100 units heparin	
Iron	Desferrioxamine 15 mg/kg/h 12–24 h if serum iron >90 µmol/l or >63 µmol/l and symptomatic	Give slowly, beware anaphylaxis
Lead	Dimercaprol (BAL) i.m. 75 mg/m^2 4 hourly 6 doses then i.v. CaNa$_2$ edetate (EDTA) 1500 mg/m^2 over 5 d if blood level >3.38 µmol/l. If asymptomatic and blood level 2.65–3.3 µmol/l infuse CaNa$_2$ EDTA 1000 mg/m^2/d 5 d or oral succimer 350 mg/m^2 8-hourly 5 d, then 12-hourly 14 d	
Methaemoglobinaemia	Methylene blue i.v. 1–2 mg/kg over several minutes	
Methanol, ethylene glycol, glycol ethers	Ethanol i.v. loading dose 10 ml/kg 10% diluted in glucose 5%, then 0.15 ml/kg/h to maintain blood level 0.1% (100 mg/dl)	
Opiates	Naloxone i.v. 0.01–0.1 mg/kg, then 0.01 mg/kg/h as needed	

Table 5.3.1 Antidotes to some serious poisons—cont'd

Poison	Antidotes	Comments
Organophosphates and carbamates	Atropine i.v. 20–50 μg/kg every 15 min until secretions dry	Blocks muscarinic effects
	Pralidoxime i.v. 25 mg/kg over 15– 30 min then 10–20 mg/kg/h for 18 h or more. Not for carbamates	Reactivates cholinesterase
Paracetamol	N-acetylcysteine i.v. 150 mg/kg over 60 min then 10 mg/kg/h for 20– 72 h or oral 140 mg/kg then 17 doses of 70 mg/kg 4-hourly (total 1330 mg/kg over 68 h)	Restores glutathione, inhibits metabolites. Give within 18 h according to serum paracetamol
Phenothiazine dystonia	Benztropine i.v or i.m. 0.01–0.03 mg/kg	Blocks dopamine reuptake
Potassium	Glucose i.v. 0.5 g/kg plus insulin i.v. 0.05 units/kg	Decreases serum potassium rapidly. Monitor serum glucose
	Salbutamol aerosol 0.25 mg/kg	Decreases serum potassium rapidly
	Sodium bicarbonate i.v. 1 mmol/kg	Decreases serum potassium slightly; beware hypocalcaemia
	Calcium chloride 10% i.v. 0.2 ml/kg	Antagonizes cardiac effects
	Resonium oral or rectal 0.5–1 g/kg	Adsorbs potassium slowly
Tricyclic antidepressants	Sodium bicarbonate i.v. 1 mmol/kg to maintain blood pH >7.45	Reduces cardiotoxicity

Table 5.3.2 Common lethal/serious poisons and substances

- Antihistamines
- Aspirin
- Barbiturates
- Carbamazepine
- Carbon monoxide
- Caustic soda
- Chloral hydrate
- Digoxin
- Disc batteries
- Dishwashing powder
- Hydrochloric acid (spirit of salts)
- Iron
- Major tranquillizers
- Opiates
- Paracetamol
- Theophylline
- Tricyclic antidepressants
- Verapamil
- Volatile substances
  In rural areas/developing countries: paraquat, chloroquine, organophosphate insecticides

Prevention

Too many poisonings are so called 'accidents', particularly among young children. Every opportunity should be taken to educate parents about the dangers of drugs and toxic substances in the home. A warning should be issued whenever a drug is prescribed and counselling given whenever poisoning occurs. It is erroneous to believe that young children cannot open drawers, cupboards and handbags or gain access to bench tops.

All drugs, however common and easily available, should be stored in a locked, child-proof cabinet. Out-of date-drugs should be discarded safely. Household cleaning substances, fuels and garden and workshop chemicals should be stored in truly inaccessible places. This applies particularly to automatic dishwasher powders and detergents and to sink and oven cleaners, all of which are highly caustic and corrosive to the gastrointestinal tract. Corrosive poisoning occurs most often when small children have access to dishwashing powder or its residue in the receptacle of an open automatic dishwasher door.

Older children should be taught at home and at school of the dangers of drug abuse, including those of 'street' and pharmaceutical drugs, and that sniffing glue or hydrocarbons imperils their lives. In the case of self-poisoning by adolescents, the provocation is often the result of complex social and psychological disharmony, making remedial action lengthy and difficult (Ch. 3.11).

All age groups are subject to iatrogenic poisoning at home and in hospital. Most iatrogenic errors result from mistakes in prescription, i.e. the dose of a drug and its interval. It is particularly important for doctors to refer always to a recognized prescription manual for children rather than relying upon memory or extrapolation from adult dosages, especially when dealing with infrequently used potent drugs. Prescriptions must be clearly written and, if abbreviations are employed, such as 'µg' or 'mcg' for microgram, they must be universally recognized. If in doubt, longhand printing should be used. Care should be taken with a decimal point. Equally, interpretation of a prescription must be with care, and the preparation checked before administration. All too often in hospitals, wrong drugs and wrong doses are given to the wrong patients.

Clinical example

Amanda, a 3-year-old girl, was brought to the emergency department by her parents. Two hours previously she had been perfectly well when they were visiting friends, but since that time had become progressively drowsy and was unconscious on presentation. On examination, her respiration was shallow and her blood pressure was low. No signs of external trauma or infection were obvious. Mechanical ventilation, intravascular volume support and vasopressor therapy were necessary. In spite of the parents' denial of drug ingestion, a high level of amylobarbital was discovered in her urine and the next day it was revealed that an opened bottle of tablets had been found in their friends' house. Amanda recovered completely.

Clinical example

Mario, a 13-year-old boy in previous good health but known to have experimented with drugs, collapsed while in the garage of a friend's house. The parents of the friend found him unconscious and summoned an ambulance, whose officers diagnosed ventricular fibrillation. They attempted to resuscitate him with mechanical ventilation and DC shock but were unsuccessful. External cardiac compression was continued, and on arrival at the hospital's emergency department he was still in refractory ventricular fibrillation. Numerous additional attempts at defibrillation using 4 J/kg of DC shock administered with amiodarone and adrenaline (epinephrine) over 45 minutes failed to achieve sinus rhythm. Eventually asystole occurred. Postmortem blood samples revealed high levels of N-butane and isobutane, constituents of cigarette lighter fluid, which presumably had been inhaled.

Practical points

- Childhood poison exposure is very common
- Most exposures carry minimal morbidity but some are serious and can be fatal
- You should know the general principles of management for poisoning
- Poison Information Centres can provide detailed management advice

Envenomation

Australia harbours a wide variety of terrestrial and marine creatures. Of these, those that cause the most frequent or serious envenomation are several species of snake, spider and jellyfish (Table 5.3.3). The reader is referred to the Further Reading list for detailed and extensive information.

Snake bite

Australia has over 100 species of snake, of which a dozen are among the world's most deadly. The average mortality from snake bite in Australia is 2–3 deaths per annum, approximately equal to the mortality from bee-sting anaphylaxis. The species that have caused mortality and significant morbidity belong to the genera of:

- tiger snakes (*Notechis*)
- brown snakes (*Pseudonaja*)
- death adders (*Acanthophis*)
- taipan (*Oxyuranus*)
- black snakes (*Pseudechis*)
- copperhead snakes (*Austrelaps*)
- rough scaled snakes (*Tropidechis*).

Tiger snakes and brown snakes account for most envenomations. All Australian snakes are elapids, which have relatively small fangs and whose venoms do not cause severe local effects.

The main components of venoms are:

- pre- and postsynaptic neurotoxins, which cause paralysis
- prothrombin activators, which cause disseminated intravascular coagulation and haemorrhage
- anticoagulants, which cause spontaneous haemorrhage
- rhabdomyolysins, which may cause renal failure
- haemolysins.

Different species have different effects but the two most common acute threats to life are neuromuscular paralysis with respiratory failure and coagulopathy causing bleeding with peripheral circulatory failure (shock).

Management

Snakes may bite but fail to inject venom on approximately 40–50% of occasions. In young children, particularly, snake bite is suspected even though a snake was not observed. In only 17–20% of such presentations has both a bite and envenomation occurred. Thus one of the difficulties in the management of snake bite is to determine whether envenomation has

Table 5.3.3 Effects of Australian venomous animals and their treatments

Animal	Main effects	Main treatments
Snakes (many terrestrial and marine species)	Paralysis (rapid) Haemorrhage	Pressure–immobilization bandage Antivenom with premedication Endotracheal intubation and mechanical ventilation
Funnel-web spiders	Paralysis (rapid)	Pressure–immobilization bandage Antivenom Endotracheal intubation and mechanical ventilation
Redback spider	Pain Paralysis (slow)	Antivenom
Australian paralysis tick	Paralysis (slow)	Remove tick Antitoxin
Bees, wasps, ants	Anaphylaxis	Adrenaline
Box jellyfish	Paralysis Hypotension	Douse with vinegar Antivenom Endotracheal intubation and mechanical ventilation
Blue-ringed octopuses	Paralysis (rapid)	Pressure–immobilization bandage Endotracheal intubation and mechanical ventilation
Stone fish	Pain	Antivenom

actually occurred, irrespective of whether or not a bite by a snake was observed.

The syndrome of envenomation is characterized by a rapid onset of paralysis accompanied by coagulopathy over minutes to several hours. However, an early diagnosis may be dependent upon subtle clinical signs and symptoms, abnormal laboratory tests of coagulation and a positive test for venom in the patient's urine or blood. The early reliable symptoms of envenomation are:

• headache
• abdominal pain
• vomiting.

Abnormal laboratory tests of coagulation are also very sensitive and reliable after bite by a species with coagulopathic effects (death adders do not cause serious coagulopathy). The onset of weakness of large muscles, including respiratory muscles, is preceded by weakness of the bulbar muscles, so that it is imperative to enquire and seek evidence of dysfunction of the external ocular muscles (double vision, ophthalmoplegia), facial muscles (ptosis) and the muscles of speech and swallowing (dysphonia, dysphagia).

The clinical diagnosis of envenomation may be confirmed with the snake venom detection kit test (CSL Diagnostics, Australia). This is a rapid two-step enzyme immunoassay designed for clinical use. It gives a result in approximately 25 minutes and is capable of detecting venom in a concentration of as little as 10 ng/ml. The test can be applied to a swab of the bite site or to the victim's blood or urine. A positive result does not necessarily identify the snake but it stipulates which antivenom to administer, if clinically indicated.

The principles of treatment for snake bite are:

• to prevent rapid absorption of the venom from the subcutaneous tissue into the circulation by application of a pressure–immobilization bandage
• to neutralize the venom by the administration of antivenom
• to treat the effects of the venom, namely respiratory failure and bleeding.

The management of suspected and definite envenomation is summarized in Figure 5.3.2.

Pressure–immobilization first aid
Limbs sustain 95% of all bites. Snake venoms gain access from the subcutaneous tissue to the circulation via the lymphatics. These channels can be effectively occluded by the application of a firm crepe (or crepe-like) bandage applied over the bite site and whole of the limb (Fig. 5.3.3). The application of a

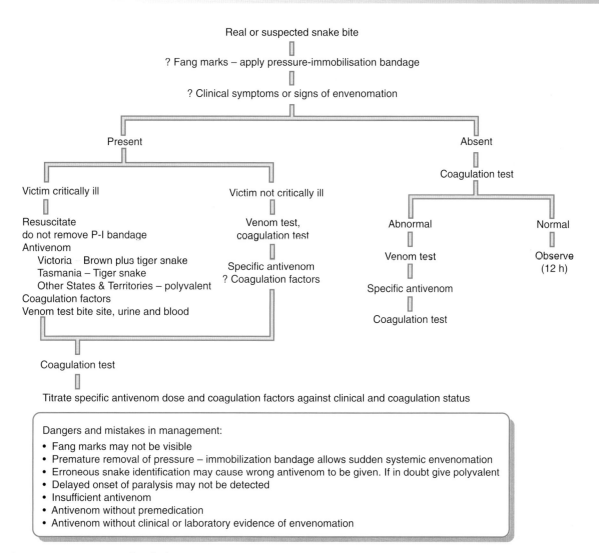

Fig. 5.3.2   Management of snake bite.

splint that includes joints on either side of the bite prevents the use of surrounding muscle groups and hence decreases lymph flow. Although the technique is a first aid measure that should be applied at the scene of the snake bite to prevent initial absorption of venom, it is also used in established envenomation in hospital to prevent additional absorption of venom while preparations are being made to administer antivenom.

The bandage can be left in place indefinitely as it should be no tighter than a bandage for a sprained ankle. However, the bandage does not allow substantial inactivation of venom in the tissues and should be removed after the asymptomatic patient reaches a hospital that has a stock of antivenom or after the envenomated patient has been given antivenom. It is dangerous to remove a bandage from an envenomated patient before administration of antivenom

because its release allows a substantial additional quantity of venom to gain rapid access to the circulation. The splint and bandage should not be removed solely to allow inspection of the bite site of an envenomated patient; instead, the splint should be removed temporarily and a window should be cut in the bandage to allow a swab of the bite site to be taken for venom testing, then the bandage should be reinforced and the splint reapplied. Bites are usually visible as scratches or puncture wounds, but their presence and appearance, or absence, does not prove or disprove envenomation and does not allow identification of the snake involved.

Antivenom
Specific monovalent antivenoms (Commonwealth Serum Laboratories Ltd, Melbourne) are manufactured against tiger, brown, taipan, black, death adder

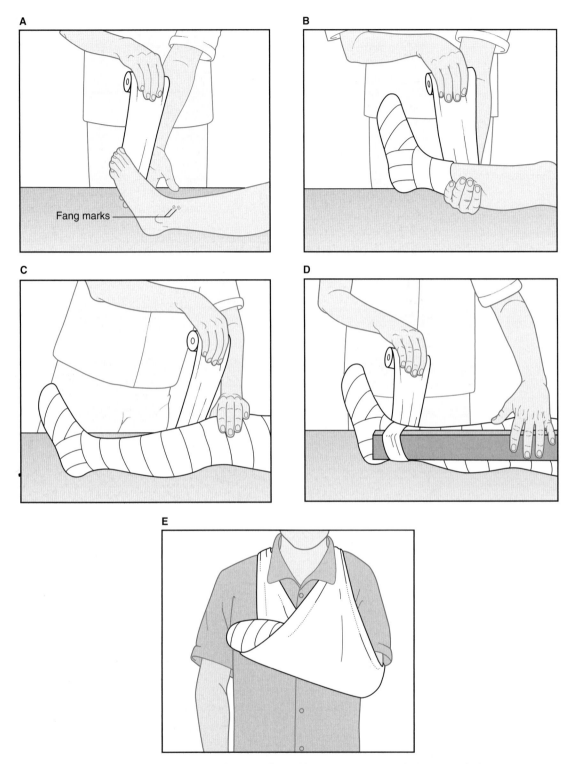

Fig. 5.3.3 Technique for applying pressure–immobilization first aid bandage. **A–D** Lower limb; **E** upper limb.

and beaked sea snake (*Enhydrina schistosa*) venoms. These are effective against all known snakes in Australia and Papua New Guinea. A mixture of the five terrestrial antivenoms is available as a polyvalent preparation. The antivenoms are highly purified equine immunoglobulins. Cross-reactivity between species is limited, so that it is essential to administer the correct antivenom according to the identity of the snake.

If the identity of the snake is not known or uncertain, the type of antivenom to be administered is based on the known geographical snake distribution or according to the result of a venom detection kit test (q.v.). In Tasmania, Australia, where the snakes are (black) tiger snakes and copperheads, the appropriate antivenom is tiger snake antivenom. In Victoria, Australia, where the dangerous species are tiger, brown, black and copperhead snakes, the appropriate antivenom therapy is tiger snake plus brown snake antivenom. Everywhere else in Australia additional species exist and the polyvalent preparation should be chosen.

Although essential and life-saving, antivenoms are foreign proteins, which may cause a life-threatening anaphylactoid reaction. However, this may be prevented by premedication with subcutaneous (not intravenous or intramuscular) adrenaline (epinephrine) 0.005–0.01 mg/kg. Additional protective agents such as a steroid (hydrocortisone) and an antihistamine may be indicated if the patient has a known allergic history. Only one premedication dose of adrenaline is required. The antivenom should be administered intravenously, diluted with a crystalloid solution, over approximately 30 minutes. However, for severe envenomation it may be delivered rapidly. If polyvalent antivenom or multiple doses of monovalent antivenom are required, a course of steroid therapy (prednisolone 1–2 mg/kg/d for 5 days) should be given to prevent serum sickness.

The dose of antivenom is never certain at the beginning of treatment because the amount of venom injected is unknown. Each ampoule of antivenom contains enough to neutralize the average yield from 'milking' – a process whereby venom is collected by inducing a snake to bite a membrane stretched tautly over a receptacle. However, the venom injected on biting is highly variable and bites may be multiple. Children are more susceptible than adults because of the larger venom-to-body-mass ratio. The majority of envenomations are treated adequately with 1–3 ampoules but this dose should never be relied upon; many more ampoules are usually required in life-threatening envenomations.

Antivenom should not be withheld if indicated, as there is no other satisfactory treatment. Antivenom should be administered either if there are clinical signs or symptoms of envenomation after snake bite or if in their absence a substantial coagulopathy is present. Occasionally, venom can be detected in the urine but there is no clinical evidence or very mild coagulopathy. In this case antivenom may be withheld, but the patient's clinical and coagulation status should be checked regularly.

Life support
In the severely envenomated patient, endotracheal intubation and mechanical ventilation may be required because of bulbar and respiratory muscle paralysis. If antivenom therapy is delayed, mechanical ventilation may be required for many days.

Coagulopathy may cause massive haemorrhage from mucosal surfaces and subsequent peripheral circulatory failure. Haemorrhage may occur into a vital organ, particularly the brain. It is essential to restore the circulatory volume with blood transfusion and to normalize coagulation with antivenom and coagulation factors (fresh frozen plasma). Antivenom neutralizes venom but it does not, per se, restore coagulation. Repeated laboratory tests of coagulation (prothrombin time, activated partial thromboplastin time, serum fibrinogen and fibrin degradation products) or bedside tests of bleeding should be performed repeatedly to determine the need for more antivenom and coagulation factors. The coagulation status is the most sensitive guide to the need for additional antivenom after bite by coagulopathic species.

Clinical example

Martina, a 2½-year-old child, collapsed with weakness, shallow respiration and weak pulses soon after playing in long grass where tiger snakes had been observed. Mechanical ventilation was necessary. A test of coagulation revealed prolonged prothrombin and activated partial thromboplastin times, a depleted serum fibrinogen level, a low platelet count and a high level of fibrin degradation products. Haematuria and melaena were observed. Venom was detected in the child's urine and blood and from scratch and puncture marks on the child's foot. Eight ampoules of tiger snake antivenom and transfusions of platelets, packed cells and fresh frozen plasma were required before her coagulation status returned to normal. Adequate spontaneous respiration was resumed after 48 hours.

Spider bite

Several thousand species of spiders exist in Australia. However, only funnel-web spiders and red-back spiders are known to be potentially lethal or to cause significant illness. However, almost all spiders have venom and a few may cause severe local injury. The white-tailed spider is often suspected of causing local tissue damage but the number of cases where it has been clearly identified as the responsible spider is very small.

Funnel-web spider bite

Several species of the genera *Atrax* and *Hadronyche* cause significant illness and are potentially lethal.

Atrax robustus (Sydney funnel-web spider) is a large, aggressive spider that has caused the deaths of more than a dozen people inhabiting an area within an approximate 160 km radius of Sydney, Australia. The male is more dangerous than the female, in contrast to other species, and is inclined to roam after rainfall. In doing so it may enter houses and seek shelter among clothes or bedding and give a painful bite when disturbed.

Bites do not always result in envenomation but envenomation may be rapidly fatal. The early features of the envenomation syndrome include nausea, vomiting, profuse sweating, salivation and abdominal pain. Life-threatening features are usually heralded by the appearance of muscle fasciculation at the bite site, which quickly involves distant muscle groups. Hypertension, tachyarrhythmias and vasoconstriction occur. The victim may lapse into coma, develop hypoventilation and have difficulty maintaining an airway free of saliva. Finally, respiratory failure and severe hypotension culminate in hypoxaemia of the brain and heart. The syndrome may develop within several hours but it may be more rapid. Several children have died within 90 minutes of envenomation, and one died within 15 minutes. The active component in the venom is a polypeptide that stimulates the release of acetylcholine at neuromuscular junctions and catecholamines within the autonomic nervous system.

Treatment consists of the application of a pressure–immobilization bandage, intravenous administration of antivenom and support of vital functions, which may include artificial airway support and mechanical ventilation. No deaths or serious morbidity have been reported since introduction of the antivenom in the early 1980s.

Red-back spider bite

This spider is distributed all over Australia and is to be found outdoors in household gardens in suburban and rural areas. Red-back spider bite is the most common cause for antivenom administration in Australia. The adult female is easily identified. Its body is about 1 cm in size and it has a distinct red or orange dorsal stripe over its abdomen. When disturbed, it gives a pinprick-like bite. The site becomes inflamed and may be surrounded by local swelling. During the following minutes to several hours, severe pain, exacerbated by movement, commences locally and may extend up the limb or radiate elsewhere. The pain may be accompanied by:

- profuse sweating
- headache
- nausea
- vomiting
- abdominal pain
- fever
- hypertension
- paraesthesias
- rashes.

In a small percentage of cases, when treatment is delayed, progressive muscle paralysis may occur over many hours and will require mechanical ventilation. Muscle weakness and spasm may persist for months after the bite. Death has not occurred since introduction of an antivenom in the 1950s. If the effects of a bite are minor and confined to the bite site, antivenom may be withheld, but otherwise antivenom should be given intramuscularly. Severe or recurrent pain should be treated with intravenous antivenom. In contrast to a bite from a snake or funnel-web spider, a bite from a red-back spider is not immediately life-threatening. There is no effective first aid but application of a cold pack or ice may relieve the pain.

Jellyfish stings

The most venomous animal in the world is the box jellyfish (*Chironex fleckeri*) and related species. It has caused at least 66 deaths in the waters off the north Australian coast. Other unrelated jellyfish species, notably the irukandji (*Carukia barnesi*), have caused significant illnesses and possibly several deaths.

Box jellyfish

This creature has a cuboid body up to 30 cm in diameter, and numerous tentacles that trail several metres. It is semitransparent and difficult to see by anyone wading or swimming in shallow water. The tentacles are lined with millions of nematocysts, which, on contact with skin, discharge threaded barbs that pierce subcutaneous tissue, including small blood vessels. Contact with the tentacles causes severe pain and envenomation that may cause death within several minutes. Death is probably due to both neurotoxic effects causing apnoea and direct cardiotoxicity, although the precise mode of action of the venom is unknown. The skin that sustains the injury may heal with disfiguring scars.

First aid, which must be administered on the beach, consists of dousing the skin with acetic acid (vinegar), which inactivates undischarged nematocysts. Adherent tentacles can then be removed safely. Cardiopulmonary resuscitation may be required on the beach. An ovine antivenom is available but prevention is of paramount importance. Water must not be entered when this jellyfish is known to be close inshore. Wet suits, clothing and 'stinger suits' offer protection.

Clinical example

A 12-year-old boy sustained a massive jellyfish sting to his legs while wading in water close to the shore. Immediately he experienced excruciating pain but managed to reach the shore, where he became apnoeic. His father gave mouth-to-mouth breathing. Vinegar was poured over the wounds, typical box jellyfish tentacles were removed and an ambulance was summoned. Shortly before arrival at hospital the boy became pulseless. Bag–mask ventilation with oxygen, external cardiac compression and intravenous adrenaline (epinephrine) were given. Spontaneous circulation was restored and he recommenced spontaneous respiration. In hospital, box jellyfish antivenom was infused. Thereafter the boy made a slow recovery but pulmonary oedema necessitated oxygen therapy and diuretic and inotropic infusion for several days. He recovered fully, but the stings healed with disfiguring scars.

Practical points

- Envenomation is a serious and potentially fatal problem
- Do not remove the pressure-immobilization bandage from a child bitten by a snake until the child is in a facility with resuscitation equipment, skilled staff and a supply of antivenom
- Many cases of suspected or confirmed snake-bite will not require antivenom
- Only treat symptomatic patients or those with significant coagulopathy
- Very large doses of antivenom may be needed for massively envenomated children

PART 6

FLUID REPLACEMENT

The child who needs fluid replacement

D. R. Brewster, T. Duke

Safe management of the fluid and electrolyte needs of unwell children requires knowledge of body water and electrolyte composition, fluid requirements, an ability to recognize signs of dehydration and over-hydration and an understanding of composition of fluids used for rehydration. Innovations in fluid management have been:

- rapid intravenous rehydration using isotonic saline solutions (Ringer's lactate or 0.9% NaCl) for severe dehydration
- rehydration with hypo-osmolar oral rehydration solution for mild or moderate dehydration
- early feeding and continued breast feeding in acute gastroenteritis
- prevention of iatrogenic hyponatraemia by giving volumes that take account of reduced free-water excretion in seriously ill children, and by avoiding hypotonic solutions
- use of zinc in the treatment of diarrhoea and dehydration.

Body composition

Body fluids are separated into two compartments, intracellular (ICF) and extracellular (ECF), with the latter subdivided into plasma and interstitial fluid. The proportion of body weight that is water falls from about 78% in a term newborn to 60% in adults (Table 6.1.1). Intracellular water accounts for about 40% of body weight and plasma for only about 5%. Interstitial fluid is proportionately higher in infants, with an interstitial to plasma volume ratio of 5:1 compared with 3:1 in adults. A 5 kg infant, for example, has approximately 3.5 l of total body water (TBW), so a loss of 500 ml as diarrhoea would represent a considerable proportion of his ECF volume. Large changes in body weight over 24 hours or less usually reflect changes in TBW, since substantial weight changes due to growth or subcutaneous tissue wasting occur over longer periods. In the first few days of life, there is a shift of water from ECF to ICF, accompanied by a 7% loss of TBW, so this is a very vulnerable period for dehydration with illness. Body fat contains only 20% water, so obesity implies a relative reduction in percentage of body weight as water. Conversely, malnourished children may have up to 80% of body weight as water. The clinical consequences are that:

- the severity of dehydration may be underestimated in obese children
- nutritional wasting is easily confused with dehydration
- fluid loads are poorly tolerated in severe malnutrition.

Water balance depends on intake (oral or parenteral), output and usage for metabolism. Water is normally lost from skin, lung, intestine and kidney. Fluid and energy requirements as a proportion of body weight decrease from infancy to adult life, so infants and children have higher metabolic requirements than adults and smaller absolute fluid stores, making them more vulnerable to dehydration.

Compared to intracellular fluid, extracellular fluid has high sodium and chloride and low potassium content (Fig. 6.1.1). Large increases in plasma lipids due to hyperlipidaemia or nephrotic syndrome may reduce the measured plasma sodium concentration but the overall ECF sodium content may remain within the normal range (artefactual hyponatraemia). In diabetes mellitus, hyperglycaemia increases ECF osmotic pressure and draws water out of cells, causing a true decrease in the plasma sodium content. ICF has high potassium, phosphate, magnesium and protein concentrations. Small intestinal secretions are high in sodium, diarrhoea fluid is high in potassium, gastric fluid is high in chloride and pancreatic secretions are high in bicarbonate (Table 6.1.2).

Cell membranes are relatively permeable to water, potassium and chloride, and relatively impermeable to sodium, phosphate and protein. Sodium is actively transported out of cells by energy-dependent sodium pumps. There is equilibrium in tonicity, hydrostatic and colloid osmotic pressure between plasma and interstitial fluid. Water leaves the arterial end of the capillary under hydrostatic pressure and is drawn into the venous end of capillary beds by plasma oncotic pressure.

Oedema is increased interstitial fluid and occurs by several mechanisms:

- increased hydrostatic pressure in the capillaries (venous obstruction, congestive heart failure)

Table 6.1.1 Body water distribution

Age group	Total body water (% of body weight)	Intracellular (% of body weight)	Extracellular (% of body weight)	ECF : ICF ratio	Blood (ml/kg)
Newborn	79	35	44	1.25	100
Infant	60	33	27	0.82	80
Child	62	41	21	0.51	70
Adult	58	39	19	0.49	60

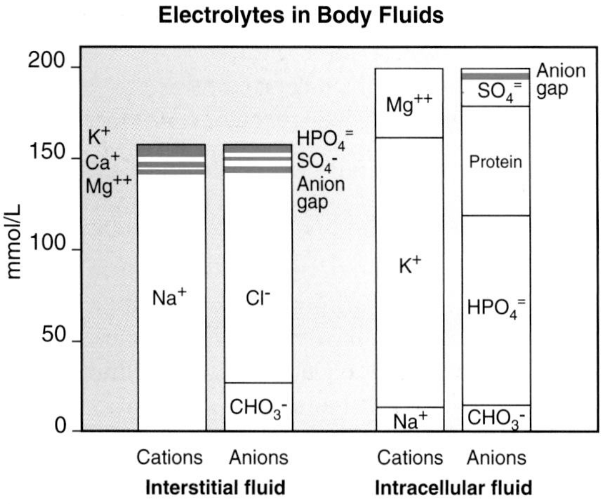

Fig. 6.1.1 Electrolytes in body fluids.

Table 6.1.2 Typical composition of body fluids in children (mmol/l)

Source	Na^+	K^+	Cl^-	HCO_3^-
Blood	140	4	100	25
Normal sweat	22	9	18	0
Bile	150	10	100	20
Gastric	50	15	125	0
Pancreatic	140	10	100	45
Small bowel	140	8	60	70
Diarrhoeal stool	40	50	25	65

These are illustrative mid-range values but there is considerable variation in individual values.

- decreased plasma oncotic pressure (hypoproteinaemic states: nephrotic syndrome, liver disease and kwashiorkor)
- increased capillary permeability (locally in insect bites, boils, general capillary leak syndrome from severe septicaemia, or cerebral oedema from traumatic brain injury).

Oedema may also occur if interstitial lymphatic vessels are poorly developed (Turner syndrome) or obstructed (e.g. filariasis, lymph node obstruction from tuberculosis).

Regulation of extracellular fluids

The plasma osmolality, which is the concentration of solute particles, remains almost constant between 285 and 300 mosmol per kg H_2O. The osmolality of plasma is controlled through a finely regulated feedback system involving osmoreceptors and volume receptors, the hypothalamus, the posterior pituitary and the collecting duct of the nephron. The intake of water is stimulated by thirst. This is regulated by a centre in the mid-hypothalamus, which responds to changes in circulating blood volume, via stretch and baroreceptors in the cardiovascular system, or changes in plasma osmolality of as little as 1–2%.

Normally water excretion through the kidneys is regulated via antidiuretic hormone (ADH). The primary action of ADH is to increase the permeability of the renal collecting ducts to water. A rise in osmolality is corrected by increased ADH secretion, resulting in a reduced volume of urine, which is concentrated. Conversely, a fall in plasma osmolality inhibits ADH secretion, resulting in excretion of an increased volume of dilute urine. Circulating blood volume is contained in arteries (10%), the venous system (55%), and heart, lungs and capillary bed (35%). The volume and distribution within the circulation is controlled by rapid feedback loops. Baroreceptors and stretch receptors in the heart and large vessels detect changes in venous tone and stimulate ADH secretion or inhibition and changes in venous tone, cardiac output and arteriolar resistance via the autonomic nervous system. Aldosterone is involved in plasma volume regulation through renal sodium retention via the renin–angiotensin system. Volume depletion is the dominant stimuli to thirst and ADH release, and so may stimulate water retention and oral intake at the expense of hypotonicity.

The kidney

In the kidney, the nephron regulates water and electrolyte excretion. The nephron comprises the proximal tubule, the hypertonic medulla and ascending loop of Henle, the distal tubule and the collecting duct. The precise regulation of fluids and electrolytes in the ECF occurs by reabsorption of the glomerular filtrate into capillaries and secretion into the lumen and eventual excretion in the urine.

The normal adult kidneys filter 25 000 mmol of sodium, 5000 mmol of bicarbonate, 700 mmol of potassium and 180 l of water daily. Under normal circumstances most of this is reabsorbed. Approximately two-thirds of the filtered sodium is reabsorbed in the proximal convoluted tubule. Another 25% is reabsorbed in the loop of Henle, which is used to create a concentration gradient for the countercurrent multiplier system, which allows the production of concentrated urine. In adults urine osmolality can vary from a maximal dilution of 100 mosmol/kg to a maximal concentration of 1400 mosmol/kg; newborns and young children have a more limited ability to concentrate and dilute urine. The distal tubule only reabsorbs 5% of the filtered sodium but the electrical gradient generated is used for potassium and hydrogen ion excretion into the distal tubule.

Assessment of dehydration

Clinical history and examination

A complete history and examination is important to ensure that the symptoms of diarrhoea or vomiting are not part of a disease other than gastroenteritis, such as intestinal obstruction, intussusception, pyloric stenosis, haemolytic–uraemic syndrome, urinary tract infection, etc. The following are some of the important symptoms and signs to elicit.

History

- *Diarrhoea*: duration, frequency, volume, consistency, blood, mucus
- *Vomiting*: duration, frequency, volume, bilious, projectile

- *Eating and drinking*: volumes, frequency, type (e.g. breast milk, oral rehydration solution, cordials)
- *Urine output*: volume, frequency, number of wet nappies (often difficult to assess)
- *Associated symptoms*: fever, cough, shortness of breath, abdominal pain, seizures, rashes, etc.
- *Nutritional status*: view the child's growth chart, check weight/height (wasting) and height/age (stunting)

Examination

- *General condition*: drowsy, restless or irritable
- *Vital signs*: temperature, pulse (or heart rate), respiratory rate, blood pressure
- *Eyes*: sunken, no tears on crying
- *Mouth and tongue*: dry mucous membranes
- *Skin*: skin turgor reduced or capillary refill time increased
- *Muscle tone*: weak, floppy or unable to hold head up
- *Chest*: deep acidotic breathing
- *Abdomen*: distended or tender, palpable masses

The signs of dehydration (Table 6.1.3) have been critically evaluated in two recent systematic reviews of published trials, using measures of validity, reliability, discriminatory power and response to change. In one review, the most useful clinical features of dehydration were: lethargic appearance, sunken eyes, dry mucous membranes and absence of tears. In another review the most useful individual signs for predicting dehydration in children were delayed capillary refill time, inelastic skin turgor and an abnormal respiratory pattern. A bicarbonate concentration of less than 16 mmol/l was associated with dehydration in acute gastroenteritis but other laboratory tests were unhelpful. Combinations of these signs of dehydration are more specific than any individual sign.

Weight change and the precision of clinical signs

If the child has been weighed accurately in the last few days, the percentage weight loss will be approximately equal to the percentage dehydration. Weight change from the immediate pre-morbid state is the most accurate way of estimating the degree of dehydration. However, the weights (premorbid and when sick) should be done using a comparable method: similar scale accuracy, unclothed, etc. If the premorbid weight was recorded more than a couple of weeks previously in young infants then the interpretation must take account of the expected weight gain

Table 6.1.3 Signs of dehydration

Degree of dehydration (approximate deficit)*	Mild, 3–5% (30–50 ml/kg)	Moderate, 6–9% (60–90 ml/kg)	Severe, ≥10% (100–150 ml/kg)
Validated signs			
General appearance	Well, alert	Thirsty, restless, irritable	Drowsy, floppy, limp ± comatose
Eyes	Normal	Slightly sunken	Very sunken
Mucous membranes	Moist tongue	Sticky tongue	Dry tongue
Tears on crying	Present	Decreased	Absent
Capillary return	Normal	Sluggish (2–3 s)	Slow (>3 s)
Respiratory rate	Normal	Increased	Fast
Skin pinch	Goes back quickly	Goes back slowly	Goes back very slowly
Other signs			
Thirst	Drinks normally, but may refuse ORS	Thirsty, drinks eagerly	Drinks poorly or not able to drink
Pulse	Normal	Fast	Fast, weak
Hands and feet	Normal	Normal	Cool, blue nail beds

* In young children.

because of growth. Additional considerations include the weight of medical equipment, e.g. an armrest for an intravenous cannula that may be absent premorbid and on admission but present on reweighing 24 hours later. However, a reliable recent premorbid weight is often unavailable. Clinical signs, if interpreted correctly, allow the estimation of dehydration range that is sufficient for clinical decision making. It is accurate to classify a child with diarrhoea (Table 6.1.3) as having no signs of dehydration (usually less than 5% dehydrated), some signs of dehydration (typically 5–9% dehydrated), or signs of severe dehydration (10% dehydrated or more).

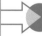

Practical points

Clinical evidence on assessing dehydration
- Capillary refill time, abnormal skin turgor and abnormal respiratory pattern are the most useful signs for detecting dehydration
- Combinations of signs perform better than individual signs, so general appearance, sunken eyes, dry mucous membranes and absence of tears are also useful
- This classification is most reliable:
  - no signs of dehydration (usually less than 5% dehydrated)
  - some signs of dehydration (typically 5–9% dehydrated)
  - signs of severe dehydration (10% dehydrated or more)
- Additional history and laboratory tests (e.g. bicarbonate) may be helpful in selected cases

Fluid requirements

The usual daily turnover of water for infants is about 25% of TBW (compared with only about 6% in adults), so infants and young children are especially susceptible to the consequences of abnormalities of fluid balance. Fluid therapy is conventionally divided into:

- maintenance
- deficit
- ongoing losses.

The fluid requirements of acutely unwell children are dynamic, and frequent monitoring of clinical signs, weight, urine output and some laboratory tests are essential so that appropriate modifications to fluid administration can be made.

Maintenance fluids

These requirements involve replacement of normal losses from urine, sweat, lungs and faeces, and assume that any fluid deficit (dehydration) has been replaced. The daily maintenance requirement can be simply calculated from the following formula:

- first 10 kg: 100 ml/kg per day
- 11–20 kg: 1000 ml + 50 ml/kg above 10 kg
- above 20 kg: 1500 ml + 20 ml/kg above 20 kg.

These volumes represent the water that is required, under normal physiological conditions, to excrete the daily production of nitrogenous wastes the body produces as urine that is isosmotic with plasma; i.e. that is neither overconcentrated or overdilute. These

Table 6.1.4   Intravenous solutions (mmol/l)

Solution	Sodium	Potassium	Chloride	Lactate	Calcium	Glucose
Ringer's lactate (Hartmann's)	130	5	110	30	2	–
4% glucose plus N/5 saline (0.18%)	30	–	30	–	–	222
2.5% glucose plus N/2 saline (0.45%)	75	–	75	–	–	139
Normal saline (0.9%)	150	–	150	–	–	–

Table 6.1.5   Conditions affecting normal fluid requirements

Condition	Response in terms of fluid requirements
Non-osmotic ADH production: bronchiolitis	(a) Decrease fluid requirements for bacterial meningitis, acute pneumonia, head injury (b) Decrease fluid requirements in stress (pain, surgery, emesis) (c) Decrease fluid requirements with certain drugs (opiates, NSAIDs*, vincristine)
Physical activity	Increase if active, decrease if inactive
Body temperature	Increase for fever, decrease for hypothermia
Metabolic rate	Increase if high, decrease if low
Respiratory rate	Increase for fast breathing
Humidity	Decrease for high humidity
Environmental temperature	Increase for sweating
*NSAID, non-steroidal anti-inflammatory drug.	

maintenance volumes are a guide only, and they cannot be directly applied to all seriously ill children, where water balance may very different from normal physiology.

Reduced free-water excretion is common in several conditions, including meningitis, encephalitis, bronchiolitis, pneumonia, perioperative states, burns, nausea and vomiting, where ADH release is stimulated by a variety of non-osmotic stimuli. In the past, hypotonic saline solutions (such as 0.18% saline plus 4–5% dextrose) (Table 6.1.4), were often used as maintenance fluid for hospitalized children. This fluid composition was based on energy expenditure and breast-milk electrolyte constituents in healthy children. However, administration of such hypotonic solutions, especially at 'maintenance' volumes or greater, have been associated with hyponatraemia, seizures, cerebral herniation and death in some patient groups. To avoid these iatrogenic complications solutions with a higher content of sodium (such as Ringer's lactate, normal 0.9% saline or half-normal 0.45% saline) should be the intravenous maintenance fluids of choice, and the volumes administered should take account of the reduced free water excretion that is common in many serious childhood conditions.

Although there is insufficient evidence from clinical trials to be certain how to avoid iatrogenic hyponatraemia and its serious consequences, after correction of signs of dehydration with isotonic saline it is essential to avoid rapid or excessive infusion of hypotonic fluids, and monitor serum sodium regularly in children on intravenous fluids, particularly in conditions associated with increased ADH release (Table 6.1.5).

Deficit therapy

Apart from severity, dehydration may also be classified as isotonic (serum sodium 130–150 mmol/l), hypotonic or hypertonic. Hypertonic dehydration may occur from osmotic diarrhoea if hypercaloric feed supplements (such as Polyjoule) or drinks with a very high glucose concentration are given while a child has diarrhoea. In hypertonic or hypernatraemic dehydration the increase in ECF osmolality results in movement of fluid out of cells. The clinical signs of dehydration in children with hypernatraemia are often not as prominent. The skin of the abdomen often has a 'doughy' feel. Because extracellular and intravascular volume is relatively well preserved, shock occurs very late. Hypernatraemia has important implications for therapy (see below).

Ongoing losses

It is difficult to quantify the amount of diarrhoea and vomiting, so it is better to review fluid balance, weight changes and clinical signs frequently and adjust fluid rates accordingly. A rough estimate for the additional volume lost in any diarrhoeal stool is:

- children under 2 years of age: 50–100 ml ($^1/_4$–$^1/_2$ large cup)
- children aged 2 up to 10 years: 100–200 ml ($^1/_2$–1 large cup).

Run the fluid rate as calculated for rehydration over 4 hours then review: weight, clinical examination including vital signs, ongoing losses, urine output and fluid intake (including breast milk). Be prepared to change the rate of administration depending on the above findings.

Rehydration

Using the guidelines for assessment of dehydration above, estimate the percentage of dehydration present:

Calculated fluid deficit (ml) =
% dehydration × weight (kg) × 10

(e.g. 10% dehydration in a 10 kg child = 1000 ml deficit).

- no signs of dehydration – <5% dehydrated, use maintenance fluids
- some signs of dehydration – calculate for 7% dehydration
- signs of severe dehydration – calculate for 10% dehydration

Intravenous

The clinical signs of *shock* or hypovolaemia are hypotension, poor peripheral perfusion, cool pale extremities, tachycardia with low-volume pulses, high blood lactate or large base deficit. Children with more than one of these signs should be given high-flow mask oxygen and 20 ml/kg of Ringer's lactate (also called Hartmann's solution) or normal saline rapidly, then reassessed. If there is no improvement give a further 20 ml/kg. If an intravenous cannula cannot be inserted, use the intraosseous route to the circulation (Ch. 3.2). If signs of hypovolaemia persist, the child should be monitored in an intensive care unit. Check for signs that are suggestive of other causes of shock (e.g. sepsis, cardiogenic, metabolic, diabetic ketoacidosis, intussusception, poisoning, etc.). In all children with meningitis, regardless of the presence of intracranial hypertension it is essential to ensure normal blood pressure and adequate circulating volume.

For the child who has signs of **severe dehydration**, replace the calculated fluid deficit with intravenous Ringer's lactate or normal saline over about 4 hours.

Table 6.1.6 Oral rehydration solutions (mmol/l of made up solution)						
Solution	Na$^+$	K$^+$	Cl$^-$	Citrate (base)	Glucose	Osmolality
WHO (standard)	90	20	80	10	111	310
WHO (hypo-osmolar)	75	20	65	10	75	245
Gastrolyte-R	60	20	50	10	(111 as rice*)	226
Repalyte	60	20	60	10	90	240
Pedialyte	45	20	35	10	126	250

* 80% amylopectin, 20% amylose.

In resuscitation of severe dehydration, crystalloids (Ringer's lactate or normal saline) are the only appropriate intravenous fluids. Similarly in resuscitation from shock from trauma isotonic crystalloids will be more effective (and much less expensive) than albumin or other colloids. In severe septic shock in adults and in severe malaria in children there is some evidence that if albumin is used outcomes are better. In general, isotonic saline or Ringer's lactate is the ideal fluid in initial resuscitation. Replacement of the fluid deficit in severe dehydration should be followed by maintenance requirements, which can usually be given enterally.

Rapid intravenous rehydration should only be carried out using Ringer's lactate or normal saline, not using hypotonic fluids such as 4% dextrose with 0.18% NaCl, which can lead to hyponatraemia, seizures and cerebral oedema. If intravenous fluids exceeding 30 ml/kg are to be administered, blood electrolytes should be measured to exclude hyponatraemia. Rapid rehydration with Ringer's lactate or normal saline is now the regimen for intravenous rehydration accepted by the World Health Organization (WHO) and the American Academy of Pediatrics. Regimens that correct the deficit over a longer period of time are usually only indicated in the setting of hypernatraemia.

Nasogastric

For nasogastric rehydration, the maximum safe rate of infusion is 20 ml/kg per hour. Nasogastric tubes can be unpleasant and carry a risk of pulmonary aspiration, so should be reserved for dehydrated children who cannot drink. Generally, refusal to drink in a conscious child means that s/he is not very dehydrated. Nasogastric fluids may not be absorbed if a child is in shock, so prompt intravascular or intraosseous infusions should be used for children in shock.

Oral

In mild to moderate dehydration, oral rehydration is usually successful. Oral rehydration solution (ORS) is a powder containing a specific balance of electrolytes and glucose, formulated for use in children with diarrhoea. ORS is based on the important principle of glucose-facilitated intestinal sodium absorption. Cereal-based solutions (e.g. rice ORS) have no advantage over glucose solutions in noncholera diarrhoea, and are no substitute for early feeding. Fluids such as soft drinks, sports beverages and fruit juices are not appropriately constituted to be an effective ORS to treat dehydration, and

may cause osmotic diarrhoea and hypernatraemic dehydration.

Oral rehydration is a highly effective means of rehydration that is greatly underused in developed countries like Australia. Doctors in teaching hospitals often have a tendency to resort too readily to intravenous and nasogastric therapies. In most developed countries severe dehydration is uncommon, yet many children with gastroenteritis are unnecessarily given intravenous fluids despite ample evidence that oral rehydration is as effective. The overall failure rate of enteral therapy from published studies is less than 5%. The main reasons for failure of oral rehydration are persistent vomiting, high purging rates (stool output), electrolyte disturbance (e.g. hypokalacmia), excessive drowsiness and shock.

The WHO ORS solution composition has been improved in keeping with the documented advantages of reduced osmolarity (75 mmol Na^+ compared with 90 mmol Na^+ per litre), but commercial solutions that have even lower sodium content (60 mmol/l) are more widely available in developed countries (Table 6.1.6). Reduced osmolarity ORS has been shown to decrease the need for intravenous therapy and not increase the risk of hyponatraemia; however, the populations of children they have been tested on have had low rates of hyponatraemia compared to what is seen in many developing countries. Reduced osmolarity ORS has not been shown to be more effective than normal osmolarity ORS in the management of cholera.

Continuation of feeding, particularly in breastfed infants, is very important in the management of diarrhoea. Continued breastfeeding, or early semisolid feeding, within 4 hours reduces weight loss during illness without worsening diarrhoea or vomiting. Probiotics may be a useful adjunct to ORS in treating acute viral gastroenteritis but may not benefit subgroups such as partially breastfed children or those with bacterial or parasitic causes of diarrhoea. Antidiarrhoeal drugs (such as opioids and binding agents) and antimicrobials have no place in the management of acute watery diarrhoea.

In recent years zinc (20 mg/d in children and 10 mg/d in infants under 6 months, for 10–14 d) has been shown to reduce the severity and duration of diarrhoea in acute diarrhoea and to reduce mortality in children with severe malnutrition and diarrhoea in developing countries. Zinc is now recommended by the WHO for the adjunctive treatment of all children with chronic or persistent diarrhoea, acute diarrhoea or severe malnutrition. When given to low birth weight babies at a dose of 5 mg/d, zinc prevents diarrhoea throughout infancy.

Clinical example

How would you manage a 2-year-old child weighing 12 kg who is assessed to be 7% dehydrated with serum Na^+ 135 mmol/l, K^+ 1.8 mmol/l, pH 7.08, bicarbonate 8 mmol/l and base excess −15?

Fluids

I.v. rehydration	Maintenance	Total fluid (24 h)

7% × 10 ml/kg × 12 kg = 840 ml
Replace over 4 h
  840 ÷ 4 = 210 ml/h as
  Ringer's lactate
	(10 kg × 100) + (2 kg × 50) = 1100 ml
	Over 20 h = 55 ml/h as Ringer's
	  lactate (or ORS, breast milk or
	  formula)
		840 + 1100 ml = 1950 ml + ongoing losses

Potassium

1. Rehydration
a. *Concentration*: 1 g KCl in 1000 ml Ringer's lactate (13.4 + 5) = 18.4 mmol/l (4 h)
b. *Flow rate*: 210 ml/h × 0.0184 mmol/ml K^+ ÷ 12 kg = 0.32 mmol K^+/kg/h for 4 h

2. Maintenance
a. *Concentration*: 2 g KCl in 1000 ml Ringer's lactate = 26.8 mmol/l (20 h)
b. *Flow rate*: 55 ml/h × 0.0268 mmol/ml K^+ ÷ 12 kg = 0.12 mmol K^+/kg/h (adjust depending on repeat K^+ and consider oral therapy)

Bicarbonate
It is not necessary to add bicarbonate to intravenous rehydration fluid. Ringer's lactate contains base as lactate and ORS contains base as citrate. Bicarbonate has not been shown to be beneficial in diarrhoeal dehydration, and acidosis generally resolves with adequate rehydration alone.

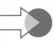

Practical points

Clinical evidence on rehydration in acute gastroenteritis
- In children admitted to hospital with non-cholera diarrhoea, reduced osmolarity ORS when compared to WHO standard ORS is associated with a reduced need for intravenous infusions, lower stool volume and less vomiting with no additional risk of developing hyponatraemia
- Standard glucose-based ORS is just as effective in reducing stool output in infants and children with non-cholera diarrhoea as rice-based ORS
- In critically ill patients with dehydration or traumatic hypovolaemia, resuscitation with crystalloids (e.g. Ringer's lactate or normal saline) is more effective than resuscitation with colloids (e.g. albumin solutions)
- Probiotics appear to be a useful adjunct to rehydration therapy in treating acute infectious diarrhoea in children but this may not be true for some settings, such as those with high rates of bacterial and parasitic causes of diarrhoea or with prolonged breastfeeding. Heat-killed lactic acid bacteria may be harmful
- Zinc reduces the severity and duration of diarrhoea and reduces mortality in children with severe malnutrition

Electrolyte disturbances

Severe electrolyte disturbances occur in up to 25% of hospitalized children in whom electrolytes are measured. Infants less than 6 months of age and children with severe dehydration or diabetes mellitus are disproportionately affected. Derangements of acid–base, sodium and potassium are the most common abnormalities. In Aboriginal children with acute gastroenteritis in northern Australia, two-thirds have metabolic acidosis and/or hypokalaemia at the time of presentation.

Hypokalaemia

Potassium can be lost from the extracellular space in diarrhoeal stools, especially with osmotic diarrhoea. In severe dehydration, rehydration and correction of metabolic acidosis may worsen hypokalaemia as ECF potassium moves intracellularly. With high aldosterone levels in dehydration, sodium and water retention by the kidney may also lead to potassium loss. Hypokalaemia may be manifest as hypotonia, irritability, intestinal ileus with distension, and cardiac arrhythmias with T wave changes. The serum potassium concentration may not reflect the degree of total body potassium depletion, as most is stored intracellularly (particularly in muscle and brain). Before giving potassium you must ensure that a child does not have renal failure (e.g. haemolytic uraemic syndrome, acute tubular necrosis, acute glomerulonephritis). In view of the cardiac effects of extremes of plasma potassium concentration, electrocardiographic monitoring is important in severe hypokalaemia (<2.5 mmol/l) and with intravenous infusions of potassium in concentrations greater than 30 mmol/l.

Management of hypokalaemia

Intravenous

Add 1 g (rapid rehydration) or 2 g (maintenance) potassium chloride to 1 l of Ringer's lactate and run at the rate calculated for rehydration. Note that *ampoules of potassium chloride must always be diluted.* 1 g of KCl = 13.4 mmol K^+, and Ringer's lactate already contains 5 mmol/l K^+, so the total concentration of the solution is 18.4 mmol/l (if 1 g KCl is added) or 31.8 mmol/l (if 2 g KCl is added). You must always calculate both the K^+ infusion rate (mmol/kg per hour) and the K^+ concentration (mmol/l). Never exceed an infusion rate of 0.4 mmol/kg K^+ per hour (as cardiac arrhythmias may occur) or an infusion concentration of 40 mmol/l K^+ (unless it is given via central vein), as it is irritating to peripheral veins.

Oral

Give 8–10 mmol/kg K^+ per day in divided doses 4–6-hourly. Large doses of oral potassium may induce vomiting, so each individual dose should not exceed 1.5 mmol/kg.

Hyponatraemia

The most common causes of hyponatraemia in young children are hypotonic dehydration and iatrogenic water overload (e.g. overestimation of the degree of dehydration, inappropriate use of hypotonic solutions for rehydration and/or too rapid administration of maintenance fluids). Other causes include the syndrome of inappropriate ADH secretion (SIADH) in meningitis (see Table 6.1.5 and Ch. 12.3), salt losing nephropathy, salt wasting in some intracranial pathologies, and the sick cell syndrome (such as in kwashiorkor). Hyponatraemia with dehydration often accompanies acute gastroenteritis and is corrected by the standard rehydration protocols, including treatment of the fluid deficit. It is unwise to infuse large volumes of hypotonic solutions in children if the serum sodium is below 138 mmol/l or if there are risk factors for ADH release such as brain infection or injury, or severe pulmonary infection.

Management

• *Reassess hydration status*: is it hyponatraemic dehydration? If the child is more than 5% dehydrated and the hyponatraemia is due to gastroenteritis, rehydrate with Hartmann's solution as above
• *Assess for signs of fluid overload*: excessive weight gain, oedema, signs of cardiac failure. If signs of fluid overload are present, then decreasing the rate of administering fluid or fluid restriction is usually all that is necessary

• The use of hypertonic saline infusions (such as 3% NaCl) to correct hyponatraemia is indicated only in severely symptomatic children (e.g. seizures when the serum sodium <120 mmol/l) and should only be given to correct the sodium to a safe level (such as 5 mmol/l more than the starting level) and until severe symptoms resolve. This should only be done after appropriate consultation
• After initial correction of any severe symptoms of hyponatraemia (e.g. convulsions) the rate of rise of serum sodium should not exceed 1 mmol/l every 2 hours. The longer the child has had hyponatraemia the slower the correction should be.

Hypernatraemia

Hypernatraemia (Na^+ >150 mmol/l) may occur with moderate or severe dehydration, especially if fluids too high in solutes have been used for rehydration. This occurred frequently when boiled skim milk and homemade salt–sugar solutions were used to treat diarrhoea and unmodified cows milk was used for infant feeding. Fortunately it is now relatively uncommon.

In children with hypernatraemia, the degree of dehydration is often underestimated because of the fluid shifts out of cells, maintaining plasma and interstitial fluid volumes; therefore the common clinical signs of intravascular dehydration (tachycardia, weak thready pulse) only occur when a child has very severe dehydration. Children with hypernatraemic dehydration may have marked irritability and a 'doughy feeling' to the skin over their abdomen, due to loss of intracellular water in the brain and soft tissues respectively. Shock occurs very late and, because of hyperosmolarity, cerebrovascular thrombosis may occur.

Management

• Avoid rapid correction of hypernatraemia, as rapidly falling serum sodium may cause cerebral oedema or seizures. Adjust fluid volume and composition to return the serum sodium to normal slowly (no more than 1 mmol/l every 2 h, or 10–12 mmol/l per 24 h). Do not use hypotonic maintenance intravenous fluids such as 4% + one-fifth normal (0.18%) saline, as this is likely to drop the serum sodium too rapidly. Use Ringer's lactate, 0.9% NaCl (normal saline) or 0.45% NaCl (half-normal saline) if intravenous fluids are necessary
• Rehydration with oral fluids is a good alternative, correcting the deficit over 24 hours
• Regardless of the method of rehydration the child's electrolytes and clinical signs need to be monitored frequently.

225

Hypocalcaemia and hypomagnesaemia

Hypocalcaemia and hypomagnesaemia often accompany hypokalaemia. There is complex interplay between these ions and changes in blood pH. Hypomagnesaemia and alkalosis lower the threshold for tetany, whereas hypokalaemia and acidosis increase this threshold. In addition, hypomagnesaemia blunts the parathyroid hormone (PTH) response to hypocalcaemia by blocking the release of this hormone, and correction of hypomagnesaemia is often necessary before correction of calcium and potassium levels can occur.

Hypocalcaemia

Clinical features of hypocalcaemia include tetany (which can manifest as irritability, lethargy, carpopedal spasm, seizures, bronchospasm, laryngospasm), the Chvostek sign (spasm of the facial muscles elicited by tapping the facial nerve in the region of the parotid gland), lengthening of QT interval on the ECG, arrhythmias and intestinal cramps.

Treatment
For oral correction:

- calcium carbonate; calcium lactate gluconate
- dose (not per kg): <4 years – 100 mg 2–5 times daily; 4–12 years – 500 mg twice daily.

For intravenous correction:

- use calcium gluconate 10% (0.22 mmol/ml Ca^{2+})
- give stat. dose i.v. 0.5 mmol/kg slowly over 10–20 min or i.m.
- follow with an i.v. infusion of 0.5 mmol/kg over 4–6 h (in fluid calculated for rehydration).

Note that intravenous calcium cannot be added to bicarbonate (precipitates as chalk); calcium is also very irritating to tissues if it extravasates or to peripheral veins, and it causes bradycardia if infused too rapidly.

Hypomagnesaemia

Hypomagnesaemia can produce tetany without hypocalcaemia and should always be measured in children with tetany, or if tetany is refractory to calcium. Other clinical features of hypomagnesaemia are hyperirritability, seizures, increased tone and reflexes, muscle fasciculations, rhabdomyolysis, cardiac arrhythmias and conduction disturbances.

Treatment
For intramuscular or intravenous correction:

- 49.3% magnesium sulphate (2 mmol/ml Mg^{2+})
- dose: 0.2 ml/kg twice daily (give i.v. slowly over 5 min).

Precautions: high doses of magnesium can cause prolongation of PR and QRS intervals and bradyarrhythmias, hypotension, neuromuscular blockade and sedation if given too quickly.

For oral treatment:

- use magnesium aspartate tablets (500 mg/ 1.5 mmol Mg).
- dose: 3–6 mg/kg/d of elemental magnesium in three divided doses.

Practical points

Electrolyte calculations
- NaCl contains 17 mmol of sodium and chloride per gram
- KCl contains 13 mmol of potassium and chloride per gram, 0.75 g/10 ml = 1 mmol/ml K+
- Sodium bicarbonate contains 12 mmol of sodium and bicarbonate per gram, and 8.4% $NaHCO_3^-$ contains 1 mmol/ml of sodium and bicarbonate per ml
- Calcium gluconate 10% = 0.22 mmol/ml Ca^{2+}
- Magnesium sulphate 49.3% = 2.465g/5 ml = 2 mmol/ml Mg^{2+}
- Magnesium chloride 0.48 g/5 ml = 1 mmol/ml Mg^{2+}
- Osmolality of serum = 2 Na^+ + glucose + urea (in mmol/l), which is normally 270–295
- Anion gap = $Na^+ + K^+ - (HCO_3^- + Cl^-)$, which is normally less than 12

Acid–base balance

Metabolic acidosis

Metabolic acidosis commonly complicates severe illness but will usually correct with treatment of the primary disorder, provided there is normal renal function and bicarbonate production. Acidosis only warrants specific treatment if the low pH is interfering with normal cellular function, often considered as a pH below 7.15 (normal range 7.35–7.45). In severe sepsis, asphyxia, multi-trauma and cardiovascular collapse, tissue oxygen delivery or cellular oxygen utilization are impaired. To produce sufficient energy for cell metabolism, adenosine triphosphate (ATP) is produced through anaerobic glycolysis. Excess hydrogen ions (H^+) in the form of lactate are produced in this process. These are initially buffered by red cells, plasma proteins or bicarbonate, or compensated for by increased removal of CO_2 by the respiratory system. The latter is manifest by Kussmaul (deep sighing) respiration. When buffers become limited, blood pH falls, causing metabolic acidosis. pH and H^+ have a logarithmic relationship, such that a fall in the pH to 7.1 means the H^+ level has doubled from 40 to 80 nmol/l (Table 6.1.7).

Table 6.1.7 Acidosis and alkalosis

Acid–base status	Clinical example	pH	Primary	Compensatory	Clinical feature
Metabolic acidosis	Diabetic ketoacidosis	↓	↓ HCO_3^-	↓ PCO_2	Deep breathing
Metabolic alkalosis	Pyloric stenosis	↑	↑ HCO_3^-	↑ PCO_2	Decreased respiration
Respiratory acidosis	Hyaline membrane disease	↓	↑ PCO_2	↑ HCO_3^-	Drowsiness
Respiratory alkalosis	Hysterical hyperventilation	↑	↓ PCO_2	↓ HCO_3^-*	Tetany

* May take several hours to develop, so will not often be present initially.

Bicarbonate reacts with hydrogen ions to produce water and carbon dioxide: $H^+ + HCO_3^- \rightarrow H_2O + CO_2$. Metabolic acidosis often accompanies diarrhoea with dehydration. There are a number of well-known causes of acidosis in diarrhoea, such as:

- bicarbonate loss in stool
- severe dehydration with decreased tissue perfusion (lactic acidosis)
- diminished renal function
- fermentation of dietary sugars from small bowel bacterial overgrowth, leading to absorption of organic acids (e.g. acetate, butyrate, propionate), may also be a factor in malnourished children.

Anion gap

Measurement of serum chloride and the anion gap (see Practical points: Electrolyte calculations) may be useful in determining the cause of metabolic acidosis:

- Causes of metabolic acidosis with normal anion gap (8–12 mmol/l)
  - gastrointestinal loss of bicarbonate (diarrhoea)
  - renal loss of bicarbonate (renal tubular acidosis)
  Note that the urine anion gap will be negative with gastrointestinal causes of acidosis and positive with renal causes of acidosis (decreased ammonia excretion)
- Causes of metabolic acidosis with increased anion gap (>12 mmol/l)
  - increased organic acid production (e.g. lactic acidosis, diabetic ketoacidosis, organic acidaemias)
  - ingestion of toxic substances (e.g. salicylates, methyl alcohol, ethylene glycol)
  - decreased excretion of acid (e.g. acute renal failure, chronic renal failure).

Acidosis is corrected by fluid replacement, correction of hypoxaemia, provision of calories and treatment of any infection. Intravenous sodium bicarbonate is rarely indicated in acidosis associated with diarrhoea and has the disadvantage of transiently worsening the hypokalaemia, and the increased sodium load may not be well tolerated, especially if the child has severe malnutrition. Persisting metabolic acidosis with diarrhoeal disease may indicate the need for further rehydration (i.e. the degree of dehydration has been underestimated) or continuing osmotic diarrhoea (e.g. lactose, sucrose, glucose polymer or monosaccharide intolerance).

Alkalosis

Although much less common than acidosis, there are a few conditions where alkalosis occurs in children. Metabolic alkalosis occurs with recurrent vomiting in pyloric stenosis and diuretic use, and respiratory alkalosis occurs in hyperventilation.

Fluid and electrolyte problems in specific illnesses

Pyloric stenosis

Severe or protracted vomiting causes a hypochloraemic hypokalaemic alkalosis. Severe intracellular depletion of potassium results in increased exchange of hydrogen ions for sodium in the distal tubule, paradoxically resulting in acid urine despite a systemic alkalosis. Infants with severe vomiting may have a serum chloride concentration below 80 mmol/l and bicarbonate above 40 mmol/l. In view of the alkalosis, Ringer's lactate is not an appropriate rehydration fluid in pyloric stenosis. Normal saline with additional potassium can be used to replace the deficit, followed by normal maintenance fluids, and formula or breast milk can be given fairly soon after surgery. It is important to correct dehydration and alkalosis before surgery. Alkalosis can result in postanaesthetic apnoea.

Adrenal insufficiency

With salt-losing manifestations, the serum sodium and chloride are low and the potassium is high with increased plasma renin activity. Intravenous administration of 5% glucose in 0.9% saline solution should be given to correct the hypoglycaemia and the sodium loss, along with hydrocortisone.

Burns

For children with a burn requiring fluid resuscitation (usually >10% body surface area burned), an appropriate starting formula is intravenous Ringer's lactate 4 ml/kg per 1% burned surface area. Half of this fluid is given in the first 8 hours and the remainder over the next 16 hours, adjusting the rate according to the patient's response. For adequate fluid resuscitation, burns cases may need to gain more than their preburn weight because of intracellular and interstitial oedema. During the second day after the burn, oedema fluid starts to be reabsorbed and urine output should increase. A rough guide to fluid requirements on day 2 is half of the first day's requirement, but as Ringer's lactate with 5% glucose. There is still controversy about whether colloid should be provided in the early period of burns resuscitation. If 0.5% silver nitrate solution is used as the topical dressing, sodium and potassium losses may be extensive and require supplements. Children with extensive burns or those involving the face or airway should be managed in specialized units.

Bacterial meningitis

Careful management of fluid and electrolyte balance is important in the treatment of meningitis since over- or underhydration are associated with adverse outcomes. Many children have increased antidiuretic hormone secretion, and some have dehydration due to vomiting, poor fluid intake or septic shock. Hyponatraemia occurs in about one-third of children with meningitis and is variously as a result of increased ADH secretion, increased urine sodium losses and excessive electrolyte-free water intake or administration. Children with meningitis require careful and regular monitoring of clinical signs of hydration state, including signs of overhydration, serum sodium and laboratory markers of hypovolaemia. The fluid rates suggested in Table 6.1.8 are starting rates only and subsequent frequent evaluation is necessary. Assessment of the clinical signs of hydration, including weight, measurement of the serum sodium and acid–base status, and clinical assessment of the neurological state should be repeated every 6–12 hours for the first 48 hours, and the total fluid intake

adjusted accordingly. Enteral feeds should be started when the child is stable but should be withheld in children who are poorly conscious, vomiting or having frequent convulsions. Children who are drinking well should have intravenous fluids running very slowly or the cannula capped.

Acute renal failure

Oliguria is defined as a urine output below 0.5 ml/kg per hour. Urine volume is determined by filtration, reabsorption and secretion, so the presence of oliguria should lead to assessment of hydration, sodium excretion and urinary osmolality. Anuria should raise suspicion of urinary obstruction. The physiological response to a decrease in intravascular volume (dehydration, septic shock) is to enhance reabsorption of tubular fluid in the proximal and distal segments of the nephron and for the posterior pituitary to release ADH. This will result in a low urinary sodium (<20 mmol/l) and high osmolarity (>500 mosmol/l). With renal tissue injury, such as in acute glomerulonephritis or haemolytic uraemic syndrome, the urinary sodium is usually above 40 mmol/l. Diuretics, especially loop diuretics such as furosemide, have been used to maintain urine output in oliguria or anuria due to renal injury. Diuretics will be further harmful in prerenal azotemia as they further reduce circulating volume and renal blood flow. While the mortality of non-oliguric renal failure is less than that of oliguric renal failure, differential mortality rates based on urine output reflect differences in severity of the underlying renal injury and overall disease processes. There is no evidence that diuretics protect renal function or prevent death in children with renal dysfunction.

Lactose intolerance

The most common carbohydrate intolerance is disaccharide intolerance, which is almost always lactose intolerance. Sucrose or glucose polymer intolerance may accompany lactose intolerance. Occasionally, transient monosaccharide intolerance may also occur, particularly in young infants with *Cryptosporidium* infection, which may necessitate grading of feeds to decrease the carbohydrate intake below the threshold level of intolerance. All carbohydrates in the diet are broken down by digestive processes into monosaccharides, of which glucose is by far the most common. Glucose and galactose are the monosaccharide end products of lactose digestion of milk; glucose and fructose of sucrose breakdown; and glucose of maltose and isomaltose digestion. Starch is the most common carbohydrate in the diet and this is converted to glucose by various steps. All carbo-

Table 6.1.8   Recommended total fluid intake (ml/h for the first 24–48 h) for children with suspected or confirmed meningitis, divided into four groups

Weight (kg)	A. Normal serum Na$^+$ *and* no dehydration, oedema or raised ICP	B. Serum Na$^+$ <135 *and* no dehydration, oedema or raised ICP	C. Signs of dehydration or hypovolaemia	D. Signs of raised ICP *or* generalized oedema
3	9	6	9	5
4	12	8	12	6
5	15	10	15	7
6	18	12	18	9
7	21	14	21	11
8	24	16	24	12
9	27	18	27	14
10	30	20	30	15
11	32	21	32	17
12	33	22	33	18
15	38	25	38	20
20	45	30	45	22
30	53	35	53	27

Group A. Normal serum Na$^+$ and no signs of hypovolaemia, dehydration or raised intracranial pressure. Fluid guideline based on giving 3 ml/kg per hour up to a weight of 10 kg (about 70% of 'maintenance fluid requirements') as normal saline +5% dextrose.

Group B. Hyponatraemia (Na$^+$ <135) but no signs of hypovolaemia, dehydration or raised intracranial pressure. Fluid guideline based on giving 2 ml/kg per hour up to a weight of 10 kg (about 50% of 'maintenance fluid requirements') as normal saline +5% dextrose. If the serum [Na$^+$] is very low (<130 mmol/l) refer to the ICU.

Group C. Signs of dehydration or hypovolaemia at presentation. Give repeated boluses of 10–20 ml/kg of normal saline until hypovolaemia is corrected. Refer to ICU if signs of hypovolaemia persist. Ongoing fluid guideline based on giving 3 ml/kg per hour up to a weight of 10 kg as normal saline +5% dextrose.

Group D. Signs of raised intracranial pressure or generalized oedema. Fluid guideline based on giving 1–2 ml/kg per hour up to 10 kg (about 25–50% of 'maintenance fluid requirements') as normal saline +5% dextrose. A child with any clinical signs of raised intracranial pressure (e.g. very bulging fontanelle, unresponsiveness to painful stimuli or papilloedema) or of overhydration (e.g. facial or generalized oedema) should have fluids restricted and be monitored in an ICU. Development of generalized oedema is a major risk factor for serious adverse outcomes in meningitis, which is due at least in part to excessive fluid administration.

hydrates are made up of monosaccharide polymers. Disaccharides contain two monosaccharides, oligosaccharides contain two to 10 monosaccharides, and polysaccharides contain more that 10 monosaccharides. Monosaccharides are absorbed by an active process and the mechanisms are different for glucose and fructose.

The enzymes that allow the breakdown of disaccharides to monosaccharides are present in the brush border of the intestinal mucosa (Ch. 20.3). Lactase is more superficial and thus more commonly reduced than sucrase or maltase with intestinal mucosal damage. When mucosal damage is more severe the absorption of monosaccharides may also be affected, particularly in non-breastfed infants with severe or intractable diarrhoea. Mucosal maltase–glucoamylase and sucrase–isomaltase and glucose cotransporter (SGLT-1) are reduced in villous atrophy. Malnourished children have a reduced mean mucosal lactase specific activity but have a compensatory increase in sucrase and SGLT-1 levels when controlled for mucosal weight. Malnutrition and

Clinical example

A 15-month-old Aboriginal boy presented with diarrhoea, floppiness and fast breathing. His mother said that he had had many watery bowel movements over a short period of time. On examination he appeared unwell and was lethargic with sunken eyes. His vital signs were: temperature 37.5°C, heart rate 120/min, respiratory rate 60/min and blood pressure 86/53. Although alert and responsive, he was noted to be floppy, with a dry mouth, absent tears on crying, weak radial pulses, a capillary refill time of over 2 seconds and slow skin pinch recoil. On auscultation his heart sounds were normal and his lung fields were clear. His abdomen was soft and slightly distended with no tenderness, masses or visceromegaly. Bowel sounds were present. Neurological examination was normal except for mild hypotonia.

He was commenced on an intravenous infusion of Ringer's lactate and blood was taken for full blood count and urea and electrolytes. His weight on admission was 6.1 kg and his height 68 cm. These are all below the 3rd centile and yield a weight for age of 56% of the median (Z-score −4.4), a height for age of 85% (Z-score −4.0) and a weight-for-height of 76% (Z-score −2.6). His head circumference was 43.6 cm, which falls well below the 2nd centile for age (Z-score −3.0).

The laboratory findings were as follows (reference ranges are given in parentheses).

Blood tests:
Full blood count
Haemoglobin (g/l): 82 (105–135)
MCV (fl): 53.9 (75–85)
RDW (%): 24.1 (11.5–14.5)
Platelets (×10⁹/l): 724 (150–450)
White cells (×10⁹/l): 15.6 (6.0–11.0)
Blood film report: Marked microcytosis and hypochromia, moderate anisocytosis and poikilocytosis, neutrophil leucocytosis with no toxic changes and moderate eosinophilia.

Electrolytes
Sodium (mmol/l): 138 (132–144)
Potassium (mmol/l): 2.0 (3.2–4.8)
Chloride (mmol/l): 111 (98–106)
Bicarbonate (mmol/l): 6 (18–27)
Anion gap: 23 (8–12)
Urea (mmol/l): 5.3 (1.4–5.4)
Creatinine (mmol/l): 44 (0–55)

Blood gases
pH: 7.12 (7.35–7.4)
$P\text{CO}_2$ (mml lg): 20.3 (35–45)
Base excess: −18 (−4 to +3)
Blood lactate (mmol/l): 1.6 (0.8–1.8)

He was rehydrated with 600 ml Ringer's lactate with 1 g/l of KCl added (17.4 mmol/l) over 4 hours, followed by maintenance fluids at 30 ml/h with breastfeeding. By 24 hours after admission he had been given 1500 ml of fluids and his condition had much improved. His weight was now 6.7 kg, which implied that he had been about 9% dehydrated on admission (6.7 − 6.1 = 0.6 kg; 0.6 ÷ 6.7 × 100 = 8.96%). His diarrhoea was settling and he was passing dilute urine.

Over the next 24 hours, however, he had six foul, watery stools containing large amounts of reducing substances. There was also a decrease in his pH, bicarbonate and magnesium compared with 24 hours previously. This relapse of osmotic diarrhoea was due to breast milk lactose overcoming the lactase threshold in the small intestinal mucosal brush border. He improved on oral lactase drops (β-D-galactosidase) with breastfeeds. The stool microscopy result reported ova of *Strongyloides stercoralis*.

This is a fairly typical case of acute gastroenteritis in an Aboriginal child from northern Australia, whose illness is frequently complicated by osmotic diarrhoea, hypokalaemia, acidosis and iron deficiency. The underlying small bowel damage could be prevented by improving hygiene, reducing overcrowding and prompt treatment of micronutrient deficiencies, which would then make community oral rehydration therapy more effective.

Table 6.1.9   Diagnosis of reducing substances in stool (osmotic diarrhoea)

For hot and cold stool testing of reducing substances you need approximately 1 ml of stool fluid. A positive test = > 0.5%

Cold test (for monosaccharide or lactose sugars)

1. Mix 1 ml stool with 2 ml water
2. Take 15 drops from that mixture and place in test tube
3. Add 1 Clinitest tablet
4. Wait until tablet stops reacting
5. Shake and compare with chart

Hot test (for sucrose, starch sugars or glucose polymers when the cold test is ≤0.5%)

1. Take 10 drops hydrochloric acid 1%
2. Add 5 drops fluid stool
3. Mix and bring slowly to boil
4. Add Clinitest tablet
5. Wait until tablet stops reacting and compare with chart

Stool water must be collected directly and tested promptly. If it is scraped from a nappy or tested after 30 minutes, it is likely to give falsely low results.

small bowel mucosal damage contribute independently to lactose malabsorption.

There is a threshold for lactose intolerance, which, when exceeded, may result in profuse osmotic diarrhoea with acidosis and hypokalaemia. Children with tropical enteropathy syndrome (asymptomatic small bowel mucosal damage from poor hygiene living circumstances) have a lower threshold, as lactase is on the tip of the brush border. Recovery of the intestinal mucosa is prompt after rotaviral gastroenteritis, so children with a normal gut before infection will usually tolerate breast milk at least by the third day of infection. However, this threshold is often exceeded in Aboriginal children during early recovery, when their intake of breast milk returns to normal or even increased volumes. The technique for testing for lactose intolerance/intolerance of other sugars is given in Table 6.1.9. Lactose intolerance in acute gastroenteritis is now uncommon in most developed country settings with good hygiene practices.

PART 7

PRINCIPLES OF IMAGING IN CHILDHOOD

Diagnostic imaging in infancy and childhood

R. Teele

Paediatric radiology became a subspecialty of radiology and of paediatrics because of two men: John Caffey, paediatrician, and Edward B. D. Neuhauser, radiologist. A quirk of fate resulted in this 'infant' subspecialty, born in the 1940s, being affiliated with radiology rather than with paediatrics – and the fact that ionizing radiation as a means of imaging was the province of radiology. Paediatric radiology has developed dramatically in the interim. Now, the tools of the radiologist include plain radiography, fluoroscopy (screening), intravenous, intracavitary and gastrointestinal contrast media, angiography, nuclear medicine, ultrasonography, computed tomography (CT) and magnetic resonance imaging (MRI).

There are many differences between imaging the child and imaging the adult. Most importantly, the diseases are different. Congenital disease as well as acquired disease must be considered in the differential list. Usually a child has a single diagnosis to explain symptoms. History taking and clinical examination is not easy for infants and children and thus information from imaging is crucial in certain situations. Radiation protection is important both for the child and for the society as a whole. The child's physical and psychological welfare during diagnostic imaging must also be considered.

Imagine yourself as a 4-month-old infant, starving hungry, being held down on a cold, hard table by strangers. A rubber nipple is being pushed into your mouth and it is full of strawberry-flavoured chalk fluid that you are supposed to swallow while a machine makes horrible noises over your head. Now imagine yourself as a 2-year-old (on the same hard, cold table), being held down and catheterized. Soon, your bladder feels like it will burst and you have to micturate all over the table (in the presence of your mother who has just started to toilet train you!).

The upper gastrointestinal series and micturating cystourethrogram are touted as both anatomical and physiological studies but, if you reread the paragraph above, you can understand why they may be lacking in their representation of normal human physiology.

Paediatric radiologists play an important intermediary role between paediatrics and radiology, both in the conduct and the interpretation of an examination. They are the clinician's friend and the patient's advocate.

Imaging has to be problem-oriented. The most important information on a requisition form, apart from the child's name and age, is the question to be answered. The next most important items are the legible name and contact number of the person asking the question. In this age of computerization, the telephone remains an invaluable instrument of technology because it allows one person to talk to another person. The paediatric radiologist should do the least possible investigation to achieve the most possible information about a child's condition.

In concluding this introductory section, it is important to recognize that there is little evidence-based information to support many of the recommendations that are in print regarding appropriate algorithms for paediatric imaging. There are few clinical situations and ethical guidelines that allow the performance of several studies on a child simply to compare their utility. Clinical information is frequently imperfect; 'comparable' studies are rarely comparable (for example, consider the problems in defining infection of the urinary tract). Furthermore, local traditions, biased by the practitioners of the area, available facilities and economic conditions, usually prevail over expert opinions and recommendations in textbooks. If you have any question about the appropriate imaging for your patient, ask a radiologist who is experienced in paediatric diagnosis for help. With these

> **Practical points**
>
> - Find out if there are clinical guidelines for your department/institution. They may include guidelines for imaging
> - Generally, in a complicated case, it is best to begin with uncomplicated imaging, such as plain radiographs. They may provide the diagnosis; if not, they can help point the way to other studies
> - Provide relevant clinical information to the radiologist when requesting examinations
> - Consult a paediatric radiologist, or one experienced in paediatric diagnosis, when you have questions about the imaging of a specific clinical problem
> - Be familiar with the preparation, immediate complications and sequelae of invasive imaging procedures

caveats, and encouragement to you, the reader, to challenge algorithms when they seem less than sensible, the following sections outline appropriate imaging considerations for particular situations, and are arranged anatomically, for easy reference.

Neurology

Newborn

- Portable ultrasonography when screening for germinal matrix/intraventricular and intraparenchymal haemorrhage in the premature infant
- CT for: suspected extra-axial collections (bleeding, infection)
- MRI for: suspected non-haemorrhagic parenchymal disease, e.g. hypoxic–ischaemic insult, neuronal migrational disorders.

Notes

Follow local protocols for timing/frequency of ultrasonographic screening for premature infants. Generally, a scan is performed at 3–4 days of age in those infants who weigh less than 1500 g unless there is clinical concern that prompts an earlier study.

Acute trauma, all ages

See Chapter 3.6.

- Include lateral cervical spine film, in collar to include the C7–T1 disc space, when injury to the neck is suspected
- CT scanning of brain when neurological signs/symptoms present
- MRI when CT scanning is negative in an infant/child with persisting abnormal neurological signs

Notes

Radiographs of the skull are poorly predictive of intracranial pathology. They are of use in the situation of suspected inflicted injury (non-accidental injury) where multiple fractures or fractures of different ages are helpful in establishing the diagnosis.

A normal lateral neck film, in collar, can be followed by anteroposterior (AP) view of the cervical spine and odontoid view. Remember that the thyroid gland is in the field of view. CT scanning of the cervical spine, often routinely acquired in adults, gives up to 15 times the radiation of plain films and is only used when there is credible utility.

Seizures

See Chapter 17.1.

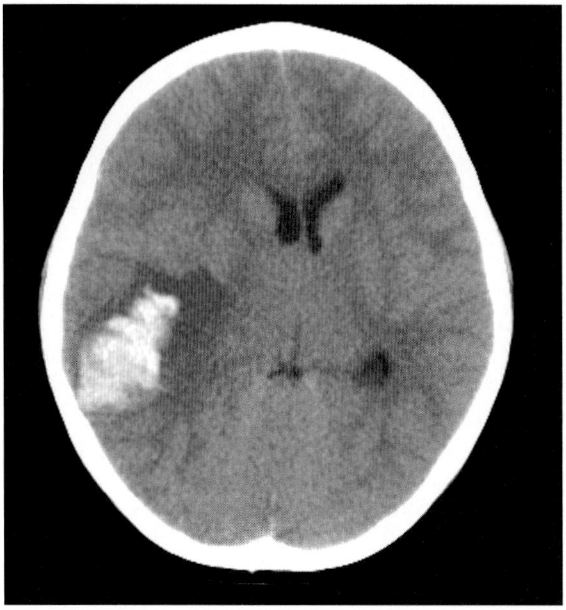

Fig. 7.1.1 CT scan without contrast following acute change in mental status associated with severe headache in this 10-year-old boy. Note the large dense lesion, representing haemorrhage, in the right posterior temporal region. The ring of lucency is surrounding oedema. Because of the strong suspicion, from clinical presentation and CT scan, that this child had a vascular aetiology for his haemorrhage, he went to angiography. This showed vessels from both anterior and posterior cerebral circulation, along with an early draining vein that identified this as an arteriovenous malformation.

CT scanning:

- without intravenous contrast media, then
- with intravenous contrast media or MRI and/or angiography if vascular etiology likely.

Altered neurological state

CT scanning:

- without intravenous contrast media, then
- with intravenous contrast media or MRI and/or angiography if vascular etiology likely (Fig. 7.1.1).

Notes

Simple febrile seizures (single or recurrent) do not usually warrant imaging.

Imaging following a single generalized afebrile seizure in children is an area of controversy. Focal afebrile seizures will usually be investigated by electroencephalography (EEG) and cerebral imaging. Because of the variable availability of MRI, local protocols should be consulted for neurologic diagnostic work-up.

Cardiology

See Chapter 15.1.

Suspected congenital heart disease

(e.g. abnormal prenatal ultrasonogram, cyanosis, murmur, unexplained oxygen requirement)

- Posteroanterior (PA) and lateral chest film to include upper abdomen
- Cardiology referral/echocardiography
- CT or MRI for anatomical detail of vascular rings as necessary

Cardiac angiography/interventional procedures are arranged by paediatric cardiologists in most centres.

Central/cardiac pain

- PA and lateral chest film to include upper abdomen
- Cardiology referral/echocardiography

Notes

Plain films of the chest can be remarkably uninformative in some infants with complex congenital heart disease; echocardiography is the gold standard. There can be clues to the presence of congenital heart disease on plain films (Fig. 7.1.2). Check the six Ss: cardiac **s**ize, cardiac **s**hape, **s**ide of aortic arch, **s**tatus of pulmonary vasculature, abdominal **s**itus and **s**keletal anomaly. Barium swallow is a very useful ancillary study for characterizing a suspected vascular ring if CT and MRI are unavailable. In most centres, echocardiography is the province of the cardiologist. Most echocardiographic examinations are time-consuming; some centres use sedation for transthoracic scanning. Transoesophageal echocardiography gives excellent detail of the heart and great vessels but the child needs sedation for the procedure.

Pulmonary/airway

See Chapter 14.5.

Cough and fever

- PA and lateral chest film

Pleuritic pain

- PA and lateral chest film

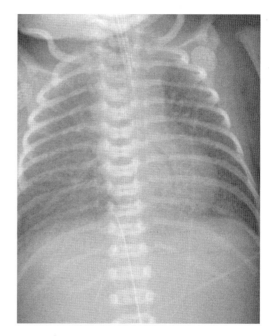

Fig. 7.1.2 The anteroposterior radiograph of this newborn who presented in severe respiratory distress has features that identify cardiac abnormality as the likely aetiology, although the heart is normal in size. Note that the nasogastric tube is entering a right-sided stomach, while the apex of the heart is left-sided. The tracheostomy tube is deviated leftward by a right-sided aortic arch and the umbilical artery catheter is in a right-sided descending aorta. This infant has heterotaxy syndrome with multiple cardiac anomalies. The venous congestion that is apparent in the lungs is from obstructed anomalous pulmonary venous return, the major cause of the respiratory distress.

Suspected sepsis in a neonate

- PA and lateral chest film

First episode of wheezing

See Chapter 14.3.

- PA and lateral chest film
- Fluoroscopy/screening if foreign body is suspected

Imaging is usually only indicated if the history is suggestive of inhaled or ingested foreign body, the child has no coryzal illness or the child doesn't get better as expected for bronchiolitis/asthma.

Unexplained stridor

See Chapter 14.2.

- PA and lateral chest film
- Lateral film of the neck
- Fluoroscopy/screening/barium swallow

Trauma to the chest

• AP supine chest film
• Computed tomographic angiography (CTA) with intravenous contrast if mediastinal injury suspected
• Angiography for rare situation of aortic injury

Thoracic mass

• PA and lateral films
• CT or MRI or, occasionally, both, depending on the organ(s) of origin and involvement
• Echocardiography for mass related to the heart

Notes

There is great debate as to whether a previously well child who has clinical symptoms and signs of pneumonia requires radiography at all. Likewise, there is argument as to whether the workup of sepsis in an infant, and the first episode of wheezing (without history of aspiration of foreign body), requires imaging. Remember that normal radiographs and fluoroscopy do not rule out the presence of an endobronchial foreign body. There has to be enough obstruction of an airway to provide radiographic evidence of its presence. Bronchoscopy should follow if there is a good history of aspiration, even if films are normal.

Some centres perform only PA films and no lateral for indications such as suspected pneumonia. There is no good prospective study that compares the utility of the PA only radiograph with PA and lateral views of the chest. There is anecdotal evidence that supports the acquisition of both views. In many cases, lower lobe pneumonia is difficult to diagnose from the PA view alone. The cardiac size is easier to judge when the shape of the chest is defined by two views. When both films are normal, the radiologist can state with certainty that the chest is normal to radiographic examination. It is just as important to document normality in some situations as to find an abnormality.

There is general consensus that follow-up radiography for an uncomplicated pneumonia is unnecessary. Follow-up films are reserved for children who have persisting symptoms of chest disease or who have had unusual radiographs on presentation.

Stridulous breathing implies narrowing of the trachea. A vascular ring, endotracheal haemangioma, tracheitis or epiglottitis are all possible causes. Imaging is not needed in children with classic croup and can be dangerous in children who are suspected of having epiglottitis from *Haemophilus influenzae*.

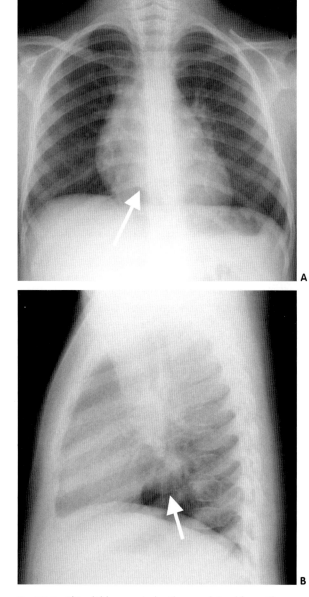

Fig. 7.1.3   This child presented with unexplained fever. The soft tissue density (arrow) on the posteroanterior film (**A**) might have been overlooked without the lateral view. The lateral film (**B**) demonstrates a smoothly outlined mass (arrow) that proved to be a bronchopulmonary foregut malformation.

No child or infant with respiratory compromise should be sent for imaging without adequate safeguards for provision of an airway.

A chest mass is usually diagnosed on a PA and lateral film after a child presents with pain, cough, respiratory compromise, etc. It may also be an incidental finding on a film. For example, a posterior mediastinal mass may be clinically silent. The diagnostic approach is tailored to the clinical situation.

An anterior mediastinal mass in the setting of T cell leukaemia needs no further imaging. A posterior mass with vertebral involvement will require MRI if available and CT for assessing the possibility of lung metastases.

Abdomen/gastroenterology

Abdominal pain

See Chapter 20.1.

- Supine and upright or decubitus plain radiography for acute abdominal pain
- No imaging, or ultrasonography only, for non-specific, periumbilical abdominal pain

Constipation

- Plain radiograph of the abdomen
- Plain radiograph then contrast enema for the neonate who fails to pass meconium

Notes

Constipation/encopresis is a clinical diagnosis but there is often a plain film obtained at the initial evaluation of a child who has constipation. The radiograph is used for assessment of the degree of distension of bowel and for examining the lumbosacral spine for occult dysraphism. Ultrasonography is often used as a means of reassuring parents, child and clinician that there is no anatomical abnormality of the liver, spleen, pancreas and kidneys. Limiting radiographs to patients who have had prior abdominal surgery, suspected ingestion of foreign body, abnormal bowel sounds, abdominal distension or peritoneal signs identifies virtually all patients with significant disease.

Constipation/encopresis is a clinical diagnosis but there is often a plain film obtained at the initial evaluation of a child who has constipation for assessment of the degree of distension of bowel and the lumbosacral spine for occult dysraphism. Rarely do plain films reveal a specific cause for chronic constipation and some question their value in this setting. Hirschsprung disease is usually diagnosed in infancy; some patients present late and are diagnosed by contrast enema and/or suction rectal biopsy.

Evaluation of transit time through the gastrointestinal tract can be performed with sequential films following ingestion of special radio-opaque markers. This study is usually at the request of a specialist paediatric gastroenterologist or surgeon.

The evaluation of a child suspected of having appendicitis (Fig. 7.1.4) is heavily reliant on the clini-

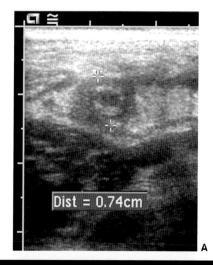

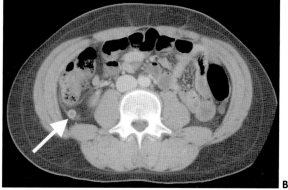

Fig. 7.1.4 Appendicitis is diagnosed on ultrasonography (**A**) when there is a blind-ending tubular structure that can be connected to the caecum, that is non-compressible, and that measures 6 mm or more in transverse diameter as shown on this scan. The presence of a shadowing appendicolith, although helpful in the diagnosis, is not a necessary feature. In another case, (**B**), retrocaecal appendicitis is evident on this slice from a CT scan. The appendix (arrow) is thick-walled, measured 8 mm in diameter and had adjacent inflammation, including thickening of the posterior peritoneum.

cal practice guidelines established at the point of care. For example, in one major centre in São Paulo, Brazil, the investigations are limited to clinical assessment then ultrasonography if the diagnosis is questionable. In many parts of the USA, CT is virtually the norm. Many institutions rely on an approach that limits CT scanning to those with negative ultrasonography or those suspected of rupture/abscess. Ultrasonography requires competent practitioners and good equipment, and is far easier in children who are not obese. CT scanning requires injection of contrast media, irradiation and good interpretation of the resultant images.

Abdominal mass

- Plain radiograph of abdomen except for adolescent female with pelvic mass
- Ultrasonography
- CT if necessary
- MRI for neurogenic tumour, soft tissue tumour, bony involvement by tumour, choledochal cyst or an unusual mass

Notes

Plain radiography provides a road map; it also provides information regarding the bases of the lungs, presence of calcification, effects of the mass on contiguous organs and/or gastrointestinal tract. Most abdominal masses in childhood are related to the retroperitoneum and, in particular, the kidney. Examples are obstructive hydronephrosis or multicystic dysplastic kidney. A mass that is gastrointestinal in origin, e.g. intussusception, requires a different approach from a mass that is hepatobiliary, such as a choledochal cyst. The plain radiograph and ultrasonography provide a means for triage to further imaging. When intussusception is diagnosed, air enema for reduction is the first therapeutic method of choice. Remember to consider pregnancy in an adolescent female who has a pelvic mass! If a malignant tumour is diagnosed, the affected child may be enrolled in treatment protocols that have very specific requirements in terms of imaging at staging and follow-up.

Abdominal trauma

- Supine radiograph, with decubitus if possible, and lateral view of lumbar spine if there has been hyperflexion of the spine, such as with a lapbelt injury
- CT with intravenous contrast

Notes

Many trauma protocols for evaluating the severely injured child have been based on the approach to adults, who have different mechanisms and types of abdominal injury. For example, a screening pelvic film is part of the 'adult' trauma series. Its use in children has not been proved to be helpful. If any screening view is considered, it should be an abdominal film, which will include the pelvis. Peritoneal lavage is not a helpful diagnostic test in paediatric trauma. Major organ injury can occur without there being free intra-abdominal fluid. Ultrasonography is not as sensitive a method of diagnosis as CT but in some remote areas may be the only tool available to search for free fluid, intraparenchymal laceration/haematoma and renal perfusion.

A child should be stabilized before being moved to a CT scanner. Cervical spine and head injury should be considered. Oral contrast medium is not usually used for the following reasons: risk of aspiration; time needed to allow contrast to pass through intestinal tract; and relative ileus in the situation of severe injury. However, some centres use positive contrast and some instil water through the nasogastric tube to outline the duodenum.

Non-bilious vomiting

See Chapter 20.1.

- Ultrasonography when pyloric stenosis is suspected but a pyloric mass is not palpated.
- Upper gastrointestinal series with barium

Bilious vomiting

- Plain films
- Upper gastrointestinal series with barium if the obstruction seems proximal

Diarrhoea

- Upper gastrointestinal series with follow-through examination of small bowel when the cause is not obvious from clinical and laboratory data, cultures and small bowel biopsy, or when idiopathic inflammatory bowel disease is suspected

Failure to thrive

- Upper gastrointestinal series with follow-through examination of small bowel when all other investigations and therapeutic interventions are unhelpful

Subacute small bowel obstruction

- CT scanning after ingestion of water soluble oral contrast may be more revealing of the site and source of obstruction than follow-through AP films after the ingestion of barium

Gastrointestinal bleeding

- Technetium-99m pertechnetate scintiscan when a Meckel diverticulum is suspected.
- Upper gastrointestinal series with follow-through examination of small bowel and antegrade evaluation of colon and/or air-contrast barium enema when all other investigations are unhelpful (e.g. upper gastrointestinal endoscopy and colonoscopy).

Notes

The availability of consultants trained in paediatric gastroenterology and their skill in endoscopy affects the role of radiology in gastrointestinal diseases. If there is no one available to perform colonoscopy, there is reliance on air-contrast barium enema for evaluation of the colon.

Normal infants vomit, spill, regurgitate or posset. If an infant younger than 6 months is 'a happy chucker', imaging is unnecessary. Pulmonary symptomatology, failure to thrive, feeding difficulty and gastrointestinal blood loss are reasons to pursue imaging with upper gastrointestinal series.

Problems in the neonatal period, such as failure to pass meconium, bilious vomiting and distension, tend to be congenital in origin and the appropriate sequence of imaging requires close cooperation between paediatric surgery and radiology. One cannot rely on ultrasonography to confirm or exclude malrotation: a contrast study of the upper gastrointestinal tract is the gold standard. Where there are appropriate ultrasonic facilities and practitioners, pyloric stenosis should be diagnosed with ultrasonography if the pyloric tumour is impalpable (Fig. 7.1.5).

Radiological studies of the child who has intermittent or chronic intestinal blood loss are rarely revealing in the absence of a Meckel diverticulum, and if endoscopy has been normal.

Hepatobiliary

Neonatal jaundice

See Chapter 11.2.

- Ultrasonography to establish anatomy
- MRC and/or radionuclide study with technetium-99m IDA derivative when biliary atresia is a consideration

Right upper abdominal pain

- Plain radiograph and often the addition of ultrasonography (Fig. 7.1.6)

Notes

Right lower lobe pneumonia may present as severe right upper abdominal pain; therefore, always look at the bases of the lungs on abdominal radiographs. Gallstones in childhood are more likely to be pigment stones than cholesterol stones and may contain enough calcium to be visible on radiography.

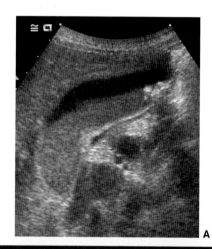

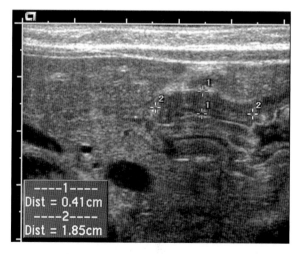

Fig. 7.1.5 Ultrasonography was performed after this 4-week-old infant presented with persistent vomiting. Scan along the long axis of the antropyloric region shows the typical features of pyloric stenosis with thickening of the muscle and elongation of the channel.

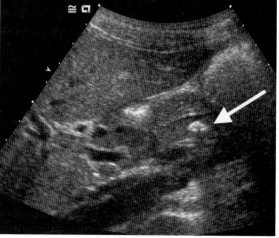

Fig. 7.1.6 Increasing jaundice and intermittent abdominal pain in this boy with sickle cell disease was evaluated with abdominal ultrasonography. Scans show sludge and stones in the gallbladder (**A**) and obstruction of the distal common bile duct by similar debris (arrow, **B**).

Juvenile/adolescent jaundice

- Ultrasonography of liver, biliary tract, pancreas and spleen
- CT or MRI, depending on the results of ultrasonography

Abnormal hepatic function

- Ultrasonography when the clinical situation is atypical for hepatitis
- Ultrasound guided biopsy if the diagnosis is uncertain

Nephrology/urology

Urinary infection

See Chapter 18.1.

- Ultrasonography of the urinary tract in neonates, at the time of infection, to rule out an obvious surgical problem, such as obstruction (The recommendation from the American Pediatric Society is that ultrasonography should also be performed in infants and young children 2 months to 2 years of age who do not demonstrate the expected clinical response within 2 days of antimicrobial therapy)
- Ultrasonography and micturating cystourethrography (MCU) in some infants and children who have had a documented urinary tract infection (Fig. 7.1.7)
- Intravenous urogram (IVU) or technetium-99m DTPA or Mag 3 scans, with furosemide, for evaluation of the child with possible obstruction at the pelviureteric junction or ureterovesical junction
- Technetium-99m DMSA or Mag 3 scans during the acute illness can support the diagnosis of pyelonephritis, and/or after infection has cleared can document renal scars
- RNC for follow-up of known reflux

Notes

The type of imaging, the timing of investigation and the age of the child requiring radiological evaluation are some of the most contentious issues in paediatrics today (Ch. 18.1). The American Academy of Pediatrics has issued guidelines regarding diagnostic imaging in young children (aged 2 months to 2 years) but has not addressed the issue of whether children up to the age of 5 years should have an MCU as part of their evaluation. The prevalence of urinary tract infection and of dilating vesicoureteric reflux varies between populations. Furthermore, the approach to imaging often depends on the services involved in a child's care. Paediatricians, paediatric urologists and paediatric nephrologists may have differing opinions. There has been a gradual change over the last

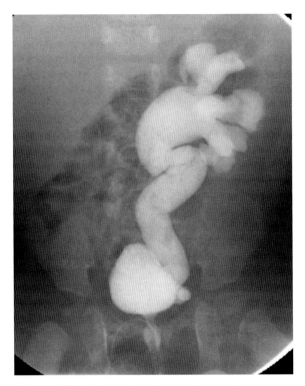

Fig. 7.1.7 Micturating cystourethrography reveals severe reflux into the left kidney in this infant who presented acutely ill with infection. Because of the degree of distension of the collecting system, this would be classified as grade 5 reflux.

25 years from performing MCU in most children who present with infection to investigating those who are younger than 5 years, or 3 years, or 6 months, depending on the institution and the other imaging that is available. There are data to suggest that reflux is just one of many factors that result in symptomatic, culture-positive urinary infection.

Radionuclide cystogram is a method of documenting reflux with far less radiation than standard MCU. The availability of this study is often limited to tertiary centres. Ultrasonographic MCU requires catheterization, the instillation of ultrasonographic contrast medium, a cooperative patient and technical expertise; it is not currently available as a routine study.

Magnetic resonance urography (MRU) with injection of gadolinium shows great promise in its ability to show parenchymal abnormalities, display split renal function and reveal anatomical abnormalities. Currently under investigation in a few centres, it has the potential to replace many of the classic investigative tools.

Renal failure

- Ultrasonography of urinary tract
- Ultrasound guided biopsy of kidney if necessary for diagnosis

Note

Ultrasonography, which does not rely on renal function for images, can usually aid in triage of the patient by determining a surgical or medical cause for renal failure.

Hypertension

See Chapter 18.2.

- Ultrasonography of urinary tract and adrenal glands
- Abdominal CT if an endocrine tumour such as phaeochromocytoma is suspected from laboratory data. Consult the radiology department regarding premedication prior to injection of intravenous contrast at the time of the study
- Nuclear medicine for quantitative, divided renal vascular flow and function (This may be superseded by MRU in the future)
- Angiography/angioplasty in the rare situation of suspected renal vascular disease

Note

Examination of the kidneys with Doppler is difficult, time-consuming and often insensitive to subtle vascular narrowing. Accessory renal vessels may be overlooked. Mid-aortic syndrome and neurofibromatosis are rare and when present, typically have other signs and symptoms. A 'negative' examination does not rule out renal vascular disease.

CTA can define renal vascularity with greater clarity than ultrasonography; MRU (discussed above) has potential for the future.

Haematuria unrelated to trauma

- Ultrasonography of urinary tract
- CT if there is strong likelihood of renal/ureteral stone that has not been identified with ultrasonography
- CT if a renal tumour is suspected
- MCU or retrograde urethrography if a distal site of bleeding is suspected and cystoscopy is unavailable

Musculoskeletal

Trauma

See Chapters 3.6, 8.1.

- Two orthogonal views of the bone or joint that has been injured (Fig. 7.1.8). Oblique/special views as needed of areas such as scaphoid, radial head, shoulder
- CT for special cases such as intra-articular fractures of ankle, pelvic fracture

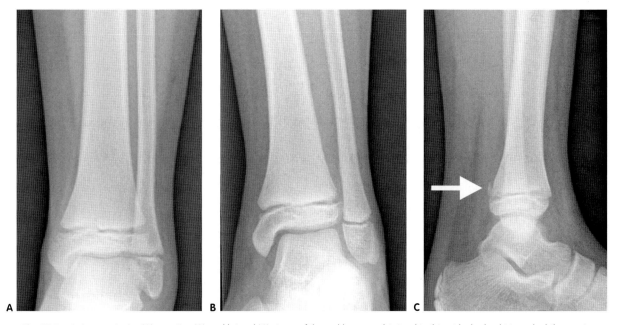

A   B   C

Fig. 7.1.8 Anteroposterior (**A**), mortise (**B**) and lateral (**C**) views of the ankle were obtained in this girl who had tripped while running. Note that the fracture of the posterior malleolus (arrow) can only be identified on the lateral view. Two or more views are often necessary for diagnosing bony injury.

Fever/pain/swelling in the musculoskeletal system

- Two orthogonal views of the symptomatic bone or joint
- Nuclear medicine technetium-99m diphosphonate bone scan
- MRI for difficult diagnoses, tumour, occult infection
- Ultrasonography for specific questions: localization of collection of fluid, joint effusion

Notes

MRI is fast replacing radionuclide studies in cases where there is localized pain or swelling and clinical concern regarding a single septic joint or focus of osteomyelitis. Follow-up studies of children with diagnosed bone tumour should be performed with MRI rather than CT; they give far more information regarding adjacent soft tissues and bone marrow.

Metabolic disease

- AP plain radiograph of wrist and/or knee

Note

Because metabolic disease such as rickets is more obvious in areas of rapid bone growth, the wrists and knees are more revealing of abnormality than other sites. Other views (hands, clavicles) may show changes of secondary hyperparathyroidism in those with renal failure.

Syndrome with potential skeletal involvement

- Plain radiographs of chest, spine, pelvis, skull, leg and arm to include hand for determination of bone age

Developmental dysplasia of the hip

See Chapter 8.1.

- Ultrasonography at 4–6 weeks of age if developmental dysplasia of the hip (DDH) suspected but not obvious on physical examination, or if risk factors (female, breech, positive family history) present *or*
- Plain radiograph at 4–6 months of age if DDH suspected but not obvious on physical examination

Notes

This is another area of contention. Ultrasonography of the infant's hips requires training and practice. Early radiography of neonates is unhelpful because so much of the anatomy is cartilaginous. Radiographs at 4–6 months are more informative and still allow intervention if necessary. In some areas of Europe, ultrasonography is used to screen all newborns. Such studies have a high false-positive rate of diagnosis of DDH. Repeated physical examination is the cornerstone of diagnosis. Infants may not have an obvious problem until after the neonatal period; hence the change in name from CDH (congenital dysplasia of the hip) to DDH. The availability of experienced paediatric orthopaedic surgeons has an effect on the local imaging protocols.

Inflicted injury (non-accidental injury)

See Chapter 3.9.

- CT or MRI of brain to assess extra-axial spaces, parenchymal injury
- Complete skeletal survey (infants) with high-detail images to search for evidence of fracture
- Nuclear medicine technetium-99m diphosphonate bone scan in unusual cases
- CT of abdomen, with intravenous contrast, if evidence of abdominal trauma

Notes

Some centres use nuclear medicine in imaging protocols for infants and young children if there is availability and local expertise in interpretation.

Often a follow up skeletal survey or limited survey may be very revealing. Periosteal reaction takes about 7–10 days to appear. The acute fracture may be occult.

Acknowledgements

The support of the Paedatric Radiologists at Starship Hospital during the preparation of this manuscript is gratefully acknowledged. Dr George Taylor of Boston Children's Hospital helped with the illustrations.

Abbreviations

The following abbreviations are in common use in imaging:

AP, Anteroposterior
PA, Posteroanterior

These terms relate to the course of the X-ray beam through the body. Anteroposterior, supine chest radiographs are much easier to accomplish in infants who cannot sit without support. Magnification of the heart is not as significant an issue as it is in adults.

CR, Computed radiography

Radiographs, films, or images are the result of X-rays passing through part of the body. 100 years ago, the images were on glass plates – hence the use of the term 'plate' by some radiologists and clinicians. You may also read of 'roentgenogram' – another relatively old-fashioned term highlighting Roentgen's contribution. With computed radiology now routine, the image is likely to be digital, and viewed on a computer screen.

CT, Computed tomography

(The older term, CAT, which is the acronym for computed axial tomography, has been dropped because, although axial scans are acquired, modern machines allow reconstruction in coronal, sagittal and three-dimensional formats.)

CTA, Computed tomographic angiography (rapid injection of contrast with imaging in the arterial phase)

IVU, Intravenous urography, synonymous with the old term of intravenous pyelogram (IVP)

MCU, Micturating cystourethrography

MRA, Magnetic resonance angiography

MRC, Magnetic resonance cholangiography

MRI, Magnetic resonance imaging

MRU, Magnetic resonance urography

MRV, Magnetic resonance venography

NM, Nuclear medicine

RNC, Radionuclide cystography

US, Ultrasound or ultrasonography

PART 8

COMMON ORTHOPAEDIC PROBLEMS

Common paediatric orthopaedic problems and fractures

8.1

P. Cundy

Skeletal variations during growth

Adult posture should not be used as a criterion for the proper posture in infancy and childhood. During development in childhood a number of different limb shapes (or postures) may be noted and these can cause parental anxiety. These transitory postures can be due to:

• *intrauterine posture*, sometimes described as 'packaging'
• *developmental variants* – i.e. not present at birth, but may appear during growth and then disappear spontaneously. These include the common conditions of bow legs, knock knees, flat feet and in-toeing. These conditions seldom require active treatment but parents do need informed reassurance, which must be based on accurate knowledge of the natural history of the variations of posture in infants and children.

Intrauterine posture

The position of the child before birth is normally one of flexion. The spine is flexed so that it forms a long curve with a concavity forward, the arms and legs are flexed, and the feet may assume a variety of postures. In the newborn the intrauterine posture can be readily reconstructed by 'folding' the baby into his or her most comfortable position, and this may indicate any postural abnormality present.

Two common foot postures are seen in newborns.

Talipes calcaneovalgus

Many babies are born with the foot turned upwards at the ankle so that the toes lie close to the front of the shin: this is known as talipes calcaneovalgus (Fig. 8.1.1). This posture can be corrected passively so that the foot can be brought down to a plantigrade position or even into equinus. The condition has a strong tendency to correct itself spontaneously over a period of 2–3 months.

Postural talipes equinovarus

Some babies are born with one or both feet in a position of plantar flexion at the ankles, and inversion of the remainder of the foot, so that the sole of the foot faces the opposite foot. This is postural talipes equinovarus and may be distinguished from true talipes equinovarus by the fact that the former condition is easily correctable, either actively by the baby's movement or passively by the attendant. The foot can be readily held in normal alignment to the leg or even in a position of calcaneovalgus, whereas in true congenital talipes equinovarus (club foot) the deformity is rigid. The fixed deformities of a true club foot require treatment by serial casting and usually surgery in the first 6 months of life.

Developmental variants

Many developmental variants are seen in early and later childhood and often cause concern for parents.

Bow legs

Bow legs (Fig. 8.1.2) are common up to 2 years of age: the parents will often be concerned that the legs are bowed and the feet turn in. The condition is not caused by bulky nappies, because the bowing is in the tibiae. It is a normal developmental process and does not require treatment apart from parental reassurance. If the bowing is in one leg only, you should investigate with plain X-rays to exclude pathological causes such as a bone dysplasia or growth abnormality.

Knock knees

A large proportion of the population between the ages of 2 and 7 years have knock knees (Fig. 8.1.3). This condition has a very strong tendency to correct itself by the age of 7 years and as a rule the only management necessary is parental reassurance that improvement will occur. There is a rare form of

249

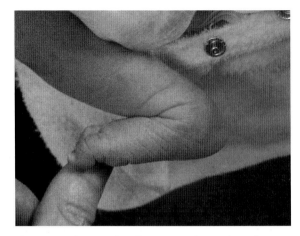

Fig. 8.1.1 Calcaneovalgus foot in a newborn – this will correct spontaneously.

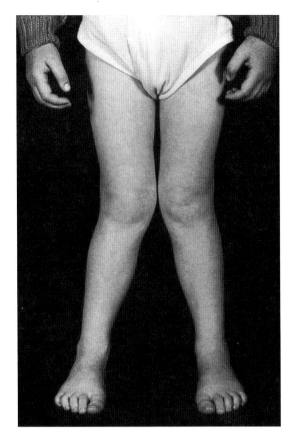

Fig. 8.1.3 A 5-year-old child with pronounced knock knees.

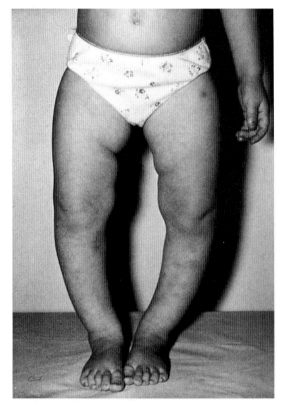

Fig. 8.1.2 Bow legs in a toddler: a normal phenomenon.

is due to physiological joint laxity and requires no treatment. The clinician can show the parents how the hind foot straightens when the child stands up on high tiptoes. This is the tiptoe test, which also demonstrates development of the medial longitudinal arch (Fig. 8.1.4).

Flat feet

Flat feet in children are a frequent cause for parental concern. Usually this concern is unwarranted and the child's foot is normal for age (Fig. 8.1.5). Often parents notice that their child's foot appears flat. Sometimes the attendant fitter at the shoe shop may comment on the shape of the child's foot. Children usually have low arches because they are loose-jointed and flexible. The arch flattens when they are standing. However, the arch can be better seen when the feet are hanging free or the child stands on tiptoes (the tiptoe test, Fig. 8.1.4).

When a child first learns to walk, the stance is usually wide to assist balance, and the feet roll. As the child grows and ankle muscles strengthen, the foot gradually develops its mature shape with some medial arch. Flat feet are common in preschoolers

knock knees that presents in obese children over the age of 12 years and which does require treatment.

Rolling in of ankles

Parents will frequently mention this, especially after it has been noticed by a concerned grandparent or shoe fitter. The rolling of the hind foot into valgus

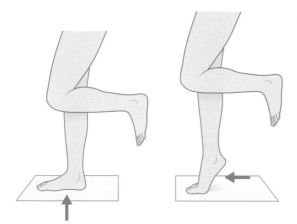

Fig. 8.1.4   If the arch appears when standing on tiptoe then the feet are flexible. The flat arch is of no significance and requires no treatment apart from explanation.

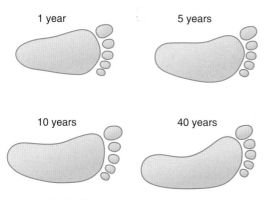

1 year   5 years

10 years   40 years

Fig. 8.1.5   Flexible flat feet are normal in infants and children. The arch develops whether the child wears shoes or goes barefoot.

but are present in fewer than 10% of teenagers. The final shape of the foot may also be influenced genetically, in that one or both parents may have low arches.

When children start walking they do so on feet that appear flat, partly because there is true flatness of the medial longitudinal arch and partly because the arch is filled in by a fat pad. Between the ages of 2 and 8 years, parents are often concerned because a 'second ankle bone' appears on the medial aspect of the foot. They are referring to prominence of the navicular bone, which is present in most children who have flat feet. Unless the prominence of this bone is causing symptoms, it can be ignored. Sometimes an accessory navicular bone (ossicle) can be seen on X-ray and this requires no treatment unless painful. If painful, the wearing of a soft 'off the shelf' arch support for a year usually helps.

Children with flat feet generally have some valgus deformity of the heel: when viewed from behind the

heels do not point straight up and down, but tend to slope outwards and downwards. The heels will correct and even swing into varus during the tiptoe test. This seldom persists into adult life.

During the first 7 or 8 years of life the majority of children develop a medial longitudinal arch but approximately 15% do not. Clearly, the results of any form of treatment for flat feet are going to be excellent, as some 85% will get better whether or not they are treated. Sometimes treatment with shoe inserts (orthotics) or other forms of arch supports/shoe modifications are recommended by therapists. These may satisfy concerned parents but do little, if anything, to correct the 'flat foot' and certainly do not make an arch where one is not present. Most of the time orthotics such as these are not necessary for children.

Other treatments, such as splints, massage or special shoes may be offered but there is little evidence that these interventions alter the foot for the better.

Shoes

The only essential is that children's shoes should be roomy enough. Shoes themselves are not necessary to promote normal foot growth and development; they are only worn for protection and need not be worn until activities demand this protection. Boots are no better than shoes, although parents may prefer boots for toddlers in that they are less likely to fall off or be taken off.

It is not harmful to use 'hand down' shoes in good condition from older children in the family provided they are roomy enough. There is no evidence that sandals, thongs or sneakers have any harmful influence on the feet. While wedging of the soles and heels has long been employed for in toeing and out toeing, such footwear modifications have no influence either on the gait itself or on the natural history. Thomas heels are of little or no value in the management of flat feet. If the child has excessive wear on the inner side of the sole of the shoes, advise parents to look for shoes that have a stiffer heel area. Some children with flexible flat feet are rather hard on their shoes and this can be dealt with by selecting shoes of stronger construction. This is usually much less expensive than elaborate and unnecessary orthotics.

Accessory navicular bone

The child with a prominent accessory navicular may have some temporary discomfort, which may be relieved by wearing arch supports for a period of a year or two. Frequently the ossicle either unites with the main navicular bone or just becomes asymptomatic. Excision of the accessory navicular bone is required only rarely.

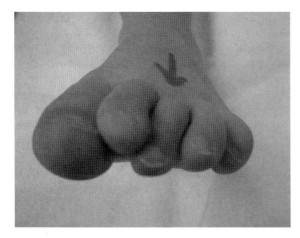

Fig. 8.1.6 Curly middle toes – flexor tenotomy is sometimes needed for severe cases.

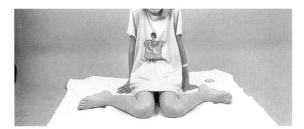

Fig. 8.1.7 'W' sitting is easy for the child with inset hips.

Curly middle toe

Sometimes the third toe curls inwards under the second toe so that the second toe tends to lie above the level of the first and third toes. Parents generally notice the abnormal posture of the second toe, but it is the third toe that is the cause of the problem. This can be safely ignored until the child is at least 2 years old. Occasionally a flexor tenotomy is required and provides excellent correction (Fig. 8.1.6).

In-toe gait (pigeon toeing)

In-toeing in childhood is common. It may appear worse when the child is running or tired. It does not cause arthritis or back problems later in life. It can be due to one or more of the following:

- inset hips
- internal torsion of the tibia
- metatarsus adductus.

Inset hips (persistent femoral neck anteversion) have internal rotation in excess of the range of external rotation. It is more common in girls and the feet seem to fly out sideways when running. The pathology lies in the top of the femur where there is a normal twist of 30° at birth, which unwinds gradually by the age of 7 years. In severe cases, when there is a major cosmetic problem unresolved by about 10 years, derotation femoral osteotomy can be performed but this is rarely required.

Children with inset hips commonly sit between their feet with their hips in full internal rotation, the knees flexed and the legs splayed outwards (the 'W' position) (Fig. 8.1.7). This is the only way they can sit comfortably as they cannot externally rotate their hips sufficiently to sit in a cross-legged fashion. There

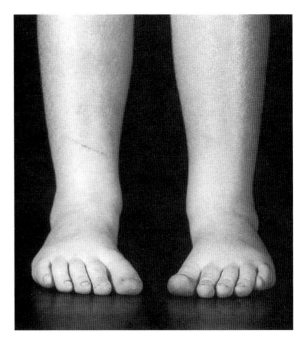

Fig. 8.1.8 A 3-year-old child with metatarsus adductus. Note the metatarsals and toes curving inwards.

is no evidence that this sitting posture should be discouraged in children and it is worthwhile remembering that it is almost unknown for an adult to present with a complaint of in-toeing.

Internal tibial torsion (a twist in the shin bone) is usually due to intrauterine pressure and can persist up to the age of 3 years and then spontaneously corrects.

Metatarsus adductus (Fig. 8.1.8) is a condition in which the feet are banana-shaped, with the convexity

---

Practical points

- Bow legs and knock knees are common normal variants
- Flexible flat feet are normal and need no treatment
- Examine the child with in-toe gait to decide cause
- Provide brochure information to reassure (see website links)

of the banana outwards and the toes directed towards each other. This may be due to intrauterine pressure; however, if it persists it is called metatarsus adductus. It is passively correctable and slowly rights itself, especially after walking commences. Very rarely, manipulation and plaster immobilization is necessary.

Congenital abnormalities

Developmental dysplasia of the hip

This condition was previously called congenital dislocation of the hip (CDH); however, developmental dysplasia of the hip (DDH) is now the preferred term as it implies that some of these hip problems may develop after birth. DDH is the most common musculoskeletal abnormality in neonates. The incidence of this condition in Australia and North America is 7 per 1000 live births. In some regions of Europe it is more common.

Clinical classification

DDH can be classified clinically as follows:

- stable
- subluxable
- dislocatable
- dislocated, reducible
- dislocated, irreducible
- teratological.

Main risk factors

Some of the important risk factors for DDH (with the degree of increased risk) are:

- breech presentation (10×)
- female baby (4×)
- oligohydramnios (4×)
- big baby >4 kg (2×)
- firstborn baby (2×)
- family history.

When diagnosed and treated from birth, it is possible to produce a normal hip joint after a few months treatment in an abduction splint. However, if the diagnosis is not made until after the child begins to walk, the treatment is long and tedious and often ends with an imperfect joint.

Diagnosis in the newborn

The Barlow and Ortolani tests are used for diagnosis (Fig. 8.1.9). Every baby should be examined for hip dislocation during the first day of life and again at discharge from the maternity ward, and at ages 6 weeks,

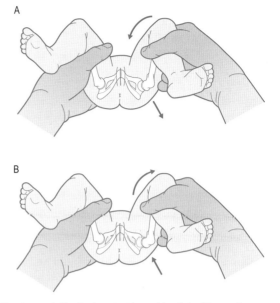

Fig. 8.1.9 **A** The Barlow test is positive if the hip can be manually dislocated. **B** The Ortolani test is positive if the hip is lying in a dislocated position and is manually reducible.

3 months, 6 months and 1 year. The baby must be relaxed for the examination to be meaningful. If the baby is crying, a bottle or pacifier is offered or the baby is examined later when relaxed. With the legs extended, any asymmetry of the legs or adductor creases is noted. The examiner then holds the leg to be examined (using the opposite hand to the side of the hip to be examined). With the knee flexed, the thumb is placed over the lesser trochanter and the middle finger over the greater trochanter. The pelvis is steadied by the other hand and the flexed thigh is abducted and adducted and any clunk or jerk is noted.

It is very important to note that frequently a fine click can be felt in the hip joint without any laxity or abnormal movement. Sometimes the click comes from the knee joint. This is very common and is of no significance. Also, it is common in the first 2 or 3 days of life for the hip to be felt to subluxate smoothly without any clunk. This is especially felt in premature babies and requires repeated examination; frequently the hip becomes normal without treatment but it must be carefully followed.

Radiography has no place in the diagnosis of developmental dysplasia of the hip in the neonatal period (Ch. 7.1). Ultrasound examination of the hips gives the clinician useful information as to the relationship of the femoral head to the acetabulum and the existence of any acetabular dysplasia during the first 6 months of life. Ultrasound has a high false-positive rate in babies under 6 weeks of age and scans should only be performed under 6 weeks either to check whether a hip is 'in joint' while in a splint or to check a 'doubtful' hip when the Barlow or Ortolani tests are equivocal. Over the age of 4 months the degree of ossification of the upper femur and acetabulum enables X-rays to be of value.

If the dislocatable or dislocated hip is held in a flexed and abducted position for 8–12 weeks, it will usually develop normally. The Pavlik harness or Denis Browne splint is used to maintain this position. Subluxable hips can be observed with a later ultrasound after 6 weeks or radiograph at 4 months. The use of double nappies is not recommended.

All abnormal or treated hips require follow-up until normal hip morphology is ascertained.

Teratological hip

If there is considerable restriction of abduction in flexion and the 'clunk' sign cannot be elicited, it usually means that the hips are dislocated and irreducible. These hips require paediatric orthopaedic surgical assessment and probably operative reduction at a later date.

Diagnosis in the older infant

The Barlow and Ortolani tests become more difficult to elicit after 3 months of age. In the abnormal hip, a new sign of limited abduction appears due to tightness of the adductor tendons. This sign is not diagnostic but an X-ray is indicated when there is asymmetry in the range of the abduction of the hips or when the range of abduction of both hips is inappropriate for the age of the child. In the first year of life the range of abduction in flexion is usually 60–90°; this arc normally lessens with age.

The physical signs of late presenting dislocation include:

- higher greater trochanter
- wide perineum
- asymmetric gluteal buttock crease
- short leg
- abnormal gait.

If a dislocation presents after walking age, an open reduction operation is usually required and these hips are rarely normal, with an increased risk of early hip osteoarthritis. Hence early diagnosis and treatment of DDH is the best way to prevent hip arthritis.

> ### Practical points
>
> - All babies should be assumed to have dislocated hips until proven otherwise
> - Re-examine babies' hips at every well-baby check
> - If in doubt, do an ultrasound when 6 weeks of age
> - Ensure that the sonographer is experienced in babies' hips

Congenital talipes equinovarus (congenital club foot)

Congenital talipes equinovarus is the commonest congenital abnormality of the foot, occurring in about 1 per 1000 live births. The male:female ratio is 2:1. The condition is bilateral in 40% of cases and there is a 2% chance of a subsequent child being affected if there is a positive family history.

The deformity is a combination of:

- equinus of the hind foot
- varus of the hind foot
- adductus of the midfoot
- cavus of the medial arch.

The degree of each deformity is variable but all are rigid and are incapable of being fully corrected manually (Fig. 8.1.10). This is distinct from the 'postural club foot', which is due to intrauterine pressure and is fully passively correctable and resolves without treatment, as described above.

Club feet should start treatment in the first week of life. Treatment involves serial plaster casting for 6–12 weeks, and surgical intervention is usually required at 3–6 months of age, with a posterior or posteromedial release of tendons and joints.

Congenital muscular torticollis

Torticollis usually presents in the first few months of life when some tilt of the head and limited lateral flexion is noted. Sometimes it can remain undetected for 1–2 years. The head is held with a lateral flexion toward the shoulder and with rotation of the face towards the opposite side. The face on that side is smaller and the eye is lower on the side of the tight sternomastoid. Most patients will have presented

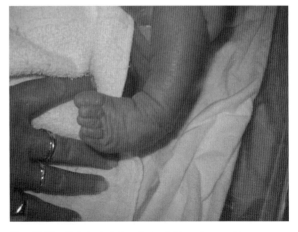

Fig. 8.1.10 Club foot deformity is rigid and cannot be passively corrected.

in the first few months of life with a sternomastoid tumour; that is, a palpable lump in the middle of the sternomastoid muscle.

The cause of this condition is unknown. Treatment in the first 6 months of life with a stretching programme supervised by a physiotherapist is usually effective, with full resolution. If the condition does not resolve then surgical correction at 2–4 years of age is required. At operation, the muscle is divided transversely and the corrected position maintained by the use of a collar.

Alexander the Great (354 BC) is reported to have had this condition, with statues showing a persistent head tilt.

Trigger thumb

This presents with the parents suddenly noticing that their 1–3-year-old child has a bent thumb. At this age children start to handle objects and the thumb deformity becomes obvious. The thumb is bent about 30° at the interphalangeal joint and cannot be passively straightened.

It is due to a constriction in the flexor tendon sheath and a nodule on the tendon itself. The cause is unknown and the treatment is surgical release of the tendon sheath under general anaesthesia. Surgery should be performed around the age of 2 years to prevent permanent joint changes.

Scoliosis

Scoliosis (lateral curvature of the spine) is most commonly seen in its adolescent idiopathic form (Fig. 8.1.11). However, there are other forms of scoliosis. The common ones are:

- *Congenital*: vertebral anomalies are responsible for the curvature. Usually the deformity is minor and may be present at birth or develop during growth. In only 5% is the deformity progressive
- *Neuromuscular*: such as Duchenne muscular dystrophy, cerebral palsy or spina bifida
- *Idiopathic*: this is usually seen as adolescent idiopathic scoliosis. Idiopathic scoliosis can be seen in younger children as:
  - *infantile idiopathic scoliosis*: most commonly seen in males and may be seen in association with congenital dislocation of the hip and other congenital anomalies. The natural history is for the curve to resolve in a high proportion of cases
  - *juvenile idiopathic scoliosis*: a curve in children between the age of 3 years and the onset of puberty; it is uncommon.

Adolescent idiopathic scoliosis

Some 90% of cases occur in girls and the scoliosis progresses during the rapid growth spurt years.

For diagnosis, the child must remove all clothing above the waist and stand with the back facing the examiner (Fig. 8.1.12). In all but very minor curves the deformity will be readily apparent. Signs to look for are:

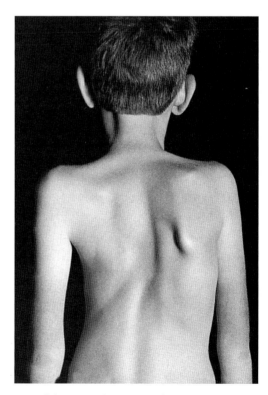

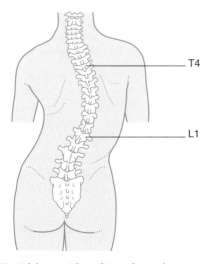

Fig. 8.1.11 Adolescent idiopathic scoliosis; the curve is usually convex to the right side.

Fig. 8.1.12 Adolescent scoliosis in a male; 90% occur in females.

255

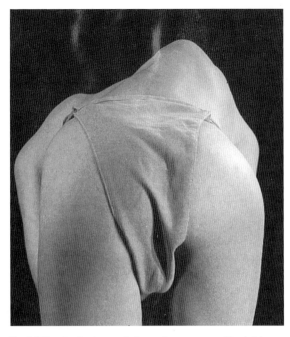

Fig. 8.1.13 On flexion, a rib hump becomes readily visible.

- uneven shoulders
- waist (flank) asymmetry
- a unilateral rib prominence when the child bends forward (Fig. 8.1.13).

If the curve disappears completely when the child bends forward, it can be labelled 'postural' and treatment is not required. Should a rib hump become visible (due to rotation of the vertebrae and consequent rib deformity; Fig. 8.1.13) the curve is labelled 'structural'.

There are three main treatment options:

- observation for curves less than 20°
- bracing for curves 20–40°
- surgery for curves greater than 40°.

These are broad guidelines only. Larger curves may not be treated if proven to be non-progressive in a skeletally mature patient. Several studies have investigated the role of exercises in improving the curve or preventing progression but there is no evidence that exercises or physiotherapy/chiropractic treatments alter the natural history of the curve.

Osteochondroses (osteochondritis)

These conditions involve the epiphysis. The pathology consists of localized areas of ischaemic bone necrosis and sometimes oedema of adjacent soft tissues. The tendency is for healing to occur but this is dependent on a number of factors, which include age, the site of the lesion, its blood supply and perhaps the method of treatment. Any bone having a cartilaginous area at the site of either the primary or secondary centre of ossification may be affected. The aetiology is uncertain.

The common osteochondroses are:

- Sever condition of the heel: 10–12 years
- Osgood–Schlatter condition of the tibial tubercle: 10–14 years
- Chondromalacia patellae: 10–20 years
- Slipped capital femoral epiphysis of the hip: 10–15 years
- Scheuermann condition of the thoracic spine: 12–16 years

Sever condition

This is an apophysitis of the os calcis (heel) bone where the tendo achillis attaches. It is seen in children aged between 10 and 12 years. It resolves over 12 months and is best treated by reassurance, calf stretches and sometimes a simple rubber heel raise. Sport is allowed within the child's level of comfort.

Osgood–Schlatter condition

This is an apophysitis of the tibial tubercle and presents with pain and swelling (Fig. 8.1.14). Children notice the pain and then an adult sees the swelling and can be concerned about a sinister cause such as malignancy. The common age of presentation is 10–14 years and the natural history is resolution over a 12–18-month period. Warn the parents that a lump will remain permanently but that it will be smaller than when first seen. Normal activities within the limits of the child's comfort are allowed. The tibial tubercle does not detach or pull off. Radiographs are not necessary for diagnosis. Simple measures such as quadriceps stretches and massage with a liniment can provide some symptomatic relief. Rarely, a small loose ossicle remains and can be excised after the child reaches 15 years.

Chondromalacia patellae

This condition has a number of other names, including:

- anterior knee pain
- lateral pressure syndrome
- maltracking of the patella.

It is particularly common over the age of 10 years. It is characterized by pain in the knee after activities that involve flexing the knee and quadriceps contraction. The child complains of aching around the patella during or especially after exercise. Stairs pre-

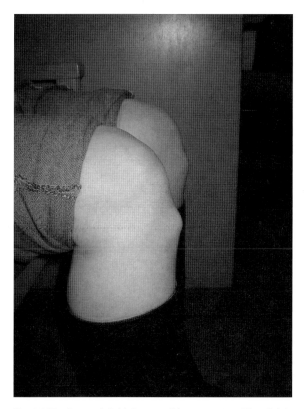

Fig. 8.1.14 Osgood–Schlatter condition presents with painful enlarged tibial tubercles.

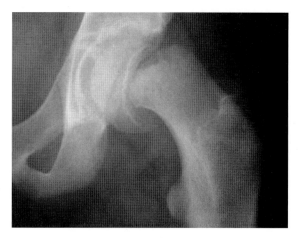

Fig. 8.1.15 Slipped capital femoral epiphysis often presents with thigh or knee pain – always exclude hip pathology when a child presents with knee/thigh pain.

Slipped capital femoral epiphysis

This is primarily a disorder of adolescents between the ages of 10 and 15 years. Approximately 40% of cases are bilateral. Its aetiology is unknown but recent reports suggest that hormonal factors may be of importance. Most cases present with pain and limp; pain is often referred to the knee and it is important to consider a hip radiograph when children present with distal thigh or knee pain.

Types of slip:

- *Acute*: the child feels the hip 'collapse' and is unable to walk. This is uncommon and needs urgent treatment
- *Acute on chronic*: the child has months of discomfort and then a worsening over a few weeks with a pronounced limp
- *Chronic*: many months of thigh ache and a mild limp.

Examination reveals limited internal rotation of the hip compared with the other side and some joint irritability. The diagnosis is confirmed radiologically, especially with a frog lateral view (Fig. 8.1.15).

All cases of slipped capital femoral epiphysis require surgery with screw fixation across the physis to prevent further slip.

cipitate discomfort, particularly walking downstairs. It is more common in adolescent females, both in those who enjoy sport and those who wish to avoid physical education lessons at school.

Clinically there is little to find, although occasionally there is some patellofemoral crepitus and rarely an effusion in the knee. Ensure that the hips are normal and that the symptoms do not relate to a slipped hip. The diagnosis is based upon obtaining the relevant history.

Some children are point tender at the inferior pole of patella (apophysis) and have a condition called jumper's knee. Treatment is massage with anti-inflammatory gels, quadriceps stretches and the expectation that symptoms will resolve over 18 months.

Treatment involves education of the child and concerned parents (explain that the 'back of the knee cap is soft' and will toughen up with time), some limitation of flexed knee/jumping activities, quadriceps stretches, elastic knee support and tincture of time. Frequently, children tolerate their symptoms and continue with their sport. The natural history suggests spontaneous resolution of symptoms over 1–2 years in 90% of patients.

> ### Practical points
>
> - Knee/distal thigh pain often comes from the hip
> - Always think of a slipped hip in adolescents with a limp
> - Know the various apophysitis pains in children
> - Anterior knee pain is common in teenagers

Scheuermann condition

The epiphyseal plates of the vertebral bodies are involved. Usually it is seen in the thoracic vertebrae but occasionally in the lumbar spine. Occurrences are almost always in the adolescent. Usually, children present in early adolescence because of pain or an increase in the normal thoracic kyphosis, so that the child appears round-shouldered. Most merely require observation, encouragement to exercise and stand straight and to be instructed in exercises by a physiotherapist. Some progress rapidly and require management in a brace. Rarely is surgery required.

The condition is frequently 'overdiagnosed' in radiology reports and causes anxiety in families, especially when the radiological changes are described as Scheuermann's 'disease'. The term 'condition' is preferred.

Injuries in infancy and childhood

Children are susceptible to injury because of their carefree play habits, and skeletal injuries are common. For practical purposes, sprains do not occur in children: 'children break bones and adults tear ligaments'. Post-trauma pain, swelling and loss of function are nearly always the result of a fracture or growth plate separation; therefore X-rays are obligatory.

Dislocations are rare in childhood, although shoulder and patella dislocations are seen in adolescents. The type of injury that may produce dislocation of an adult joint usually gives rise to a fracture or growth plate separation in a child.

Fractures are the commonest type of skeletal injury in childhood; these generally unite in less than half the time the equivalent injury would take to heal in an adult, and non-union is almost unknown. Childhood fractures may unite in a position of deformity, with the deformity correcting itself spontaneously over the ensuing 6–12 months, especially if the fracture is near the ends of the bone where there is most growth. Some shortening of bones also can be expected to correct spontaneously following childhood fractures.

Child abuse is an important cause of childhood injury; it is important because, if unrecognized, further abuse is likely to occur and might even be fatal. When assessing a child after trauma, ensure that you check the whole child, using the principles of emergency management of severe trauma (EMST), and look for hidden injuries.

Clavicle fractures

These are the most common fractures seen in children. The fracture is usually midshaft and of green-stick type. Complete fractures with overlap of the ends are seen in older children and unite well. It is important to warn the parents at the beginning that they must expect to see a large lump develop: this is healing callus, which will remodel over 6–12 months without any cosmetic or functional deficit.

Treatment is with a triangular sling inside the clothes to support the elbow, regular analgesia and rest. The clavicle will start to join within a week and the sling can usually be discarded by 4 weeks.

Forearm fractures

Children's bones can break in several ways, namely:

- bend
- buckle
- greenstick
- complete, with/without displacement and overlap.

Most forearm fractures are of the buckle or green-stick variety and if there is minimal tilt or deformity they can be treated in an above elbow cast for 5 weeks. It is important to do a check radiograph after 7–10 days to ensure that the fracture has not tilted more. If it has tilted to an unacceptable position, the fracture can still undergo a closed reduction before firm union occurs.

Fractures with visible deformity or significant tilt/displacement (Fig. 8.1.16) require closed reduction and a similar time of cast immobilization.

Ensure that you complete and document a neurovascular examination of the limb initially. Provide the parents with written instructions for neurovascular observations at home and provide them with emergency contact details if excessive swelling or symptoms develop. Look for the five Ps:

- excessive *Pain*
- *Paraesthesia* (compression of the sensory nerves)
- *Paleness* of the fingers
- *Plum*-coloured (venous congestion)
- *Pulseless.*

Approximately 30% of children's fractures involve the growth plate (physis). If the physis suffers permanent damage, the bone can end up:

- short (all physeal growth stops), or
- angulated (one side of the physis stops growing).

The Salter–Harris classification is used for growth plate fractures (Fig. 8.1.17). Type I is often seen in the distal fibula as the childhood equivalent of the adult ankle sprain. Type II is the commonest variety and frequent in the distal radius. Types III and IV have a much higher risk of growth disturbance and

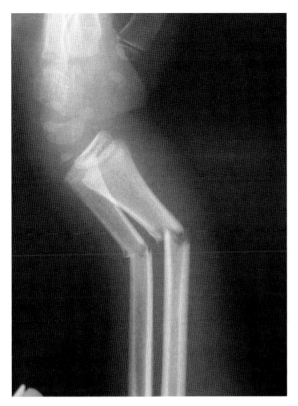

Fig. 8.1.16   Forearm fractures usually have dorsal tilt.

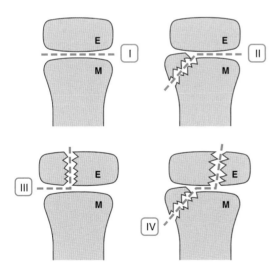

Fig. 8.1.17   Salter–Harris fracture: type I, the fracture passes directly through the physis; type II, a corner of the metaphysis (M) is broken off; type III, the fracture passes through the physis and the epiphysis (E); type IV, the fracture passes through the epiphysis and the metaphysis, causing a high risk of growth arrest.

usually require accurate reduction and internal fixation to minimize the risk of growth arrest.

Supracondylar fracture of the humerus

This fracture is often seen in children of 4–10 years after a fall from a height, such as from monkey bars, or when running. The mechanism is usually hyperextension of the elbow joint with the olecranon acting as a fulcrum lever to cause the fracture.

Neuropraxia of the radial, median, ulnar nerve is common. Occasionally displaced fractures cause damage to the brachial artery. Again, neurovascular assessment is mandatory. Minimally tilted fractures can be treated in a collar and cuff under the clothes for the first 2 weeks, then outside the clothes for a further 2 weeks. Warn the parents to expect elbow stiffness, especially loss of elbow extension for several months.

Displaced fractures require accurate reduction to avoid later deformity. Often the fracture will be held with K wires, which are removed at 4 weeks (Fig. 8.1.18).

Toddler fracture of the tibia

This distal shaft fracture may not be visible on initial radiographs and often perplexes clinicians faced with a toddler who refuses to walk for days after a seemingly minor trauma. The fracture can be diagnosed clinically by twisting the good leg first and then noting the cry or facial expression when twisting the affected side. Warn the parents what you are going to do first!

Treat the fracture in an above knee cast and allow weight bearing as the child dictates. Most will walk after 1 week in the cast and the cast can be removed at 3 weeks. Warn the parents to expect a limp for 1–2 months: the limp will resolve spontaneously.

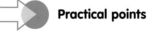

Practical points

Rules of 2 for fractures
- 2 views (anteroposterior and lateral X-ray)
- 2 joints (X-ray the joint above and joint below to exclude dislocation)
- 2 joints (immobilize the joint above and below the fracture in a cast)
- 2 times (ensure the fracture has not shifted after 1 week)
- 2 sides (you can X-ray the contralateral side for comparison if needed)

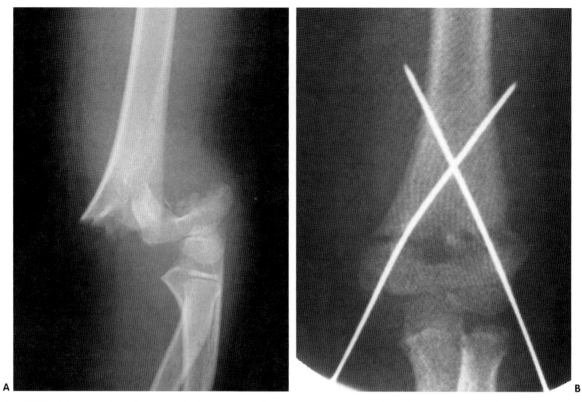

Fig. 8.1.18 **A** Supracondylar fracture of the humerus may have a nerve injury. **B** Displaced fractures require reduction and K-wire fixation.

Pulled elbow

The patient is usually a child aged 1–4 years who has been pulled along or up by the hand or treated to a 'whizzy'. The child presents with 'pseudo-paralysis' of the upper limb with the limb held by the side with the elbow extended and pronated. (Note that most elbow fractures present differently, with the elbow flexed and held across the body.)

The history is typical in all cases. The pathology is believed to be a minor stretch of the annular ligament around the radial head. It is treated by forced full flexion and simultaneous full supination of the elbow. Sometimes a satisfying click can be felt. A collar and cuff sling in flexion is worn overnight with the expectation of ready return to full function. Warn parents that it can recur and that it is best to avoid pulling on the hand.

COMMON PAEDIATRIC SURGICAL PROBLEMS

Common surgical conditions in children

S. W. Beasley

The penis and foreskin

The glans of the uncircumcised penis is protected by a layer of loose skin called the foreskin or prepuce. The amount of foreskin present varies among boys. At birth, and for many years afterwards, it is normal for part or all of the undersurface of the foreskin to be adherent to the glans penis. This adherence slowly separates during childhood. Forcible retraction of the foreskin before it is ready can damage the glans and may cause secondary phimosis. Therefore, the foreskin should not be retracted forcibly unless a circumcision is being performed. Spontaneous separation of these adhesions is normally complete by puberty.

Smegma

Smegma accumulates beneath the adherent foreskin. It appears as asymmetrical accumulations of yellow-tinged material predominantly in the coronal groove beneath the foreskin (Fig. 9.1.1). There may be sufficient smegma to produce a noticeable swelling, which may be misdiagnosed as a dermoid cyst or tumour. It is often misinterpreted as being mid-shaft because a small child's coronal groove may be a long way from the tip of the foreskin. Smegma is normal, and is released spontaneously as the foreskin separates from the glans penis. When it is released, it may be associated with some redness and irritation of the foreskin for a day or so: this, too, is a normal process.

Balanitis

Infection can develop beneath the foreskin and, if severe, pus may appear from the end of the foreskin. Balanitis is often associated with phimosis. Infection may cause considerable redness and swelling of the penile shaft, necessitating treatment with either topical or oral antibiotics.

Phimosis

In phimosis the opening at the tip of the foreskin has narrowed down to such a degree that the foreskin cannot be retracted (Fig. 9.1.2). The external urethral meatus is not visible. Phimosis must be distinguished from the normal adherence of the foreskin to the glans. In most boys, phimosis can be treated by application of steroid ointment (e.g. betamethasone valerate ointment) to the tight, shiny part of the foreskin. This usually obviates the need for circumcision. However, marked previous inflammation, infection, skin splitting and balanitis xerotica obliterans can lead to marked scarring of the foreskin and phimosis, and in many of these children the only reasonable treatment is circumcision. Sometimes the severity of phimosis is such that there is ballooning of the foreskin on micturition, and on rare occasions it may even cause urinary retention with a distended bladder. A degree of phimosis is common in infancy but tends to resolve spontaneously in the first few years of life, and is not considered abnormal in this age group.

Paraphimosis

Paraphimosis occurs when a mildly phimotic foreskin has been retracted over the glans and has become stuck behind the coronal groove, causing oedema of itself and the glans penis (Fig. 9.1.3). It is a painful and progressive process. Treatment involves gentle manipulation of the foreskin forwards, which may require a general anaesthetic. Circumcision is not performed at this time, but a few children may need it subsequently if the phimosis does not respond to topical application of steroid ointment.

Hypospadias

It is important to recognize hypospadias when it is present (Fig. 9.1.4). The foreskin looks square and hangs off the penis, and the shaft of the penis is bent ventrally. The two main problems in hypospadias are:

- the location of the urethra (which can be found on the ventral side of the shaft of the penis, proximal to its correct position)
- chordee (ventral angulation of the shaft and glans)

Correction of chordee to straighten the penis is required to allow later successful sexual function.

263

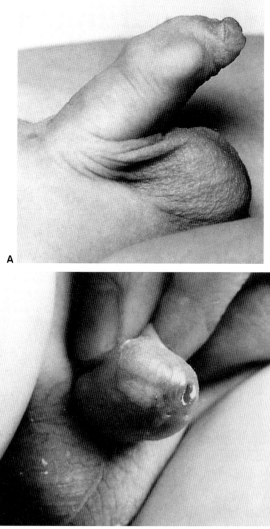

A

B

Fig. 9.1.1 A. The normal foreskin with accumulation of smegma beneath it. The swellings caused by the smegma are in the region of the coronal groove. B. On retraction, smegma appears as accumulations of material beneath a foreskin that has not yet separated from the glans.

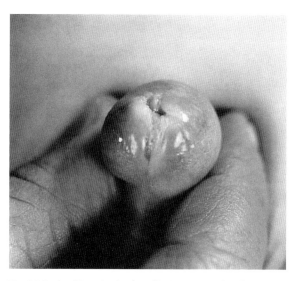

Fig. 9.1.2 In phimosis, the foreskin is narrowed and cannot be retracted.

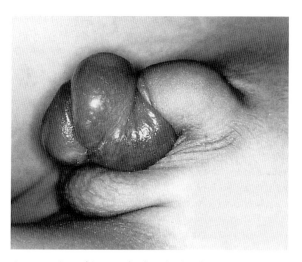

Fig. 9.1.3 Paraphimosis: the foreskin has become stuck behind the coronal groove.

The operation is usually performed as a single-stage procedure at 9–12 months of age, often as day surgery.

Circumcision is absolutely contraindicated in hypospadias because the skin of the prepuce is used during repair of the hypospadias. Severe hypospadias may be indicative of an intersex abnormality. For example, when there is penoscrotal hypospadias and a bifid scrotum, the scrotum should be examined carefully for testes, because some of these children may be females with congenital adrenal hyperplasia; the labioscrotal folds are labia rather than scrota,

and the presumed urethral opening may in fact be the entrance to the vagina (Ch. 19.3).

Circumcision

The indications for circumcision remain controversial. In many countries, circumcision has been abandoned in the neonatal period because of its relatively high complication rate. Apart from the risk of septicaemia and meningitis when performed in the relatively immunologically immature neonate, there are a number of problems that may occur during circumcision at any age. These include removal of too much or too little foreskin, postoperative bleeding and infection. Haemorrhage postoperatively occa-

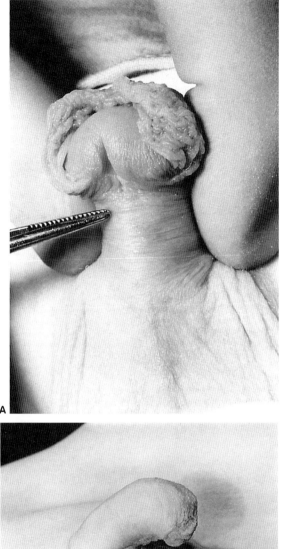

A

B

Fig. 9.1.4 In hypospadias the ventral shaft of the penis is angulated and shortened (chordee), the urethral meatus is ventrally placed and the foreskin is deficient on the underside. A. Ventral aspect. B. Appearance from above.

sionally requires surgical reintervention. The most troublesome and common complication of circumcision is abrasion and ulceration of the sensitive glans penis, particularly near the urethral meatus. As the meatal ulceration heals it may produce meatal stenosis and require a meatotomy to re-establish an adequate urinary stream.

Epispadias

In epispadias, the urethra opens on to the dorsal aspect of the base of the penis. Epispadias is part of a spectrum of lower abdominal wall defects in which ectopia vesicae (bladder exstrophy) and cloacal exstrophy are the most severe forms. Boys with epispadias are often incontinent of urine because the sphincter of the bladder neck is also deficient.

Clinical example

James was a 7-year-old boy who presented following two episodes of balanitis. He also complained of discomfort on micturition. Examination revealed a tight foreskin that could not be retracted; the urethral meatus could not be seen. After 1 month of topical application of betamethasone ointment four times a day to the tight part of the foreskin, he was able to fully retract it. Circumcision was not necessary.

The inguinoscrotal region

Inguinal hernia

After the testis has descended into the scrotum during the seventh month of pregnancy, the canal down which it migrates, the processus vaginalis, should obliterate. Failure of obliteration of the processus vaginalis may produce an inguinal hernia, a hydrocele or an encysted hydrocele of the cord.

A widely patent proximal processus vaginalis allows bowel (and, in girls, the ovary as well) to enter the inguinal canal, producing a reducible lump in the groin called an indirect inguinal hernia (Fig. 9.1.5). This occurs in about 2% of live male births but is less frequent in girls. The greatest incidence is in the first year of life.

The usual presentation is that of an intermittent swelling, overlying the external inguinal ring, that has been noticed by a parent. At times it may appear to cause discomfort. It is most likely to be obvious during an episode of crying or straining, and in infants may be seen during nappy changes. Inguinal hernias should be repaired as soon as practicable.

Strangulation of inguinal hernias is common, particularly during the first 6 months of life. Strangulation can be recognized when the groin swelling becomes irreducible. If left untreated, a strangulated hernia may damage the incarcerated bowel and, occasionally, by compressing the testicular vessels may lead to testicular atrophy. For this reason, an immediate attempt should be made to reduce the hernia manually. This is done by first disimpacting

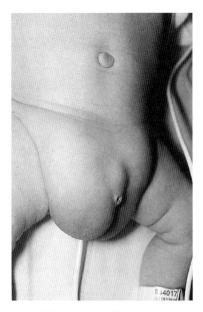

Fig. 9.1.5 Large bilateral inguinal hernias.

the hernia at the external inguinal ring, and then reducing it along the line of the inguinal canal.

Fortunately, most hernias that become stuck can be reduced manually; the hernia can then be repaired as an elective procedure within a few days. This is best done in a specialist paediatric surgical centre.

Hydrocele

A hydrocele presents as a painless cystic swelling around the testis in the scrotum (Fig. 9.1.6). It contains peritoneal fluid that has tracked down a narrow but patent processus vaginalis. It transilluminates brilliantly. When the hydrocele is lax, the testis can be felt within it. The upper limit of the hydrocele can be demonstrated distal to the external inguinal ring, distinguishing it from an inguinal hernia, where the swelling extends through the external inguinal ring. There is no impulse on crying or straining.

Hydroceles are common in the first few months of life, do not cause discomfort and usually disappear spontaneously. Surgery is only indicated if the hydrocele persists beyond 2 years of age.

Undescended testis

Undescended testis (or cryptorchidism) is a term used to describe the testis that does not reside spontaneously in the scrotum. Undescended testes occur in about 2% of boys, being more common in premature infants. Spontaneous descent of the testis is unlikely beyond 3 months post-term. Cryptorchidism is important to detect because it will result in

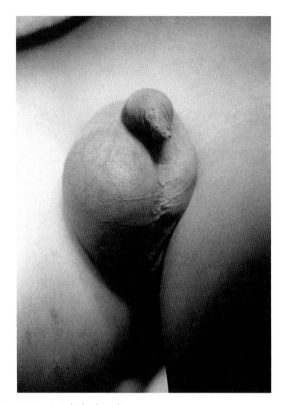

Fig. 9.1.6 A right hydrocele.

reduced fertility if left untreated. It is suspected that the higher temperature to which an undescended testis is subject impairs spermatogenesis.

The diagnosis is made by examining the inguino-scrotal region. Normally, the testis should be found within the scrotal sac. In cryptorchidism the scrotum looks empty (Fig. 9.1.7). The testis is 'milked' down the line of the inguinal canal towards the scrotum and is pulled gently towards the scrotum. If the testis cannot be brought into the scrotum or will not remain there spontaneously it is considered undescended.

Clinically, it may be difficult to distinguish a retractile testis from an undescended testis. In most normal boys the testis resides in the bottom of the scrotum, but the cremasteric reflex, which is prominent during mid-childhood, may cause it to move upwards, sometimes completely out of the scrotum. A retractile testis found outside the scrotum initially can be brought down into the normal position and should stay there spontaneously, at least until the cremasteric reflex is stimulated (Table 9.1.1). An undescended testis will not stay in the scrotum spontaneously and usually cannot even be coerced beyond the neck of the scrotum. It is often smaller than a normal testis on the other side.

Undescended testes should be brought down into the scrotum surgically between 9 and 12 months of

Table 9.1.1 Comparison of undescended and retractile testes

Feature	Undescended testis	Retractile testis
Can be brought fully to bottom of scrotum	No	Yes
Remains in scrotum spontaneously for a period before retracting	No	Yes
Resides spontaneously in scrotum at times	No	Yes
Normal size	Normal or small	Normal

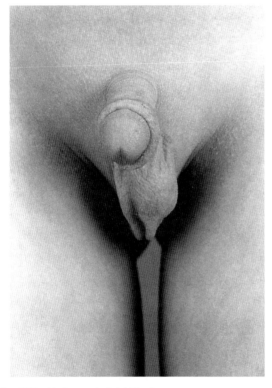

Fig. 9.1.7 Undescended right testis.

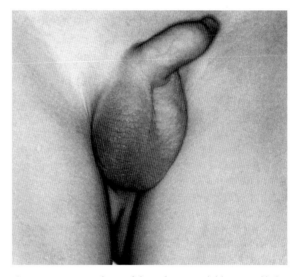

Fig. 9.1.8 An acutely painful scrotum in a child is most likely to be caused by torsion of an appendix testis or torsion of the testis.

age. Unfortunately, in many boys the diagnosis is not made until the child is older. The later the testis is brought down, the more likely it is that there will be damage to spermatogenesis. Orchidopexy is performed as a day case procedure. In general, the results are excellent when the procedure is performed by a specialist paediatric surgeon.

The acutely painful scrotum

There are a number of conditions that cause an acutely painful or enlarged scrotum (Fig. 9.1.8), of which torsion of a testicular appendage is the most common, and torsion of the testis itself the most important (Table 9.1.2). In both conditions the boy complains of severe pain in the scrotum. In the early stages of torsion of a testicular appendage, a blue-black 'pea-sized' swelling which is extremely tender to touch may be seen through the skin of the scrotum near the upper pole of the testis. Palpation of the testis itself causes no discomfort. Later, a reactive hydrocele develops, the tenderness becomes more generalized and the clinical features may make it difficult to distinguish from torsion of the testis. Where torsion of the testis has occurred, both the testis and the epididymis are exquisitely tender (unless necrosis has already occurred) and the testis may be lying high within the scrotum. In older boys the pain radiates to the ipsilateral iliac fossa and may be associated with nausea and vomiting, producing symptoms similar to those of appendicitis, which highlights the importance of always examining the scrotum in boys presenting with lower abdominal pain.

Table 9.1.2 Causes of an acutely painful scrotum

Condition	Comment	Frequency
Torsion of testicular appendix	Peak age 11 years Unilateral tenderness	>75%
Torsion of testis	Peaks in neonatal and adolescent age groups Surgical emergency	20%
Epididymo-orchitis	Usually in infancy Association with urinary tract abnormalities	Rare
Idiopathic scrotal oedema	Usually in young child Bilateral oedema Testes not tender	Rare

Treatment

Urgent surgical exploration of the scrotum is required to untwist the testis and epididymis and to suture both testes to prevent subsequent torsion. A completely necrotic testis should be removed. A torted and infarcted testicular appendix should be removed. In this situation the testis should be checked to make sure that it has not twisted but otherwise it requires no treatment. When a testis has twisted the contralateral testis should also be examined and 'pexed' to prevent it from twisting at a later date.

Other causes of scrotal pathology

Epididymo-orchitis is unusual in children: it is most often seen during the first year of life, where it may signify an underlying structural abnormality of the urinary tract. For this reason investigation involves a renal ultrasound and micturating cystourethrogram. Examination of the urine may show leukocytes and bacteria. Mumps orchitis is extremely rare prior to puberty. In idiopathic scrotal oedema there is painless boggy oedema of the whole scrotum and the testes are completely non-tender. Testicular malignancy is occasionally seen in leukaemia or with a primary testicular neoplasm.

Abnormalities of the umbilicus

The umbilical cord desiccates and separates several days after birth, allowing the umbilical ring to close. Sometimes the stump of the cord may become infected, the umbilical ring may not close, or there may be remnants of the embryonic channels that pass through the umbilicus before birth (Table 9.1.3).

Table 9.1.3 Abnormalities of the umbilicus

Abnormality	Comment
Exomphalos	See Chapter 11.5
Gastroschisis	See Chapter 11.5
Umbilical hernia	Common, most resolve Asymptomatic Skin covered
Umbilical sepsis ('omphalitis')	Neonatal, serious condition
Umbilical granuloma	Common, treat with silver nitrate Often pedunculated
Ectopic bowel mucosa	Treat with silver nitrate
Patent vitellointestinal duct	Sinus opening at umbilicus Communication with ileum Discharges faecal fluid and gas
Patent urachus	Communication with bladder Discharges urine

Umbilical hernia

Failure of the umbilical ring to close after birth produces an umbilical hernia (Fig. 9.1.9). Umbilical hernias are common in neonates but most close spontaneously in the first year of life. The skin overlying the umbilical hernia never ruptures and strangulation of the contents is virtually unknown. The swelling will become tense when the infant cries or strains. Umbilical hernias normally do not cause pain. No treatment is required during the first few

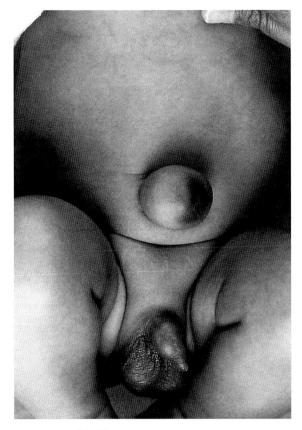

Fig. 9.1.9 Umbilical hernia.

years of life. If the hernia is still present after the age of 3 years it can be repaired as a day surgical procedure.

Discharge from the umbilicus

Discharge from the umbilicus may be pus, mucus, urine or faeces. An umbilical granuloma is a common lesion that first becomes evident after separation of the umbilical cord. There is a small accumulation of granulation tissue in the umbilicus, accompanied by a seropurulent discharge. If it has a definite stalk it can be ligated without anaesthesia, but most often it is treated by topical application of silver nitrate. Ectopic bowel mucosa has a similar appearance but has a smooth, red, glistening surface and discharges mucus. It is treated in the same way. Persistence of part or all of the vitellointestinal (omphalomesenteric) duct produces one of a number of abnormalities, which usually present in early infancy but may not be evident for some years. Complete patency of the tract allows ileal fluid and air to discharge from the umbilicus. Persistence of one part produces a sinus or cyst, which may become infected to form an abscess and may discharge pus. A vitellointestinal

band attaching the ileum to the deep surface of the umbilicus may cause intestinal obstruction. A Meckel's diverticulum represents persistence of the ileal part of the duct. Vitellointestinal duct remnants are excised.

Urinary discharge from the umbilicus suggests a persistent communication with the bladder in the form of a patent urachus. Sometimes it may produce a cystic mass or abscess in the midline just below the umbilicus. Urachal remnants should be excised.

The anus and perineum

A variety of unrelated conditions affect the anus and perineum in children.

Anal fissure

These are usually seen in infants and toddlers when passage of a hard stool splits the anal mucosa, causing sharp pain and often a few drops of bright blood. The condition is of little consequence and the fissure usually heals within days. Examination of the anal margin shows a split in the epithelium anteriorly or posteriorly in the midline. An anal fissure may occur in an older child, in which situation it tends to be related to constipation. The child gets severe pain on defaecation and becomes reluctant to defaecate, further worsening the constipation. Treatment is directed at overcoming the underlying constipation. A stool softener and lubricant, e.g. paraffin oil, may be helpful. A chronic indolent, often non-painful, fissure away from the midline may indicate inflammatory bowel disease, such as Crohn disease.

Perianal abscesses

These are most likely to occur in the first year of life from infection of an anal gland. The abscess points superficially, a centimetre or two from the anal canal. The abscess should be drained and the fistula between the abscess and the anal canal laid open to reduce the likelihood of recurrence.

Rectal prolapse

Rectal prolapse tends to occur in the second and third years of life in otherwise normal children. The rectum prolapses during defaecation and returns spontaneously afterwards. In some, manual reduction is required. The prolapsed mucosa may become congested and bleed but causes little discomfort. Clinically, it needs to be distinguished from prolapse of a benign rectal polyp (a benign hamartomatous lesion seen in children) and the apex of an intussusception (the child would have other symptoms of intussusception). The passage of time, and treatment of any underlying constipation, is all that is required in the majority of toddlers. Occasionally, a sclerosant is injected into the submucosal plane of the rectum for persistent cases.

In a few patients there is an underlying organic cause for the rectal prolapse. Usually the reason is obvious, as in paralysis of anal sphincters in spina bifida and sacral agenesis, undernourished hypotonic infants, bladder exstrophy, cloacal exstrophy, following surgery for imperforate anus, or malabsorption.

Labial adhesions

This common condition is often detected on routine examination in infant girls, or noted incidentally by parents. The epithelium of the labia minora has fused in the midline; this may sometimes cause discomfort on micturition and may be associated with urinary infection. Labial adhesions are never present at birth. Asymptomatic adhesions require no treatment and resolve as the girl gets older as a result of rising levels of oestrogen. Gentle lateral traction on the labia may assist their separation if this is necessary because of problems with micturition or urinary infection. Adhesions have a tendency to recur after separation.

The neck

Lesions of the neck fall into two broad groups: developmental anomalies and acquired lesions. The exact location of the lesion will usually provide a clue as to its nature.

Midline neck swellings

The most common midline neck swelling in children (Table 9.1.4) is a thyroglossal cyst. Typically, there is a swelling overlying and attached to the hyoid bone that moves on swallowing and tongue protrusion. It may become infected to form an abscess with overlying erythema of the skin. The thyroglossal cyst and the entire thyroglossal tract is best excised before it becomes infected. Excision must include the middle third of the hyoid bone (Sistrunk operation), otherwise recurrence is common. Ectopic thyroid tissue is a less common cause of a midline neck swelling. Clinically, it may be difficult to distinguish from a thyroglossal cyst. If suspected preoperatively, a thyroid isotope scan will clarify the distribution of all functioning thyroid tissue.

Table 9.1.4 Midline neck swellings	
Cause of swelling	Comment
Thyroglossal cyst	Most common (80% of midline neck swellings) Moves with tongue protrusion and swallowing Attached to hyoid bone
Ectopic thyroid	May be only thyroid tissue present Do thyroid isotope scan
Submental lymph node/abscess	Check inside mouth for primary infection Other cervical lymph nodes may be enlarged
Dermoid cyst	Small, mobile, non tender Yellow tinge through skin In subcutaneous layer
Goitre	Lower neck
Cystic hygroma	Hamartoma Usually evident from birth May be extensive

Congenital dermoid cysts can occur along any line of fusion, including the neck, where they are situated in the midline. A midline cervical dermoid is occasionally mistaken for a thyroglossal cyst. It contains sebaceous material surrounded by squamous epithelium. The most common congenital dermoid cyst is the external angular dermoid, which is found at the orbital margin. Dermoid cysts enlarge slowly and it is appropriate for them to be removed.

Cystic hygromas are congenital hamartomas of the lymphatic system. They vary greatly in size and may involve the front of the neck or extend to one or both sides asymmetrically. Some complex cystic hygromas may contain cavernous haemangiomatous elements and may extend upwards into the floor of the mouth or downwards into the thoracic cavity. They may enlarge rapidly from viral or bacterial infection, or from haemorrhage. Depending on their extent and location, the airway may be compromised, leading to life-threatening respiratory obstruction. Surgery involves excision or debulking of the lesion. In some situations they are injected with sclerosants.

Lateral neck swellings

Most lateral neck swellings are acquired, being due to infection of one or more of the cervical lymph nodes. Persistently enlarged cervical lymph nodes are normal in children with frequent upper respiratory infections: they represent a normal response to infection (i.e. reactive hyperplasia) and require no treatment. Lymph nodes may enlarge rapidly and become tender during active infection but usually settle with rest, analgesia and antibiotics as required. In children aged 6 months to 3 years lateral cervical lymphadenitis may progress to abscess formation: the lymph nodes enlarge over 4–5 days and become fluctuant, although deeper nodes may not exhibit fluctuation. The overlying skin becomes red. Treatment involves incision and drainage of the abscess under general anaesthesia.

MAIS lymphadenitis

Cervical lymphadenitis due to atypical mycobacterial infection is common in preschool children. The MAIS (*Mycobacterium avium, intracellulare, scrofulaceum*) infection produces chronic cervical lymphadenitis and collar stud abscesses (so called MAC or *Mycobacterium avium* complex) and usually affects the jugulodigastric, submandibular or preauricular lymph nodes. The involved lymph node increases in size over several weeks before erupting into the subcutaneous tissue as a collar stud 'cold' abscess. Eventually, if untreated, it may cause purple discoloration of the overlying skin and will ulcerate through the skin to produce a chronic discharging sinus. MAIS infections respond poorly to antibiotics. Treatment involves surgical removal of the collar stud abscess and excision of the underlying infected lymph nodes.

Lymph node tumours

Primary tumours involving the lymph nodes occur in older children. Both Hodgkin and non-Hodgkin lymphomas may involve cervical lymph nodes. Rarely, other tumours may metastasize to the cervical lymph nodes, e.g. neuroblastomas and nasopharyngeal tumours.

Branchial remnants

Branchial remnants arise from the branchial arch system. A variety of abnormalities occur, including branchial cysts, branchial sinuses, branchial fistulas and persistent cartilaginous remnants. Branchial fistulas are present from birth but, because the opening is so tiny, they may not be noticed for some years. A drop of mucus or saliva may be observed leaking from the external orifice near the anterior border of the sternomastoid muscle in the lower neck. Branchial cysts present later in childhood with a mass

beneath the anterior border of the sternomastoid near its upper third. They may become infected and should be removed. Sinuses or fistulas usually arise from the second branchial cleft, although sometimes the first and third clefts are responsible.

Torticollis

Torticollis, or wry neck, has many causes in childhood (Table 9.1.5). A sternomastoid tumour presents in the third week of life when the parents notice a hard lump in the neck or that the head cannot be turned to one side. The head is flexed slightly to the side of the shortened sternomastoid muscle, and is turned to the contralateral side. There may be a history of breech delivery or forceps delivery. There is a hard, painless swelling, usually 2–3 cm long, in the shortened sternomastoid muscle (Fig. 9.1.10). Sometimes the whole muscle may be involved.

Table 9.1.5   Causes of torticollis

Cause	Comment
Sternomastoid tumour	Not present at birth Present at 3 weeks of age Tight, shortened sternomastoid muscle Most resolve without treatment
Postural torticollis	Present at birth Disappears in months From intrauterine position
Cervical hemivertebrae Imbalance of ocular muscles (strabismus) Lateral cervical lymphadenitis Tumours Atlanto-occipital subluxation Benign paroxysmal torticollis of infancy	

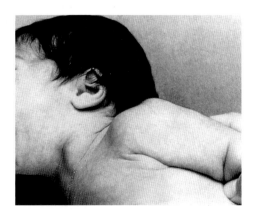

Fig. 9.1.10   Sternomastoid tumour in torticollis.

Rotation of the head to the side of the tumour is limited. Plagiocephaly and hemihypoplasia of the face may develop in subsequent months. The 'tumour' disappears within 9–12 months in the vast majority of affected infants. Where fibrosis persists and causes permanent shortening of the muscle with persistent torticollis, the sternomastoid muscle should be divided. Occasionally, older children present with torticollis due to a short, tight and fibrous sterno-mastoid muscle; the ipsilateral shoulder is elevated, there may be compensatory scoliosis, and the child has difficulty rotating the head towards the affected side. These children require surgical division of the muscle.

PART 10

INHERITED AND METABOLIC PROBLEMS

Birth defects, prenatal diagnosis and teratogens

J. Liebelt, N. J. Hotham

Birth defects

A birth defect is any abnormality, structural or functional, identified at any age, that began before birth, or the cause of which was present before birth. Examples of structural birth defects include spina bifida, congenital heart malformations and cleft lip. Phenylketonuria, Duchenne muscular dystrophy and Huntington disease are examples of functional birth defects.

With continued advances in obstetric and paediatric medicine, birth defects have become the most important cause of perinatal and postneonatal mortality in developed countries.

Birth defects:

- are the leading cause of perinatal death (20–25% of deaths)
- are now the leading cause of postneonatal deaths (25–30%), as deaths due to sudden infant death syndrome continue to decline
- are responsible for a major proportion of the morbidity and disability experienced by children and young adults
- are the cause for 20–30% of the admissions to a tertiary paediatric hospital
- have an immense impact on the emotional and physical wellbeing of the children and their families
- have a significant financial cost for the community.

Types of structural birth defect

Structural birth defects may be classified on the basis of the mechanism by which they arise:

- *Malformations* arise during the initial formation of the embryo and fetus as a result of genetic and/or environmental factors during organogenesis (2–8 weeks postconception). Malformations may include failure of formation, incomplete formation or abnormal configuration. Examples include spina bifida, cleft palate and hypospadias
- *Disruptions* result from a destructive process that alters structures after formation. Examples include early amnion rupture causing amputation defects of digits, or an abdominal wall defect

- *Deformations* result from moulding of a part by mechanical forces, usually acting over a prolonged period. Examples include talipes, congenital hip dislocations and plagiocephaly associated with oligohydramnios.

Causes of birth defects

Birth defects can be caused by a wide variety of mechanisms. These range from genetic abnormalities, both monogenic and polygenic, through presumably accidental events within the developing embryo, e.g. vascular accidents, to environmental factors, including teratogens generated by the mother, e.g. maternal phenylketonuria and maternal diabetes, and those originating outside the fetomaternal unit, e.g. medications, infectious agents and high-dose X irradiation. Table 10.1.1 provides a framework for thinking about causes of birth defects. Most have a multifactorial basis, reflecting interaction between genes, environment and chance events within the developing embryo and fetus.

Genes and birth defects

Early human development from fertilized ovum to fetus involves numerous processes controlled by genes, expressed sequentially in a defined cascade. The processes and developmental phases include such things as definition of polarity, cell division, formation of the germ layers, segmentation of the embryo, cell migration, organ formation, cell differentiation, interactions between cells, tissues and organs and programmed cell death.

There has been a recent rapid increase in knowledge of the genes that determine or predispose to birth defects. This has resulted from technological advances in molecular genetics, in phenotype delineation, gene mapping and gene discovery in humans and other species, and an understanding of the cascade of sequential gene expression during embryonic development in other species.

Examples of these genes include the homeotic (HOX) and paired box (PAX) gene families. HOX genes are involved in the formation of structures developing from specific segments of the embryo and PAX genes have an important role in eye develop-

Table 10.1.1 Causes of birth defects

Mechanism	Example	Cause
Whole chromosome missing or duplicated	Down syndrome Turner syndrome	Trisomy 21 Monosomy X
Part of chromosome deleted or duplicated	Cri du chat syndrome Cat eye syndrome	Deletion 5p Duplication 22q
Submicroscopic deletion or duplication of chromosome material	Williams syndrome Velocardiofacial syndrome Charcot–Marie–Tooth disease IA	Deletion 7q Deletion 22q Duplication 17p
Mutation in single gene	Smith–Lemli–Opitz syndrome Holt–Oram syndrome Apert–Crouzon–Pfeiffer syndrome	7-dehydrocholesterol reductase TBX5 Fibroblast growth factor receptor 2
Consequence of normal imprinting	Prader–Willi syndrome	Maternal uniparental disomy or paternal deletion for 15q12
Imprinting errors	Beckwith–Wiedemann syndrome Angelman syndrome	Multiple mechanisms resulting in overexpression of IGF2 Mutations in UBE3A gene
Multifactorial/polygenic: one or more genes and environmental factors	Isolated heart malformations, neural tube defects and facial clefts	Complex interactions between genes and environmental factors not yet defined
Non-genetic vascular and other 'accidents during development'	Poland anomaly Oculoauriculovertebral dysplasia	Subclavian artery ischaemia Stapedial artery ischaemia
Uterine environment	Talipes, hip dysplasia, plagiocephaly	Oligohydramnios, twins, bicornuate uterus
Maternal environment	Mental retardation Caudal regression	Maternal phenylketonuria Maternal diabetes mellitus
Wider environment	Fetal rubella syndrome Fetal alcohol syndrome Microcephaly Limb deficiency	Rubella infection in pregnancy Maternal alcohol ingestion High-dose X-irradiation Thalidomide

ment. Birth defects caused by mutations in selected developmental genes are shown in Table 10.1.2.

Frequency of birth defects

Major birth defects

Major birth defects:

- are those with medical and social consequences
- are present with the highest prevalence among miscarriages, intermediate in stillbirths and lowest among liveborn infants
- are recognized at birth in 2–3% of liveborn infants.

The birth prevalences of the more common birth defects are shown in Table 10.1.3. They represent the frequency with which the defect occurred during development (its incidence), less the spontaneous loss of affected fetuses during pregnancy. An almost equal number of additional major abnormalities, particularly heart defects and urinary tract abnormalities, will be recognized by 5 years of age during clinical examinations or because of symptoms.

Minor birth defects

Minor birth defects:

- are relatively frequent but pose no significant health or social burden
- are recognized in approximately 15% of newborns
- are important to recognize, as their presence prompts a search for coexistent, more important abnormalities.

Table 10.1.2 Some developmental genes that, when mutant, cause birth defects in humans

Gene	Disorder	Features
CBP	Rubinstein–Taybi syndrome	Mental retardation, broad thumbs/toes, facial features
DAX1	X-linked adrenal hypoplasia	Adrenal insufficiency
ENDR3B	Hirschsprung disease	Megacolon
FGFR2	Apert–Crouzon–Pfeiffer syndrome	Craniosynostosis, faciostenosis, ± brachysyndactyly
FGFR3	Achondroplasia	Short-limbed dwarfism, macrocephaly
GLI3	Grieg cephalopolysyndactyly	Polysyndactyly, frontal bossing
HOXD13	Dominant polysyndactyly	Polysyndactyly
L1 CAM	X-linked hydrocephalus	Aqueduct stenosis, mental retardation, adducted thumbs
MITF	Waardenburg syndrome type 2	Deafness, pigmentary disturbance
MSX2	Craniosynostosis (Boston type)	Craniosynostosis, short metatarsals
Myosin 7A	Usher syndrome type 1B	Congenital deafness, prepubertal retinitis pigmentosa
PAX2	Coloboma	Coloboma, urinary tract abnormalities
PAX3	Waardenburg syndrome type 1	Deafness, pigmentary disturbance, dystopia canthorum
PAX6	Aniridia	Aniridia
SHH	Holoprosencephaly	Holoprosencephaly
SOX9	Campomelic dysplasia	Short-limbed dwarfism, bowed bones, abnormal brain development, sex reversal, cleft palate
TBX5	Holt–Oram syndrome	Variable upper limb defects, heart malformations

Infants free of minor defects have a low incidence of major malformations, approximately 1%. Those with one, two or three minor defects have risks of major malformations of 3%, 10% and 20%, respectively.

Practical points

Birth defects
- Birth defects are the leading cause of perinatal and postneonatal deaths, and result in substantial morbidity and disability in developed countries
- There is a wide variety of mechanisms including genetic, environmental and multifactorial
- Major birth defects affect 2–3% of liveborns, and minor birth defects affect 15%
- Preventive strategies remain limited, but include maternal folic acid supplementation, reduction in teratogen exposure, alternative reproductive options, prenatal detection and neonatal screening

Multiple birth defects

Various terms have been used to classify multiple birth defects in the hope that the terminology will convey information about aetiology, pathogenesis and the relationship between the birth defects. However, no system of naming meets all these criteria or is able to meet all the situations encountered in clinical practice. Some commonly used terms are *syndrome*, *association*, *sequence* and *developmental field defect*: these are defined in Chapter 10.3. *Phenotype* is a useful general term that makes no assumptions about aetiology or pathogenesis but registers the fact that multiple birth defects are present and are related in some way. *Complex* and *spectrum* are alternative terms that have been used in this context.

Diagnosis of birth defects

Hundreds of patterns of multiple birth defects have been defined and the diagnosis for a child with multiple birth defects is often not obvious.

Table 10.1.3 Prevalence of some common birth defects	
Defect	Rate
Malformations of heart and great vessels	12.0
Developmental hip dysplasia	6.9
Hypospadias	3.7
Talipes equinovarus	2.2
Hypertrophic pyloric stenosis	1.9
Down syndrome	1.8
Cleft lip with or without cleft palate	1.1
Spina bifida	0.9
Anencephaly	0.7
Renal agenesis and dysgenesis	0.6
Tracheo-oesophageal fistula, oesophageal atresia and stenosis	0.4
Abdominal wall defects: exomphalos and gastroschisis	0.6

Rate per 1000 births including terminations of pregnancy, stillbirths and livebirths.
Source: South Australian Birth Defects Register 1986–2003.

The primary reasons for pursuing a diagnosis are that a specific diagnosis allows:

- discussion with the parents about the prognosis for their child
- parents to develop an understanding of how the birth defect arose
- counselling of the parents regarding recurrence risk and possibilities for reduction of this risk.

Thorough investigation, including autopsy if the child dies, may lead to a diagnosis, and referral to a clinical geneticist should be considered. Diagnosis is aided by computerized syndrome identification systems such as POSSUM and the London Dysmorphology Database. In spite of the large number of known syndromes, clinicians continue to encounter many children with birth defects the cause of which cannot be diagnosed or ascertained.

Birth defect/congenital malformation registers

Birth defects registers were established in many countries following the 'thalidomide tragedy' in which hundreds of children were born with a range of anomalies following maternal use of thalidomide in pregnancy as an antiemetic.

Clinical example

Susan and Craig's first child Anna was diagnosed soon after birth with a significant congenital heart defect (tetralogy of Fallot) that required surgery. No concerns had been raised at the midtrimester ultrasound, which had been performed in the regional centre for the region in which they lived. Anna was also noted to have a number of minor birth defects, including unusually shaped ears, and a hemivertebra in the thoracic spine, seen on a chest X-ray.

The family were referred to a clinical geneticist for an opinion regarding the possibility of an underlying genetic condition to account for Anna's health issues. The geneticist also noted that Anna had relatively long, slender fingers and that her mother reported frequent nasal regurgitation of milk during feeds, suggesting palatal dysfunction. This combination of issues raised the possibility of a condition called velocardiofacial syndrome, caused by a microdeletion on chromosome 22q. A chromosome analysis was arranged, including a specific fluorescent in situ hybridization (FISH) test for this microdeletion, which confirmed the diagnosis.

90% of children with this condition are the first person in their family to be affected. However, 10% have inherited the condition from a parent, who may be unaware they are affected, as the medical issues it has caused them have been mild. As the recurrence risk for further pregnancies differs significantly between these two situations, blood tests were arranged for Susan and Craig. Craig was found also to have the microdeletion on chromosome 22q and,

when his medical history was taken, he reported having required serial plastering for talipes as an infant and that he had had recurrent ear infections as a child, had struggled academically at school and was now being treated for depression, all of which can be features of this condition.

Given the wide variability of potential medical issues associated with velocardiofacial syndrome, a number of screening tests were arranged for Anna and Craig to detect any previously unrecognized birth defects. This included renal ultrasounds, immune function tests, serum calcium levels, thyroid function tests, eye and hearing reviews, and spine X-rays and cardiology review for Craig. Anna was found to have only one normally functioning kidney. The potential long-term consequences of the condition were discussed with the family and they were put in touch with the local support group. Anna was referred to a general paediatrician for ongoing medical and developmental follow-up. It was discussed with the family that there would be a 50% chance that any further children they conceived would also inherit the condition, but that they might experience more or less severe medical issues.

A range of reproductive options were discussed with the couple, including sperm donation, prenatal diagnosis and preimplantation genetic diagnosis. Anna required multiple hospitalizations in the first few years of life related to her condition, which placed a great deal of stress on the family. Subsequently in the couple's second pregnancy they chose to have a CVS with FISH for the microdeletion to assess whether the fetus had inherited velocardiofacial syndrome. The results showed that the fetus had not inherited the condition and a healthy boy was subsequently born.

Registers serve a number of purposes, including:

- provision of early warning of new environmental teratogens
- provision of precise prevalence figures for individual birth defects and syndromes
- monitoring of geographical and temporal trends in birth defects
- comparison of birth defect prevalence in different populations
- assessment of the impact of population-based prevention strategies and prenatal diagnosis
- research into the epidemiology of birth defects.

Prevention of birth defects

Despite considerable research efforts there are very few preventive strategies that effectively reduce the incidence of birth defects. Some effective population-based examples include:

- oral folic acid supplementation at least 1 month prior to and in the early months of pregnancy can reduce the incidence of neural tube defects by up to 70%
- education and legislation to reduce potential exposure to teratogens:
  - public health policy on rubella immunization
  - restrictions on prescribing of known teratogens such as thalidomide and retinoids
  - education about avoidance of foods in pregnancy that may predispose to maternal infection with known teratogenic agents, e.g. toxoplasmosis and uncooked meat
- genetic counselling and the development of alternative reproductive options, including donor gametes and embryos, to allow avoidance of the risk of conception of a child with a birth defect related to a specific genetic condition
- neonatal screening to detect children with those types of birth defect which do not cause permanent damage before birth, with a view to early treatment and improved prognosis. Neonatal screening for phenylketonuria, hypothyroidism and cystic fibrosis, and clinical examination for hip dislocation are examples of highly successful screening programmes.

At present, the primary approach to the prevention of the birth of children affected by birth defects is prenatal diagnosis.

Prenatal diagnosis

Prenatal diagnosis refers to testing performed in pregnancy aimed at the detection of birth defects in the fetus. Depending on the type of birth defect identified, the gestation of the pregnancy and the perception of the parents, prenatal detection of a birth defect may allow:

- termination of an affected fetus
- potential treatment in utero or postnatally to improve prognosis related to the defect
- preparation for the birth of a child with a specific medical condition.

The number of prenatal tests available and the range of birth defects that may be detected are expanding rapidly. Many chromosome abnormalities, structural anomalies, enzymatic and single gene defects are already potentially detectable prenatally. Advances in knowledge regarding the aetiology of birth defects and technical aspects of testing will expand this range further. Despite these advances, the majority of birth defects remain undetected until after birth.

In our society, it is an individual decision whether or not to utilize prenatal testing in a pregnancy. The provision of antenatal care must therefore ensure that parents are able to make informed decisions about testing and are supported throughout the testing process.

Types of prenatal test

Prenatal tests fall into two main categories:

- screening tests
- diagnostic tests.

These are discussed further below.

Screening tests

Prenatal screening tests:

- are aimed at all pregnant women
- assess whether an individual pregnancy is at increased or low risk of a particular birth defect
- generally pose no risk to maternal or fetal wellbeing
- are followed by an offer of a diagnostic test if an increased risk is identified
- are aimed primarily at the detection of structural anomalies and chromosomal abnormalities, in particular Down syndrome.

Screening tests in pregnancy are evolving rapidly, with the aim being earlier, more accurate and more accessible tests.

Screening tests available

Currently, screening tests are either performed on a serum sample from the mother, or utilizing ultrasound.

Maternal serum screening

• maternal serum screening (MSS) is primarily aimed at the detection of Down syndrome and, in some programmes, trisomy 18
• MSS involves measuring the levels of a number of different analytes produced by the fetus in a blood sample from the mother
• the analytes have been selected on the basis that large population studies have shown that the levels of the analytes in maternal serum differ significantly between pregnancies in which the fetus does or does not have Down syndrome
• MSS is most commonly offered in the second trimester (around 15–18 weeks) using various combinations of three or four analytes. These may include, estriol, alphafetoprotein (AFP), inhibin and the alpha and beta subunits of human chorionic gonadotrophin (hCG)
• a computer based algorithm, which takes into account the mother's age-related risk, the gestation of the pregnancy and the analyte levels, is used to calculate a risk figure for Down syndrome in that pregnancy
• if the risk figure is greater than a predetermined 'cutoff' risk, the risk is considered to be increased and a diagnostic test is offered to clarify the situation
• most programmes are designed so that 5% of women having the test will receive an increased risk result. The majority of these women will go on to have healthy babies
• if all these women chose to have a diagnostic test, the screening programme would be expected to detect about 60–70% of cases of Down syndrome
• if AFP is one of the analytes used in second trimester MSS, then the test can also be used to screen for open neural tube defects, as AFP will be elevated if neural tissue is exposed to the amniotic fluid. If it is elevated, then the diagnostic test is a tertiary level ultrasound to examine the fetal spine
• first-trimester maternal serum screening programmes are being developed using inhibin and pregnancy-associated protein A (PAPP-A) as analytes

Ultrasound

Ultrasound uses sonar waves to allow real-time, two-dimensional visualization of the fetus in utero. The fetus can be examined in different views and fetal movements can be studied. Improved technology and training allow excellent views to be obtained to allow detection of many specific structural anomalies. Most antenatal care programmes now offer an ultrasound between 18 and 20 weeks gestation to screen for fetal anomalies.

Ultrasound is usually considered a screening rather than a diagnostic test as:

• some structural anomalies may not be readily detected, e.g. cleft palate
• interpretation of a possible anomaly and its impact on fetal development may be limited
• the detection rate of anomalies is dependent on the skill of the operator, equipment and fetal views obtained.

Potential advances that may enhance the value of fetal imaging as a screening test in pregnancy include three-dimensional ultrasound and alternative imaging techniques such as fetal magnetic resonance imaging (MRI).

Nuchal translucency screening

During the last decade, a new form of ultrasound-based screening for Down syndrome in the first trimester has been developed, based on the MSS model. This depends on the assessment of the nuchal (posterior neck) region of the fetus:

• All fetuses have a collection of fluid in the nuchal region that can be visualized as a translucent area and can be measured by ultrasound at the end of the first trimester (11–13 weeks gestation)
• Large population studies have shown that on average this nuchal translucency measurement is increased in pregnancies in which the fetus has Down syndrome
• As with MSS, a computer algorithm that takes into account the mother's age-related risk, the gestation and the thickness of the nuchal translucency measurement is used to calculate a risk for that individual pregnancy
• If the risk is above a predetermined 'cutoff risk' a diagnostic test is offered
• The detection rate of a nuchal translucency screening programme is dependent on the skill of the operator; however, detection rates of up to 70–80% of cases of Down syndrome have been reported
• Other chromosome abnormalities, in particular Turner syndrome (45,XO) and triploidy are also often associated with an increased nuchal translucency measurement
• An increased nuchal translucency measurement in the presence of normal chromosomes may be an indicator of other types of fetal anomaly, such as cardiac malformations or skeletal dysplasias. Detailed ultrasound follow-up is then recommended.

Combined screening

In order to increase the detection rates of screening tests, combinations of the different tests are being explored. The most promising is the combination of a nuchal translucency measurement with the measurement of two first-trimester maternal serum analytes to give a combined first-trimester risk. This allows increased detection rates for Down syndrome of up to 90%, with a 5% false-positive rate, and is increasingly replacing second-trimester maternal serum screening as the screening test of first choice, with the added advantage of allowing an earlier diagnostic test to be offered. The best combination of screening tests is yet to be firmly established and a number of large multicentre trials are in progress to address this issue.

Diagnostic tests

Prenatal diagnostic tests:

- arc aimed at pregnant women who have been identified to be at increased risk of having a baby with a particular birth defect (see below)
- allow accurate clarification of whether an individual fetus is affected or not
- usually pose a small risk of fetal loss; this risk relates to the need to sample fetal tissue for testing
- are primarily aimed at the detection of chromosomal abnormalities, enzymatic and single gene defects.

New diagnostic tests continue to be developed, with the principal aim of increasing both the safety of the tests and range of conditions that may be tested for.

Practical points

Prenatal diagnosis
- Prenatal diagnosis is aimed at detection of birth defects prior to birth to allow options for parents
- There are two main categories, diagnostic and screening
- There is a move towards earlier, less invasive testing options such as preimplantation genetic diagnosis and combined screening tests
- The majority of birth defects remain undetected by current prenatal diagnostic methods
- Prenatal diagnosis for specific genetic conditions usually requires significant prepregnancy workup

---

Indications for diagnostic prenatal tests

Although all women are at risk of conceiving a baby with a birth defect, for an individual woman there are a number of risk factors that increase the risk above the background population risk. In general, diagnostic prenatal tests are offered to women whose risk of conceiving a baby with a specific birth defect is considered to be above an arbitrary level. This 'cutoff' level takes into account the

risk of fetal loss related to the test and economic issues relating to the number of women who would be offered testing.

Some of the reasons why a woman may be offered a prenatal diagnostic test include:

- advanced maternal age (see below)
- increased risk identified by a screening test, e.g. maternal serum screening
- a previous child with a birth defect for which a prenatal test is available and an increased risk of recurrence is recognized, e.g. chromosome abnormality, neural tube defect, single-gene disorder such as cystic fibrosis
- a parent or couple known to carry a genetic mutation for which testing is available and that poses a risk of abnormality in offspring, e.g. chromosome translocation or single-gene defects
- other factors known to increase the risk of birth defects, e.g. exposure to teratogens such as maternal infection.

Advanced maternal age

As maternal age increases, there is an increased risk of conception of a fetus with some specific chromosomal anomalies, primarily trisomies (an additional copy of a single chromosome). Most fetuses conceived with a trisomy miscarry. However, trisomy 21, 13 and 18 are potentially viable chromosomal anomalies leading to the potential birth of a baby with specific constellations of birth defects (Ch. 10.3). Maternal age is not associated with an increased risk of other birth defects.

Trisomy 21 (Down syndrome) is the most common chromosome abnormality seen at live birth in our population. Many screening and diagnostic prenatal tests are therefore aimed at detection of this condition. Population data exist that can be used to counsel women regarding their 'age-related' risk in order that they may make informed decisions about prenatal testing (Table 10.1.4).

Diagnostic tests available

Most diagnostic tests involve sampling of fetally derived tissue, which can then be directly analysed for abnormalities. The most common test performed is chromosomal analysis. However, tissue may also be used as a source of DNA for molecular genetic tests, for metabolic tests or more rarely to look for evidence of fetal infection or histological confirmation of abnormality of a specific tissue, e.g. the skin for the diagnosis of epidermolysis bullosa.

Amniocentesis and chorionic villus sampling (CVS) are the two principal diagnostic tests used. However, fetal blood samples, skin, liver or kidney

Table 10.1.4 Age-specific risks for a liveborn child with Down syndrome	
Maternal age (years)	Risk (1 in) at expected time of delivery
20	1441
25	1383
30	959
34	430
35	338
36	259
37	201
38	162
39	113
40	84
42	52
44	38
46	31

The risk of any chromosome abnormality is approximately double these risks.
Source: after Gardner & Sutherland 2004.

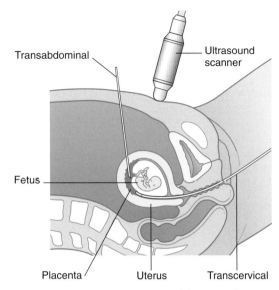

Fig. 10.1.1 Schematic representation of chorionic villus sampling showing transabdominal and transcervical routes. Courtesy of Ultrasound Department, Royal Women's Hospital, Melbourne.

biopsies may be required in very specific, rare circumstances. Amniocentesis, CVS and fetal blood sampling are performed as outpatient procedures under ultrasound guidance (Fig. 10.1.1). Each of these tests has advantages and disadvantages in certain situations (Table 10.1.5).

Imaging techniques

In some circumstances, ultrasound or other forms of fetal imaging such as MRI, or even plain X-rays, are considered diagnostic and may be the only tool available for diagnosis of genetic conditions that do not have a chromosomal, enzymatic or known molecular basis. Examples include neural tube defects, skeletal dysplasias and congenital heart defects. Imaging techniques, however, are dependent on gaining adequate views and appropriate interpretation of the views and are limited by the gestation at which some defects may be identifiable; for example, hydrocephalus may not become apparent in a fetus until the third trimester.

Future options

Hope for 'non-invasive' diagnostic testing previously rested on the concept of isolation of fetal cells found within the maternal circulation during pregnancy. More recently, recognition of 'free fetal DNA' within the maternal circulation during pregnancy, and the fact that fetal cells can be isolated from cervical swabs during pregnancy, has raised the potential for future options that would allow collection of fetal tissue for the purpose of testing without risk to fetal wellbeing. Current techniques do not yet allow this option to be used in a clinical setting; however, research continues and clinical trials are pending.

Prenatal diagnosis for specific genetic conditions

Rapid progress in knowledge of the underlying molecular genetic aetiology of specific conditions allows an increasing number of genetic conditions to be diagnosed prenatally by utilizing specific DNA-based technology. In order that this can occur for any individual couple known to have an increased risk of conceiving a child with such a disorder, a number of conditions must be satisfied:

- accurate diagnosis of the condition in the affected family member
- confirmation of the aetiology of the condition by identification of a mutation in the causative gene

Table 10.1.5 Prenatal diagnostic tests

	Chorionic villus sampling (CVS)	Amniocentesis	Fetal blood sampling or fetal biopsies
Tissue sampled	Chorionic villi derived from the same initial fertilized ovum as the fetus	Amniotic fluid containing fetal cells	Fetal blood, liver skin or skin
Indications for test	1. Increased risk of fetal chromosomal anomaly 2. Increased risk of specific genetic conditions for which a molecular or enzymatic test exists	1. As for CVS 2. Increased risk of fetal infection 3. Other less common indications, AFP measurements to assist in diagnosis of neural tube defects	1. Increased risk of fetal chromosome anomaly when rapid results are required 2. Diagnosis of fetal haemoglobinopathy 3. Diagnosis of fetal conditions by tissue histology (e.g. some skin disorders)
Gestation at which test is performed	Can be performed safely after 10 weeks gestation; most often done between 11 and 13 weeks gestation	Can be performed safely after 15 weeks, gestation; most often done at 16–18 weeks gestation	Can be performed after 18 weeks gestation
Risks	0.5–1% rate of miscarriage related to the test	0.5% rate of miscarriage related to the test	1–5% rate of miscarriage related to the test, depending on the indication for the test
Other issues	1% risk of a discrepant result between fetal and placental tissue (confined placental mosaicism), requiring amniocentesis to clarify	1% risk of failure of the amniocytes to culture, requiring a repeat test	Potentially difficult access
Timing of results	Rapid chromosome analysis by FISH 24–48 hours.* Final chromosome, DNA or enzyme test results 7–21 days	As for CVS	Dependent on test performed

* FISH (fluorescent in situ hybridization) involves the use of labelled DNA probes designed to bind to specific regions of individual chromosomes. This allows the number of a specific chromosome in an interphase cell to be ascertained within 24–48 hours.

or an enzymatic defect that can be tested for accurately in fetal tissue (a process that may take many months and may not be possible in some cases)
- appropriate pretest (preferably prepregnancy) counselling regarding the process of testing and implications and options relating to the potential results of testing
- appropriate support throughout the process.

Prenatal diagnosis in these circumstances is best provided by an experienced multidisciplinary team consisting of an obstetrician, a clinical geneticist, a genetic counsellor and experienced laboratory staff. Chorionic villus sampling is usually the preferred method for DNA-based and enzymatic prenatal tests, as it often allows direct testing rather

than a need for culturing of tissue prior to testing. Examples of conditions that DNA-based prenatal diagnosis may be available for include: Duchenne and Becker muscular dystrophy, fragile X syndrome, cystic fibrosis, haemoglobinopathies and metabolic defects such as maple syrup urine disease.

In some families, although the specific mutation causing the condition in the family has not been identified, linkage studies using polymorphic DNA markers close to or within the gene may be possible. This requires further testing of family members and has a margin of error related to the possibility of genetic recombination. For X-linked conditions in which the gene has not yet been identified or a mutation cannot be identified, identification of the gender of the fetus by chromosome analysis and termination of males (50% of whom would be unaffected) may be the only available option.

Preimplantation genetic diagnosis

Prenatal diagnosis in an already established pregnancy may not be an option for some couples, for ethical and moral reasons. Following advances during the last two decades in both reproductive and molecular genetic technology, the technique of pre-implantation genetic diagnosis (PGD) has become a potential alternative option.

The principle of this technique is the genetic analysis of an embryo produced by in vitro fertilization (IVF) technology, in order to select those embryos free of a specific genetic condition for transfer to the woman's uterus to establish a pregnancy.

A single cell can be removed for genetic analysis on day 3 postconception from an embryo cultured in vitro. Genetic analysis may consist of specific mutation detection or a limited analysis of chromosomes. The limited amount of material and the limited time frame available for analysis have provided the impetus for the development of specialized techniques to prevent misdiagnosis. Thousands of babies have now been born worldwide following PGD in a number of highly specialized centres. Continual improvements in genetic techniques and pregnancy rates following IVF will mean that PGD will continue to become a more common alternative to the well established methods of CVS and amniocentesis.

Teratogens

A teratogen is an environmental agent that can cause abnormalities of form or function in an exposed embryo or fetus. It is estimated that between 1% and 3% of birth defects may be related to teratogenic exposure.

A teratogen may cause its effect by a number of different pathophysiological mechanisms, including:

- cell death
- alteration of cell division and tissue growth, including cell migration
- interference with cellular differentiation.

Examples of the different ways in which teratogens may have their effects are seen with alcohol and sodium valproate, which are believed to cause dysmorphic facial features with underdevelopment of the mid-face and philtrum due to cell death in these areas, whereas syndactyly can result from failure of programmed death of cells between the digits.

Factors modifying the effects of a teratogen

In theory, to produce a malformation a teratogen must be present in a sufficient amount, at the appropriate time, in a genetically susceptible individual, where other conditions do not prevent the effects occurring. In other words, there are a number of factors that can modify the effects of a teratogen, including:

- timing of exposure
- dose to the fetus
- genetic susceptibility
- access of the drug to the fetus
- interaction between teratogens
- maternal folic acid supplementation.

Timing of exposure

The effect of an environmental agent may differ depending on the gestational age at which exposure occurs:

- exposure very early in embryogenesis, prior to organogenesis (<2 weeks after conception) is likely to cause embryonic death rather than malformations. This is seen as an 'all or nothing' effect
- during organogenesis (2–8 weeks after conception), malformations may occur if the exposure is not lethal
- each organ develops during a specific time period and will be susceptible to the malforming effects of teratogens only during that critical period
- during fetal development (after organogenesis) functional effects, such as mental retardation, are most likely, although malformations can still occur, e.g. in slowly forming organs such as the brain and kidney. Teratogens such as vasoactive drugs may also damage structures that have already formed.

An example of this effect is seen with thalidomide, which affects limb development only at the time when limb buds are developing, between 27 and 41 days, and causes ear abnormalities between 21 and 27 days. Another example is the effect of tetracycline, which only causes tooth discoloration with fetal exposure after about 16 weeks from conception. Angiotensin converting enzyme (ACE) inhibitors in the third trimester can affect fetal kidneys and may cause anuria.

Dose

The harmful effects of teratogens are dose-dependent. A dose threshold is reached where the rate of abnormalities rises. For example, there is no observed effect of X-rays at doses routinely used in diagnostic radiology, while doses associated with nuclear explosions cause microcephaly, mental retardation and growth failure.

Genetic susceptibility

There are marked differences in genetic susceptibility to environmental agents, both between species and between individuals of one species. It is likely that the susceptibility to the harmful effects of many teratogens depends on the genetically determined efficiency of both the mother's and fetus's detoxifying metabolic pathways. Thalidomide again forms an example of this, in that it is not teratogenic in a large number of species but is teratogenic in some rabbits and some primates, including humans. Phenytoin metabolism by a fetus with low epoxide hydrolase activity may put the fetus at risk of fetal phenytoin syndrome.

Access

In order to have an effect, a teratogen must gain access to the fetus. Some potentially harmful agents are not teratogens because their molecular size, means of transport or binding properties prevent or restrict them from crossing the placenta. Clinically this is seen with heparin and pancuronium.

Practical points

Teratogens
- Timing of exposure to teratogens is important: there may be an 'all or nothing effect'
- The 'dose' received by the fetus may be critical. All teratogens have a threshold dose, after which abnormalities increase
- Risk–benefit ratios need considering, e.g. maternal wellbeing versus teratogenic risk
- Genetic susceptibility may be important in exposure to some teratogens
- Access of the drug to the fetus should be considered: is it absorbed by the mother? Does it cross the placenta?
- Interaction between teratogens may increase risk: polypharmacy of antiepileptic drugs

---

Interaction between teratogens

The ingestion of multiple medications can have additive effects. An example is that the risk of fetal effects is greater if a mother with epilepsy is taking multiple anticonvulsants (polypharmacy) rather than a single one.

Some important teratogens

Selected teratogens that cause common clinical issues are discussed below; a more extensive list is provided in Table 10.1.6.

Rubella virus

Infection of the fetus by the rubella virus in the first trimester can cause devastating birth defects, including mental retardation, short stature, deafness, blindness and congenital heart defects.

- The risk is greatly reduced if the mother has been immunized prior to pregnancy.
- Many countries have implemented preventive public health programmes to immunize either adolescent girls or all children.
- Affected children can be born to previously immunized mothers, due to initial failure of seroconversion or waning immunity with age; therefore, immune status of women planning pregnancy should be reviewed.

Alcohol

The harmful effects of ethanol on the developing human are well documented:

- Teratogenic effects of alcohol are dose-related, ranging from clinically inapparent effects to the fetal alcohol syndrome of prenatal and postnatal growth failure, microcephaly, intellectual disability, a characteristic facial appearance, cleft palate, microphthalmia and heart defects.
- Heavy drinking throughout pregnancy is associated with a 10% risk of fetal alcohol syndrome and a 30% risk of observable fetal alcohol effects.
- No minimum safe dose has been defined.
- Consumption of a significant amount of alcohol prior to diagnosis of pregnancy is a frequent clinical scenario. It is difficult to estimate the risk of harm to the baby because of lack of good data.
- Women should be advised to avoid alcohol during pregnancy.

Antiepileptic medication

Women with epilepsy receiving treatment with anticonvulsant medication have a two- to threefold risk of giving birth to a child with a birth defect.

- most anticonvulsants have not been shown to be safe in pregnancy, and specific teratogenic effects have been defined for phenytoin, sodium valproate, carbamazepine and trimethadione, particularly for neural tube defects.
- the risk to the fetus increases if multiple anticonvulsants are needed to prevent seizures.

Table 10.1.6   Environmental agents that can adversely affect human development
Infectious agents *Viruses*: rubella, cytomegalovirus, varicella-zoster, Venezuelan equine encephalitis, herpes simplex, [parvovirus B19] *Bacteria*: syphilis, [*Listeria*] *Parasites*: toxoplasmosis
Physical agents Ionizing radiation, carbon monoxide, (heat)
Drugs and chemicals *Environmental chemicals*: organic mercury compounds, (polychlorinated biphenyls, i.e. PCBs) *Non-prescription drugs*: ethanol, cocaine, (amphetamines), [tobacco smoking, marijuana smoking] *Prescription drugs*: *Anticancer drugs*: aminopterin, busulfan, chlorambucil, cyclophosphamide, plicamycin, methotrexate, cytarabine, (dacarbazine, fluorouracil, procarbazine) *Anticonvulsants*: phenytoin, sodium valproate, carbamazepine, trimethadione, (primidone, phenobarbital, lamotrigine) *Hormones*: diethylstilbestrol, male sex hormones, strongly androgenic progestogens *Antibacterials*: tetracyclines, streptomycin, (gentamicin, quinolones, fluconazole (high doses 400–800 mg daily), trimethoprim) *Antivirals*: ribavirin, (ganciclovir. zalcitabine) *Anthelmintics*: (albendazole) *Antimalarials*: (chloroquine when used to treat malaria but not when used for prophylaxis) *Retinoids*: systemic isotretinoin, acetretin, (vitamin A, topical tretinoin and isotretinoin) *Immunomodifiers*: (methotrexate), [interferon beta-1b] *Miscellaneous*: thalidomide, misoprostol, penicillamine, warfarin, phenindione, lithium, intra-amniotic methylthioninium chloride {methylene blue}, (diazepam, antithyroid drugs, paroxetine, statins, mycophenolate, ACE inhibitors, angiotensin II receptor antagonists)
Maternal disorders Insulin-dependent diabetes mellitus, maternal phenylketonuria
The above list should be considered illustrative only and may change in the light of new knowledge. No brackets, teratogen; ( ), possible teratogen; [ ] not known to be teratogenic but may cause other effects, including embryonic/fetal death and/or growth retardation.

• it is likely that individual susceptibility exists, based on the activity of genetically determined detoxifying metabolic pathways for disposal of the drug and/or its metabolites.

• epileptic women must accept some additional risk of birth defects in their infants, but the risk can be minimized if epileptic control can be achieved with a single drug at the lowest possible dose.

• periconceptional folic acid supplementation at a dose of 5 mg daily should be recommended for women on anticonvulsant medication because of the increased risk of neural tube defects in their offspring.

Vitamin A analogues: isotretinoin and acetretin

These highly potent analogues of vitamin A are extremely teratogenic.

• their systemic use in early pregnancy is associated with a high (25–30%) risk of birth defects, including serious abnormalities of brain development, with microcephaly, hydrocephalus, cortical blindness and intellectual disability, cranial nerve palsies, dysmorphic facial features, microtia, cleft palate, heart defects, thymic hypoplasia and genitourinary abnormalities.

• there is no 'safe' period in early pregnancy from the teratogenic effects of these drugs.

• the teratogenic dose has not been determined.

• many countries have restricted the right to prescribe these drugs to particular groups of doctors and recommend that women should have a pregnancy test before commencing treatment and should use effective contraception for 1 month before treatment begins, throughout treatment and for a period after treatment stops.

• oral isotretinoin is used to treat severe cystic acne. Although it has a short elimination half-life for most women, it is recommended that pregnancy should be avoided for at least 1 month after the last dose.

• acetretin is used to treat psoriasis and other disorders of keratinization. It has a relatively short half-life, but is converted to etretinate during therapy. Etretinate is readily taken up into adipose tissue, is slowly released from it and has a long elimination

Clinical example

Kylie, a 25-year-old woman, had just found out that she was 4 weeks pregnant. She had an artificial heart valve and had taken warfarin for the past 6 months. She had been advised not to become pregnant and had used medroxyprogesterone depot for contraception. However, she had not recently renewed it because of side effects experienced after her first dose 4 months ago. Now condoms had failed. Kylie also had a urinary tract infection and treatment with trimethoprim was a being considered as one of the possible options. Her partner Adam had taken large doses of vitamins, including vitamin A, prior to conception and had read that vitamin A can be harmful in pregnancy. They sought advice about risks to their unborn baby.

First, reassurance was be given about the paternal exposure to vitamin A. Drugs and chemicals taken by men have not been proved to increase the incidence of abnormalities in their offspring. Vitamin A should not be confused with vitamin A analogues, which are potent teratogens when used by the mother.

It was important to treat the urinary tract infection; however, trimethoprim, being an antifolate antimicrobial, was not a suitable antibiotic and another antibiotic was used. Warfarin treatment during Kylie's pregnancy was of concern. At 4 weeks of pregnancy, Kylie's fetus was prior to the time of greatest fetal susceptibility, 6–9 weeks gestation (6–9/40). However, Kylie needed to be counselled that her medical condition required anticoagulation with warfarin, which crosses the placenta, and that there was approximately a 5% chance of fetal warfarin syndrome. Unfortunately, although heparin does not cross the placenta and is not teratogenic, it is inadequate prophylaxis for pregnant patients with artificial heart valves. In spite of negative product information, the medroxyprogesterone depot was not a cause for concern even if she had received the dose while in early pregnancy.

---

half-life of 120 days. It is, therefore, recommended that pregnancy be avoided for 2 years following the use of acetretin.

Warfarin

Warfarin is used in the treatment of thromboembolic disease and for individuals with artificial heart valves.

- warfarin crosses the placenta, is teratogenic and may cause haemorrhage in the fetus
- the teratogenic effects appear to result from inhibition of vitamin K and/or arylsulphatase E activity during skeletal development
- the fetal warfarin syndrome comprises nasal hypoplasia, short fingers with hypoplastic nails, low birth weight, stippling of epiphyses on X-ray and intellectual disability

- recent estimates indicate that the risk of fetal warfarin syndrome in the babies of women who require warfarin throughout pregnancy is low, around 5%
- the period of greatest embryonic susceptibility is between 4 and 7 weeks after conception, although it is recommended that the drug should be avoided throughout the first trimester, if possible
- it has been suggested that warfarin exposure limited to the second and third trimesters can cause brain and eye damage, presumably as a result of haemorrhage but, if so, the risk also appears low
- heparin is not a teratogen. It is used in the treatment of thromboembolic disease but does not cross the placenta
- use of heparin instead of warfarin may be appropriate when the indication is venous thrombosis but not when it is used for artificial heart valves. Low-dose heparin carries a significant risk of valve thrombosis, and high-dose heparin in the outpatient setting carries a risk of serious maternal and retroplacental haemorrhage.

Ionizing radiation

Very high doses of X-rays can affect the developing fetus, resulting in growth failure, microcephaly, intellectual disability and ocular defects.

- the sensitive period for these effects appears to be between 2 and 4–5 weeks after conception.
- the doses delivered to the appropriately shielded uterus by modern X-ray equipment in the course of standard diagnostic radiology are well below the level that is teratogenic.
- women who are inadvertently exposed to diagnostic X-rays in early pregnancy can usually be reassured, although they may find it hard to understand that, while public health policy strongly recommends avoidance of diagnostic X-rays in pregnancy, the absolute risk to the baby of an exposed woman is negligible.
- if an undiagnosed pregnancy is irradiated during radiotherapy, the dose must be calculated and the risk assessed.
- ionizing radiation is not only potentially teratogenic but also potentially mutagenic and carcinogenic. It is likely that even low-dose irradiation of the fetus, as with the child and adult, does have mutagenic and carcinogenic potential but the absolute size of the risk increase is very small.
- in general, if there is a good clinical reason for performing diagnostic radiology in pregnancy, it can be done, knowing that the risks to the fetus are very low.

Diethylstilbestrol

This drug (diethylstilboestrol USP), widely used in the 1950s and 1960s in the belief that it prevented miscarriage, is both a teratogen and a prenatal carcinogen.

• exposure, especially before 10 weeks gestation, can cause vaginal adenosis in girls and these areas of epithelium have an increased risk of progressing to vaginal adenocarcinoma years later.
• this knowledge highlights the fact that there can be a delay of many years before the effects of fetal exposure to environmental agents become apparent, and absence of birth defects in the earliest years of life is not sufficient evidence to declare a drug safe in pregnancy.
• exposed girls also appear to have an increased risk of cervical abnormalities and uterine malformations.
• exposed boys appear to have an increased risk of testicular abnormalities, infertility and, possibly, testicular malignancy.

Paternal exposures

To date, there has been no convincing evidence that preconception paternal exposures to environmental chemicals are teratogenic, although paternal drugs may affect fertility. For paternal exposure to be teratogenic, it would have to involve mutagenesis of paternal DNA. A mutagenic agent could affect any part of the genome, resulting in the spread of risk of mutation across a very large number of individual genes. While new dominant and X-linked mutations could potentially occur, one would not expect a consistent pattern of birth defects in the children of exposed men. At present, any teratogenic risk from paternal exposures should be considered negligible, although it is admitted that it would be very hard to see an effect against the significant background prevalence of birth defects in humans. It is theoretically possible that environmentally induced mutations could contribute to the known paternal-age-related risk of new dominant mutations, e.g. for achondroplasia.

Teratogen advisory services

Appropriate public concern about the possible effects of exposure to environmental agents in pregnancy, as a result of the thalidomide experience and a more general uneasiness about environmental agents and health, has resulted in the establishment of services to provide information to health professionals and women with concerns. Teratogen advisory services have access to online databases such as TERIS and OTIS, containing the most recent distillation of information about individual agents, have experience in assessing the significance of an exposure and counselling skills, and can usually be contacted by phone when the need arises.

Modern genetics

G. Suthers, N. Poplawski

Most of the content of this book describes the management of abnormalities of structure or function in children, that is, the ways that such abnormalities present in clinical practice, how to identify the underlying cause and how to correct or ameliorate the abnormality. These abnormalities may reflect a problem that is intrinsic to the child or due primarily to external factors. More usually an abnormality reflects a combination of both intrinsic and extrinsic factors.

The cells of the human body need a source of information to direct those activities that are primarily intrinsic in nature. Errors in this intrinsic information may result in abnormalities that occur independently of any external factor such as infection or trauma. For example, certain errors may cause congenital abnormalities despite the developing fetus being nurtured in a healthy uterine environment. On the other hand, the cells also need a source of information to regulate their responses to external factors. Variations in this information may account for one child developing a life-threatening infection while the same microorganism is tolerated by another child without apparent effect. Furthermore, both types of information must be passed from parent to child (during reproduction) and from cell to cell (during development) so that the next generation will benefit from the information that allowed the parents (or cells) to survive and reproduce successfully.

The study of this information is called genetics. There has been an explosion in the amount of information available about human genetics in the last few decades. Most medical practitioners are unable to keep abreast of all the advances in genetic knowledge pertinent to their field. A clinical geneticist, a medical specialist with an expert knowledge of this information, can assist a patient or medical colleague to obtain the genetic information that is relevant in a specific situation. However, genetic information underlies the development and responses of every individual and an understanding of human genetics is essential for every medical practitioner.

The pervasive and complex nature of human genetics cannot be encompassed in a single component of this textbook. This chapter will provide a brief overview of the principles of genetics as they pertain to paediatrics, but the reader is cautioned that there is much that is both important and fascinating that cannot be covered in the space available. It is strongly recommended that the reader utilize other resources, such as those listed in the Further Reading relevant to this section. Readers should also bear in mind that genetics is a rapidly developing field, and detailed information derived from any source may become outdated within a matter of months.

The nature of genetic information is reviewed briefly in the next part of this chapter. Although many technical terms are used, most of them will be familiar from courses in genetics or biochemistry (also refer to the glossary in Useful Links). Readers will need to be familiar with these terms to ensure that their genetic education keeps pace with the advances in genetic knowledge in the years ahead. The focus of the remainder of the chapter is genetic errors, or mutations.

The nature of genetic information

Genetic information is encoded in DNA, a double strand of simple molecules

Genetic information is encoded in the structure of a chemical within the nucleus of each cell. The chemical is deoxyribonucleic acid (*DNA*). A DNA molecule consists of a long chain made up of four simple molecules, *adenosine* (A), *thymidine* (T), *cytosine* (C) and *guanidine* (G); these molecules are collectively termed *nucleotides*. Each nucleotide is linked to its immediate neighbour by a sugar molecule, *deoxyribose*. The bonds between these molecules dictate a polarity or direction to the sequence of nucleotides such that information is coded in only one direction along the length of the DNA strand. The sequence of nucleotides along this chain provides a basic but robust code to record all the genetic information needed by the cell. The genetic information or instructions required to run a human cell are encoded by approximately 3 billion (3×10^9) nucleotides. The entire DNA sequence is called the human *genome*.

Each of the four nucleotides has chemical affinity for one of the other nucleotides, and will form non-covalent hydrogen bonds with that nucleotide. Adenosine consistently pairs with thymidine, and cytosine pairs with guanidine. As a result, the entire chain of 3 billion nucleotides has an adjacent and complementary strand of paired nucleotides. DNA can be viewed as a double-stranded chain in which one strand encodes the information and the second represents the complementary sequence (Fig. 10.2.1). The polarity of the nucleotide sequence on one DNA strand is the opposite of the polarity of its complementary sequence, that is, the two strands are anti-parallel. The attraction between the nucleotide pairs of A–T and C–G can be represented as rungs on a very long ladder. The entire ladder is twisted along its length and the end result is often referred to as a 'double helix' of DNA. This long double-stranded sequence of nucleotides is copied and passed on to the next cell during cell division, ensuring that the next cell benefits from the survival of its predecessor.

The process of accurately copying (or replicating) such a large number of nucleotides is somewhat simplified by the duplex structure of DNA. If the strands of DNA are separated, each nucleotide in each strand will attract an unattached complementary nucleotide. With assistance from a variety of enzymes, each strand of the original DNA molecule can act as a template for the production of its own complementary strand and two double-stranded DNA molecules will be formed from the original double helix.

A gene is a single item of genetic information encoded in the DNA sequence

A unit of genetic information is called a *gene*. A gene usually encodes a particular *protein*, or it may provide a regulatory function within the nucleus. Each gene

The double-stranded structure of DNA is represented as a series of squares and rectangles representing the four nucleotides. The molecular forces between A-T and C-G (shown as dashed lines) provide a template for accurate copying of the DNA strand.
This long thin strand is twisted lengthwise to form a double helix.

A triplet of nucleotides (or codon) represents the genetic code for a single aminoacid. A sequence of three codons is shown (with the corresponding aminoacids indicated below). A typical gene has a few hundred codons encoding a protein of the same number of aminoacids.

A gene consists of regions of codons (called exons; shown as grey boxes) separated by regions of non-coding DNA called introns (white boxes). An exon may consist of 100 or so codons. A gene is transcribed into RNA and the introns are spliced out to form messenger RNA (mRNA). The spliced mRNA then directs the formulation of the specified protein.

The DNA required to encode all the genes in the human genome is present as 23 fragments of varying length. The total length of these fragments is approximately 1 m.

Each DNA fragment is coiled into a short bundle called a chromosome. The chromosomes are numbered in decreasing order of size (except for the X and Y chromosomes). With the exception of sperm and ova, all cells have two copies of each chromosome. One chromosome of each size is inherited from each parent (as shown by the different shading). Each cell has a total of 23 pairs of chromosome (46 in all).

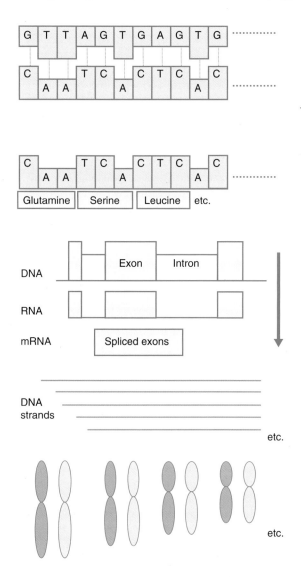

Fig. 10.2.1 The packaging of DNA.

consists of a sequence of between several hundreds and many thousands of nucleotides. There are specific DNA sequences that define the beginning and end of a gene. It has been estimated that there are approximately 30 000 genes encoded by the 3 billion paired nucleotides of human DNA. Overall, only 5% of the human genome consists of genes, and adjacent genes are often separated by long stretches of non-coding DNA. These regions of intergenic, non-coding DNA have a variety of structural, regulatory and evolutionary roles that are only slowly becoming evident.

By international convention, each human gene is known by a sequence of capital letters and numbers. The choice of characters is idiosyncratic and often reflects the history of the research that led to the isolation of the gene. Typical gene symbols include *HBA*, *F8C*, *FRAXA* and *COL2A1* (see GeneCards in Useful links). The convention is mentioned here because this nomenclature frequently appears in laboratory reports.

The DNA sequence of most genes is broken up into modules (*exons*), which are separated from each other by short regions of non-coding DNA (*introns*) (Fig. 10.2.1). Exons are usually a few hundred nucleotides long, while introns may be many thousands of nucleotides in length. Like the non-coding DNA lying between genes, introns have regulatory and evolutionary roles that are poorly understood. The order of exons along the DNA strand reflects the linear structure of the protein that will be encoded. With rare exceptions, the exon of one gene is not embedded between the exons of another gene, and an intron is flanked only by adjacent exons of one gene.

To access the information encoded in a gene, the enzyme *RNA polymerase* generates a short-lived single-stranded transcript of the gene made from the chemical ribonucleic acid (*RNA*). RNA is similar in structure to single-stranded DNA but has the great advantage that it is degraded rapidly within the cell. If a cell is to react quickly to its environment it must be able to regulate the level of RNA (and hence the synthesis of specific proteins) with speed and precision.

The RNA initially contains both exons and introns. The introns are carefully *spliced* out of the message by a family of molecules within the nucleus. Usually the spliced RNA strand of transcribed exons (called messenger RNA or *mRNA*) is then moved from the nucleus to ribosomes in the cytoplasm, which direct the synthesis of the protein encoded by the mRNA (and the gene). Importantly, some intronic RNA fragments are further processed to produce short sequences (called *small interfering RNAs*, or siRNA) that can bind to specific RNA or DNA sequences and regulate the transcription and splicing of one or more genes.

An amino acid is encoded by a triplet of DNA nucleotides

Proteins are made of many amino acids joined end to end in a long chain. This chain of amino acids then folds to form a specific three-dimensional shape that is the essential feature of each protein. Each amino acid of the protein is encoded in DNA as a triplet of nucleotides (or *codon*). For example, the codon ATG encodes the amino acid methionine and the codon CGC encodes the amino acid arginine. During protein synthesis, each successive codon of the mRNA directs the addition of the appropriate new amino acid to the growing sequence of amino acids. There are also specific *stop codons* (such as TAG) that indicate the end of a gene.

There is no gap or boundary between adjacent codons. For example, the DNA sequence . . . AATC-GCTATGGC . . . could be interpreted as . . . –AAT–CGC–TAT–GGC– . . . or . . . A–ATC–GCT–ATG–GC . . . or . . . AA–TCG–CTA–TGG–C . . . and each codon sequence would encode a different sequence of amino acids. In practice, the sequence of codons in a DNA sequence (or *reading frame*) is simply determined by the point from which the first codon is 'read', and this starting position is dictated by the specific sequence that identifies the start of a gene.

A gene is regulated by DNA sequences that lie adjacent to the gene

The amount of protein synthesized from a gene is regulated by molecules that interact with DNA sequences lying to one side or other of the gene. Regulatory regions may also be chemically altered by the addition of methyl groups ($-CH_3$) to nucleotides of the sequence. These methyl groups interfere with the binding of regulatory molecules and the net effect is inactivation of the gene. The methyl groups may also be removed and so provide a means for varying gene activity. A gene may be inactivated by this process of *methylation* in normal cells in a specific tissue or at certain times during development.

The activation or silencing of a gene is usually independent of whether the gene was paternally or maternally inherited. However, certain genes are selectively inactivated (by methylation) when transmitted by sperm and selectively activated (by removal of methylation) when transmitted by an ovum; other genes demonstrate the reciprocal pattern of (in)activation. This is a normal process that persists for the life of the individual and results in there being just one active copy of the gene in the cell. The selective inactivation of specific genes by methylation according to the parental gender is called *imprinting*.

Chromosomes are tightly coiled lengths of DNA

A DNA double helix of 3 billion nucleotides is approximately 1 nanometre (10^{-9} m) wide and 1 m long. This represents an enormous length of DNA within the tiny volume of a cell's nucleus (10^{-5} m in diameter). The metre of DNA is packaged into 23 fragments of varying length. During cell division each of these fragments is tightly coiled into a short bundle (or *chromosome*), which is visible down the light microscope. The division of the genetic code into these fragments is very consistent between individuals. As a result a gene that is located at a specific point on a chromosome will be found at the same location on the equivalent chromosome in any other individual.

Evolutionary processes have dictated that virtually all human cells have two copies of the entire genetic code, with one copy being inherited from each parent. Thus the nucleus of each cell contains two copies of the metre-long DNA sequence, and this DNA is packaged into a total of 23 pairs of chromosomes.

The only cells that have less DNA are sperm and ova. These cells contain just a single copy of the genetic code, that is, 1 m of DNA packaged as 23 chromosomes. The fertilization of an ovum by a sperm cell restores the amount of DNA to the usual 2 m (46 chromosomes).

The chromosome pairs can be ranked according to length, and 22 of the pairs are identified by their relative size (i.e. each copy of chromosome 1 is slightly longer than each copy of chromosome 2, which is longer than chromosome 3, etc.). These 22 pairs of chromosomes are collectively called *autosomes*.

Men and women have different types of sex chromosome

Two of the chromosomes are referred to as *sex chromosomes* and they are the important exception to the concept of pairs of chromosomes within the cell. In women the sex chromosomes consist of two equivalent chromosomes that are relatively long (similar in size to chromosome 6); for historical reasons these two chromosomes are referred to as *X chromosomes*. In men the sex chromosomes consist of one X chromosome and a very small *Y chromosome*. The Y chromosome is the smallest of all the human chromosomes. It encodes a few genetic instructions that trigger a cascade of other processes, which result in the developing embryo becoming male.

All human embryos inherit an X chromosome from their mothers; the inheritance of an X or Y chromosome from the father determines whether the embryo will develop as a female (XX) or as a male (XY). Sex is one of the few elements of human variation that is visible at the chromosomal level; almost all the genetic variation in the population occurs at the level of individual genes and cannot be identified by examining the chromosomes.

Women compensate for the presence of two X chromosomes by inactivating one X chromosome

The difference in the number of X chromosomes between men and women represents a profound difference in the amount of genetic information in the cell. A woman has two copies of the thousands of genes located on the X chromosome, but the fact that men survive as well as they do indicates that a single copy is sufficient. Although this genetic information is duplicated in half the human race, it is made functionally equivalent in both sexes by an intriguing process in women. At the time of conception both X chromosomes in a female conceptus are active, but at a very early stage (after just a few cell divisions) one of the X chromosomes is rendered inactive in each cell by extensive methylation. Hence men and women have only one active X chromosome in each cell. This process was first described by Mary Lyon and is called *lyonization*. The choice of X chromosome is usually random and the same X chromosome remains inactive in all the cells derived from that ancestral cell. On average, one of the two X chromosomes will be active in half of the cells of a woman's body. But the proportion in different women can vary markedly because X inactivation is initiated when the conceptus consists of a small number of cells. By chance alone, approximately 10% of women have skewed X inactivation such that one of the two X chromosomes is active in 90% of cells.

Each mitochondrion contains its own DNA strand

Mitochondria are small organelles within the cell that have an essential role in many metabolic processes including the beta-oxidation of fat, urea detoxification and calcium homeostasis. Mitochondria are also responsible for oxidative phosphorylation, the metabolic process that generates ATP via aerobic metabolism.

Mitochondria contain more than 1000 different proteins, including a complex array of over 60 proteins directly involved in oxidative phosphorylation. As one might expect, most mitochondrial proteins are encoded by genes located on chromosomes within the nucleus of the cell. However, each mitochondrion also has its own DNA strand that encodes 13 proteins involved in oxidative phosphorylation, as well as 22 transfer RNAs and two ribosomal RNAs. The *mitochondrial DNA* (*mtDNA*) is a double-stranded loop that is 16 569 nucleotides long and is joined end to end in a circle. Each mitochondrion has five to 10 copies of this mtDNA loop and, depending on the type of tissue, a single somatic cell contains up to 1000 mitochondria. The number of mitochondria within a single cell varies with tissue type. In general, tissues that are highly dependent on oxidative phosphorylation for normal function (e.g. neurones) have more mitochondria per cell than tissues that are less dependent (e.g. some epithelial cells).

Mitochondria (and their DNA) are copied independently of the process of copying DNA within the cell's nucleus. The number of mitochondria within a cell can vary without the need for cell division. When a cell does divide into two, approximately half of the mitochondria present are distributed to each new cell.

The mitochondria in all the cells of a person are *maternally* inherited, i.e. all the mitochondria are derived from the original ovum. A sperm has mitochondria that provide energy to the cilium that propels it, but these mitochondria usually do not enter the ovum at fertilization. The exclusive maternal inheritance of the mitochondrial DNA is in marked contrast to the inheritance of the DNA in the cell's nucleus, which is inherited from both parents.

Genes and networks

A single gene does not produce its effect independent of the action of other genes. All processes within a single cell are regulated by an interacting network of many genes. For example, a network of several hundred different genes is involved in intracellular galactose metabolism. This leads to a degree of biological robustness because a mutation in a single gene will not necessarily result in cellular dysfunction if the remainder of the genetic network is able to compensate for the abnormal gene.

This network of genes is embedded within a network of interacting cells within a single tissue or organ, which is embedded in a network of interacting tissues and organs within single individual. Individuals, in turn, are embedded in social and environmental networks. The interplay and variation within and between these genetic, cellular, biological, social, and environmental networks helps explain why the clinical features of a specific disorder can vary from one individual to another.

Clinical example

Genes function within genetic, cellular, biological, social, and environmental networks (see text).

Cystic fibrosis (CF) is a common autosomal recessive disorder that affects approximately 1 in 2000 Caucasian children. Approximately 1 in 20 healthy Caucasian adults are carriers of a mutation that can cause CF and over 1000 different mutations have been identified in the CF gene. One mutation accounts for ≈80% of all mutations; the other mutations are much less common.

The classical form of CF has three major features; chronic respiratory infections leading to bronchiectasis, malabsorption of fat due to exocrine pancreatic dysfunction, and elevated sweat sodium and chloride concentrations. Children with classical CF die during infancy unless they receive intensive therapy. At least 50% of these children will still be alive in their mid 40s, and this outlook will probably improve in the future.

Despite having the same CF gene mutations, the survival of individuals (including siblings) affected by CF can vary by years or even decades. Mutations in the CF gene are also well documented in individuals with non-classical forms of CF including typical CF-respiratory disease without pancreatic dysfunction, mild respiratory disease with recurrent pancreatitis, and (in men) infertility due to congenital bilateral absence of the vas deferens without other clinical features of CF.

Networks help explain the clinical heterogeneity seen in individuals with *CF* gene mutations:

- The different mutations that can occur in the *CF* gene have different effects on the function of the protein. In general, mutations that severely disturb the function of the CF protein are associated with more severe disease.
- Variations in other genes that determine a child's susceptibility to respiratory infection, such as genes encoding proteins in the immune system, could modulate the severity of the respiratory infections in a child with cystic fibrosis
- Social factors such as access to health care and the degree of support by family and friends are associated with longer survival
- Environmental factors such as aerobic fitness, nutritional status, smoking and the colonization of the respiratory tree by certain bacteria can all have an impact on disease severity and survival.

Detailed information about the human genome is accumulating very rapidly

Within the last few years, the entire DNA sequence of the human genome was defined as part of the *Human Genome Project*. With the availability of this DNA sequence, the genes responsible for an increasing number of diseases have been identified. But our understanding of the ways in which this genetic information is regulated and integrated within a cell (or an individual) is still rudimentary. The study of how an entire genome functions in health and disease has been described as 'genomics', distinguishing this endeavour from the study of individual genes and diseases.

Defining the sequence of the human genome was only one of the goals of the Human Genome Project. The project encompasses many issues, including the genetic variation within and between ethnic groups, the ethical use of genetic knowledge, the development of new computational methods for analysing the sequences and interactions of billions of nucleotides, and the development of new genetic therapies. There are many technical and general resources dealing with the Human Genome Project available on the internet.

What causes mutations?

DNA replication consists of accurately copying the 6 billion nucleotides that are spread along the 2 m of DNA within the few microns of space within the nucleus of a cell. The resulting 4 m of DNA must be carefully separated into two equivalent portions and normal cellular functions must be maintained all the while. The process of copying DNA and dividing into two equivalent cells is called *mitosis.*

The penalty for failing to copy DNA accurately is the generation of new genetic errors (or *mutations*), which are transmitted to all of the cell's progeny. The enzyme *DNA polymerase* is very good at copying DNA accurately, having an error rate of only one wrong nucleotide pair per million processed. This is impressive, but it would amount to thousands of new mutations at every cell division. There is an additional proofreading mechanism that compares the original with the copied strand and corrects any mismatched nucleotides on the new strand. This mechanism reduces the overall mutation rate to approximately one wrong nucleotide per billion processed. As a consequence, the division of any cell results in approximately six new mutations in the DNA sequence.

The accumulation of these new mutations is relentless. Each person consists of billions of cells, each of which is derived from the original fertilized egg. Every mutation that was generated during any cell division will be present in the descendants of that cell. By the time we reach adulthood, every cell in the body has accumulated hundreds of new mutations that were not present at the moment of conception.

Despite the frequency of mutations, most of them have no adverse effect on the information encoded in the DNA. Genes account for only 5% of the human genome, and the majority of mutations occur in non-coding DNA and do not affect genes or the proteins they encode. These mutations are usually referred to as *polymorphisms* (meaning 'many forms') because they do not reduce an individual's ability to survive. Polymorphisms are very common. On average the sequences of non-coding DNA in two individuals differ by one nucleotide pair in every 300. These polymorphisms have played a central role in identifying and analysing genes because they can act as landmarks along the DNA within a cell.

Mutations in genes are much less common than polymorphisms. They may interfere with the function of a gene, compromise the cell's function, and so cause a disorder. Subtle variation in certain DNA sequences (and hence in the functions of certain genes) is also the basis for much of the variation in human structure that makes us individually different.

The different versions of a specific gene that are present in a population are referred to as *alleles*. This term includes mutations which cause disease as well as polymorphisms. Some genes have only one allele. The role of such a gene is so critically dependent on the specific DNA sequence that any change results in the death of the cell and loss of the mutant gene. Other genes demonstrate many alleles. For example, the *MC1R* gene has a role in the regulation of melanocytes. It has nine alleles which are present in the normal Caucasian population; some of these alleles are usually found in healthy people with red hair or fair skin, while others are usually noted in healthy dark-haired people.

What types of mutation cause disease?

It is convenient to divide mutations into groups according to the scale of the mutation (a portion of DNA sequence versus entire chromosomes) and the type of mutation (affecting primarily the structure versus the function of the gene). This distinction is artificial, but it provides a basis for classifying various mutations (as summarized in Table 10.2.1).

Structural mutations of genes

The simplest mutation is the loss (or *deletion*) of all or part of a gene's DNA sequence. A deletion could involve as little as one or two nucleotides. Such a deletion would alter the sequence of codons (or reading frame) of the gene, which would result in disruption of the information encoded by the gene.

A deletion of three nucleotides could involve the loss of a single codon and the consequent absence of a single amino acid from the mature protein. The

Table 10.2.1 Types of mutations that occur during DNA replication

Scale and type of error	Mutation	Description	Examples of diseases due to these mutations*
Structural errors	Deletion of genes	Loss of all or part of a gene, resulting in little or no protein product	Duchenne muscular dystrophy
	Duplication	Duplication of all (or part) of a gene resulting in excess (or deficiency) of the protein product	Charcot–Marie–Tooth disease
	Nonsense/ truncation	Mutation involving one or more nucleotides that prevents the cell from generating a complete RNA strand	Hurler syndrome
	Missense	Mutation involving one codon that causes a critical alteration in the protein sequence	Achondroplasia
	Splicing error	Mutation involving the nucleotides which identify the junction between exons and introns resulting in generation of an abnormal RNA strand	Crouzon syndrome
Functional errors of genes	Regulatory mutation	Mutation in the regulatory region of a gene causing inappropriate activation or silencing of gene	Thalassaemia
	Abnormal imprint	Reversal of the normal silencing or activation of specific genes in the maternal or paternal germline	Beckwith–Wiedemann syndrome
	Unstable triplet repeat	Increase in the number of copies of a repeated triplet of nucleotides causing impairment of function of gene or protein	Fragile X syndrome
Structural errors of chromosomes	Monosomy (deletion)	Loss of whole (or part) of a chromosome	Turner syndrome
	Trisomy (duplication)	Excess of the whole (or part) of a chromosome	Down syndrome
	Triploidy	Presence of an extra copy of each chromosome	Miscarriage
Functional errors of chromosomes	Uniparental disomy	Both copies of all or part of a chromosome inherited from just one parent	Prader–Willi syndrome

* Note that different patients with the same genetic disorder may have different types of mutation in the same gene.

impact of such a mutation would depend on the role of the specific amino acid. For example, the most common mutation in the familial disorder cystic fibrosis is the loss of the three nucleotides that encode the 508th amino acid, phenylalanine. The absence of this one amino acid renders the protein inactive.

Another type of mutation is *duplication* of the DNA sequence. A small duplication of one or two nucleotides will disrupt the reading frame of the gene and, as with a small deletion, will render the gene inactive. Larger duplications may also disrupt the reading frame.

Very large deletions or duplications may encompass one or more genes. The presence of one or three active copies of a gene (instead of the normal two copies) may be sufficient to cause a disorder.

A change in the DNA sequence may not alter the overall length of the sequence but may introduce a new stop codon. For example, an alteration in just one nucleotide would change the codon TAC (which encodes the amino acid tyrosine) to TAG (which is one of the stop codons). The presence of a premature stop codon results in a shortened (or *truncated*) protein. This type of mutation is called a *nonsense* mutation.

A small change in DNA sequence also may alter the amino acid encoded by the codon. For example, achondroplasia is a common familial bone dysplasia that causes short stature; the underlying mutation is a change in DNA sequence from GGG to AGG. The effect of this mutation is that the 380th amino acid in the protein is arginine rather than glycine. The total length of the protein is normal but the altered amino acid sequence at this point causes a major change in the function of the encoded protein and hence in bone formation. This type of mutation is called a *missense* mutation.

The transition of genetic information from numerous exons to a single, spliced mRNA molecule represents a major change in the structure of this genetic information. A *splicing mutation* is an abnormality in the DNA sequence of an intron that indicates its boundary with an adjacent exon. A splicing mutation will cause the splicing process to fail, with the result that an intron may be left inappropriately in the mRNA or an exon may be spliced out inappropriately. In either case the end result is a structurally abnormal mRNA molecule and the synthesis of an abnormal protein.

Functional mutations of genes

The activity of a gene is controlled by proteins that bind to regulatory regions of DNA close to the gene. A mutation in a regulatory sequence may interfere with the binding of regulatory molecules and so may interfere with the normal control of gene activity. A *regulatory mutation* can lie thousands of nucleotides away from the nearest exon of the gene that is affected, and the DNA sequence of all the exons and introns of the gene would be normal.

Most genetic variants occurring within the introns are polymorphisms and are of no clinical significance. However, as noted above, mutations at the extreme boundaries of an intron can result in a splicing mutation. Mutations within an intron that corrupt the sequence of small interfering RNAs (siRNAs) may interfere with the regulation of expression of one or more genes.

Imprinting involves the selective methylation (and hence inactivation) of a regulatory region according to the gender of the parent. A failure of the imprinting process will cause problems. For example, the maternal copy of the *IGF2* gene is normally imprinted, leaving the paternal copy as the only active copy in the cell. Failure to imprint the maternal *IGF2* gene results in there being two active copies of the gene, producing excess growth in the developing baby (Beckwith–Wiedemann syndrome). The specific cause of abnormal methylation and *imprinting mutations* is not known.

Triplet repeat mutations are a special class of mutation that have features of both structural and functional mutations, as well as having unique characteristics of their own. Throughout the genome there are many locations at which pairs or triplets of nucleotides are present as multiple adjacent copies. Most of these nucleotide repeats occur in non-coding

DNA and are of no clinical consequence. However, some occur within genes (in exons or introns) or within nearby regulatory regions. A number of genes contain the DNA sequence CAG–CAG–CAG repeated many times within an exon. The codon CAG encodes the amino acid glutamine and the proteins synthesized from these genes contain regions of polyglutamine. Other genes have the sequence CCG repeated many times in the regulatory region of the gene.

The number of CAG repeats may vary widely (approximately five to 40 copies) in the normal population. An abnormal expansion outside this range in an exon will result in an increased length of polyglutamine in the protein and usually interferes with protein function or degradation. An increase in the number of repeats in a regulatory region may inactivate the gene. Larger degrees of expansion tend to be associated with more severe disruption of normal function of the gene or protein.

One of the most striking features of these expanded triplet repeat mutations is that they tend to increase in size during cell division. The increase may occur during ovum or sperm formation such that an expanded mutation is passed from parent to child, or it may occur during normal cell division during development (mitosis). The effect of this increase in size over time is that a genetic disorder due to a triplet repeat mutation may become more severe when passed from parent to child, or during the lifetime of the individual.

Structural mutations of chromosomes

With the exception of the sex chromosomes, chromosomes are normally present in the nucleus as pairs. The presence of two copies of a chromosome in a normal cell is called *disomy*. A deletion involving all or part of one chromosome is equivalent to the loss of hundreds or thousands of genes and is called *monosomy*. Conversely, the duplication of part or all of a chromosome results in the cell having three copies of many genes (*trisomy*). The commonest cause of moderate intellectual disability in children is Down syndrome; this condition is due to the presence of an extra copy of chromosome 21 (trisomy 21).

Monosomy and trisomy interfere with a multitude of cellular functions. The majority of developing embryos that have monosomy or trisomy will have such severe abnormalities that the pregnancy will miscarry. The surviving children with monosomy or trisomy always have major developmental problems but they represent the relatively mild end of the spectrum. Approximately 1 in 200 babies is born with a chromosome abnormality, and structural chromosome abnormalities are a major cause of morbidity and mortality in childhood.

It is important to note that these concerns do not necessarily apply to abnormalities in the number of sex chromosomes within the cell. The observation that normal men and women have different numbers of X and Y chromosomes highlights the fact that alterations in the number of sex chromosomes are of less significance than monosomy or trisomy involving autosomes. The Y chromosome is very small and boys with an extra Y chromosome usually demonstrate normal growth and development. The X chromosome is much larger. Children with abnormalities in the number of X chromosomes may have abnormalities of pubertal development and growth but their intellectual development is frequently normal.

An extreme form of trisomy frequently occurs in early pregnancy. The cells of a developing embryo may contain an extra copy of each chromosome, that is, 23 chromosome triplets, or 69 chromosomes in all. This condition is called *triploidy*. It is compatible with survival during the first (and even second) trimester of pregnancy but inevitably results in a miscarriage.

Functional mutations of chromosomes

Occasionally a child will inherit two copies of a particular chromosome from one parent and none from the other, rather than having one copy from each parent. This is called *uniparental disomy* (the normal situation of a chromosome being inherited from each parent could be described as 'biparental disomy'). Despite the total number of chromosomes being normal in this situation, a child may have a genetic disorder if the uniparental disomy involves a chromosome with imprinted genes (genes that are inactivated by methylation when inherited from a male parent but remain active when inherited from a female parent – or vice versa).

If any genes on a chromosome are usually imprinted, uniparental disomy for that chromosome results in there being either zero or two copies of the active gene instead of the normal single active copy. If both copies of the gene are inherited from the parent of the gender associated with imprinting (inactivation by methylation) uniparental disomy of that imprinted gene results in zero active copies of the gene. In contrast, if both copies of the gene are inherited from the parent of the gender not associated with imprinting there are two active copies of the gene. This alteration in the number of active copies of the gene may result in congenital abnormalities. For example, the Prader–Willi syndrome is a cause of intellectual disability and obesity in chil-

dren. It is due to an abnormality involving a gene on chromosome 15. In normal children the maternal copy of the Prader–Willi gene is imprinted; only the paternal copy is active. Some children with this condition have inherited two copies of chromosome 15 from their mothers. The total number of chromosomes and genes is normal but they have no active (paternal) copy of this essential gene.

When do mutations occur?

Conception is the time when the genetic code is most vulnerable

The significance of any mutation depends on when it occurs during development. The moment of conception could be regarded as the time when the genetic code is at its most vulnerable. Any mutation present at that time will be replicated in all the cells of the body. The significance of each mutation will be tested again and again in billions of cells in various stages of growth and differentiation.

Many of the mutations present at conception are new mutations that occurred during the formation of the individual ovum or sperm (or *germ cell*). The process of DNA replication during germ cell formation (*meiosis*) is even more challenging than that confronting a cell undergoing normal cell division. A germ cell contains just one copy of each chromosome rather than the pair of chromosomes present in other cells. To create such a cell the germ cell's precursor first duplicates the initial 23 chromosome pairs and then parcels the resulting 92 chromosomes into four equivalent sets of 23 each.

The error rate during meiosis is higher than during mitosis. Approximately 10% of sperm and over 20% of ova have new chromosome errors, and many more are presumed to have errors in the DNA sequence. The frequency of new mutations in germ cells accounts for much of the high failure rate of human conception. It is estimated that three-quarters of all human conceptions fail to survive longer than the first 6 weeks of a pregnancy; the majority of these miscarriages occur before a woman is aware that she is pregnant. Furthermore, many birth defects are due to new mutations that had occurred during the formation of the egg or sperm from which the baby developed.

If a mutation is present at conception, the gonads of the developing baby will also consist of cells with this mutation. This mutation can then be passed on to the child's progeny. In this way a *sporadic mutation* that occurred during the formation of a germ cell in one generation can be transmitted to the next generation and can become a *familial mutation*.

Mutations occurring during embryogenesis are limited to specific lineages of cells

Embryogenesis encompasses the first 12 weeks of a pregnancy. It is the period when the organs of the body are formed. A new mutation that occurs during embryogenesis may affect the structure, function or even survival of tissues in that cell lineage; the other cells of the body that lack this mutation will function normally. A mixture within the body of normal cells and cells with a defined mutation is called *somatic mosaicism*; the term 'somatic' refers to the cells of the body other than germ cells. The clinical hallmark of somatic mosaicism is a focal birth defect or (in the skin) a birthmark.

If a mosaic mutation is not present in the gonads it will not be transmitted to the next generation and hence will not be familial. However, if a new mutation occurs in a cell that contributes to the formation of an ovary or testis the mature gonad will contain a mixture of germ cell precursors that either have or lack the mutation; this situation is called *gonadal mosaicism*. This can result in a healthy person having a number of children with the same 'new' mutation. For example, the condition osteogenesis imperfecta type II is a severe bone dysplasia that is fatal in the newborn period. Each affected baby has a new mutation that occurred in one of the germ cells from which the baby developed. Although each affected baby has a new mutation, the parents are at a 5% risk of having a second affected child. These familial cases are due to one parent having a mixture of mutant and normal germ cells in their testes or ovaries, i.e. gonadal mosaicism. The mutant germ cells had been derived from a single mutant precursor cell in the parent.

It is important to recognize that the focal effects of a mosaic mutation can be mimicked by a non-mosaic phenomenon. As noted above, all women inactivate one X chromosome in each cell of the body (lyonization). In healthy females there is little to distinguish cells that have inactivated different X chromosomes. However, a mutation on one X chromosome can result in patchy birth defects. If a girl is conceived with a mutation in an essential gene located on one X chromosome, the mutation will interfere with the development of cells in which the mutant X chromosome is left active; cells that *in*activate the mutant X chromosome will function normally. This patchwork of functionally normal and abnormal cells is not due to a mutation which has occurred during embryogenesis but reflects the patchy inactivation of an abnormal gene that is present in every cell of the girl's body. The cells in the girl's ovaries will also have the mutation and the mutation may be transmitted to her children.

Mutations occurring after embryogenesis cause many of the features of ageing

After embryogenesis is completed, the impact of new mutations becomes less apparent. A new mutation cannot wind back the developmental clock and cause a malformation in a previously normal organ or tissue. However, new mutations continue to be generated, and these are transmitted to all the progeny of a cell. These mutations accumulate within a cell's genetic code and eventually interfere with cellular function. If the cellular dysfunction results in cell death, the loss of an individual cell will probably go unnoticed. If a cell accumulates mutations in a number of growth-limiting genes, the consequence will be failure to regulate cell division. Unregulated cell division arising from one cell is clinically evident as cancer.

The progressive accumulation of mutations in the nuclear DNA is compounded by a similar process occurring in mitochondrial genes. The rate at which mutations accumulate in mitochondrial DNA is 10–20 times faster than the rate in nuclear genes. This is due to the relatively high exposure of mitochondrial DNA to oxygen radicals (a byproduct of ATP synthesis) and the lack of protective proteins and effective DNA repair mechanisms in mitochondria. The mitochondrial mutation rate is increased even further by hypoxia, which may be a consequence of coronary or cerebral vascular disease. Mitochondrial DNA is replicated independently of nuclear DNA and, as a result, mitochondrial mutations accumulate in cells (such as neurones) that are not actively dividing.

We are usually unaware of our accumulating mutation load but at some point the mutations must inevitably cause problems. The mitochondrial mutations may be so widespread that energy production in many cells is compromised and causes problems such as cardiac failure or dementia, or accumulated mutations in nuclear genes may cause a cell to become malignant.

How are mutations inherited?

The fact that an individual's genetic code is not static but is accumulating mutations constantly from the moment of conception has been highlighted above. Mutations that are present only in cells outside the gonads are not familial. These mutations may account for the development of clinical problems in an individual, but they will not result in a familial disorder. On the other hand, mutations that are present in the cells of the gonads may be transmitted to a fertilized egg in the next generation. A mutation that is present at conception will subsequently be present in the ovaries or testes of the developing child. If these children then survive to have children of their own, the mutation may be transmitted again to the next generation.

An autosomal recessive disorder is due to mutations in both copies of a gene

With the exception of sperm and ova, the cells of the body have two copies of the genes present on the autosomes (i.e. on chromosomes other than the sex chromosomes). If a mutation interferes with the function of one copy of a gene, the presence of the other normal copy of the gene may be sufficient to prevent the development of a medical problem. This type of mutation could be inherited by many family members who remain healthy and are unaware that they are carrying the mutation. It is called an *autosomal recessive* mutation. We all have at least two or three different genes with recessive mutations affecting just one copy. A person who has a recessive mutation in a particular gene is called a *carrier* of that mutation.

It is much more serious if a person has recessive mutations in both copies of a particular gene. This situation could arise if both parents are carriers of mutations in the gene and the child has inherited the mutant gene from each parent (Fig. 10.2.2). In the absence of a normal copy of the gene the child will develop an autosomal recessive disorder related to the absence of the specific protein encoded by that gene. Autosomal recessive disorders affect both males and females.

The hallmark of autosomal recessive inheritance is the presence of affected siblings, with other members of the extended family being unaffected. Some of the unaffected family members will, of course, be carriers, but if their partner is not a carrier of the same disorder they will not have affected children and their carrier status will not be revealed.

Thousands of autosomal recessive disorders have been identified. The frequency of an autosomal recessive disorder will be determined by the frequency of carriers in the population. The carrier frequencies for many autosomal recessive conditions vary in different ethnic groups and may be quite high. For example, the carrier frequency for mutations causing cystic fibrosis (among Caucasians) and beta-thalassaemia (in some Mediterranean populations) is approximately 5–10%. As a consequence, these disorders are relatively common in those populations. However, the carrier frequency of most autosomal recessive disorders is approximately 1%, and the chance of both parents being carriers for the same disorder is very small. Consanguinity repre-

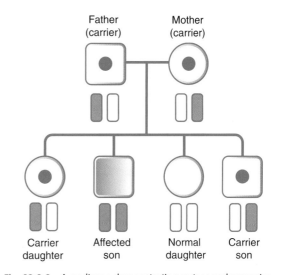

Fig. 10.2.2 A pedigree demonstrating autosomal recessive inheritance. Both parents are carriers of mutations in a particular gene and hence have one normal and one abnormal copy of the gene (indicated as white and grey rectangles, respectively). There is a 50% (1/2) chance that a child will inherit the mutant gene from one parent, and a 50% (1/2) chance that the mutant gene will be inherited from the other parent. The chance that the child will inherit the mutant genes from both parents and develop the disorder in question is 25% ($1/2 \times 1/2 = 1/4$). By similar reasoning, the chance of this couple having a child with no mutations (i.e. two normal genes) is also 25%; the risk of the child being a carrier is 25% + 25% = 50%. The symbols used for males, females, carriers and affected people are those in common use.

sents an important exception; a couple who are biologically related are more likely to be carriers of the same disorder than a couple picked at random from the general population, and parental consanguinity increases the chance of a child having an autosomal recessive disorder.

An autosomal dominant disorder is due to a mutation in one copy of a gene

For certain autosomal genes and mutations, the presence of one abnormal gene may be sufficient to cause a clinical disorder. In this situation most of the family members who have the mutated gene will be affected. This type of mutation is called an *autosomal dominant* mutation. Dominant mutations are less common than recessive mutations. Autosomal dominant disorders affect both males and females.

In contrast to an autosomal recessive disorder, an autosomal dominant disorder may be evident in successive generations (Fig. 10.2.3). In some large families with an autosomal dominant disorder it may be apparent that an individual has the mutation, yet is

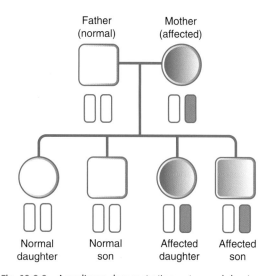

Father
(normal)

Mother
(affected)

Normal
daughter

Normal
son

Affected
daughter

Affected
son

Fig. 10.2.3 A pedigree demonstrating autosomal dominant inheritance. One parent has a mutation in a particular gene and hence has one normal and one abnormal copy of the gene (indicated as white and grey rectangles, respectively). A child will inherit a normal gene from the unaffected parent. The child could inherit a normal gene from the affected parent (as shown for the first and second children; 50% (1/2) chance for each child) or the abnormal gene from the affected parent (third and fourth children; 50% (1/2) chance for each child). The symbols used for males, females and affected people are those in common use.

unaffected. The reasons why some individuals remain healthy despite having a dominant mutation are usually unknown.

An autosomal dominant disorder may be due to a new mutation that occurred for the first time in the egg or sperm from which the affected person developed. For this reason a child may have a dominant disorder yet may be the only affected person in the family. In this situation, the recurrence risk of the disorder in the siblings of the affected child would be very low, but the recurrence risk among the offspring of the affected child would be 50%. A new dominant mutation may cause such a severe disorder that the affected child does not survive to reproduce. Many abnormalities of chromosome structure fall into this category. These disorders are never familial because the severity of the dominant mutation precludes the possibility of reproduction.

It is often not clear why some genes or mutations cause a recessive rather than a dominant disorder. Some genes produce an abundance of the particular protein from each copy of the gene, and the presence of one normal gene is more than sufficient to meet the cell's needs. Mutations in these genes will cause a recessive disorder. For other genes it may be essential that both are active for sufficient protein to be produced. A mutation in just one gene may cause

such a reduction in protein production that cell function is compromised. A mutation in this type of gene would result in a dominant disorder. A dominant disorder may also be due to abnormal interactions between different proteins. Certain proteins bind together in the normal cell to form a complex of proteins that has a particular function. A mutant gene may produce a protein of abnormal structure that interferes with the function of the protein complex even though the other proteins in the complex are normal.

An X-linked recessive disorder is due to a recessive mutation on the X chromosome

Mutations on the X chromosome demonstrate an important and common mode of inheritance. If a girl has a recessive mutation on one X chromosome the presence of the normal gene on the other X chromosome usually prevents the development of a severe genetic disorder. The girl would be a carrier of the mutation. On the other hand, a boy has just one X chromosome and a mutation on the X chromosome will result in a genetic disorder. A disorder due to a recessive mutation on the X chromosome is referred to as an *X-linked recessive* disorder. A family with an X-linked disorder will have affected males and carrier females (Fig. 10.2.4).

If there is only one boy in the family with an X-linked recessive disorder, his mother may be a carrier and the absence of affected male relatives may be due to chance. In this situation the recurrence risk among the boy's brothers would be 50% (1/2). On the other hand, the absence of affected male relatives could indicate that the boy has a new mutation that occurred for the first time during the formation of the egg from which he developed. In this situation the recurrence risk among his brothers would be very low. The distinction between these two possibilities is usually of great concern to the parents and represents a major task for the clinical geneticist.

It is important to note that some female carriers of an X-linked recessive disorder may be mildly affected. This is in contrast to the situation with carriers of an autosomal recessive disorder. A woman inactivates one X chromosome in every cell (lyonization). The normal and mutant X chromosomes within a cell are usually equally likely to be inactivated. On average, 50% of the cells will have inactivated the normal X chromosome. The other cells will have inactivated the mutant X chromosome and the woman is unlikely to demonstrate any features of the X-linked recessive disorder. But some women tend to inactivate their normal X chromosome, and the mutant X chromosome may be left activated in the majority of cells. In this situation a woman may dem-

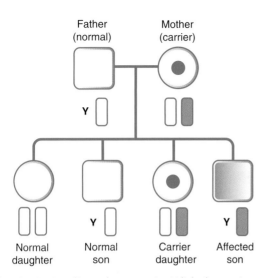

Fig. 10.2.4 A pedigree demonstrating X-linked recessive inheritance. The mother is a carrier of a mutant gene on the X chromosome. She has one normal and one abnormal copy of the gene (indicated as white and grey rectangles, respectively). Her husband has a single normal X chromosome (white rectangle) and a normal Y chromosome (as shown). A child could inherit the normal gene from the mother (as shown for the first two children; 50% (1/2) chance for each child) or inherit the abnormal gene from the mother (as shown for the third and fourth children; 50% (1/2) chance for each child). Each child could inherit the father's normal X chromosome (and be female, as shown for the first and third children; 50% (1/2) chance for each child) or his Y chromosome (and be male, as shown for the second and fourth children; 50% (1/2) chance for each child). Overall there is a 25% (1/2 × 1/2 = 1/4) chance of each of the following outcomes: normal daughter, normal son, carrier daughter and affected son.

onstrate mild features of an X-linked recessive disorder.

A polygenic disorder is due the interaction of a number of different genes

Many common genetic disorders cannot be attributed to a mutation in a single gene but are due to the interaction of a number of genes. Examples of such *polygenic* disorders include common congenital malformations, such as cleft lip, and disorders of later life, such as asthma, diabetes and schizophrenia. These conditions result from the interaction of a number of genes, each of which has some mutation or polymorphism that increases the risk of the condition. Any one of these mutations or polymorphisms is unlikely to cause the disorder on its own.

Even if a fetus has inherited a number of mutations that place it at increased risk of a birth defect, non-genetic factors, such as maternal nutrition or chance,

may ultimately determine whether the malformation occurs. A disorder due to the interaction of multiple genes and non-genetic factors is called a *multifactorial* disorder. An example is spina bifida in which a nutritional deficiency of the vitamin folate and variations in genes responsible for folate metabolism are associated with an increased risk of this major malformation.

Polygenic and multifactorial disorders typically affect between 0.1% and 1% of the population. The recurrence risk among close relatives is usually 10–20 times higher. Few of the genes responsible for polygenic disorders have been identified, and this remains a major objective in genetic research.

Disorders due to mutations in mitochondrial DNA exhibit maternal inheritance

Mitochondria are essential for providing chemical energy to the cell. Some mitochondrial proteins are encoded by genes within the nucleus, while the remainder are encoded by a small loop of DNA within the mitochondrion itself. Mutations in either the nuclear or mitochondrial genes will result in impairment of normal energy production by the mitochondrion. An abnormality of mitochondrial function due to a mutation in a nuclear gene demonstrates autosomal recessive or X-linked inheritance (Figs 10.2.2 and 10.2.4). A mutation in a nuclear gene will affect all the mitochondria and all the affected children in a family will have similar problems.

A mitochondrial abnormality due a mutation in a mitochondrial gene will be maternally inherited, i.e. the abnormal mitochondria will always have been inherited from the child's mother (Fig. 10.2.5). A child with such a mutation may have a mixture of normal and mutant mitochondria in each cell. The impact of the mutation on cell function will depend on the proportion of mitochondria that are affected. A small number of mutant mitochondria may have little impact on cell function in a woman and she may be asymptomatic. The distribution of mitochondria to new cells during cell division is random and it is possible that an ovum could have a relatively high proportion of mutant mitochondria. During subsequent development, the many cells of the fetus could inherit varying proportions of mutant mitochondria. Those tissues that have a high proportion of mutant mitochondria will not function correctly, while other tissues with comparatively low proportions of mutant mitochondria may function normally. For this reason disorders due to mutations in mitochondrial genes demonstrate marked variability in both severity and the type of tissue involved within the one family. Disorders due to mitochondrial mutations affect both boys and girls.

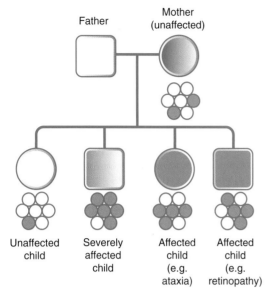

Father

Mother (unaffected)

Unaffected child

Severely affected child

Affected child (e.g. ataxia)

Affected child (e.g. retinopathy)

Fig. 10.2.5 A pedigree demonstrating mitochondrial inheritance. The cells of the mother have a mixture of normal and mutant mitochondria (shown as a mixture of white and grey circles, respectively); the majority of the mitochondria are normal and the woman is unaffected. Her husband has normal mitochondria; these are not transmitted to his children and are not shown. A child could inherit predominantly normal mitochondria from the mother and be unaffected (first child); a child could inherit predominantly abnormal mitochondria and be severely affected (second child); or the child could inherit an intermediate proportion of mutant mitochondria and the manifestations of the disease would depend on the proportion of mutant mitochondria in various tissues (third child moderately and fourth child mildly affected). Usually the probabilities of each of these outcomes cannot be predicted.

Practical points

Modern genetics
- The genetic information in cells is a key determinant of both the development of children and their responses to external stressors
- The genetic code is complex and is degraded by errors during cell division and over time
- These genetic errors account for many congenital abnormalities and disorders of ageing. If these errors are present in testes or ovaries, they may be passed on to offspring and become familial
- Examination of a child's family history of disease can provide essential clues regarding the type of genetic error that may be responsible for a child's disorder and the recurrence risk among relatives
- Genetic testing may identify the underlying cause of a child's disease, but may also highlight the potential risks to family members. Testing of unaffected relatives may clarify their risk of developing a certain disease long before the disease becomes apparent. These outcomes from genetic testing raise significant ethical issues that must be considered prior to initiating testing

Clinical example

The genetic basis for many common diseases has been identified in recent years, and this has raised a number of ethical issues.

Preamble

Hereditary haemochromatosis is an autosomal recessive condition caused by mutations in the *HFE* gene. The condition is characterized by abnormal storage of iron in a range of body tissues resulting in progressive organ damage and complications including cirrhosis of the liver, cardiomyopathy, diabetes mellitus and arthritis. The clinical features of this disorder are usually manifest in adulthood.

A simple genetic test can identify the mutation responsible for the majority of cases of hereditary haemochromatosis. Approximately 10% of people of Caucasian descent carry this mutation. A significant proportion of people with two abnormal *HFE* genes will never develop signs of organ damage. The factors known to increase the risk of developing iron overload include male gender, older age and mutations in other iron metabolism genes. Iron overload can be readily prevented by regular phlebotomy.

Proposal

It has been proposed that all babies born in Caucasian communities be screened for the presence of the common *HFE* mutation. The aim would be to identify individuals with two abnormal genes who are at increased risk of developing iron overload in adult life, and to prevent the development of this disease by regular phlebotomy.

Some arguments in favour are:
- Hereditary haemochromatosis is a common, life-threatening, yet preventable disease provided regular phlebotomies are initiated before organ damage is established
- Neonatal screening programmes have already been established for a number of disorders, and the inclusion of *HFE* gene screening would be practically and psychologically straightforward
- The identification of a mutation in a baby would trigger investigation of family members and might identify relatives with two abnormal *HFE* genes prior to the development of iron overload.

Some arguments against are:
- A newborn infant cannot give consent for testing or retain privacy regarding the test result, and there may be a risk of discrimination in the long term (e.g. in relation to life or health insurance)
- The identification of two abnormal *HFE* genes is of limited clinical relevance during childhood because regular phlebotomies to prevent iron overload are usually deferred until adulthood
- Newborn screening would equate the presence of two abnormal *HFE* genes with disease, but a significant and ill-defined proportion of those with two abnormal genes never develop iron overload.

Similar arguments could be made for (and against) screening for carriers of other autosomal recessive disorders. Do you think that such screening programmes should be established?

The practical application of genetics

The application of the genetic principles outlined in this section will primarily be found in the other components of this book. The pattern of inheritance of a child's disorder is clearly a major issue in counselling parents about their child's condition. An understanding of the different types of mutation will become essential for interpreting laboratory reports from a laboratory genetics service. The ability to define the molecular basis of a disorder may also make prenatal diagnosis in subsequent pregnancies an option for the parents.

The ability to define specific mutations may also raise ethical issues. Should there be widespread screening for carriers of common autosomal recessive disorders? Should children be tested to determine carrier status at a young age so that they can grow up mindful of this knowledge, or should genetic testing be deferred until a child can give informed consent to have the DNA test performed?

The parents of a child who has a genetic disorder due either to a new mutation or to inherited mutations are usually stunned. They may be angry or confused, blaming themselves for causing the problem, or they may search for some environmental agent to blame. It can be very difficult for them to accept the genetic basis of the disorder. It is often helpful to highlight the universality of mutations. We are all conceived with mutations inherited from both our parents, and we all create new mutations throughout development and postnatal life. The processes that caused the mutations responsible for the child's condition are the same processes that ultimately cause our own demise.

10.3 The dysmorphic child

E. Thompson

Dysmorphic, which literally means 'abnormal form', refers to an unusual appearance, usually of the face. A dysmorphic child may have an underlying diagnosis that could have implications for the health not only of the child but also of other family members if the condition is inherited. The child may present as a neonate with one or more birth defects, such as a missing hand, or with developmental delay or intellectual disability, an organ defect such as congenital heart disease, failure to thrive or obesity, short or tall stature, a behavioural disturbance or a metabolic problem.

Birth defects can be classified as deformations, disruptions, dysplasias or malformations (Ch. 10.1). It is important to distinguish between abnormalities and minor variants that are common in the general population. These can, however, appear in syndromes. For example, a unilateral single transverse palmar crease is seen in 4% of normal people but is more common in Down syndrome. Some physical traits, such as an unusually shaped nose, are a harmless family variant but, again, could be part of an undiagnosed syndrome in the family.

Making an overall diagnosis relies on recognizing a pattern of problems. The types of pattern include:

• *Syndrome*. This is from the Greek 'running together' and refers to a cluster of physical and other features occurring in a consistent pattern, with an implied common specific cause that may be unknown. The word syndrome is often used loosely to describe any of the other diagnostic patterns described below
• *Association*. This is a group of physical features that tends to occur together but the link is not consistent enough to allow the term syndrome to be used. An example is the VATER association (see below). The distinction between a syndrome and an association may be artificial. For example, the CHARGE association (Coloboma, Heart defects, Atresia choanae, Retardation of growth and development, Genital and Ear anomalies) is now commonly accepted as a syndrome, particularly since the finding in 2004 of mutations in a gene called *CHD7* on chromosome 8 in some patients with the condition

• *Sequence*. This refers to a group of abnormalities caused by a cascade of events beginning with one malformation. An example is the Potter sequence, which can result from any cause of severe oligohydramnios, such as renal agenesis. For example: renal agenesis means no fetal urine, leading to severe oligohydramnios, with the consequence of lung hypoplasia and intrauterine constraint, and therefore the development of limb deformities, such as talipes and a compressed facial appearance
• *Developmental field defect*. This refers to a group of malformations caused by a harmful influence in a particular region of the embryo. Abnormalities of blood flow are thought to underlie many of these. An example is hemifacial microsomia with unilateral facial hypoplasia and ear anomalies relating to an abnormality in development of first and second branchial arch structures.

Why is it important to recognize an underlying diagnosis? Some important reasons are:

• avoiding unnecessary investigations
• providing information about prognosis for doctors and family
• recognizing complications that need to be looked for prospectively
• determining the pattern of inheritance and recurrence risk
• enabling support from other families. Individual syndromes are rare and parents become the experts in day-to-day management of the child and can share this with other families.

Are there any pitfalls in making a diagnosis? Some areas for consideration are:

• the diagnosis must be correct. Often the diagnosis is based on clinical assessment alone with no confirmatory tests. Diagnosis must not be undertaken lightly as it can be difficult to remove or alter a diagnosis once it has been made, with harmful consequences for the child and family
• parents do not wish their child to be labelled, especially if the child is young and they do not yet perceive any problems themselves
• doctors may attribute all new problems to the syndrome.

Practical points

- Syndromes are individually rare but collectively common
- Accurate syndrome diagnosis is important to give information about prognosis, associated problems, recurrence risk and support groups for families
- Diagnoses are made by thorough clinical assessment followed by use of aids such as computerized syndrome databases
- Even an experienced clinical geneticist may not make a syndrome diagnosis in a child with dysmorphic features
- It is better to make no syndrome diagnosis than to make an incorrect diagnosis

How to assess the dysmorphic child

Instant recognition

A 'waiting room diagnosis' based on the facial 'gestalt' might be made if the doctor has seen a person with the particular syndrome before, just as most people are able to recognize whether a person in the street has Down syndrome. Often, however, the diagnosis is not apparent initially, and the following approach is recommended.

History

A detailed medical history is important. Special points to note include:

- antenatal history:
  - teratogens, such as drugs, viruses, maternal diabetes, maternal hyperthermia (Ch. 10.1)
  - fetal movements – a neuromuscular disorder may cause reduced fetal movements, resulting in arthrogryposis (multiple fixed deformities of joints)
  - prenatal screening and diagnostic tests
- perinatal history, weight, length and head circumference and Apgar scores at birth
- growth and development, behaviour, sleep patterns
- family history; draw a family tree noting the following:
  - miscarriages, stillbirths and deaths of siblings
  - information about other family members with the same features.

Examination

Observe the child before undressing or disturbing her/ him. On the other hand, the examination is not complete until the child has been fully undressed. Especially note:

- behaviour and alertness
- body size and proportions, relative head size, asymmetry, chest shape and spinal curvature
- height, weight, head circumference, arm span, upper and lower body segments
- always plot measurements on standard normal charts. Charts are available for many different body parts, e.g. hand measurements, foot and ear length. Special charts are available for certain disorders, e.g. Down syndrome, and various bone dysplasias, e.g. achondroplasia
- facial features:
  - shape of the head and face
  - spacing of the eyes (hyper- or hypotelorism, i.e. wide or closely spaced); slant of the palpebral fissures (up or down)
  - shape and size of the nose and mouth
  - structure and position of the ears
- proportions of the limbs, muscle bulk and tone, joint contractures and mobility
- structure of hands and feet (shape, length, number of digits, dermal ridges, nails)
- skin pigmentary or vascular markings
- external genitalia
- any birth defects (e.g. cleft palate)?
- auscultate the chest for any cardiac murmurs
- palpate the abdomen for organomegaly.

A *photograph* (with parental consent) is useful for:

- comparing later on to see how the face has changed
- consulting colleagues.

Examining the family of a child with unusual facial features:

- parents and siblings should be examined to see if this is a family characteristic
- photographs of them at a younger age and of other family members may be helpful
- in the event of a syndrome being diagnosed, the family should also be examined for its specific features.

Putting it all together

- ***Check textbooks of syndromes*** by trying to match the most important dysmorphic features and comparing the photographs with those of the patient
- ***Consultation***:
  - *Paediatricians* will recognize the more common syndromes, e.g. Down syndrome
  - *Clinical geneticists* have experience in identifying many more syndromes. Some have a special interest and expertise in syndrome diagnosis (*dysmorphologists*)

- it's not easy! A skilled dysmorphologist makes a syndrome diagnosis in a dysmorphic child in only 20% of cases referred from an experienced paediatrician
  - if an overall diagnosis is not made, the recognized problems must still be managed.
- *Review* in a few years time may allow a diagnosis to be made, as the features of many syndromes evolve with time and new information or laboratory techniques may be available for specific diagnoses
- *Computerized databases*
  - several thousand syndromes are published, and many are individually rare
  - computerized databases combine pictures and descriptions of syndromes
  - searches are made using a few key dysmorphic features and a number of possible diagnoses are suggested that can be compared with the patient
  - occasionally, a match will be achieved
  - success is more likely if relatively rare features are used for the search. For example, a common feature such as hypertelorism (wide-spaced eyes) would give a long list of suggested syndromes, whereas imperforate anus would give a more manageable list to consider
  - training and experience are needed to use these databases effectively
- Examples of these databases are:
  - POSSUM (Pictures Of Standard Syndromes and Undiagnosed Malformations), developed by the Genetic Health Services, Victoria, Australia
  - the Winter–Baraitser Dysmorphology Database (previously called the London Dysmorphology Database)
  - REAMS (a Radiological Electronic Atlas of Malformation Syndromes and Skeletal Dysplasias)
  - the Baraitser–Winter Neurogenetic Database (previously called the London Neurogenetics Database)
  - the London Ophthalmic Genetics Database (GENEYE)

Investigation

Investigations are necessary in many instances of attempted assessment of the child with a dysmorphic appearance. The most common of these is a chromosome analysis.

Chromosome analysis

- a routine chromosome study (karyotype) on blood lymphocytes should be done on all children with an intellectual disability, especially when dysmorphic features and birth defects are present
- submicroscopic deletions or duplications of a gene or cluster of genes underlie some syndromes. These may be detected by fluorescence in situ hybridization (FISH). Examples of these are Williams syndrome, with an elastin gene deletion.
- subtelomeric rearrangements detectable by FISH occur in about 7% of children with an unexplained intellectual disability, often with dysmorphic features. The subtelomeres are just next to the ends of the chromosomes and are prone to structural rearrangement.

New methods of chromosome analysis such as 'molecular karyotyping', using microarray technology, analyse the chromosomal DNA at a much higher resolution than established methods. Early studies suggest that the detection rate of chromosomal alterations in the population of intellectually disabled people may double that offered by routine karyotyping and subtelomere FISH. Parental chromosomes may need to be examined if a structural alteration is found, in order to clarify the abnormality and to facilitate genetic counselling in the family.

Other investigations

Other investigations such as metabolic studies or radiology should be done as clinically indicated.

Common chromosomal disorders

Children with chromosome disorders, particularly of the autosomes (chromosomes 1–22), tend to be small, dysmorphic and have an intellectual impairment.

Numerical chromosome disorders

Trisomy 21 (Down syndrome)

Down syndrome (Fig. 10.3.1) is the commonest chromosome disorder in liveborn babies and is the commonest genetic cause of intellectual disability:

- birth incidence is about 1 in 1200 live births; the overall incidence rises after maternal age of 35 years
- maternal serum screening and ultrasound can be offered to all pregnant women to identify those at high risk, who may then opt for prenatal diagnosis by amniocentesis (Ch. 10.1).
- features include:
  - flat midface, flat occiput, upward slanting eyes with medial epicanthic folds, Brushfield spots in

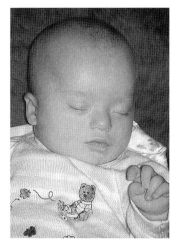

Fig. 10.3.1 Down syndrome. Note round face, small mouth, upward-slanting palpebral fissures.

the iris, palpebrae 'purse' on laughing or crying, small, down-turned mouth and protruding tongue, small ears, excess nuchal skin in the neonate
• short fingers, clinodactyly of the fifth fingers (short middle phalanges lead to incurving), single palmar creases, widened gap between 1st and 2nd toes
• birth defects may be present, e.g. congenital heart disease in 40–50%, duodenal atresia, anal atresia and many others
• intellectual disability of varying degree, mean IQ less than 50, up to about 70 and declines with age; all have neuropathological changes of Alzheimer disease by 35–40 years with clinical onset in early 50s; is an important cause of death in adults
• slightly reduced life span (around 60 years if no organ defects)
• follow-up is necessary for children with Down syndrome to monitor for:
  • cataracts, strabismus (30–40%), leukaemia, hypothyroidism, obesity, infections, constipation, obstructive sleep apnoea, dental problems and atlantoaxial instability, but only a minority develop neurological complications from this.
  • behaviour: often happy, affectionate, friendly but anxiety and depression often occur with age
• cause:
  • 95% have trisomy for chromosome 21 with a low recurrence risk
  • the rest have either a robertsonian translocation (a chromosome 21 attached to another similar chromosome, usually chromosome 14) or mosaicism (some cells with trisomy 21 and some with a normal karyotype)
  • half of the translocation cases are inherited from a parent, so parental chromosomes should

be checked only if there is a translocation. An inherited translocation is associated with an increased risk of recurrence.

Trisomy 18 (Edwards syndrome)

The birth incidence of trisomy 18 is about 1 in 8000 live births:

• many have prenatal ultrasound abnormalities and are then detected at amniocentesis
• low birth weight, prominent occiput, dysplastic low set ears, micrognathia (small chin), short palpebral fissures, small mouth
• characteristic clenched hand posture (5th and 2nd fingers overlap 4th and 3rd); prominent heels
• malformations are common, e.g. heart, brain, exomphalos, kidney
• behaviour: poor feeding and neurological development, about one-third die in the first month, less than 10% live beyond 1 year
• most have trisomy for chromosome 18, which is associated with advanced maternal age; a few have translocations
• recurrence risk for trisomy or non-inherited translocation is low and prenatal diagnosis is available for the next pregnancy.

Trisomy 13 (Patau syndrome)

The birth incidence of trisomy 13 is about 1 in 30 000 live births:

• many have prenatal ultrasound abnormalities and are then detected at amniocentesis
• low birth weight, microcephaly with sloping forehead, scalp defects, cleft lip and palate, broad flat nose, polydactyly (extra digits)
• birth defects such as holoprosencephaly and heart defects are common
• very poor neurological status and 50% of babies die within the first month
• most have trisomy 13 associated with advanced maternal age; some have translocations
• recurrence risk for trisomy is low and prenatal diagnosis is available.

Turner syndrome

Turner syndrome is one of the commonest chromosome defects at conception but the majority miscarry, usually at an early stage of pregnancy:

• birth incidence is around 1 in 3000 liveborn girls
• lymphoedema of the hands and feet and redundant nuchal skin are common in neonates
• may present in childhood with short stature, or in adolescence with failure of onset of puberty

- variable features, which include: webbed neck, increased carrying angle of elbows, broad chest, pigmented naevi, narrow, deep-set hyperconvex nails, coarctation of the aorta, idiopathic hypertension, renal anomalies
- intelligence usually normal but specific learning problems are common. One in 10 have a generalized learning disability
- most are infertile because the ovaries are dysplastic
- pregnancy has been achieved by in vitro fertilization using donor eggs
- the mean untreated adult height is around 140 cm. Refer early for assessment regarding growth hormone treatment
- cause: 60% have 45,X, others have a structural defect in which one X chromosome is missing all or part of the p (short) arm, or there is mosaicism 46,XX/45,X
- not associated with advanced maternal age; recurrence risk not increased.

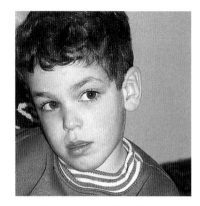

Fig. 10.3.2 Fragile X syndrome. Note long face, macrocephaly, big ears.

Klinefelter syndrome

Klinefelter syndrome is a disorder of males where there is an additional X chromosome:

- birth incidence is about 1 in 700 liveborn males
- many present as adolescents with delayed puberty, or as adults with infertility
- may present in childhood with developmental delay, especially of speech or with learning disabilities, often involving reading and mathematics
- overall, IQ is reduced compared to siblings but can be normal
- features: tall stature, long limbs, small testes, undescended testes, gynaecomastia and female fat distribution with age, infertility, behaviour problems
- treatment with testosterone at puberty will bring about a more normal virilization
- cause: 47,XXY karyotype
- recurrence risk is low.

Triple X syndrome

This is a syndrome where females have an extra X chromosome:

- birth incidence is about 1 in 1500 liveborn females
- features: tall stature, few dysmorphic features
- intellect: can be normal, but overall the IQ is lower than that of siblings. Learning difficulties, delayed speech and motor milestones, poor coordination and behaviour problems are common

- pubertal development and fertility are generally normal
- cause: 46,XXX karyotype
- recurrence risk to siblings and offspring is low.

Structural chromosome disorders

Fragile X syndrome

Fragile X syndrome (Fig. 10.3.2) is the commonest familial form of intellectual impairment, affecting 1 in 4000 males and 1 in 10 000 females.

The features of fragile X syndrome are:

- intellectual disability of varying degree, usually more severe in males than females
- mild dysmorphism with macrocephaly, high forehead, long face, large jaw, big ears, postpubertal macro-orchidism (large testes)
- soft skin, joint laxity
- shy personality, autistic features.

The cause of fragile X syndrome is a mutation called an 'unstable triplet repeat' in the *FMR1* gene on the X chromosome:

- a normal *FMR1* gene contains a sequence with five to 55 copies of a CCG triplet
- a *premutation* contains 55–230 CCG repeats. Male and female carriers of this are clinically normal (note that normal male carriers are unusual in X linked disorders). Some premutation carriers are very shy and have significant social difficulties
- a *full mutation* contains more than 230 CCG repeats. All males and about 60% of females with a full mutation show clinical features of the syndrome. The full mutation in males and some females is associated with the appearance of a 'fragile site' on light microscopy when cells are cultured in folate-deficient medium

- when the CCG repeat is passed from a carrier mother to a child (but not from a carrier father), it is unstable and tends to enlarge
- intellectual impairment increases with CCG repeat number
- female carriers pass the abnormal gene to 50% of their children but only males with the full mutation and 60% of females with the full mutation will be affected with the syndrome
- male premutation carriers pass the premutation unchanged to their daughters and both are clinically normal
- male premutation carriers are at risk after their 50s of the FXTAS syndrome with ataxia, Parkinsonian features and cognitive defects
- DNA testing can identify carriers of the pre- and full mutation. Female premutation carriers are at risk of premature menopause. Prenatal diagnosis on chorionic villus sampling or amniocentesis is available but is complicated by the uncertainty of clinical outcome in a female fetus carrying a full mutation.

The above syndrome is called fragile XA syndrome. There is also a much less common fragile XE syndrome, which is similar clinically and at the DNA level but involves a CCG repeat in the *FMR2* gene on the X chromosome.

Velocardiofacial syndrome

The estimated birth incidence of the velocardiofacial syndrome (also called VCFS, Shprintzen, 22q deletion, DiGeorge, Cayler and Sedlacková syndrome) (Fig 10.3.3) may be as high as 1 in 2000. It is a very variable syndrome, with more than 180 clinical features described. The diagnosis should be suspected if a child has the following two features:

- cleft palate – VCFS is found in 8% of children with cleft palate and 5% with cleft lip and palate

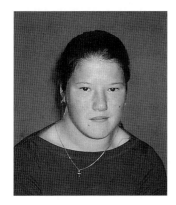

Fig. 10.3.3 Velocardiofacial syndrome. Note long mid-face, prominent nose with a squared-off nasal tip and notched alae nasi.

- conotruncal congenital heart defects (aortic arch defects, ventricular septal defect, pulmonary atresia/stenosis, tetralogy of Fallot and truncus arteriosus) – VCFS is found in about 5% of children with a congenital heart defect.

The facial appearance is variable but often there is a prominent nasal bridge, narrow nostrils, and a bulbous nasal tip. Older children often have developmental delay and learning disabilities, social immaturity, anxiety and phobias. Up to 20% of adults with the syndrome have psychiatric illness:

- cause: deletion of 22q11, visible in only 15%, detectable by FISH in the others
- up to 5% who clinically appear to have the syndrome have no detectable deletion
- parents should be tested, as features can be mild and risk to each child of a carrier is 50%.

Prenatal diagnosis is available.

Other common disorders

VATER association

VATER is an acronym for **V**ertebral anomalies, **A**nal malformations, **T**racheo-(O)**E**sophageal fistula with (o)esophageal atresia (American spelling), **R**adial and **R**enal anomalies.

- **c**ardiac and non-radial **L**imb abnormalities are common and the association is sometimes enlarged to **VACTERL**
- no particular facial appearance is associated and mental development is usually normal
- cause is unknown
- recurrence risk is low.

Noonan syndrome

The birth incidence of Noonan syndrome (Fig. 10.3.4) is 1 in 1000–2500 live births. It may present in utero with fetal nuchal oedema.

- main features:
  - short stature. Some have growth hormone deficiency
  - short neck with webbing or redundancy of skin
  - cardiac defect, especially pulmonary stenosis, atrial septal defect, ventricular septal defect, patent ductus arteriosus, hypertrophic cardiomyopathy
  - characteristic chest deformity with pectus carinatum superiorly and pectus excavatum inferiorly
  - broad chest with wide-spaced nipples
  - characteristic facial appearance, which changes with age: hypertelorism, broad forehead, ptosis,

309

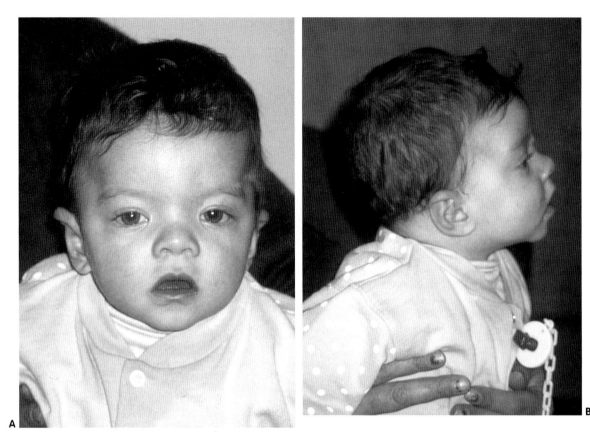

Fig. 10.3.4A, B Noonan syndrome. Note widely spaced eyes, mild ptosis, downward slanting palpebral fissures, medial epicanthic folds, broad forehead, posteriorly rotated ears, slightly coarse facial appearance.

down-slanting eyes in infancy, epicanthic folds, posteriorly rotated ears; similar facial appearance to Turner syndrome but affects both sexes and chromosomes are normal
- developmental delay is common and mild intellectual disability occurs in about one-third of cases
- look for:
  - hearing loss (one-third of cases)
  - a bleeding diathesis (one-third of cases)
  - visual problems (in most children with the syndrome)
- many are sporadic but is transmitted to offspring as an autosomal dominant
- mutations in a gene called *PTPN11* on chromosome 12q24.1 have been identified in about 50% of 22 Noonan syndrome patients (other loci may be involved)
- prenatal diagnosis is not routinely available.

Marfan syndrome

This is a syndrome associated with tall stature and a number of other features:

- incidence 1–2 in 10 000 individuals
- connective tissue disorder caused by mutations in the fibrillin gene (at chromosome 15q21.1)
- diagnosis is clinical and is based on established criteria (the Ghent criteria, 1996)

Features include:

- musculoskeletal:
  - tall stature, long limbs with significantly increased arm span and reduced upper to lower body segment ratio
  - long fingers (arachnodactyly)
  - joint laxity and flat feet
  - chest deformity and kyphoscoliosis
  - long narrow face with deep set eyes, a high narrow palate and dental crowding
- cardiovascular:
  - mitral valve prolapse
  - dilatation of the ascending aorta in 50% of children, which requires drug therapy to prevent or delay development of aortic dissection and rupture
- eye:
  - ectopia lentis (dislocation of the lens, often upward)

- myopia
- retinal detachment.

Other problems such as spontaneous pneumothorax, striae (stretch marks of the skin) and hernias can occur:

- mental development is normal
- autosomal dominant, 25% of cases are new mutations (i.e. parents are normal)
- prenatal diagnosis is possible in some families in which the fibrillin mutation has been identified.

Achondroplasia

This is the commonest and most widely recognized skeletal dysplasia, affecting about 1 in 26 000–28 000 newborns:

- main features:
  - short stature – mean adult height is 130 cm in males and 125 cm in females
  - short limbs, most marked in the upper segments of the limbs (rhizomelic shortening)
  - short fingers with 'trident' hand shape
  - relatively large head, depressed nasal bridge
  - small chest
- the radiological features are also characteristic and allow a firm diagnosis to be made soon after birth
- length can be within the normal range at birth. Occasionally the diagnosis is unrecognized for a few months

- regular follow-up is required throughout childhood to monitor for complications such as:
  - hydrocephalus
  - constriction of the cervicomedullary junction, mainly in the first 2 years
  - upper airway obstruction, especially during sleep, due to small upper airway size
  - middle ear dysfunction and hearing loss
  - kyphosis
  - lumbosacral spinal stenosis causing symptoms in older children and adults
  - hypermobile joints, knee instability
  - varus deformity (bow legs)
  - dental crowding
  - adverse psychosocial impact of the disorder on the child and family.
- treatment:
  - growth hormone transiently increases growth velocity but it is not known if final adult height is increased
  - limb lengthening by cutting and stretching the long bones with an external distractor is controversial. Recently, a radio-operated internal distractor device has been developed with reduced risk of infection compared to the external one. Many families believe it is better to modify the environment rather than the child
- autosomal dominant inheritance is usual but most cases result from a new mutation in the *FGRF3* (fibroblast growth factor receptor 3) gene.

10.4 Genetic counselling

M. B. Delatycki

Genetic counselling is what happens when an individual, a couple or a family asks questions of a health professional about a medical condition or disease that is, or may be, genetic in origin. Genetic counselling is not always provided by genetic specialists (clinical geneticists or genetic counsellors). It is appropriate for paediatricians and disease-oriented specialists to counsel in their own area of expertise. It may be difficult, however, for the doctor who looks after a child with a genetic condition to challenge a family to look at their feelings in the genetic counselling context. Even when another practitioner provides genetic counselling to the immediate family, the genetic specialists will often be involved in counselling the broader family.

The provider of counselling for any particular condition or situation tends to evolve with time. As new technology arises it is often the genetic specialist who will counsel the family, but with time this often falls to the disease-oriented specialist and general practitioner. An example is counselling for advanced maternal age and tests to diagnose Down syndrome prenatally. In the 1980s medical geneticists and some specialized obstetricians largely undertook this. It is now done by obstetricians and general practitioners in most instances.

Genetic specialists

Clinical geneticists are medical practitioners who undertake specialist training in this discipline. Their primary training is usually in paediatrics or adult internal medicine but can be in other areas, such as obstetrics and gynaecology.

Genetic counsellors come from a range of different backgrounds, such as science, nursing and teaching. They undertake a basic training programme in both genetics and counselling, followed by on the job training.

Areas that are covered by genetic specialist practice include:

- dysmorphology
- prenatal counselling and testing
- neurogenetics
- cancer genetics

- bone dysplasias
- metabolic diseases.

As can be seen, it covers a wide age range of patients – preconception to postmortem! Traditionally a paediatric specialty, the genetic specialist is increasingly involved in diagnosis and counselling for adult-onset diseases as more and more genes are discovered for these conditions.

Indications for formal genetic counselling

Anybody who suspects that there might be an increased risk of a genetic condition or producing a child with a genetic condition or birth defect may wish to receive formal genetic counselling. This includes:

- individuals who themselves have a genetic disorder
- couples who have had a stillbirth
- couples who have had a child with a birth defect
- couples who have had a child with intellectual disability
- family history of any of the above
- family history of known genetic disorders, such as Huntington disease, muscular dystrophy
- multiple miscarriages
- exposure to radiation or drugs during pregnancy
- advanced maternal age
- consanguinity
- chromosome anomalies, including translocations and inversions
- cancers, particularly where there are multiple affected family members and/or where there is a very young age at disease onset.

For appropriate genetic counselling, the following are essential:

- diagnostic precision
- knowledge of risk
- knowledge of burden
- knowledge of reproductive options
- knowledge of scientific advances
- counselling skills.

Process of genetic counselling

The genetic specialist needs to allow each family sufficient time in quiet surroundings. Medical records and doctors' reports are best obtained before undertaking counselling as this will make the consultation more efficient.

Detailed histories or records of probands (the affected individual through whom a family with a genetic disorder is ascertained) need to be obtained. A pedigree is drawn with a minimum of three generations. This should include information about stillbirths, deaths and health problems. Probands and other members of the family are examined carefully and investigated as necessary. Only then can counselling be undertaken properly.

Genetic counselling is generally non-directive. A genetic specialist will not tell the family what they should do but will help them reach an informed and reasoned decision based on the family's own sets of values. Thus, when a family asks 'Should we have another child?', instead of a direct answer the geneticist might ask 'How would you feel about having another child with cystic fibrosis?' In this way families are encouraged to explore their own feelings. For many families it is possible to be counselled in a single visit, but some families need to return for further discussions.

It is excellent practice to write to all families seen for counselling, restating the advice given to them at the time. This letter should be written in simple, clear language and outline the discussion that has taken place. A copy of this letter is sent to the family doctor and other specialists so that everybody involved has the same information. This document then serves as a valuable family record, can be shown to other professionals and overcomes the problem of selective recall.

Diagnostic precision

A critical element in genetic counselling is establishing the correct diagnosis. When considering the need for investigations, a precise diagnosis may not influence treatment but appropriate genetic counselling may be of extreme importance to the patient and his or her family. An example is muscular dystrophy. There are many different forms of muscular dystrophy. The principles of management are similar for these, e.g. appropriate splints, physiotherapy and occupational therapy. The risk for other family members, however, varies considerably between these disorders because muscular dystrophies may be autosomal dominant, autosomal recessive, X-linked recessive or mitochondrial. To counsel a family appropriately, the exact diagnosis must be known.

A postmortem examination may be necessary to establish a precise diagnosis. This can be of particular importance in a child with malformations or retardation when a diagnosis is not possible, and in adults with neurological disorders. Postmortems need to be planned in advance so that specific tissues can be obtained for biochemical study, electron microscopy or histochemistry. When death can be anticipated, it is best to raise the issue of a postmortem before death occurs. In practice this works better than asking permission immediately after the death, when families are bound up in their own grief. When permission for a postmortem has been granted, it is of the greatest importance that the parents return to fully discuss the autopsy findings.

Clinical example

Anne and her partner Bob were planning to start a family. They sought genetic counselling because Anne's sister had a son with muscular dystrophy. They were told that it is an X-linked condition and that there was therefore a significant risk that they could have a son with the same condition. After gaining permission from Anne's sister, a muscle biopsy from the affected child revealed the diagnosis of limb girdle muscular dystrophy 2B, an autosomal recessive condition. Anne and Bob were reassured that the risk for their own children was low.

Collection of samples for DNA

With advances in DNA technology it has become essential to store samples of DNA from family members with the condition in question who are likely to die, as well as relatives such as grandparents. This enables subsequent family members to benefit from advancing knowledge. Such samples can also be obtained at the time of postmortem if not collected earlier. Appropriate samples to allow DNA to be stored include blood and fibroblasts from a small skin biopsy.

Diagnostic precision may require the help of specialists who are expert in differentiating various neuromuscular diseases, retinal dystrophies and other complex problems. Dysmorphic and intellectually disabled children often require investigation before counselling can be given. An underlying chromosomal or metabolic basis should always be excluded and specific dysmorphic syndromes identified where possible (Chs 10.1, 10.3 and 10.5).

Clinical example

Andrew died from Hunter syndrome at 10 years of age in 1975. Hunter syndrome is a rare X-linked recessive neurodegenerative disorder. In 2005 his sister Jane came for advice about her risk of having a son with Hunter syndrome. Fibroblasts from Andrew had been stored. A gene mutation was found in DNA extracted from the fibroblasts, even though the gene was cloned 15 years after Andrew's death. Jane was shown not to carry the mutation. She could therefore be reassured that her risk of having a son with Hunter syndrome was no higher than any couple's without a family history of the condition.

Genetic counselling without a diagnosis

Of children presenting with intellectual disability or dysmorphic features, approximately half will not have a precise diagnosis. There is a large body of empirical data that can be used for counselling in this group. The only caveat is that appropriate examination and investigation should be done by an experienced clinician to exclude known disorders. While an inability to label a child with a specific diagnosis is disappointing and frustrating for both parents and doctors, it should not disadvantage the child, as management can be based on periodic assessment and planning.

The evolution of knowledge and new techniques make it necessary to look again at old problems. Thus patient review is of the greatest importance. For example, when the underlying chromosomal fragile site in fragile X syndrome became recognized as a major cause of intellectual disability, many families required further study using new chromosome techniques. This required further repetition using DNA studies when the triplet repeat abnormality was recognized as the cause. Also, new approaches using DNA for diagnosis and identification of carriers will require recall and further study of affected families. In addition, the clinical features making up a syndrome may become more apparent with increasing age and thus allow for better diagnostic precision.

Counselling for risk

Following diagnostic evaluation, an estimate of risk can be made. Risk is a numerical estimate of the likelihood of a particular disorder occurring in a current or future pregnancy.

Risk in specific situations

Mendelian disorders

These are conditions that are autosomal dominant, autosomal recessive or X-linked. Some 6500 mendelian disorders have been described in humans. They are comprehensively catalogued in Online Mendelian Inheritance in Man (OMIM, http://www.ncbi.nlm.nih.gov/entrez/query.fcgi?db=OMIM). Where the disorder follows mendelian inheritance, risk calculation is based on the mode of inheritance and other factors, such as carrier testing. DNA testing has improved the precision of counselling in some cases.

Polygenic or multifactorial inheritance

There are many common disorders in which there is a genetic component and where the inheritance pattern cannot be explained simply in terms of mendelian inheritance or chromosomal rearrangement. It appears that these disorders are due to the cumulative action of a number of genes together with environmental influences. This is called polygenic or multifactorial inheritance and numerically is the commonest pattern of inheritance responsible for the familial tendency or predisposition to various disorders. The recurrence risk of multifactorial disorders after a single affected child or with a single affected parent depends on the condition and can often be estimated from empirical data. The following are examples of conditions that generally follow multifactorial inheritance:

- congenital cardiac anomalies
- asthma

Clinical example

Lara's brother James had recently had a child, Craig, who was diagnosed with cystic fibrosis by newborn screening. Lara and her partner Ivan were planning a family and sought advice about their risk of having a child with this condition. Based on a community carrier rate of 1 in 25, Lara and Ivan were informed that their risk was 1 in 200. Mutation testing of the *CFTR* gene revealed that Craig was homozygous for the deltaF508 mutation, the commonest mutation that leads to cystic fibrosis. Lara was tested and was shown to carry this mutation. Ivan was then tested and was shown to carry another cystic fibrosis mutation, G551D. This meant that they had a 1 in 4 risk of having a child with cystic fibrosis and that it was possible for them to have prenatal or preimplantation testing by DNA analysis for this condition.

- neural tube defects, such as spina bifida and anencephaly
- coronary artery disease
- cleft lip and cleft palate
- congenital dislocation of the hip
- pyloric stenosis.

Clinical example

Sonya and her partner Joe had a child with anencephaly, a neural tube defect. This is an invariably fatal condition where the skull and brain do not fully form. They sought counselling about the risk of recurrence and what could be done to avoid this and detect it if it did recur. They were informed that the risk of a neural tube defect (anencephaly, spina bifida, encephalocele) in Sonya's next pregnancy was about 1 in 25. This risk could be reduced by Sonya taking folate 5 mg daily for 3 months prior to conception and during the first 3 months of pregnancy. Sonya and Joe were told that detailed expert ultrasound at about 11 and 18 weeks gestation are the best tests to detect a neural tube defect.

Unknown diagnosis

The commonest example here is where one child in a family has a syndrome with dysmorphic features and intellectual disability. Despite expert evaluation and investigation, no diagnosis is made. Again here empiric data are used, with the recurrence risk usually being in the order of 1 in 20 (5%).

Interpretation of risk

Many families do not have a good grasp of probability and careful discussion is needed to give meaning to any risk estimate. It is important to emphasize to families that chance has no memory. Simple illustrations and a concrete example such as tossing two coins are often helpful. Describing the risk in more than one way can also be helpful for some people. Thus some may understand a 25% recurrence risk more readily than one in four.

It can be helpful to put risk into the perspective of how their risk compares with that of other families. There is approximately a 1 in 30 risk that any child will be born with a major defect. This is the risk that any family either accepts or ignores and is a useful point of comparison. While genetic counselling does not aim to tell a person what to do, it is important for a counsellor to see that parents understand the meaning of any numbers used.

From the nuclear to the extended family

Where a disorder is identified in a family that puts other family members at significant risk of either a problem themselves or of having a child with a problem, the extended family needs to be offered the opportunity to discuss this and have testing. An example of this is the clinical example of Lara and Ivan (above), where their risk of having a child with cystic fibrosis only came to light because a child was born into the family with this condition. This form of testing is called cascade testing. Examples of conditions where the extended family may be at risk are a chromosome translocation, an autosomal dominant disorder such as Marfan syndrome, common recessive disorders such as cystic fibrosis and haemochromatosis, or sex linked disorders such as Duchenne muscular dystrophy. Where members of the extended family need to be informed that there is a risk to them or their offspring of having a genetic disorder, a letter from the genetic specialist can be very helpful in conveying this sensitive information.

Clinical example

John had symptoms of lethargy, joint pain and abdominal pain. Extensive medical evaluation eventually revealed that the underlying cause for this was iron overload due to hereditary haemochromatosis. He was shown to be homozygous for the common C282Y mutation in the *HFE* gene. John had a brother, George. George was found to be C282Y-homozygous and iron studies showed a moderately raised ferritin and transferrin saturation. He had had no symptoms referable to haemochromatosis. He had regular venesections to return his iron indices to normal. By doing this George was avoiding the risk of developing symptomatic haemochromatosis.

Predictive testing

Predictive or presymptomatic testing is defined as a test on an asymptomatic person that allows that individual to know whether or not s/he will go on to develop the condition in question. The test may be genetic (e.g. testing for the CAG triplet repeat expansion in Huntington disease) or may involve other types of investigation (e.g. nerve conduction studies in an asymptomatic person at risk of Charcot–Marie–Tooth disease).

Predictive testing is available mainly for neurodegenerative diseases (e.g. Huntington disease, autosomal dominant spinocerebellar ataxia) and some cancers (familial breast/ovarian cancer, familial bowel cancer). It is conducted in the setting of a counselling protocol to give those undertaking the testing the opportunity to understand what a gene positive or negative result would mean for them. Where no preventative treatment is available (e.g. Huntington disease), the majority of those at risk choose not to be tested. Predictive testing for conditions where the onset is generally in adulthood and where no preventative treatment is available is not generally undertaken on minors.

Clinical example

Sue and David were 12-year-old twins and had a 50% risk of having familial polyposis coli (FAP). FAP results in a sufferer having hundreds or thousands of bowel polyps, which, if untreated, invariably leads to malignant change in one or more polyps. Sue and David's mother, uncle and grandfather, as well as a number of other relatives, had suffered from FAP. The causative mutation in the *APC* gene in Sue and David's family was known. Because polyposis and malignant change may occur in the teens, it was recommended that surveillance by lower gastrointestinal tract endoscopy begin in the early teens. Sue and David underwent predictive testing. It was found that Sue did not have the familial mutation but David did. David was therefore recommended to have yearly colonoscopies but Sue did not need to do so. Prior to the availability of molecular diagnosis, Sue would have had yearly colonoscopies until she reached her 30s before a confident diagnosis that she did not have FAP could be made.

The burden

The burden of an actual or possible genetic diagnosis is of great importance in genetic counselling. This can be considered in two contexts: in prenatal diagnosis and a diagnosis in a child. Where a diagnosis is made prenatally, the couple need to be fully informed about the problems a child with that condition may face. This is to allow an informed decision about pregnancy termination but also allows couples who choose not to terminate the pregnancy to prepare for that child's birth. Where there is a strong family history of a condition, the couple may be well aware of the burden. An example is a woman who has grown up with a brother with Duchenne muscular dystrophy who has prenatal testing that reveals that the male she is carrying has this condition. More difficult is where a diagnosis is made that was not specifically being looked for. An example is the diagnosis of Klinefelter syndrome (47,XXY) on a prenatal chromosome test done to look for Down syndrome. Here much time is often required to help the couple

understand what that diagnosis will mean for their child and the rest of the family.

Similar issues exist where a child is diagnosed with a particular condition. For example, parents of a baby recently diagnosed as having cystic fibrosis or intellectual disability may have little idea of what lies ahead for the child and themselves. It is necessary to give parents an understanding of what is going to be involved in the care of a child with that particular disorder, including the life expectancy, the quality of life, treatment and variability that exists for that disorder. Just as importantly, it is vital that, in situations where the prognosis cannot be predicted, this uncertainty is conveyed to the parents. For instance, an individual with a genetic mutation in one of the two genes in which mutations occur resulting in tuberous sclerosis may present with hypsarrhythmia and profound intellectual disability, s/he may be unaffected or may have problems that fall between these two extremes.

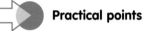

Practical points

- Accurate diagnosis is critical to enable the most accurate advice to be provided
- Thorough assessment and investigation is essential to give the best chance of a specific diagnosis
- All reproductive options should be discussed so individuals and couples can make an informed choice about the best choice for them
- Sensitivity to the emotional impact of genetic disease is critical and should be sought and addressed in all consultations

Alternatives for families at risk

Where a couple have a child, or they know they are at risk of having a child, with a genetic condition, there are a number of reproductive options available to them. These include:

- childless lifestyle
- acceptance of risk
- adoption
- intrauterine diagnosis
- donor sperm
- donor ova
- donor embryo
- preimplantation genetic diagnosis.

Childless lifestyle

A family may choose not to have children where there is a risk of a genetic condition or where a child has been born with a genetic condition.

Acceptance of risk

For some couples the risk of the disorder may be acceptable compared to the burden of other alternatives. This may relate to the perceived severity of the disorder. Thus prenatal diagnosis is requested much more often when the disorder is lethal in childhood (e.g. Duchenne muscular dystrophy) than when it frequently leads to many years of health before its onset (e.g. Huntington disease) or where its severity is unpredictable and it is often relatively mild (e.g. neurofibromatosis type I). Religious and cultural factors may contribute to this decision.

Adoption

The number of young babies available for adoption is very limited because of the increase in single-parent families and termination of pregnancies. Thus adoption is much less common and less easily arranged than in the past.

Intrauterine diagnosis

Intrauterine diagnosis provides an option for many couples. This can be offered to families who feel that termination of pregnancy is acceptable. The range of disorders that can be recognized by intrauterine diagnosis is constantly increasing (Ch. 10.2).

Donor sperm

Artificial insemination by donor (AID) is of limited appeal. Many couples and ethnic groups find it unacceptable. This, however, should never be assumed and couples should be informed about this option to determine whether or not it is acceptable to them. Artificial insemination by donor can provide an alternative when the father has an autosomal dominant disorder, carries a chromosome translocation or produces a child with an autosomal recessive disorder.

Donor ova

In vitro fertilization (IVF) using donor ova can be offered when a woman carries a sex-linked disorder, has an autosomal dominant disorder, carries a chromosome translocation, has a mitochondrial DNA mutation or produces a child with an autosomal recessive disorder. Parents may find this more acceptable, as the mother still experiences the pregnancy.

Donor embryo

Donor embryos are usually donated by couples who have utilized IVF and have stored residual embryos but do not require them as they have completed their family. Some couples prefer this to donor sperm or ova, as they feel uncomfortable about one partner being genetically related to their offspring but the other partner not being related.

Preimplantation genetic diagnosis

In preimplantation genetic diagnosis, cells from an embryo produced by IVF are tested for the disorder in question. This may be through DNA analysis or chromosome examination by fluorescence in situ hybridization (FISH). Only those embryos where the disorder is excluded are returned to the uterus. The advantage of preimplantation genetic diagnosis is that termination of pregnancy is not required. The disadvantages are that it is expensive, labour-intensive with often long delays before it can be offered for the specific disorder in a particular family and for each cycle of IVF the completed pregnancy rate is well below 50%, even in fertile couples.

Emotional impact of genetic counselling

Patients often feel very vulnerable when referred for genetic counselling. This may be because of the recent birth of a child with a disability, a stillbirth or a neonatal death. People might be concerned about details of their family history and worry that they might be blamed for the problem that lead them to seek genetic counselling.

In counselling, the emotional impact of a birth defect, and the risk of producing a child with a birth defect, are carefully explored. People need an opportunity to vent their fears and anxieties. Discussions of emotional issues are of equal importance to discussions of risk, burden and alternatives. Families who have recently lost a child may need understanding and reassurance about the process of mourning and may need to allow time before they are ready for a further pregnancy.

Acknowledgements

I wish to thank Dr John Rogers for teaching me about the practice of genetic counselling. Dr Rogers was the author of this chapter in the first four editions of *Practical Paediatrics* and the current chapter draws much from that work.

Inborn errors of metabolism

J. McGill

Inborn errors of metabolism, or metabolic disorders, are clinical conditions that result from a block in one of the metabolic or biochemical pathways in the body.

Metabolic disorders, particularly those presenting acutely, remain seriously underdiagnosed. This is because the presentation is often precipitated by or mimics infection and so the possibility of an inborn error of metabolism is overlooked. Diagnostic clues such as:

- hypoglycaemia
- presence or inappropriate absence of ketosis
- metabolic acidosis (usually with a high anion gap)
- lactic acidosis
- respiratory alkalosis

are often overlooked or are misinterpreted as being due to the precipitating infection. The possibility of a metabolic disorder needs to be considered so that specific diagnostic tests such as plasma acylcarnitine profile, urine organic acids, plasma amino acids and ammonium are ordered. Rapid diagnosis and institution of appropriate therapy are essential to avoid death or permanent neurological damage.

Although individually uncommon, collectively metabolic disorders are frequent. The main forms of presentation are:

- acutely: in the neonatal period or later in infancy

or childhood associated with intercurrent illness or dietary changes
- neurodegeneration
- multisystem disorders with organ dysfunction.

Acute metabolic decompensation

Neonatal

In the neonatal period, metabolic disorders can be grouped into those that become symptomatic because of:

- the accumulation of a toxin, or
- an energy deficiency.

Those neonates with toxin accumulation are usually well until 2–5 days of age, as the placenta has usually cleared the toxin in utero. Poor feeding and lethargy are frequent early symptoms, followed by a decreased conscious state, biochemical disturbances and abnormalities of tone and movement.

The neonate with energy deficiency can present at any time from birth with seizures, acidosis, hypertrophic cardiomyopathy, hypotonia and malformations being common features.

The history can be helpful and questions asked should include possible consanguinity, family history of similar presentations, previous neonatal deaths or stillbirths, particularly on the maternal side (X-linked or mitochondrial inheritance), and dietary exposures such as galactose (breast or cow's milk) or fructose (fruit, honey on dummy). Most of the disorders are due to an enzyme deficiency, and autosomal recessive inheritance is far more common than X-linked or maternal mitochondrial inheritance.

A very useful approach to diagnosis in the newborn period has been devised by Saudubray et al (see Further Reading) based on the measurement of glucose, ketones, lactate, ammonium and acidosis.

Older children

Acute metabolic presentations in children beyond the neonatal period are normally precipitated by a viral illness associated with loss of appetite or

---

Practical points

Inborn errors of metabolism
- Inborn errors of metabolism, particularly those presenting acutely, remain significantly underdiagnosed
- Presence of hypoglycaemia, presence or inappropriate absence of ketoacidosis, metabolic or lactic acidosis, or respiratory alkalosis should raise suspicion of a disorder of metabolism
- Early diagnosis is essential to prevent death or major morbidity
- Inborn errors of metabolism frequently have effects on many body systems
- Neonatal screening programmes exist for early detection of some inborn errors of metabolism

vomiting. This causes catabolism and the gluconeogenic, fat and protein catabolic pathways are stressed. Ingestion of large amounts of protein or deliberately fasting (e.g. for surgery) can also precipitate an acute decompensation in some disorders.

For all age groups the presentation can be as decreased conscious state, hypoglycaemia, metabolic acidosis or seizures.

Decreased conscious state

A decreased conscious state may be the result of:

- metabolic encephalopathy
- hypoglycaemia
- hyperammonaemia
- aminoacidopathies, e.g. maple syrup urine disease.

Diagnosis of the latter is based on plasma and urine amino acids, which show elevated branched chain amino acids: valine, leucine and isoleucine.

Hyperammonaemia

Hyperammonaemia often causes a respiratory alkalosis. The absence of ketosis can be important in distinguishing these disorders from the secondary hyperammonaemia of patients with an organic acidosis.

Findings and possible causes of hyperammonaemia may be:

- normal anion gap – high amino acids:
  - urea cycle disorders, e.g. citrullinaemia, argininaemia, argininosuccinic aciduria
- normal anion gap – low/normal amino acids:
  - urea cycle disorders, e.g. ornithine transcarbamylase (OTC) deficiency, carbamyl phosphate synthetase (CPS) deficiency
  - lysinuric protein intolerance
  - transient hyperammonaemia of newborn (premature babies with respiratory distress)
- increased anion gap:
  - liver disease/failure
  - organic acidaemias, e.g. methylmalonic acidaemia, propionic acidaemia.

The presence of a raised urine orotic acid distinguishes OTC from CPS deficiency. OTC deficiency is an X-linked disorder so an extended family pedigree on the maternal side may be useful. Females heterozygous for the gene may be symptomatic.

Children with milder or partial deficiencies of urea cycle enzymes, including some females who are heterozygous for OTC deficiency, present later in life, usually after a high protein intake or with catabolism with an intercurrent illness. Abdominal pain and vomiting are early symptoms.

Clinical example

Joseph was born at term to non-consanguineous parents. He fed well on the breast initially and was discharged to home on day 2 of life. On day 3 he was noted by his mother to be sleepy and feeding poorly. By that afternoon he could not be roused for feeds and he presented to the Emergency Department. He was afebrile and a septic workup was negative. Blood gases revealed a respiratory alkalosis and the alert paediatric registrar ordered a plasma ammonium, which was 830 mmol/L (NR <60). Plasma amino acids and urine orotic acid were collected and Joseph was transferred to intensive care, where a repeat ammonium was 1546 mmol/L. He was treated with peritoneal dialysis, sodium benzoate, sodium phenylbutyrate (alternative pathways to excrete nitrogen) and arginine and his ammonium gradually returned to normal. Plasma amino acid analysis showed high glutamine and low citrulline concentrations, and his urine was positive for orotic acid. DNA studies confirmed ornithine transcarbamylase deficiency and testing of his mother showed that she was a carrier. There was no family history of the disorder. Joseph was managed with a low protein diet in combination with the above medications.

Hypoglycaemia

The causes of hypoglycaemia can be grouped according to the presence or absence of ketones, hepatomegaly, lactic acidosis and the rapidity of onset after the last feed.

Tests to be performed at the time of hypoglycaemia (i.e. before it is corrected):

- glucose
- insulin
- C-peptide
- growth hormone
- cortisol
- ACTH
- free fatty acids
- beta-hydroxybutyrate
- acylcarnitine profile
- lactate
- ammonium
- plasma amino acids
- organic acids (the first urine passed after the episode).

Findings and causes of hypoglycaemia

There are many causes of hypoglycaemia. The following list provides a guide to potential diagnoses according to specific findings at presentation:

- hypoketotic hypoglycaemia:
  - hyperinsulinism – fat mobilization inhibited (congenital hyperinsulinism (previously called nesidioblastosis), transient hyperinsulinism of infancy, Beckwith–Wiedemann syndrome, congenital disorders of glycosylation types 1a and 1b, small for gestational age infants, infants of diabetic mothers, or insulinoma)
  - fatty acid oxidation disorders producing a block in ketone production, e.g. medium chain acyl CoA dehydrogenase (MCAD) deficiency
  - growth hormone deficiency
- hypoketotic hypoglycaemia and hyperammonaemia:
  - glutamate dehydrogenase upregulation (hyperinsulinism–hyperammonaemia syndrome) (note that hypoglycaemia in this disorder occurs after a protein meal)
- ketotic hypoglycaemia:
  - recurrent ketotic hypoglycaemia of childhood – commonly occurs in mornings before breakfast or with prolonged fasting as with a vomiting illnesses. It is usually not a problem after 6–8 years of age. This is a diagnosis of exclusion
  - adrenal insufficiency
  - hypopituitarism
  - organic acidurias, e.g. methylmalonic acidaemia
- persisting hepatomegaly with liver dysfunction:
  - galactosaemia
  - tyrosinaemia type 1
  - neonatal haemochromatosis (now known to be an alloimmune disease)
  - alpha-1-antitrypsin deficiency
  - respiratory chain disorders
  - hereditary fructose intolerance (postprandial after fructose ingestion)
- hepatomegaly without liver dysfunction:
  - glycogen storage diseases types I and III
- transient hepatomegaly:
  - fatty acid oxidation disorders
  - gluconeogenic disorders, e.g. fructose 1,6 bisphosphatase deficiency
- onset within 2–6 hours postprandially:
  - hyperinsulinism
  - glycogen storage diseases
- associated lactic acidosis:
  - glycogen storage disease type 1
  - glycogen synthetase deficiency (lactic acidosis occurs postprandially)
  - gluconeogenic disorders.

Some babies with hypopituitarism present with hypoglycaemia and obstructive jaundice.

> **Practical points**
>
> **Sample collection and other points of note**
> - Plasma ammonium values increase markedly if the specimen is allowed to sit around – collect the sample on ice and analyse it quickly
> - Glucometers are often unreliable for measuring hypoglycaemia and all children in whom there is a suspicion of hypoglycaemia should have it confirmed by a formal blood glucose measurement
> - When investigating hypoglycaemia of unknown cause, collect 6 ml of blood in total: 4 ml lithium heparin tube on ice, 1 ml in a serum tube and 1 ml in EDTA tube at time of insertion of drip. If there are problems collecting blood, don't delay correcting the hypoglycaemia
> - Children with disorders of hyperinsulinism can be identified by the higher glucose requirements needed to control the hypoglycaemia and because they become hypoglycaemic on maintenance intravenous fluids containing dextrose
> - Ketones are normal in a child with vomiting or starvation from other causes. Their presence in less than expected amounts is abnormal and warrants further investigation
> - In a child presenting acutely with a metabolic acidosis and where an inborn error of metabolism is a possibility, it is essential that the first urine passed is analysed for organic acids, as the diagnostic metabolites can clear quickly once intravenous glucose is given

Metabolic acidosis (excluding lactic acidosis)

These infants and children are severely ill but symptoms and signs are similar to severe infection and that is the usual initial diagnosis. The associated tachypnoea can be mistaken for respiratory disease. The metabolic acidosis has a high anion gap (metabolic acidosis plus normal anion gap can occur with renal tubular acidosis). Associated laboratory abnormalities can include neutropenia, thrombocytopenia, hypoglycaemia or hyperglycaemia, hypocalcaemia and moderate hyperammonaemia. The diagnosis is reached by the examination of urine organic acids or plasma acylcarnitine profile, both of which are most likely to be diagnostic if the specimen is collected during the acute decompensation. Common disorders in this group are methylmalonic, propionic and isovaleric acidaemias.

Lactic acidosis

These patients have an energy deficiency. The main symptoms are due to the high anion gap acidosis. In neonates, ketosis is an important clue and increases the likelihood of a metabolic disease as it is not

Clinical example

A 2-year-old boy, Gareth, presented with a 2-day history of vomiting and diarrhoea. He was noted to have a reduced conscious state and to be tachypnoeic. A blood gas revealed a compensated metabolic acidosis. His urine had large amounts of ketones on standard urine dipstick testing, and was positive for Phenistix, indicating aspirin ingestion. His parents denied giving him aspirin but were not believed and were warned of the dangers of aspirin in children. He made a good recovery with intravenous fluids and was discharged. Six months later he represented after a more severe vomiting illness and was again acidotic with a pH of 7.1, and the anion gap was 28 mmol/L (NR 4–13). He required ventilation in ICU and after recovery was found to have dystonia. A magnetic resonance image of his brain showed basal ganglia changes. A urine sample collected when he was acidotic and sent for analysis of urine organic acids showed large amounts of methylmalonic acid. Gareth was not responsive to vitamin B$_{12}$ injections. In retrospect, the positive Phenistix was due to the methylmalonic acid and not aspirin as suspected initially. Not only had the parents been falsely accused but an opportunity to diagnose methylmalonic aciduria before it caused permanent disability had been lost.

Clinical example

Rebecca, aged 18 months, was noted to have a protuberant abdomen. Hepatomegaly was present, but there was no splenomegaly. Liver function tests were normal. Four months later she was noted not to be using her left arm and further testing revealed a left hemiplegia. Investigations at that time revealed marked hyperlipidaemia and an appropriate diet was introduced. A further 5 months later, she represented with anorexia due to an upper respiratory tract infection. She was tachypnoeic and sweating but was conscious. Her blood glucose was 0.8 mmol/l and her bicarbonate was 12 mmol/l (NR 22–33) with a high anion gap. Further testing showed a lactate of 15.0 mmol/l (NR 0.7–2.5) With correction of the blood glucose the lactate returned to normal.

Glycogen storage disease was suspected and was confirmed by a liver biopsy, which showed glycogen accumulation in the liver and a deficiency of glucose-6-phosphatase (glycogen storage disease type 1b). The hyperlipidaemia is a feature of this disorder and, in retrospect, the stroke was probably due to unrecognized hypoglycaemia. In this condition, the brain can learn to use lactate as an alternate fuel and that is why Rebecca was conscious with such a low blood glucose value. To maintain her blood glucose, she required cornstarch with feeds, which were given every 4 hours, and overnight feeds with Polyjoule.

usually present with hypoxia. Some of the disorders causing lactic acidosis have associated dysmorphic features and malformations.

Findings and causes of lactic acidosis may be:

- high lactate:pyruvate ratio:
  - respiratory chain defects
  - pyruvate carboxylase deficiency type B (+ hyperammonaemia and citrullinaemia)
- normal lactate:pyruvate ratio:
  - pyruvate dehydrogenase deficiency
  - pyruvate carboxylase deficiency type A
  - glycogen storage disease type 1 (hepatomegaly)
  - fructose 1,6 bisphosphatase deficiency (hepatomegaly)
- abnormal organic acids:
  - organic acidaemias, e.g. methylmalonic acidaemia
  - fatty acid oxidation disorders.

Seizures

Seizures may be present from birth in infants with one of the energy-deficiency disorders, may occur at any time with hypoglycaemia and may be seen as a late sign in patients with metabolic encephalopathy due to toxin accumulation. The most common disorders in the group with energy deficiency are non-ketotic hyperglycinaemia (diagnosed by an elevated cerebrospinal fluid (CSF):plasma glycine ratio), sul-

phite oxidase deficiency (diagnosed by urine metabolic screen), peroxisomal disorders (diagnosed by plasma very-long-chain fatty acids and phytanic acid) and disorders of the mitochondrial respiratory chain. This last group is usually dysmorphic and hypotonic. Pyridoxine-dependent seizures are important to identify and the diagnosis should be confirmed by improvement of the electroencephalogram (EEG) during injection of pyridoxine.

An uncommon but increasingly recognized cause of difficult to control seizures is due to glucose transporter 1 deficiency, which causes reduced transport of glucose across the blood–brain barrier. It is diagnosed by a low CSF:plasma glucose ratio. A ketogenic diet is very effective in controlling the seizures in this disorder.

Treatment

The basis of treatment in the disorders of fat and protein metabolism is to reverse the catabolism. This is usually achieved by intravenous 10–20% dextrose with maintenance salts. Sometimes it is necessary to remove the toxins by dialysis or haemoperfusion. Many of the enzymes have vitamin cofactors, and in a small proportion giving pharmacological doses of the vitamin can overcome the defect, e.g. vitamin B$_{12}$

for methylmalonic acidaemia and biotin for biotinidase deficiency. A secondary carnitine deficiency may develop in many of these disorders and correction of that is essential.

Long term, the disorders of protein metabolism require a low protein diet supplemented by amino acid formulas lacking the amino acid(s) that accumulate(s) proximal to the block and boosted in those amino acids that are deficient distal to the block.

High glucose infusions may exacerbate disorders of the mitochondrial respiratory chain and pyruvate dehydrogenase deficiency. In these disorders a high proportion of calories needs to come from fats.

Neurodegeneration

Metabolic disorders are high in the differential diagnosis for children who have a loss of acquired skills following a period of normal development. This is termed regression and the disorders causing it are termed neurodegenerative disorders. Seizures are a frequent associated symptom. Lysosomal storage disorders, peroxisomal disorders and disorders of the mitochondrial respiratory chain can all be associated with neurodegeneration.

Multisystem disease

With these disorders, many different organ systems can be involved. Although involvement of the nervous system is common, it is not present in all disorders. The liver, gastrointestinal tract, heart, kidney, skeletal system, hearing and the eye can be involved. The skeletal changes can be either abnormalities of skeletal formation (bone dysplasia) or progressive destruction of skeletal structures due to accumulating material. Some lysosomal storage disorders, disorders of the mitochondrial respiratory chain, peroxisomal disorders and congenital disorders of glycosylation can all have multisystem involvement.

Lysosomal storage disorders

In these children the lack of one of the lysosomal enzymes results in the accumulation of the structural substrate, usually metabolized by that enzyme, in a variety of tissues. Presenting features include developmental regression, hepatomegaly, splenomegaly, coarsening of the facial features and clouding of the cornea. Radiological examination often reveals changes in the spine (dysostosis multiplex) and long bones. Not all types have CNS involvement. Storage bodies may be seen in white blood cells on a blood film. Disorders in this group include the mucopolysaccharidoses (e.g. Hurler and Sanfilippo syndromes), Gaucher, Krabbe and Niemann–Pick diseases. Diagnosis is made by urine screens for mucopolysaccharides and oligosaccharides and confirmed by white cell, plasma or fibroblast lysosomal enzyme analysis.

A new form of therapy is available for this group of disorders. Enzyme replacement therapy (ERT) is already commercially available for Gaucher disease types I and III, Fabry disease, Hurler–Scheie and Scheie syndromes (the milder end of the spectrum of mucopolysaccharidosis (MPS) type 1), and Maroteaux–Lamy syndrome (MPS VI). The enzymes are produced by recombinant DNA technology and are then modified so that they are delivered to the target tissues. Trials of ERT are currently under way for Pompe disease (glycogen storage disease type II) and the mild form of Hunter syndrome (MPS type II). The ERT does not effectively cross the blood–brain barrier and so disorders that involve the central nervous system (CNS) will need different approaches (intrathecal injections of the enzymes are being trialled).

Bone marrow transplantation has been an effective treatment for several lysosomal disorders with CNS involvement. The outcome depends on the neurological status at the time of transplant. More recently, cord blood stem cell transplantations have replaced bone marrow for this form of therapy. The transplanted cells can cross the blood–brain barrier and therefore can stabilize brain pathology. Substrate inhibition therapy is also being trialled for disorders with CNS involvement.

Mitochondrial respiratory chain disorders

Respiratory chain disorders are increasingly being recognized as a cause of progressive neurological disease and multisystem disease. The range of symptoms is vast and mitochondrial disorders can present at any age and with any combination of symptoms. Tissues that most depend on mitochondrial adenosine triphosphate (ATP) production, such as brain, skeletal muscle and heart, are more frequently affected in disorders of the mitochondrial respiratory chain. Common presentations in childhood include seizures, developmental delay, regression, strokes, lactic acidosis, myopathy, endocrine disorders, cardiomyopathy, liver failure, renal disorders, ophthalmoplegias, retinitis pigmentosa and deafness. There are mitochondrial mutations that predispose to aminoglycoside toxicity and many of the patients who developed liver failure after sodium valproate therapy had a mitochondrial disease.

The diagnosis should be suspected in any child with a combination of symptoms, particularly if they are unrelated, e.g. CNS and liver disease or renal tubular acidosis and a neurodegenerative disease. The basal ganglia are often seen to be involved on magnetic resonance imaging (MRI) and are a useful marker for this group of disorders.

Mitochondria have their own DNA and mitochondria are inherited from the mother via the egg (maternal inheritance). Some mitochondrial diseases are inherited as mutations in the mitochondrial DNA, e.g. MELAS (Mitochondrial Encephalopathy, Lactic Acidosis and Stroke-like episodes), MERRF (Myoclonic Epilepsy, Ragged Red Fibres), NARP (Neurogenic muscle weakness, Ataxia and Retinitis Pigmentosa) and Leigh disease. Others, such as complex IV and polymerase gamma (POLG) deficiencies, are inherited from nuclear genes, mainly autosomal recessive. The latter form of inheritance is more common in childhood.

The diagnosis of mitochondrial diseases is difficult. The screening tests include elevated lactate in the blood or CSF and histological changes on muscle biopsy including ragged red fibres. Only a small proportion of children have one of the common mutations of mitochondrial DNA and these may only be present in some tissues such as muscle. The next stage of investigation is to assay the enzyme complexes of the respiratory chain in muscle, liver or skin. Because the investigations are of enzyme complexes, the results are often suggestive rather than diagnostic of a respiratory chain disorder. It is important to realize that, at present, there is no test that can exclude a disorder of the mitochondrial respiratory chain.

There are a variety of treatment regimes for mitochondrial respiratory chain disorders, but only a small proportion of patients have clearly benefited. A 'cocktail' of cofactors of the mitochondrial respiratory chain, including co-enzyme Q10, thiamine, riboflavin, vitamin C and vitamin K are usually trialled.

Congenital disorders of glycosylation

This group of disorders is being increasingly recognized and delineated. Glycoproteins are those proteins that require the attachment of specific sugars for their function. Clinical presentations include multiorgan failure, neuropathies, strabismus, dysmorphic features (facial changes, inverted nipples, fat pads), coagulation disorders, cardiomyopathy, ataxia, psychomotor retardation, strokelike episodes, gastrointestinal symptoms and hormonal disorders. Cerebellar hypoplasia is found on cerebral imaging in the common type 1a form. Recently, mild forms have been identified in individuals who are able to participate in the open work force.

The disorders are grouped into type I (a–l) in which the assembly defect occurs mainly in the endoplasmic reticulum, and type II (a–e) in which the defect is mainly within the Golgi apparatus.

The most useful diagnostic test is to look for abnormalities in transferrin isoforms. Transferrin is a glycoprotein. The diagnosis is confirmed by enzyme analysis or DNA techniques.

Therapy is symptomatic for most forms. Mannose has been successful in the treatment of type 1b.

Peroxisomal disorders

Peroxisomes are subcellular organelles involved in the metabolism of many compounds including very-long-chain fatty acids, phytanic acid, etherlipids and bile acids. Disorders in this pathway often involve assembly problems and therefore affect all the enzymes that normally function within the peroxisomes. Children with these biogenesis defects usually present in infancy.

Profound hypotonia is a common problem but other features include seizures, cataracts, retinitis pigmentosa, liver disease, renal cysts and dysfunction, and dysmorphic features.

X-linked adrenoleukodystrophy (XALD) is the most common peroxisomal disorder in older children. It usually presents at 4–10 years of age with behavioural disturbances, motor problems, regression and adrenal insufficiency. It is rapidly progressive over a few years. A milder disorder of the same gene, adrenomyeloneuropathy (AMN), occurs later in life with spasticity and peripheral neuropathy as well as adrenal insufficiency. The adrenal insufficiency, Addison disease, may be the only symptom in some males. The different forms can all occur within the one family.

Clinical example

A 3-year-old girl, Roberta, presented to a general paediatrician because of her mother's concern regarding her gait. She had been seen by another paediatrician when she was aged 18 months. At that time an ataxic, broad-based gait had been noted but no cause had been found. Her gait had deteriorated and was associated with poor muscle bulk and low tone. There were no fasciculations. An MRI scan showed changes in the basal ganglia and posterior white matter. Her plasma lactate was 4.2 mmol/L (NR 0.7–2.5),the CSF lactate was 4 mmol/L (0.7–2.5) and the lactate:pyruvate ratio was 24 mol/mol (NR 10–16).

A disorder of the mitochondrial respiratory chain was confirmed by muscle and liver biopsies, which showed low complex IV activity. By age 3½ years Rebecca was unable to walk or crawl and was having swallowing difficulties. Following placement of a gastrostomy allowing improved nutrition, she became stronger but still could not walk. She remained mentally normal.

Table 10.5.1 Non-acute presentations of metabolic disorders

Sign	Common metabolic causes
Cataract	Galactosaemia, galactokinase deficiency, peroxisomal disorders, CDG
Cardiomyopathy	Respiratory chain disorders, CDG, carnitine deficiency, disorders of fatty acid oxidation
Strokes	Homocystinuria, CDG, MELAS
Retinal haemorrhages	Glutaric aciduria type 1
Retinitis pigmentosa	Peroxisomal disorders, NARP, CDG
Abnormal hair	Menke syndrome, argininosuccinic aciduria
Dislocated lenses	Homocystinuria, sulphite oxidase deficiency
Endocrine abnormalities	Respiratory chain defects, CDG
Liver failure	Galactosaemia, fructosaemia, tyrosinaemia type 1, mitochondrial respiratory chain disorders, neonatal haemochromatosis
Obstructive jaundice	Panhypopituitarism, peroxisomal disorders, alpha-1-antitrypsin deficiency
Renal cysts	Glutaric aciduria II, CDG, peroxisomal disorders
Dysmorphic face	Smith–Lemli–Opitz syndrome, peroxisomal disorders, CDG
Movement disorders	Mitochondrial respiratory chain, neurotransmitter disorders
CDG, congenital disorders of glycosylation.	

Bone marrow or stem cell transplantation remains the treatment of choice for XALD. The role of Lorenzo's oil in the treatment of this group of disorders remains unclear.

Table 10.5.1 lists other non-acute presentations of metabolic disorders.

Newborn screening

Newborn screening is performed from a blood sample collected onto a blotting paper at 2–4 days of age. Tests are performed to identify disorders that are difficult to recognize clinically and for which early treatment is beneficial. The first and most successful disorder so diagnosed is phenylketonuria (PKU). Prior to newborn screening, children with PKU were not diagnosed until they presented in childhood with intellectual impairment. With treatment in the neonatal period, intelligence is normal.

All Australian states and New Zealand screen for PKU, cystic fibrosis and hypothyroidism, and most screen for galactosaemia. A new form of screening based on tandem mass spectroscopy has commenced in all Australian states and this allows the diagnosis of organic acidaemias (e.g. methylmalonic acidaemia), aminoacidopathies (e.g. maple syrup urine disease) and disorders of fatty acid oxidation (e.g. MCAD) in addition to the above disorders. Trials have started for detection of lysosomal storage disorders by newborn screening and techniques for identifying other disorders, such as the peroxisomal disorders, are also being investigated. Congenital adrenal hyperplasia is also likely to be added to newborn screening protocols in the near future.

Phenylketonuria

Phenylketonuria is usually diagnosed by newborn screening. Untreated, it causes mental retardation, eczema and behavioural problems. It occurs in about 1 in 10 000 newborns and is an autosomal recessive disorder. It is due to a deficiency of the enzyme phenylalanine hydroxylase. About 1% of cases are due to a deficiency of the cofactor, tetrahydrobiopterin (BH_4). These are more severe, as BH_4 is a cofactor for two other enzymes in the neurotransmitter pathway.

Treatment is by a very restrictive low-protein diet that is essentially a vegan diet with some further restrictions and the need to weigh and measure all protein-containing food. This is supplemented by special amino acid formulas that lack phenylalanine and are boosted in tyrosine (e.g. XP Analog, XP Maxamaid, PKU gel, XP Maxamum, PKU Express, Easiphen and Phenex 1 and 2). Recently, a subgroup of patients with hyperphenylalaninaemia (a mild form of PKU) have been found to respond to high doses of BH$_4$.

Perimortem protocol

If the possibility of a metabolic disorder is considered in an infant or child who is terminal it is impor-

tant that arrangements are made to collect appropriate samples either before or as soon as possible after death (within 1–2 h but the sooner the better). This should be discussed with the parents before death (Ch. 10.4) and the parents must be allowed some time with their child after death before the procedure occurs.

Samples of blood (plasma and serum), CSF and urine should be collected and frozen. Muscle, liver and, if indicated, heart tissue should be collected. This is best achieved by a right upper quadrant incision taking liver tissue, rectus muscle and cardiac muscle. The tissue samples should be no greater than 1 cm^3 and should be wrapped in aluminium foil, labelled and put into dry ice until storage at −70°C. A small sample of each tissue should be collected into glyceraldehyde for electron microscopy.

PART 11

NEONATAL PROBLEMS

The newborn infant: stabilization and examination

B. A. Darlow

Dr Neil Campbell began this chapter in the 5th edition of this book, thus:

> Most babies are born at term gestation (37–42 weeks), following normal pregnancy and labour, and are healthy. Having a baby is for most people one of life's most joyous and enriching experiences. Health professionals should keep these matters in mind and be as unobtrusive as possible with medical interventions, remembering we are, in a way, privileged to share in this special experience.

Introduction

Currently, annually, approximately 255 000 babies are born in Australia and 57 000 in New Zealand. In both countries the average age of the mother having her first baby has been increasing in recent years and is now around 28 years. Approximately 92% of all births are at term (≥37 completed weeks gestation). Around 25% of all births are now by caesarean section, although in many other countries this figure is much lower.

It is worth being aware that the outcome from pregnancy in developed countries does not always conform to parental expectations:

- around 1 in 5 pregnancies end in an early miscarriage
- about 6–8% of infants are born preterm (<37 completed weeks)
- 1% of infants still die around the time of birth
- up to 5% of infants will have some form of birth defect.

Neonatal transition

Much of the adaptation of the fetus to life ex utero takes place over a few days and may bring to light congenital disorders. If the process is disrupted, serious disease may result.

Circulation

In utero there is high pulmonary vascular resistance such that only 10–15% of the cardiac output goes through the pulmonary circulation. Most of the cardiac output bypasses the lungs by flowing right to left across the foramen ovale or through the ductus arteriosus (Fig. 11.1.1). With the infant's first breath the pulmonary vascular resistance falls and blood flows to the lungs; with cord clamping the peripheral vascular resistance rises and the foramen ovale is kept shut; and with the rise in partial pressure of oxygen (P_aO_2) and withdrawal of prostaglandins produced by the fetoplacental unit, the ductus closes. In some babies with persistent pulmonary hypertension (PPHNB), these changes do not occur and there continues to be a right-to-left shunt at the atrium and ductus. Such infants are tachypnoeic and remain cyanosed.

Respiration

The fetal lungs are filled with fluid, which has been secreted by the pulmonary epithelium. There is a net outward movement of this fluid into the amniotic fluid with breathing movements during fetal life. Hormonal changes, including a rise in catecholamines, occurring with the onset of labour, lead to the reabsorption of some of this fluid from the alveolar sacs. Most remaining fluid is squeezed out of the lungs during passage of the chest through the birth canal (and can be seen as clear fluid around the nose and mouth at birth). With normal chest recoil the infant's lungs fill with air, surfactant is released from the type II pneumocytes, lowering surface tension in the alveoli, and the residual lung volume is established with the first few breaths. Infants born by caesarean section, prior to labour, are more likely to have retained lung fluid (transient tachypnoea of the newborn, see Ch. 11.3).

Temperature control

Newborn infants have a larger surface area compared with their weight than do adults and can

Normal foetal circulation

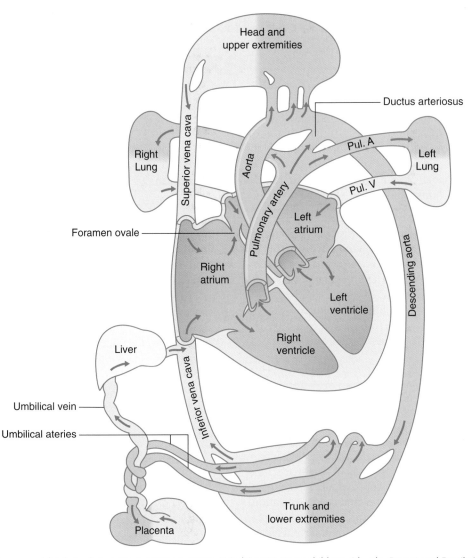

Fig. 11.1.1 The normal fetal circulation. From: Davies L, Mann M (eds) 2000 Heart children, 4th edn. Parent and Family Resource Centre Inc., Auckland.

become cold rapidly. They are wet at birth and lose heat through water evaporation, as well as via radiation, conduction and convection if not clothed. After birth, hormonal changes lead to heat production from non-shivering thermogenesis in the brown adipose tissue. Core temperature is normally maintained at 36.5–37°C. Hypothermia will increase oxygen consumption required for basal metabolism and is a not uncommon cause of tachypnoea (Ch. 11.3). Hypothermia may also occur in conditions such as sepsis.

Metabolism

The fetus is dependent on the maternal supply of glucose via the placenta and glycogen stores are laid down in the liver, muscle and heart as gestation increases. At birth the maternal glucose supply ceases and the infant's glucose levels fall over the next 1–2 hours before hormonal mechanisms bring about a rise from mobilized stores. Infants who have delay in feeding, preterm, growth retarded and sick infants, as well as infants of diabetic mothers are all at increased risk of significant hypoglycaemia (Ch. 11.2).

Fluid balance

The fetal urine contributes significantly to the amniotic fluid volume. The fetal urine is dilute and the placenta is responsible for fluid and electrolyte haemostasis. After birth a transition is made to water and salt conservation by the kidneys. In the first 2–3 days there is a negative sodium and fluid balance, contributing to much of the infant's weight loss, as well as a shift in fluid from the extracellular to the intracellular compartments.

Gastrointestinal

The fetus does swallow amniotic fluid, which is rich in growth factors. After birth, coordination of sucking and swallowing is readily established on day 1, and healthy term infants demand to feed from the breast eight or more times a day. Meconium should be passed by all infants by 48 hours of age. Before birth, unconjugated bilirubin is excreted by the placenta. During the transition to hepatic conjugation and excretion of bilirubin all infants have a raised serum bilirubin to some degree (Ch. 11.2). All newborn infants have low levels of vitamin-K-dependent clotting factors. Intrinsic vitamin K production follows bacterial colonization of the gut. This occurs in the first few days but the vitamin-K-deficiency state carries with it a risk of haemorrhage (see below).

Neonatal stabilization and resuscitation

More than 5 million neonatal deaths occur worldwide every year – with the World Health Organization estimating that 19% of these are from birth asphyxia. In developing countries, nearly 1 in 4 infants who fail to initiate and sustain breathing at birth will die. Yet easily acquired skills and simple equipment can help the majority of these babies.

It is estimated that 5–10% of newborns need some stimulation to breathe at birth. But population-based surveys in developed countries suggest that only 1–2% of term or near-term infants need active resuscitation with inflation breaths from a bag and mask. Only 20% of these (2 per 1000 births) progress to intubation.

Resuscitation of the newborn infant follows the same principles as resuscitation at other times (A, B, C, D: Airway, Breathing, Cardiac, Drugs). At the same time there are important differences resulting from the unique physiological changes associated with the infant's transition from in utero to ex utero existence, as well as pathological states presenting at birth. In most cases it is better to talk of neonatal stabilization rather than resuscitation, and delayed onset of respiration rather than birth asphyxia.

Advanced resuscitation skills can readily be learned with the aid of manikins and teaching scenarios. There are a number of different neonatal resuscitation guidelines and courses. Because neona-

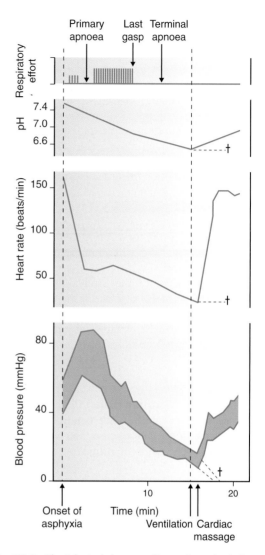

Fig. 11.1.2 Physiological changes after acute asphyxia in a newborn monkey. From: Roberton NRC 1968 A manual of neonatal intensive care, 2nd edn. Edward Arnold, London, and adapted from Dawes GS et al 1963 Journal of Physiology 169: 167–184.

tal resuscitation demands a team approach, it is essential to be familiar with local equipment and protocols.

Animal experiments carried out in the 1960s looked at the effects of acute, total asphyxia on heart rate and breathing (Fig. 11.1.2). At delivery by caesarean section (simply to control the situation), air breathing was totally prevented by occlusion of the airway. There was an initial period of gasping followed by cessation of breathing (*primary apnoea*), then a further period of gasping and finally no breathing (*terminal apnoea*).

Primary apnoea usually lasted for 1–2 minutes, with heart rate maintained at 80–120 bpm. It could

331

be prolonged by commonly used obstetric analgesic or anaesthetic agents. Simple tactile stimulation shortened the time to further gasping. In terminal apnoea, the time from the start of active resuscitation (ventilation) to further gasping and regular breathing reflected the degree of acidosis from asphyxia.

In the human situation, acute total asphyxia may always occur, although rarely, for example with shoulder dystocia and a tight cord around the neck (nuchal cord), abruption or cord accidents. However, most peripartum hypoxia is in the context of prolonged, partial insults and many of these can be predicted by the obstetric situation and fetal monitoring. At birth most such infants will not have progressed to terminal apnoea and will promptly respond to resuscitation.

Because the extent of the asphyxial insult will be reflected by the pH and lactate in the arterial cord blood, resulting from anaerobic metabolism, a segment of cord can be clamped at each end and sampled up to 20 minutes later.

Apgar scores

Since the 1950s the Apgar score (Table 11.1.1) has been used to assess the infant's condition at birth and to differentiate those who are vigorous or depressed. Many health jurisdictions require the Apgar score at 1 and 5 minutes to be recorded.

Historical note

Virginia Apgar was an American obstetric anaesthetist. Her score, based on the five signs typically used by anaesthetists to monitor their patients, was first published in 1953 as a method of assessing the effect of obstetrical and maternal anaesthetic management on the newborn.

There are many problems with the Apgar score:

- different observers will record slightly different scores
- there are clearly many routes to a score of 5 or 6 (for example) and both this and the infant's condition should be fully described
- vigorous infants should not be suctioned (as this may lead to vagus-induced bradycardia or even vocal cord occlusion) and so a score of 2 is awarded for 'reflex irritability' by inference. Such infants will all have scores of 9–10
- the score is much less satisfactory in very preterm or ventilated infants
- for an individual infant there is little correlation between the Apgar score and pH or lactate. And unfortunately neither are good at predicting the long-term outcome.

However, the 1-minute Apgar, if low, does indicate the need for stimulation, and the 5-minute Apgar indicates the response to earlier resuscitation.

Which births to attend?

All births do need someone capable of looking after the mother and a separate person capable of looking after the infant. Anyone involved in the practice of childbirth does have a duty to be competent in neonatal resuscitation and a responsibility to see that the appropriate equipment is available and in working order.

Resuscitators should become familiar with their equipment, or that provided in the health facility in which they practise. The main tools to deliver positive pressure ventilation, short of intubation, are self-inflating bags (Laerdal) or T-piece resuscitators (Neo-puff), and appropriate-sized face masks. The wearing of gloves is recommended.

Table 11.1.1 The Apgar score			
Score	0	1	2
A Appearance (colour)	Pale or blue	Body pink, extremities blue	Pink
P Pulse rate	Absent	<100	>100
G Grimace (reflex irritability, i.e. the response to nasal suction)	None	Some, e.g. grimace	Vigorous, cry
A Activity (tone)	Floppy	Some flexion	Good flexion
R Respiratory rate	Apnoeic	Irregular, weak	Active crying

Basic care and stabilization (Fig. 11.1.3)

- Check the maternal and obstetric history
- Anticipate problems
- Check the equipment: infant overhead warmer, oxygen supply, suction apparatus, bag and appropriate size masks and/or pressure device and T-piece, intubation equipment, umbilical catheter, drugs
- Start stop-watch when the infant's body is free from the mother
- Assess the infant rapidly; colour, tone, breathing and heart rate (use stethoscope on chest):
  1. *The infant is vigorous and crying.* Leave them alone (but dry and wrap, or place in skin-to-skin contact with mother)
  2. *Infant cyanosed, irregular respirations, HR > 100.* Gentle stimulation, gentle airway suction, check head in neutral position (avoid neck flexion and hyperextension) to open the airway. Most respond
  3. *Still inadequate respirations or apnoea, or HR <100 (30 s from birth).* Five slow (3 s) breaths then bag and mask at 40–60/min. Have pop-off valve or manometer set at 30 cm H_2O but probably lower pressures adequate. Check the response: should be visible chest movement and increase in HR.
  either
  4. *HR >100 and becoming pink, but inadequate respirations.* Has mother had pethidine injection in previous 2–3 hours? If yes, consider naloxone 0.25 ml of 0.4 mg/ml solution. Preferred route is via umbilical venous catheter (see below), i.m. may take several minutes to be effective (NB. Do not give naloxone to infant if mother is opioid-dependent)
  or

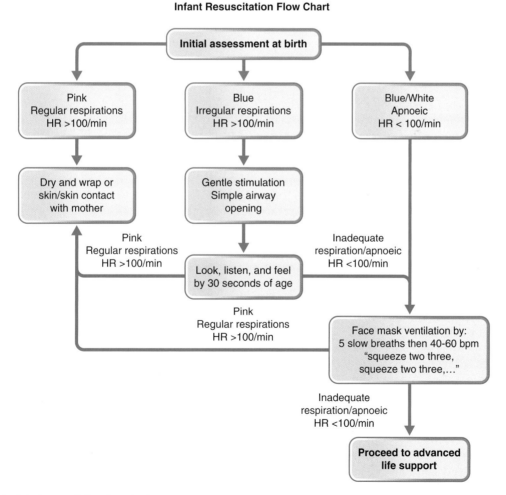

Infant Resuscitation Flow Chart

Fig. 11.1.3   Infant resuscitation flow chart.

5. *HR < 60 and not increasing, inadequate respirations or apnoea*. Proceed to *advanced* resuscitation:
   - intubate if skilled. Otherwise continue with bag and mask, check head in neutral position with jaw thrust, check chest movement and air entry. Call for help
   - give three cardiac compressions (see below) to one breath
   - consider drugs (ET or i.v. adrenaline (epinephrine))

Practical points

Neonatal resuscitation
- It is essential to be familiar with the equipment in the birthing location and with the local resuscitation protocols
- The vast majority of term or near-term infants do not need active resuscitation
- Apgar scores are useful to assess the infant's condition at birth but do not predict long-term outcome or the cause of any future disability
- Resuscitation with air is at least as good as 100% oxygen for term or near-term infants

Additional notes

Caesarean sections

The Royal Australasian College of Physicians (RACP) now recommends that paediatricians (or the designated person for neonatal resuscitation, such as a trained nurse practitioner) do not need to attend elective caesarean sections under regional anaesthesia, although, as with all births, there must be a person present whose role it is to care for the infant.

Chest compressions

Newborn infants generally experience bradycardia secondary to respiratory problems rather than primary cardiac arrest:

- it is essential that chest compressions follow a period of adequate lung inflation – which is generally the most effective
- chest compressions must not divert attention from ongoing lung inflation, or compromise adequate ventilation
- the correct method is with hands encircling the chest and thumbs on the lower third of the sternum, compressing about one-third of the depth of the chest
- one large survey of over 30 000 births suggested that only around 1 in 1000 infants 'need' cardiac compressions. It is likely that chest compressions are probably greatly overused.

Resuscitation in air or 100% O₂?

The time-honoured practice of using 100% oxygen in neonatal resuscitation has recently been challenged in a number of ways, including trials comparing resuscitation in air or 100% oxygen in term infants. A recent meta-analysis of these studies concluded that for term infants room air should be used for initial resuscitation with oxygen as backup if resuscitation fails. Exactly how to interpret these studies is uncertain but one message is that if oxygen is not available for a 'flat' baby, bagging with air is likely to lead to as good an outcome. Further studies may lead to new recommendations in the future.

Meconium exposure

Up to 10–20% of deliveries are accompanied by meconium-stained liquor:

- with delivery of the head it is possible to suction the mouth and the nose if the meconium is thick and particulate, although a recent study found no benefit from this practice
- following birth, if the infant is vigorous and crying, no further suctioning is required
- if the infant is floppy and has no or inadequate respirations, the upper airway should be aspirated under direct vision using a laryngoscope.

Umbilical vein cannulation

This is easy to achieve (Fig. 11.1.4). Place a cord tie around the cord to control any bleeding by tying tight. Cut the cord 1 cm from the skin. The vein is oval and flush with the cord; the two arteries usually project slightly from the surface. An umbilical catheter, or other sterile catheter, filled with 0.9% saline and attached to syringe, should be inserted 3–5 cm. There should be no obstruction.

Clinical example

Baby Aloisi was born at term following a ventouse-assisted delivery because of a delayed second stage. He cried briefly at birth but at 30 seconds there was noted to be clear fluid coming from both his nose and mouth, which was vigorously suctioned. The heart rate was the noted to fall to 80 bpm and he was apnoeic. The senior midwife immediately positioned the baby on his back with his head in a neutral position and pushed the jaw forward to make sure his airway was open. Baby Aloisi cried, his heart rate rose to 120 bpm and he became fully pink. He was placed on his mother's chest and covered to keep him warm.

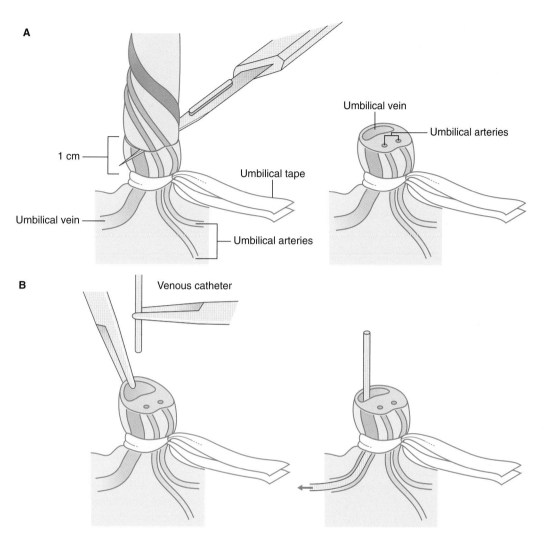

A

1 cm

Umbilical vein

Umbilical tape

Umbilical arteries

Umbilical vein

Umbilical arteries

B

Venous catheter

Fig. 11.1.4 **A** Applying cord tie and cutting cord 1 cm from skin, and view of umbilical vein and arteries. **B** Inserting catheter into umbilical vein (bottom pictures). From: Gomella TL (ed.) 1992 Neonatology, 2nd edn. Prentice-Hall International, New York. © The McGraw-Hill Companies, Inc.

Newborn examination

It takes time to get to know the range of normality and to feel comfortable examining newborn babies. New parents spend many hours looking at (examining) their offspring and may have concerns that are easily put to rest by a compassionate professional.

Purpose of newborn examination

- To check successful perinatal transition achieved and that the infant is healthy
- To screen for significant anomalies
- To establish baseline for further assessments (weight, length, head circumference)
- To address any parental concerns and provide reassurance

- To continue provision of health advice (e.g. supine sleeping, breast feeding, etc.).

Excellent comprehensive guidelines are to be found in textbooks of neonatology.

As in all medicine, the newborn examination must be seen in the context of medical history and family background. Some knowledge of family history, pre-pregnancy maternal history, obstetric history, details of this pregnancy (e.g. any antenatal scans) and birth must be elicited either from the notes and/or the mother. Patient-held obstetric notes greatly facilitate this process.

Who should do the examination?

Anyone with appropriate training: midwife, nurse practitioner, general practitioner, paediatrician or junior doctor as part of the paediatric team. Training will consist of some or all of tutorials, visual aids that can be reviewed repeatedly, observation of an experienced practitioner and fully observed examination by the student. It will still take some time to become fully familiar with the wide range of normality and people should not be shy of seeking another opinion *and* telling the parents this is being done and why.

When should it be done?

The traditional and still the ideal, if possible, is a three-tiered approach:

- a fairly quick examination at birth to establish the sex, identify major anomalies and to check that the infant is well and kept warm. Most newborns are alert and responsive for some time after birth and this is often a special time for new parents and their infant to get to know each other
- a full and thorough examination in the next 48 hours, in the presence of one or both parents
- a repeat examination sometime later in the first week to particularly check on feeding, weight gain or loss, jaundice and other aspects of the original exam.

This approach, however, is clearly tempered by early discharge policies and will depend to some extent on the place of birth and the domiciliary facilities, and will often mean there is one main examination in the first 24 hours.

Frequency of anomalies

Several series suggest that as many as 10–20% of newborn infants will have some anomaly, although the great majority are of no importance, with 1–1.5% of all infants having a more significant congenital anomaly. The difference between a normal phenotypic variation (common in the population and often familial, for example partial syndactyly of the second and third toes) and an anomaly occurring in less than 4% of the population may be a matter of definition. The presence of three or more minor anomalies greatly increases the risk of there also being a major malformation.

Whether born by vaginal delivery or caesarean section, around 3% of infants may have some form of birth trauma, such as bruising or a transient nerve palsy. Mostly this quickly resolves.

Outline of general examination

Ideally, the examination should be when the infant is quietly alert and the parents are present. Clarify

that the parents think their child is well or whether they have concerns. Usually a review of feeding and passage of urine and bowel motions, plus inquiry into mother's health, can establish rapport. The room should be warm and the lighting good.

Check that the infant has been weighed and the length and head circumference measured, and these values plotted on an appropriate centile chart.

Well infants have a minor objection to being undressed but settle easily. Unwell infants are often either unduly irritable or lethargic. Most infants have somewhat flexed limbs and spontaneous movements of all four limbs.

Check that the baby is not unduly pale. The hands and feet are sometimes rather blue but the tongue and mucous membranes should be pink. If there are any doubts as to cyanosis, check with a saturation monitor: healthy term infants should normally have a S_aO_2 of 95% or more.

Chest and heart

The *respiratory rate* is normally 40–60 breaths per minute and frequently somewhat irregular, faster and slower with brief pauses. Infants with respiratory distress have rapid and often regular breathing, and may have sub-costal recession and an expiratory grunt (Ch. 11.3).

Inspiratory stridor, more obvious when the infant is crying, is common and self-limiting and should be distinguished from inspiratory or expiratory stridor at rest or in the presence of other symptoms.

The *heart rate* varies from 90 to 160 or more with crying. Sinus arrhythmia and occasional ectopic beats are common. Feel the brachial and femoral pulses.

With coarctation of the aorta there may be absent femoral pulses, not always an easy thing to be sure about. If there any doubts, check the blood pressure in the arm and leg, a difference in pressure of 20 mmHg being significant for possible coarctation.

When the infant is quiet listen for *heart murmurs*. The chance of detecting a murmur will depend upon the timing of this examination, up to 50% of infants having a praecordial murmur within 6 hours from birth from ductal or other flow. Later in the first week the incidence of murmurs is closer to 1–2%. Although there are reported features that increase the probability that a murmur is innocent in the newborn (soft, grade 1–2/6 systolic murmur at left sternal edge, normal pulses and no other abnormalities) it is recognized that significant heart disease can occur with no murmur or seemingly innocent murmurs. If the murmur persists at a second examination within 24 hours, our policy, in common with others, is to carry out an echocardiogram; this is almost certainly cost-effective and greatly reassuring for parents.

Most examiners then generally prefer to carry out a top to toe method of review but take the opportunity to examine out of sequence as it arises. For example, if the infant cries then look in the mouth. Various reflexes can be elicited as the exam proceeds. The *Moro*, or startle, reflex is when the infant's head is lifted a few centimetres off the bed and then allowed to fall back suddenly on to the examiner's hand. In a normal Moro reflex the infant cries, the arms extend and then adduct across the chest. The Moro adds little to the rest of the examination, is upsetting for the infant and can usually be left out.

Look for the presence of any skin lesions or rashes.

A majority of infants will have faint pink lesions over the eyelids, temples, upper lip, nape of the neck or elsewhere on the face. These *capillary naevi*, also called salmon patches or stork marks, are benign and those on the front of the face nearly always fade completely.

Many infants also will have tiny white spots on the forehead, nose or cheeks. These are inclusion cysts in the epidermis called *milia*, and are of no consequence. Similar are small white to yellow papules from *sebaceous hyperplasia* on the nose and face.

Head and scalp

A *caput* is oedema over the presenting part of the scalp and will resolve in a day or two (Fig. 11.1.5).

A *cephalohaematoma* is a haemorrhage under the periosteum of a skull bone, most commonly the parietal, and so will not cross the suture lines. As this large bruise will organize from the margins it may feel firm at the edges with a soft, fluctuant, centre before fully resolving.

A *subgaleal haemorrhage*, bleeding into the scalp in the subaponeurotic space, is much rarer and more serious because significant hypovolaemia and anaemia can result. All the scalp feels boggy and loose.

There is often considerable *moulding* of the skull, i.e. movement of skull bones to allow passage through the birth canal, and sutures may be overriding but should move separately. A clear ridge over the suture, most commonly of the metopic (anterior part of the sagittal) suture, may indicate *craniosynostosis* or premature fusion and will need neurosurgical referral. The anterior fontanelle may vary hugely in size but should move with respirations and not be tense when the infant is quiet.

Face

Many syndromes have several minor anomalies affecting the facies (e.g. Down syndrome, fetal alcohol syndrome) (Ch. 10.3).

Facial asymmetry when the infant cries is most commonly a temporary facial palsy affecting eye closure caused by pressure on the facial nerve during delivery. There is lack of creasing by the nose and side of the mouth and lack of mouth movement on the side affected with crying. Function usually recovers within a few days but in a few cases the defect is more protracted. There may also be a congenital nerve palsy as opposed to trauma and isolated congenital hypoplasia of the depressor anguli oris muscle.

Elicit a rooting reflex by stroking the infant's cheek. The infant's suck can be assessed by letting him/her suck on a clean finger and the roof of the mouth can then be palpated for a submucous cleft.

Cleft lips and palate may be isolated or syndromic. *Pierre Robin* sequence comprises micrognathia and

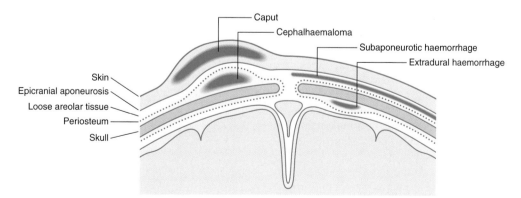

Fig. 11.1.5 Sites of extracranial and extradural haemorrhage in the newborn. From: Pape KE, Wigglesworth JS 1979 Haemorrhage, ischaemia and the perinatal brain. Clinics in Developmental Medicine Nos 69/70. Spastics International Medical Publications, London.

Caput
Cephalhaemaloma
Subaponeurotic haemorrhage
Extradural haemorrhage
Skin
Epicranial aponeurosis
Loose areolar tissue
Periosteum
Skull

cleft palate and requires careful assessment that the infant can protect his/her airway.

Mucus retention cysts of the gums are common and benign. Occasionally an infant will be born with a (natal) tooth present. These are loose and easily dislodged so should be removed.

Many infants open their eyes when sucking or may do so spontaneously. It should be easy to see that the infant focuses on the examiner's face (about 50 cm away) and can follow movement visually. *Subconjunctival haemorrhages* are common and resolve without problems. Elicit a normal red reflex with a small torch. An ophthalmoscope is needed to look for *cataracts* (most cannot be seen with the naked eye). Hold the ophthalmoscope about a foot away from the infant.

If the there are *sticky eyes* and the conjunctiva are red and swollen, an urgent Gram stain and culture are required to look for gonococcal ophthalmitis. Unilateral sticky eyes are more likely to be a bacterial infection, or blocked tear duct if no redness or swelling is present. Bilateral mildly sticky eyes with no redness is often a chlamydial infection and requires special swabs and a course of oral erythromycin.

Pre-auricular skin tags and pits are common and, together with more major aural defects, such as microtia, should mean the infant has a formal hearing test (see below).

Abdomen and genitalia

There is often *divarication of the rectus abdomini*, leading to a soft midline bulge above the umbilicus; this is normal.

Check the *umbilicus*. The cord separates by a process of low-grade inflammation over several days. In the past, various regimens, including anointing the stump every 4 hours with antiseptic or alcohol, have been used to try to minimize bacterial colonization. It is doubtful whether such practices are useful or necessary, and they may delay cord separation.

Feel for any *masses*. The liver edge is usually palpable 1–2 cm below the right costal margin. A spleen tip may be felt in normal babies and the lower pole of both kidneys may be felt on deep bimanual palpation. A distended bladder, such as with posterior valves, can be felt up to the umbilicus.

Bile-stained vomitus is always abnormal and urgent investigations and possible surgical referral are required (Ch. 11.5).

Ambiguous genitalia should have been detected in the labour ward. There are many causes and urgent investigations are required. The parents should be clearly told that it is not possible to tell whether their infant is a boy or a girl just now, and a phrase such as 'because the genitalia are immaturely formed' may be useful.

Hypospadias can be subtle and it may be necessary to see the infant micturate to detect the urethral opening.

Hydroceles, demonstrated by transillumination, are common and need no action. Other scrotal swellings and undescended or maldescended testes require surgical referral (Ch. 11.5).

The *foreskin* is not retractile in the newborn.

Tiny *epithelial pearls*, white papules, are common.

There is no medical indication for *circumcision* of the healthy male newborn.

Checking for *anal agenesis* requires parting the buttocks and fully examining the perineum. It is not uncommon to be fooled by observing some meconium on the perineum or the nappy if there is an associated fistula connected to the bowel.

Vaginal mucoid discharges are common; as is a small *vaginal bleed* in the first few days of life, which needs no treatment (but check that vitamin K has been given – see below). *Vaginal mucosa skin tags* are also common and benign.

Limbs

Extra digits may be parts of syndromes or isolated and sometimes familial.

Is there a *grasp reflex* on placing a finger in the open palm? A similar plantar reflex can be found by placing a finger on the sole of the foot.

Erb's palsy occurs in 1–2 per 1000 births, being more common following shoulder dystocia or instrumental deliveries. It is the most common brachial plexus injury and the arm is flaccid by the side or in a 'waiter's tip' position. Most are very transient, with improvement over a few days, otherwise physiotherapy is indicated. Sometimes there is also a *fractured clavicle*, usually detected by crepitus over the bone, but no specific treatment is required.

Infants who have been in a *breech presentation* with extended legs may sometimes still prefer to lie in this position after birth for a few days. For examination for congenital dislocation of the hip see Chapter 8.1.

Talipes calcaneovalgus with the dorsum of the foot pressed against the front of the shin is nearly always positional and the ankle can be moved through a full range of movements. *Talipes equinovarus* with the foot inverted is more likely to have restricted ankle movements and requires orthopaedic referral (Ch. 8.1). There may be associated or isolated *metatarsus varus* in which the forefoot is twisted relative to the heel.

Other

Check the infant's tone. Placed prone, the infant will lie with flexed limbs and can just move his/her head, at least to the midline. On pulling the infant up by the arms from supine there will be some flexion of the elbows and resistance and tone in the shoulders but quite marked head lag. On holding the infant in ventral suspension the hips and shoulders and head will raise up a little in contrast to the 'rag-doll' feel if there is significant hypotonia.

Check limb reflexes. One or two beats of clonus at the ankle on sudden dorsiflexion of the foot is normal.

The walking reflex consists of walking movements of the legs stimulated by the soles of the feet touching a surface when the baby is held vertical. It is not necessary to elicit this reflex if the baby otherwise appears normal, but it is often of great interest to parents.

Gestational age scoring. A time-honoured occupation of paediatricians has been estimation of gestational age but this is now rarely indicated (such as a concealed pregnancy):

- many more pregnancies have early ultrasound examinations that can confirm mother's dates
- the time of conception is not a fixed time from the first day of the last menstrual period so two infants of the same gestation may not be the same physiological maturity
- at best a Dubowitz or Ballard score will estimate the gestational age ±2 weeks.

There is little point in the exercise, fun though it is!

Clinical example

Baby Jane was born at term following a spontaneous vaginal delivery in a community hospital. Baby Jane's mother was 26 years old and had been well in this first pregnancy but smoked 10 cigarettes a day. A 19-week ultrasound scan agreed with her dates and showed normal growth and anatomy. The birthweight was 2780 g, length 48.5 cm and head circumference 30.2 cm. The birthweight plotted on the 3rd centile on appropriate growth charts and the length on the 10th centile, but the head circumference was not plotted. Baby Jane was thought to be well after birth, with normoglycaemia, and went home on day 3. On day 7, she was seen at home, when the domiciliary midwife plotted the head circumference and found it to be 4 cm below the 3rd centile. Baby Jane was immediately referred for a paediatric opinion and an MRI scan a few days later showed significant intracranial anomalies.

Common minor anomalies and debated importance

More recent series have confirmed earlier evidence that *simple sacral dimples or pits* are not markers for occult spinal dysraphism (such as a tethered cord or

dermal sinus). Simple sacral dimples are defined as less than 5 mm deep and less than 2.5 cm from the anus in the gluteal fold. Lesions outside these limits or if there are two or more cutaneous markers should be investigated by ultrasound (up to 2–3 months of age).

A *single umbilical artery* (SUA), detected antenatally or at the time of birth, occurs in about 1 in 200 infants and 1 in 5 of these have an associated malformation, which is often multiple and chromosomal. A recent review suggests that, if the SUA occurs without obvious associated anomalies, there will only be a very small yield from further investigation of the urinary tract, with the majority of findings being self-limiting conditions such as minor degrees of vesicoureteric reflux. Despite this, other authors do recommend a renal ultrasound scan if a SUA is detected.

Tongue tie (ankyloglossia), describes a short frenulum with relative tethering of the tongue, After many years of leaving such infants alone unless they have significant feeding difficulties or later speech problems, both rare, there has been a recent increase in recommendations that the tongue should be 'released'. The change seems to stem from lactation consultants believing the short frenulum may affect breastfeeding and lead to maternal pain from poor latching, views that have been supported by several small studies. If frenectomy is being considered, rather than a 'quick snip' at the cot side, there should be a surgical referral and appropriate anaesthesia and surgical technique.

Later examination

If there is a later examination at around 1 week or beyond, the focus is a little different. It will include a history of feeding and bowel movements, and measurement of weight gain. The five 'Hs' are:

- *Head.* Congenital hydrocephalus may now present with a full fontanelle, widened sutures and abnormally increasing head circumference

---

Practical points

Neonatal examination
- All infants must have a thorough examination within 48 hours of birth
- Clear and accurate records must be kept of all examinations
- The findings will to some extent depend upon the timing of the examination
- Weight, length and head circumference must be accurately recorded on an appropriate centile chart

- *Heart.* Some murmurs may now be apparent, or signs of heart failure (tachypnoea, hepatomegaly)
- *Hepar.* Jaundice may need assessment (Ch. 11.2)
- *Hips.* Another opportunity to examine for congenital dislocation of the hips (Ch. 8.1)
- *Hearing.* Does the baby hear, shown by a sudden quieting to his/her mother's voice or a rattle shaken out of view?

Other issues

Analgesia

Newborn infants may be subjected to a number of painful procedures, e.g. heel pricks, and have a right to effective analgesia. The RACP has issued recent comprehensive guidelines on this topic.

Use of a pacifier with 0.5–1.0 ml of 24% sucrose in 0.25 ml aliquots 2 minutes prior to venepuncture or heel pricks reduces discomfort from these. Some mothers may prefer to breastfeed and swaddle the baby during the procedure.

Vitamin K

Vitamin-K-deficiency bleeding is an uncommon but potentially fatal disorder that presents with spontaneous bruising or internal, including intracranial, haemorrhage. There are three recognized forms:

- *Early.* This is very rare, occurs on the first day of life, and is usually associated with maternal medication such as anticonvulsants
- *Classic.* Bleeding occurs from day 2–3 of life. Without vitamin K prophylaxis it may occur in 1 in 400 breastfed infants
- *Late.* Between 1 week and 6 months of age, almost exclusively in breastfed infants and often in association with unrecognized liver disease or malabsorption syndrome.

In both Australia and New Zealand a mixed micelle form of vitamin K is used (Konakion MM). The guidelines state that:

- the recommendations about vitamin K should be discussed with parents before the infant's birth
- the preferred route is intramuscular, 1 mg, following birth
- should parents not agree to an intramuscular injection (and most do), three oral doses of Konakion can be given over several weeks, although this may be less effective prevention.

Hearing screening

In the past, referrals for hearing tests have been based on a number of factors conferring increased risk, including congenital deafness in a close relative, malformations of face or ear, very low birth weight, high serum bilirubin (>340 µmol/l), hypoxic–ischaemic encephalopathy, bacterial meningitis, congenital infection with rubella or cytomegalovirus, or exposure to aminoglycosides. However, such criteria only detect a minority of affected infants and many countries, including Australia and New Zealand, are now moving to universal neonatal screening, with either otoacoustic emissions or automated auditory brain stem responses, or a combination of these tests.

Immunization

There is a high risk of vertical transmission of hepatitis B during delivery for mothers who are hepatitis B carriers (HBsAg-positive). The risk of the infant acquiring the virus remains high during the first 5 years of life. Infection in early life is associated with a high risk of chronic hepatitis (Ch. 20.5).

Infants born to such mothers should be given:

1. an early bath with 1% chlorhexidine obstetric cream to remove maternal blood and fluids

Within 12 hours of birth and as early as possible:

2. hepatitis B immunoglobulin 100 IU i.m.
3. hepatitis B vaccine i.m.

Metabolic screening

Following informed parental consent, all infants should have a heel prick performed at 48–72 hours of age for metabolic screening (commonly called the Guthrie card). Different diseases are screened for in the various states of Australia and in New Zealand but they usually include phenylketonuria, hypothyroidism and cystic fibrosis. The introduction of tandem mass spectrophotometry will mean that it will also be possible to screen for a range of other conditions (Ch. 10.5).

Normal infant matters

Weight

Normal infants lose up to 8% of their birth weight in the first 3–5 days and regain birth weight by 7–10 days.

Micturition

Normal infants often pass urine soon after birth, then infrequently for the next 24 hours. As feeding is established urine is passed more often, usually every 3–4 hours. Normal newborn urine is clear and colourless, although in the nappy there may be a pink colour from the presence of urates exposed to the air.

Bowel actions

20% of infants pass meconium before delivery or during the first 4 hours afterwards, 96% pass meconium by 24 hours and 99.9% by 48 hours. Failure to pass meconium by 48 hours is almost always abnormal and may indicate Hirschsprung disease, meconium plug syndrome or other bowel obstruction.

Vomiting

Small-volume (<5 ml) occasional vomits are common, as all infants have some degree of gastro-oesophageal reflux in the first week of life. 'Possets' are tiny 1–2 ml vomits. Larger, more frequent vomits may be a normal variation but also may be the first signs of illness, e.g. a bacterial infection. Vomits containing bile (which is green, not yellow) are almost always abnormal, strongly suggesting bowel obstruction, and should always be investigated even if other indicators of bowel obstruction (distension and constipation) are absent.

Waking, sleeping, crying

Normal infants are usually awake and active for 30 minutes or so after birth. Thereafter patterns of sleep, wakefulness and crying are extremely variable. On average, infants sleep for at least 18 hours a day in the first week, with sleep evenly distributed throughout the 24 hours. By 6 weeks of age most infants are sleeping more at night than during the day, and by 12 weeks of age much more sleep occurs at night. Acquisition of this circadian rhythm is clearly affected by various care practices, as well as by endogenous hormone production. Newborn infants also may cry for an average of 4 hours or more per 24 hours.

Newborn infants will look at objects within a focal distance of 20–45 cm and preferentially focus on the edges of objects, lines and shapes. They can distinguish the human face from other objects. They can hear and distinguish their mother's voice from other sounds. They have a sense of smell and can distinguish their mother's smell from others. They distinguish between several tastes. They move in characteristic ways to different rhythms of speech and they mimic adult facial movements, including tongue protrusion.

We attribute many human experiences, emotions and moods to newborn infants, and rightly so, but no one really knows what it is like to be a newborn. Health workers should strive to make this episode in life as rewarding as possible for infants and their parents. The rewards for health workers who achieve these goals are also great.

List of (normal) newborn topics in other chapters

- Breastfeeding and nutrition – Chapter 3.3
- General resuscitation – paediatric emergencies, Chapter 5.2
- Congenital dislocation of the hip – Chapter 8.1
- Surgical issues (e.g. hydroceles) – Chapters 9.1, 11.5 and 20.1
- Birth defects – Chapter 10.1
- Dysmorphic child – Chapter 10.3
- Newborn (metabolic) screening – Chapter 10.5
- Jaundice – Chapter 11.2
- Group B streptococcus and other infections – Chapter 11.4
- Antenatal pelvicaliceal dilatation – Chapter 18.1
- Skin disorders – Chapter 21.1
- Hearing screening – Chapter 22.1

Low birth weight, prematurity and jaundice in infancy

J. E. Harding

Principles of care

Care of the sick newborn is often complex and requires specialized training and equipment. However, remembering the basic principles will allow you to provide emergency care for the sick newborn, regardless of diagnosis, until specialized help is available:

• *Keep the baby pink*. Initial resuscitation should follow the usual ABC guidelines (Chs 5.1, 5.2 and 11.1). After that, many babies will maintain breathing with supplemental oxygen until more sophisticated respiratory support is available. The right amount of oxygen is the least amount that is needed to keep the baby pink
• *Keep the baby warm*. Cooling increases the baby's oxygen and glucose requirements and is associated with increased mortality. Dry the baby and put a hat on to reduce heat loss while you are assessing other problems. Use a radiant heater, electric blanket or incubator if available
• *Keep the baby fed.* Sick babies are at risk of hypoglycaemia, which can cause brain damage. If milk feeds are not possible, give intravenous 10% dextrose 60 ml/kg/d (2.5 ml/kg/h)
• *Consider infection*. Almost any signs and symptoms of illness in the newborn can be caused by infection, and untreated septicaemia can cause death within hours. If specialized care is likely to be delayed by more than an hour or two, take blood cultures if possible and give intravenous or intramuscular antibiotics.

Definitions

Babies are commonly classified into groups associated with different disease patterns and different outcomes (Fig. 11.2.1). These include:

• Gestation
  • term: ≥37 completed weeks gestation
  • preterm: <37 completed weeks gestation
  • post-term: >42 completed weeks gestation

• Birth weight
  • low birth weight (LBW): <2500 g
  • very low birth weight (VLBW): <1500 g
  • extremely low birth weight (ELBW): <1000 g
• Weight for gestational age
  • appropriate for gestation (AGA): birth weight between 10th and 90th centiles for gestation
  • small for gestational age (SGA): birth weight <10th centile for gestation
  • large for gestational age (LGA): birth weight >90th centile for gestation.

The premature infant

Causes of preterm birth

Although there are many risk factors for preterm birth (Table 11.2.1), approximately half of preterm births occur in the absence of recognized risk factors. Survival rates increase and the incidence and severity of complications all decrease with increasing gestational age and birth weight (Figs 11.2.2, 11.2.3, Table 11.2.2).

Short-term complications of prematurity

Respiratory

See also Chapter 11.3.

Respiratory distress syndrome
Respiratory distress syndrome is also called hyaline membrane disease or surfactant deficiency syndrome. Immaturity of the respiratory system with surfactant deficiency results in respiratory distress. This is managed with oxygen, nasal continuous positive airway pressure (NCPAP) or, when more severe, surfactant administration and mechanical ventilation. Corticosteroids given to the mother before preterm birth reduce the incidence and severity of respiratory distress syndrome.

Periodic breathing, apnoea of prematurity
Premature babies commonly experience periodic breathing due to immaturity of the respiratory centres of the brain. Cessation of breathing persisting

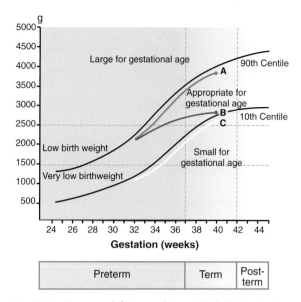

Fig. 11.2.1 Common definitions of size at birth, illustrating the difference between intrauterine growth restriction (IUGR) and small for gestational age (SGA). Baby A is an appropriately grown term baby. Baby B is also born appropriate size for gestational age (AGA), but has suffered reduced intrauterine growth compared to baby A and thus has intrauterine growth restriction (IUGR). Baby C has had normal intrauterine growth, but is born small for gestational age (SGA).

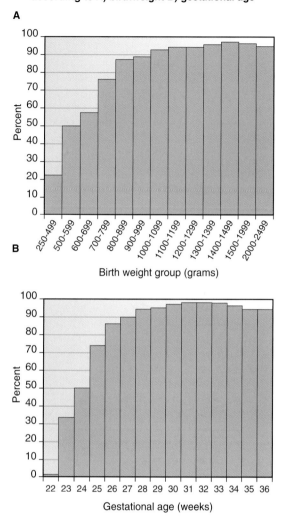

Fig. 11.2.2 Survival of preterm infants admitted to neonatal units according to (**A**) birthweight and (**B**) gestational age. Data from: Donoghue DA for the ANZNN 2004 The report of the Australian and New Zealand Neonatal Network, 2002. ANZNN, Sydney.

for more than 20 seconds is termed apnoea. This often results in bradycardia and desaturation, so premature babies require cardiorespiratory and pulse oximetry monitoring. Apnoea of prematurity occurs in almost all extremely premature babies and usually improves around 34–36 weeks postmenstrual age. Pharmacological treatment includes methylxanthines such as caffeine or theophylline, which improve diaphragmatic contraction and stimulate the respiratory centres. Nasal continuous positive airway pressure (NCPAP) is also helpful, partly by reducing any obstructive component to the apnoea and reducing the work of breathing. If apnoea is severe the baby may have to be ventilated mechanically. Apnoea can also be caused by many other complications of prematurity, such as infection, neurological problems, anaemia, hypoxia, patent ductus arteriosus and upper airway obstruction, so these need to be considered in babies experiencing apnoea.

Cardiac

Patent ductus arteriosus

Before birth the ductus arteriosus diverts blood from the right ventricle away from the lungs to the aorta. After birth it normally closes functionally within a few days. In premature babies, closure may be delayed, leading to left to right shunting of blood from the aorta through the ductus to the lungs. This results in pulmonary congestion, worsening lung disease and decreased blood flow to the gastrointestinal tract and brain. These changes have been implicated in the pathogenesis of necrotizing enterocolitis and intraventricular haemorrhage. A significant patent ductus arteriosus (PDA) is often clinically silent, or there may be a continuous heart murmur, hyperdynamic precordium, bounding pulses and widened pulse pressure. Diagnosis is made by echocardiogram. Treatment is by giving prostaglandin inhibitors (indomethacin or ibuprofen). If these are unsuccessful, surgical ligation may be necessary.

343

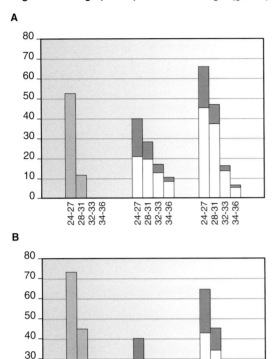

Frequency of complications of prematurity in babies admitted to neonatal units according to A gestational age (weeks) and B birth weight (grams)

A

B

Chronic Lung Disease — Intraventricular Haemorrhage — Retinopathy of Prematurity

■ 1-4 years   ■ 5-9 years   □ 10-14 years

Fig. 11.2.3 Frequency of complications of prematurity in babies admitted to neonatal units according to (**A**) gestational age (weeks) and (**B**) birth weight (grams). Data from: Donoghue DA for the ANZNN 2004 The report of the Australian and New Zealand Neonatal Network, 2002. ANZNN, Sydney.

Table 11.2.1   Risk factors associated with preterm birth

Maternal
- Previous preterm birth
- Extremes of maternal age
- Low prepregnant weight
- Acute illness, e.g. pyelonephritis
- Uterine anomalies
- Cervical incompetence
- Preeclampsia/eclampsia
- Prior miscarriage or termination of pregnancy
- History of infertility

Fetal
- Multiple gestation
- Fetal anomalies
- Polyhydramnios
- Fetal demise
- First trimester threatened abortion

Placenta and membranes
- Placenta praevia
- Abruptio placentae
- Premature rupture of membranes
- Chorioamnionitis

Social
- Low socioeconomic status
- Smoking
- Alcohol abuse
- Illicit drug abuse
- Heavy physical work
- Psychological stress

Neurological

Intraventricular haemorrhage
This is due to bleeding from the immature capillary bed of the germinal matrix lining the ventricles, often within the first 48 hours after birth. Risk factors include asphyxia and changes in cerebral blood flow due to hypotension or rapid intravenous fluid infusion. Intraventricular haemorrhage is diagnosed by cranial ultrasound and varies in severity from grade I intraventricular haemorrhage (germinal matrix haemorrhage) to grade IV (intraparenchymal haemorrhage). Although lower grades have a good prognosis, grades III and IV intraventricular haemorrhage are often associated with later hydrocephalus and neurological abnormalities such as cerebral palsy.

Periventricular leukomalacia
This is an uncommon problem, characterized by ischaemic necrosis of the white matter surrounding the lateral ventricles. Periventricular leukomalacia is diagnosed on head ultrasound, usually at 4–6 weeks of age. It often results in cerebral palsy.

Hepatic

Hypoglycaemia is common because of decreased glycogen stores and increased glucose requirements in premature babies.

Hyperglycaemia can also occur in VLBW babies because of high glucose infusion rates, reduced insulin secretion and impaired insulin sensitivity.

Hyperbilirubinaemia is common and due to hepatic immaturity coupled with a shorter half-life of red blood cells. Premature babies require treatment at

Table 11.2.2 Complications of preterm birth

	Common	Rare except in very low birth weight
Early		
Respiratory	Respiratory distress syndrome Apnoea	
Cardiac		Patent ductus arteriosus
Neurological		Periventricular haemorrhage Periventricular leukomalacia
Hepatic	Hypoglycaemia Hyperbilirubinaemia	Hyperglycaemia
Renal	Hyponatraemia	Hyperkalaemia Metabolic acidosis
Gastrointestinal	Feeding problems	Necrotizing enterocolitis
Other	Anaemia Infection Poor thermoregulation	
Late		
	Delayed growth	Retinopathy of prematurity Chronic lung disease Neurodevelopmental delay

lower bilirubin levels than term babies because their low albumin levels and immaturity of the blood–brain barrier place them at greater risk of bilirubin encephalopathy.

Renal

Immaturity of the kidneys results in a poor ability to concentrate or dilute the urine. This may be aggravated by immature skin leading to high insensible water losses, contributing to:

- *dehydration*
- *hyper-* and *hyponatraemia*
- *hyperkalaemia*
- *metabolic acidosis* due to inability to conserve bicarbonate.

Gastrointestinal

Necrotizing enterocolitis
This is an uncommon inflammatory process in the bowel wall that can lead to necrosis. Fluctuating gut blood flow, hypotension, hypoxia, infection and feeding practices have all been implicated but their exact contribution remains unclear. Presentation of necrotizing enterocolitis can be non-specific, including apnoea, bradycardia and temperature instability, then with more focal abdominal signs such as distension, tenderness, feed intolerance, bloody stools and bilious gastric aspirates. Occasionally there may be rapid progression to sepsis, shock and death. Classic X-ray findings are air in the bowel wall (pneumatosis

intestinalis) and perforation of the gut. Treatment is by withholding of feeds, antibiotics and, if necessary, surgery.

Feeding problems
Premature babies have weak and uncoordinated suck and swallow reflexes, delayed gastric emptying and immature gut motility. Feed intolerance and gastro-oesophageal reflux are common. Parenteral nutrition is usually required initially in extremely premature babies, with gradually increasing volumes of milk given by tube. Once full milk feeds are established, supplemental vitamins, minerals, protein and calories may also be required to allow adequate growth. Sucking feeds are usually established at 34–36 weeks postmenstrual age.

Haematological

Anaemia
Anaemia of prematurity is almost universal, as a result of low iron stores and red cell mass at birth, rapid growth, reduced erythropoiesis and decreased survival of red blood cells, aggravated by repeated blood sampling. Treatment is supportive with transfusion in the early period, iron supplementation and sometimes erythropoietin.

Immunological

Infection
Premature babies have increased susceptibility to infection due to impaired cell-mediated immunity

and reduced concentrations of complement and immunoglobulins, together with exposure to invasive procedures and monitoring. Signs of sepsis are extremely non-specific, including lethargy, temperature instability, apnoea, tachypnoea, feed intolerance and jaundice. Investigation usually requires a full blood count, blood culture, chest X-ray, bladder tap urine and lumbar puncture. Because deterioration can be rapid, early treatment with antibiotics is essential pending culture results.

Thermoregulation

This is a significant problem in the premature baby due to a relatively large body surface area, thin skin and subcutaneous tissues and lack of a keratinized epidermal barrier.

Late-onset complications of prematurity

Retinopathy of prematurity

Retinopathy of prematurity (ROP) results from disruption of the normal process of vascularization of the retina, with new vessel formation and fibrous scarring. Although ROP can result from excessive oxygen exposure, most cases occur in extremely premature babies with multiple other problems even when oxygen monitoring has been meticulous. Severity is classified on the basis of the location and extent of ROP, from grade 1 (mild changes) to grade 4 (retinal detachment). Most mild ROP regresses spontaneously; however, regular eye examinations are required to detect progressive ROP requiring laser therapy to reduce the chances of myopia and blindness.

Chronic lung disease

This is usually defined as the need for supplemental oxygen at 36 weeks postmenstrual age. It results from a combination of lung immaturity, oxygen toxicity, barotrauma, volutrauma, inflammatory and free-radical-mediated lung injury. Babies with chronic lung disease may require supplemental oxygen for months or even years, and are at increased risk of respiratory infections in the first year and adverse developmental outcome.

Growth

Because premature babies often do not grow for 2–3 weeks after birth, most are still below birth centiles at discharge; however, steady catch up growth is usual during the first 2 years of life. Permanent growth failure is more likely in premature babies who were also small for gestational age.

Neurodevelopmental impairments

Severe impairments (cerebral palsy, mental retardation, blindness, deafness) occur in 10–15% of VLBW babies. More subtle delays in language, attention deficits and social/behavioural difficulties are common. Regular developmental assessment is recommended for all VLBW babies.

Growth and developmental expectations

Growth according to centiles and developmental achievements are usually corrected for prematurity up until the end of the first year of life.

Immunizations

Immunizations should be administered according to the baby's chronological age and the timing should not be adjusted for prematurity.

Small for gestational age

Terminology

Smallness for gestational age (SGA) is usually defined as birth weight below 10th centile for gestation. The distinction between SGA babies and those with intrauterine growth restriction (IUGR) would be useful but is difficult to make clinically (Fig. 11.2.1). SGA is measured by birth weight because this is easy and accurate, but babies with IUGR suffer a variety of complications even if birth weight is in the normal range. Similarly, some SGA babies are small normal babies; for example, the small infant of a small mother in some ethnic groups. This problem is reduced by the use of centile charts specific for the relevant population.

Causes and complications

It is useful to think of the causes and complications of SGA in two main groups (Table 11.2.3):

• *Intrinsic fetal problems*: altered fetal potential for growth, such as chromosomal anomalies, intrauterine infection and congenital anomalies. Management and outcome in this group depend on the underlying cause
• *Extrinsic problems in fetal supply*: the baby is undernourished in utero as a result of factors limiting nutrient supply at one or more places along the fetal supply line. Complications and outcome can be thought of as those of intrauterine starvation (Table 11.2.4).

However, in a large proportion of cases (perhaps 30%), no cause is identified.

Treatment

No specific treatments have been shown to improve growth before or after birth. Treatment is directed to preventing and managing complications (Table 11.2.2).

Prognosis

• *General*. Prognosis depends on the cause of growth restriction. For the intrinsic group, outcome is that of the underlying problem. For the extrinsic group, outcome depends on severity and time of onset of the growth restriction. In general, the earlier the onset in gestation and the more severe the growth restriction, the greater the likelihood of permanent growth and developmental problems.

• *Growth*. Most SGA babies catch up in the first 6 months after birth. However, babies born short tend to remain short, and account for approximately 20% of short adults.

• *Neurodevelopment*. If growth restriction is of late onset and head size is normal, outcome may be good. However, many of the complications of growth restriction impair developmental outcome, and on average performance is reduced (Table 11.2.2).

• *Adult disease*. Babies born small are at increased risk of a number of chronic diseases in adulthood, particularly coronary heart disease, stroke, hypertension and non-insulin-dependent diabetes. This is thought to be because fetal adaptations to under-nutrition in utero result in both small size at birth and permanent resetting of homeostatic mechanisms (programming) that increase risk of later disease (the developmental origins of adult disease or Barker hypothesis).

Jaundice

See also Chapter 20.5.

Jaundice is the visible yellow coloration of the skin due to elevated bilirubin levels. It is extremely common, affecting approximately 50% of all new-borns. In most babies jaundice is physiological. However, it should always be taken seriously, as it is a common sign of illness, and at high levels bilirubin can cause permanent brain damage (kernicterus).

Bilirubin synthesis

Bilirubin is derived from haemoglobin, and to a lesser degree from myoglobin and the cytochromes.

Table 11.2.3 Causes of being small for gestational age
Intrinsic: altered growth potential
• Chromosomal
• Congenital anomalies
• Dysmorphic syndromes
• Congenital infections
Extrinsic: reduced fetal nutrient supply
• Reduced substrates in maternal blood (e.g. severe maternal undernutrition, eating disorders, chronic illness)
• Reduced uterine blood flow (e.g. hypertension, renovascular disease, vigorous exercise)
• Reduced placental transfer of substrates to the fetus (e.g. placental infarcts, abruption)
• Factors acting at all these points (e.g. drugs, smoking, alcohol)

Table 11.2.4 Pathophysiology of intrauterine growth restriction

Fetal nutrient limitation	Consequences for the fetus	Possible clinical consequences for the newborn	Long-term consequences
Reduced supply of glucose	Reduced body fat Reduced glycogen stores	Hypothermia Hypoglycaemia	Increased mortality Neurological damage
Reduced supply of oxygen	Stillbirth Asphyxia Increased haematopoiesis Redistributed cardiac output Cardiac failure	Meconium aspiration Hypoxic ischaemic encephalopathy Coagulopathy Polycythaemia Jaundice Relatively big head (head-sparing) Pulmonary haemorrhage	Neurological damage
Reduced supply of amino acids	Impaired immune function Delayed bone maturation Reduced muscle mass	Infection Hypocalcaemia Insulin resistance	Poor growth

347

These haeme proteins are oxidized in the reticuloen-dothelial system to form biliverdin and then *unconjugated bilirubin*. Because unconjugated bilirubin is not water-soluble, most of it circulates bound to albumin. Circulating bilirubin is taken up by the liver, bound to intracellular proteins Y and Z and conjugated in the endoplasmic reticulum by the enzyme glucuronyl transferase to form bilirubin mono- and diglucuronides. *Conjugated bilirubin* is excreted via the biliary tree into the gastrointestinal tract and then into the faeces. However, some of the conjugated bilirubin is converted back to unconjugated bilirubin and is reabsorbed into the circulation by a process known as *enterohepatic circulation.*

Evaluation of jaundice

Jaundice usually becomes visible at serum bilirubin levels of 85–120 mmol/l; however, the depth of jaundice is an extremely unreliable guide to the bilirubin level. Unconjugated hyperbilirubinaemia is the most common type and can be physiological or pathological. Conjugated hyperbilirubinaemia, defined as a serum conjugated bilirubin above 35 mmol/l, always requires urgent evaluation (Ch. 20.5).

The extent of evaluation required in a jaundiced baby depends on the wellness of the baby and the pattern of jaundice (Fig. 11.2.4). As a minimum, all jaundiced babies should have a history taken, physical examination and measurement of the serum bilirubin level.

History

• *Family history*: previous sibling, other family members with jaundice (hereditary causes?)
• *Maternal history*: history of splenectomy, haemolytic anaemia, gallstones, blood type

• *Pregnancy history*: gestational diabetes, illnesses (polycythaemia, infections?)
• *Delivery history*: type of delivery (forceps, vacuum extraction, trauma?), medications, length of rupture of membranes (sepsis?), delay in cord clamping (polycythaemia?), Apgar score (asphyxia?)
• *Newborn history*: feeding history (dehydration, starvation?) stool pattern (Hirschsprung disease?), vomiting (intestinal obstruction, pyloric stenosis?)

Physical examination

• *Measurements*: small for gestational age or infant of a diabetic mother (polycythaemia?)
• *Colour*: plethora (polycythaemia?) pallor (anaemia?)
• *Wellness*: activity, tone, cry (sepsis?)
• *Presence of bruising*, petechiae, cephalhaematoma
• *Umbilical cord*: infection or umbilical hernia (hypothyroidism?)
• *Hepatosplenomegaly* (haemolysis, intrauterine infection?)
• *Neurological examination*: evidence of bilirubin encephalopathy

Laboratory evaluation

Early jaundice (<24 hours of age)

Always pathological.
 Evaluate for haemolysis and sepsis:

• Full blood count
• Maternal and infant blood type
• Coombs test
• Assess risk for hereditary haemolytic diseases
• Consider cultures for infection.

Jaundice at more than 24 hours of age

Is it physiological? (Normal history and examination, normal pattern of jaundice.)

• Monitor, no further investigations.

Not definitely physiological?

• Assess for haemolysis and sepsis as above
• Assess feeding and weight gain/loss
• Assess for gastrointestinal obstruction.
• Urinalysis for reducing substances (galactosaemia).

Persistent or late jaundice (>1 week in term baby, >2 weeks in preterm baby)

• Confirm bilirubin is unconjugated (conjugated requires immediate investigation)
• Breast milk jaundice?
• Thyroid function tests
• Liver function tests.

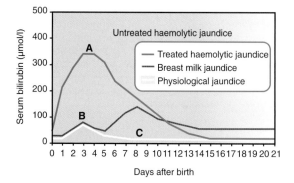

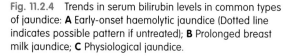

Fig. 11.2.4 Trends in serum bilirubin levels in common types of jaundice: **A** Early-onset haemolytic jaundice (Dotted line indicates possible pattern if untreated); **B** Prolonged breast milk jaundice; **C** Physiological jaundice.

Physiological jaundice

Physiological jaundice begins after 24 hours of age, peaks on approximately day 3 and resolves around the end of the first week (Fig. 11.2.4). It is unconjugated and caused by a number of factors, including increased bilirubin load and impaired excretion (Table 11.2.5). The infant is healthy with a relatively slow rise in serum bilirubin (<85 mmol/d), which does not generally exceed 250 mmol/l. In the premature baby the bilirubin peaks towards the end of the first week and resolves in the second week.

Physiological jaundice is a diagnosis of exclusion. In a well baby whose jaundice is following the predicted course, no further investigation or treatment is required; however, any signs of illness in the baby or alterations in the pattern of jaundice require immediate investigation.

Breast milk jaundice

Breast milk jaundice is a prolonged unconjugated hyperbilirubinaemia common in breastfed babies. The jaundice peaks in the second week but resolves only very slowly and may last up to 3 months (Fig. 11.2.4). The infant is healthy and thriving. Breast milk jaundice is thought to be due to factors in breast milk that cause increased enteric absorption of bilirubin.

Diagnosis is based on the pattern of jaundice and wellness of the baby. As for any prolonged jaundice, conjugated hyperbilirubinaemia must be excluded. The diagnosis can be confirmed by improvement of the jaundice on temporary interruption of breastfeeding, but this is rarely required.

Pathological unconjugated jaundice

Haemolysis

The onset of jaundice before 24 hours of life is always pathological and usually caused by haemolysis (Table 11.2.6). Haemolytic jaundice is most commonly immune-mediated and due to blood group incompatibilities, such as ABO and rhesus incompatibility. If investigations for immune-mediated haemolysis are negative then further investigations are necessary to determine whether haemolysis is due to other causes such as glucose-6-phosphate dehydrogenase (G6PD) deficiency, an X-linked disorder seen in Mediterranean and Asian ethnic groups, or hereditary sphcrocytosis, an autosomal dominant disorder affecting the cell membrane.

Non-haemolytic jaundice

Unconjugated hyperbilirubinaemia can be caused by increased production or decreased clearance of bilirubin, or sometimes by a combination of these factors (Table 11.2.7).

Complications of jaundice

Unconjugated bilirubin is lipid-soluble, so can cross cell membranes and is toxic to cells, especially the brain. *Kernicterus* is a term used to describe the yellow staining of the brain and the associated neuronal death seen on histology. The cerebellum, basal ganglia and cranial nerve nuclei tend to be most severely affected. *Bilirubin encephalopathy* refers to the clinical manifestations of bilirubin injury to the central nervous system. These can include abnormalities

---

Table 11.2.5 Causes of physiological jaundice
Increased bilirubin load
• Increased red blood cell volume
• Decreased red blood cell survival
• Increased enterohepatic circulation
Defective hepatic uptake
• Low levels of protein Y, protein Z
• Relative hepatic uptake deficiency
Defective bilirubin conjugation
• Decreased synthesis and activity of glucuronyl transferase
Defective bilirubin excretion
• Higher concentration of β-glucuronidase in intestinal mucosa increasing bilirubin breakdown
• More alkaline pH in proximal small intestine causing breakdown of conjugated bilirubin
• Lack of intestinal flora

Table 11.2.6 Causes of haemolytic jaundice
Immune mediated
• ABO incompatibility
• Rhesus disease
• Minor blood group incompatibilities
• Drug induced
• Maternal autoimmune haemolysis
Acquired, non-immune
• Congenital intrauterine infection
• Bacterial sepsis
Hereditary
• *Membrane defects*: hereditary spherocytosis, elliptocytosis, and others
• *Enzyme abnormalities*: G6PD deficiency, pyruvate kinase deficiency
Haemoglobinopathies

Table 11.2.7 Other causes of unconjugated hyperbilirubinemia

Increased haem load
- Haemorrhage
  - Haematoma (especially cephalohematoma), pulmonary haemorrhage, cerebral haemorrhage, birth trauma, occult
- Polycythaemia
- Swallowed blood

Increased enterohepatic circulation
- Bowel obstruction or ileus
- Pyloric stenosis

Impaired hepatic uptake and conjugation
- Inborn errors of bilirubin metabolism
  - Non-haemolytic inherited disorders: type I, type II, Gilbert disease
  - Metabolic disease: galactosaemia, tyrosinosis, hypermethionaemia
- Endocrine
  - Hypothyroidism, hypopituitarism, drugs
- Inhibitors
  - Lucey–Driscoll syndrome, breast milk

Mixed
- Asphyxia
- Prematurity
- Sepsis
- Infants of diabetic mothers

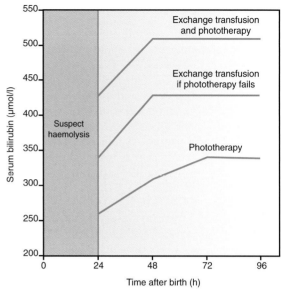

Fig. 11.2.5 Example of nomogram for treatment of jaundice in healthy term infants.

of muscle tone, lethargy, seizures, opisthotonus (arching of back), cerebral palsy and deafness. The risk of brain damage can be increased by:

- high serum unconjugated bilirubin concentration
- reduced binding of bilirubin to albumin, due to prematurity with low serum albumin concentrations, acidosis and displacement of bilirubin by fatty acids (e.g. intralipid) or certain drugs
- impairment of the blood–brain barrier due to prematurity, asphyxia, meningitis.

Treatment of jaundice

The aim of treatment is to prevent encephalopathy by reducing bilirubin levels.

- *General.* Ensure adequate calorie and fluid intake and adequate stool production to reduce enterohepatic circulation. Treat with antibiotics if sepsis is suspected
- *Phototherapy.* The baby is nursed under blue light at wavelengths of 450–460 nm. This transforms bilirubin near the skin into a water-soluble form through photoisomerization. Bilirubin can then be excreted

in the bile and urine. This is a safe, simple treatment, designed to avoid exchange transfusion
- *Exchange transfusion.* The baby's blood is replaced with donor blood in order to rapidly decrease the bilirubin levels. The procedure carries a small risk of morbidity and mortality and is now rarely undertaken.

The levels at which phototherapy and exchange transfusion are performed are usually determined using standard hospital nomograms. An example is illustrated in Figure 11.2.5. The threshold for treatment is lower if the infant is premature, asphyxiated, ill or haemolysing.

Intravenous immunoglobulin may be helpful in the treatment of immune-mediated haemolytic disease, probably by blocking the Fc receptors on the red blood cells and thereby inhibiting haemolysis.

Practical points

Jaundice
- History and physical examination – is the baby well and feeding?
- Jaundice on day one is not physiological – think haemolysis, sepsis
- Jaundice in the first week – baby well? pattern of jaundice appropriate? – think physiological jaundice
- Late jaundice – conjugated or unconjugated? Conjugated always requires investigation

Breathing problems arising in the newborn period

D. Tudehope

The establishment and maintenance of respiratory function is one of the most important features of the perinatal period. It is at this time that transition from dependence on placental function occurs.

Fetal circulation

During pregnancy, the fetal circulatory system works differently from after birth (Figs 11.3.1, 11.3.2):

- the fetus is connected by the umbilical cord to the placenta, the organ that develops and implants in the mother's uterus during pregnancy
- through the blood vessels in the umbilical cord, the fetus receives all the necessary nutrition, oxygen and life support from the mother through the placenta
- waste products and carbon dioxide from the fetus are sent back through the umbilical cord and placenta to the mother's circulation to be eliminated.

The placenta is a fetal organ with two major functions: transport and metabolism. Its transport role of gaseous exchange of oxygen and carbon dioxide, maintenance of acid–base status, diffusion of nutrients and excretion of waste products is essential for fetal homeostasis.

The fetal circulation consists of two umbilical arteries and an umbilical vein. Pulmonary blood flow is kept to a minimum by high pulmonary vascular resistance and three right-to-left shunts:

- ductus venosus shunts blood away from the liver from the umbilical vein to the inferior vena cava
- foramen ovale shunts oxygenated blood from right to left atrium
- ductus arteriosus protects the lungs against circulatory overload by shunting blood from the pulmonary artery to the aorta.

The fetal lungs are not used for gas exchange and breathing.

Cardiopulmonary adaptations for extrauterine life

- Removal of fetal lung fluid by expulsion into trachea and absorption into pulmonary capillaries and lymphatics and inflation of lung with air
- Extrauterine breathing is initiated by the bombardment of the baby with physical stimuli
- Decrease in pulmonary vascular resistance and increased pulmonary blood flow and drop in pulmonary, and right ventricular and atrial blood pressures
- Cessation of R $\rightarrow$ L shunting of blood and closure of fetal shunts.

Maladaptation at birth

Conditions that interfere with normal oxygenation and lung expansion after birth may delay the physiological drop in pulmonary vascular resistance. This results in persistence of the fetal circulation, leading to severe hypoxia and acidosis.

Other clinical sequelae of maladaptation at birth are:

- perinatal asphyxia
- excessive placental transfusion – hypervolaemia, polycythaemia, hyperviscosity
- transient tachypnoea of the newborn
- meconium aspiration syndrome
- respiratory distress syndrome
- patent ductus arteriosus.

Respiratory disorders in the newborn

Respiratory problems are perhaps the commonest of all disorders in the newborn period and present clinically in three different ways:

- respiratory distress
- upper airways obstruction
- apnoea and bradycardia.

Respiratory distress

Many infants exhibit transient signs of respiratory distress in the first hours after birth. Rarely, an infant with a life-threatening perinatal infection exhibits signs of respiratory distress at birth.

Fetal circulation

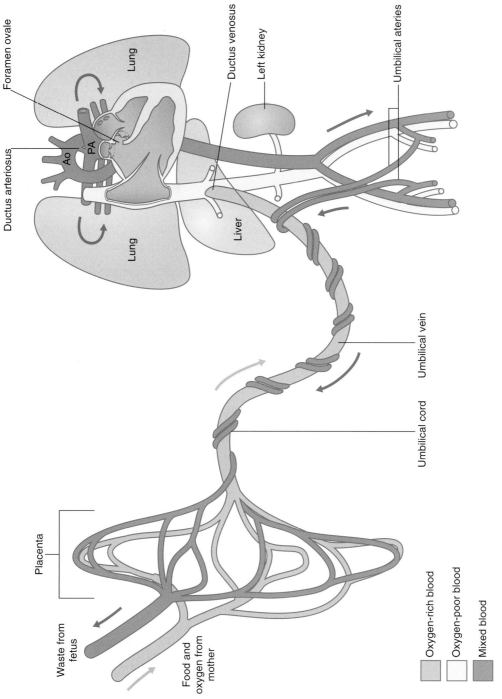

Foramen ovale

Lung

Ductus venosus

Left kidney

Umbilical ateries

Ductus arteriosus

Ao

PA

Lung

Liver

Umbilical vein

Umbilical cord

Placenta

Waste from fetus

Food and oxygen from mother

Oxygen-rich blood

Oxygen-poor blood

Mixed blood

Fig. 11.3.1 Placental–umbilical fetal circulation. Adapted with permission from: Levene M I, Tudehope D I, Thearle M J 2000 Essentials of neonatal medicine, 3rd edn. Blackwell Science, Oxford.

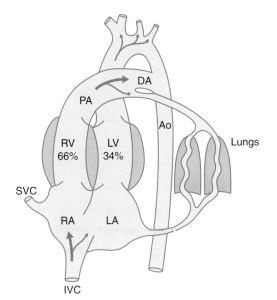

Fig. 11.3.2   Fetal heart.

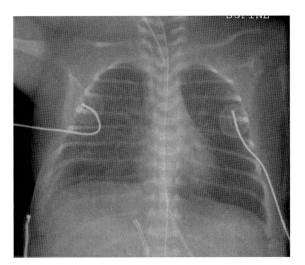

Fig. 11.3.3   Chest X-ray of transient tachypnoea of the newborn showing cardiomegaly, perihilar cuffing, fluid in the horizontal fissure and coarse streaking in the lungs.

Respiratory distress is the generic term used to describe the following clinical signs persisting for more than 4 hours:

- tachypnoea – respiratory rate in excess of 60 per minute
- chest retraction or recession – intercostal, subcostal, sternal or substernal
- cyanosis in room air – central
- flaring of ala nasae – use of accessory respiratory muscles
- expiratory grunt – particularly in preterm infants.

The specific diagnosis is made by taking an appropriate perinatal history, physical examination and investigations. The perinatal history should include gestational age, the presence of poly or oligohydramnios, anomalies detected on ultrasound, risk factors for sepsis, the passage of meconium, duration of membrane rupture and depression at birth. Investigations include:

- chest X-rays – anteroposterior and sometimes lateral films
- bacteriology – deep cultures: blood, urine, cerebrospinal fluid, gastric aspirate
- virological studies – nasopharyngeal aspirate, blood
- haematocrit and full blood count – ancillary evidence for sepsis
- chest transillumination with cold light source – diagnosis of pneumothorax
- passage of nasogastric catheters – diagnosis of choanal atresia, oesophageal atresia
- hyperoxia or nitrogen washout test – to distinguish cyanotic heart disease from respiratory disorders.

There are many causes of respiratory distress in the newborn.

Transient tachypnoea of the newborn

Retained fetal lung fluid occurs when either there is an excess of lung fluid or clearance mechanisms are inefficient.

- Benign disorder in 1–2% of newborn infants
- Onset of tachypnoea, cyanosis and grunt in first 1–3 hours
- Usually responds to 30–40% oxygen and settles in 24–48 hours but may persist for 3–5 days
- Term or near term infant, caesarean section, breech delivery, male sex, birth asphyxia, heavy maternal analgesia
- Chest X-ray reveals coarse streaking, fluid in fissures giving 'wet lung' appearance (Fig. 11.3.3)
- When managing an infant with suspected transient tachypnoea of the newborn observe for signs of clinical deterioration that suggest other diagnoses and fatigue.

Respiratory distress syndrome (RDS)

Epidemiology
The incidence and chances of survival are directly related to birth weight and gestational age (Table 11.3.1) and are affected by antenatal corticosteroid treatment and surfactant replacement therapy.

RDS, also known as hyaline membrane disease, is a specific entity in preterm infants; it is caused by a lack of surfactant (a surface tension lowering agent) in the alveoli. It has a characteristic clinical picture and chest X-ray shows hypoaeration, a diffuse granuloreticular pattern, air bronchograms and, in its most severe form, a diffuse 'white out' (Fig. 11.3.4).

353

Table 11.3.1 Incidence and survival rates for respiratory distress syndrome (RDS) in the intensive care nursery, Mater Mothers' Hospital, Brisbane, Australia 1996–2000

Birth weight (g)	Incidence of RDS (%)	Survival rate with RDS (%)	Gestational age (weeks)	Incidence of RDS (%)	Survival rate with RDS (%)
500–999	79	71	23–27	82	65
1000–1499	48	95	28–30	65	95
1500–1999	25	97	31–33	28	99
2000–2499	12	95	34–36	12	97
≥2500	Not available	99	≥37	Not available	96

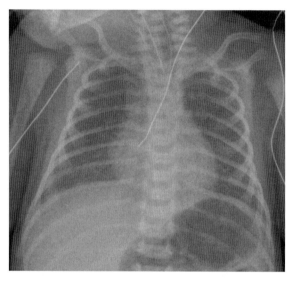

Fig. 11.3.4 Chest X-ray of respiratory distress syndrome with hypoaeration, air bronchograms and diffuse granuloreticular pattern – almost a 'white out'.

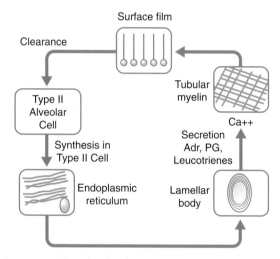

Fig. 11.3.5 Life cycle of surfactant.

Clinical features
- Diagnosed at birth or first 4 hours
- Signs of respiratory distress:
  - tachypnoea, cyanosis
  - nasal flaring, expiratory grunt
  - harsh, diminished breath sounds
- Oedema
- Apnoea
- Course of RDS:
  - classically increases for 24–72 hours, then baby has a diuresis and recovery is seen over the next 48–96 hours (Table 11.3.1)
  - if severe and requiring mechanical ventilation, slow recovery over weeks to months.

Pathophysiology
Surfactant is a phospholipid secreted by the type II alveolar cells of the fetal lung from about 28–32 weeks gestation. The major phospholipid is lecithin but other phospholipids and surfactant proteins A, B and C must be present for full activity (Fig. 11.3.5).

The action of surfactant can be understood by the La Place equation:

$$P = 2\gamma/r$$

where P = pressure, γ = surface tension and r = radius. The equation explains why, in the presence of high surface tension, large alveoli tend to get larger and small ones remain collapsed.

When the lungs of an infant who has survived for several hours are examined at autopsy, hyaline membranes are demonstrated lining respiratory bronchioles and alveolar ducts.

Prognosis
Acute, subacute and chronic complications are summarized in Table 11.3.2. The prognosis for RDS relates to severity and gestational age but has improved since the availability of exogenous surfactant.

Neurosensory disabilities may be divided into major handicaps (spasticity, posthaemorrhagic hydrocephalus, blindness, deafness, mental retardation) and minor handicaps (attention deficit/hyperactivity disorder, incoordination, speech and language delay).

Table 11.3.2 Complications of respiratory distress syndrome

Acute	Subacute	Chronic
Cardiopulmonary		
Perinatal asphyxia	Encephalopathy	Neurosensory disability
Pulmonary air leak	Consolidation/collapse	Bronchopulmonary dysplasia
Patent ductus arteriosus	Lung oedema	Sudden infant death syndrome
Pulmonary hypertension	Opportunistic infection	Subglottic stenosis
Pulmonary haemorrhage		Chronic obstructive pulmonary disease
Cerebral		
Cerebroventricular haemorrhage	Ventricular dilatation	Hydrocephalus
Periventricular leukomalacia	Cysts	Porencephaly
		Cerebral atrophy
Gastrointestinal tract		
Necrotizing enterocolitis	Bowel obstruction	Malabsorption

Clinical example

Baby Chyle was born by caesarean section to a 17-year-old single primigravida who had no antenatal care and who spontaneously ruptured her membranes at 29 weeks gestation. His mother was given one dose of betamethasone, in an attempt to accelerate fetal lung maturity but, despite an infusion of tocolytics, she delivered 4 hours later. At birth Chyle weighed 1250 g and had Apgar scores of 3 and 6 at 1 and 5 minutes of age.

Septic workup and full blood count were performed and Chyle was commenced on amoxicillin and gentamicin. Umbilical and venous catheters were inserted. Despite being commenced on nasal CPAP shortly after birth he developed early-onset respiratory distress with increasing work of breathing and oxygen requirements increased to 60% by 6 hours of age. After a premedication he was intubated with a 3.0 mm endotracheal tube and ventilated with synchronous intermittent positive pressure ventilation. Following the administration of exogenous surfactant at 7 and 13 hours his condition improved, with a diuresis at 48 hours and then extubation to nasal CPAP on day 4. He remained oxygen-dependent for a further 21 days.

Pneumonia

Presentation

Pneumonia in the newborn may be contracted in utero and be present at birth or during the first 48 hours of life (congenital), or acquired after birth (nosocomial).

In the presence of risk factors there is a high index of suspicion and low threshold for septic workup and antibiotic therapy.

Perinatal acquisition or congenital pneumonia

- Usually pulmonary component of severe, early septicaemic illness

- Often non-specific with lethargy, apnoea, bradycardia, temperature instability and feed intolerance
- Sometimes isolated neonatal pneumonia
- Often not easy to differentiate from other causes of respiratory distress such as RDS, transient tachypnoea of the newborn (TTN) and meconium aspiration syndrome.

Predisposing factors
- Prolonged rupture of membranes – group B beta-haemolytic streptococcus, Gram-negative bacilli
- Colonization; ascending infection; chorioamnionitis; fetal and neonatal infection
- Transplacental infection; group B beta-haemolytic streptococcus, *Listeria monocytogenes*
- Maternal bacteraemia.

Late-onset (usually nosocomial) pneumonia

Late-onset nosocomial infection occurs in ventilated infants who exhibit ventilatory deterioration, worsening chest X-ray, mucous plugging and increased secretions. Diagnosis is by isolation of pathogenic organisms cultured from endotracheal tube or nasopharyngeal aspirate and toxic full blood count.

Diagnosis
- Diminished air entry, increased crepitations, consolidation and effusions
- Chest X-ray essential for diagnosis but appearance often non specific. Lobar pneumonia rarely occurs, sometimes widespread diffuse or patchy coarse changes (Fig. 11.3.6).

Organisms
- Bacteria
  - Gram-negative bacilli (*Escherichia coli, Klebsiella* spp., *Pseudomonas* spp.)
  - Group B beta-haemolytic streptococcus
  - *Staphylococcus aureus*
  - *Listeria monocytogenes*

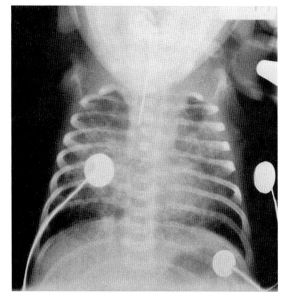

Fig. 11.3.6 Chest X-ray of group B streptococcus pneumonia, showing diffuse, coarse pulmonary opacification.

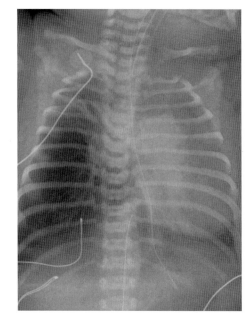

Fig. 11.3.7 Chest X-ray showing right tension pneumothorax with underlying pulmonary interstitial emphysema.

- Non-bacterial pathogens
  - *Chlamydia trachomatis*, *Ureaplasma urealyticum*, *Candida albicans*, *Pneumocystis jiroveci* (formerly *carinii*)
  - Viral pneumonitis is rare but may occur with cytomegalovirus, Coxsackie virus, respiratory syncytial virus and rubella.

Pulmonary air leaks

Pulmonary air leaks are more common in the neonatal period than at any other time of life. There are several types:

- *pneumothorax*: air in the pleural cavity
- *pneumomediastinum*: air in the mediastinum
- *pneumopericardium*: air in the pericardial space
- *pulmonary interstitial emphysema (PIE)*: air in the interstitial lung spaces
- *pneumoperitoneum*: air in the peritoneal cavity
- *air embolus*: air dissecting into pulmonary veins and disseminating through the bloodstream.

The pathophysiology of these conditions is similar, in that the alveoli become hyperinflated and rupture. Air escapes into the lung interstitium (PIE) or tracks along the perivascular spaces and ruptures into the mediastinum (pneumomediastinum), through the visceral pleura (pneumothorax) (Fig. 11.3.7) or rarely into the pericardial space (pneumopericardium).

Predisposing factors

- Spontaneous pneumothorax occurs in 1% of vaginal and 1.5% of caesarean section deliveries. Usually asymptomatic

- Active resuscitation at birth
- Other lung disorders – RDS, hyperinflated lungs, hypoplastic lungs, meconium aspiration syndrome, transient tachypnoea of the newborn.

Treatment of RDS with exogenous surfactant decreases the likelihood of a pulmonary air leak.

Presentation

- Respiratory distress
- Sudden deterioration with mediastinal shift to the opposite side, asymmetrical chest expansion, cardiorespiratory collapse
- Prominent sternum suggests pneumomediastinum.

Diagnosis

- Aided by chest transillumination with powerful cold light source
- Confirm by chest X-ray
- In an emergency, 'needle' aspiration and then drainage with an intercostal catheter

Meconium aspiration syndrome

- Meconium staining of liquor occurs in 10–15% of births, especially breech, post-term and fetal distress
- Staining may be mild, moderate or severe (with oligohydramnios)
- Aspiration into the lungs occurs within a few breaths of birth
- Once spontaneous respirations occur, meconium migrates into distal airways

Table 11.3.3   Interaction of clinical and pathological features of meconium aspiration syndrome

Fetal compromise	Neonate	Pathological effects	Complications
Fetal heart rate irregularity	Meconium-stained	Plugging → collapse	
→			
Meconium passage	Asphyxia →	→ Ball valve → pulmonary air leaks	Pulmonary hypertension
	Retained lung fluid	Irritant → pneumonitis; bacterial contamination	Encephalopathy

- Clinical and pathological features interact (Table 11.3.3)
- Decreased incidence relates to obstetric induction of labour to prevent post maturity
- Increased incidence with fetal distress, low Apgar scores and Pacific Islander or indigenous ethnicity (Table 11.3.3).

Chest X-ray reveals hyperinflated lungs with widespread, coarse pulmonary infiltrate and collapse (Fig. 11.3.8).

Presentation

- Severe birth asphyxia requiring active resuscitation
- Early onset of respiratory distress – often mild at first but worsening
- Infant covered in meconium with staining of cord, skin and nails
- Progressive respiratory failure with pulmonary hypertension.

Management

Morbidity and mortality from meconium aspiration syndrome can be prevented or minimized by optimal perinatal management. Treatment for established meconium aspiration syndrome is as for respiratory distress, with emphasis on humidification of inspired gases, postural drainage and airway suction, and antibiotics. Other management strategies include surfactant, paralysis with non-depolarizing muscle relaxant, inhaled nitric oxide, high-frequency oscillator ventilation and extracorporeal membrane oxygenation.

Pulmonary hypoplasia

Normal fetal lung development requires adequate amniotic fluid volume and fetal breathing movements. Although unilateral lung hypoplasia may be an isolated developmental anomaly, bilateral hypoplasia is secondary to other factors, such as:

- oligohydramnios, e.g. prolonged membrane rupture, severe renal disease; the baby may exhibit

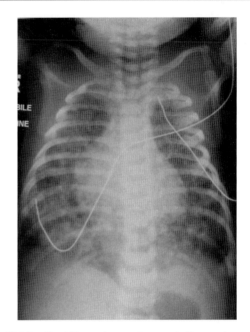

Fig. 11.3.8   Chest X-ray of meconium aspiration syndrome. Hyperinflated lungs with widespread coarse pulmonary infiltration.

additional features of Potter syndrome, with facial dysmorphism, joint contractures and amnion nodosum of the placenta
- decreased intrathoracic space, e.g. diaphragmatic hernia, hydrops fetalis, cystic adenomatoid malformation of the lung
- chest wall deformities, e.g. skeletal dysplasia.

Clinical features

- Progressive respiratory failure from birth, with marked hypoxia, hypercarbia and metabolic acidosis
- Pneumothorax is common
- Death, ventilator dependence or bronchopulmonary dysplasia may result.

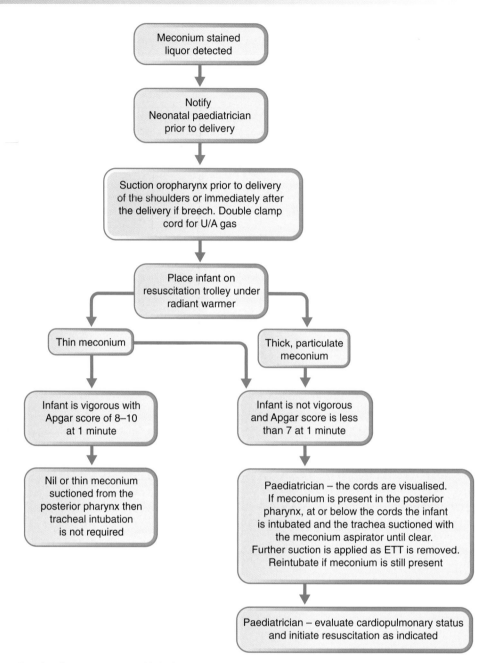

Fig. 11.3.9 Algorithm for management of baby born through meconium liquor.

Pulmonary haemorrhage

• Usual presentation is haemorrhagic pulmonary oedema coming up the endotracheal tube, compromising ventilation and resulting in cardiovascular collapse

• Complicates severe perinatal asphyxia, coagulation disturbances, severe intrauterine growth restriction, hypothermia or congenital heart disease and occasionally following exogenous surfactant therapy for RDS

• Additional treatment is required for shock, metabolic acidosis, coagulation disturbance, pulmonary oedema (furosemide/morphine) and positive end-expiratory pressure to splint lungs.

Pulmonary collapse

• Pulmonary collapse or atelectasis may be segmental or lobar, most commonly of the right upper lobe after extubation from ventilation (Fig. 11.3.10)

• It occurs after aspiration of meconium, blood or milk and is common following muscle paralysis for surgery and when an endotracheal tube is inadvertently pushed down into right main stem bronchus.

Clinical example

Andrew was born to a 38-year-old multigravid mother after induction of labour at 41 weeks' gestation. Continuous intrapartum fetal heart rate monitoring initially revealed type I decelerations, followed by type II decelerations, with thick meconium-stained liquor. A Neville Barnes forceps delivery under epidural anaesthesia was performed to deliver a 2.8 kg infant who was heavily meconium-stained. The obstetrician suctioned his airways as the head crowned. Apgar scores were 3 and 6 at 1 and 5 minutes, with an umbilical cord pH of 7.12, Po_2 15 mmHg and a base excess of –12.

The paediatrician suctioned meconium from the oropharynx and intubated the trachea on three occasions for suctioning of meconium with the aid of a meconium aspirator. There was early-onset respiratory distress requiring 40% head box oxygen. The chest X-ray revealed hyperinflation and some coarse opacification. Andrew responded well to active chest physiotherapy and humidified oxygen, and the respiratory distress, consistent with mild meconium aspiration, slowly abated during the next 4 days.

Clinical example

Mrs T's fetus was diagnosed as having a left diaphragmatic hernia on her routine ultrasound scan at 17 weeks gestation. Serial ultrasound examinations revealed progressive polyhydramnios, with a gastric shadow in the left chest and mediastinal displacement. Lucas was born at 36 weeks gestation after spontaneous rupture of membranes. He was in good condition at birth, with an Apgar score of 7 at 1 minute and an umbilical cord pH of 7.3, but there was rapid deterioration, with cyanosis and bradycardia.

An orogastric tube was passed and Lucas's stomach was aspirated. He did not receive bag and mask ventilation but was intubated at 1 minute of age and given positive pressure ventilation with 100% oxygen. He was paralysed with a muscle relaxant and commenced on an infusion of morphine. Intratracheal exogenous surfactant was given but inhaled nitric oxide did not improve oxygenation. Intravascular volume replacement and a dopamine infusion improved blood pressure and oxygenation. Corrective surgery was delayed until Lucas was more stable on day 6. After a stormy postoperative period he was finally extubated on day 16 but required continuous low-flow intranasal oxygen for 3 months and marked delay in achieving full oral feeding.

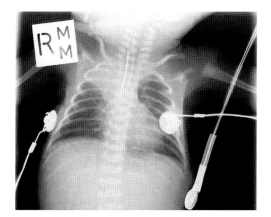

Fig. 11.3.10 Chest X-ray of right upper lobe collapse. Endotracheal tube located too far down trachea with associated right upper lobe collapse.

• Thick pulmonary secretions → mucous plugs → migratory pulmonary collapse
• Prevention is by adequate humidification, postural drainage, chest physiotherapy and exogenous surfactant therapy.

Congenital diaphragmatic hernia

See also Chapter 11.5.

Abdominal contents herniate through a muscular defect in the diaphragm into the chest. The incidence is 1 in 3800 births, with 60% isolated and 40% associated with other anomalies or chromosomal defects. The hernia is usually a posterolateral (Bochdalek) type with 85% occurring on the left side. The defect in the diaphragm permits bowel or liver (right-sided) to herniate into thorax with lung compression and pulmonary hypoplasia.

Clinical presentation

• Most cases are diagnosed by routine obstetric ultrasound at 17–19 weeks gestation or following investigation for polyhydramnios
• Typically rapidly progressive respiratory failure after birth
• Less acute cases present in the nursery with respiratory distress, dextrocardia or scaphoid abdomen.

Diagnosis

Diagnosis is confirmed by demonstration of bowel loops in the thorax on chest X-ray (Fig. 11.3.11).

Management

Management involves gastric decompression, cardiorespiratory support and avoidance of hypoxia. Surgical repair is typically delayed 3–7 days to enable maximum stabilization. Overall only 40–60% of children with an isolated lesion survive. All infants with other anomalies die.

Prognosis

Prognosis depends on age at presentation, degree of pulmonary hypoplasia, presence of polyhydramnios and development of persistent pulmonary hypertension.

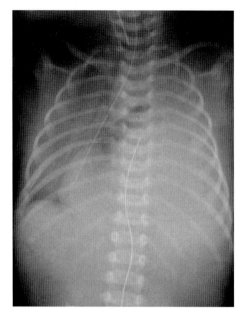

Fig. 11.3.11 Chest X-ray of left diaphragmatic hernia with mediastinal shift to the right and gas pattern within the thorax.

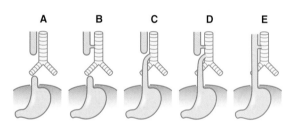

Fig. 11.3.12 Anatomical types of oesophageal atresia; 85% of all cases are type C.

Oesophageal atresia and tracheo-oesophageal fistula

See also Chapter 11.5.

With this congenital anomaly, there is usually complete interruption of the lumen of the oesophagus, resulting in a blind upper pouch. This generally is associated with a tracheo-oesophageal fistula. The various types are shown in Figure 11.3.12.

Maternal hydramnios occurs in 60% of cases and is largely responsible for the high frequency of premature births.

The outlook for oesophageal atresia is good but complications and sequelae from surgery are frequent. These include a brassy cough associated with coexistent tracheomalacia, oesophageal stricture, breakdown of anastomosis, recurrence of the tracheo-oesophageal fistula and gastro-oesophageal reflux. Preterm birth worsens prognosis.

Congenital lobar emphysema

- Rare anomaly due to cartilaginous deficiency in lobar bronchus (left upper lobe 50%, right middle lobe 24%, right upper lobe 18%)
- Insidious onset of respiratory distress over 2–3 weeks
- Hyperinflated lobe causes surrounding pulmonary collapse and mediastinal displacement
- Surgical lobectomy is usually curative
- Associated with congenital heart disease in 30% of cases.

Acquired lobar emphysema may be secondary to an extrinsic or intrinsic bronchial obstruction, such as a mucous plug.

Cystic adenomatoid malformation

Often diagnosed on antenatal ultrasound. Polyhydramnios, hydrops fetalis, prematurity or stillbirth may result. There are three types:

- type 1 (70%) – single or multiple large cysts in one lobe
- type 2 (18%) – multiple medium sized cysts
- type 3 (10%) – large cysts containing smaller cysts.

Differential diagnosis is from lobar emphysema, sequestration of lung and pulmonary lymphangiectasia. Surgical resection is usually curative.

Other lung diseases

Other disorders presenting in the newborn include sequestration of lung, pulmonary lymphangiectasia, lung cysts (especially bronchogenic), pleural/chylous effusions and eventration of the diaphragm.

Treatment of the neonate with respiratory distress

The supportive care of the infant with respiratory distress is similar regardless of aetiology.

Observation and monitoring

- Observation for colour, chest recession, expiratory grunt, flaring of ala nasae
- Continuous monitoring – heart rate, respiratory rate, skin temperature, blood pressure
- Fluid balance chart
- Thermoregulation in servocontrolled incubator (open or closed)
- Maintain mean BP >30 mmHg using volume expanders and inotropic support.

Oxygen

- Monitor percentage delivered continuously with analyser or use of O_2 blender. Monitor oxygenation continuously with pulse oximetry and transcutaneous $PO_2 + PCO_2$ monitor
- Warm to 36–37°C and humidify to 90–100%
- Delivery into head box (if >30%) or servocontrolled incubator
- Indwelling arterial catheter enables sampling for blood gas analysis and continuous BP monitoring.

Fluids

- Avoid oral feeding; gavage feed if mild respiratory distress
- Intravenous fluids and electrolytes (added after 24 hours) for moderate/severe distress
- Total parental nutrition after 72 hours of no feeding.

Venous/arterial access

- Reliable venous access is provided by insertion of umbilical venous catheter or peripheral intravenous central line
- Insertion of an umbilical or peripheral arterial line will facilitate blood sampling for analysis of blood gases and electrolytes and continuous blood pressure monitoring.

Acid–base balance

- Normal range of blood gases (Table 11.3.4)
- Metabolic acidosis – volume replacement, inotropic support, $NaHCO_3$
- Respiratory acidosis – pH < 7.20 and PCO_2 > 60 mmHg infant needs assisted ventilation.

Assisted ventilation

Assisted ventilation usually consists of continuous positive airway pressure (CPAP) via nasal prongs or face mask or mechanical ventilation (CPPV) via an endotracheal tube. Rarely ventilation is given non invasively via nasal prongs or a face mask. The need for assisted ventilation at birth is determined by condition at birth, birth weight and gestational age and whether mother received antenatal steroids.

An approach to assisted ventilation after birth is:

- 24–26 weeks gestation – intubation, CPPV and prophylactic exogenous surfactant
- 27–31 weeks gestation – CPAP for airway stabilization and careful monitoring and assessment if establishes adequate spontaneous (especially if antenatal steroids) respirations.

All infants – intubation, CPPV and surfactant if:

- F_iO_2 > 0.6 to maintain P_aO_2 > 60 mmHg
- moderate to severe apnoea
- marked chest retractions on CPAP with increasing oxygen requirements
- rising P_aCO_2 > 60 mmHg with pH < 7.20.

Techniques of mechanical ventilation vary between neonatal units and include intermittent mandatory ventilation, patient triggered ventilation, volume ventilation and high-frequency oscillation. Large infants often struggle or 'fight' the ventilator and benefit from analgesia and sedation or paralysis with a non-depolarizing muscle relaxant.

Surfactant replacement

Exogenous surfactant (natural, synthetic, partially synthetic) administered via endotracheal tube, both in prophylactic (infants < 30 weeks) and rescue modes, has resulted in a 40% reduction in mortality from RDS. Pulmonary air leaks have been dramatically reduced but not so bronchopulmonary dysplasia or patent ductus arteriosus. Exogenous surfactant may benefit selected infants with meconium aspiration, congenital pneumonia and congenital diaphragmatic hernia.

Management and prevention of infection

- Bacteriological investigation, which includes cultures of blood, tracheal and gastric aspirate, is essential before commencing antibiotics
- A penicillin (penicillin G or amoxicillin) and an aminoglycoside (gentamicin or tobramycin) are used when infection is suspected
- Prevention of infection involves meticulous hand washing for all procedures, the use of gloves for tracheal toilets and routine bacteriological surveillance and swabbing of all infants in intensive care nurseries
- Active chest physiotherapy may be required for pneumonia, collapsed segments of lungs and aspiration syndromes

Table 11.3.4 Normal ranges for arterial blood gases in term and preterm infants		
Parameter	Term	Preterm
PO_2 (mmHg)	60–90	50–80
PCO_2 (mmHg)	35–42	40–50
pH	7.35–7.42	7.30–7.40
Base excess (mmol/l)	−2 to 0	−4 to 0
Bicarbonate (mmol/l)	22–26	18–24

- All infants with respiratory distress require correct positioning with frequent changes to facilitate ventilation and lung drainage.

Specific treatment

- Tension pneumothorax: drainage with intercostal catheter
- Pleural/chylous effusion: thoracentesis or indwelling pleural drain
- Symptomatic polycythaemia (venous haematocrit >66%): dilutional exchange transfusion
- Diaphragmatic hernia, oesophageal atresia, lobar emphysema, choanal atresia, lung cysts, and sometimes Pierre Robin sequence require surgery.

Chronic neonatal lung disease

Two definitions of chronic neonatal lung disease (CNLD) are in common usage:
- preterm infant with parenchymal lung disease requiring increased inspired oxygen more than 28 days from birth
- preterm infant requiring increased or assisted ventilation beyond 36 weeks postmenstrual age.

In spite of the numerous advances in respiratory care of the preterm infant including antenatal steroids, exogenous surfactant therapy and refinements in assisted ventilation there has been minimal impact on the incidence of CNLD in surviving preterm infants.

Bronchopulmonary dysplasia

The classification of chronic neonatal lung disease is given in Table 11.3.5; the most common type is characteristically associated with the healing phase of severe RDS in extreme prematurity but it may complicate meconium aspiration, diaphragmatic hernia, apnoea or congenital pneumonia.

Clinical features

Wide spectrum of severity, from prolongation in plateau phase of wean from mechanical ventilation to failure to wean 24–28-week infant from O_2, to progressive respiratory failure and death.

Infants with bronchopulmonary dysplasia (BPD) have persistent chest retractions, gross lung hyperinflation, increased work of breathing, episodes of O_2 desaturations and crepitations/rhonchi on auscultation of the chest.

Complications

- Pulmonary – collapse, pneumonia, gastro-oesophageal reflux, aspiration

Table 11.3.5 Classification of chronic neonatal lung disease

- Bronchopulmonary dysplasia
- Wilson–Mikity syndrome
- Chronic pulmonary insufficiency of prematurity
- Recurrent aspiration
  - Pharyngeal incoordination
  - Gastro-oesophageal reflux
  - Tracheo-oesophageal fistula
- Interstitial pneumonitis
  - Cytomegalovirus
  - *Candida albicans*
  - *Chlamydia trachomatis*
  - *Pneumocystis jiroveci*
- Chronic pulmonary oedema due to a left to right shunt
- Rickets of prematurity

- Apnoea – central, obstructive
- Systemic hypertension
- Bronchospasm – wheezing
- Progressive pulmonary hypertension
- Cor pulmonale
- Postnatal growth failure
- Sudden, unexpected death in infancy
- Developmental delay and sensorineural disability.

Pathogenesis

Bronchopulmonary dysplasia is a multifactorial disease relating to the severity of RDS and degree of prematurity. Other factors in its causation are patent ductus arteriosus, positive pressure ventilation, high inspired O_2 concentration and pulmonary complications such as air leaks, oedema, mucous plugging, recurrent aspiration and infection. Ventilatory risk factors are baro- (pressure), volume and atelectatic trauma.

Chest X-ray

Radiological appearances of BPD are staged as 1–4. Stage 4 has an irregular honeycomb appearance with overinflated lung fields, extensive fibrosis and lung cysts (Fig. 11.3.13). Most infants with BPD have less severe changes consisting of a fine, homogeneous pattern of abnormality with some dense streaks.

Management

The stratagem of modern mechanical ventilation is to obtain acceptable blood gases with the minimum of barotrauma and volutrauma to preterm lungs. Exogenous surfactant for RDS reduces pulmonary air leaks and duration of assisted ventilation but produces only a modest reduction in BPD. Low-dose

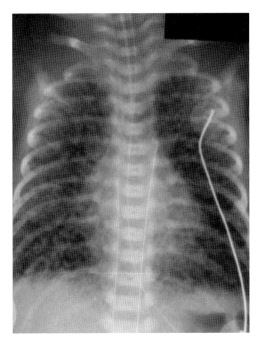

Fig. 11.3.13 Chest X-ray of stage 4 bronchopulmonary dysplasia showing gross hyperinflation, large cysts and bullae and fractured ribs.

dexamethasone for ventilated infants accelerates extubation. Diuretics may reduce interstitial lung fluid and inhaled bronchodilators decrease airway reactivity. For established BPD the mainstay of therapy is prolonged supplemental O_2 to maintain high O_2 saturations, adequate nutrition, physiotherapy and parental support.

Prognosis

Death from BPD is now rare, and occurs in infants with multiple complications of extreme prematurity or following respiratory syncytial virus infection. The healing stage is associated with continued lung growth and may take 2–3 years. Survivors are prone to recurrent wheezing episodes associated with viral infection in the first 2 years of life. The incidence of oxygen dependence at 36 weeks for infants of birth weight 500–749 g, 750–999 g and 1000–1499 g was 72.7%, 45.2% and 15.1%, respectively, in Australian and New Zealand intensive care nurseries in 2002.

Wilson–Mikity syndrome (or pulmonary dysmaturity)

This syndrome used to be common in preterm infants of less than 32 weeks gestation but is now rarely diagnosed. It occurred in the absence of RDS and had an insidious onset in the second and third weeks of life.

Upper airway obstruction

Frequently, upper airway obstruction presents in the delivery room or nursery as a result of foreign material in the airway. This can be readily relieved by suction to the airway. Upper airway obstruction not relieved by suction is unusual and may be mild, occurring only at times of stress or during feeds, or may be life-threatening, presenting acutely in the delivery room.

Clinical features

The cardinal signs of upper airway obstruction are:

- stridor (inspiratory if obstruction is extrathoracic or expiratory if obstruction is intrathoracic)
- suprasternal retraction
- a croupy cough
- a hoarse cry.

With severe increasing upper airway obstruction, the infant may develop cyanosis followed by a secondary apnoea and bradycardia.

Aetiology

The causes of upper airway obstruction may be classified according to the site of obstruction.

- *Intraluminal obstruction* from foreign material, such as mucus, blood, meconium or milk, may be relieved by suction. Vocal cord paralysis is a rare complication of traumatic birth
- *Intramural obstruction* in the larynx is due to subglottic stenosis, laryngeal oedema, a laryngeal web, diaphragm, papilloma or haemangioma. Transient stridor is a frequent consequence of neonatal resuscitation in the delivery room. The most common cause of persistent upper airway obstruction is subglottic oedema/stenosis following prolonged intubation of the trachea
- *Extramural obstruction* may occur with a goitre, vascular ring or cystic hygroma. Nasal obstruction may be due to choanal atresia or nasal congestion.

Infants with Pierre Robin sequence (micrognathia, cleft palate and glossoptosis) are prone to severe upper airway obstruction, especially when asleep, and require careful nursing in the prone position or insertion of a long nasopharyngeal tube. Stridor due to an infantile larynx (laryngomalacia) usually improves after 6 months of age but requires careful medical supervision, particularly during intercurrent respiratory tract infection.

Investigations

Persistent or progressive stridor especially with an expiratory component requires ENT or paediatric respiratory physician consultation. The definitive investigation is bronchoscopy performed with a flexible, fibreoptic bronchoscope. Other investigations such as X-ray or ultrasound of the neck, cine barium swallow and angiography are helpful on occasion.

Treatment

• An airway for acute stridor may be achieved with suction, a Guedel airway, intubation, tracheostomy or even intravenous cannula though the first and second tracheal rings

• Reversible mucosal damage and oedema may respond to dexamethasone 0.5 mg/kg 8-hourly for 48 h or inhaled nebulized adrenaline (epinephrine).

Apnoea and bradycardia

Apnoea is defined as a cessation of breathing lasting for 20 seconds or more. Apnoea lasting for less than 20 seconds is also significant if accompanied by colour change, bradycardia of less than 100 beats per minute or hypotonia.

Physiology

The control of breathing in the neonate is complicated and poorly understood. The regulation of breathing in premature infants is unstable and shows a variety of patterns. These may be regular, irregular or periodic, in which cycles of hyperventilation alternate with periods of hypoventilation, with eventual apnoea lasting between 3 and 10 seconds. With advancing gestation to term, the proportion of time the infant is breathing regularly increases and phases of irregular, periodic and apnoeic periods decline. Further maturation occurs in the months after birth. Infants revert to shorter periods of regular respiration and longer periods of less stable forms of breathing during rapid eye movement (REM) sleep.

Infants, particularly preterm, have less well developed chemoreceptor responses to hypoxia and hypercapnia. A low PO_2 initially stimulates respiratory effort for only a short time before irregular respiration and apnoea occur, which induce further hypoxia. Hypercapnia may also fail to stimulate respiration, particularly in the presence of hypoxia.

Aetiology

All babies who suffer from apnoea must be fully investigated. In the term infant the aetiology is usually identified, whereas in the preterm infant it is unusual to find a cause. Recurrent apnoea of prematurity is presumed to be due to immaturity of the respiratory centre in the brainstem and immaturity of the chemoreceptor response to hypoxia and acidosis. Apnoea is common in more immature babies, occurring in 25% of infants under 2500 g and in over 80% of infants under 1000 g birth weight.

Central apnoea

Central apnoea is due to factors affecting the respiratory centre in the brain stem or higher centres in the cerebral cortex.

Causes include:

• prematurity
• hypoxia/acidosis
• drugs (e.g. maternal narcotics, tromethamine (THAM), prostin, magnesium sulphate)
• metabolic (e.g. hypoglycaemia, hypocalcaemia, hypomagnesaemia, hypermagnesaemia)
• sepsis – generalized or a specific infection
• intracranial haemorrhage
• polycythaemia with hyperviscosity
• necrotizing enterocolitis
• patent ductus arteriosus
• convulsions
• brain maldevelopment
• temperature instability (e.g. incubator temperature too high, hypothermia, too rapid warming or cooling).

Obstructive apnoea

Babies are obligatory nose breathers and if their nares are obstructed, especially while sleeping, they are prone to severe apnoea. Obstructive apnoea occurs with some congenital malformations, such as choanal atresia and the Pierre Robin sequence. Preterm infants with small upper airways may have apnoea when lying in the supine position, especially during active (REM) sleep. Babies who have milk, mucus or meconium lodged in the airways are likely to have episodes of obstructive apnoea.

Mixed apnoea

This is difficult to diagnose clinically. It resembles central apnoea, initially, with the cessation of respiration, but then the baby makes intermittent respiratory efforts without achieving gas exchange.

Reflex apnoea

Reflex or vagally mediated apnoea may be due to suction of the pharynx or stomach or from passage of a nasogastric tube, physiotherapy or even in response to defaecation. Apnoea associated with gastro-oesophageal reflux may be reflex and/or obstructive.

Investigation of apnoea

Initially the infant must be examined carefully to exclude respiratory or remote disease. Investigations will depend to a large extent on the suspected cause but at times may be extensive.

Apnoea monitoring

A variety of monitors are available but none will detect obstructive apnoea until the baby stops fighting for breath. The use of an electrocardiogram (ECG) monitor together with an apnoea monitor is recommended in order to recognize bradycardia occurring with an obstructed airway.

Treatment of apnoea and bradycardia

Prevention and early detection
Infants at risk should have continuous heart rate and respiratory monitoring with appropriate set alarms. Low-birth-weight infants must be carefully handled and attention must be paid to feeding techniques, with avoidance of stomach distension and rapid feeding. Temperature must be maintained in the thermal neutral range. Nursing the infant in the prone position and careful suctioning of the airway will minimize obstruction to the airway.

Treatment of the underlying cause
This will depend on the findings on examination and of relevant investigations.

Management of the acute apnoeic episode
• *Stimulation of the infant.* This may be all that is required. Suction of the upper airways is indicated when obstruction is the likely cause
• *Manual ventilation with a facemask and bag.* Intubation and intermittent positive pressure ventilation will be necessary when the baby fails to respond to bag and mask ventilation or when severe apnoeic attacks occur frequently.

Treatment of recurrent apnoea
Recurrent apnoea usually occurs in preterm babies and may be very difficult to manage; however, before undertaking sophisticated therapy the potential hazards of therapy need to be carefully balanced against the brain damaging effects of the apnoeic episodes.
  Pharmacological treatment
• Methyl xanthines
  • aminophylline
  • theophylline
  • caffeine – the neonate methylates theophylline to caffeine and caffeine may be used to treat apnoea

• Doxapram – adding a doxapram infusion to an infant with apnoea resistant to methyl xanthines can sometimes bring additional benefit. Severe jitteriness is a well recognized side effect.
  Continuous positive airway pressure (CPAP). May be effective in treating or preventing apnoea. The use of nasal prongs to administer CPAP may produce additional effects by local stimulation.
  Stimulation. Tactile stimulation, which has been shown to be effective in reducing the number of apnoeic episodes, cannot be used as a routine; however, a variety of rocking mattresses have been devised for use as a means of stimulation and appear to reduce the number of apnoeic episodes in some infants.

Prognosis
This will depend on the underlying cause of the apnoea. Although modern management has decreased the incidence and severity of apnoea, in very low-birth-weight infants, the long-term outlook has not yet been fully evaluated.

Recurrent apnoea of prematurity usually resolves by 37 weeks postmenstrual age but in some instances it may persist beyond the expected date of delivery and no cause can be found. In some cases, discharge home on methyl xanthine drugs is recommended and home apnoea monitors may be of some benefit.

Home apnoea monitors
The parents of a preterm infant may request a monitor for use at home. There is no evidence that home monitoring reduces the risk of a life-threatening event occurring out of hospital, nor does it prevent death; babies have died despite being monitored. One consensus view for indications for home monitoring includes the following:

• one or more apparently life-threatening events associated with apnoea and requiring vigorous resuscitation
• symptomatic preterm infants
• siblings of two or more victims of sudden infant death syndrome (SIDS) – the consensus view is that monitoring of subsequent infants after a single case of SIDS cannot be justified
• infants with hypoventilation conditions.

Most paediatricians believe that the use of monitors at home for less rigorous indications than those listed above is justified if it is felt that it will reduce parental anxiety. It is essential that, before parents are given an apnoea monitor, they are shown how to apply basic resuscitation skills to the infant in case the baby is found apnoeic or collapsed at home. Most important of all is the education of parents in the strategies to reduce the risk of SIDS.

Congenital and perinatal infections

M. Starr

Introduction

Infections in the fetus and newborn (perinatal infections) may be acquired in utero (congenital infection), around the time of delivery, or in the neonatal period. Neonatal sepsis generally refers to acute infection in the first 2 months of life and is often caused by an organism acquired from the maternal genital tract (Table 11.4.1).

Modes of acquisition of infection

- In utero
  - haematogenous – placental infection and/or transplacental transmission
  - ascent from the maternal genital tract – across intact membranes, or after the membranes rupture
- During delivery
  - from maternal genital secretions
  - from maternal blood
- After birth
  - from breast milk
  - by conventional (horizontal) routes from mother or other contacts.

The route by which the fetus or newborn acquires the infection has important implications for management during pregnancy and the neonatal period, and for the development of appropriate intervention strategies to prevent mother-to-child transmission.

The outcome of perinatal infection may include particular constellations of congenital abnormalities, spontaneous abortion or stillbirth or acute neonatal infection. Common clinical manifestations include:

- growth retardation
- prematurity
- hepatitis, thrombocytopenia
- meningoencephalitis
- microcephaly
- intracerebral calcifications
- rash
- chorioretinitis
- deafness
- neurological defects.

For some congenital infections, there may be no symptoms or signs in the neonatal period and it may be weeks, months or even years before the effects first become evident.

Many organisms can cause infection in the fetus and newborn. Table 11.4.1 lists some of the more common or clinically significant.

Risk assessment

The risk of fetal damage can be estimated, based on:

- the likelihood of maternal exposure and infection
- the likelihood of transmission to the fetus
- the stage in gestation at which infection occurs – this influences the risk of vertical transmission and/or the fetal or perinatal consequences.

Only a small number of exposed infants are infected and, of these, a minority will have adverse effects. Many infections that can damage the fetus are mild or asymptomatic in the mother and diagnosis may depend on routine antenatal screening. Whether this is appropriate depends on the frequency and severity of fetal or neonatal disease and the availability of a suitable screening test and effective intervention.

> ### Practical points
>
> **Congenital infections**
> - Some common viral infections (e.g. cytomegalovirus, parvovirus, rubella, varicella-zoster virus) can cause fetal infection with severe consequences if acquired during pregnancy by a non-immune woman
> - Ensuring that a woman has antenatal testing and is immunized with all recommended vaccines is an important part of planning for pregnancy
> - Management of a pregnant woman exposed to relevant viral infections depends on a careful risk assessment, which includes knowledge of the woman's immune status, history of the exposure, stage in the pregnancy, and clinical presentation in the woman

Table 11.4.1 Organisms commonly associated with perinatal infection

Associated with congenital abnormalities
- Cytomegalovirus
- Parvovirus B19
- Rubella
- *Toxoplasma gondii*
- *Treponema pallidum* (syphilis)
- Varicella zoster virus

Associated with acute neonatal infection
- *Chlamydia trachomatis*
- *Escherichia coli*
- Enterovirus
- Herpes simplex virus
- *Listeria monocytogenes*
- Group B streptococcus

Associated with chronic infection
- Hepatitis B virus
- Hepatitis C virus
- Human immunodeficiency virus

Organisms associated with perinatal infection

Cytomegalovirus

Primary cytomegalovirus (CMV) infection is usually asymptomatic or causes a non-specific illness with fever, atypical lymphocytosis and mild hepatitis. The virus remains in a latent state with periodic asymptomatic reactivation and excretion in urine, saliva or genital secretions. Primary maternal infection or reactivation can result in fetal CMV infection, although fetal damage is generally associated with primary infection only. CMV can infect the fetus transplacentally to cause congenital infection.

Cytomegalovirus can also be transmitted during or after delivery when the neonate comes in contact with maternal genital secretions or with breast milk. However, it appears that there are no hearing or neurodevelopmental sequelae.

Cases of congenital CMV born without overt symptoms are also clinically important. There is a risk of developing hearing loss or mental retardation that continues for years. Overall, approximately 15% of cases born without symptoms will develop disease on follow-up.

The best evidence for primary maternal infection is seroconversion but this may not be demonstrable if investigation is delayed. Specific IgM may indicate recent infection but is unreliable: it may be detectable for months; can rise after reactivation, and false-positive results are not uncommon.

Primary infection

- 50% of young women are seronegative (susceptible). In developing countries and lower socioeconomic groups, primary infection occurs at a younger age and fewer women are susceptible
- 1% of women seroconvert during pregnancy
- 30% of fetuses of women with primary infection are infected
- The risk of congenital CMV infection after primary maternal CMV infection remains elevated for up to 4 years following seroconversion, with the highest risk being in the first 2 years
- Infection is transplacental; severe fetal damage is more likely early in gestation
- 10% of infants infected during primary maternal infection are symptomatic at birth: 90% have significant long-term handicap
- 90% of infants infected during primary maternal infection are asymptomatic at birth: 10% go on to develop deafness or intellectual handicap
- Overall incidence of congenital infection due to primary maternal infection is 1 in 1000.

Reactivation

- 20–30% of seropositive women reactivate latent infection during pregnancy
- 2–5% of their infants are infected in utero but significant CMV disease is rare; mild sequelae (unilateral deafness) occur infrequently (<10%)
- Overall incidence of congenital infection is 1–2% – the majority are unaffected.

Clinical features

The clinical features of severe intrauterine CMV infection include:

- intrauterine growth restriction
- hepatosplenomegaly, hepatitis
- anaemia, thrombocytopenia
- pneumonitis
- microcephaly, encephalitis, cerebral calcification and chorioretinitis
- sensorineural hearing loss (SNHL) in congenital CMV affects 50% of symptomatic infants and 10% of asymptomatic infants. It is the most common long-term consequence. It ranges from mild unilateral to profound bilateral hearing loss. In asymptomatic infants it may be underdiagnosed because the SNHL is detected too late to prove congenital infection
- cerebral palsy, intellectual disability, epilepsy and visual impairment.

Diagnosis

If primary maternal infection is suspected or cannot be excluded, fetal infection can be diagnosed by culture and/or polymerase chain reaction (PCR) analysis of amniotic fluid at 18 weeks gestation. Depending on when maternal infection occurred, the risk of fetal damage may justify termination of pregnancy.

Congenital CMV infection is diagnosed by a positive culture of urine or saliva collected in the first 2 weeks of life; after that it is difficult to distinguish congenital from postnatal infection. Testing for CMV IgM in the infant's serum is less sensitive and specific.

Treatment

Antiviral drugs active against CMV are too toxic for use during pregnancy but have been used with limited success in congenitally infected infants. The potential side effects and social cost of 6 weeks of intravenous ganciclovir therapy in an individual child must be weighed against a possible, but yet unproven long-term benefit. There is currently no indication for systemic antiviral therapy for infants with asymptomatic infection at birth.

Clinical example

A 32-year-old delivered a small-for-gestational-age baby boy at 38 weeks gestation. On examination at birth, he weighed 2400 g. His head circumference was smaller than expected for his weight and he had hepatosplenomegaly. He also had thrombocytopenia.

Rubella, CMV, *Toxoplasma* and syphilis serology were performed on the baby and compared with the mother's antenatal serological results. The baby had urine collected for viral culture. The baby had CMV IgG and IgM present and CMV was cultured from the urine, confirming CMV infection.

Ganciclovir has been used with limited success in congenitally CMV-infected infants. The potential side effects and social cost of 6 weeks of intravenous ganciclovir therapy in an individual child must be weighed against a possible but yet unproven long-term benefit. Affected neonates should have baseline audiology testing and this should be repeated in the first 6 months of life. They should also be monitored for developmental delay.

Parvovirus B19

Most cases of parvovirus B19 infection are asymptomatic. The most common clinical presentation of infection is erythema infectiosum, or 'slapped cheek disease' in children.

Parvovirus B19 can also cause:

- asymptomatic infection
- mild respiratory tract illness without rash
- atypical rash, which is rubelliform or petechial
- arthritis in adults
- chronic bone marrow failure in immunodeficient patients
- transient aplastic crisis in patients with haemolytic anaemia (e.g. sickle cell disease).

Approximately 60% of adult women are immune. The risk of infection in seronegative women is greatest in women exposed to an infected child at home (≈50%). The risk for childcare and primary school teachers exposed is 20–30% and the risk overall depends on exposure to children but is approximately 10–20%.

Fetal risks following maternal infection

In 50% of cases of maternal infection, the fetus is unaffected. Fetal damage only occurs if maternal infection occurs before 20 weeks gestation. The complications include:

- fetal loss in the first 20 weeks of pregnancy (15% compared with 5% in controls, i.e. 10% excess fetal loss)
- congenital abnormalities: <1% (anecdotal reports only)
- hydrops fetalis: following maternal infections at 9–20 weeks' gestation (incidence is approximately 3%). May result in:
  - spontaneous resolution (one-third of cases)
  - fetal death (usually without intrauterine transfusion; occasionally despite it)
  - resolution after intrauterine transfusion (most cases in which it is attempted)
- long-term sequelae: chronic congenital anaemia after intrauterine transfusion is rare.

See also Table 11.4.2.

There are no specific congenital abnormalities associated with maternal parvovirus infection.

Diagnosis

Diagnosis in children is mainly clinical. In potentially infected women, serology and PCR can be performed. IgM is detectable within 1–3 weeks of exposure and usually remains detectable for 2–3 months. IgG indicates previous infection and immunity. Parvovirus DNA can be detected in serum after the acute viraemic phase for up to 9 months in some patients, so it does not necessarily indicate acute infection.

Table 11.4.2 Risk assessment – parvovirus B19		
	Any pregnant woman exposed to parvovirus (%)	Pregnant woman with proven recent infection (%)
Excess fetal loss in first 20 weeks	0.4–1 (1 in 100–1 in 250)	5 (1 in 20)
Death from hydrops or its treatment	0.05–0.1 (1 in 850–1 in 2000)	0.6 (1 in 170)

Management

Pregnant school teachers or childcare workers do not need to be excluded from work, even during an epidemic (nor do infected children). It is certainly not practicable to prevent exposure at home. Pregnant women who have been exposed to parvovirus, and those with an illness consistent with parvovirus, should be tested serologically. If maternal infection is confirmed, the pregnancy should be monitored with serial ultrasounds.

Clinical example

A 24-year-old primary school teacher was 12 weeks pregnant. She had a 3-year-old who was well at the moment. She was concerned because there was a boy in her class with 'slapped cheek disease'. What advice should be given to her?

The likelihood is that she was immune – 60% of women of child-bearing age are seropositive. She should have her serology done to check. Even if she's not immune, there's no point in her staying away from school. The boy with slapped cheek disease is probably no longer infectious – once the rash is apparent, children are not infectious; and there may well have been others in the class with asymptomatic infection. If there have been many cases of parvovirus infection around, her 3-year-old may have had it too, and the greatest risk of infection for a pregnant mother is from her own children.

If she is seronegative when checked, she should be offered repeat serology in 2 weeks. If the serology is negative at this time, nothing further needs to be done. If she has evidence of seroconversion, there is a 50% chance that the fetus will be infected and a very small risk that she will lose the pregnancy or that the fetus will develop hydrops. She should have ultrasounds at 1–2-week intervals for the next 8 weeks, checking for the development of fetal hydrops. Even if this develops, at least 60% of fetuses will have a good outcome.

Rubella

The teratogenic effects of rubella were first noted in 1941 by an Australian ophthalmologist, who recognized several cases of congenital cataract following a large outbreak of rubella. Maternal rubella is now rare in many industrialized countries that have rubella vaccination programmes. However, in many developing countries, congenital rubella syndrome remains a major cause of developmental anomalies, particularly blindness and deafness.

Clinical features

The risk of fetal infection and damage is greatest during the first 8 weeks of pregnancy and damage is rare after 16 weeks. Congenital rubella syndrome may include a number of clinical features, some of which may not present until adolescence or adulthood:

- intrauterine growth restriction
- neonatal purpuric rash and hepatosplenomegaly
- microcephaly and developmental delay
- cardiac: pulmonary artery hypoplasia, patent ductus arteriosus
- eye: cataract, retinopathy; microphthalmia
- deafness – develops later
- diabetes mellitus – develops later.

Diagnosis

Congenital rubella is confirmed by:

- isolation of rubella virus from saliva, tears, urine, cerebrospinal fluid (CSF) or tissue during the first 3 months of life
- demonstration of specific IgM antibody or persistence of IgG antibody beyond 6 months of age.

Prevention

Congenital rubella is preventable by immunization in childhood (Ch. 3.5). Routine antenatal screening and postpartum immunization of susceptible women provides additional protection. If rubella infection or contact is suspected during pregnancy, investigation to detect or exclude infection (specific IgM or IgG seroconversion) should be done even in women with known past immunity, as reinfection occasionally occurs. Termination of pregnancy may be recommended after proven infection during the first trimester.

Toxoplasma gondii

Toxoplasma gondii is a protozoan parasite that infects up to a third of the world's population. Infection is mainly acquired by ingestion of food or water that is contaminated with oocysts shed by cats or by eating undercooked or raw meat containing tissue cysts. Primary infection is usually subclinical but may cause lymphadenopathy or ocular disease. Infection acquired during pregnancy may cause severe damage to the fetus. The risk of fetal infection increases but that of fetal damage decreases with advancing gestation (Table 11.4.3). There is geographical variation in the incidence of congenital infection; in Australia it is estimated to be fewer than 1 in 1000 births.

Clinical features

- Most congenitally infected infants are asymptomatic at birth
- Many later develop signs and sometimes symptoms of chorioretinitis (up to 80%, with some visual impairment in about half)
- ≈10% develop neurological sequelae and/or hearing deficit
- Signs of severe symptomatic congenital toxoplasmosis include:
  - anaemia, hepatosplenomegaly, jaundice, lymphadenopathy
  - thrombocytopenia, petechial rash
  - central nervous system damage – intracranial calcification, hydrocephalus and microcephaly
  - neurological and/or visual impairment in most survivors.

Diagnosis and management

Toxoplasmosis during pregnancy is ideally diagnosed by showing seroconversion. More commonly it is suspected because specific IgM is detected in serum by antenatal screening. IgM can remain detectable for many months and, in the absence of symptoms, further testing is needed. Tests for the avidity of IgG antibodies can discriminate between recently acquired and previous infection. If recent infection is confirmed or cannot be excluded, treat-

ment of the mother with spiramycin can reduce the risk of vertical transmission.

Appropriate management depends on diagnosis of intrauterine infection by amniotic fluid PCR at about 18 weeks gestation. If fetal infection occurs during the first trimester, termination of pregnancy is often recommended. If infection occurs during the second or third trimester, treatment of the mother with a combination of pyrimethamine and a sulphonamide is likely to reduce sequelae of the disease in the newborn.

Specific IgM in the infant's serum or persistence of IgG beyond the first few months of life are evidence of congenital toxoplasmosis. *T. gondii* may be detected in tissue by histological examination or PCR, or in CSF by PCR. Treatment of a congenitally infected infant with spiramycin, pyrimethamine and a sulphonamide can reduce progressive damage after birth.

Treponema pallidum (syphilis)

Syphilis is a sexually transmitted infection caused by *Treponema pallidum*. Congenital syphilis is now a rare disease in most countries but it remains a severe, adverse pregnancy outcome in many less developed countries. Untreated syphilis in pregnancy can cause stillbirth, preterm labour and intrauterine growth restriction. Later in life, a range of neurological disorders can occur, including paretic neurosyphilis; all these manifestations respond poorly to treatment.

Fetal infection is a result of haematogenous spread from an infected mother, although transmission at the time of delivery can occur from direct contact with infectious genital lesions. Transmission from mother to fetus can occur at any stage of pregnancy, particularly during early (primary, secondary or early latent) syphilis. Maternal syphilis is often asymptomatic and recognized only because of a positive routine antenatal serological test. Early antenatal screening and treatment of maternal syphilis can prevent most cases of congenital infection.

The fetal outcome of untreated maternal syphilis depends on the stage of the disease:

- primary or secondary: premature delivery or perinatal death ≈50%; congenital syphilis ≈50% (few normal infants)
- early latent syphilis (or indeterminate): at least 50% normal, 20–40% congenital syphilis; increased risk of perinatal death and preterm birth.

Clinical features

At least 50% of infants with congenital syphilis are asymptomatic, so diagnosis may rely on serology. Clinical features typical of congenital syphilis include:

Table 11.4.3 Risk assessment – *Toxoplasma gondii*		
	Fetal infection (%)	Fetal damage (%)
1st trimester	5–15	60–80
2nd trimester	25–40	15–25
3rd trimester	30–75	2–10

- an abnormally bulky placenta – histological examination should be done
- hydrops fetalis due to severe anaemia and/or severe liver disease
- lymphadenopathy, hepatosplenomegaly, jaundice
- osteochondritis with typical radiological changes; arthropathy or pseudoparalysis
- rhinitis ('snuffles')
- vesiculobullous rash on back, legs, palms and soles, followed by desquamation
- condylomata lata – fleshy lesions in moist areas of skin.

The diagnosis is confirmed by serological tests on the mother and infant: neonatal IgG antibody titres that are significantly higher than the mother's and/or the presence of specific IgM in the infant. A lumbar puncture should be performed on the infant. Neurosyphilis is suggested by CSF pleocytosis, raised protein level and positive CSF serology.

Treatment

Congenital syphilis is treated with parenteral penicillin. Serological and clinical follow-up is needed to confirm successful treatment and exclude neurological or ophthalmological abnormality or deafness.

Congenital syphilis may present in a variety of ways. It is important to screen for maternal syphilis following stillbirth or if an unusual lesion or condition consistent with syphilis is present in the newborn infant. Routine antenatal screening for syphilis is cost-effective and still recommended, although the prevalence in Australia is low. Adequate treatment of an infected mother during pregnancy will prevent fetal damage.

Varicella-zoster virus

At least 90% of adults are immune to varicella but exposure during pregnancy is common. Fetal outcomes following maternal infection early in pregnancy include:

- uncomplicated self-limiting infection ($\approx$10%)
- herpes zoster (shingles) in the first year of life (2–3%)
- fetal varicella syndrome (2–3% of cases), manifestations of which include:
  - growth restriction
  - skin scarring over a dermatomal distribution
  - ipsilateral limb or other skeletal hypoplasia
  - encephalopathy and abnormalities of various organs.

The risk of fetal varicella syndrome in children exposed to varicella-zoster virus (VZV) in utero is around 0.5% after maternal infection at 2–12 weeks of pregnancy, 1.4% after infection at 12–28 weeks, and does not occur after infection from 28 weeks onwards. It occurs in around 1.6 per 100 000 births in the population. Shingles in the mother does not carry a risk of fetal varicella syndrome.

Varicella-zoster virus infection of the newborn results from transmission from a mother with chickenpox to her infant around the time of delivery, in circumstances where the infant lacks the protection of maternal antibodies. The likelihood of such infection depends on the timing of delivery in relation to when the mother develops the chickenpox rash. If the rash develops more than 7 days before delivery, this generally allows time for the development and transfer of protective maternal antibodies. However, since transfer of antibodies from the mother to the infant is limited before around 26–28 weeks of gestation, maternal immunity to VZV does not usually protect preterm infants delivered before 28 weeks gestational age.

If maternal VZV infection occurs during the week from 5 days before delivery until 2 days afterwards, infection of the infant may be complicated by pneumonia, hepatitis or encephalitis and a high mortality.

Clinical example

A 19-year-old intravenous drug user had a past history of a stillbirth at 36 weeks gestation, for which no cause was found. She was known to be hepatitis-C-positive, but her human immunodeficiency virus (HIV) status was unknown. She was now pregnant and presented at term, having had no antenatal care. She delivered a baby boy who was noted to have hepatosplenomegaly. What tests should be done?

With no antenatal care and a baby with hepatosplenomegaly, the concern is that the baby may have a congenital infection. Given the history that she was an intravenous drug user and hepatitis-C-positive, particular concerns would include syphilis, hepatitis C, hepatitis B and HIV.

Mother and baby should have serological tests for syphilis: rapid plasma reagin test (RPR) and *Treponema pallidum* haemagglutination test (TPHA) reactive. If the neonatal antibody titres were significantly higher than the mother's, the baby's IgM should be tested. A lumbar puncture should also be performed on the baby. Neurosyphilis is suggested by CSF pleocytosis, raised protein level and positive CSF serology.

The mother should have other serological testing: HIV antibodies, hepatitis B surface antigen and hepatitis C antibody and viral load. The baby should have hepatitis C antibody testing no earlier than 12 months, and preferably at 18 months of age. If performed earlier, a positive result may simply reflect the mother's antibody.

When maternal infection occurs more than 5 days before delivery, infection in the infant is usually mild. Infants exposed to varicella after the first few days of life also usually have mild disease, although this is variable and depends on, among other factors, the mother's immune status.

Prophylaxis and treatment

Zoster immune globulin (ZIG) can prevent or modify varicella if given within 4 days (preferably 48 hours) of exposure to:

- pregnant women with no past history of chickenpox who are seronegative or whose immune status is unknown
- newborn infants of women who develop varicella within 5 days before or 2 days after delivery.

Severe varicella in mother or infant should be treated with acyclovir.

Varicella vaccine is now a component of the routine immunization schedule (Ch. 3.5). Immunization of susceptible women of child-bearing age will protect the fetus from the risk of congenital varicella.

Clinical example

A 30-year-old mother of two had just had her third baby. The day after delivery, her 2-year-old developed chickenpox. She had cuddled and kissed her mother and the new baby. The 4-year-old had not had chickenpox and the mother was not sure whether she had had it herself. The father had chickenpox as a child. What should be done for this family?

The mother should have her VZV serology checked immediately. If she was found to be seronegative, the baby should be given zoster immune globulin within 96 hours of exposure. ZIG may not abrogate the risk of fetal infection, so the baby should be watched for development of vesicles, and aciclovir should be given if she develops chickenpox.

The mother and 4-year-old should be offered VZV vaccine, as postexposure administration of the vaccine within 5 days of exposure can prevent or limit severity of disease.

If the mother was found to be seropositive, nothing needs to be done for her or the baby.

Neonatal sepsis

The bacterial pathogens that classically cause neonatal sepsis are:

- *Streptococcus agalactiae* (group B streptococcus, GBS) – the most common
- *Escherichia coli*
- *Listeria monocytogenes* – uncommon but often occurring in clusters

Numerous other bacteria can cause neonatal infection, including other Gram-negative bacilli, other streptococci, anaerobes, *Staphylococcus aureus*, *Chlamydia trachomatis* and genital mycoplasmas.

Neonatal infection with herpes simplex virus and enterovirus may mimic bacterial sepsis.

Risk factors for neonatal sepsis include premature rupture of the membranes, chorioamnionitis and maternal fever.

Clinical features

Intrauterine infection can cause premature labour or fetal distress with or without maternal fever. The clinical manifestations of perinatal sepsis are non-specific:

- respiratory distress, tachypnoea, apnoea
- temperature instability, irritability
- feeding difficulty, vomiting, diarrhoea and jaundice
- haematological changes – neutrophilia or neutropenia, increased proportion of immature neutrophils, thrombocytopenia and coagulopathy.

Focal disease such as pneumonia, meningitis or urinary tract, bone, soft tissue or middle ear infections may complicate disseminated sepsis or occur alone, often with only non-specific systemic symptoms.

Diagnosis

Investigations for suspected neonatal sepsis may include:

- full blood examination and acute phase reactants such as C reactive protein.
- culture of blood, CSF or urine (collected by suprapubic bladder aspiration)
- CSF examination (if indicated): typical findings in bacterial meningitis are pleocytosis, with a

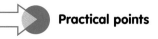

Practical points

Neonatal sepsis
- Newborn infants can develop bacterial sepsis from the same postnatally acquired infections as older infants (e.g. *Streptococcus pneumoniae*, *Staphylococcus aureus*, *Haemophilus influenzae*), but in addition are at risk of infection from perinatally acquired organisms
- These organisms include group B streptococcus, *Escherichia coli* and *Listeria monocytogenes*
- Herpes simplex virus and enterovirus infection in the newborn can mimic bacterial sepsis
- Investigations and empiric antibiotic treatment for sepsis in the neonatal period must take account of these organisms

predominance of polymorphonuclear leukocytes, a raised protein and decreased glucose level; in viral meningoencephalitis the cell counts are lower, mononuclear cells usually (not always) predominate and glucose levels are normal
- Chest X-ray

Organisms associated with acute neonatal infection

Chlamydia trachomatis

Chlamydia trachomatis is a sexually transmitted organism that causes cervicitis, pregnancy complications and secondary infertility in women and can be vertically transmitted during delivery. Neonatal chlamydial infection, which manifests principally as ophthalmia neonatorum or pneumonia, is a significant cause of neonatal morbidity. *C. trachomatis* is the most common infectious cause of ophthalmia neonatorum in industrialized countries and is a significant cause of neonatal conjunctivitis in developing countries.

The incidence of chlamydial infection varies widely according to geography and socioeconomic group. The incidence is relatively high in young, single women with multiple sexual partners, in socially disadvantaged groups and in developing countries. Additional risk factors include presence of another sexually transmitted infection or a partner with urethritis.

Most infants of infected women are normal at delivery but about 60% of those exposed are infected and, of these, about half develop symptoms: 18–50% develop conjunctivitis, 15–20% nasopharyngeal colonization and 5–20% pneumonia.

Clinical features

- Conjunctivitis:
  - may develop a few days to several weeks postpartum, typically between 5 and 14 days after delivery
  - severity ranges from mild conjunctival injection to severe conjunctivitis with purulent discharge
  - usually begins in one eye with progressive involvement of the other eye after 2–7 days
  - symptoms are often persistent but are eventually self-limiting
- Pneumonia:
  - usually occurs between 2 and 19 weeks postpartum, typically around 6 weeks of age
  - associated with conjunctivitis in only half of all cases
  - subacute onset and insidious course

- paroxysmal cough, vomiting and weight loss; often misdiagnosed as pertussis
- systemic symptoms are minimal and fever absent
- prolonged but eventually self-limited course.

Diagnosis

Culture, immunofluorescence or PCR analysis of conjunctival scrapings or nasopharyngeal aspirate.

Treatment

Infection in an infant is a marker of maternal infection; if untreated, it can cause postpartum salpingitis with a risk of secondary infertility. Thus, it is important for both mother and infant that a specific diagnosis be made, even if mild conjunctivitis is the only symptom. The mother and her sexual partner(s) should be treated. Treatment of chlamydial pneumonia should reduce the duration of illness.

Conjunctivitis or pneumonia should be treated with oral erythromycin for 2 weeks. Topical therapy does not eradicate *C. trachomatis* from the nasopharynx or prevent pneumonia. Newer macrolides, such as azithromycin, may also be used.

Escherichia coli

Escherichia coli causes bacteraemia, urinary tract infection and meningitis in the first week of life. However, there is a continued risk up to 2 months of age. Premature infants are more commonly affected.

Treatment is with intravenous antibiotics for 3 weeks.

Enterovirus

Enteroviruses, which include Coxsackie A, B and echoviruses, cause hand, foot and mouth disease, gastroenteritis and meningitis. Neonatal infection may be acquired from maternal infection in the 2 weeks prior to delivery or postnatal exposure. In newborn infants, enteroviral disease may be particularly severe and is associated with high morbidity and mortality. During summer and autumn, neonatal enteroviral disease may be more common than diseases caused by group B streptococci or herpes simplex virus. Despite this, it is frequently unrecognized as a cause of neonatal sepsis.

Clinical features

- Meningoencephalitis
- Thrombocytopenia

- Disseminated intravascular coagulopathy
- Cardiomyopathy
- Hepatitis.

Diagnosis

Viral culture or PCR analysis of CSF, stool or throat swab.

Treatment

Intravenous immunoglobulin has been used to treat neonatal enteroviral disease, but there is insufficient evidence to recommend this routinely.

Herpes simplex virus

Perinatal herpes simplex virus (HSV) infection can be acquired in one of three ways:

- in utero – maternal viraemia during primary infection (HSV-1 or HSV-2) – 5%
- peripartum – maternal genital tract during delivery (usually HSV-2) – 85%
- postpartum (postnatal) – contact after birth with cold sores, infected saliva or hands (usually HSV-1) – 10%.

Primary maternal HSV infection can cause fever, systemic symptoms and severe mucocutaneous lesions, but is often asymptomatic (and diagnosed by seroconversion). Transplacental infection is rare but spontaneous abortion or preterm labour can occur.

Risk factors for vertical transmission

- Type of maternal infection – recurrent genital herpes infections are the most common form of genital HSV during pregnancy. However, women with primary genital HSV infections who are shedding HSV at delivery are 10–30 times more likely to transmit the virus to their babies than women with a recurrent infection. The difficulty is that approximately 66% of women who acquire genital herpes during pregnancy remain asymptomatic
- Maternal (and neonatal) antibody status – transplacental passage of anti-HSV neutralizing antibodies reduces the risk of transmission and of disseminated disease
- Prolonged rupture of membranes
- Poor integrity of mucocutaneous barriers (e.g. use of fetal scalp electrodes)
- Mode of delivery – caesarean section reduces risk of HSV transmission in women shedding HSV at the time of birth, particularly in women with first-time infections who are HSV-type-specific-antibody-negative.

Clinical features

Perinatal HSV infections can be classified as:

- disseminated disease
  - involving multiple visceral organs, including lung, liver, adrenal glands, skin, eye and the brain
  - 25% of perinatal HSV disease (with early treatment)
  - usually presents at 10–12 days of life
  - fever, disseminated intravascular coagulation, shock, hepatitis, pneumonia, encephalitis
  - 80% mortality untreated
  - high incidence of sequelae in survivors
- CNS disease
  - meningoencephalitis
  - one-third of perinatal HSV disease
  - usually presents at 16–19 days of life
  - 60% have skin lesions at some point
  - seizures, lethargy, irritability, poor feeding
  - presentation may be indistinguishable from neonatal sepsis
- Skin, eye, mouth (SEM) disease
  - disease limited to the skin, eyes and/or mouth
  - 45% of perinatal HSV disease (with early treatment)
  - usually presents at 10–12 days of life
  - infants with apparently localized mucocutaneous HSV infection may have neurological sequelae from unrecognized encephalitis.

Diagnosis

Neonatal HSV infection is diagnosed by isolation or detection of HSV by immunofluorescence or PCR in skin lesions, blood, CSF, saliva, urine or tissue biopsy.

Treatment

Early treatment with high-dose intravenous acyclovir reduces the mortality and morbidity and should be given for suspected neonatal HSV infection. Treatment must be continued for 3 weeks if HSV is proved (or cannot be excluded).

Prevention

- Caesarean delivery in a woman with active genital lesions can reduce the risk of perinatal HSV infection.
- Prophylactic aciclovir beginning at 36 weeks gestation reduces the risk of clinical HSV recurrence at delivery, caesarean delivery for recurrent genital herpes and the risk of HSV viral shedding at delivery. However, it is not clear whether there is a reduction in perinatal disease.

- There may be a role for the use of condoms and oral antivirals in a seronegative women with a seropositive sexual partner.

Listeria monocytogenes

- Listeriosis is usually acquired from contaminated food such as dairy products and processed meats.
- Pregnant women, neonates, the elderly and the immunocompromised are most at risk.
- Maternal infection is often asymptomatic or mild.
- Spontaneous abortion, stillbirth or premature delivery and neonatal sepsis or meningitis can occur.

Diagnosis

Culture of blood and CSF.

Treatment

High-dose intravenous penicillin.

Group B streptococcus

Streptococcus agalactiae or group B streptococcus (GBS) is the most common cause of neonatal sepsis. GBS is carried in the vaginal flora of 25% of healthy women. Less than 1% of the infants of carriers are infected. The overall incidence of neonatal GBS sepsis is 0.25 in 1000.

Clinical features

Group B streptococcus can cause neonatal sepsis, pneumonia, meningitis and, less frequently, focal infections such as osteomyelitis, septic arthritis or cellulitis.

- Early-onset disease occurs within the first week of life; most occur on day of birth or within 72 hour
- Late-onset disease occurs after the first week, and cases are relatively evenly distributed through the fist 3 months of life
- ≈50% of infections begin in utero; associated with preterm labour, prolonged rupture of membranes and chorioamnionitis
- Mortality varies with gestational age at infection:
  - 2% after 37 weeks
  - 10% for neonates between 34–36 weeks
  - 30% for neonates less than 33 weeks.

Risk factors for early-onset disease

- Maternal GBS colonization
- Prolonged rupture of membranes

- Preterm delivery
- GBS bacteriuria during pregnancy
- Birth of a previous infant with invasive GBS disease
- Maternal chorioamnionitis
- Young maternal age
- Low levels of serotype specific IgG antibody against GBS

These factors often coexist, but maternal age and gestational age have been shown to be independent predictors of early-onset disease risk.

Risk factors for late-onset disease

- Preterm gestation
- Young maternal age
- Maternal GBS colonization

Intrapartum antibiotic prophylaxis

Intrapartum penicillin given to carrier mothers has been shown to decrease early-onset neonatal GBS sepsis. However, there is no consensus as to the best way of identifying which women should receive intrapartum chemoprophylaxis. The two strategies that have been used are routine antenatal screening for vaginal GBS carriage and identification of clinical risk factors during labour. Recent data suggest that screening programmes for the detection of GBS carriage may be more effective than risk-based strategies to prevent early-onset neonatal GBS sepsis. Combined vaginal and rectal swabs, collected between 35 and 37 weeks gestation either by a healthcare worker or by the patient herself and inoculated on to selective media after enrichment provide the optimum conditions to detect carriage. Increasingly erythromycin and clindamycin resistance is being described overseas, which may influence the choice of antibiotics used in those allergic to penicillin. Widespread antibiotic use, particularly with broad-spectrum agents, may lead to increasing neonatal sepsis with ampicillin-resistant organisms. While rates of non-GBS neonatal sepsis are generally stable there is evidence suggesting that *E. coli* sepsis in premature infants is increasing.

Diagnosis

Culture of blood and CSF, plus chest X-ray if indicated.

Treatment

High-dose intravenous penicillin plus synergistic gentamicin.

Organisms associated with chronic infection

Hepatitis B virus

Women who are chronic carriers of hepatitis B virus (HBV) (i.e. have persistently detectable hepatitis B surface antigen (HBsAg) in serum) or who have acute hepatitis B late in pregnancy often transmit the virus to their infants. The three main modes of transmission from the mother to the infant are:

- in utero infection – unusual except in the setting of acute hepatitis B infection during the third trimester
- direct inoculation during delivery – most common mode of transmission. As the fetus passes through the vaginal canal, blood present there is swallowed by the fetus. Up to 95% of infants born to mothers who are HbsAg-positive have the antigen in their gastric fluid
- postnatal (horizontal) transmission.

The risk and the outcome depend on the amount of live virus in maternal serum. A relatively high level of infectivity is indicated by the presence in serum of the hepatitis B e antigen (HBeAg) or DNA polymerase, both of which are associated with active viral replication. About 90% of infants of HbeAg-positive carriers are infected during delivery and will become chronic carriers; they are at risk from chronic liver disease, cirrhosis and hepatocellular carcinoma, which does not usually occur before early adulthood. Children who are HBsAg carriers are a potential source of horizontal transmission of HBV to other young children.

The risk of becoming a carrier is much lower (approximately 5%) for infants of HBsAg carriers with antibody to HBeAg (indicating lower infectivity) but these infants can develop acute HBV infection.

The risk of chronic infection and subsequent liver disease is inversely proportional to age at the time of infection:

- 90–95% of HBV infections under 1 year of age result in chronic liver disease
- 25–50% of HBV infections in 1–5-year-olds result in chronic liver disease
- 6–10% of HBV infections in adults result in chronic liver disease.

Prevention

Universal HBV immunization is the most effective means of preventing HBV transmission (Ch. 3.5). Routine antenatal screening and immunization of infants of HBsAg carriers can prevent neonatal HBV infection. The infant should be given hepatitis B immune globulin (HBIG) as soon as possible after birth (no later than 48 hours) and a course of HBV vaccine starting in the first week. Three further doses should be given at 2, 4 and 6 or 12 months (the timing depends on the combination vaccine used). This prevents HBV infection in more than 95% of infants at risk.

Lamivudine has been used to prevent the transmission of HBV to neonates in mothers with high viral load.

Hepatitis C virus

Approximately 1% of pregnant women are infected with hepatitis C virus (HCV). Perinatal transmission has been shown to be the leading cause of HCV infection among infants and children. However, the risk of vertical transmission is low (approximately 5%). There is an increased risk with high maternal viral load and maternal coinfection with HIV.

Perinatally acquired HCV infection has a slower, more indolent course than infection in older children and adults. Approximately 20% of children appear to clear the infection, 50% develop chronic asymptomatic infection and 30% develop chronic active infection.

The general recommendation for testing a child after perinatal HCV exposure is to test for HCV antibody at or beyond 18 months of life. Passively transferred maternal anti HCV antibody will have cleared by this age. When follow-up cannot be guaranteed, however, testing by HCV RNA PCR should be performed opportunistically, but not at less than 1 month of age, as the sensitivity of the test is low (22%). A positive PCR result should be always be confirmed on a separate occasion.

There is no evidence that HCV transmission occurs during breastfeeding, nor that caesarean delivery reduces the risk of transmission.

Human immunodeficiency virus

The rates of mother-to-child transmission of HIV around the world vary according to availability of antenatal care, antiretroviral drugs and background prevalence rates. In the absence of antiviral and obstetric interventions, the risk overall of mother-to-child transmission is reported as 15–20% in Europe, 15–30% in USA and 25–35% in Africa.

There are three routes of vertical transmission of HIV:

- in utero
- during labour and delivery – 70%

- breastfeeding – transmission risk is highest in the first few months of life.

Measures that have been shown to reduce mother-to-child transmission of HIV:

- antiretroviral therapy (for the mother during pregnancy and labour) and to the infant for the first 6 weeks of life
- elective caesarean section (it is generally thought that interventions to minimize infant contact with maternal vaginal secretions and infected blood during passage through the birth canal is important to reduce the risk of vertical transmission)
- avoidance of invasive obstetric procedures
- avoidance of breastfeeding.

The Royal Australian and New Zealand College of Obstetricians and Gynaecologists recommends that all pregnant women should be assessed for risk of HIV infection and should be offered HIV antibody testing following appropriate counselling.

Acute neonatal surgical conditions

S. W. Beasley

The majority of the conditions discussed in this chapter will present initially to the paediatrician, general practitioner or obstetrician as emergencies. Delay in diagnosis may seriously compromise recovery and will almost certainly increase morbidity. Disorders that are obvious at birth but do not require urgent surgical referral have not been included in this chapter. For information on these, the reader is referred to paediatric surgical texts.

Oesophageal atresia

Any newborn infant who appears to salivate excessively at birth (drooling) should be suspected of having oesophageal atresia. This is a congenital abnormality where the mid-portion of the oesophagus is missing. In most there is an abnormal communication between the lower oesophageal segment and the trachea, called a distal tracheo-oesophageal fistula.

The diagnosis is confirmed by passing a large, firm catheter, for example a 10 French gauge orogastric tube, through the mouth and finding that it cannot be passed more than about 10 cm from the gums. The child must not be fed; otherwise, aspiration of feeds into the lungs is likely to occur. A plain X-ray of the torso will show gas in the bowel, confirming the presence of a distal tracheo-oesophageal fistula. About 50% of these infants have other congenital abnormalities, most of which form part of the VATER association (vertebral, cardiac, renal, anorectal and radial abnormalities; Ch. 10.3). Major chromosomal abnormalities are seen in 5%, of which trisomy 18 and trisomy 21 are the most frequent. Many are premature and a history of maternal polyhydramnios is common.

Initial management involves regular suctioning of the upper oesophageal pouch to prevent aspiration until the tracheo-oesophageal fistula has been divided. The oesophageal ends are anastomosed at the time of thoracotomy to close the fistula.

Duodenal obstruction

Bile-stained vomiting starts soon after birth. The obstruction may be:

- intrinsic, as in duodenal atresia
- extrinsic, when it is the result of malrotation with volvulus.

In duodenal atresia there may be other abnormalities such as Down syndrome and imperforate anus (see Ch. 10.3). In the absence of birth asphyxia these infants are usually alert and feed well but they vomit bile-stained material almost immediately. There may be epigastric distension. The diagnosis of duodenal atresia is made on plain X-ray of the abdomen, which reveals a characteristic 'double bubble' due to gas in the stomach and proximal duodenum (Fig. 11.5.1). Little or no gas will be visible distal to the obstruction. Duodenoduodenostomy is performed after resuscitation and correction of any fluid and electrolyte disturbance.

Bile-stained vomiting may also be an indication of malrotation in which volvulus has supervened. The midgut twists around the superior mesenteric vessels and the small bowel mesentery has a narrow attachment to the posterior abdominal wall, the so-called 'universal mesentery'. This is a true surgical emergency as the blood supply to the midgut may be cut off as the midgut twists around this axis. The diagnosis can be confirmed with an urgent barium meal. If signs of peritonitis with abdominal distension and guarding are already present, the infant should be taken immediately to theatre.

Distal bowel obstruction

In more distal bowel obstructions, vomiting remains a major feature but tends to occur later and is associated with abdominal distension. The more distal the obstruction, the later the vomiting and the more pronounced the distension (Fig. 11.5.2). The vomitus may become faeculent. An erect film of the abdomen will show distended loops of bowel and fluid levels (Fig. 11.5.3). The number of loops is dependent on the level of obstruction. The radiological appearances of ileal atresia, meconium ileus and Hirschsprung disease may be similar, and a contrast study, rectal biopsy or laparotomy may be required to make the definitive diagnosis.

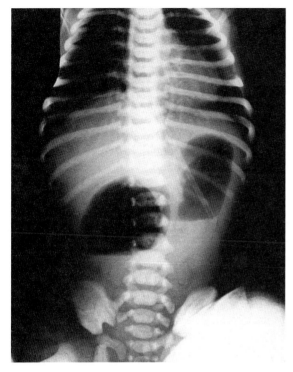

Fig. 11.5.1 X-ray of the abdomen in a neonate demonstrating the 'double bubble' sign. Note the absence of gas in the bowel distal to the second bubble. This child had duodenal atresia.

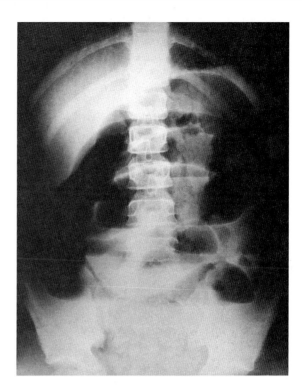

Fig. 11.5.3 Erect plain X-ray of the abdomen, showing marked dilatation of multiple loops of bowel and several fluid levels. The most likely diagnoses include Hirschsprung disease, meconium ileus and ileal atresia.

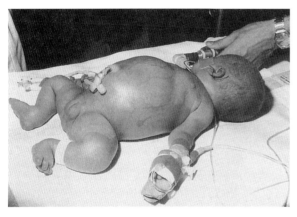

Fig. 11.5.2 Distal bowel obstruction in a neonate. Gross abdominal distension is evident and was associated with vomiting of faeculent material.

Hirschsprung disease

Hirschsprung disease (congenital megacolon) is the most common cause of neonatal bowel obstruction. There is an absence of ganglion cells for a variable distance proximal to the anus. Peristalsis is abnormal in the aganglionic segment and results in severe constipation and an incomplete lower intestinal obstruction. The bowel proximal to the aganglionic segment becomes dilated and hypertrophied. The diagnosis is confirmed on rectal suction biopsy. Most of these infants present at 3 or 4 days of age with increasing abdominal distension and delay in the passage of meconium. Surgical correction involves:

- excision of the aganglionic segment
- anastomosing ganglionated bowel to the anus.

It is often performed as a single-stage procedure at diagnosis but in certain circumstances requires staging.

Meconium ileus

Meconium ileus occurs in infants with cystic fibrosis. In this condition meconium becomes excessively thick and tenacious, causing obstruction, and the distal ileum is jammed with hard pellets of inspissated meconium. The colon is empty and no meconium is passed after birth. The infant has a distended abdomen and commences vomiting shortly after birth. A contrast enema will demonstrate a microcolon.

Sometimes the impacted pellets can be dislodged with a Gastrografin enema but usually surgery is required. A temporary ileostomy allows the bowel to be irrigated. The diagnosis of cystic fibrosis is confirmed subsequently (Ch. 14.6).

Small bowel atresias

Atresias of the jejunum are often multiple (Fig. 11.5.4). There is gross distension of the proximal jejunum followed by multiple short segments of jejunum and normal bowel distally. Ileal atresia tends to be an isolated lesion. Colonic atresia is extremely rare.

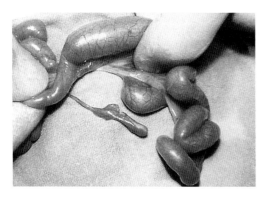

Fig. 11.5.4 Intraoperative photograph showing multiple areas of jejunal atresia in a neonate who presented with vomiting after the first two feeds after birth.

Neonatal necrotizing enterocolitis

Neonatal necrotizing enterocolitis is an acquired condition that predominantly afflicts the premature infant who has undergone severe perinatal stress (Ch. 11.2). The infant becomes lethargic and unwell, usually between 2 days and 2 weeks after birth. There is bile-stained vomiting and the abdomen becomes distended. Loose stools are passed, which may contain blood. As the disease progresses, signs of peritonitis develop: there is redness and oedema of the abdominal wall and increasing abdominal tenderness. Both small and large bowel may be involved.

Plain X-rays of the abdomen show:

- dilated loops of bowel
- intramural gas (pneumatosis intestinalis). Gas may outline the portal venous system and, if full-thickness perforation has occurred, free gas within the peritoneal cavity will be evident.

Initial management involves cessation of all oral feeds, decompression of the gastrointestinal tract by nasogastric aspiration, fluid resuscitation and antibiotics. Where there is continued clinical deterioration despite appropriate resuscitation, or there is evidence of full-thickness bowel necrosis (e.g. free intraperitoneal gas on X-ray), surgery is indicated.

Necrotic bowel is excised and a defunctioning stoma may be required. Malabsorption, short gut syndrome and colonic strictures may complicate the condition.

Anorectal malformations

There is a spectrum of abnormalities that affect the anorectum, loosely called 'imperforate anus' (Fig. 11.5.5). They fall into two main groups: high lesions, where the rectum stops at or above the pelvic levator ani musculature (Fig. 11.5.5A), and low lesions, where it continues beyond this point. Low lesions usually have a fistulous communication with the skin as an anocutaneous fistula (Fig. 11.5.5B). High lesions tend to be more complicated and are more likely to be associated with other congenital abnormalities, particularly of the urinary tract. In the male with a high lesion there is either no opening at all or the rectum communicates with the urinary tract via a rectourethral or rectovesical fistula (Fig. 11.5.5C). In the female the rectum usually communicates with the vestibule or vagina as a rectovestibular or rectovaginal fistula respectively (Fig. 11.5.5D). In addition, a rare but even more severe group of abnormalities may occur in the female: in these cloacal malformations there is only one opening for the rectum, vagina and urinary tract.

In general, low lesions are treated by cutback anoplasty on the day of birth. High lesions require an anorectoplasty – a considerably more complicated procedure, performed either at birth or as a staged procedure later.

Clinical example

Thomas was born normally after an uneventful pregnancy and labour. Meconium was first passed at 36 hours. At the age of 4 days he was noted to be feeding poorly and his abdomen was becoming increasingly distended but no mass was palpable. He vomited twice. On rectal examination a 'squirt' of meconium was passed. A plain upright film of the abdomen revealed several fluid levels suggestive of intestinal obstruction. A provisional diagnosis of Hirschsprung disease was made. This was confirmed on suction rectal biopsy, which demonstrated the absence of ganglion cells in the submucosa. A primary pull-through procedure via the perineum was performed with the transition zone being determined by frozen section.

Abdominal wall defects

The two main major abdominal wall defects are:

- exomphalos (omphalocele)
- gastroschisis.

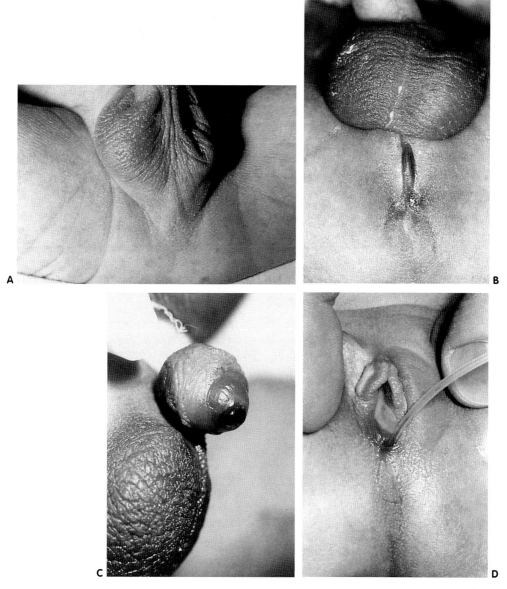

Fig. 11.5.5 Anorectal anomalies presenting as imperforate anus in the neonatal period. **A** High imperforate anus, the lesion being above the levator ani musculature. **B** Imperforate anus due to a low lesion. Meconium is visible behind the distended skin of the median raphe. **C** Passage of meconium from the urethra. This has occurred in a neonate with a high imperforate anus and an associated rectourethral fistula. **D** Anorectal anomaly in a newborn girl. The catheter has been passed into the rectum.

Frequently, both diagnoses are made on antenatal ultrasonography; this may influence the location and timing of delivery but does not influence the mode of delivery. It also provides an opportunity for antenatal counselling.

Exomphalos

This is a large defect at the umbilicus with herniation of bowel and liver into a sac covered by fused amniotic membrane and peritoneum (Fig. 11.5.6). The sac is translucent at birth but quickly becomes opaque as it desiccates. Coexisting abnormalities are common and usually involve the heart and kidneys. Beckwith–Wiedemann syndrome may also be present and must be recognized as it is associated with severe hypoglycaemia that requires immediate correction at birth (Ch. 10.3).

The early management of exomphalos involves placing the baby in a warm Humidicrib incubator and wrapping the entire torso, including the exposed viscera, in clear plastic wrap to prevent evaporative

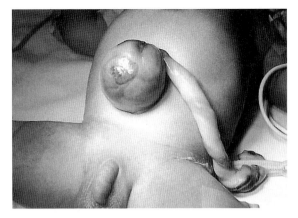

Fig. 11.5.6 Exomphalos, showing the site of the defect at the umbilicus. In some affected neonates the lesion is much larger and may contain most of the bowel and liver.

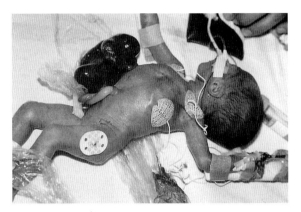

Fig. 11.5.7 Gastroschisis, with herniation of abdominal contents through an abdominal wall defect lateral to the umbilicus.

heat loss. A nasogastric tube keeps the stomach empty, aiding subsequent closure of the defect. The defect can usually be repaired at birth but the largest defects, particularly those that contain liver, may require a staged procedure.

Gastroschisis

In gastroschisis there is a small defect immediately to the right of the umbilicus through which bowel (and sometimes the gonads) herniate (Fig. 11.5.7). The eviscerated small and large bowel is thickened and densely matted with exudate as a result of amni-

otic peritonitis before birth. These infants have a significant risk of hypothermia and exposed bowel should be wrapped in a plastic sheet to avoid evaporative heat loss. Surgery is directed at returning the bowel to the peritoneal cavity and repairing the defect. Where the peritoneal cavity is too small to accept the bowel it may be necessary to create a temporary prosthetic silo. After surgical repair the bowel may take many weeks to function normally. Coexisting abnormalities are normally confined to the gastrointestinal tract.

Diaphragmatic hernia

In the most common type of congenital diaphragmatic hernia (Bochdalek hernia) there is a defect of the left posterolateral part of the diaphragm that allows the contents of the abdomen to herniate into the left thoracic cavity. This limits the space available for the lungs to develop in utero. The resulting pulmonary hypoplasia creates severe respiratory distress within minutes of birth and in some infants is not compatible with long-term survival. The more severe the lung hypoplasia the earlier the infant becomes symptomatic and the poorer the prognosis. Diagnosis of the condition may be made antenatally on routine ultrasonography.

The diagnosis is confirmed after birth by a plain chest X-ray, which shows loops of bowel in the left chest. The heart is displaced to the contralateral side and there is little room available for the lungs. Right-sided diaphragmatic hernias account for only 15% of such lesions. Early treatment involves aggressive cardiorespiratory support and decompression of the bowel. When the child is stable, operative repair of the diaphragm is undertaken.

Sacrococcygeal teratoma

This is a rare tumour that is usually evident at birth; the baby is born with a large mass protruding from the lower back and arising from the tip of the coccyx or sacrum. In other infants it may expand predominantly into the pelvis. It may be extremely large and cause obstetric difficulties. A few become malignant. Malignant change is more likely if surgery is delayed or where the tumour is uniformly solid and devoid of cysts. They are removed soon after birth.

PART 12

INFECTIONS IN CHILDHOOD

Infectious diseases of childhood

D. Isaacs

Infectious diseases of childhood are still a significant cause of illness in children, especially in the first years of life. Although immunization has resulted in a very marked reduction in many of the childhood infections that in previous times caused significant morbidity and mortality (Ch. 3.5), some of these infections are still seen and others have yet to have effective vaccines developed. This chapter describes the features of some of these infections.

Measles (rubeola, morbilli)

Measles virus is a paramyxovirus, one of the RNA viruses. It causes measles, one of the most important of the childhood exanthems, due to its high infectivity and virulence. At the end of the twentieth century measles still caused a million childhood deaths a year worldwide.

The rash of measles is mediated by T cells: infected subjects with defective T cells (cellular immunity) get little or no rash, but classically develop a giant cell pneumonia. Measles infection also causes significant suppression of host T cell immunity, resulting in anergy to tuberculin (negative Mantoux test) and increased susceptibility to diarrhoeal and respiratory illness.

Epidemiology

- Respiratory droplet spread, highly infectious, causing outbreaks every 2 years in unimmunized populations
- From 1978–1992 in Australia over 10 children a year died from measles, as a result of acute encephalitis or pneumonia
- As immunization levels improved, the number of deaths fell to 1–2 per year from 1992, and there have been none since 1995, when a second dose of measles vaccine was introduced at 4–5 years of age
- In developing countries, the high mortality is mainly due to pneumonia, often with bacterial (staphylococcal or pneumococcal) superinfection
- Children in developing countries who recover from measles have increased mortality for a year afterwards because of the resultant suppression of cellular immunity

- Measles is highly contagious and over 98% of adults in unimmunized communities are seropositive.

Clinical features (Figs 12.1.1, 12.1.2)

- Incubation period 10–14 days
- Prodromal period (symptoms before rash) 3–5 days, with high fever, irritability, cough, exudative conjunctivitis, otitis media, and white spots on buccal mucosa (Koplik spots)
- Rash starts behind ears and descends: blotchy, raised rash, confluent in places
- Child miserable and febrile when rash present
- Cervical lymphadenopathy, conjunctivitis, otitis media and wheeze commonly accompany rash.

Complications

See Table 12.1.1.

Differential diagnosis

- In roseola infantum (see below) the rash can be identical to measles but appears as the fever subsides, and the child looks well
- Other viruses causing morbilliform (measles-like) rash on occasions: enteroviruses, Epstein–Barr virus (EBV), influenza, parinfluenza
- Antibiotics, especially amoxicillin or ampicillin, may cause a rash
- Kawasaki disease
- Scarlet fever.

Laboratory diagnosis

- Rapid antigen detection: immunofluorescent antibody stain on nasopharyngeal secretions
- Serology: measles-specific IgM or fourfold or greater rise in IgG titre.

Treatment

- Mainly symptomatic in industrialized countries
- Vitamin A therapy recommended for severe cases and malnourished children
- Antibiotics for bacterial complications, particularly pneumonia.

385

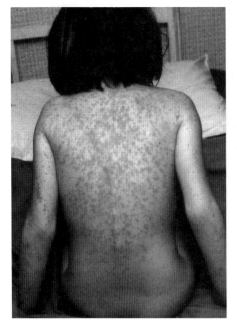

Fig. 12.1.1 Measles: blotchy, raised rash.

Prevention

- Measles is a *vaccine-preventable disease*
- There are effective live, attenuated vaccines
- There is only one serotype of measles
- Humans are the only host
- It should be possible to eradicate measles from the world by immunization
- In developing countries, routine vitamin A supplementation reduces the mortality of measles. In Australia measles–mumps–rubella (MMR) vaccine is given at 1 year of age and a

Clinical example

Harriet, 3 years old, was in preschool with a friend who 2 weeks earlier (1) had a cough and fever (2) and later came out in a rash. Neither had been immunized against measles (3). Harriet developed a high fever, runny nose and cough (4) and was irritable. Her eyes became red and weepy (5) and her ears were sore (6). After 3 days (2) her doctor found bilateral otitis media (6) and white spots on a red background on her buccal mucosa (7). Next day she remained miserable and hot, and developed a rash behind her ears, which spread over the next 2 days to her face, trunk and limbs, and was pink to red and blotchy (8). In some areas the rash joined up and was raised. She had scattered wheezes bilaterally (4). She remained febrile and unwell for 3 days, then the rash faded, leaving a brown discoloration of the skin with desquamation of the fingers and toes (9).

The following are features typical of measles infection:
- Incubation period 10–14 days (1)
- Infectious during the prodromal period, which lasts 3–5 days (2)
- Immunization over 95% protective (3)
- Bronchitis (4), exudative conjunctivitis (5) and otitis media (6) almost invariable features
- Enanthem called Koplik spots (7)
- Rash is classically descending, blotchy to confluent, papular (8), with desquamation, often more marked in children from developing countries (9).

Fig. 12.1.2 The development of measles.

Day of illness	1	2	3	4	5	6	7	8	9	10
Temperature 40.0 39.4 38.8 38.3 37.7 37.2 36.6										
Rash										
Koplik										
Conjunctivitis										
Coryza										
Cough										

Table 12.1.1 Major complications of measles in industrialized countries			
	Incidence	Clinical features	Outcome
Neurological			
Acute encephalitis	1 in 1000 to 1 in 5000	Onset usually day 4–7 after rash, i.e. postinfective	10–15% die, 15–40% brain damage
Subacute sclerosing panencephalitis (SSPE)	1 in 25 000	Intellectual deterioration, myoclonic jerks	Invariably fatal
Respiratory			
Pneumonia	1 in 25	Viral pneumonitis or secondary bacterial infection	Occasional deaths
Otitis media	1 in 40	During prodrome	Transient hearing loss

second dose at 4–5 years of age (note that maternal antibody is generally protective before 1 year and interferes with immunogenicity if vaccine is given earlier)
- Measles vaccine is contraindicated for immunosuppressed children. If exposed to measles, they should be given normal human immunoglobulin, as 'passive' protection.

Roseola infantum (exanthem subitum)

- Caused by infection with human herpesvirus 6 (HHV-6) and occasionally HHV-7
- Affects infants aged 6–18 months
- Morbilliform (measles-like) rash appears as high fever subsides
- Child well and afebrile when rash appears (in contrast to measles)
- May get febrile convulsions in acute phase

Clinical example

Mark, a 9-month-old baby who was previously well, developed a runny nose, fever and irritability (1) and went off his feeds. After 2 days, he had a generalized, tonic–clonic seizure (2), which stopped after 2 minutes. He was admitted to hospital, where he was found to have a fever of 40°C, cervical lymphadenopathy (3) but no rash or enanthem (4). A lumbar puncture was normal. After 24 hours observation in hospital his fever subsided but he developed a diffuse papular rash on his trunk, thought at first to be measles (5). He was well and was discharged home. Serology for HHV-6 revealed positive specific IgM.
   The following are features typical of roseola infantum. (1), (3) Usual presenting features, lasting 2–3 days. Febrile convulsion (2) is a recognized complication. No enanthem (4). Rash often misdiagnosed as measles but the child with roseola is well and the fever falls as the rash appears (5), in contrast to measles.

Rubella (German measles)

The main importance of rubella virus is its teratogenic effect on the fetus, causing congenital rubella syndrome.

Epidemiology

- Respiratory droplet spread
- Causes spring and summer epidemics in unimmunized communities
- Mainly affects children aged 5–10 years but also non-immune pregnant women
- Less infectious than measles: 15–20% of adults in unimmunized populations (including south-east Asia) are non-immune
- Most rubella infections are subclinical.

Clinical features (Figs 12.1.3, 12.1.4)

- Incubation period 14–21 days
- Rash much fainter and less florid than measles, not raised
- Rash often starts on face in young children, spreads to neck, trunk and extremities
- Lymphadenopathy usual, particularly suboccipital, postauricular and cervical

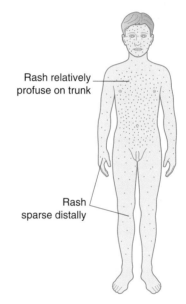

Rash relatively profuse on trunk

Rash sparse distally

Fig. 12.1.3   The distribution of rash in rubella.

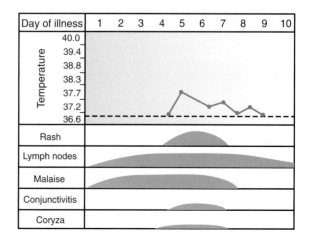

Fig. 12.1.4   The development of rubella.

- Adolescents and adults often get more constitutional symptoms: conjunctivitis, arthralgia or arthritis, malaise, fever
- Encephalitis, purpura are rare complications
- Congenital rubella syndrome results from first-trimester rubella infection (Ch. 11.4).

Diagnosis

Non-immune pregnant woman exposed to possible rubella: send acute serum for rubella-specific IgM and IgG (usually measured by enzyme-linked immunosorbent assay (ELISA)) and a convalescent serum 2–4 weeks later, looking for rubella IgM and/or a rising IgG titre.

Clinical example

Rosie, 7 years old, was off colour for 2 days with headache and low grade fever to 38°C (1). Several of her school-friends had been unwell with fever and rash in the past few weeks, including her best friend 2 weeks ago (2). Rosie then developed a fine rash on her body, a sore throat and a cough, but no joint symptoms (3). Her neck was sore on the day the rash appeared and lymph nodes could be seen in her neck, behind her ear and at the back of her head. Her eyes were slightly red (3). The next day she felt better, and the day after was almost back to normal (4). A clinical diagnosis of rubella was made.

Her mother was 10 weeks pregnant and went to see the doctor (5). The doctor found she had been rubella-seronegative when she booked for her pregnancy with Rosie (her only child), but had not been immunized against rubella after delivery (6). The doctor took blood from Rosie's mother for rubella IgM and IgG and made an appointment for 2 weeks for repeat serology (7).

(1) The prodromal period of rubella is short for children aged 5–9 years (the peak age), who may have no symptoms prior to the rash. Adolescents and adults, in contrast, may have a preceding 1–5 days of fever, headache, sore throat, cough, and often arthralgia or arthritis. The incubation period is 14–21 days (2). The rash and lymphadenopathy (3) are characteristic but not diagnostic and other infections such as erythema infectiosum (slapped cheek disease) can cause clinically similar outbreaks in schoolchildren. The symptoms improve rapidly (4). The major concern is close contact with women in the first trimester of pregnancy (5). In most countries, women are screened for rubella antibodies at booking (6). If they are seronegative, they should be immunized with rubella vaccine (usually in the form of MMR vaccine) after delivery (6). A non-immune pregnant woman in contact with a child with clinical rubella should have serology performed, because women may develop asymptomatic rubella (7). The serology should be repeated 2 weeks later, to look for seroconversion, i.e. the appearance of rubella IgM or a fourfold or greater rise in IgG (7).

Differential diagnosis

- Many other viruses cause rubelliform rashes
- Clinical diagnosis of rubella is notoriously unreliable
- Rubella is very rare in infancy: other viruses, e.g. enteroviruses, HHV-6 are much more likely to cause infantile rashes.

Prevention

- Live attenuated rubella vaccine is usually given universally as MMR in industrialized countries
- Congenital rubella syndrome is rare in industrialized countries such as Australia but common in developing countries.

Erythema infectiosum (slapped cheek disease, fifth disease)

- Caused by human parvovirus B19 (parvo = small)
- Spread by respiratory route
- Causes epidemics in school aged children, which mimic rubella outbreaks
- Initial presentation is with fever, cervical lymphadenopathy and facial rash resembling sunburned cheeks (viraemic phase)
- Subsequently develop lacy, reticular rash on limbs and trunk, sometimes with arthralgia or arthritis (immune-complex-mediated) (Figs 12.1.5, 12.1.6)

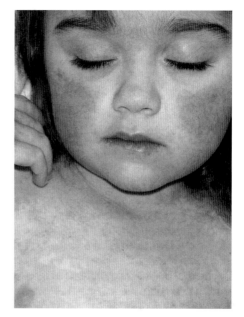

Fig. 12.1.5 Fifth disease: slapped cheeks and lacy rash (With permission of Bernard Cohen, Dermatlas: http://www.dermatlas.org).

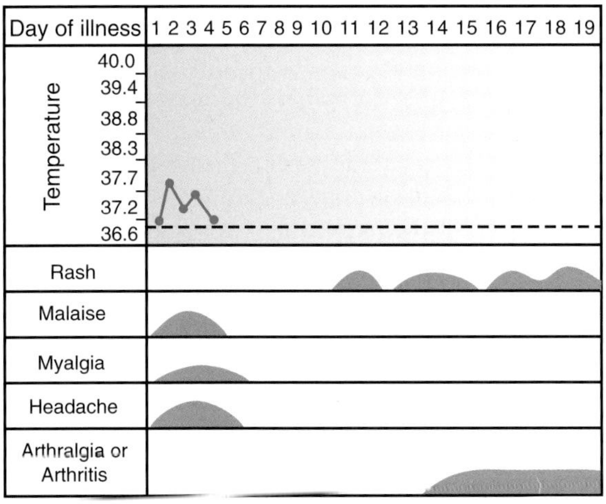

Day of illness	1 2 3 4 5 6 7 8 9 10 11 12 13 14 15 16 17 18 19
Temperature	40.0 39.4 38.8 38.3 37.7 37.2 36.6
Rash	
Malaise	
Myalgia	
Headache	
Arthralgia or Arthritis	

Fig. 12.1.6 The development of erythema infectiosum (fifth disease).

- The virus infects red cell precursors in the bone marrow, causing no effect in normals (haemoglobin drops by 1 g/dl) but severe anaemia in those with shortened red cell survival (e.g. children with abnormal haemoglobin or fetus)
- In sickle cell disease and other hereditary anaemias, infection causes aplastic crises due to red cell aplasia
- Infection during the second or third trimester of pregnancy can cause fetal hydrops due to fetal anaemia.

Varicella (chickenpox)

Chickenpox (Figs 12.1.7, 12.1.8) is a highly infectious disease causing a bullous (pox-like) rash. The DNA virus responsible, varicella-zoster virus (VZV), is a herpesvirus and has the ability to remain dormant in the dorsal root ganglia and reactivate as herpes zoster (shingles).

Epidemiology

- Occurs worldwide, although spreads less readily in tropical countries
- Highly infectious, spread by respiratory route, due to infectious particles from burst vesicles and from respiratory tract
- Incubation period 10–21 days, short prodromal period of 1–2 days
- Peak age incidence is 2–8 years.

Complications

- Bacterial superinfection of skin
- Pneumonia/pneumonitis:

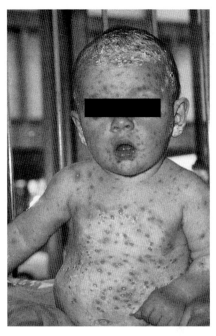

Fig. 12.1.7 Chickenpox: vesicles and pustules on trunk and scalp.

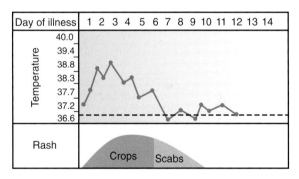

Fig. 12.1.8 The development of chickenpox.

- varicella pneumonitis occurs in immunocompromised children but also in pregnant women and normal adults
- bacterial pneumonia (pneumococcal or staphylococcal) can rarely complicate varicella pneumonitis
- Encephalitis:
  - incidence about 1 in 1000 cases
  - most common form is pure cerebellar ataxia, with complete recovery over days to weeks
  - severe form is acute disseminated encephalomyelitis (ADEM), a postinfectious demyelinating illness with high morbidity and mortality
- Haemorrhagic chickenpox – severe illness in subjects with profound defect in cellular immunity (e.g. oncology patients), indicating

importance of T cells in recovery from VZV infection
- Congenital varicella syndrome – affects up to 2% of babies whose mothers develop chickenpox in pregnancy.

Diagnosis

- Usually clinical
- Can grow virus from blister fluid in tissue culture or detect antigen by immunofluorescence on vesicle fluid
- Can use serology (IgG, IgM).

Prevention

- Live attenuated VZV vaccines are now available and are highly protective
- Varicella zoster immune globulin (ZIG or VZIG) is an immunoglobulin preparation with a high titre of anti-VZV IgG antibodies. It is used for passive prophylaxis of immunocompromised patients (e.g. oncology patients, neonates) exposed to VZV.

Treatment

The antiviral drug acyclovir inhibits viral thymidine kinase and can be used to treat children with severe varicella.

Clinical example

Charles, aged 6, had been in contact with a schoolfriend who was off school 2 weeks ago with chickenpox. Charles had a sore throat and fever of 38°C but no spots. Next day, a few small red spots like mosquito stings appeared on his trunk and limbs and on his scalp under the hair. These became raised, then developed into small, fluid-filled blisters surrounded by a small area of erythema. They were intensely itchy and when scratched readily became superinfected and left a scar. These spots crusted over within hours but fresh crops of vesicles kept appearing on Charles's face, trunk and limbs. He had difficulty swallowing and his eyes were red and sore. He was miserable but not unwell and was troubled by the intense pruritus. After a week, the last spot had crusted and the scabs disappeared over the next 2 weeks.

The following are features typical of varicella. Incubation period 10–21 days. Short 1–2 day prodrome during which infectious (not infectious during the incubation period). Spots under hairline characteristic and distinguish from insect bites. Start as macules, then progress to papules, vesicles or pustules. If scratched they may become infected, the commonest complication, and leave a scar or pockmark. They come in crops, and can infect the pharynx, palate and conjunctivae of the lids. The child is infectious until the last spot crusts.

Zoster (herpes zoster, shingles)

- VZV can remain dormant in the dorsal root ganglia of sensory nerves after primary infection and reactivate many years later as zoster. Zoster follows a dermatome distribution and was the means by which the distribution of the sensory nerves was mapped. Vesicles form a band and do not usually cross the midline. They can occur on the trunk and limbs or follow cranial nerves. The Ramsay Hunt syndrome presents with vesicles on the pinna of one ear and facial nerve palsy due to zoster of the geniculate ganglion.
- Zoster infection in a previously well child is almost always benign and not suggestive of underlying malignancy.
- About 10% of children whose mothers developed chickenpox during pregnancy will develop zoster in early childhood: if a young child gets zoster, ask about chickenpox in pregnancy.
- Immunocompromised children are at increased risk of zoster.
- Neuralgia before, during and after zoster is very uncommon in children, in contrast to adults.
- Most childhood zoster does not need specific treatment but intravenous acyclovir is indicated for ophthalmic zoster (to prevent eye damage) or if the child is immunocompromised (to prevent life-threatening disseminated infection).

Mumps (epidemic parotitis)

- Infectious disease of childhood, 90% before adolescence
- Preventable by immunization with live attenuated virus (usually given as MMR vaccine)
- Causes swelling, pain and tenderness of the parotid glands
- Can rarely be unilateral but unilateral neck swelling more suggestive of alternative diagnoses (e.g. lymphadenopathy, autoimmune parotitis)
- Other salivary glands, sublingual and submandibular, may be involved
- Complications include viral meningitis (symptomatic in 10% of children with mumps, asymptomatic in over 50%), encephalitis, orchitis, oophoritis, pancreatitis, thyroiditis, deafness and rarely ophthalmitis, arthritis, myocarditis and nephritis.

Scarlet fever and scarlatina

- Scarlet fever (Figs 12.1.9, 12.1.10) is a toxin-mediated disease caused by exotoxins elaborated by

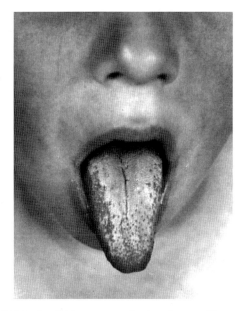

Fig. 12.1.9   Scarlet fever: generalized erythema with circumoral pallor.

Day of illness	1	2	3	4	5	6	7	8	9	10

Fig. 12.1.10   The development of scarlet fever.

group A streptococcus (*Streptococcus pyogenes*) and coded by plasmids
• These toxins act as 'superantigens', causing widespread T-cell activation because they can bind to the edge of the T-cell receptor and bypass its usual highly specific recognition of antigens
• Analogous superantigen-mediated diseases include toxic shock syndrome and Kawasaki disease.

Scarlatina is a mild form of scarlet fever, often affecting preschool age children, whereas scarlet fever is commonest at age 5–10 years.

In both, the primary site of group A streptococcal infection is the throat, causing exudative tonsillitis and/or pharyngitis.

In preantibiotic days, scarlet fever, and the related erysipelas, was a quarantinable disease, highly contagious and with a high mortality. Although scarlet fever became less common after the 1940s, it has re-emerged, perhaps due to the re-emergence of strains producing virulent exotoxins.

Diagnosis

Positive throat swab or positive serology: high or rising titre to streptolysin O (ASOT) or deoxyribonuclease B (anti-DNAase B).

Clinical example

Anna, 7 years old, presented with fever and sore throat for 2 days, followed by a rash. Her tonsils were red and covered in spots of white exudate. Her tongue had prominent red papillae. Her face looked red but was white around the mouth, like a clown. The rash was red, patchy and rough to the touch, and covered her whole body. In the axillae and groins there were lines of petechiae. Her cervical lymph nodes were enlarged and tender. She was treated with penicillin and rapidly improved. Two weeks later she had extensive peeling of her hands and feet.

The following are features typical of scarlet fever. Exudative tonsillitis; strawberry tongue; circumoral pallor; sandpaper rash; Pastia's lines; tender cervical lymphadenitis; peripheral desquamation.

Glandular fever (infectious mononucleosis)

Classical glandular fever is caused by Epstein–Barr virus (EBV) and is associated with atypical mononuclear cells in the blood, giving the name infectious mononucleosis. A similar syndrome can be produced by infection with cytomegalovirus (CMV) and *Toxoplasma gondii* (toxoplasmosis).

Adolescence is a common time of presentation, with transmission from infected saliva by the oral route ('kissing disease'). However, EBV can also present in infancy and early childhood with an 'anginose' form, mainly affecting the tonsils.

Diagnosis

• Serological: specific IgM or rising IgG titre to EBV. The Paul–Bunnell test and monospot test detect non-specific antibodies produced because of the polyclonal B cell proliferation caused by EBV. They have low sensitivity in children
• The blood film is often strongly suggestive, showing many atypical mononuclear cells.

Clinical example

Beth, 6 years old, presented with fever, sore throat and malaise. She was treated with amoxicillin for exudative tonsillitis. Two days later, she developed a florid rash. When reviewed, she had marked tonsillar enlargement and large matted nodes in the neck, which were moderately tender. She had petechiae on the soft palate. Her eyelids were puffy and her spleen was palpable 2 cm below the costal margin. Pulse oximetry, performed overnight to exclude significant upper airways obstruction, was normal, so dexamethasone was withheld and she was sent home.

'Purulent' exudative tonsillitis may be due to group A streptococcus or EBV at this age. Ampicillin or amoxicillin causes a dramatic rash in EBV infection. Tender lymphadenitis occurs in both but palatal petechiae, puffy eyelids and splenomegaly are typical features of EBV infection. There is no specific treatment but steroids are sometimes used to reduce upper airway obstruction.

Herpes simplex virus

- Herpes simplex virus (HSV) is a DNA herpesvirus, with two serotypes, HSV-1 and HSV-2
- HSV-1 is primarily oropharyngeal
- HSV-2 is primarily genital
- Neonates can catch HSV around delivery, usually (about 90%) HSV-2, although neonatal HSV-1 infection is increasing
- The commonest childhood HSV infection is gingivostomatitis, due to primary HSV-1 infection: it causes nasty ulceration of the gums (gingivae), buccal mucosa (stoma = mouth) and pharynx
- HSV infection can disseminate in the skin of children with eczema (eczema herpeticum, Kaposi varicelliform eruption) if not treated promptly with aciclovir
- Neonatal HSV infection may be localized to skin, eye (conjunctivitis) and/or mouth, may cause isolated encephalitis or isolated pneumonitis or, if not treated with acyclovir, will usually disseminate to cause hepatitis, disseminated intravascular coagulation, encephalitis and death
- Herpes encephalitis can occur at any age, may be primary or secondary, due to HSV-1 or HSV-2, and has a poor prognosis, even if treated with acyclovir
- As a herpesvirus, local recurrences of HSV are common, often at the mucocutaneous junction of the lip ('cold sores') but can be on the finger ('whitlow') or on the skin anywhere
- Try to avoid the child inoculating virus into the genital area.

Diagnosis

Rapid diagnosis by immunofluorescence of blister fluid or polymerase chain reaction (PCR) of blister fluid and/or cerebrospinal fluid is preferred to culture or serology (IgM).

Enteroviruses

- The enteroviruses, as the name suggests, are gut viruses, usually transmitted mainly faecal-orally, although respiratory spread can occur
- They are picornaviruses (from pico = small + RNA)
- They can affect the central nervous syndrome, causing a variety of syndromes
- The major groups of enteroviruses are:
  - Coxsackieviruses (Coxsackie is a town in New York State where an outbreak occurred)
  - echoviruses (from *e*nteric *c*ytopathic *h*uman *o*rphan)
  - polioviruses types 1–3
  - enterovirus 71 (EV 71)
- *Fever*: common cause of isolated fever in infancy
- *Rashes*:
  - hand, food and mouth disease: blistering rash on palms, soles and palate caused by Coxsackievirus A16 and other enteroviruses, including enterovirus 71
  - various non-specific rashes: macular, papular, papulo-urticarial, vesicular, morbilliform, rubelliform, etc.
- *Enanthem*: herpangina (= ulcerative pharyngitis) due to Coxsackievirus A
- *Neurological*:
  - paralytic: poliomyelitis due to infection of anterior horn cells by poliovirus, but similar syndrome can be caused by other enteroviruses
  - monoplegia: EV 71, other enteroviruses
  - aseptic meningitis, meningoencephalitis: Coxsackieviruses, echoviruses, EV 71
- *Cardiac*: myocarditis – mainly Coxsackievirus B
- *Liver*: hepatitis – mainly echoviruses
- *Eyes*: epidemic conjunctivitis – EV 71
- *Muscles*: Bornholm disease (epidemic pleurodynia) due to Coxsackie virus B.

Spread

Swimming and wading pools, direct contact, mainly in summer and autumn.

Treatment

The antiviral drug pleconaril has activity against enteroviruses, but is not widely available.

Prevention

Immunization against polio with oral polio vaccine (live, attenuated) or inactivated polio vaccine (injected, killed).

Adenoviruses

• Multiple serotypes
• In infancy, adenoviruses are an important cause of exudative tonsillitis with high fever (at this age, group A streptococcal infection is rare)
• Can cause epidemics of conjunctivitis, often with red throat (pharyngoconjunctival fever)
• Can cause disseminated infection with pneumonia, hepatitis and encephalitis (particularly adenovirus 7 and 21): rare but may be fatal
• Enteric adenoviruses can cause gastroenteritis.

Diagnosis

Viral culture or immunofluorescence on throat swab.

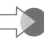

Practical points

• Measles is a severe vaccine-preventable childhood infection
• Children with measles are sick when the rash appears: children with roseola infantum are sick until the rash appears
• Rubella is usually mild but can cross the placenta in the first trimester to cause congenital rubella syndrome
• Chickenpox and measles can be devastating in children with impaired cell-mediated (T-cell) immunity
• Scarlet fever is a toxin-mediated disease caused by an exotoxin produced by group A streptococci

Bone and joint infections

J. R. Carapetis, A. C. Steer

Introduction

Infections of bones (osteomyelitis) and joints (septic arthritis) can occur at any age but are much more common in children than adults. They are often difficult to diagnose, can be difficult to treat and if improperly diagnosed and treated can lead to permanent disability. Many children and adults have shortened or deformed limbs, fused joints or even amputations because osteomyelitis or septic arthritis was diagnosed too late or treated inadequately. Almost all these poor outcomes need not have happened; with careful history taking and examination, prudent use of investigations – particularly imaging – and close observation, virtually all bone and joint infections can be diagnosed and treated before permanent damage ensues.

Pathogenesis

The area around the growth plates of children's bones is particularly prone to infection. Although the metaphysis has a plentiful blood supply from nutrient arteries, blood flow through capillary loops and sinusoidal veins at the metaphyseal-epiphyseal junction is slow, which allows blood-borne bacteria to deposit in this region (Fig. 12.2.1). This area also has poor penetration of white blood cells and other immune mediators, so that deposited bacteria are relatively protected. As the infection progresses, pus accumulates under pressure, which further limits the blood supply to the region. Increased stasis and activity of cytokines encourages clots to form in these vessels, leading to ischaemic bone necrosis. Infection then spreads to the cortex through the Volkmann canals and Haversian system, and subsequently into the subperiosteal space.

If the infection remains untreated, bone necrosis may lead to development of a sequestrum – an area of dead cortical bone separated from normal bone. Sometimes the infection becomes walled off by granulation tissue that forms a fibrous capsule; the so-called Brodie abscess. These are usually located in the metaphysis and present subacutely with pain and tenderness but rarely fever.

Chronic osteomyelitis is usually the result of untreated or inadequately treated acute osteomyelitis. Sequestra and Brodie abscesses are sometimes found in chronic osteomyelitis. Most cases of chronic osteomyelitis, like acute osteomyelitis, are caused by *Staphylococcus aureus*, but chronic presentations increase the likelihood of unusual organisms, including *Mycobacterium tuberculosis*, fungi and *Kingella kingae*.

Septic arthritis may occur de novo, as a result of deposition of bacteria in the joint. Alternatively there may be extension of an adjacent osteomyelitis, which is more common in children than adults, possibly because of transport of bacteria through blood vessels that cross the epiphyseal plate. In some joints, the metaphysis is intra-articular, which means that osteomyelitis can transform directly into septic arthritis. These joints are:

- proximal femur → hip joint
- proximal humerus → shoulder joint
- proximal radius → elbow joint
- distal lateral tibia → ankle joint.

Synovial joints are poor at clearing infection and the connective tissue may be damaged by enzymes released by bacteria. Initially, the inflammation results in a joint effusion, which may be purulent, but if left untreated the articular and growth cartilage can be destroyed. Longer-term complications may include dislocation, avascular necrosis of intra-articular epiphyses and joint destruction.

Microbiology

Although occasionally caused by fungi, and rarely by parasites or viruses, osteomyelitis and septic arthritis are predominantly bacterial infections, most often caused by *Staphylococcus aureus*. The major bacterial pathogens are:

- *Staphylococcus aureus* (80–90% of culture positive cases). Usually methicillin-susceptible but community acquired MRSA (CA-MRSA) is on the rise in many places
- *Streptococcus pyogenes* (group A streptococcus). Sometimes associated with varicella infection

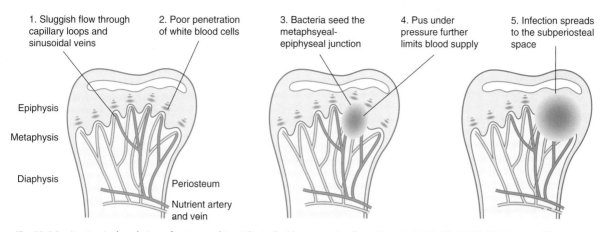

Fig. 12.2.1 Anatomical evolution of osteomyelitis. Adapted with permission from Krogstad P, Smith A L 2004 Osteomyelitis and septic arthritis. In: Feigin R D, Cherry J D, Demmler G J, Kaplan S L (eds) Textbook of pediatric infectious diseases, 5th ed. W B Saunders, Philadelphia, PA, pp 683–703.

- *Streptococcus pneumoniae.* Mainly in children aged less than 2 years
- *Pseudomonas aeruginosa.* Immunocompromised patients, or traumatic (classical cause is a nail through a tennis shoe causing calcaneal osteomyelitis)
- group B streptococcus or *Escherichia coli.* Especially in neonates
- *Haemophilus influenzae* type B. In unimmunized populations (mainly in developing countries)
- *Mycobacterium tuberculosis.* Mainly developing countries or immigrant populations. 50% of cases affect the spine. Often subacute presentation
- *Salmonella* spp. Particularly in people with sickle cell anaemia
- *Neisseria gonorrhoea.* Mainly in developing countries. May cause multifocal septic arthritis in neonates or sexually active adolescents.

Clinical presentation

Although osteomyelitis and septic arthritis are usually considered distinct entities, in paediatric practice they are sometimes difficult to distinguish and may occur together. Children with septic arthritis are more likely than adults to have osteomyelitis in the adjacent bone. In neonates and infants, osteomyelitis and septic arthritis coexist so commonly that the preferred term is 'osteoarticular infection'.

The typical child with osteomyelitis or septic arthritis is aged less than 5 years – approximately 50% of cases occur under the age of 5 and of these 25% are under the age of 1. Usually the symptoms have been present for 2–3 days prior to presentation.

Early in the illness, when bacteraemia is present, the child may be unwell with fever and malaise. Later, as the infection establishes itself, the symptoms relate to the main site of infection. Both diseases usually present with fever and limb pain – in younger children this will most often manifest as a limp, or disuse of a limb or other body part. Septic arthritis is more likely than osteomyelitis to have obvious localized clinical signs.

Osteomyelitis

In osteomyelitis, there is pain, which may be poorly localized, especially in young children. Neonates may present with a generalized febrile illness, without any localizing features. The precise location of the infection can often be elicited with careful physical examination, particularly looking for metaphyseal tenderness. Erythema and swelling are signs of abscess formation, which occurs late in the illness. In one-third of cases there is a history of mild preceding trauma to the affected area so such a history should increase rather than reduce the suspicion of osteomyelitis.

Osteomyelitis most commonly affects, in order:

1. femur
2. tibia
3. humerus
4. calcaneus.

Pelvis and vertebrae are less commonly affected but more likely to present with advanced disease because of delayed presentation (in vertebral osteomyelitis) or delayed diagnosis (in pelvic osteomyelitis). The diagnosis of osteomyelitis in long bones may also be

Labels within Fig. 12.2.1:
1. Sluggish flow through capillary loops and sinusoidal veins
2. Poor penetration of white blood cells
3. Bacteria seed the metaphsyeal-epiphyseal junction
4. Pus under pressure further limits blood supply
5. Infection spreads to the subperiosteal space

Epiphysis
Metaphysis
Diaphysis
Periosteum
Nutrient artery and vein

delayed – and hence subacute or chronic – because of formation of a Brodie abscess or the presence of low-grade infection, sometimes due to unusual organisms. In these cases, diffuse pain or tenderness are prominent and fever may be absent.

Septic arthritis

Differentiating septic arthritis from osteomyelitis can be difficult. Children with osteomyelitis may not want to move the adjacent joint because of either pain or muscle spasm. In addition to fever and limb pain, the hallmark of septic arthritis is a warm, tender joint with a dramatically restricted range of movement and an effusion. However, these signs are not always present. Septic arthritis of the shoulder or hip is very difficult to diagnose early, because of the lack of visible joint swelling in the early stages.

The following features should raise suspicion that there is coexistent osteomyelitis and septic arthritis:

- osteomyelitis in a bone with an intra-articular metaphysis (proximal femur, proximal humerus, proximal radius, distal lateral fibula)
- slow clinical response to therapy
- slow response of inflammatory markers (e.g. C-reactive protein) to therapy
- age less than 18 months
- delayed presentation
- prior antibiotic therapy.

Differential diagnosis

The most important diagnosis to exclude in possible osteomyelitis is malignancy. Bone tumours can cause local bone destruction, and leukaemia may present with fever and bone pain. Cellulitis may mimic the focal tenderness and erythema of late-presenting osteomyelitis. Patients with sickle cell disease may develop bone infarction, which can be difficult to differentiate from osteomyelitis.

Chronic recurrent multifocal osteomyelitis (CRMO) is a rare, non-infectious inflammatory syndrome of unknown pathogenesis that affects children and young adults and is most common in girls. Affected children have prolonged symptoms of pain and swelling that relapse and recur. A classical site of involvement is the clavicle. Treatment with antibiotics does not alter the course of the disease but steroids and anti-inflammatory medication may provide symptomatic relief. CRMO usually resolves, although it may relapse and recur over a prolonged period (up to 15 years) and there is a danger of premature epiphyseal closure.

Septic arthritis of the hip can present similarly to transient synovitis ('irritable hip'), which usually occurs following minor injury or a viral illness. Children with transient synovitis are usually not unwell and their joint signs are not as severe as children with septic arthritis but in the early stages of either illness the diagnoses can be confused. Sometimes the only way to be sure of the diagnosis is to aspirate the joint and observe the child. It is important not to treat empirically with antibiotics without first obtaining a diagnostic specimen.

Acute joint swelling may be caused by inflammatory arthritis (e.g. juvenile chronic arthritis, inflammatory bowel disease, other connective tissue diseases), reactive arthritis (which may occur in association with a wide range of pathogens including *Mycoplasma*, cytomegalovirus, Epstein–Barr virus, parvovirus, hepatitis, rubella vaccination, *Yersinia*, *Salmonella* and *Shigella* spp.), rheumatic fever, and Henoch–Schönlein purpura.

Rarely, osteomyelitis or septic arthritis may affect multiple bones or joints at the same time. This should raise the suspicion of a distant source of persistent bacteraemia such as endocarditis or occult abscess and should lead to a thorough investigation for other sites of infection (e.g. in heart, liver, spleen, brain, eyes). It should also raise suspicion of unusual organisms (e.g. *Neisseria gonorrhoea* as a cause of multifocal septic arthritis) or an alternative diagnosis if an organism cannot be identified (e.g. CRMO, inflammatory or reactive arthritis or rheumatic fever).

Confirming the diagnosis

As a minimum all patients with suspected bone or joint infections should have a blood culture, blood count and film, C- reactive protein (CRP) measurement and plain radiograph. Other investigations are tailored to the likelihood of bone or joint infection (Fig. 12.2.2).

Osteomyelitis

Diagnosis depends upon the presence of two of the following:

- clinical signs (fever, localized tenderness, erythema, oedema)
- pus aspirated from bone
- positive blood or bone culture
- evidence of osteomyelitis on plain radiograph, bone scan or magnetic resonance imaging (MRI) scan.

Approach to the management of osteomyelitis and septic arthritis in children

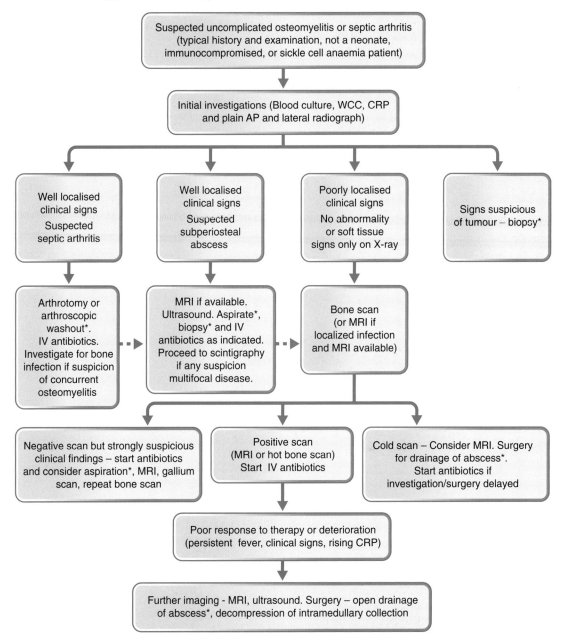

Fig. 12.2.2 Approach to the management of osteomyelitis and septic arthritis in children. AP, anteroposterior; CRP, C reactive protein; IV, intravenous; MRI, magnetic resonance imaging; WCC, white cell count. Adapted with permission from Steer A C, Carapetis J R 2004 Acute hematogenous osteomyelitis in children: recognition and management. Pediatric Drugs 6: 333–346.

Other laboratory tests can provide supportive evidence for the diagnosis:

- the peripheral white cell count (WCC) is normal in half or more of osteomyelitis cases. However, WCC and blood film examination should be performed to exclude leukaemia
- erythrocyte sedimentation rate (ESR) and CRP are elevated at presentation in more than 90% of cases. CRP is preferred to ESR because it rises faster (within 6 h compared to 24 h for ESR) and responds more quickly to treatment (returning to normal in 2 weeks compared to 3–4 weeks for ESR in typical cases).

Pus aspirated from bone

Although some advocate diagnostic bone aspiration or biopsy as a routine, the majority of children do not need these invasive tests. A diagnostic specimen should be obtained in any of the following situations:

- delayed presentation
- a child with any predisposing condition (e.g. immunocompromise, sickle cell disease and other haemoglobinopathies)
- unusual radiographic findings (e.g. lucency on plain radiography at presentation)
- geographical region where there is a high likelihood of CA-MRSA
- reason to suspect a complication such as an abscess
- reason to suspect an alternative diagnosis such as malignancy
- delayed response to antibiotics.

Positive blood or bone culture

Bone aspiration and bone biopsy cultures are positive at admission in 50–70% of osteomyelitis cases and culture-negative cases may have a positive Gram stain or typical histological features of acute osteomyelitis. However, as stated above, this procedure is usually not needed. Blood cultures are positive in 30–50% of cases.

Imaging

Plain radiography
Plain radiographs should be performed routinely to exclude a fracture or malignancy. There are no changes of osteomyelitis in the first 3 days. From days 3–10 there may be non-specific deep soft tissue swelling followed by poor distinction of muscular planes. From days 10–21 periosteal elevation or lytic lesions may be seen (Fig. 12.2.3). Because these changes

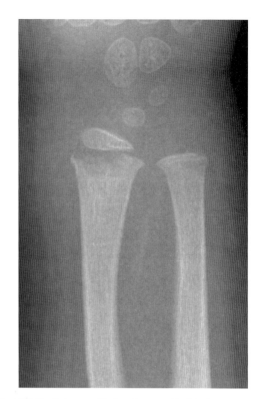

Fig. 12.2.3 Osteomyelitis in a 3-year-old girl who presented with pseudoparalysis. Radiographs at presentation were normal. This radiograph, taken 2 weeks after presentation, shows early abscess formation in the distal radius with erosion of the radial metaphysis and loss of fat plane definition. Courtesy of Professor Kerr Graham; reproduced with permission from Steer A C, Carapetis J R 2004 Acute hematogenous osteomyelitis in children: recognition and management. Pediatric Drugs 6: 333–346.

indicate longer-standing disease, if they are seen on radiographs at presentation the child should not be treated as having acute, uncomplicated osteomyelitis (i.e. s/he requires more prolonged courses of initial intravenous and subsequent oral antibiotics).

Bone scan
The typical bone scan uses technetium-99m-labelled phosphates or phosphonates, which bind to hydroxyapatite crystal as they flow through bone. Uptake is increased with increased blood flow, inflammation and altered osteoblastic activity. The sensitivity of bone scans in the diagnosis of osteomyelitis is more than 90% but a negative bone scan does not exclude the diagnosis. False-negative bone scans in osteomyelitis can be caused by focal ischaemia due to compression from abscess formation, leading to a 'cold' rather than the typical 'hot' scan. There is a 5–30% false-positive rate of bone scans, usually due to the difficulty in differentiating infection in surrounding soft tissue or joints from bone. Bone scans are considered the investigation of choice by many people

Clinical example

Michael, aged 15 months, was noted by his parents to be reluctant to weight bear on his right leg and had a low-grade fever. He was seen by his general practitioner and referred immediately to the emergency department, from where he was admitted with 'possible osteomyelitis' of the right distal femur because of mild metaphyseal tenderness and refusal to weight bear. Osteomyelitis was confirmed by positive blood culture (*S. aureus*) and a positive bone scan. Plain radiographs were normal. Michael was managed with intravenous flucloxacillin for 3 days, followed by oral flucloxacillin for 3 weeks. He was followed for 6 months and had no long-term sequelae.

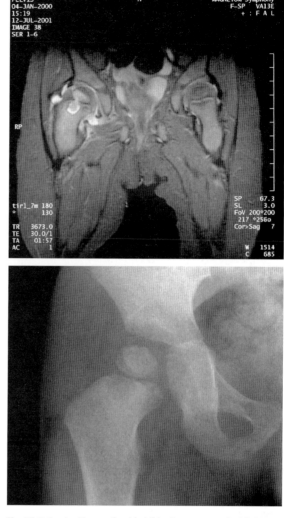

Fig. 12.2.4 An 18-month-old child who presented with fever and limp. **A** MRI shows an abscess that originates in the metaphysis of the right proximal femur crossing the physeal cartilage to the epiphysis. **B** Plain radiograph shows an abscess in the proximal femur. Courtesy of Professor Kerr Graham; reproduced with permission from Steer A C, Carapetis J R 2004 Acute hematogenous osteomyelitis in children: recognition and management. Pediatric Drugs 6: 333–346.

for osteomyelitis because they are sensitive, cheap, usually positive within 48 hours of onset of symptoms, rarely require sedation and allow for the detection of multifocal disease (because the whole skeleton is visualized). However, bone scans give a relatively high radiation dose (equivalent to 100 chest X-rays, or half that of a computed tomography (CT) scan of the chest) and don't give any detailed anatomical information particularly relating to collections of pus.

Ultrasonography

Ultrasound is mainly used to guide aspiration of subperiosteal fluid collections. There may be other changes that suggest osteomyelitis (e.g. cortical breaches and soft tissue swelling), but ultrasound is rarely used by itself for diagnosing osteomyelitis. It may also detect fluid collections in adjacent joints suggestive of septic arthritis.

Magnetic resonance imaging

MRI is the best test for osteomyelitis in cases where symptoms and signs are localized (Fig. 12.2.4). A finding of dark bone marrow intensity on T1-weighted images has almost 100% sensitivity. The specificity is not quite as high, although the use of fat-suppressed contrast-enhanced imaging improves specificity. The other advantages of MRI are that it will show abscesses and sinus tracts and is particularly useful in planning surgery in complex cases. MRI is often used in vertebral osteomyelitis because of the risk of epidural abscess, and in the pelvis, where there is a higher risk of abscess formation. However, it is often not easy to obtain an MRI scan at short notice, scans are expensive and younger children may need to be anaesthetized for a scan. MRI may also be useful in cases where there is high clinical suspicion of localized osteomyelitis but a negative (and therefore possibly false-negative) bone scan.

Septic arthritis

Septic arthritis can usually be diagnosed more easily than osteomyelitis because the signs are more obvious and a diagnostic specimen more easily obtained. Any child with a possibly infected joint requires urgent surgical intervention. This should be done as a formal arthroscopic washout or arthrotomy in the operating theatre under general anaesthetic. Joint aspiration alone should only be performed to obtain a specimen when the diagnosis is in doubt – with the intention of proceeding to the operating theatre if the diagnosis is confirmed – or if there is an unavoidable delay before getting the child to the operating theatre.

Joint fluid should be sent immediately to the laboratory for Gram stain and culture. The Gram stain is not a reliable method of microbiological diagnosis, so Gram stain results should not be used as a reason to cease antistaphylococcal antibiotics in favour of other antimicrobials. Instead, a Gram stain suggesting other organisms (e.g. Gram-negative bacilli) is an indication to add broader-spectrum cover to the antistaphylococcal antibiotic. The antimicrobial treatment can be rationalized when definitive culture and susceptibility results are known.

Occasionally, pus from an obviously infected joint may not grow organisms on culture, even if a child has not received prior antibiotics. This is probably because of the high levels of natural cytokines and other antibacterial agents in the effusion. Most of these cases can be managed as *S. aureus* infections but sometimes the negative culture result is because the joint is not actually infected. A number of patients with juvenile chronic arthritis and rheumatic fever present initially with culture-negative 'septic arthritis'. Therefore, a negative culture of synovial fluid should lead to a thorough re-evaluation of the patient and exclusion of other diagnoses.

Treatment

The choice of empirical antimicrobial therapy is similar for septic arthritis and osteomyelitis. The duration of treatment is identical for uncomplicated cases. Osteomyelitis is more likely than septic arthritis to be complicated and then require longer courses of initial parenteral and subsequent oral therapy. Surgery is always required for septic arthritis but only occasionally required for osteomyelitis.

Antibiotic choice

Because *S. aureus* is the most common cause of bone and joint infections in all age groups, empirical antibiotic therapy should always contain an antistaphylococcal antibiotic such as a beta-lactamase-resistant penicillin (e.g. flucloxacillin) or first-generation cephalosporin (e.g. cephalothin or cefazolin). Clindamycin is a good choice in patients allergic to beta-lactam antibiotics or in areas with high rates of CA-MRSA infection (unless clindamycin resistance is also a problem, in which case vancomycin is usually needed).

The following patients should have other antibiotics added to (not substituted for) the antistaphylococcal antibiotic regimen:

- *neonates*: add gentamicin or a third-generation cephalosporin (e.g. cefotaxime, ceftriaxone)
- *sickle cell anaemia*: add a third-generation cephalosporin (e.g. cefotaxime, ceftriaxone)
- *puncture wounds to the feet*: add an antipseudomonal antibiotic (e.g. ceftazidime, piperacillin, ticarcillin)
- *immunocompromise*: add an antipseudomonal antibiotic, as above. If there is no response, consider also adding an antifungal (e.g. amphotericin or voriconazole)
- children aged less than 5 years and not immunized against *Haemophilus influenzae* type b (Hib): add a third-generation cephalosporin (e.g. cefotaxime, ceftriaxone).

Following identification of the organism antibiotic choice is dictated by susceptibility testing. If cultures are unable to be taken or if cultures are negative then the initial empirical choice should be continued, provided the clinical response is adequate.

Duration of antibiotic therapy

Adult patients are usually treated for osteomyelitis or septic arthritis with 4–6 weeks of intravenous antibiotics. By contrast, children can often be treated for a shorter time and most of the treatment course can be given orally. The typical child with acute, uncomplicated osteomyelitis or septic arthritis who responds quickly to initial therapy can be treated with 3 days of intravenous antibiotics followed by 3 weeks of oral antibiotics. However, this regimen should be used only in otherwise healthy children with classical acute presentations, no evidence of chronicity on initial radiography and a rapid response to treatment. Children with atypical presentations, underlying illness, evidence of chronicity, complications or delayed response to treatment should all be treated with longer initial courses of intravenous antibiotics and longer total duration of therapy. When the switch is made from parenteral to oral antibiotics, they should be used at two to three times higher doses than normally given to achieve adequate serum and bone concentrations. Children usually tolerate this well, with few side effects.

Surgical management

As mentioned above, all children with septic arthritis require a formal arthroscopic washout or arthrotomy as a diagnostic and therapeutic procedure. Splinting an infected joint may be useful to reduce pain in the first few days but joint mobility should be encouraged once the acute signs have settled. An infected hip may require abduction bracing to prevent or treat septic dislocation in the younger child.

The main place for surgery in osteomyelitis is to confirm the diagnosis or manage complications such as abscesses, chronic osteomyelitis, sequestra, pseudarthroses or growth defects. In chronic osteomyelitis, both long-term antibiotics and surgical debridement are needed. Deformities that result from chronic osteomyelitis or growth plate damage may require limb reconstruction techniques. Destruction to articular cartilage causes lifelong problems that are not correctable by surgery.

Monitoring therapy and follow-up

The child should be followed clinically to ensure that pain, tenderness, mobility and systemic symptoms all respond quickly and do not relapse on or after antibiotic treatment. Inflammatory markers are usually also followed. The CRP is the best marker in bone and joint infections – it is almost always elevated initially, unlike the WCC, and responds more quickly to treatment than the ESR. It is not necessary to wait for the ESR to normalize before ceasing antibiotic treatment, provided the child has fully responded clinically and the CRP has normalized or dramatically improved. A rise in CRP after antibiotics have been started may indicate the presence of complications or septic arthritis in addition to osteomyelitis.

If there is persistent fever or local symptoms and/or the CRP has not begun to fall 2–3 days after commencing intravenous antibiotics, there may be a complication such as an abscess, coexistent septic arthritis or a sequestrum. In these cases, re-imaging is usually needed with MRI or ultrasound. Any collection should be drained and, if no collection is present, aspiration at the site of infection should be undertaken for histology and culture/Gram stain.

Typical cases that respond well to initial treatment and can be switched to oral treatment in the first week can be discharged from hospital shortly after commencing oral antibiotics. They should be assessed clinically and with CRP measurement for 3 weeks and reviewed occasionally (e.g. every 6 months) for the next 2 years to monitor for relapse.

Prognosis

In affluent countries, children almost never die from osteomyelitis but some children develop recurrent infection (which may occur many months or even

Clinical example

Jennifer, aged 6 months, was admitted to hospital with a diagnosis of 'pyrexia of unknown origin'. She was investigated extensively. Eventually she was treated with oral antibiotics for a 'possible urinary tract infection'. This made her afebrile, but her fever returned within 2 days of completing the antibiotic course. Septic arthritis of the right hip and proximal femoral osteomyelitis was diagnosed 3 weeks after the onset of fever. She progressed to develop septic dislocation of the right hip, avascular necrosis of the femoral capital epiphysis and growth arrest. She required more than 20 hospital admissions for orthopaedic operations throughout childhood. At the age of 15 years, she is a very troubled teenager with a painful hip, short leg and severe limp.

years later) or chronic osteomyelitis. Other rare complications include pathological fractures and bone deformities, including growth arrest, and leg-length discrepancy. The outcome of septic arthritis is also usually good but delayed or inadequate treatment can lead to joint damage or destruction, with long-term problems of poor function and osteoarthritis. All of these complications are more common in children whose diagnosis is not made sufficiently early or who receive inadequate initial treatment.

Discitis and vertebral osteomyelitis

Musculoskeletal infection of the spine is uncommon but does occur in children. There are two distinct entities of spinal infection – vertebral osteomyelitis and discitis. In their initial phases both present with poorly localized back pain and absent or only low-grade fever.

Children with vertebral osteomyelitis are usually older (>8 years) and eventually become febrile and toxic, developing localized back pain that may affect any part of the spine. The cause is usually *S. aureus* infection and, because of delayed presentation, complications such as paraspinal abscesses are often found. These children require prolonged antibiotics and frequently also need surgical drainage of abscesses to prevent spinal cord or nerve compression.

Discitis tends to occur in the lower lumbar spine and in younger children (<5 years) who present with less specific symptoms such as a limp or refusal to

Practical points

Osteomyelitis
- Fever and limb pain is a common presentation of osteomyelitis in older children, with the femur and the tibia being the most commonly affected bones
- Osteomyelitis in neonates and infants presents non-specifically with fever – neonates are more likely to have multifocal disease and Gram-negative organisms
- Bone malignancy is an important differential diagnosis and must be excluded (usually by X-ray at presentation)
- A bone scan or MRI is indicated in the investigation of suspected osteomyelitis – MRI is the best test where symptoms are clearly localized, because of the detailed information it provides
- Treatment of simple, uncomplicated cases is with an antistaphylococcal antibiotic given intravenously for 3 days followed by a high-dose oral antistaphylococcal antibiotic for 3 weeks
- In cases that are not simple or have a delayed response to treatment, further investigation, obtaining a surgical specimen and longer and broader-spectrum antibiotic therapy are indicated

Practical points

Septic arthritis
- Most cases of uncomplicated acute septic arthritis are due to *Staphylococcus aureus*
- A Gram stain result of aspirated fluid that suggests organisms other than *S. aureus* is an indication to add broader-spectrum antibiotic therapy
- Septic arthritis is more likely to coexist with osteomyelitis when the joint involved has a metaphysis that is intra-articular (hip, shoulder, elbow and ankle), when there has been slow response to therapy, in infants and when there is delayed presentation
- Every child with septic arthritis requires urgent surgical intervention – this means a washout of the joint
- Treatment of uncomplicated cases following joint washout is with an antistaphylococcal antibiotic given intravenously for 3 days followed by a high-dose oral antistaphylococcal antibiotic for 3 weeks

weight bear. The ESR is usually raised and by 4 weeks plain radiographs of the spine reveal narrowing of one or more disc spaces. MRI may provide further detailed anatomical information. In many cases of discitis no clear evidence of infection can be found, and surgery is usually not recommended when the diagnosis is clear from history, examination and imaging.

It is generally accepted that the treatment is prolonged empirical antistaphylococcal antibiotics such as flucloxacillin.

Meningitis and encephalitis

K. Grimwood

Meningitis and encephalitis are potentially life-threatening disorders that demand prompt recognition and treatment. They must be considered in all ill-appearing infants and children and in those with an impaired conscious state.

Bacterial meningitis

Bacterial meningitis is a medical emergency requiring rapid diagnosis and treatment. Equal attention must be paid to specific antimicrobial and supportive therapy, including the immediate treatment of:

- circulatory collapse
- convulsions
- cerebral oedema.

Epidemiology

The annual incidence of bacterial meningitis is 30–50 cases per 100 000 children aged 0–5 years. Rates are highest in infants and indigenous populations and during late winter and spring. Most cases are sporadic, with only meningococci leading to epidemics. The events that cause meningitis are incompletely understood but most probably include interactions between microbial, host and environmental factors:

- Microbe
  - polysaccharide capsule
- Host
  - young age
  - recent respiratory infection
  - ? genetic predisposition
- Environment
  - household crowding and poverty
  - tobacco smoke exposure
  - season
  - daycare attendance
  - sharing food, drink, pacifiers.

Factors that increase the risk of meningitis include:

- Impaired immunity
  - human immunodeficiency virus (HIV) infection, asplenia

- terminal complement or immunoglobulin deficiencies
- Neuroanatomical defects
  - penetrating head injuries, neurosurgical procedures
  - cerebrospinal fluid (CSF) leak
  - congenital dural defect (dermal sinus or myelomeningocele)
  - cochlear implants.

Aetiology

The most common pathogens in each age group are:

infants and children
- *Neisseria meningitidis* (meningococcus)
- *Streptococcus pneumoniae* (pneumococcus)
- *Haemophilus influenzae* type b (Hib)

children older than 5 years
- *Neisseria meningitidis*
- *Streptococcus pneumoniae*.

Both Hib and *S. pneumoniae* are uncommon in countries that have introduced routine immunization.

Pathogenesis

As outlined in Figure 12.3.1, the development of bacterial meningitis follows (1) the colonization of the nasopharynx by encapsulated bacteria, (2) invasion of the host with infection of the meninges, (3) bacterial multiplication and induction of inflammation within the subarachnoid space and (4) neuronal injury.

Clinical presentations

Infants and toddlers

Symptoms and signs of serious infection within this age group are often non-specific:

- fever, poor feeding, vomiting
- irritability, drowsiness
- neck stiffness or a bulging fontanelle.

Both neck stiffness and a bulging fontanelle may be absent, especially during infancy and early in the illness.

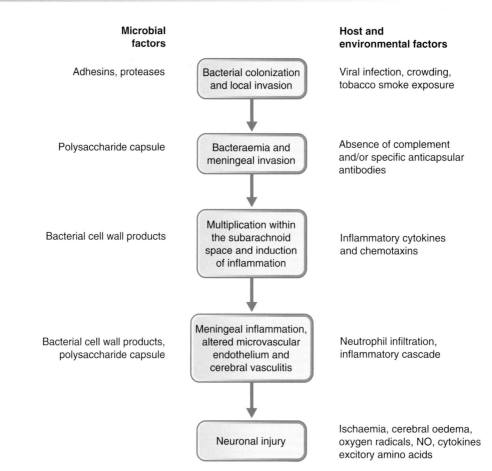

Microbial factors		Host and environmental factors
Adhesins, proteases	Bacterial colonization and local invasion	Viral infection, crowding, tobacco smoke exposure
Polysaccharide capsule	Bacteraemia and meningeal invasion	Absence of complement and/or specific anticapsular antibodies
Bacterial cell wall products	Multiplication within the subarachnoid space and induction of inflammation	Inflammatory cytokines and chemotaxins
Bacterial cell wall products, polysaccharide capsule	Meningeal inflammation, altered microvascular endothelium and cerebral vasculitis	Neutrophil infiltration, inflammatory cascade
	Neuronal injury	Ischaemia, cerebral oedema, oxygen radicals, NO, cytokines excitory amino acids

Fig. 12.3.1 The pathophysiological cascade of meningitis.

Children over the age of 3 years

The signs of meningeal irritation are more obvious:

- fever, severe headache, vomiting, photophobia
- neck stiffness
- delirium or deteriorating consciousness follow rapidly.

Convulsions are a presenting feature in 20–30% of infants and children with bacterial meningitis. Those with meningococcal meningitis may have a petechial or purpuric rash over the trunk and limbs (Fig. 12.3.2).

Diagnosis

Immediate tests should include:

- lumbar puncture for microscopy, culture, biochemistry and molecular diagnostic testing
- blood culture, whole blood for molecular diagnostic studies and (if necessary) clotted blood for baseline serology
- suprapubic aspirate or catheter urine specimen (if less than 6 months old)

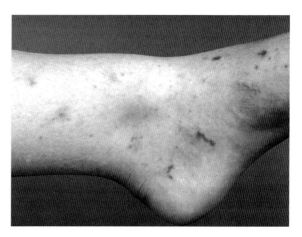

Fig. 12.3.2 The purpuric rash of meningococcal disease.

- full blood count, including white blood cell differential, C-reactive protein or procalcitonin
- serum electrolytes, glucose and creatinine
- needle aspirate of any focal areas of infection.

Molecular diagnostic testing by amplification of bacterial DNA by polymerase chain reaction (PCR) of whole blood and CSF helps identify the cause of meningitis in patients pretreated with antibiotics.

Lumbar puncture establishes the diagnosis and aids identification of the causative organism and its antibiotic sensitivities. It is postponed when there are signs of cerebral herniation, circulatory compromise or disseminated intravascular coagulation (DIC). A lumbar puncture is delayed for patients with any of the following:

- absent or non-purposeful responses to pain
- focal neurological signs
- abnormal pupil size or reaction
- decerebrate or decorticate posturing
- irregular breathing, hypertension or bradycardia despite peripheral vasoconstriction
- papilloedema.

In these situations, blood cultures and whole blood for PCR testing are collected and antibiotics started immediately. Such patients require intensive care management and the necessary measures to reduce intracranial pressure.

The typical CSF changes in bacterial meningitis are outlined in Table 12.3.1. Organisms are often seen on Gram stain of the CSF and a presumptive diagnosis may be made.

Occasionally the CSF examination is difficult to interpret, especially when antibiotics have been given before lumbar puncture. The decision to treat a child for bacterial meningitis is a clinical one and antibiotics are continued at least until the CSF is found to be sterile on culture and molecular diagnostic testing is negative. Parameningeal foci, such as brain abscess or subdural empyema, and tuberculous meningitis can have a similar CSF profile to partially treated bacterial meningitis and should be considered. However, if they are not ill, it is reasonable to observe some children closely in hospital without specific therapy until the pattern of illness becomes apparent.

Cerebral imaging by either computed tomography (CT) or magnetic resonance imaging (MRI) is not routinely recommended unless conditions that may mimic meningitis, such as intracranial mass lesions, are suspected and a lumbar puncture is contraindicated.

Table 12.3.1 Cerebrospinal fluid: normal values and typical changes in some pathological conditions

	Total WCC ($\times 10^6$/l)*	Predominant cell type	Glucose (mmol/l)	Protein (g/l)
Normal	<5	Lymphocytes	2.5	<0.4
Normal neonate	<20	Lymphocytes	Normal	Mildly elevated
Bacterial meningitis	1000s	Neutrophils	Reduced or undetectable	Moderately elevated
Partially treated bacterial meningitis[†]	100–1000s	Neutrophils	Reduced or undetectable	Moderately elevated
Tuberculous meningitis	50–100s	Neutrophils/mononuclear cells	Reduced or undetectable	Moderately to markedly elevated
Viral meningitis	<10–100s	Lymphocytes[‡]	Usually normal	Normal to <1 g/l
Encephalitis	<10–100s	Lymphocytes	Usually normal	Mildly to moderately elevated
Brain abscess and other mass lesions[§]	Normal to mild increase	Variable neutrophils	Normal	Normal to mildly elevated

* A traumatic tap is the commonest cause of bloodstained cerebrospinal fluid; for every 1000×10^6/l of red blood cells add 2×10^6/l of white blood cells and 0.01 g/l of protein to normal values. [†] Partially treated meningitis is seen when children in the early phase of illness are thought to have other infections, e.g. an upper respiratory infection, and receive oral antibiotics before the diagnosis of meningitis is made. [‡] Neutrophil predominance may be present in enterovirus meningitis. [§] Lumbar puncture is not done if a mass lesion is suspected. CSF changes depend on the site of the lesion, for example if near the cerebral surface pleocytosis occurs.
WCC = white cell count.

Table 12.3.2 Antibiotic therapy for bacterial meningitis

Pathogen	Antibiotic	Dose (mg/kg)	Duration (days)
Streptococcus pneumoniae			
Penicillin-susceptible	Penicillin G	60 i.v. 4 h	7–10
Penicillin non-susceptible	Cefotaxime*	50 i.v. 6 h	7–10
Penicillin + third-generation	Vancomycin +	15 i.v. 6 h	10–14
cephalosporin non-susceptible	cefotaxime*	75 i.v. 6 h	
Neisseria meningitidis	Penicillin G	60 i.v. 4 h	4–7
Haemophilus influenzae b and non-b species			
Non-beta-lactamase	Amoxicillin	50 i.v. 4 h	7
Beta-lactamase producer	Cefotaxime*	50 i.v. 6 h	7
Unknown pathogen	Cefotaxime* ±	50 i.v. 6 h	7
	Vancomycin	15 i.v. 6 h	

Maximum doses of penicillin G 2.4 g, amoxicillin 2 g, cefotaxime 3 g, ceftriaxone 2 g, vancomycin 500 mg.
* Ceftriaxone 50 mg/kg 12 h can be substituted for cefotaxime.

Antibiotic treatment

Antibiotics are selected that are effective against commonly encountered causative bacteria. The emergence of strains of *S. pneumoniae* not susceptible to penicillin and cephalosporin means that vancomycin is often added to a third-generation cephalosporin for the initial empiric treatment of bacterial meningitis. Subsequent therapy is adjusted according to culture and sensitivity results. Dosage and duration of antibiotic treatment are outlined in Table 12.3.2.

Supportive treatment

Clinical observations

Regular recording of the pulse, respiratory rate, blood pressure, temperature and conscious state is required. The head circumference in infants with meningitis should be measured daily as part of the neurological assessment.

Fluid therapy

Intravenous fluids are administered initially to restore circulating blood volume, to correct glucose or electrolyte disturbance and to minimize the risk of aspiration.

As meningitis is frequently accompanied by increased secretion of antidiuretic hormone (see below), once any dehydration or shock has been corrected, overhydration is avoided by moderate fluid restriction, e.g. to 50–70% of calculated maintenance fluid requirements. This reduces the risk of cerebral oedema and hyponatraemic convulsions (for discussion, see Chs 5.1 and 6.1). Fluid administration is then adjusted according to the serum sodium levels, adequacy of circulation and improvement in the clinical state. Hypotonic intravenous fluids should be avoided.

Corticosteroids

As inflammatory mediators contribute to the pathophysiology of bacterial meningitis, a role for dexamethasone when treating meningitis has been raised. Nevertheless, this is controversial and has not been universally adopted. Children with Hib meningitis may have a reduced risk of deafness if dexamethasone is administered before the first dose of antibiotics. However, benefit from dexamethasone in children for either pneumococcal or meningococcal meningitis remains unproven. Concerns over its effectiveness for treating beta-lactam-resistant pneumococcal meningitis and its putative role in neuronal apoptosis suggest a need for caution before making broad recommendations.

Acute complications

During meningitis, complications from central nervous system infection or systemic effects of infection are common. Children with frequent or protracted convulsions, circulatory instability or signs of cerebral oedema should be managed in an intensive care unit.

Convulsions

About 30% of children with bacterial meningitis have convulsions. These are more common with pneumococcal or Hib meningitis than meningococcal meningitis. Benzodiazepines such as diazepam or midazolam will control most convulsions but if these recur or are prolonged they raise intracranial pressure, worsening the cerebral ischaemic injury. Administration of phenytoin or phenobarbital and mechanical ventilation may be necessary. It is important to suspect hyponatraemia or hypoglycaemia as a cause of convulsions in any child with meningitis.

Cerebral oedema

Careful observations for signs of increased intracranial pressure are essential. These include:

- progressive loss of consciousness
- irregular breathing, hypertension or bradycardia when peripheral vasoconstriction exists
- pinpoint pupils
- respiratory arrest.

Management involves fluid restriction and circulatory and respiratory support.

The syndrome of inappropriate antidiuretic hormone secretion (SIADH) occurs often in meningitis. This results in dilution of the extracellular fluid compartment and fluid shift into cells. When it involves the brain, cerebral oedema develops. Careful fluid management, avoiding overhydration (facial or generalized oedema), by regular monitoring of the serum sodium concentration usually prevents cerebral oedema in meningitis. The diagnosis of SIADH is made when the serum sodium concentration is less than 130 mmol/l and is accompanied by urine sodium concentrations greater than 20 mmol/l. When SIADH is present and is complicated by cerebral oedema the treatment is fluid restriction, but intravenous hypertonic saline, mannitol or furosemide are used in an emergency.

Circulatory shock

Approximately 5–10% of children with bacterial meningitis present in shock and initially require large-volume fluid resuscitation to maintain tissue perfusion and blood pressure. Sustaining adequate cerebral perfusion is critical but care is required to avoid worsening cerebral oedema and provoking hyponatraemic convulsions. Inotropic agents are used to support the circulation.

Neurological lesions

Neurological deficits, such as hemiparesis, persistent hypotonia, ataxia and isolated cranial nerve palsies, are present in 10–20% of children during the acute illness and at the time of hospital discharge but are often reversible.

Subdural effusions

These are accumulations in the subdural space, usually of sterile fluid with high protein content. Common and generally asymptomatic, subdural effusions can occasionally be associated with:

- persistent or recurring high fever
- focal or generalized convulsions
- persistent vomiting
- increasing head circumference or fontanelle tension
- development of a focal neurological deficit.

Most subdural effusions resolve spontaneously but a very large symptomatic effusion may require surgical drainage. Subdural empyema is uncommon but should be suspected when the above features are accompanied by persistent irritability and sustained elevation of systemic inflammatory indices, such as C-reactive protein or procalcitonin. Cerebral CT (Fig. 12.3.3) or MRI establishes the diagnosis of subdural effusion or empyema.

Persistent (>7 days) or secondary fever

Frequently this results from:

- viral nosocomial infection
- subdural effusion
- thrombophlebitis
- other suppurative lesions

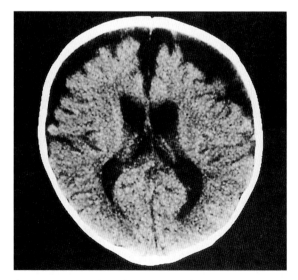

Fig. 12.3.3 Cranial CT of a 5-month-old boy with pneumococcal meningitis who developed secondary fever and generalized convulsions on his 7th day in hospital. It shows subdural effusions over both frontal lobes. He received anticonvulsant therapy and the effusion resolved spontaneously.

- immune mediated disease – reactive arthritis or pericarditis.

Uncommonly, fever may also result from:

- inadequately treated meningitis
- a parameningeal focus (e.g. abscess or subdural empyema)
- drugs.

Cerebral imaging

Cranial CT or MRI is useful in identifying:

- subdural collections
- brain abscess
- cerebral vascular thrombosis
- hydrocephalus.

These tests are considered for patients with:

- prolonged coma
- sustained irritability or convulsions
- persistent focal neurological deficits
- enlarging head circumference
- recurrent disease.

Outcome

- Mortality 2–15%, which is lowest in meningococcal and greatest in pneumococcal meningitis
- Intellectual disability, spasticity, convulsions, hydrocephalus, deafness 10–25%
- Later learning and behaviour disorders 25–30%.

Meningitis in infancy, delayed diagnosis, persistent or late-onset convulsions and focal neurological signs are independent risk factors for severe neurological or intellectual disability. Mild–moderate neurocognitive deficits are more common in children with meningitis in the first 12 months of life.

All children should have their hearing tested following meningitis, either by brain stem (auditory) evoked potentials or formal audiometry. Regular review should be continued in children with persisting auditory and neurological abnormalities.

Primary prevention

Antibodies directed against the capsular components of Hib, *S. pneumoniae* and *N. meningitidis* play an important role in developing protective immunity against these pathogens. Protein conjugated vaccines have been successfully developed against:

- Hib
- *S. pneumoniae*
- *N. meningitidis* A, C, Y W135.

Clinical example

Bridgette, a 5-month-old, infant presented after a 15-minute right-sided focal convulsion. She had been unwell for 12 hours and had been feeding poorly. Her past medical history, growth and development were normal. She had received her primary immunizations and there was no family history of convulsions. Her temperature was 39.3°C; she was pale and very irritable when handled. Neck stiffness, bulging fontanelle and rash were absent. No focal neurological signs were present.

A lumbar puncture revealed turbid CSF. Numerous Gram-negative coccobacilli were seen in the CSF, and non-typeable *H. influenzae* was isolated. Bridgette's course was complicated by a secondary fever, a tense fontanelle with increasing head circumference, recurrent focal and generalized convulsions, right hemiplegia and persistently elevated peripheral white blood cell counts and C-reactive protein concentrations. Subdural pus was surgically drained after MRI scans demonstrated a left-sided empyema. This was followed by a rapid clinical improvement. Subsequent testing found no signs of underlying immunodeficiency.

Fewer than 1% of children with febrile convulsions have meningitis. Infants and those with complex febrile convulsions are at greatest risk. It is important that all children are carefully evaluated for signs of meningitis following a febrile convulsion. The successful introduction of protein conjugate vaccines means that rare causes of bacterial meningitis will become relatively more important. Although the incidence of non-typeable *H. influenzae* meningitis remains unchanged, in fully immunized children it has become a more common cause of meningitis than Hib. Such children often have an underlying medical condition and compared with Hib infection they have a more severe illness with greater mortality.

Cases of Hib, pneumococcal and meningococcal serogroup C meningitis have decreased by approximately 90% in countries where these vaccines are part of the national immunization schedule (Ch. 3.5).

The quadrivalent A, C, Y, W135 meningococcal conjugate vaccine offers additional prospects of reducing meningitis in adolescents, while future maternal immunization with a polyvalent *Streptococcus agalactiae* conjugate vaccine could decrease neonatal meningitis. The success of these vaccines is due to their capacity not only to induce immunity in young children and establish immunological memory but also to develop herd immunity. Challenges remain over the cost and delivery of these vaccines to children in developing nations. The important, but poorly immunogenic, meningococcal polysaccharide serogroup B strains remain an important challenge for safe and effective vaccine development. In New Zealand, a sustained epidemic of meningococcal disease from a single clonal strain of serogroup B resulted in the introduction of a monovalent vaccine. This was prepared from bacterial cell wall outer membrane proteins instead of the polysaccharide capsule and is immunogenic only for the epidemic strain.

Chemoprophylaxis

Transmission of Hib and meningococci is by oral and respiratory secretions. Those at increased risk of infection are:

- household members
- childcare contacts
- persons intimately exposed to oral secretions.

At-risk contacts of a case of meningococcal meningitis should each immediately receive oral rifampicin, 10 mg/kg (neonates 5 mg/kg) (maximum 600 mg) twice daily for 2 days. Alternatively a single dose of intramuscular ceftriaxone (125 mg for children under 12 years of age, 250 mg for older children and adults) is given, or adults may receive 500 mg of oral ciprofloxacin. The index case does not require further prophylaxis if treatment has included a third-generation cephalosporin. Parents must be warned that, if they or their children are unwell, immediate medical attention should be sought.

Because of the increased risk of Hib infection in young contacts, rifampicin 20 mg/kg (maximum 600 mg) as a single daily dose for 4 days is prescribed for the index case of Hib meningitis and all household contacts, if the child is aged less than 2 years or if the household contacts include unimmunized children younger than 4 years. Unlike *N. meningitidis*, single doses of ceftriaxone do not eradicate Hib from the nasopharynx. In contrast, chemoprophylaxis is not required in cases of pneumococcal meningitis.

Special circumstances

Neonatal meningitis

Neonates, particularly if premature, are at increased risk of meningitis. The responsible pathogens are mainly:

- *S. agalactiae*
- *Escherichia coli* and other Gram-negative bacilli
- *Listeria monocytogenes*.

As in infants, the symptoms and signs of meningitis can be non-specific. Approximately 5–20% of septic neonates have concomitant meningitis. Initial therapy is with amoxicillin and cefotaxime until culture and antibiotic sensitivities are available. Antibiotic treatment is at least 2 weeks for Gram-positive meningitis, and 3 weeks for Gram-negative bacillary cases.

Infants aged 1–3 months and the immunocompromised

These patients may have meningitis from pathogens common to both neonates and older children. Empiric therapy (usually with amoxicillin and cefotaxime) must be capable of treating a wide range of pathogens. When the CSF Gram stain or PCR testing suggests *S. pneumoniae* as the causative agent, vancomycin should replace amoxicillin.

Meningococcaemia

While *N. meningitidis* serogroup A is associated with epidemics in parts of sub-Saharan Africa, serogroups B and C are endemic in industrialized countries where serogroup B causes 30–70% of sporadic meningococcal disease. Large increases in disease caused by meningococcal clones have been observed in several European and other countries in recent years. The important, but poorly immunogenic, meningococcal polysaccharide serogroup B strains remain an important challenge for safe and effective vaccine development.

Approximately 60% of invasive meningococcal disease is acute meningococcaemia. Although nearly 70% have concomitant meningitis, signs of sepsis dominate the clinical course. Half the cases occur in children aged less than 5 years where serogroup B strains predominate. Many older patients present critically ill with a rapid progression of symptoms and signs:

- fevers and rigors
- severe pain in the limbs, neck or back
- vomiting, especially with headache or abdominal pain.

The presenting features of meningococcal disease in infants and young children are more non-specific:

- fever, irritability or drowsiness
- pallor with cool extremities
- grunting or moaning respirations.

A rash is present in most cases irrespective of age. Initially it may be a blanching macular or maculopapular rash before evolving into the characteristic petechial or purpuric rash of meningococcaemia (Fig. 12.3.2). The clinical course can be rapidly progressive, with the time from onset of fever until death as short as 12 hours. While overall mortality for invasive meningococcal disease is 10%, case fatality reaches 20% for fulminant forms of the disease and from infection with serogroup C, Y or W135 in adolescents and young adults.

The clinical features of meningococcaemia are initiated by the release of cell wall products, which activate proinflammatory cytokines and complement leading to endothelial injury with capillary leak and loss of vasomotor tone. The major cause of death in meningococcaemia is circulatory collapse from capillary leak, intravascular volume depletion, vasodilatation and myocardial failure. Haemodynamic collapse in combination with DIC leads to multiorgan dysfunction.

Treatment is urgent and is commenced immediately the diagnosis is suspected, and ideally after taking blood cultures. Penicillin G is the drug of choice, the recommended dose being 60 mg/kg i.v. 4-hourly. The patient is managed in respiratory isolation during the first 24 hours of treatment. Management of those with signs of septic shock should be in an intensive care unit and includes aggressive fluid resuscitation to restore the circulating blood volume, cardiac and respiratory support, and careful management of blood electrolytes and glucose. Short term, physiological doses of corticosteroids may benefit those in septic shock unresponsive to fluid resuscitation or inotropic support. The role in children of other adjunctive therapies, such as recombinant human activated protein C, awaits further evaluation. While prehospital treatment with penicillin has reduced the number of culture-confirmed cases, the use of molecular techniques such as PCR to detect meningococcal DNA in sterile fluids has greatly aided diagnosis.

Tuberculous meningitis

This is most common in children younger than 5 years. The onset is gradual, with malaise, fever and irritability, progressing over 1–2 weeks to drowsiness, neck stiffness, convulsions, cranial nerve palsies and coma. Typical CSF changes are listed in Table 12.3.1. There may be no history of infectious contacts. Mantoux testing is often normal and a chest X-ray abnormality is present in only half of cases. Gastric aspirates, urine and CSF are sent for culture, while some centres induce sputum with hypertonic saline and offer PCR testing for *Mycobacterium tuberculosis* DNA. Cranial CT or MRI may detect hydrocephalus and basilar meningeal inflammation, while basal ganglia infarction is a late radiographic sign. Treatment is with isoniazid, rifampicin and pyrazinamide. A fourth drug is added if there are concerns over potential drug resistance. High-dose steroids are also used during the first weeks of therapy.

Recurrent meningitis

This is uncommon and underlying causes should be sought:

- immunodeficiency (Ch. 13.2)
- neuroanatomical defects – intracranial or lumbosacral.

Consider neuroanatomical defects when enteric bacteria or *Staphylococcus aureus* are cultured from the CSF. Cranial and spinal MRI, or high-resolution CT of the temporal and frontal bones, may be indicated.

Viral meningitis and encephalitis

Many viruses are capable of invading the central nervous system and, depending upon the primary site of involvement, the clinical designations used are meningitis and encephalitis (Table 12.3.3).

Viral meningitis

Non-polio enteroviruses cause 80–90% of identifiable cases. The onset is acute with:

- fever
- headache
- vomiting
- neck or spine stiffness.

The absence of an altered sensorium and focal neurological findings generally helps to distinguish viral meningitis from encephalitis.

Abdominal pain is common and occasionally a macular rash appears, suggesting an enterovirus as the causative agent. Parotid or mandibular swellings

Clinical example

Tom, aged 14 years, had developed chills on the day of presentation and complained of pain in his head, neck and limbs. He rapidly became confused, agitated and started to vomit. When seen by his family doctor Tom was pale and a faint red macular rash had appeared over his buttocks and legs. A diagnosis of possible meningococcaemia was made and he received 1.2 g of penicillin intramuscularly before immediate transfer to hospital. On arrival he was pale and shocked, was difficult to arouse and had an evolving purpuric rash. He received aggressive fluid resuscitation, inotropes, assisted ventilation and cefotaxime. He gradually improved and a delayed lumbar puncture showed 150 white blood cells only. Although cultures were sterile, PCR testing of whole blood collected upon arrival at hospital confirmed meningococcal infection and he completed his treatment with intravenous penicillin G.

Table 12.3.3 Viruses and non-bacterial infecting agents that may commonly cause meningitis and encephalitis
Acute disseminated encephalomyelitis without direct invasion of CNS
• Measles, rubella, varicella, Epstein–Barr virus, mumps, influenza, *Mycoplasma pneumoniae*
Meningitis and/or encephalitis with viral CNS infection
• Enteroviruses – ECHO, Coxsackie, enteroviruses and polio viruses. These usually cause meningitis but can occasionally cause encephalitis • Mumps – usually meningitis, less often meningoencephalitis • Herpes simplex virus type 1 can cause focal (usually temporoparietal) encephalitis (HSV-1 or -2 can cause encephalitis in neonates) • Other herpes group viruses – human herpes virus 6, Epstein–Barr virus, varicella, cytomegalovirus (neonates, immunocompromised) • Other viruses – adenoviruses, influenza, measles, rubella • Arbovirus (arthropod-borne virus) – e.g. flaviviruses such as Japanese encephalitis, West Nile encephalitis or Australian encephalitis viruses
Progressive encephalitis
• For example, subacute sclerosing panencephalitis due to measles virus infection, or human prion disease

implicate mumps. Signs of meningism indicate the need for lumbar puncture. Typical CSF findings in viral meningitis are presented in Table 12.3.1.

PCR testing of CSF specimens for enterovirus genetic material has become an important diagnostic tool. Other disorders that may present in a similar fashion and need to be considered include:

• partially treated bacterial meningitis
• tuberculous meningitis
• cryptococcal meningitis
• cerebral abscesses
• cerebral tumour.

A repeat lumbar puncture or cerebral imaging may be required to further clarify the diagnosis.

Viral meningitis is a benign disease, and requires symptomatic treatment only. Complete recovery without sequelae is expected within a few days.

Viral encephalitis and myelitis

Encephalitis means inflammation of the brain. Acute viral encephalitis results from direct infection of neural tissue affecting mainly grey matter, while acute disseminated encephalomyelitis (ADEM) results in white matter demyelination and is thought to be immune-mediated after a variety of viral and bacterial infections or rarely immunization (Table 12.3.3). Viral encephalitis typically presents with fever, headache, altered conscious state and often with convulsions. ADEM usually presents after a non-specific respiratory or gastrointestinal illness. It is characterized by multifocal neurological signs and fever is often absent. Clinically the distinction between acute encephalitis and ADEM can be difficult unless the demyelinating illness complicates an exanthema such as measles, rubella or chickenpox.

Encephalitis presents with an array of neurological signs:

• headache, vomiting and altered conscious state
• confusion and disorientation
• behaviour or speech disturbance
• generalized or focal convulsions
• ataxia or other movement disorders
• focal neurological deficits.

Meningism is frequently absent. The involvement of the spinal cord (transverse myelitis) may develop in isolation and can lead to flaccid paralysis, loss of tendon reflexes, neurogenic bladder and a definable sensory level. When it occurs, acute cord compression from a spinal extradural abscess or some other cause must also be considered and urgently excluded by MRI or CT myelogram.

Causes of acute encephalitis may be suggested by:

• the season
• recent travel history
• prior personal or family illness
• animal exposures
• drug and immunization history
• presence of lymphadenopathy, parotitis, rash or pneumonia.

Investigations to identify the aetiological agent include:

• PCR of CSF, blood, respiratory secretions
• viral culture of CSF, blood, respiratory secretions, faeces and urine
• serology.

The CSF profile of encephalitis is outlined in Table 12.3.1, although many patients may have normal CSF parameters. However, PCR analysis provides a rapid and accurate diagnosis for a wide range of pathogens. Electro-encephalographic (EEG) abnormalities are seldom specific but may be helpful in herpes simplex virus (HSV) encephalitis. MRI is more sensitive than cranial CT and helps differentiate encephalitis from ADEM (Fig. 12.3.4). MRI T2-

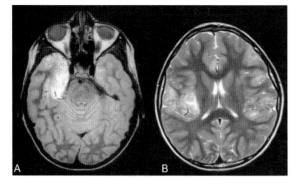

Fig. 12.3.4 MRI T2-weighted axial images. **A** A 6-year-old girl with HSV encephalitis (see text for clinical details), which shows an increased signal in the right temporal lobe. **B** A 4-year-old boy with focal convulsions and dysphasia following a respiratory illness. The bilateral and asymmetric multifocal increased signal in the white–grey junction and subcortical white matter is characteristic of acute disseminated encephalomyelitis.

weighted images in viral encephalitis demonstrate one or more diffuse areas of hyperintensity involving the grey matter of the cerebral cortex and the underlying white matter, with involvement of the basal ganglia, brain stem and cerebellum to a lesser extent. In contrast, ADEM is characterized by multiple asymmetric areas of increased focal signal in the white matter of both hemispheres, basal ganglia, cerebellum and, on occasions, the spinal cord. Other treatable causes of acute encephalopathy should also be sought.

Initially, acyclovir is given until a diagnosis of HSV encephalitis can be excluded by clinical, radiological and PCR criteria. Treatment of viral encephalitis and ADEM is supportive, involving:

- careful fluid and electrolyte management
- control of convulsions
- monitoring for signs of raised intracranial pressure
- circulatory support to maintain cerebral perfusion
- assisted ventilation for respiratory failure
- maintenance of nutrition.

Corticosteroids should be considered when the MRI shows striking enhancement of multifocal white matter lesions consistent with ADEM.

Almost 10% of children with encephalitis die and long-term studies suggest that nearly half of the survivors have neurological or educational disabilities. Young age, coma, delayed presentation, high CSF protein and infection with HSV or *Mycoplasma pneumoniae* are associated with a poor prognosis. However, patients can also make excellent recoveries, even after prolonged coma.

Herpes simplex encephalitis

Herpes simplex virus causes a severe, sporadic focal encephalitis. Unlike most other causes of encephalitis it is amenable to treatment with the antiviral agent acyclovir, which reduces the mortality to below 20%. However, most survivors still have severe neurological or behavioural sequelae. More than 95% of postneonatal cases are caused by HSV-1 and one third result from a primary infection.

The course described in the clinical example is typical of HSV encephalitis. PCR is the diagnostic test of choice. While frontal and temporal lobe localization is characteristic, PCR and MRI testing have shown that the disease can be diffuse in neonates who have mainly HSV-2 disease and in young children.

Clinical example

Rachael, aged 6 years, was hospitalized with a 3-day history of fever, headache, intermittent confusion and progressive lethargy. On presentation she had several left-sided focal convulsions. Her temperature was 40.1°C; she was drowsy with mild neck stiffness and left hemiparesis.

Her CSF had $100 \times 10^6/l$ lymphocytes. The protein content of the CSF was mildly elevated and the glucose concentration was normal. HSV encephalitis was suspected and acyclovir (500 mg/m² i.v. 8-hourly) was started. Phenytoin controlled Rachael's convulsions. An EEG demonstrated periodic discharges localized to the right temporal lobe and an MRI scan showed increased signal in T2-weighted images of this region (Fig. 12.3.4a). PCR of the CSF was positive for HSV-1 DNA.

She gradually improved over several days, but was still febrile after 2 weeks of treatment. A repeat lumbar puncture at 3 weeks revealed persisting HSV-1 DNA. Acyclovir was continued for a total of 4 weeks. Her fever settled, but the hemiparesis remained and she was left with major behaviour and learning disabilities.

Arthropod-borne encephalitis viruses

Viruses transmitted to humans by biting arthropods (mainly mosquitoes and ticks) are a major cause of encephalitis. Flaviviruses are the most common and include Japanese encephalitis (Asia), West Nile encephalitis (Africa/Middle East/North America) and Australian encephalitis (Australia). West Nile encephalitis has recently become established in North America following its introduction into New York in 1999, while Japanese encephalitis has expanded throughout Asia and into Australia.

Most infections are mild or subclinical, with fewer than 1% developing neurological symptoms. However, when symptomatic the disease is often severe with fever, headache, vomiting, altered consciousness, convulsions, tremor and dystonia. Both Japanese encephalitis and West Nile encephalitis may present with acute flaccid paralysis. Mortality for Japanese encephalitis and Australian encephalitis is 20–30%, with 50% of survivors experiencing severe neurological and intellectual sequelae. Vector control programmes and personal protection are important prevention measures, while there is a vaccine for Japanese encephalitis.

Slow virus infection

Some viruses can cause a subacute or chronic neurodegenerative disorder. The major example in childhood is subacute sclerosing panencephalitis, a rare late complication of measles, especially if measles occurs early in life. Rubella is a less common cause. The disorder is manifest by:

- deterioration of behaviour, personality and intellect
- myoclonic convulsions
- motor disturbance.

The onset is usually several years after measles. As the disease progresses, spastic paresis, tremors, athetosis and ataxia develop. The disease runs a variable but progressive course and is usually fatal within 2 years. Initially, the EEG shows a typical 'suppression-burst pattern'. The typical clinical picture and high-titre CSF measles antibody establish the diagnosis.

Transmissible spongiform encephalopathies

Transmissible spongiform encephalopathies (TSE) are a group of clinical syndromes in animals and humans characterized by a slowly progressive neurodegenerative course. All are caused by toxic accumulation within the CNS of an abnormal cell surface protein, the prion protein, which has undergone a physiochemical transition from an original normal host cellular glycoprotein. New variant Creutzfeldt–Jakob disease has attracted considerable attention as it represents the first instance where an animal TSE has jumped the species barrier to infect humans. Several cases have been reported in adolescents. The first symptoms are those of depression and dysaesthesia, then ataxia, involuntary movements, spasticity and cognitive decline quickly follow, leading to death within 3 years. MRI shows abnormal enhancement of the thalamus. Distinctive amyloid plaques are seen on brain biopsy.

> **Practical points**
>
> - Meningitis and encephalitis should always be considered in ill-appearing infants and children and in those with an impaired conscious state
> - Unless contraindicated by signs of raised intracranial pressure or haemodynamic instability, lumbar puncture should be performed when meningitis is suspected to establish the diagnosis and to help identify the causative organism
> - Restoration of the circulating blood volume, treatment of convulsions and rapid sterilization of cerebrospinal fluid are the immediate treatment goals for bacterial meningitis
> - Once any dehydration or shock are corrected, overhydration and accompanying risk of hyponatraemic convulsions and cerebral oedema are avoided by moderate fluid restriction
> - Bacterial meningitis that is recurrent, caused by an unusual pathogen or vaccine failure in a fully vaccinated child raises the possibility of an underlying disorder, including immunodeficiency or a neuroanatomical defect
> - The absence of an altered sensorium and focal neurological findings helps distinguish viral meningitis from acute encephalitis

12.4 Infections in tropical and developing countries

D. R. Brewster, M. J. Robinson

Most of the world's population lives in the tropics and subtropics in developing countries where health outcomes tend to be much poorer than in developed countries such as Australia and New Zealand. In addition, educational standards are lower, with a high rate of illiteracy, particularly for women, which is an important determinant of child survival. Personal hygiene, water and sanitation standards are also poor in the developing world, placing individuals at higher risk of infectious diseases, particularly enteric infections in a tropical climate. In addition, poor developing countries are characterized by high under-5 child mortality, with rates of 150–284 per 1000 in 25 African countries and Afghanistan compared to 3–6 per 1000 in the 30 lowest-mortality countries. Rather than exotic tropical diseases, the main causes of morbidity and mortality are common conditions such as malaria, diarrhoeal diseases, acute respiratory infections, malnutrition and acquired immune deficiency syndrome (AIDS). Paediatric practice is probably more influenced by economic factors than by geography or climate, so paediatrics in the developing world is above all a medicine of poverty. It deals with children from poor families with heavy burdens of disease and health care resources for the task are very limited.

Of the seven Millennium Development Goals (MDG) for 2015, three have direct relevance to childhood infections:

- MDG 4: Reduce by two-thirds the mortality rate among children under 5 years of age
- MDG 6: Halt and begin to reverse the spread of HIV/AIDS and the incidence of malaria and other diseases
- MDG 7: Reduce by half the proportion of people without sustainable access to safe drinking water and basic sanitation.

As with the previous World Health Organization (WHO) goal of 'health for all by the year 2000', there are serious doubts about whether the MDGs can be achieved, particularly in Africa. However, a positive development is the initiative on Public–Private Partnerships (PPP), which brings together government, industry, academia, not-for-profit organizations, philanthropists and other donors for product development, improved access and global coordination for improvements in health in the developing world (see *Transactions of the Royal Society for Tropical Medicine and Hygiene* 2005; 99: suppl. 1).

The WHO has developed treatment protocols for the common diseases, based upon simple clinical indicators such as fast breathing, chest wall retractions, inability to drink, drowsiness, convulsions, pallor, etc., which could be assessed by health workers with minimal training. The Integrated Management of Childhood Illness (IMCI, see http://www.who.int/child-adolescent-health/integr.htm) initiative aims to reduce child morbidity and mortality in developing countries by improved management of common illnesses (Table 12.4.1). This integrated horizontal approach is in marked contrast to the vertical single-disease approaches such as control of malaria, tuberculosis and diarrhoeal disease.

Evaluation studies of the quality of care at hospitals and health centres in the developing world have found major deficiencies in triage, emergency care, monitoring, drug availability, staffing levels and the use of protocols. This suggests that more emphasis needs to be placed upon on-site supervision of health workers. Although protocols are useful, they are no substitute for clinical experience in a supervised setting. In addition to acute care protocols, there are a number of important child health programmes, such as breastfeeding promotion, immunizations, malaria control (e.g. insecticide-treated bednets), supplementary feeding and control of diarrhoeal disease (e.g. handwashing with soap). Poor nutrition is an important contributor to the high childhood mortality from infectious diseases in the developing world. Over half of child deaths are due to the potentiating effect of malnutrition on infections, most of which is due to mild to moderate malnutrition.

The ease of air travel and the frequency of people of all ages visiting the tropics has made it essential for the student and practising doctor to have an appreciation of tropical medicine. Migration, for both personal and humanitarian reasons (refugees), makes it almost certain that some will carry disease undetected by the medical screening process. It is of

Table 12.4.1 Diagnostic classifications and clinical signs for referral to hospital

Young infants (0–2 months)
1. Possible serious bacterial infection
Seizures, tachypnoea (≥60 breaths/min), severe chest indrawing, nasal flaring, grunting, bulging fontanelle, perforated eardrum, omphalitis, fever or hypothermia (≥38°C or <30°C), many or severe skin pustules, difficult to wake up or cannot be calmed within 1 hour

2. Diarrhoea with severe dehydration
Lethargic or unconscious, sunken eyes and skin pinch goes back very slowly

3. Severe persistent diarrhoea (≥14 days)

4. Not able to feed

Children (2 months–5 years)
1. General danger signs
Not able to drink or breastfeed, vomits everything, convulsions, or lethargic or unconscious

2. Severe febrile disease
Fever (rectal temperature ≥38°C) and any general danger sign, or stiff neck

3. Severe pneumonia
Cough or difficult breathing and any general danger sign, chest indrawing, or stridor when calm

4. Diarrhoea with severe dehydration
Abnormally sleepy or difficult to wake up, sunken eyes, not able to drink or drinking poorly, skin pinch goes back very slowly

5. Severe persistent diarrhoea (≥14 days) with dehydration
Restless/irritable, sunken eyes and skin pinch goes back slowly

6. Severe malnutrition or severe anaemia
Visible severe wasting, oedema of both feet, or severe palmar pallor

Adapted from WHO Integrated Management of Childhood Illness: http://www.who.int/child-adolescent-health/New_Publications/IMCI/WHO_FCH_CAH_00.40/WHO_FCH_CAH_00.12.4.pdf

the greatest importance in any unusual illness, particularly a febrile one, that a history of overseas travel is sought. The purpose of this chapter is to give an overview of common infections in tropical regions of Australia and developing countries. It is not possible to discuss in detail all of the many disorders endemic to these areas, so readers are urged to look elsewhere for more specific advice. This section deals only with bacterial infections, malaria, dengue, parasitic diseases, and infections of tropical Australia.

Bacterial infections

Serious bacterial infections are much more common in children in tropical and developing countries than in temperate and developed countries, and bacteraemia is found in 25% or more of hospital deaths. *Haemophilus influenzae* type b (Hib) and *Streptococcus pneumoniae* (pneumococcus) have been considered to be the main causes of bacterial sepsis in children, but multiresistant Enterobacteriaceae (e.g. *Salmonella* species, *Escherichia coli*, *Klebsiella pneumoniae*, *Citrobacter freundii*) are also important causes of sepsis, especially in infants. *Staphylococcus aureus* bacteraemia may be found in approximately 5% of positive blood cultures in children and has a 20–35% mortality.

About half of cases are associated with one or more foci (e.g. abscess, cellulitis, osteomyelitis, pyomyositis, omphalitis), with a much higher mortality rate in those without a known focus, who tend to be younger and/or malnourished. Good-quality studies from Kilifi, Kenya have documented that syndromic protocols (Table 12.4.1) in hospitalized children identified the need for antibiotics in about half of admissions, in whom they had a 12% case fatality rate and 11% had an invasive bacterial infection. Malaria parasitaemia did not justify withholding empirical antibiotics when indicated by syndromic presentation, since 4.0–8.8% of these also had a documented invasive bacterial infection.

The new conjugate vaccines have reduced the prevalence of bacterial infections in developed countries but are still not widely available in developing countries because of their cost, although some initiatives to address this through aid programmes are under way, as well as research on less expensive regimens. However, the new conjugate pneumococcal vaccines only reduce the rate of X-ray-proven pneumonia in hospital by about 20% in most settings.

Salmonella infections occur worldwide but are particularly important in tropical and developing countries. There are over 200 species of *Salmonella* and common sources of human infection include shellfish, poultry, fish, meat and dairy products. Three clinical syndromes are associated with *Salmonella* infection:

- acute gastroenteritis (e.g. *Salmonella enteritidis)*
- septicaemia (e.g. *Salmonella choleraesuis)*
- enteric fever (e.g. *Salmonella typhi* and *Salmonella paratyphi*).

A systematic review of the use of antibiotics in non-typhoid *Salmonella* infections found no evidence of a clinical benefit in non-severe cases, and antibiotics appeared to increase adverse effects and prolong the period of stool carriage.

Typhoid fever is confined to humans and occurs where standards of hygiene, water supply and sanitation are poor. Carriers of *S. typhi*, particularly those working in the food industry, are an important reservoir of infection. The typical presentation is fever, malaise, headache, abdominal discomfort and sometimes vomiting and diarrhoea. In severe disease, toxaemia is profound and complications such as small bowel perforation occur in older children.

Although typhoid fever was widely considered a disease of school age, it may also affect younger children, with a clinical picture of sepsis and milder and atypical manifestations compared with older children. The diagnosis is established from cultures of blood, stools or even urine, but cultures are negative in up to 50% of cases. The Widal test is an unreliable test because of the effects of previous vaccination and the delay in seroconversion. Antibiotic resistance to ampicillin and co-trimoxazole is common, so chloramphenicol is the drug of choice in the developing world unless there is resistance to it as well. Third-generation cephalosporins (e.g. ceftriaxone) or quinolones (e.g. ciprofloxacin) are highly effective and are the drugs of choice, if affordable.

In recent years there has been a resurgence of tuberculosis (TB) in tropical and developing countries, with the epidemic of human immunodeficiency virus (HIV) infection, which has been accompanied by the emergence of resistant strains of the tubercle bacillus. The accurate diagnosis of tuberculosis in young children in the developing world is often difficult because of the unavailability of sputum, the unreliability of gastric aspirates and Mantoux testing, and the overlap in clinical presentation with malnutrition, respiratory infections and AIDS. Treatment is expensive, with even short-course chemotherapy taking 6 months and requiring drug combinations (e.g. isoniazid, rifampicin, pyrazinamide), making compliance problematic. Most recurrences are related to relapse of the same strain due to poor adherence, multi-drug-resistant TB and/or HIV, although reinfections with another strain may also occur in high TB prevalence settings and in HIV-infected TB cases on antiretroviral therapy.

Finally, although bacterial pneumonia is still highly prevalent in most developing countries, it is important to recognize that virus-induced airways disease (acute bronchiolitis, asthma) is increasingly emerging as the major cause of acute respiratory infections in the Asia–Pacific region, with important implications for IMCI protocols, which currently focus on bacterial infections.

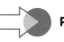

Practical points

Bacterial infections
- Serious bacterial infections in children tend to be more common causes of hospital admissions in developing countries
- In addition to pneumococcus and *Haemophilus influenzae*, multiresistant *Enterobacteriaceae* (e.g. *Salmonella*, *E. coli*) are also important causes of sepsis
- IMCI protocols with training and supervision can help primary care health workers to identify children needing antibiotic treatment

Malaria

Malaria is a major global health problem, with an estimated 50% of the world's population in 88 countries (3.4 billion people in 2010) exposed to various degrees of risk, almost exclusively in tropical regions (Fig. 12.4.1). Severe and complicated malaria is caused by *Plasmodium falciparum* infection. The two forms of severe malaria in children are cerebral malaria and severe anaemia. Cerebral malaria tends to be in older children (mean age 3–4 years) in areas with seasonal and moderate transmission, compared with severe anaemia malaria, which is most frequent in younger children (mean 1–2 years) with high malarial transmission, especially if there is resistance to standard antimalarials in use. The interval between symptom onset and death is short, averaging less than 3 days. Unlike adults, renal failure, pulmonary oedema, shock, jaundice and disseminated intravascular coagulation (DIC) are uncommon in childhood malaria, as are the classical malarial paroxysms with cold shivers, burning heat and drenching sweats.

Parasites are not synonymous with disease so in 1000 children bitten by an infected mosquito there might be 400 asymptomatic infections, 200 cases of clinical malaria, 12 cases of severe malaria and one death. Not only do many children have parasitaemia without disease, but the density of peripheral blood parasitaemia bears little relationship to mortality, as infected red cells cytoadhere and sequester in the microvasculature. Clinical algorithms for malaria diagnosis are not useful as they tend to be age- and site-specific and perform poorly in identifying a need for treatment. Thick blood film microscopy remains the gold standard for malaria diagnosis but new rapid diagnostic tests are available using immunochromatographic methods to detect *Plasmodium*-specific antigens. Their main disadvantages at present are cost, inability to quantify parasite density,

The distribution of global child mortality

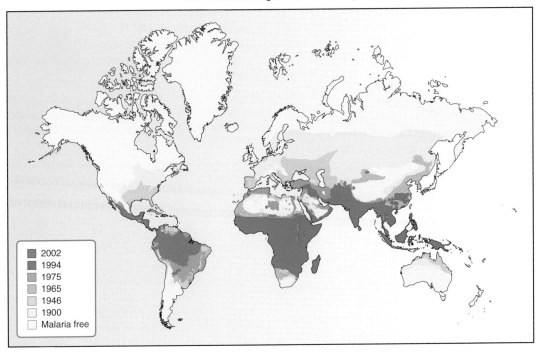

Fig. 12.4.1 The global distribution of malaria 1900–2002 (after Hay SI, Guerra CA, Tatem AJ et al 2004 The global distribution and population at risk of malaria: past, present, and future. Lancet Infectious Diseases 4: 327–336).

persistently positive tests after adequate treatment, and lack of species and sexual–asexual (e.g. gametocytes) stage differentiation. Tests under development are likely to improve rapid malarial diagnosis further and may even be able to detect sequestered parasites.

Cerebral malaria has been defined as unrousable coma not attributable to any other cause in a patient with falciparum malaria. The level of consciousness (Table 12.4.2) is confounded by convulsions and the postictal state, so coma must persist for 30 minutes after a convulsion for a diagnosis of cerebral malaria to be made. In Africa, cerebral malaria has a mortality of around 15%; neurological sequelae occur in 20% of survivors with profound coma on admission. However, nearly all survivors have fully recovered 6 months after admission. The main features of severe disease are prolonged unresponsive coma, decerebrate posturing and hypoglycaemia. Other features that may increase mortality are seizures, cerebral oedema, an abnormal breathing pattern due to metabolic acidosis, dehydration or bacteraemia. Routine phenobarbital in cerebral malaria is associated with fewer convulsions but more deaths. Corticosteroids have no documented benefit in cerebral malaria.

Severe malarial anaemia presents to hospital with respiratory distress due to lactic acidosis and/or heart failure from an abrupt drop in haemoglobin.

Table 12.4.2	Modified Blantyre Coma Score as used for cerebral malaria
Coma score	Responses to painful fingernail and sternal pressure
0	No response or decerebrate/decorticate or opisthotonic postures
1	Non-specific response (e.g. moans or moves)
2	Withdraws the limb
3	Localizes the painful stimulus
4	Responds and cries momentarily but relapses into coma
5	Normal or fully conscious

The need for blood transfusion can be confirmed on blood film by heavy parasitaemia and lack of a reticulocyte response. However, it may be possible to avoid transfusion in a child with malaria pigment with few or no parasites, many reticulocytes and nucleated red cells (marrow response) but without overt cardiac failure, as rapid clinical improvement can usually be expected within 24 hours. There is insufficient evidence for routinely giving blood to clinically stable children (without respiratory distress) with severe malarial anaemia in terms of either reduced mortality or higher haematocrit at 1 month. Excessive transfusion is a significant risk, particularly in infants, so it is important to monitor volumes, give packed cells where possible and limit transfusions to 10–15 ml/kg over 4–6 hours.

The most effective malaria control measures available to clinicians are insecticide-treated bednets (e.g. permethrin), personal protection with mosquito repellents (e.g. DEET) and effective malaria treatment. Because of widespread resistance of antimalarial drugs to *P. falciparum*, chloroquine and sulfadoxine–pyrimethamine are no longer effective treatment in many parts of the world, yet persist as primary treatment in many countries because of the high cost of newer drugs, lack of data and poor decision making. The most effective treatment of *P. falciparum* malaria is artemether combination therapy (ACT), which has the potential to significantly reduce the high mortality rates from malaria in the developing world. A recent adult study from south-east Asia showed a mortality reduction of over one-third (14% vs 23%) in severe falciparum malaria with artesunate compared to quinine, which needs to be confirmed in children in different settings. Artesunate is an artemisinin derivative (qinghaosu), which is better absorbed parenterally than artemether and (unlike quinine) kills circulating ring-stage parasites and helps prevent sequestration of parasites, which obstructs the microcirculation.

The WHO has formulated a global strategic plan (2005–15) called Roll Back Malaria (http://www.rollbackmalaria.org/docs/gsp_en.pdf). Its priorities include:

- locally appropriate vector control methods, such as insecticide-treated bednets
- prompt diagnosis and treatment with effective antimalarial medicines (e.g. ACT)
- pregnant women receive intermittent preventive treatment.

Although there have been major international efforts to develop malaria vaccines, an effective, affordable vaccine is at least a decade away from implementation.

Dengue virus infection

A number of viruses are capable of producing haemorrhagic disease in humans (Table 12.4.3). They are mainly arthropod-borne, the most common vectors being ticks and mosquitoes. Dengue is the most widespread vector-borne viral infection in humans, with 50–100 million cases annually, being particularly common in tropical countries where the mosquito vector *Aedes aegypti* is present. Most dengue cases are sporadic but it is endemic in south-east Asia and recent epidemics have occurred in our region (e.g. East Timor, Fiji, New Caledonia). The incubation period is 2–7 days and asymptomatic infections are common. The clinical features are abrupt onset of high fever with generalized aches and pains and a macular skin eruption. The flu-like illness lasts 2–6 days and then may relapse a day or two later with fever and rash, followed by fatigue for several weeks.

Severe dengue is characterized by the two syndromes:

- dengue haemorrhagic fever (DHF)
- dengue shock syndrome (DSS).

Practical points

Malaria

- Malaria affects 50% of the world's population in 88 countries
- In addition to clinical activities, there need to be malaria control activities in endemic areas such as the use of insecticide-treated bednets
- Clinical algorithms for malaria diagnosis perform poorly, so diagnosis should be based upon thick blood film or rapid diagnostic tests
- Cerebral malaria and malarial anaemia are the two forms of severe falciparum malaria in children.
- Artemether combination therapy (ACT) is the most effective falciparum malaria treatment now that chloroquine and sulfadoxine–pyrimethamine resistance is widespread.
- Parenteral artesunate is the drug of choice for severe malaria.

Table 12.4.3 Agents causing viral haemorrhagic fever

Disease	Viral agent
Yellow fever	Flavivirus
Dengue	Flavivirus
Chikungunya	Alphavirus
Rift Valley fever	Bunyavirus
Kyasanur virus disease	Flavivirus
Hantaan virus disease	Bunyavirus
Lassa fever	Arenavirus
Marburg virus	Filovirus
Ebola virus	Filovirus

In DHF, a petechial rash appears on about the third day, with bleeding from the gums, nose, gastrointestinal tract and venepuncture sites. After the initial phase, when the fever is beginning to subside, signs of circulatory failure appear, with restlessness, pallor, diaphoresis and cool peripheries. There is evidence of T-cell activation with a rapid increase in cytokines and chemical mediators leading to malfunction of vascular endothelial function and of the haemocoagulation system. Typical laboratory findings include thrombocytopenia, elevated haematocrit, raised liver enzymes and abnormal coagulation tests (e.g. partial thromboplastin time (PTT) and tourniquet test).

Shock in DSS results from marked plasma leakage due to a diffuse vasculitis, often with features of DIC. It usually progresses from haemorrhagic fever, but some develop signs of shock earlier in the illness.

The management of dengue fever is symptomatic and supportive. This means an adequate fluid intake, the use of plasma expanders, the replacement of coagulation factors, paracetamol (not aspirin) and careful clinical observation. Most children will recover and proper management of severe disease is

crucial for reducing case fatality rates, but a mortality of 2% remains even in sophisticated centres. It is still not clear why about 6% of children with dengue progress to shock or haemorrhagic syndromes, but the key immunopathological mechanisms are viral strain virulence and host immune responses, which augment the severity of infection (antibody-dependent enhancement). Host genetic factors may also be important but have not been well documented. A notable risk factor for DHF is the existence of heterotypic dengue virus antibodies before a new infection, which increases the level of viraemia in secondary infections, indicating the importance of the immune response in the pathogenesis of severe disease and complicating vaccine development. Epidemics can only be contained by vector control until a vaccine is available in the (hopefully) near future.

Parasitic infections

Human parasites are classified into five major divisions:

- protozoa (e.g. amoebae, sporozoans)
- platyhelminths (cestodes, trematodes)
- acanthocephala (thorny headed worms)
- nematodes (roundworms)
- arthropods (spiders, tics).

Geohelminths are a subgroup of soil-transmitted intestinal nematodes such as *Strongyloides*, hookworm, *Ascaris* and *Trichuris* (Table 12.4.4). The WHO estimates that some 3.5 billion people are infected by intestinal parasitic and protozoan infections and that 450 million have disease, the majority being children. In China, for example, a nationwide survey, including stool microscopy on 1.5 million people, found a prevalence of 63%, of whom 43% had multiple parasites. The five most common parasites were *Ascaris lumbricoides* (47%), *Enterobius vermicularis* (26%), *Trichuris trichiura* (19%), *Giardia lamblia* (2.5%) and *Entamoeba histolytica* (0.9%). This compares to prevalence estimates in sub-Saharan African schoolchildren of 32% for hookworms, 30% for *Ascaris* and *Trichuris* and 14% for *Schistosoma mansoni*.

Giardiasis

Giardia lamblia is one of the most common parasitic infections in humans, with a prevalence of 20–30% in many developing countries. *Giardia* accounts for about 5% of traveller's diarrhoea and is more common in children with immunodeficiency, although not HIV infection. The clinical manifestations of *Giardia* vary from asymptomatic passage of cysts to chronic diarrhoea with malabsorption and

Clinical example

Fatimah, a 10-year-old Malay girl, presented with a 2-day history of fever, headache, muscle aches and pains and a sore throat. She was generally unwell and toxic and was admitted to hospital for observation, diagnosis and management. Over the next 24 hours she deteriorated with continuing high fever (39°C), persisting symptoms and the appearance of a diffuse erythematous rash involving her face, limbs and trunk. On close inspection, scattered petechiae were seen within the erythema. At this stage her liver was enlarged 4 cm below the right costal margin but the spleen was not palpable. Her blood pressure was normal but the Hess test was positive.

Results of investigations revealed an elevated haemoglobin level, low white cell count and a platelet count of 30 000/m³. The haematocrit was grossly elevated, indicating haemoconcentration. Several blood cultures were negative. Liver function studies revealed slightly elevated transaminase levels. The prothrombin concentration was low and the PTT was prolonged.

A diagnosis of Dengue haemorrhagic fever was made on clinical grounds. Management involved careful observation of pulse and temperature, maintenance of blood pressure with saline and plasma infusions as indicated, correction of haemoconcentration and replacement of coagulation factors. Despite the initial severe bruising and bleeding from the venepuncture sites, she gradually improved and was discharged 7 days later completely recovered. Serology sent off on admission later confirmed the diagnosis when IgM antibodies to Dengue type 4 were noted to be highly elevated.

Table 12.4.4 Common intestinal parasites

Infection	Other name	Symptoms	Transmission	Treatment of choice	Alternative treatments
1. Protozoa					
Entamoeba histolytica	Amoebiasis	Dysentery	Faecal–oral	Metronidazole	
Entamoeba dispar		Asymptomatic	Faecal–oral	Nil	
Giardia lamblia (duodenale or intestinalis)	Giardiasis	Chronic diarrhoea, malabsorption	Faecal–oral	Tinidazole	Metronidazole or nitazoxanide
Cryptosporidium parvum	Cryptosporidiosis	Persistent diarrhoea	Faecal–oral	Nitazoxanide*	
Cyclospora cayetanensis	Cyclosporiasis	Diarrhoea	Faecal–oral	Co-trimoxazole	
Isospora belli	Isosporiasis	Diarrhoea with AIDS	Faecal–oral	Co-trimoxazole	
2. Nematodes					
Ascaris lumbricoides	Roundworm	Intestinal obstruction	Faecal–oral	Albendazole†	Levamisole, pyrantel
Enterobius vermicularis	Pinworm or threadworm	Nocturnal anal pruritus	Faecal–oral	Albendazole	Levamisole, pyrantel
Ancylostoma duodenale	Hookworm	Iron deficiency anaemia	Percutaneous	Albendazole	Levamisole, pyrantel
Necator americanus	Hookworm	Iron deficiency anaemia	Percutaneous	Albendazole	Levamisole, pyrantel
Strongyloides stercoralis	Strongyloidiasis	Diarrhoea	Percutaneous	Ivermectin	Albendazole
Trichuris trichiura	Whipworm, trichuriasis	Dysentery, rectal prolapse (rare)	Faecal–oral	Albendazole	Levamisole, pyrantel
3. Cestodes					
Hymenolepis nana	Dwarf tapeworm	Asymptomatic	Faecal–oral	Nitazoxanide*	Praziquantel
4. Trematodes					
Schistosoma mansoni	Bilharzia	Melaena, portal hypertension	Percutaneous	Praziquantel	Oxamniquine
Fasciolopsis buski	Giant intestinal fluke		Percutaneous	Praziquantel	

* Nitazoxanide is the drug of choice (if available) where treatment is indicated. † Or mebendazole.

weight loss. The usual clinical syndrome is characterized by watery diarrhoea, foul-smelling stools, bloating and abdominal cramps. Only about half of patients develop symptoms following ingestion of cysts, with 15% passing cysts asymptomatically and the remainder showing no trace of infection. The course of giardiasis is frequently prolonged and, although many eventually resolve without treatment, some go on to syndromes of chronic diarrhoea or frequent relapses. Children in the developing world with chronic diarrhoea and malnutrition often have giardiasis but it is not always clear how much *Giardia* is contributing to the illness, since they are often co-infected with other enteric pathogens. The control of giardiasis could be important in programmes to combat anaemia for children in high-prevalence settings. The diagnosis of giardiasis relies upon stool microscopy finding trophozoites or cysts. The sensitivity of a single stool sample is only 50–70% but increases to 90% if three stools are examined. Giardia is waterborne and cysts are highly resistant to chlorine and ozone, so filtration provides the best protection against transmission through tap water.

Amoebiasis

Although this organism is commonly found in stools in children in the tropics, recent molecular and immunological techniques have demonstrated two distinct species of *Entamoeba* that are morphologically identical. *Entamoeba histolytica* is pathogenic, causing symptomatic disease in 10% of infections, whereas *Entamoeba dispar* causes only asymptomatic colonization. In addition to the *E. histolytica* strain, other risk factors for invasive disease are interaction with bacterial flora, host genetic susceptibility, malnutrition, male sex, young age and immunodeficiency. *Entamoeba coli* and *Entamoeba hartmanni* are other non-pathogenic morphologically distinct members of the genus.

Abdominal discomfort may be the only symptom of amoebiasis but an acute attack may provoke severe diarrhoea, cramps, tenesmus and toxaemia, with stools containing blood and mucus but little pus. Amoebic liver abscess, a well-known complication in adults, is rare in childhood.

Schistosomiasis (bilharzia)

There are seven human species of this trematode, including *Schistosoma haematobium*, which affects the renal tract and *Schistosoma mansoni*, which affects the gastrointestinal tract. It has been estimated that 220 million people are infected by schistosomiasis in 74 countries and that 20 million have severe disease. Eggs of *S. mansoni* are passed in the faeces that hatch in warm water; the ciliated larvae swim and penetrate fresh water snails (*Biomphalaria*). After a sporocyst stage, by 4–5 weeks of infection the larval phase results in thousands of tiny cercariae, which penetrate human skin in water, enter peripheral lymphatics or veins and are carried to the lung and mature in portal vessels. Adult worms migrate to the liver and mesenteric veins, where they may survive 2–5 years or longer, producing eggs 25–28 days after cercarial infection.

Eggs cause granuloma formation, resulting in localized colitis and hepatitis. The acute phase of *S. mansoni* may cause allergic symptoms (Katayama syndrome), which are rarely recognized in children. Most chronic infections are light and asymptomatic but with heavy infections up to half of the eggs become trapped in the mucosa and submucosa of the colon, resulting in granulomatous reactions with significant blood loss. The host's inflammatory reaction to eggs carried to the liver in the portal veins leads to portal hypertension. Severe disease with hepatosplenomegaly affects about 10% of *S. mansoni* cases in endemic areas, taking 5–15 years to develop.

With *S. haematobium* the key early feature is terminal haematuria due to the granulomatous response in the bladder, which untreated may progress over years of heavy exposure to obstructive uropathy, hydronephrosis and pyelonephritis. With *S. mansoni*, diarrhoea with blood and mucus and abdominal discomfort may be occasional presenting features, but most infected children have few specific symptoms and complain only of tiredness, lack of energy, anorexia and weight loss. This can present later in life after chronic exposure as hypersplenism, portal hypertension and bleeding oesophageal varices from hepatic granulomas with fibrotic changes.

Diagnosis is based on finding eggs in the faeces but stool concentration methods and numerous immunological techniques (enzyme-linked immunosorbent assay (ELISA), immunoblotting) are more sensitive for milder infections. Treatment is with praziquantel 40 mg/kg as a single dose. Prevention involves avoidance of water sources containing cercariae and promotion of latrine use. Control programmes for schistosomiasis involve mass chemotherapy, destruction of snails, environmental sanitation, prevention of water contact and health education.

Ascariasis

Ascariasis is one of the most prevalent infections in the world, affecting approximately 1400 million people (23% of the world's population), with 59 million, mostly children, at risk of morbidity. Highest prevalences are found in countries where sanitation is deficient, affecting particularly children. Morbidity is directly related to worm load. Geophagy (eating soil) is a significant risk factor for ascariasis and trichuriasis but not for schistosomiasis or hookworm. *Ascaris* infection is not associated with mucosal damage and 85% of infected individuals have light infections that remain asymptomatic. Heavy infection may induce a pneumonitis from migrating pulmonary larvae, with cough, wheeze, eosinophilia and transient patchy infiltrates, which may be difficult to differentiate from pneumonia, asthma or bronchitis. This syndrome of tropical pulmonary eosinophilia (Loeffler) is rarely recognized clinically in children with *Ascaris* or hookworm but is more often symptomatic with filariasis or toxocara infections.

The most common clinical feature of ascariasis is intestinal obstruction from a bolus of worms, which occurs in 0.2% of infections in children but accounts for 72% of all complications of *Ascaris*. Surgical management can invariably be avoided with experience with this syndrome, using daily nasogastric administration of anthelminthics with supportive therapy until the bolus is passed. Worms are often vomited or passed in stools on presentation of sick children. The diagnosis is based upon identification of the characteristic eggs on microscopy of stool or identification of the adult worm passed spontaneously or after treatment. Eggs are plentiful in faeces, since each female produces a mean of 200 000 eggs daily. A lack of latrines and soap for handwashing are risk factors for infection.

Hookworm

The two major species of hookworm are *Ancylostoma duodenale* and *Necator americanus*, which have similar life cycles and disease. The gravid female hookworm produces about 5000–30 000 eggs/day in faeces. The eggs require a moist shady environment to hatch into rhabditiform larvae, which grow to become infective larvae and enter the host's venules or lymphatics, usually when walked upon with bare feet. The larvae then migrate into the lungs and ascend the respiratory tract and descend to the small intestine, where they attach and mature in the jejunum. The time from infection to egg production is almost 2 months.

Hookworms are probably the second most prevalent intestinal parasite after ascariasis, with 1200 million people infected worldwide (two-thirds by *Necator*), including 90–130 million with morbidity. *Necator* predominates in Central and South America (New World), and *Ancylostoma* in India, China, North Africa and tropical Australia, but mixed infections occur in many regions. Unlike *Ascaris* and *Trichuris*, hookworm transmission is closely associated with rural farming settings rather than urban slums. There are several other species of dog and cat helminth (e.g. *Toxocara* species) that can cause eosinophilic enteritis, cutaneous larva migrans or viscera larva migrans in humans. For example, studies in tropical Australia have described eosinophilic enteritis with abdominal pain caused by *Ancylostoma caninum*, a dog hookworm.

Hookworm larvae entering the skin can result in a papulovesicular rash at the site of entry (ground itch) or cutaneous larvae migrans for animal hookworms. Although eosinophilia accompanies the larval migration phase, pneumonitis is mild and is rarely recognized in children. The main morbidity from hookworm is iron deficiency anaemia, particularly with heavy infections. The diagnosis of hookworm is based upon identifying hookworm eggs on microscopy of faeces. Eosinophilic enteritis due to animal hookworm may require endoscopy for definitive diagnosis, since stool microscopy will be negative. Charcot–Leydan crystals in the stools reflect breakdown of eosinophils, which is a non-specific feature of early infection.

Measures to prevent hookworm include ceasing the use of human faeces as fertilizer, use of toilets, wearing shoes and generally improving living standards. In high prevalence areas of hookworm and schistosomiasis, regular mass deworming campaigns with albendazole and praziquantel are effective in reducing anaemia rates.

Whipworm

Trichuris trichiura, meaning 'hairy tail', is actually a misnomer, since it is the proximal end for the worm that is hairlike. A mature female worm produces up to 20 000 eggs/day, which are not infectious until the larval stage develops in warm dark soil over 2–4 weeks. Once ingested, larvae penetrate the epithelium of the mucosal crypt in the cecum, where they moult and the hairlike stichosome remains attached while the broader distal end extends into the lumen. The adult worm is 4 cm long and survives 1–2 years in the host. Trichuriasis is a very common infestation with an estimated 1049 million cases worldwide, including 114 million preschool and 233 million school-age children. Most infections in children are light (<20 adult worms) and asymptomatic with symptoms developing in fewer than 10% of infected children. Occult blood in faeces is uncommon even with heavy infestations, although even light infections incite a local inflammatory response involving eosinophils and neutrophils in the colon. With heavy infestations, frequent watery or mucus stools occur, sometimes with frank blood. Rectal prolapse can occur with heavy infestations and occasionally heavily infected children develop a dysentery syndrome characterized by chronic dysentery, stunting, anaemia and finger clubbing.

The diagnosis is based on finding eggs on stool microscopy. The use of proper latrines, good hygiene with handwashing and washing vegetables will interrupt the life cycle. Overcrowded urban slums with limited water supply and heavily faecally contaminated soil for growing vegetables place children at particular risk. Mass chemotherapy is highly effective but reinfection occurs rapidly in high exposure settings.

Cryptosporidiosis

The protozoa *Cryptosporidium parvum*, *Isospora belli*, *Cyclospora cayetanensis* and *Sarcocystis hominis* all belong to the group of intestinal coccidial infections, which cause diarrhoea. They have come into prominence in recent years through causing severe and protracted diarrhoea in AIDS and infecting piped water supplies as a result of the chlorine resistance of oocysts. However, *Cryptosporidium* also causes persistent diarrhoea and proximal small intestinal enteropathy in children with normal immune function.

Transmission is person to person and from animals to people by ingestion of fecally contaminated food or water. Cryptosporidial infection causes watery diarrhoea with low-grade fever, vomiting and often cramps, severe dehydration and hypokalemia. Among Aboriginal children in Darwin, cryptosporidium was found in the stool of 7.4% of admissions with diarrheal disease, with a mean age of 12 months and mean admission serum potassium of 2.7 mmol/l. It was associated with the most severe and prolonged mucosal damage and inflammation on permeability and nitric oxide testing, but caused less lactose intolerance than rotavirus.

Cryptosporidiosis is diagnosed by finding oocysts in stool using an acid-fast stain, which is only sensitive in diarrhoeal cases. Immunofluorescent and ELISA techniques are more sensitive, and PCR may be even more sensitive for detecting low numbers of oocysts in stool specimens. The high infectivity and ubiquitous oocysts in the environment make prevention by water, hygiene and sanitation programmes very difficult, indeed, impossible in the developing world, where up to 95% of children in some areas have positive serology by age 2 years. Precautions for travellers include handwashing, boiling water, avoiding animals, proper cooking of food, peeling fruit and avoiding uncooked food in contact with unboiled water (e.g. salads).

Strongyloidiasis

Although not a major cause of morbidity worldwide, the nematode *Strongyloides stercoralis* is unique in its ability to persist indefinitely within the host through autoinfection and to cause disseminated disease with the prolonged use of corticosteroids or other causes of immunosuppression.

S. stercoralis is present in virtually all tropical and subtropical regions but estimates of worldwide prevalence vary widely (3–100 million), with the best estimate 30 million people in 70 countries. Strongyloidiasis accounts for about 8% of acute diarrhoeal admissions in Australian Aboriginal children in Darwin, with a mean age of 23 months, this group being significantly older than for other children with diarrhoeal admissions. Prevalence rates vary with climate, geographical region, environmental conditions, soil characteristics and socioeconomic status, but also with modifiable risk factors such as quality of housing, hygiene standards and crowded population density.

Malabsorption and small bowel bacterial overgrowth occur with strongyloidiasis and symptoms of abdominal pain, diarrhoea and weight loss. As with hookworm, larval migration may affect the lungs (eosinophilic pneumonitis) or skin ('ground itch' on the foot or 'larva currens' on the buttocks) but these are not usually recognized in children. Larvae from other mammal species may penetrate the skin of humans, causing only local irritation, but cannot complete their life cycle. The most common manifestation of *S. stercoralis* infection in children is an acute diarrheal illness with foul stools with a typical musty odour. Severe dehydration is uncommon, but hypokalaemia and malabsorption occur commonly. Eosinophilia (5–15% of total white blood cell count) is a common but not universal finding. A syndrome of partial intestinal obstruction with strongyloidiasis has been described in Aboriginal children in the Northern Territory. *Strongyloides fulleborni* is a more virulent infection affecting young children in Papua New Guinea, which may be transmitted via breastmilk, and is characterized by abdominal swelling, ascites, pleural effusions and a high mortality.

Disseminated strongyloidiasis (hyperinfection) occurs with impaired cell-mediated immunity, such as children treated with prolonged courses of steroids (although not from short courses of steroids for asthma) or malignancy (e.g. lymphoma, leukaemia) on immunosuppressive drugs (except cyclosporin, which is antiparasitic). Eradication of *Strongyloides* is essential before immunosuppressive therapy is commenced. Disseminated infection is always a serious complication with high mortality, usually affecting bowel, lungs and central nervous system and often accompanied by sepsis.

The diagnosis is established by identification of larvae on stool microscopy, which is very reliable with acute diarrhoea but less reliable with chronic or

423

asymptomatic infection because rhabditiform larvae excretion is irregular and the parasite load is often low, so a single stool examination may only detect larvae in 30% of cases of latent infections. The agar plate technique is more sensitive, by identifying larval tracks. Because of the unreliability of stool microscopy and the importance of detecting even low levels of infection, various serological tests are available. Disposal of human excreta, wearing shoes, treatment of cases and improved hygiene reduce the risk of transmission of strongyloidiasis in communities. Regular mass chemotherapy programmes against all geohelminths (e.g. albendazole) may have a modest impact on strongyloidiasis, but less than for the other helminths.

Drug treatments for parasitic diseases

The benzimidazoles albendazole and mebendazole have broad-spectrum activity against roundworm, whipworm, hookworm, pinworm and wireworm species. The action of albendazole on the parasite is to bind to tubulin, inhibit microtubule assembly, decrease glucose absorption and inhibit fumarate reductase. Albendazole 400 mg (200 mg if <10 kg) as a single dose or mebendazole 200 mg (100 mg if <10 kg) daily for 3 days is the treatment of choice for ascariasis. The first line treatment for hookworm is albendazole 400 mg as a single dose (200 mg if <10 kg) or mebendazole 100 mg twice daily for 3 days (or single dose of 500 mg if >2 years of age). For clinically significant *Trichuris* infections, the treatment of choice is albendazole 400 mg (or mebendazole 200 mg) daily for 3 days. Half of these doses are used for children under 10 kg but clinical judgement must be used to assess risk-benefit in this age group. Albendazole 400 mg daily for 5 days is an alternative treatment for giardiasis. Albendazole 400 mg daily for 3 days and repeated a week later is also highly effective in acute strongyloidiasis in children but parasitological cure rates are only 45–75% so all larvae may not be eradicated. The benzimidazoles are usually very well tolerated, with occasional gastrointestinal symptoms. Worm migration is uncommon with albendazole treatment. Albendazole should be avoided in pregnancy and used with caution in young infants.

Pyrantel is a depolarizing neuromuscular blocking agent that paralyses worms until they are expelled in faeces. Pyrantel pamoate is active against *Ascaris* and *Enterobius*, only partially effective against hookworm and ineffective against *Trichuris* and *Strongyloides*. It is given as a single dose of 20 mg/kg up to 750 mg orally (repeat after 7 d if heavy infection) or 10 mg/kg daily for 3 days for hookworm.

Levamisole is an immune stimulant that is effective against *Ascaris* and hookworm, and may be more effective for intestinal obstruction from roundworms, since it acts by paralysing the myoneural junction of the worm. The dosage is 3 mg/kg as a single dose.

Ivermectin has broad-spectrum activity against helminths and filariasis but is the drug of choice against strongyloidiasis. Ivermectin is well absorbed orally, accumulates in adipose tissue, is metabolized in the liver, is highly protein-bound with a serum half-life of 12 hours and is excreted in the stools. It is generally well tolerated, with occasional abdominal distension, chest tightness or wheezing. Ivermectin is more effective than albendazole for curing *Strongyloides*, equally effective for *Ascaris*, less effective for *Trichuris* and ineffective against hookworm. Ivermectin 200 µg/kg as a single dose has a reported cure rate of 83% for *Strongyloides*. In complicated or disseminated infection, ivermectin should be repeated on days 2, 15 and 16 to decrease relapse. In immunosuppressed patients, treatment is not always successful and may need to be repeated at monthly intervals or a longer course given. Disseminated disease has a high mortality, so may require ivermectin over 3–4 weeks.

Metronidazole is used for giardiasis and amoebiasis. It is activated by reduction of its 5-nitro group, is concentrated in anaerobic organisms and interacts with DNA to cause microbial death. Amoebic colitis or dysentery should be treated with metronidazole plus a luminal agent for eradicating cyst passage, such as diloxanide furoate, paromomycin or iodoquinol. Although improvement usually occurs within 3–4 days of treatment, metronidazole should be continued for a minimum of 10 days to eliminate intestinal colonization with risk of relapse. The dosage for treatment of acute amoebic colitis is metronidazole 35–50 mg/kg per day in three divided doses for 10 days. The dose of metronidazole for giardiasis has been controversial but a computer simulation study using the conventional 30 mg/kg per day regime calculated that steady state was reached at 24 mg/kg per day in rehabilitated children and at 12 mg/kg per day in severely malnourished children using twice-daily dosage. Metronidazole is not well tolerated, with anorexia and gastrointestinal upset occurring after several days treatment. Patients with immunodeficiency may require treatment for 6–8 weeks for giardiasis. Asymptomatic *Giardia* infections (cyst excreters) should not be treated. Treatment of asymptomatic cyst passers may be warranted for *E. histolytica,* but not for *E. dispar.*

Tinidazole is another 5-nitroimidazole with similar mechanism of action to metronidazole but in a convenient single dosage. Tinidazole 50 mg/kg in a single dose has a higher clinical cure rate than short-course treatment with metronidazole.

Nitazoxanide is a new broad-spectrum antimicrobial agent with activity against nematodes, trematodes,

Clinical example

Ali, aged $2^1/_2$ years, presented with persistent watery diarrhoea of several weeks' duration. On questioning, his parents gave a history of eating dirt (pica). His parents were obviously poor and Ali had three older and one younger siblings. None of the children had attended a child health clinic.

On physical examination there was obvious pallor of the mucous membranes and abdominal distension. Ali's height and weight were both below the 3rd centile and there was finger clubbing and slight ankle oedema. He also had rectal prolapse and was grossly malnourished, with signs of early kwashiorkor.

Endoscopic examination revealed hyperaemic and oedematous rectal mucosa with some ulceration. Many whipworms were attached to the inflamed rectal mucosa. Characteristic ova were seen and the morphology of the worm confirmed the diagnosis of *Trichuris trichiura*. Mucosal ulceration strongly suggested co-infection with *Entamoeba histolytica*.

There was an excellent response to albendazole given over a period of 3 days. A course of metronidazole was also given to eliminate the amoebae. Treatment of the parasitic infestation was the easiest part of the total management. Management of the anaemia and the gross nutritional deficiency was a much greater problem, bearing in mind the very deprived social circumstances of this family. Dietary supplements with vitamins and minerals were supplied in hospital but without health education and financial assistance, Ali's problems were thought likely to recur.

Practical points

Intestinal parasites
- Intestinal parasitic and protozoan infections are highly prevalent, with 3.5 billion people infected and 450 million having disease
- Roundworms, whipworms and protozoa are transmitted faecally–orally (poor hygiene), hookworms and *Strongyloides* percutaneously (walking barefoot) and schistosomiasis from water (bathing, wading)
- Amoebic organisms in stool are most likely to be *Entamoeba dispar*, which is not pathogenic
- Only *Cryptosporidium* and *Strongyloides* are significantly associated with diarrhoea; *Giardia* can cause chronic diarrhoea but is found more commonly in stools of children without diarrhoea
- Nitazoxanide is a new broad-spectrum antihelminthic that treats *Cryptosporidium*, *Giardia*, common helminths and dwarf tapeworm

---

Table 12.4.5   Common infections in Aboriginal community children in tropical Australia

Respiratory infections
- Otitis media – especially chronic suppurative otitis media (CSOM)
- Airways disease – acute bronchiolitis, chronic mucopurulent bronchitis progressing to *bronchiectasis
- Bacterial pneumonia (N.B. pneumococcal and Hib infections now uncommon because of the use of conjugate vaccines)

Infectious diarrhoea
- *Enteropathogenic *Escherichia coli* (EPEC) and enteroaggregative *E. coli* (EAEC)
- Rotavirus (*complicated by metabolic acidosis and secondary lactose intolerance)
- *Strongyloides stercoralis*
- *Cryptosporidium parvum*
- Salmonella (N.B. clinical dysentery uncommon)

Intestinal nematodes
- *Whipworm – *Trichuris trichiura* (N.B. *Ascaris* or roundworm is very rare)
- *Strongyloides*, which causes diarrhoea and occasionally disseminated infection
- *Hookworm – *Ancylostoma duodenale* (less common now because of widespread use of albendazole)

Skin infections
- Impetigo and cellulitis – usually *Streptococcus pyogenes*
- Boils and abscesses – usually *Staphylococcus aureus*
- *Scabies, often with pyoderma
- Tinea corporis – usually *Trichophyton rubrum*

Bone, joint and muscle infections
- Septic arthritis, osteomyelitis and *pyomyositis, usually *Staphylococcus aureus*

Other
- *Rheumatic fever (group A streptococcus)
- *Acute poststreptococcal glomerulonephritis (group A)
- *Epidemic gonococcal conjunctivitis (occasionally)
- *Trachoma (*Chlamydia trachomatis*)
- Hepatitis A (usually anicteric)

* Predominantly occurs in Aboriginal children.

---

anaerobic bacteria and protozoal parasites such as *Cryptosporidium*. It inhibits the key enzyme pyruvate ferredoxin oxidoreductase of target organisms, and is excreted in urine and faeces. Adverse effects tend to affect the gastrointestinal tract appear to be mild and transient. A 3-day course of 100–200 mg 12 hourly in children (adults 500 mg) is effective against giardiasis (equivalent to metronidazole), amebiasis, *Blastocystis hominis*, *Balantidium coli*, *Isospora belli*, *Ascaris*, *Trichuris* and hookworm and is the drug of choice for cryptosporidiosis and *Hymenolepis nana* (dwarf tapeworm) when therapy is indicated. In view of this wide spectrum of action, single-dose therapy in combination with other drugs is under investigation for community treatment programmes.

Specific infections of the Australian tropics

Table 12.4.5 lists the common infections in hospitalized children in the Top End of Australia. Murray Valley encephalitis is endemic in north-west Australia, with significant rates of exposure but a low clinical attack rate of about 0.1% of those infected. However, those who develop clinical illness develop a devastating encephalitis with fever, coma, seizures and neurological signs of cerebellar, spinal cord and brain-stem involvement, and there is a mortality of 20% and neurological sequelae in up to 40% of survivors. While more common in the tropical north of Australia, Ross River and Barmah Forest viruses cause outbreaks throughout Australia. Infection in children is usually asymptomatic and it is likely that infection in childhood accounts for the very low incidence of clinical disease in Aboriginal communities in northern Australia despite high rates of seropositivity.

Melioidosis is caused by the bacterium *Burkholderia pseudomallei*, which is ubiquitous in soil and water in northern Australia and is even more common in Thailand. Disease in children is relatively uncommon compared with adults (e.g. only 4% of cases at Royal Darwin Hospital are in children) because predisposing chronic disease risk factors, such as diabetes and alcoholism, are less common. Although pneumonia is the commonest presentation of melioidosis, there is a wide spectrum of manifestations, from mild cutaneous lesions to fulminant disease with multiple visceral abscesses. Prolonged treatment is required, usually with the antibiotics ceftazidime or imipenem and co-trimoxazole.

PART 13

ALLERGY, IMMUNITY AND INFLAMMATION

M. Gold

General principles

Definition, prevalence and burden of disease

Atopy is defined as the ability of an individual to form specific IgE antibodies to one or more common inhaled aeroallergens such as animal dander, pollen, mould or house dust mite. The clinical expression associated with this immune dysregulation may be an atopic disease, which includes:

* atopic dermatitis
* asthma
* allergic rhinoconjunctivitis.

Interestingly, some atopic individuals do not express clinical disease and the reasons for this variable disease expression are not known. For example, 30–40% of individuals in developed countries can be shown to be atopic yet only 5–20% may manifest an atopic disease.

There is a marked variation in the global prevalence of atopic disease. This variation occurs not only between countries but also regionally within countries. The prevalence is highest in countries that are Westernized, industrialized and/or urbanized. In these countries atopic diseases are now the commonest ailments of childhood, and Australian and New Zealand children have the fifth highest global rates of atopic disease (Table 13.1.1).

The prevalence of atopic disease has been increasing in most communities for reasons that are not yet apparent. Environmental factors are thought to account for the variable and increasing prevalence of atopic disease. A commonly cited hypothesis is that the lack of early childhood exposure to recurrent infections, possibly gastrointestinal infections and viral infections, may predispose to atopy in genetically susceptible individuals. Such a hypothesis can be supported by epidemiological and possibly immunological evidence.

Because atopic diseases are common, often chronic and usually begin in early childhood, the burden to the community, family and individual is considerable. The cost burden of asthma to the Australian community is estimated to range from $585–720 million per annum, with the cost of allergic rhinitis being only marginally less. Importantly, the impact of severe atopic disease such as atopic dermatitis, on a family may exceed that of other chronic childhood disorders such as diabetes mellitus.

Pathogenesis

Although atopy is defined by an excessive production of IgE, this is only one of many immunological changes that characterize the condition, which is associated with a complex dysregulation of the humoral and cellular immune systems (Fig. 13.1.1). For this to occur, both a genetic predisposition and early life environmental allergen exposure are important. Central to this understanding is that naive T helper lymphocytes respond in a particular way to an allergen by secreting specific cytokines that regulate the production of IgE. Continued allergen exposure initiates the allergy cascade, in which there is an early and late response. This occurs in cells located in the skin, respiratory tract, gastrointestinal tract and the vascular system; the end result in some individuals is an atopic disease.

Approach to diagnosis, investigation and management

History and examination

The history and examination should cover the following aspects:

* Specific symptoms
  * nature, timing (seasonal, perennial, episodic), situational (specific site or circumstance)
* Severity of symptoms and degree of disability
  * medication required to control symptoms, medical visits and hospitalization, school absenteeism, interference with sleep, sport or play
* Use of medication
  * current and past medications, efficacy, compliance, technique of use and side effects
* Environmental history – identification of triggers
  * exposure to common allergens (Table 13.1.2) and non-allergen (e.g. cigarette smoke) triggers should be considered

Table 13.1.1 Prevalence (%) of atopic disorders among Australian children

Disorder	6–7-year-olds (%)	13–14-year-olds (%)
Eczema ever (current eczema)	23 (11)	16 (10)
Asthma ever (current wheeze)	27 (25)	28 (29)
Hayfever ever (current rhinitis)	18 (12)	43 (20)

Data obtained from the International Study of Asthma and Allergy in Childhood questionnaire based survey of 10 914 children in Melbourne, Sydney, Adelaide and Perth (see Further reading).

Table 13.1.2 Allergens that may trigger symptoms in atopic children

Inhaled allergens
- Animal dander – cat, dog, horse, rabbit
- Pollen – grass (rye, couch, timothy), weed (plantain), tree (olive, plane)
- Mould – *Alternaria, Aspergillus, Cladosporium, Penicillium* spp.
- House dust mite – *Dermatophagoides pteronyssinus, Dermatophagoides farinae*
- Cockroach

Ingested allergens
- Food – cows' milk, egg, nuts, fish, shellfish, soy, wheat, fruit
- Medication – antibiotics (penicillin) and non-antibiotic medication

Miscellaneous
- Latex contained in balloons and surgical gloves

Clinical example

Michaela, aged 10 years, had severe persistent asthma. She presented for follow-up after a recent admission to the intensive care unit for acute respiratory symptoms diagnosed as status asthmaticus. In passing, her mother mentioned that immediately prior to her most recent episode she had inadvertently eaten a chocolate containing peanuts. She did not usually eat peanuts because she said that they made her mouth 'feel funny'. Her mother recalled that as an infant Michaela experienced two episodes of generalized skin rash immediately following peanut ingestion.

The history is suggestive of an IgE-mediated peanut anaphylaxis. Children with asthma are at increased risk of mortality from anaphylaxis. Additional questions in the history should ascertain whether Michaela had experienced any urticaria, angio-oedema, abdominal pain or vomiting with the most recent episode, as this would confirm the recent presentation as being due to anaphylaxis rather than status asthmaticus. A skin or RAST test to peanut should be obtained. Management should include the complete dietary exclusion of all nuts, an anaphylaxis action plan, adrenaline (epinephrine) for first aid use (Epipen) and a Medic Alert bracelet. Michaela's parents and other carers (including those at school) should be trained to use the anaphylaxis action plan. At this age, nut allergy is likely to be lifelong.

atopic disease. However, since many children manifest more than one atopic disease, it is important to consider whether any other of the atopic conditions is present. A differential diagnosis should be considered, as uncommon disorders may be missed and may assumed to be due to an atopic disease (Table 13.1.4).

Investigations

Investigations in the atopic child are limited. Total IgE is elevated in the majority of children with atopic disease but there is substantial overlap with non-atopic children. Measurement of total IgE is seldom indicated. Allergen-specific IgE (ASE) is more useful and can be determined using both in vivo (skin testing) and in vitro (serological) methods (Table 13.1.5). Measurement of ASE may be helpful in identifying a specific allergen trigger. However, interpretation of the ASE result is critical:

- The presence of specific IgE to an allergen is only one factor in establishing if the allergen is a clinically significant trigger
- The predictive value of a negative result is higher than the predictive value of a positive result
- The result should always be correlated with the history and/or a trial of allergen avoidance with or without subsequent challenge

- a trigger may be easily identified if the onset of symptoms is acute and occurs soon after exposure, if symptoms occur in a specific geographic location, are seasonal, or occur repeatedly following similar exposures
- a trigger may be difficult to identify when continuous exposure results in chronic symptoms
- identification of possible triggers requires knowledge of the likely circumstances of allergen exposure.

On examination atopic children may have a typical appearance (Table 13.1.3).

Assessment

Once the history and examination are completed, there is seldom difficulty in diagnosing the presenting

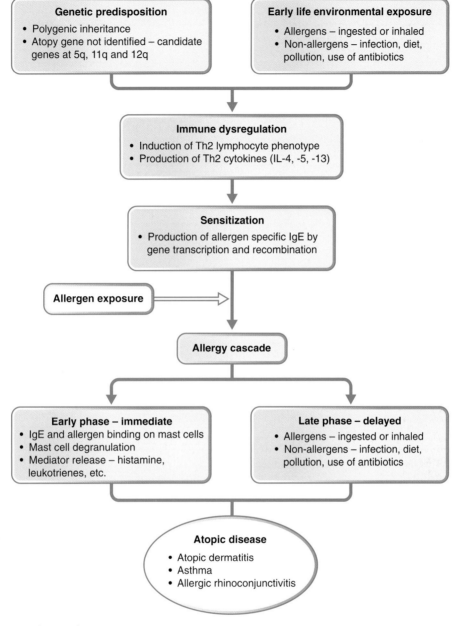

Fig. 13.1.1 Pathogenesis of atopic disease.

• An ASE result should always be discussed with the parent or caregiver to avoid misinterpretation. Failure to do this often leads to inappropriate avoidance measures, which is particularly important when foods are excluded from the diets of children solely on the basis of a positive ASE result.

Management

The aims of management in atopic disease may vary depending on the clinical context.

Prevention of atopic disease

The offspring of families at high risk because either or both parents and/or siblings have an atopic disease have been targeted for the primary prevention of atopy. Current primary preventative strategies have recommended reduced exposure to environmental allergens and irritants perinatally, during infancy and in early childhood. The hypothesis is that reduced exposure during this critical period will prevent (or delay) the onset of atopic disease in genetically susceptible individuals.

431

Table 13.1.3   Examination of the atopic child

Growth	Weight Height
Facies	Facial pallor Allergic shiners – infraorbital dark circles due to venous congestion Dennie–Morgan lines – wrinkles under both eyes Mouth breathing Dental malocclusion – from long-standing upper airway obstruction Sinus tenderness
Skin	Atopic dermatitis White dermatographism – white discoloration of skin after scratching Xerosis – dry skin Urticaria and/or angio-oedema
Nose	Horizontal nasal crease Inferior nasal turbinates – pale and swollen Clear nasal discharge
Respiratory	Chest deformity – Harrison sulcus, increase in anteroposterior diameter Respiratory distress Wheeze and/or stridor
Eyes	Conjunctivitis Subcapsular cataracts associated with conjunctivitis
Ears	Tympanic membrane dull and retracted
Throat	Tonsillar enlargement Postpharyngeal secretions and cobblestoning of mucosa
Cardiovascular	Blood pressure

Table 13.1.4   Differential diagnosis of atopic disease

Atopic disease	Differential diagnosis
Atopic dermatitis	Seborrheic dermatitis Psoriasis Wiskott–Aldrich syndrome* Hyper IgE syndrome*
Asthma	Infection – viral, bacterial, mycobacterial Congenital anomaly, e.g. vascular ring Cystic fibrosis Immunodeficiency disease Aspiration syndrome secondary to gastro-oesophageal reflux, incoordinate swallowing or tracheo-oesophageal fistula Inhaled foreign body Cardiac failure
Allergic rhinitis	Infective rhinitis Non-allergic rhinitis Vasomotor rhinitis Rhinitis medicamentosa Sinusitis Adenoidal hyperatrophy Nasal polyps Nasal foreign body Choanal atresia (unilateral, bilateral)

* These immunodeficiency diseases may have atopic dermatitis as a component.

Table 13.1.5 Determination of allergen-specific IgE		
	Skin testing	Serology
Method	Skin puncture test	RAST
Availability	Limited	Widely available
Expense	Cheap	Expensive
Results	Immediate	Delayed
Risk of anaphylaxis	Rare	Nil
Interference	Antihistamines Extensive atopic dermatitis Dermatographism	High total IgE
Sensitivity	++++	++
Specificity	++++	++

Table 13.1.6 Methods to reduce house dust mite exposure
Definitely useful   • Encase bedding in impermeable covers (dust mite covers): most important measure, since the bed is the major source   • Hot water washing of bedding and clothes (>56°C): will destroy house dust mite and remove allergens
Probably useful   • Replacement of fitted carpets with smooth flooring   • Hard-surface cleaning with a damp cloth, at least once a week
Possibly useful   • Air filtration, ionizers and air conditioning
Unlikely to be useful   • Acaricides (dust mite sprays) for the carpet and mattress

Although further studies are awaited to assess the role of early avoidance of allergens in the prevention of atopic disease, it would appear sensible to advise families who have infants at high risk of atopy to:

• avoid exposing the infant to tobacco smoke
• prolong breastfeeding (12 months if possible)
• delay the introduction of solids (4–6 months)
• consider use of a hypoallergenic formula if breastfeeding is not possible
• restrict the maternal intake of allergenic proteins (such as nuts, eggs, cows' milk) during breastfeeding. This measure is controversial and if this is prescribed it should be done in conjunction with a dietitian.

Since approximately 50% of infants with atopic dermatitis may progress to develop asthma and allergic rhinoconjunctivitis, strategies are being considered to prevent the progression of atopic disease. A recent double-blind placebo-controlled study has shown that the daily use of a non-sedating antihistamine may prevent the development of asthma in infants with atopic dermatitis who have been sensitized to either house dust mite or grass pollen.

Management of symptomatic atopic disease

Once the child has developed symptomatic atopic disease, management involves allergen identification and avoidance, and symptomatic treatment. Immunotherapy may be appropriate for selected children.

Allergen identification and avoidance
When possible, this remains an important component of management. Avoidance measures may involve considerable parental education, effort and expense. Note that:

• with ingested allergens identification and avoidance are particularly important when atopic disease is associated with a food allergy, as this is the only means of therapy
• with inhalant allergens, methods have been evaluated to reduce exposure to indoor allergens, most importantly the house dust mite (Table 13.1.6). A number of studies in sensitized individuals have demonstrated improvements in atopic dermatitis and allergic rhinitis following house dust mite reduction measures. The benefit of house dust mite avoidance in asthma is much more controversial
• other indoor allergens (cat, cockroach, mould) and outdoor allergens are less easily avoided and alternative forms of therapy may be required.

Symptomatic treatment
When allergen avoidance is difficult, the response is partial or the allergen cannot be identified, symptomatic treatment is indicated. A number of medications are available, including antihistamines, sympathomimetics, mast cell stabilizers, corticosteroids and leukotriene antagonists (Table 13.1.7).

Induction of tolerance: immunotherapy
Allergen immunotherapy was first used for grass-pollen-induced allergic rhinitis almost 100 years ago and is only effective for IgE-mediated inhalant allergic disease. Although the exact mechanism is not

Table 13.1.7 Medications for the symptomatic treatment of allergic disease

	Important mechanisms of action in allergic disease	Examples
Antihistamines	**1st and 2nd generation** H_1-receptor antagonism **2nd generation** Above plus antiallergic effects Decrease mediator release Decreased migration and activation of inflammatory cells Reduced adhesion molecule expression	Diphenhydramine Promethazine Hydroxyzine Cetirizine Loratadine Terfenadine
Sympathomimetics	**Beta agonists** Bronchial smooth muscle relaxation Reduce mast cell secretion **Alpha and beta agonists** Bronchial smooth muscle relaxation Vasoconstriction – skin and gut Inotropic and chronotropic effects Reduce mast cell secretions Glycogenolysis	Salbutamol Albuterol Terbutaline Adrenaline (epinephrine)
Theophylline	Phosphodiesterase inhibition Improved respiratory muscle function Respiratory stimulant Improved ciliary function Anti inflammatory effects	Theophylline
Cromolyn	Mast cell stabilizer Inhibits chemotaxis of eosinophils Inhibits pulmonary neuronal reflexes	Cromolyn sodium Nedocromil sodium
Corticosteroids	Reduce T cell cytokine production Reduce eosinophil adhesion, chemotaxis Reduce mast cell proliferation Reduce vascular permeability Reverse adrenoreceptor downregulation	Hydrocortisone Beclomethasone Budesonide Fluticasone/flunisolide Triamcinolone acetonide
Leukotriene antagonists	5-lipoxygenase enzyme inhibition or LTD4 receptor antagonist	Zileuton Montelukast Zafirlukast

known, the induced state of tolerance to an allergen is associated with the production of blocking antibodies, downregulation of T-helper-2 (Th2) lymphocytes and a decrease in ASE.

Immunotherapy should be initiated and supervised by an experienced allergist. Pollen-induced allergic rhinoconjunctivitis remains the main indication for immunotherapy and should be considered in children who have intractable and disabling symptoms that have failed to respond to allergen avoidance and to symptomatic treatment. Immunotherapy for children who present primarily with asthma is controversial. Not only is the risk of an adverse reaction higher in these children but they are often sensitized to both seasonal and perennial allergens. No form of immunotherapy is currently available for atopic dermatitis.

Future prevention and management of atopic disease

A number of novel approaches and therapies may become available to prevent and manage atopic disease in the future:

• Specific methods of allergen avoidance are being studied in large prospective studies for the primary prevention of atopic disease
• An alternative approach is to expose high risk infants to an 'allergy vaccine' which would induce a Th1 rather than Th2 lymphocyte response. Measures under current laboratory investigation include the use of novel vaccines and adjuvants
• For those children with symptomatic atopic disease a number of trials are investigating ways to prevent disease progression or to reduce the long-term

consequences, such as airway remodelling in chronic asthma. Of particular interest is the role of pharmacotherapy (antihistamines, cromolyn and corticosteroids) or immunotherapy
• A number of novel immunopharmacological agents are under investigation for symptomatic disease. These include an anti-IgE monoclonal antibody that binds IgE, thereby preventing IgE binding to mast cell receptors. Other agents under investigation include cytokines and cytokine antagonists
• There is renewed interest in immunotherapy, as a number of new developments are likely to enhance this form of therapy for symptomatic disease. These measures include the use of recombinant allergens, novel adjuvants, combinations of allergens and modulatory cytokines, naked plasmid DNA vaccines and peptide vaccines.

Specific atopic disorders

The majority of children who develop atopic dermatitis or asthma present by 6 years of age, with most individuals manifesting symptoms of allergic rhinoconjunctivitis by 20 years of age. However, there is a predictable pattern of disease expression, which is called the 'allergic march':

• Expression of atopy usually starts with atopic dermatitis, which presents in the first 6 months of life and improves in the second year of life
• Approximately 50% of children with atopic dermatitis will then develop asthma in early childhood
• With resolution of asthma in late childhood some children then develop allergic rhinitis, which may be lifelong
• Importantly, in a number of children all forms of atopic disease may be expressed concurrently. For this reason, although one atopic disease may be predominant at a particular age, it is always important to consider which other atopic conditions may be present.

Atopic dermatitis

See also Chapter 21.1.

Definition and clinical presentation

Atopic dermatitis is a chronic inflammatory skin disorder that is associated with overproduction of IgE and eosinophils due to a systemic Th2 cytokine response. Histamine, neuropeptides, proinflammatory cytokines, mast cells, eosinophils and antigen-presenting cells are all increased in skin affected by atopic dermatitis. The cardinal features of atopic dermatitis include:

• intense pruritus
• a relapsing course
• a typical distribution of skin rash
• a personal or family history of an atopic disease
• additional features that may be present:
 • dry skin (xerosis), skin infection, white dermatographism
 • other atopic diseases and atopic facies (Table 13.1.4)
 • food allergy and intolerance.

Clinical example

Hannah, aged 8 months, had severe atopic dermatitis. Her skin was permanently excoriated and erythematous. She had been breastfed and was on solids, which included rice, vegetables and wheat. A dietary history revealed that she also had food that contained small amounts of egg and cows milk protein. A RAST performed by her GP showed specific IgE antibodies to egg of more than 100 KUA/l (very high) and to cows milk of 30 KAU/l (moderate). No specific IgE had been detected to wheat and rice.

The treatment of atopic dermatitis involves avoidance of skin irritants, use of skin moisturization, topical anti-inflammatories and the identification and avoidance of triggers. Approximately 50% of infants with atopic dermatitis have IgE sensitization to one or more of the common food proteins. Some of these infants may have an IgE-mediated food allergy and ingestion of these food proteins may trigger atopic dermatitis. Dietary exclusion of egg and cows milk protein should occur in this infant and the affect of this on atopic dermatitis should be assessed. If possible, this should occur under the supervision of a dietitian and alternative sources of protein and calcium should be included in the diet. Egg and cows' milk allergy usually resolves by 5 years of age.

The main symptom of atopic dermatitis is intense pruritus, which when severe may be associated with disruption of sleep, school and social interactions and can profoundly affect the quality of life. In older children and adolescents, disfigurement and teasing may be important. The appearance of the skin in atopic dermatitis may be variable:

• In infants with an acute presentation the lesions are erythematous, papulovesicular and mostly occur on the face, scalp, extensor surfaces of the limbs and trunk
• With increasing age the lesions localize to the hands, feet and the antecubital and popliteal flexures
• Chronic changes include lichenification of the skin, which is a skin thickening resulting from persistent rubbing and scratching

- The skin is almost invariably dry and the appearance of the skin may be altered by intense excoriation and secondary bacterial infection.

Investigations

Determination of specific IgE to inhaled or ingested allergens should be considered if the atopic dermatitis is extensive and has not responded to measures of general skin care and symptomatic treatment.

Most affected children above 2 years of age have a raised total IgE concentration and have measurable specific IgE to common inhaled and ingested allergens. This is a marker of atopic status rather than indicating that a specific allergen may be a trigger for atopic dermatitis. Response to withdrawal of the allergen is currently the only way to determine the significance of these results.

Management

A number of triggers may exacerbate atopic dermatitis, including:

- skin irritants (e.g. soap, heat)
- viral infection
- food allergens
- allergens such as house dust mite, animal dander, mould and pollen
- bacterial (*Staphylococcus aureus*) or viral (herpes simplex type I) skin infection
- stress.

The aim of management is to reduce as many of these triggers as possible and to provide symptomatic relief until the disorder improves, which fortunately occurs in most children.

The majority of children respond to general measures of skin care, which include:

- avoidance of skin irritants – soaps, shampoo, woollen clothing, hot baths
- frequent use of topical moisturizers (at least twice daily)
- antiseptic measures – antiseptic bath oil, topical antiseptic cream (intermittent)
- wet wraps – wet dressings (bandages) applied to the affected skin.

If symptoms persist despite these general measures then medication should be considered:

- Topical corticosteroids are used commonly:
  - the least potent steroid should always be used for maintenance therapy
  - if possible steroids should be used intermittently
  - potent steroids must be avoided on the face and creases

- Sedating antihistamines may be useful intermittently particularly for night time itch
- Antibiotics may also be useful for secondary bacterial infection of the skin.

If symptoms persist and are severe despite general measures of skin care and topical steroids, an allergy review would be appropriate; the aim would be to identify allergens that could be significant triggers. Allergen avoidance is particularly important in infants and children who have associated food allergies and those who have been sensitized to house dust mite.

Unfortunately, there are a small number of children who, despite all these measures, have severe and disabling atopic dermatitis and these children may require intermittent hospitalization for intensive topical therapy, phototherapy and immunosuppressive medication.

Asthma

See also Chapter 14.3.

Definition and clinical presentation

Asthma is defined as a chronic inflammatory lung disorder that is usually associated with bronchial hyperactivity and presents as a symptom complex of cough, wheeze and shortness of breath. Since asthma is discussed elsewhere (Ch. 47), this section will review asthma in the context of the atopic child.

Although the exact cause of asthma is not known, the two most significant risk factors are a family history and atopy. Specifically, between 60% and 80% of asthmatic children are atopic. Furthermore, sensitization to indoor allergens (house dust mite and cockroach) combined with exposure to high levels of these allergens is an important risk factor associated with symptomatic asthma. The implication is that exposure to indoor allergens may contribute to the development of asthma and that ongoing exposure or intermittent exposure may be a trigger factor for asthma.

Role of inhaled allergens in the development of asthma
One of the important features of asthma is airway inflammation, which is characterized by infiltration of the airways with mast cells, lymphocytes and eosinophils. It is postulated that this chronic inflammatory response may be initiated by allergen exposure in a genetically susceptible individual.

Allergen triggers and asthma
Asthma has multiple triggers, the most important of these being viral infections and physical factors such

as cold air and exercise. However, in individuals who have become sensitized to inhaled allergens, further allergen exposure may act as a trigger for asthma:

- Bronchial challenge studies show that acute bronchospasm can be induced in atopic asthmatics by inhalation of aeroallergens
- Epidemics of asthma have been documented in association with airborne allergens
- The level of exposure to indoor allergens has been correlated with the extent of asthma severity
- In controlled settings asthmatic symptoms, peak expiratory flow rate and bronchial hyperresponsiveness improve when individuals avoid allergens to which they are allergic.

Investigations

Demonstration of ASE may be useful in children who:

- present with the symptom complex of cough and/ or wheeze and in whom the diagnosis of asthma may not be clear, as atopy is commonly associated with asthma
- have persistent asthma. Determination of ASE to inhaled allergens could be considered part of routine asthma management in children with persistent asthma. Identification of those individuals sensitized to animal dander and house dust mite may be useful.

Determination of ASE is not indicated in episodic asthma because viral infection is the most frequent trigger. However, if a specific inhaled allergen trigger is suspected from the history, ASE may be helpful.

Management

The management of asthma depends on the frequency and severity of the condition. Episodic asthma may require intermittent treatment, while persistent asthma may require continuous treatment (Ch. 14.3). Asthma education is critical and includes an explanation of the disease, education about techniques of using the inhalers and spacers, home monitoring, an explanation of the side effects of medications, an action plan for home treatment, and education about allergen avoidance.

Allergen identification and avoidance in asthma

Studies of house dust mite reduction in atopic asthmatics with persistent asthma have had variable results. It is clear that studies that have markedly reduced the exposure of asthmatics to house dust mite (e.g. by hospitalization) have shown an improve-

ment in asthma. However, clinical trials that have aimed to reduce dust mite exposure in patients' homes have had more variable results, which probably correlate with the effectiveness of dust mite reduction methods. Although effective methods have been evaluated to reduce house dust mite levels, these are expensive and time-consuming and often not adhered to by patients (Table 13.1.6). Removal of pets from the homes of sensitized asthmatics should be recommended but occurs uncommonly.

Ingested allergens rarely trigger asthma as a sole manifestation. Other features in relation to episodes of asthma are:

- acute bronchospasm, which may be part of anaphylaxis in asthmatic children but occurs with other manifestations of anaphylaxis, such as skin rash or vomiting
- cows' milk ingestion, which is not uncommonly implicated by parents as a cause of upper respiratory tract symptoms, including asthma; however, empiric removal of cows milk from the diets of children with asthma is not justified
- in some asthmatics, ingestion of metabisulphite, which can result in an immediate bronchospasm. This is because of a pharmacological intolerance to metabisulphite, possibly as a result of direct irritation of the airway. Metabisulphite is a commonly used preservative in a number of food substances including meat, dried fruit, fruit juices and hot chips.

Allergic rhinoconjunctivitis

See also Chapter 22.1.

Definition and clinical presentation

Allergic rhinoconjuctivitis is rare in infants under 6 months old. Perennial allergic rhinoconjuctivitis may occur at any age in childhood and seasonal allergic rhinoconjuctivitis often develops in older children.

The primary functions of the nose are olfaction and air filtration and humidification. This is achieved by the nasal structure, which ensures that inhaled air is in contact with an extensive and highly vascular mucosal membrane. In sensitized individuals, mucosal contact with inhaled allergens in the nose and conjunctiva elicits IgE-mediated mast cell degranulation and a chronic inflammatory response.

The history should determine the specific symptoms, as the presentation is quite variable, with either rhinitis or conjunctival symptoms predominating:

- The symptoms of rhinitis are nasal obstruction, itch, sneezing and rhinorrhoea
- Conjunctival symptoms include itching and an increase in tear fluid.

The timing of symptoms provides important information concerning possible triggers. Symptoms may be seasonal, perennial, a combination of perennial and seasonal or episodic:

- Symptoms during spring, summer or autumn indicate seasonal allergic rhinoconjunctivitis, which may be triggered by pollen (grass, weed or tree) or mould
- Perennial symptoms may be due to indoor allergens (house dust mite, animal dander, cockroach)
- Episodic symptoms are most often due to exposure to animal dander but may occur in response to other allergens.

Examination of the nose and eyes is important (Table 13.1.4):

- The inferior nasal turbinates can be visualized with a light source (using an otoscope), with the diagnostic features being pallor and swelling. When severe, the swollen nasal turbinates may extend to the nasal septum and may be mistaken for nasal polyps, which are uncommon in children. Typical findings may not be present
- Conjunctival injection and oedema affect both the bulbar and tarsal conjunctiva and appear as redness and swelling.

Rhinitis symptoms may occur without evidence of an allergic cause (Table 13.1.5). If nasal obstruction is the main symptom, it is important to exclude an anatomical cause. If symptoms such as sneezing, rhinorrhoea and/or obstruction are predominant, alternative diagnoses such as vasomotor or infective rhinitis need to be considered.

Investigations

Determination of ASE is not indicated in seasonal allergic rhinitis unless symptoms are intractable and immunotherapy is being contemplated. ASE is indicated in perennial allergic rhinitis if symptoms are troublesome because, if specific IgE to an indoor allergen(s) can be demonstrated, a trial of allergen avoidance measures would be justified.

Management

In children sensitized to indoor allergens a trial of avoidance measures should be instituted. The choice of symptomatic treatment depends on the nature, severity and timing of symptoms. Intermittent and infrequent symptoms can be treated with antihistamines. Prolonged symptoms are best treated with topical steroids combined with antihistamines if control is inadequate. For seasonal allergic rhinoconjunctivitis treatment should be commenced prior to the onset of spring:

- Topical nasal corticosteroids are most effective for nasal obstructive symptoms but also reduce rhinorrhoea, sneezing and conjunctival symptoms. Steroids may take up to a week to work and may require prior use of a decongestant to allow adequate nasal delivery. In general, nasal steroids have been shown to be safe in children but epistaxis may be a problem in some children. This can be reduced by directing the nasal spray away from the nasal septum
- Cromolyn is a safe alternative for both nasal and conjunctival application but needs to be given frequently because of the short duration of action
- Antihistamines (oral or topical) are useful for symptoms of rhinorrhoea, nasal or eye itch, and watery eyes but are not effective for nasal obstruction. When given orally, non-sedating and long-acting antihistamines are preferred but often are more expensive
- Use of nasal decongestants (vasoconstrictors), either topical or oral, for longer than 5 days should be discouraged.

Immunotherapy should be considered in children with pollen-induced seasonal allergic rhinoconjuctivitis who have failed to respond to symptomatic treatment, provided the selection criteria have been fulfilled.

Complications of atopic disease and important associated conditions

A number of important conditions occur more commonly in children with atopic disease and complicate management. Interestingly, medication and insect venom allergy is not more common in atopic children.

Food allergy and intolerances

Adverse reactions to food are often reported in children with atopic disease. The important reactions to consider are food allergies and intolerances, particularly in infants and young children with atopic dermatitis (Table 13.1.8). Conversely, food is an uncommon trigger for asthma and allergic rhinitis. Food allergy and intolerance may occur in children without any atopic disease.

Food allergy

IgE-mediated food allergy
It is important to recognize IgE-mediated food allergy in children with atopic disease:

Table 13.1.8   Food allergy versus food intolerance

	Food allergy	Food intolerance
Mechanism	Immune-mediated IgE-mediated Non-IgE-mediated – cell mediated	Non-immune-mediated Pharmacological

Food triggers	**Food proteins**
	Cows' milk
	Egg
	Nuts
	Fish and shellfish
	Soy
	Wheat
	Fruits
		Food chemicals
		Food additives
		  Preservatives
		  Food colourings
		  Monosodium glutamate
		Natural constituents
		  Salicylates
		  Amines
		  Monosodium glutamate

• The condition is more common in infants and children with atopic dermatitis. In some studies of children presenting with atopic dermatitis up to one third may have an IgE mediated food allergy
• Those children who have asthma and IgE mediated food allergy are at greater risk of experiencing more severe reactions, and rarely mortality from anaphylaxis may occur in this group of children.

Diagnosis. The diagnostic hallmark of IgE-mediated food allergy is that symptoms usually occur immediately (minutes to hours) after ingestion of the food. Although the most severe manifestation of IgE-mediated food allergy is anaphylaxis, a generalized or facial skin rash may be the sole manifestation. Anaphylaxis is a multisystem disorder characterized by respiratory and/or cardiac involvement usually in combination with involvement of another system, most often the skin. The following symptoms and/or signs may occur with a generalized allergic reaction, including anaphylaxis:

• skin – generalized skin erythema, urticaria or angio-oedema
• respiratory system – rhinorrhoea, sneezing, cough, wheeze, stridor, respiratory distress
• gastrointestinal system – abdominal pain, vomiting, diarrhoea
• cardiovascular system – hypotension if severe collapse with loss of consciousness.

Up to 60% of children who have an IgE-mediated allergy to one food protein may have an allergy to another, with the majority having reactions to cows' milk, egg, nuts, soy, fish and wheat. Hence, if an infant presents with reaction to one food it is always important to exclude others.

Clinical example

John, aged 12 years, had asthma. While swimming he was stung by a bee on his hand. Within 5 minutes he developed generalized urticaria, facial angio-oedema, cough, wheeze and difficulty breathing. An ambulance was called and intramuscular adrenaline (epinephrine) was administered, with resolution of John's symptoms.

Anaphylaxis is defined as a multisystem and generalized allergic reaction with involvement of the cardiorespiratory system. The emergency treatment is adrenaline, which initially is easily administered by the intramuscular route. The occurrence of bee venom anaphylaxis is not increased in asthmatics. However, asthma is a risk factor for more severe episodes of anaphylaxis in anyone with a food, medication or insect venom allergy. For this reason, in someone who has asthma and anaphylaxis, first aid measures should be in place, including access to an adrenaline autoinjector device (Epipen). This should be prescribed together with an anaphylaxis action plan. Immunotherapy is recommended for the long-term treatment of bee venom anaphylaxis.

Non-IgE-mediated food allergies
Non-IgE-mediated food allergies are thought to be mediated by cellular mechanisms, probably involving T lymphocytes. Cow or soy milk protein is the usual trigger but other food proteins may be involved:

• The most common reaction is an exacerbation of underlying atopic dermatitis, which usually presents as a delayed reaction 1–2 days after exposure to the offending food

• A number of gastrointestinal manifestations of non IgE mediated food allergy may occur:
  • cows'-milk-protein-induced colitis presents as a well infant with fresh blood in the stools, which resolves once cows' milk is excluded from the infant's diet or from the diet of the mother if breastfeeding
  • food-protein-induced enterocolitis may present as sudden vomiting, dehydration and collapse, which may be mistaken for a gastroenteritis or bowel obstruction and occurs within hours of exposure to the food trigger
  • other manifestations include an enteropathy, which may present as failure to thrive, irritability, chronic diarrhoea and anaemia, or eosinophilic eosophagitis, which presents with abdominal pain, recurrent vomiting and dysphagia and may be mistaken for gastro-oesophageal reflux.

Food intolerances

Food intolerances are thought to be pharmacological in nature. Important food intolerances in atopic children include:

• metabisulphite, a commonly used preservative, which may trigger acute wheeze in selected children with asthma
• facial skin rashes due to contact irritation from foods such as tomato and citrus are common in children with atopic dermatitis
• generalized exacerbations of eczema may occur in children with atopic dermatitis that are due to a food intolerance.

Investigation of food allergy and intolerance

The investigation of food allergy and intolerance is limited:

• If an adverse food reaction is thought to be IgE-mediated, determination of ASE is indicated. However, foods should not be excluded from the diet solely on the basis of a skin or RAST test
• There are no validated tests for non-IgE-mediated food allergy or food intolerances. The only investigation is to demonstrate an improvement of symptoms following withdrawal of the food trigger and recurrence of symptoms with rechallenge. Double-blind and placebo-controlled challenges are preferable but are seldom available except in specialized facilities. An open and non-blind challenge is more practical but is less accurate
• Empirical use of a diet that eliminates a number of naturally occurring food substances should never be instituted for more than 4 weeks and should be used as a diagnostic trial. If the child responds this should be followed by appropriate challenges to identify food triggers
• Unsubstantiated tests, e.g. Vega or Cytotoxic tests, should never be used to diagnose food allergy or intolerance.

Management

The only management available for food allergy or intolerance is exclusion of these foods from the child's diet. Additionally:

• Education of the parents and other carers, particularly when young children attend child care and kindergarten, is essential and may require the advice of a dietitian
• In breastfed infants with atopic dermatitis and food allergy, exclusion of food triggers from the maternal diet may also be tried but this is best done with the support of a dietitian and may not be beneficial in all infants
• With any exclusion diet it is important to ensure that the diet is nutritionally adequate. This is particularly important as regards calcium intake when milk products are excluded
• In atopic children who have had food anaphylaxis the following points are important:
  • anaphylaxis is a medical emergency and requires prompt recognition and treatment (Table 13.1.9)
  • all children should undergo subsequent specialist review
  • appropriate dietary advice is essential to avoid recurrent episodes
  • adrenaline (epinephrine) for first aid use by parents and other carers should be considered. This is most conveniently prescribed in the form of an autoinjector device (Epipen). Appropriate training and documentation in the form of an anaphylaxis action plan is essential.

Table 13.1.9 Emergency management of anaphylaxis

1. Remove the trigger
2. Administer adrenaline (epinephrine) by deep intramuscular injection: 0.01 ml/kg of 1 : 1000 adrenaline (max. dose 0.5 ml)
3. Establish an airway if required and administer oxygen
4. Assess circulation. If hypotensive: administer i.v. adrenaline dose 0.1 ml/kg of 1 : 10 000 (max. dose 3 ml); administer i.v. fluids, normal saline 10–20 ml/kg as a bolus
5. Repeat doses of adrenaline can be administered every 5 minutes until clinical improvement occurs
6. Antihistamines and steroids are not administered for the initial management but should be given as second-line therapy

Clinical example

Justine was 6 months old and was known to have atopic dermatitis. She had been otherwise well and her weight was 10.0 kg. She was breastfed and because her mother was about to return to work Justine was offered her first bottle feed containing a cows' milk protein formula. Immediately after drinking a small amount she became irritable, vomited and then developed generalized urticaria, a persistent cough, difficulty breathing and stridor.

Justine had experienced an anaphylactic reaction to cows' milk protein. Although this was the first apparent exposure, she was likely to have been exposed to cows' milk protein in maternal breast milk.

Adrenaline (epinephrine) is required for the emergency management and is most easily administered by deep intramuscular injection (0.01 ml/kg of 1:1000, i.e. 0.1 ml at Justine's weight of 10.0 kg). The response is usually rapid but the dose can be repeated until a clinical response is obtained.

It was important to ensure that the family was educated regarding subsequent exclusion of cows' milk from Justine's diet. In addition, other allergenic food proteins, including egg, nut, soy, fish, shellfish and wheat should be excluded if these had not yet been ingested and tolerated. Determination of specific IgE to these food proteins and an allergy review would be indicated. Tolerance to cows' milk develops by school age in the majority of children.

Practical points

- The atopic diseases of childhood are eczema, asthma, and allergic rhinitis. The majority of children who have these conditions will be atopic (have allergen-specific IgE (ASE) to one or more common allergens)
- The presence of ASE does not always indicate an allergen trigger and should be interpreted together with the history and/or a trial of allergen avoidance with or without subsequent challenges
- The management of atopic disease includes identification and avoidance of allergens (if possible), symptomatic treatment and immunotherapy for selected children
- Anaphylaxis is a generalized multisystem allergic reaction, which includes cardiorespiratory involvement
- The emergency treatment of anaphylaxis is adrenaline (epinephrine), which, unless hypotension is present, can be administered via the intramuscular route
- All children with anaphylaxis should undergo a specialist review so that the trigger can be identified, avoidance strategies implemented and first aid measures established, including use of injectable adrenaline (Epipen).

Prognosis

The natural history of food allergy and intolerances is to improve with increasing age. IgE-mediated nut, fish and shellfish allergies are an exception, since these allergies may be lifelong, although tolerance may develop in up to 10% of children. Therefore carefully supervised challenge with the implicated food at 12-month intervals is recommended. Determination of ASE may predict when it is appropriate to consider a challenge.

Recurrent or chronic sinusitis in allergic rhinitis

Allergic rhinitis should be considered as a possible predisposing factor in children who:

- have recurrent or chronic sinusitis. The orifices of the frontal, ethmoid and maxillary sinuses are located in close proximity to the nasal turbinates and rhinitis may predispose to ostial obstruction. Symptoms of sinusitis in older children and adults are typical and include facial pain, toothache, headache and fever (Ch. 22.1). However, young children may present with rhinorrhoea, cough, postnasal discharge, periorbital swelling and otitis media

- have secretory otitis media, in whom the incidence of atopy is increased. However, it remains unclear whether allergic rhinitis is a significant underlying factor because of eustachian tube obstruction. If indicated, allergic rhinitis should be treated in such children but this may not improve the secretory otitis media.

Obstructive sleep apnoea in allergic rhinitis

Nasopharyngeal obstruction in children may present with snoring and, if severe, obstructive sleep apnoea (OSA). Obstructive sleep apnoea may present in children with early morning headache, daytime sleepiness and poor concentration. Children who present with allergic rhinitis should be questioned about these symptoms and those children presenting with upper airway obstruction should be evaluated and, if needed, treated for allergic rhinitis.

Skin infection in atopic dermatitis

Bacterial, viral and fungal skin infection is an important complication of atopic dermatitis:

- *Staphylococcus aureus* is detected almost universally in atopic dermatitis. The organism produces exotoxins, which may potentiate the inflammatory process. Topical antiseptic measures are important but oral antibiotics may be required
- Herpes simplex virus (HSV) type I may infect lesions and present as vesicular lesions which soon ulcerate. Generalized HSV skin infection may be

441

severe and would be an indication for hospitalization and parenteral aciclovir

• Dermatophyte infections may occur in atopic dermatitis and should be considered in resistant lesions.

Spasmodic croup

Spasmodic croup is a condition of recurrent sudden upper airway obstruction that presents as stridor and cough, usually in the early hours of the morning (Ch. 14.2). Typically the condition is short-lived and there are no features to suggest an infective laryngo-tracheobronchitis such as fever or coryza. Approximately 50% of these children have an atopic disease. The condition is managed symptomatically and there is no evidence to suggest that measures such as allergen avoidance or symptomatic treatment with antihistamines are useful.

Immunodeficiency and its investigation

M. Wong

The child who 'is always sick' is a common scenario, creating concerns for parents and doctors about underlying immunodeficiency. Primary immunodeficiencies are rare but the genetic defects responsible are being increasingly identified. Susceptibility to infection varies and is influenced by age, genetic and environmental factors, including atopy, siblings, day care, exposure to cigarette smoke and anatomical variations.

The aim of this section is to provide an approach for differentiating primary immunodeficiency from other factors predisposing to real or apparent increased risk of infection, based on history, examination and appropriate investigation.

Host factors and resistance to infection

Immune defence is provided by multiple components, which can be categorized as two main groups.

- *Innate, non-antigen-specific mechanisms*:
  - barriers: epithelial surfaces, mucosal barriers
  - secretions: saliva, respiratory secretions, tears, urine
  - normal microbial flora: gastrointestinal, genital tract
  - phagocytic cells: neutrophils, macrophages
  - natural killer cells
  - proteins: complement, mannose-binding lectin, antimicrobial peptides
- *Adaptive, antigen-specific immune responses*: these are the basis of immunological memory and are essential for maturation of protective immune responses and efficacy of vaccination. The components are:
  - T cells
  - B cells and antibody.

Deficiencies or disruption of any of these components can predispose to infection. These defects may be the result of immaturity, primary or acquired deficiency, influencing age and severity of presentation as well as management and prognosis. Some defects will result in localized disease while others predispose to infection with specific microorganisms, as shown in Figure 13.2.1.

The influence of atopy

When recurrent respiratory infections are the sole infectious manifestation, allergy must be considered. Distinguishing features that suggest an allergic or atopic disorder rather than infection include absence of fever, clear, non-purulent discharge, personal and/or family history of atopic conditions such as eczema, food allergies, asthma and allergic rhinitis, seasonal or exposure related pattern, variable response to antibiotics and good response to antihistamines, bronchodilators and/or topical steroids. In addition, atopic tendencies can prolong and adversely modify the severity of otherwise minor, often viral, infections for which antibiotics may be prescribed, contributing to the perception of frequent severe infection.

Acquisition of immunological memory

The adaptive immune response develops with recurrent exposure to infection. Primary exposure often results in clinically evident infection and occurs most frequently in infancy and early childhood. Secondary exposure in the presence of an intact adaptive immune system results in a more rapid and efficient response, and avoidance of subsequent infection and clinical symptoms in older children and adults. In association with increasing exposure, this results in the peak number of infections between the ages of 2 and 4 years of life, with an average of six infections a year. Existence of siblings, day care attendance and exposure to cigarette smoke further increases this number.

Age of onset of infective complications and diagnosis

Deficiencies of humoral immunity present in the second half of the first year of life, when maternally derived antibody has waned. Significant deficiencies of T-cell function present within the first few months of life. Many primary immunodeficiencies present in infancy with dermatological manifestations such as severe or atypical eczema, thrombocytopenic purpura, recalcitrant candidiasis and abscesses, or are diagnosed in association with other conditions

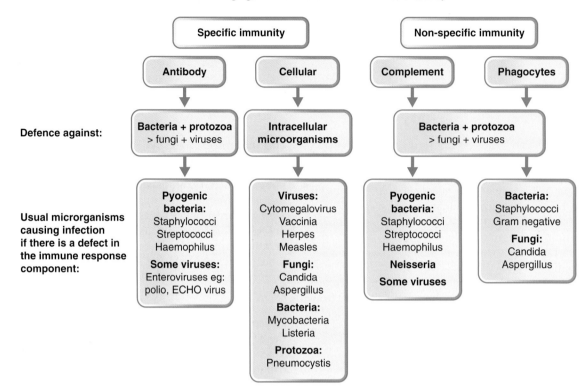

Common infecting agents associated with immunodeficiency

Specific immunity		Non-specific immunity	
Antibody	**Cellular**	**Complement**	**Phagocytes**

Defence against:

| **Bacteria + protozoa** > fungi + viruses | **Intracellular microorganisms** | **Bacteria + protozoa** > fungi + viruses | |

Usual microrganisms causing infection if there is a defect in the immune response component:

| **Pyogenic bacteria:** Staphylococci Streptococci Haemophilus **Some viruses:** Enteroviruses eg: polio, ECHO virus | **Viruses:** Cytomegalovirus Vaccinia Herpes Measles **Fungi:** Candida Aspergillus **Bacteria:** Mycobacteria Listeria **Protozoa:** Pneumocystis | **Pyogenic bacteria:** Staphylococci Streptococci Haemophilus **Neisseria** **Some viruses** | **Bacteria:** Staphylococci Gram negative **Fungi:** Candida Aspergillus |

Fig. 13.2.1 Common infecting agents associated with immunodeficiency.

such as cardiac, endocrine and neurological anomalies, such as DiGeorge syndrome and ataxia telangectasia.

Defects associated with prematurity and delays in immunological development

In the absence of intrauterine infection, the fetus exists in a sterile environment until birth, at which time specific immune responses begin to develop. Active transplacental transport of IgG (but not IgA, IgM or IgE) occurs during the third trimester, providing humoral protection to the newborn.

Physiological hypogammaglobulinaemia of infancy occurs between 3 and 6 months of life as the nadir of waning maternal IgG is balanced by increasing infant production of IgG (Fig. 13.2.2). This can be accentuated and prolonged in premature infants because of a reduced store of maternally derived IgG. In other infants, there may sometimes be a delay in IgG production, this being termed transient hypogammaglobulinaemia of infancy.

In most cases, these measurable abnormalities are asymptomatic and resolve completely, usually by

Clinical example

Thomas presented at 12 months of age with a history of six episodes of otitis media associated with a green nasal discharge since the age of 6 months. Each episode of infection responded to antibiotics but there was recurrence soon after cessation. There was a discharge from the left ear on two occasions, from which *Streptococcus pneumoniae* and non-typeable *Haemophilus influenzae* were isolated. Thomas was thriving and had no other symptoms. He was an only child, his immunizations were up to date and there was no significant family history.

Examination revealed a perforated left tympanic membrane. Tonsillar tissue was present. A full blood count was unremarkable. Serum IgG (2.5 g/l; normal 3.41–11.62 g/l) and IgA (0.1 g/l; normal 0.15–1.24 g/l) were moderately reduced but Thomas's serum IgM concentration was normal for age. Both IgG1 and IgG2 were slightly below the normal range. T and B cell numbers were normal. Levels of antibodies to vaccine antigens (tetanus, diphtheria and conjugated *H. influenzae* b and pneumococcal vaccines) were acceptable.

A provisional diagnosis of transient hypogammaglobulinaemia of infancy was made. A trial of prophylactic daily low-dose co-trimoxazole successfully prevented further recurrences of ear infection, until an attempt to cease therapy after a year. Antibiotic prophylaxis was ceased uneventfully at 3 years of age. Serum IgG and IgA concentrations gradually rose into the lower end of the normal range by the age of 2 and 5 years respectively.

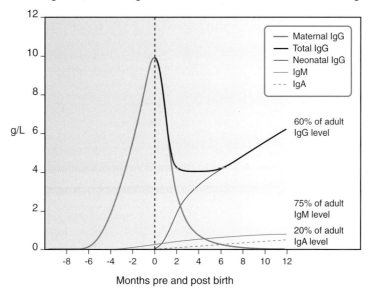

Evolution of serum IgG, IgA and IgM levels in utero and during the first year following birth, illustrating the contribution of maternal and neonatal IgG

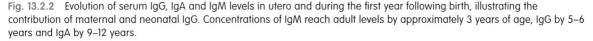

Fig. 13.2.2 Evolution of serum IgG, IgA and IgM levels in utero and during the first year following birth, illustrating the contribution of maternal and neonatal IgG. Concentrations of IgM reach adult levels by approximately 3 years of age, IgG by 5–6 years and IgA by 9–12 years.

9–15 months of age. However, in some cases, low IgG concentrations may persist until 5 years of age. Rarely, immunoglobulin replacement therapy is required in affected infants experiencing significant infections despite prophylactic antibiotics such as co-trimoxazole. If commenced, a trial of cessation of intravenous immunoglobulin (IVIG) should be undertaken after a period free of significant infection. A small number of these children continue to have immune abnormalities and continue to depend on IVIG, the diagnosis evolving to one of common variable immunodeficiency (CVID). This diagnosis cannot be made definitively before the age of 2 years.

T-cell-independent responses, such as to polysaccharide antigens, which are important for humoral protection from encapsulated microorganisms such as the pneumococcus, *Haemophilus* spp. and the meningococcus, are poor in infants less than 2 years of age. Protein-conjugated vaccines induce T-cell-dependent antibody production in younger infants, enabling immunization from 2 months of age (Ch. 3.5).

Maturational delay of T-cell-independent antibody responses may prolong susceptibility to infections (particularly sinopulmonary infections) with encapsulated bacteria, even in the presence of quantitatively 'normal' levels of IgG, IgA and IgM. This is termed specific antibody deficiency (SAD) in children over the age of 2 years. Approach to management of these children, like those with probable transient hypogammaglobulinaemia, includes ready access to antibiotic therapy, trials of antibiotic prophylaxis and in a small subset, IVIG with periodic reassessment of ongoing requirement.

Neonates have relatively low levels of complement and impairment of neutrophil chemotaxis, both of which rapidly mature during early infancy. T-cell proliferative responses are reasonable but cytokine production, particularly of proinflammatory (Th1) cytokines such as interferon-gamma, is immature, which may compromise T cell help. Although generally maturing during the first couple of years, this pattern may persist in infants with an atopic tendency.

Primary and secondary immunodeficiency disorders

More than 100 primary immunodeficiency disorders have been identified and characterized. An expert international committee of the International Union of Immunological Societies (IUIS) meets regularly to continually update the known primary immunodeficiencies and, where identified, the underlying genetic cause. The most recent publication by Bonilla et al in 2005 is shown in Table 13.2.1. More detailed tables summarizing clinical features and laboratory findings were published by Notarangelo et al in 2004 (see Further reading).

Table 13.2.1   Classification of primary immunodeficiencies

Disease	Gene	Disease	Gene
Humoral immunodeficiency		**Combined immunodeficiency**	
Known genetic basis		MHC class II gene transcription complex	
X-linked (Bruton) agammaglobulinaemia		CIITA (complementation group A)	MHC2TA
Bruton tyrosine kinase	BTK	RFXANK (complementation group B)	RFXANK
Autosomal recessive agammaglobulinaemia		RFX5 (complementation group C)	RFX5
IgM heavy chain	IGHM	RFXAP (complementation group D)	RFXAP
Igα	CD79A	MHC class I	
Surrogate light chain	CD179B	Transporters of antigenic peptides 1 and 2	TAP1, TAP2
B-cell linker protein	BLNK	TAP-binding protein (tapasin)	TAPBP
Leucine-rich repeat containing 8	LRRC8	CD3 complex components	
Autosomal recessive hyper-IgM syndrome		CD3δ	CD3D
Activation-induced cytidine deaminase	AICDA	CD3ε	CD3E
Uracil-DNA glycosylase	UNG	CD3γ	CD3G
Late-onset hypogammaglobulinaemia		ζ associated protein of 70 kDa	ZAP:70
Inducible T-cell costimulator	ICOS	CD45	PTPRC
Immunodeficiency, centromeric instability,		Adenosine deaminase	ADA
and facial anomalies syndrome		Purine nucleoside phosphorylase	NP
DNA methyltransferase 3B	DNMT3B	Wiskott-Aldrich syndrome	
Unknown genetic basis		Wiskott-Aldrich syndrome protein	WASP
Common variable immunodeficiency		Ataxia telangectasia and related disorders	
Selective IgA deficiency		Ataxia telangectasia mutated	ATM
IgG subclass deficiency		Ataxia telangectasia related disorder	HMRE11
Specific antibody deficiency		Nijmegen breakage syndrome	NBS1
Transient hypogammaglobulinaemia of		DNA ligase iV	LIG4
infancy		DNA ligase I	LIG1
Hypogammaglobulinaemia, unspecified		DiGeorge syndrome	22q11 del
Cellular immunodeficiency			(TBX-1)
Known genetic basis			10p13 del
Defects of the IL12/IFN-γ axis			other
IFN-γ receptor α chain	IFNGR1	Hyper-IgM syndrome	
IFN-γ receptor β chain	IFNGR2	Tumour necrosis factor superfamily	TNFSF5
IL-12 p40	IL12B	member 5 (CD40L, CD154)	
IL-12 receptor β1 chain	IL12RB1	Tumour necrosis factor receptor	TNFRSF5
Signal transducer & activator of	STAT1	superfamily member 5 (CD40)	
transcription 1		X-linked lymphoproliferative syndrome	
Chronic mucocutaneous candidiasis		SH2D1A/SLAM-associated protein (SAP)	SH2D1A
Autoimmune regulator	AIRE	Warts, hypogammaglobulinaemia, infections	
CD16 deficiency	FCGR3A	and myelokathexis syndrome	
Unknown genetic basis		CXC chemokine receptor 4	CXCR4
Idiopathic CD4+ T lymphocytopenia		Defects of NF-κB regulation	
Chronic mucocutaneous candidiasis due to		IκB kinase γ chain (IKKγ) or NF-κB essential	IKBKG
unknown defect		modifier (NEMO)	
Natural killer cell deficiency due to unknown		IκBα chain	IKBA
defect		Defects of Toll-like receptor signalling	
Cellular immunodeficiency, unspecified		IL-1 receptor-associated kinase 4	IRAK4
Combined immunodeficiency		Caspase 8 deficiency	CASP8
Known genetic basis		Unknown genetic basis	
Severe combined immunodeficiency		Severe combined immunodeficiency with	
X-linked SCID		unknown defect	
Cytokine receptor common γ chain (γc)	IL2RG	Combined immunodeficiency with unknown	
Janus kinase 3	JAK3	defect	
IL-7 receptor α chain (CD127)	IL7RA	**Phagocytic cell disorders**	
IL-2 receptor α chain (CD25)	IL2RA	Known genetic basis	
Recombinase activating genes 1 and 2	RAG1,RAG2	Chronic granulomatous disease	
(includes Omenn syndrome)		X-linked due to mutation of gp91phox	CYBB
Artemis	DCCRE1C	(cytochrome b₅₅₈ β chain)	

Table 13.2.1 Classification of primary immunodeficiencies

Disease	Gene	Disease	Gene
Phagocytic cell disorders		**Complement deficiencies**	
Autosomal recessive		C1	
P22^{phox} (cytochrome b$_{558}$ α chain)	CYBA	C1q	
P47^{phox}	NCF1	C1q β chain	C1QB
P67^{phox}	NCF2	C1q γ chain	C1QG
Chediak-Higashi syndrome		C1r	C1R
Lysosomal transporter	LYST	C2	C2
Griscelli syndrome	RAB27A	C3	C3
Hermansky-Pudlak syndrome type 2	AP3B1	C4	C4A, C4B
Leukocyte adhesion deficiency		C5	C5
Type 1, CD18 (integrin β2)	ITGB2	C6	C6
Type 2, GDP-fucose transporter 1	FLJ11320	C7	C7
Neutrophil specific granule deficiency		C8	
Transcription factor C/EBPε	CEBPE	C8α	C8A
Congenital cyclic or chronic neutropenia		C8β	C8B
(Kostmann syndrome)		C9	C9
Elastase 2 deficiency	ELA2	Factor D	DF
X-liked neutropenia due to WASP mutation	WASP	Factor H	HF1
Unknown genetic basis		Factor I	IF
Hyper-IgE syndrome		Properdin	PFC
		Mannose binding lectin-associated protease 2	MASP2

Table 13.2.2 Warning signs of primary immunodeficiency

Patients are advised to seek medical review if affected by two or more of the following ten warning signs of primary immunodeficiency (Jeffrey Modell Foundation, New York):

1. Eight or more new ear infections within 1 year
2. Two or more serious sinus infections within 1 year
3. 2 or more months on antibiotics with little effect
4. Two or more pneumonias within 1 year
5. Failure of an infant to gain weight or grow normally
6. Recurrent, deep skin or organ abscesses
7. Persistent thrush in the mouth or on the skin, after age 1 year
8. Need for intravenous antibiotics to clear infections
9. Two or more deep seated infections such as meningitis, osteomyelitis, cellulitis or sepsis
10. A family history of primary immunodeficiency

to be amenable to gene therapy. Gene therapy for X-linked severe combined immunodeficiency has been the most successful to date, but remains experimental in view of ongoing safety and technical concerns.

Secondary immunodeficiency, usually as a result of suppression, reduced production or loss of components of the immune system, is much more common. Important causes, listed in Table 13.2.3, include prematurity, metabolic diseases, infiltrative diseases and their treatment, malnutrition, infection, trauma, immunosuppressive therapy and ageing.

The necessity to consider a primary immunodeficiency disorder may be indicated by the frequency, severity and type of infections, the response or lack of response to antimicrobial therapy, associated failure to thrive and the existence of a significant family history (Table 13.2.2). Some primary immunodeficiency disorders have been shown

Practical points

- Recurrent infections are common in early childhood
- Resistance to infection is provided by non-specific mechanisms and through the adaptive immune response
- A small number of children with recurrent infections will have a primary immunodeficiency disorder
- Some components of the immune response are immature at birth
- A blood count, blood film and measurement of serum immunoglobulin concentrations can be a useful screen for primary immunodeficiency disorders

Table 13.2.3 Secondary immunodeficiency
Premature and newborn infants
Hereditary and metabolic diseases • Chromosomal abnormalities (e.g. Down) • Uraemia • Diabetes mellitus • Malnutrition • Vitamin and mineral deficiencies • Protein losing enteropathies • Nephrotic syndrome • Myotonic dystrophy • Sickle cell disease
Immunosuppressive agents • Radiation • Immunosuppressive drugs • Corticosteroids • Antilymphocyte or antithymocyte globulin • Anti-T-cell or anti-B-cell monoclonal antibodies
Surgery and trauma • Burns • Splenectomy • Anaesthesia • Head injury
Infectious diseases • Congenital rubella • Viral exanthema – measles, varicella • HIV infection, AIDS • Cytomegalovirus • Infectious mononucleosis • Bacterial infections • Mycobacterial, fungal or parasitic diseases
Infiltrative and haematological diseases • Histiocytosis • Sarcoidosis • Hodgkin disease and lymphoma • Leukaemia • Myeloma • Agranulocytosis and aplastic anaemia • Lymphoma in immunocompromised transplant recipients
Miscellaneous • Lupus erythematosus • Chronic active hepatitis • Alcoholic cirrhosis • Ageing

Investigations

In most registries of primary immunodeficiency, disorders that are primarily antibody deficiencies account for 50%, combined antibody and cellular deficiencies for 20%, disorders of phagocytic cells for 18%, primarily cellular deficiencies for 10% and complement defects for 2% of all reported cases.

Since 70% of primary immunodeficiencies affect humoral immune responses, screening of antibody concentrations will detect a large proportion of cases. A blood count and examination of the blood film will identify patients with asplenia, neutropenia, neutrophil granule abnormalities and thrombocytopenia associated with small platelet size, the latter features being pathognomonic of Wiskott–Aldrich syndrome.

Second tier investigations (Table 13.2.4), some of which are available only from specialized laboratories, will depend on clinical suspicion of either humoral, cellular, phagocytic or complement abnormalities. Genetic testing may be available to confirm some primary immunodeficiency disorders and/or may be used for genetic counselling and future prenatal testing.

Consideration of age-related reference ranges is essential for interpretation of serum immunoglobulin concentrations (particularly IgG subclass concentrations), lymphocyte numbers and subset analyses. However, there is significant variability in the rate of rise in these values as well as biological fluctuations over time. The division of age groups for each reference range is arbitrary, such that values for children at the boundaries of age groups may be interpreted erroneously. This may not be obvious to the requesting clinician, since reference ranges are usually reported without information regarding the actual age range or the reference range of adjacent age groups. Thus normal screening tests, particularly at the lower end of the reference range, in the presence of a suspicious clinical picture, should not prevent specialist referral.

Treatment

Management will depend on the diagnosis but may include:

• awareness of the types of infection most likely to be associated with a particular primary immunodeficiency disorder
• early appropriate antibiotic treatment
• prophylactic therapy: e.g. co-trimoxazole for chronic granulomatous disease (CGD) and severe combined immunodeficiency (SCID), antifungals for CGD and mucocutaneous candidiasis (MCC), γ-interferon for CGD
• awareness and management of autoimmune and atopic disease complications: e.g. in common variable immunodeficiency (CVID) and Wiskott–Aldrich syndrome (WAS)
• immunoglobulin replacement therapy, usually as a monthly intravenous infusion in hospital, but increasingly via subcutaneous infusion at home

Table 13.2.4   Investigations for immunodeficiency

Test	Suspected deficiency
Screening	
Blood count and film	
Immunoglobulin G, A and M levels	
Second tier dependent on clinical suspicions	
Immunoglobulin G subclass titres (IgG 1, 2, 3, 4)	H, Comb
Immunoglobulin E	H, Comb, N
Isohaemagglutinins	H, Comb
Specific antibody titres	H, Comb
– after routine vaccinations – tetanus, diphtheria, Hib, pneumococcal	
– after pneumococcal polysaccharide vaccine – non-conjugate vaccine serotypes	
Lymphocyte subsets (T, B and natural killer (NK) cell)	H, C, Comb
Check chest X-ray for thymus (neonates and young infants)	C, Comb
Lymphocyte proliferation to mitogen e.g.: PHA, Con A (non-specific)	C, Comb
Lymphocyte proliferation to specific antigen e.g.: candida	C, Comb
Adenosine deaminase and purine nucleotide phosphorylase measurements	C, Comb
Neutrophil function testing	N
– nitroblue tetrozolium (NBT)/equivalent dihydro-rhodamine (DHR)-based assay	
– more extensive testing of chemiluminescence, chemotaxis	
– surface expression of CD11 and CD18	
NK cell cytotoxicity	NK
Complement testing	Complement
C3, C4, CH50 (AH50, specific complement components)	
C1 esterase inhibitor and function	C1INH
HIV testing	C, Comb
Genetic studies	

H: humoral, Comb: conbined; C: cellular; N: neutrophil; NK: natural killer cell; C1INH: C1 esterase inhibitor.

- bone marrow transplantation: e.g. in SCID, WAS
- gene therapy, although this is still considered to be experimental, even for X-SCID
- avoidance of live vaccines where a T-cell defect is suspected, and live polio vaccination in hypogammaglobulinaemia. Routine immunization is unnecessary when receiving immunoglobulin replacement therapy and any potential response may be inhibited.

Specific primary immunodeficiency disorders

Examples of some important primary immunodeficiency disorders are provided as follows.

Humoral immunodeficiency disorders

X-linked agammaglobulinaemia

Affected boys have a defect in the *BTK* (Bruton tyrosine kinase) gene on the X chromosome. The gene product, Btk, has a major role in activated B-cell receptor signalling and is required for normal B-cell development. In X-linked agammaglobulinaemia (XLA), precursor cells in the marrow fail to develop into mature circulating B cells. Absence of peripheral mature B cells is also a feature of several rarer autosomal recessive forms of early onset hypogammaglobulinaemia with clinical features similar to XLA but also affecting girls (Table 13.2.1).

Most boys with XLA are asymptomatic for the first 4–6 months of life. Nearly all develop symptoms by 18 months of age and the diagnosis is usually made within the first 3 years of life. The commonest manifestations are recurrent mucopurulent otitis media, upper and lower respiratory tract infections with common respiratory tract organisms (in particular *Streptococcus pneumoniae* and *Haemophilus influenzae* b, despite vaccination), and *Staphylococcus aureus* infections. Resolution is often slow and incomplete, eventually leading to bronchiectasis in the absence of intervention. Meningitis, septicaemia, diarrhoea, aseptic mono- or oligoarticular arthritis, septic arthritis, osteomyelitis, chronic or recurrent conjunctivitis and chronic or disseminated enteroviral infections occur more frequently.

The most useful clinical feature is absent or markedly hypoplastic tonsils and lymph nodes. Serum IgG concentrations are markedly reduced and IgA and IgM are undetectable. Circulating B cells are absent and there are no functional/specific antibody responses to immunization antigens such as tetanus and diphtheria.

Absent Btk expression can be demonstrated on flow cytometry and *BTK* mutations are found on genetic testing, both of which can also be useful for detection of female carrier status. If prenatal diagnosis is not undertaken, newborn males with a family history can be screened non-invasively for absent cord blood B cells. Early diagnosis allows institution of therapy before the development of infective complications.

Early commencement of lifelong immunoglobulin replacement therapy will minimize complications, significantly reducing the incidence of chronic lung disease and prolonging life expectancy. However, since these infusions replace only IgG, recurrent conjunctivitis and diarrhoea may not be eliminated because secretory IgA function is not restored. The usual dose of intravenous immunoglobulin (IVIG) is 400 mg/kg every 4 weeks but the dose administered needs to be varied to maintain adequate trough IgG levels and to prevent infection. The interval for administration of IVIG is based on the half life of IgG in normal individuals of between 21 and 28 days. Home administration by more frequent subcutaneous infusions is an alternative form of administration of immunoglobulin replacement therapy.

Specific infections are treated with appropriate antibiotics. Prophylactic antibiotics are not generally required.

Common variable immunodeficiency

The term common variable immunodeficiency (CVID) is used for a heterogeneous group of disorders that are due either to an intrinsic B-cell defect or to B-cell dysfunction secondary to abnormal T cell–B cell interaction. Underlying genetic defects are being now being identified, some of which are shared by other well defined immunodeficiencies such as mutations in genes for Btk in XLA, CD40 ligand in hyper-IgM syndrome and SLAM-associated protein (SAP) in X-linked lymphoproliferative disease. The majority of patients with CVID have no family history of related disease, although in 10–20% there may be a relative with selective IgA deficiency.

CVID is an acquired hypogammaglobulinemia, with onset usually in the second and third decades of life. However, the presentation may sometimes be in childhood and the symptoms may be more insidious. The spectrum of respiratory infections is similar to that observed in XLA. Uncommonly, pneumonia has been associated with *Pseudomonas aeruginosa* or *Pneumocystis jiroveci* (formerly *carinii*). Occasionally, lymphoid interstitial pneumonitis develops, presenting with cough, dyspnoea, weight loss and an interstitial infiltrate, causing a restrictive lung disease pattern. Diarrhoea due to *Campylobacter jejuni* and *Giardia lamblia* is common. Other manifestations include hepatosplenomegaly, autoimmune haemolytic anaemia, thrombocytopenia, neutropenia and thrombocytopenia, non-caseating granulomas of lungs, spleen, skin and liver, and atypical lymphoid hyperplasia. The incidence of lymphoma is increased in patients with CVID.

The diagnosis of CVID depends on excluding other well-defined syndromes. There are reduced serum IgG concentrations (although the values are usually higher than in XLA) and usually significantly reduced IgA and IgM concentrations. There are defective specific antibody responses. T- and B-cell numbers are variable, as are T-cell proliferative responses. A diagnosis of CVID cannot be made in children less than 2 years of age, although a small number of children followed with presumed transient hypogammaglobulinaemia, selective antibody, IgA or IgG subclass deficiency may subsequently develop definitive features of CVID.

Treatment consists of IVIG replacement therapy and appropriate antibiotic treatment of specific infections. Autoimmune phenomena may need corticosteroid therapy and in those considered at risk of *Pneumocystis* infection, co-trimoxazole prophylaxis should be considered.

Selective IgA deficiency

Selective IgA deficiency is defined as a serum IgA concentration of less than 0.05–0.07 g/l (the lower limit of detection of most commercial assays), with normal IgG and IgM levels. This probably occurs secondary to impaired switching from IgM to IgA production. No specific underlying genetic defect has been identified and there is usually no family history. It is the commonest primary immunodeficiency, with a reported prevalence ranging from 1:200–1:1000 in the normal population. Most individuals with selective IgA deficiency are asymptomatic but there is an increased incidence of recurrent infections, particularly bronchitis and otitis media. More severe suppurative sinopulmonary disease is less common and is often associated with IgG2 subclass deficiency. Secretory IgM is thought to compensate for IgA deficiency in asymptomatic individuals.

Serum IgA concentrations are low in normal infants, eventually reaching adult concentrations by 9–12 years of age. IgA deficiency may be transient, reflecting a maturational delay. The detection of salivary IgA may help distinguish this group, as salivary IgA concentrations reach normal adult levels by 6 months of age. The clinical significance of detectable serum IgA, but at a level below the normal reference limit, is uncertain but in most it is likely to eventually increase to the normal range. Infants and children with transient IgA deficiency seem unlikely to be predisposed to an increased frequency or severity of infections.

IgA deficiency is associated with an increased incidence of autoimmune diseases, allergic disorders and malignancy. Acute reactions, including anaphylaxis, to residual IgA in blood transfusions and intravenous immunoglobulin can occur due to the development of anti-IgA antibodies.

IgG subclass deficiency and specific antibody deficiency

There are four subclasses of IgG. These subclasses are named IgG1, 2, 3 and 4. They contribute varying proportions of the total IgG concentration (IgG1 65%, IgG2 25%, IgG3 7%, IgG4 < 5%). Antibody responses to peptides are predominantly IgG1 and IgG3, while responses to polysaccharides are predominantly IgG2, but with an IgG1 component also. Deficiency may occur in one or more subclasses. However, the diagnosis is hampered by technical issues in relation to measurement of IgG subclass concentrations, and difficulties in establishment of age-related normal ranges.

There is a poor correlation between the diagnosis of IgG subclass deficiency and susceptibility to infection. The functional activity of antibody is of more relevance, particularly specific antibody responses to polysaccharide antigens, such as unconjugated pneumococcal vaccine in children more than 2 years of age.

Defective antibody responses can be associated with IgG subclass deficiency, particularly IgG2 subclass deficiency. However, there may be quantitatively normal IgG and IgG subclass concentrations in specific antibody deficiency. A response to conjugated vaccine may be of therapeutic benefit but does not negate the diagnosis.

Clinical features of IgG subclass deficiency and of specific antibody deficiency include chronic otitis media with discharge, bronchitis and sinusitis. Presentation of symptomatic disease is usually in the first 7 years of life.

Management of symptomatic children with defective antibody responses with or without IgG subclass deficiency includes ready access to antibiotic therapy, a trial of antibiotic prophylaxis and, in a small subset, intravenous immunoglobulin therapy with periodic reassessment of ongoing requirement. In many, the defect will resolve with age, whilst in a smaller proportion, the defect is permanent or evolves into CVID.

T-cell immunodeficiency disorders

Chronic mucocutaneous candidiasis

Chronic mucocutaneous candidiasis is characterized by persistent or recurrent *Candida* infections of the skin, mucous membrane and nails. In most, isolated defects in cell-mediated immunity to *Candida* can be demonstrated by delayed hypersensitivity skin tests or in vitro techniques. There are several distinct clinical syndromes. The autosomal recessive form, secondary to mutations in the *AIRE* gene, is associated with autoimmune polyendocrinopathies (APECED), which may present at any age. Long-term oral antifungal therapy is usually required to prevent recurrence.

Defects of the interleukin 12/interferon-gamma axis

A number of gene defects of the interleukin 12 (IL12)/interferon gamma (IFNγ) axis have been identified (Table 13.2.1), which appear to predispose affected individuals to atypical mycobacterial and salmonella infections.

Combined immunodeficiency disorders

Severe combined immunodeficiency

The term severe combined immunodeficiency (SCID) encompasses a heterogeneous group of conditions associated with a profound deficiency of both T- and B-cell function. The genetic basis of these disorders is being increasingly identified (Table 13.2.1). X-linked SCID secondary to a mutation in the common gamma chain of the IL2 receptor accounts for over half of all cases. Autosomal recessive forms include defects of recombinase activating genes (*RAG1* and *RAG2*), signalling components after T-cell receptor activation such as ZAP-70 and Jak3, and enzymes essential for lymphocyte metabolism such as adenosine deaminase (ADA) and purine nucleoside phosphorylase (PNP).

Severe combined immunodeficiency usually presents within the first 6 months of life. Diarrhoea, lower respiratory tract infections, failure to thrive, candidiasis and rash are common. *Pneumocystis* pneumonia is common and its occurrence in an infant or child should always prompt investigation to exclude SCID. Pneumonia due to *Pneumocystis* is often insidious in onset, with cough and pulmonary infiltrates that progress over several weeks (Fig. 13.2.3). Children with SCID have a severe susceptibility to bacterial, viral and fungal infection. Without marrow transplantation, death usually occurs within the first 2 years of life.

Clinical example

Daniel presented to the emergency department of his local hospital at 4 months of age with a 2-week history of increasing cough and respiratory distress. He also had persistent oral and napkin area thrush associated with chronic loose stools, irritability and poor weight gain during the preceding 2 months. He had received his routine vaccinations at 2 months of age. There was no known family history of immunodeficiency.

On physical examination, Daniel had evidence of failure to thrive, with reduced subcutaneous fat. His weight was significantly below the 3rd percentile for his age. Lymph nodes were not palpable and no tonsils were seen. He was tachypnoeic and there was generally reduced air entry. Chest X-ray revealed hyperinflated lung lungs with a diffuse interstitial infiltrate. There was no thymic shadow visible on the chest X-ray.

Daniel was found to be lymphopenic (0.2×10^9/l) on full blood count. The serum IgG was very low (0.4 g/l; normal 1.63–7.78 g/l) and IgA was undetectable The serum IgM concentration was mildly reduced (0.26 g/l; normal 0.33–1.05 g/l). Isohaemagglutinins were not detected. Analysis of lymphocyte subsets demonstrated an absence of T and natural killer cells but some B cells were present. There were no detectable antibodies to the routine immunizations that had been given at age 2 months and no T-cell proliferative response to the mitogen phytohaemagglutinin (PHA). Stool culture detected vaccine-associated poliovirus. *Pneumocystis* was isolated from bronchoalveolar lavage sampling.

The diagnosis of X-linked severe combined immunodeficiency was made. Daniel commenced treatment with high-dose intravenous co-trimoxazole and steroids for the *Pneumocystis* pneumonia and replacement monthly intravenous immunoglobulin. On recovery from his respiratory illness, his co-trimoxazole was reduced to a prophylactic dose to prevent recurrence of *Pneumocystis* infection. He underwent a successful HLA-matched unrelated bone marrow transplant from cord blood 3 months later, having no suitably HLA-matched relatives. Daniel is now well, with no detectable immune abnormality.

Genetic testing confirmed the diagnosis of X-SCID and Daniel's mother's carrier status. This enabled prenatal diagnosis in subsequent pregnancies.

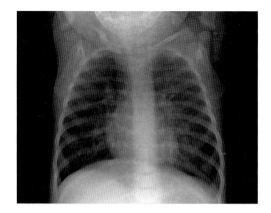

Fig. 13.2.3 Chest X-ray of a 6-month-old child with *Pneumocystis* pneumonia associated with severe combined immunodeficiency. The mediastinum is narrowed by absence of the thymic shadow. The lungs are hyperinflated and there is bilateral diffuse pulmonary infiltrate.

Pneumocystis infection. Live viral vaccines should be avoided and blood products need to be irradiated to prevent graft versus host disease from transferred T cells. Definitive therapy is bone marrow transplantation. Early transplantation from an HLA-identical sibling has a success rate of over 90%; the success rate is lower with matched unrelated donors. ADA deficiency can be treated with ADA replacement. Patients with X-SCID have been treated successfully with gene therapy, but this remains experimental due to technical and safety concerns.

Hyper-IgM syndrome

Most cases of hyper-IgM syndrome (HIM) are X linked and are characterized by defective B-cell switching from IgM to IgG and IgA production. There are abnormalities of T-cell function due to mutations in the CD40 ligand gene. An autosomal recessive form, secondary to mutations in the CD40 gene, has similar clinical features, while there is no T-cell dysfunction in the three other known recessive forms.

The spectrum of respiratory infections is similar to that observed in XLA. However, *Pneumocystis* pneumonia is a frequent presentation. Intermittent or persistent neutropenia commonly causes oral and upper gastrointestinal tract ulceration. Haemolytic anaemia, thrombocytopenia, nephritis and arthritis also occur. Infection with *Cryptosporidium* is common and may lead to sclerosing cholangitis.

Serum IgA and IgG concentrations are low in HIM, with a normal or elevated IgM. B- and T-cell numbers are normal. Primary and secondary antibody responses are reduced and are limited to the

Immune abnormalities vary but usually include lymphopenia with markedly reduced T-cell numbers and reduced serum IgG, A and M concentrations. T-cell proliferative responses to mitogens are abnormal, and specific antibody responses, including isohaemagglutinins, are absent. Molecular diagnosis should be undertaken where available to aid genetic counselling and future prenatal diagnosis.

Supportive treatment involves protective isolation, specific antimicrobial therapy, intravenous immunoglobulin replacement and prophylaxis to prevent

IgM isotype. X-linked hyper-IgM syndrome can be confirmed by demonstration of absent CD40 ligand expression on activated T cells or by identification of mutations in the CD40 ligand gene.

Treatment consists of intravenous immunoglobulin replacement therapy, appropriate antibiotic treatment of specific infections and prophylaxis for *Pneumocystis* infection. Granulocyte–macrophage colony-stimulating factor (GM-CSF) may be required if neutropenia is severe. Measures to avoid cryptosporidial infection may prevent liver disease.

Wiskott–Aldrich syndrome

Wiskott–Aldrich syndrome is an X-linked condition that usually presents with refractory atopic dermatitis and thrombocytopenic purpura. Otitis media and pneumonia are common and are associated with defective antibody responses to polysaccharide antigens. There is a variable T-cell defect, and there is a risk of *Pneumocystis* infection. Serum IgA concentrations are usually high with low or normal IgG and IgM concentrations. There is a variable reduction in T-cell numbers and function that progressively worsen with age.

Platelets are typically small and this is a useful diagnostic feature. Definitive diagnosis can be made by demonstrating a mutation in the *WASP* gene.

Treatment consists of intravenous immunoglobulin for demonstrated antibody deficiency, appropriate antibiotic treatment of specific infections and prophylaxis for *Pneumocystis* infection. Life expectancy is reduced by infection, haemorrhage and a high incidence of malignancy, often B-cell lymphoma, in early adult life. Splenectomy can reduce the risk of life-threatening haemorrhage but increases the risk of serious infection with encapsulated organisms. Definitive treatment is by bone marrow transplantation.

Ataxia telangectasia

Ataxia telangiectasia is an autosomal recessive chromosomal breakage syndrome. Most cases present with ataxia in infancy or early childhood, then develop telangiectasia of the skin and bulbar conjunctivae associated with hyperpigmented and depigmented cutaneous patches.

The degree of immune dysfunction is variable. Suppurative sinopulmonary infections occur in half of patients. Aspiration may contribute to correlations between the severity of respiratory tract disease and the severity of neurological impairment. Pneumonia is a major cause of death. There is a high incidence of lymphoreticular malignancy. IgA deficiency is common and is often associated with IgG2 subclass deficiency. IgE is often absent. Defects in T-cell function and number are variable. Serum alpha-fetoprotein is raised in virtually all cases. Defects in DNA repair lead to an increased incidence of chromosome breaks. Infections should be treated early with appropriate antibiotics and intravenous immunoglobulin may be indicated if a significant antibody defect is present.

DiGeorge syndrome (velocardiofacial syndrome, Sprintzen syndrome)

DiGeorge syndrome is the result of interrupted embryonic development of the third and fourth pharyngeal pouches. Deletions of chromosome 22q11.2, detectable by fluorescent in situ hybridization (FISH) are found in over 85% of affected individuals, while deletions of chromosome 10p13–14 are found in a smaller number.

There is a great phenotypic variability but the syndrome is characterized by conotruncal cardiac defects (e.g. interrupted aortic arch or truncus arteriosus), symptomatic neonatal hypocalcaemia secondary to parathyroid hypoplasia, characteristic facies with palatal dysfunction leading to feeding difficulties and speech delay, behavioural and developmental problems and thymic absence or hypoplasia, resulting in T-cell-mediated immunodeficiency.

Complete absence of the thymus is rare, resulting in a SCID phenotype. Most patients have mild immune impairment. Susceptibility to otitis media and sinusitis is usually more a result of anatomical and functional airways compromise than of systemic immunodeficiency. The commonest finding is a mild reduction in total numbers of T cells (CD3), particularly of the CD4+ subset, which is usually of no clinical significance. Occasionally there is inadequacy of T-cell-regulated antibody production requiring antibody replacement therapy. Live vaccines should not be given until the degree of immune impairment is determined.

> ### Practical points
>
> - Primary immunodeficiency disorders may present with severe or unusual infections
> - Many of the primary immunodeficiency disorders are associated with specific gene mutations
> - Treatment of a primary immunodeficiency disorder depends on a specific diagnosis, treatment and prevention of a variety of infections, and therapies such as intravenous immunoglobulin and bone marrow transplantation
> - Demonstration of a specific genetic defect is important information for genetic counselling

Phagocytic cell disorders

Chronic granulomatous disease

This disorder is caused by a defect of one of the four subunits of phagocyte NADPH oxidase (phox). This enzyme complex is necessary to produce the respiratory burst that generates reactive oxygen intermediates, such as superoxide and hydrogen peroxide, that are used for killing of phagocytosed pathogens. The majority (60–70%) of cases of chronic granulomatous disease (CGD) are due to an X-linked mutation of the gp91^{phox} gene. The remaining cases are due to autosomal recessive mutations of p22^{phox}, p47^{phox} or p67^{phox}.

Failure to thrive, bacterial adenitis, and abscesses or osteomyelitis occur within the first year of life. Pneumonia and lymphadenitis due to catalase-positive organisms such as *Staphylococcus* and *Serratia*, or fungi such as *Candida* and *Aspergillus*, are the most common infections. Intestinal or urinary tract obstruction can be caused by granuloma formation. Gingivitis (Fig. 13.2.4), inflammatory bowel disease, hepatosplenomegaly and lymphadenopathy are other features.

The diagnosis is made by demonstrating absence of an oxidative burst in activated neutrophils on nitroblue tetrazolium (NBT) testing or an equivalent flow cytometric assay. These tests can detect female carriers of X-linked CGD but not autosomal recessive carriers. Chronic granulomatous disease can be confirmed on formal neutrophil function testing and/or by molecular testing.

Early diagnosis and co-trimoxazole prophylaxis has dramatically reduced the incidence of infections and has improved survival. Additional antifungal and/or IFN-γ prophylaxis is also beneficial. Development of invasive fungal infections is associated with poorer prognosis. Bone marrow transplantation is limited to patients with more severe disease, preferably where there is a related HLA-matched donor, and is associated with significant mortality. Promising results have been reported in preliminary trials of gene therapy.

Leukocyte adhesion deficiency (LAD) disorders

These rare conditions are secondary to abnormalities of cell-surface expression of proteins that are responsible for the adhesion, activation and movement of phagocytes out of blood vessels into areas of inflammation. The most common defect (LAD type II) is due to an autosomal recessive deficiency of β-integrins (CD18). Affected children suffer from recurrent severe infections and usually die in the first few years of life without bone marrow transplantation.

The characteristic features are delayed separation of the umbilical cord, a significantly elevated peripheral blood neutrophil count and a paucity of neutrophils in areas of infection. Diagnosis is confirmed by flow cytometry, which shows absence of CD18 and associated molecules (CD11a, CD11b and CD11c) on stimulated neutrophils.

Hyper-IgE syndrome

Hyper-IgE syndrome is characterized by recurrent infections, an eczematous or vesicular rash from infancy and markedly elevated serum IgE levels. There is progressive development of coarse facial features, osteopenia and skeletal abnormalities. Inheritance can be autosomal dominant, recessive or sporadic.

Subcutaneous cold abscesses and suppurative lower respiratory tract disease caused by *Staphylococcus*, *H. influenzae*, pneumococcus, *Candida* and *Pseudomonas* are common. Persistent pneumatoceles following infection occur in most patients. Extremely high IgE levels can be detected in infants with severe atopic dermatitis, which can be differentiated from hyper-IgE syndrome by the localization of infection to superficial skin and the distribution and characteristics of the rash. The immunological defect is unknown. There are variable defects in neutrophil chemotaxis. Some subjects have a defective functional antibody response to polysaccharide antigens.

Management consists of long-term antistaphylococcal antibiotic prophylaxis and appropriate treatment of acute infections. Surgical intervention may be required and intravenous immunoglobulin may reduce the incidence of infection if a functional antibody deficiency is demonstrated.

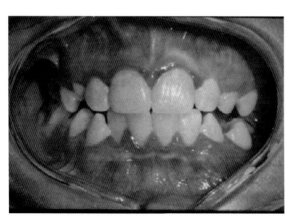

Fig. 13.2.4 Gingival inflammation secondary to infection in an individual with cyclic neutropenia. Symptoms included halitosis and bleeding gums with minor trauma.

Complement disorders

Deficiencies of early classical complement components are associated with an increased incidence of immune-complex-mediated autoimmune disease, particularly systemic lupus erythematosus (SLE). Patients with a deficiency of terminal complement components are at increased risk of recurrent neisserial infections, while deficiency of some components of the alternate pathway, e.g. properdin, predispose to overwhelming/fatal neisserial and pneumococcal infection. C3 deficiency predisposes to severe recurrent bacterial infection and there is a high mortality.

Integrity of the classical and alternate complement pathways is tested by the classical (CH50) and alternate (AH50) pathway haemolytic complement assays respectively. Although CH50 and the complement components C3 and C4 are readily available, AH50 and assays of other individual components are usually only available from specialized laboratories.

13.3 Arthritis and connective tissue disorders

K. J. Murray, D. M. Roberton

The term arthritis is used here to describe an inflammation of one or more joints of the body for some period of time. The term connective tissue disorder is used to describe an inflammatory process that may involve the joints but commonly involves other internal organs and non-organ-specific tissues or tissue components. The events that initiate and sustain the inflammation are unknown but research has revealed that complex genetic interactions with the environment are likely to lie at the heart of these and all autoimmune conditions.

Table 13.3.1 lists some of the important forms of arthritis and connective tissue disorders of childhood.

Pathology and laboratory findings

Common findings on investigation in a child with one of the arthritis or connective tissue disorders are:

- hypochromic microcytic anaemia
- elevated erythrocyte sedimentation rate (ESR) and C-reactive protein (CRP)
- autoantibodies, e.g. antinuclear antibody (ANA) or rheumatoid factor
- inflammatory synovial fluid (elevated white cell count and protein)
- histological evidence of chronic inflammation in tissues such as synovium, kidney, blood vessels or muscle.

Incidence

The chronic arthritis and connective tissue disorders in childhood are generally uncommon. The most common are the various forms of childhood chronic inflammatory arthritis or juvenile idiopathic arthritis (JIA). Most population studies suggest that chronic arthritis of childhood occurs at a rate of 1–5 new cases per year per 10 000 children under the age of 16 years. As these forms of arthritis have a duration of several years, there may be as many as 1 in every 1000 children with some form of persisting inflammatory arthritis, and mild forms may be even more common. Far more commonly seen in general are the mechanical disorders of growing pains or symptoms related to ligamentous laxity or hypermobility.

Other connective tissue disorders are much rarer. Systemic lupus erythematosus (SLE) is uncommon, but is seen more frequently in some ethnic groups, e.g. in those from some Asian countries, and it is more common in females. In Australia, SLE is up to four times more common in indigenous people than in those of Caucasian origin. Juvenile dermatomyositis and scleroderma are rare.

Arthritis in children

The term arthritis means inflammation in a joint. Symptoms of arthritis may include:

- pain in or around the joint
- warmth
- swelling
- occasionally erythema
- loss of function, particularly loss of range of movement
- stiffness, particularly early-morning.

The acute onset of inflammation in a joint in any child must be considered to be due to infection or trauma until proven otherwise. Infection may occur as a primary septic arthritis or as extension of infection into the joint space from a nearby osteomyelitis (Ch. 12.2). Infection in a joint may be seen also in association with other systemic infections. Staphylococcal infections probably overall remain the commonest. Meningococcal and *Haemophilus influenzae* type b meningitis may be followed by joint infection with these organisms, or by sterile effusions in joints. Trauma may be responsible for joint symptoms in association with a fracture, or disruption of soft tissue elements in or near to the joint. Inflammation in a joint may occur as a result of bleeding into the joint in haemophilia (Ch. 16.2), or rarely may be due to foreign body penetration.

Juvenile idiopathic (chronic) arthritis in children

Inflammation in a joint for which no infective or other cause is found, and which persists for more

Table 13.3.1 Chronic inflammatory arthritis and connective tissue disorders of childhood (including the new ILAR classification system for juvenile idiopathic arthritis)

- Juvenile idiopathic arthritis:
  - oligoarticular
  - extended oligoarticular
  - polyarticular rheumatoid-factor-negative
  - polyarticular rheumatoid-factor-positive (rheumatoid arthritis)
  - systemic arthritis
  - psoriatic arthritis
  - enthesitis-related arthritis
  - unclassified
- Systemic lupus erythematosus
- Juvenile dermatomyositis
- Scleroderma
- Overlap syndromes
- Primary vasculitis disorders

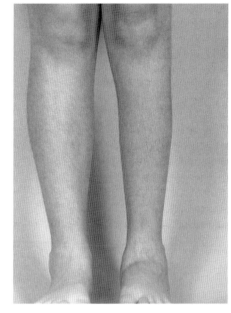

Fig. 13.3.1 8-year-old with oligoarthritis of both ankles and the right knee, with marked swelling of the left ankle and calf muscle wasting.

than 6 weeks, is known as juvenile arthritis. The point of this definition is that other forms of arthritis (largely acute reactive arthritis) will have been diagnosed and/or resolved during this time. Stiffness of joint movement, particularly in the mornings and after inactivity is common in inflammatory arthritis, and in most cases the involved joint will have visible swelling, be warm to touch and the joint will have some limitation of motion. By arbitrary definition JIA starts earlier than 16 years of age but in reality there is a continuum into adult years of several forms of JIA.

International efforts to harmonize the clinical classification of juvenile onset forms of chronic arthritis have led to a new classification which is widely recognized and clinically useful. This classification is under the heading juvenile idiopathic arthritis in Table 13.3.1.

Practically, however, there are three major clinical patterns of juvenile arthritis, which may evolve over time. The three major categories in order of prevalence are:

- oligoarthritis
- polyarthritis
- systemic arthritis.

Oligoarthritis

This is the most common form of JIA, accounting for over 60% of all cases. By definition, four or fewer joints are involved during the first 6 months after onset. Oligoarthritis is more common in early childhood, with onset being seen most often between the ages of 1 and 4 years. Girls are affected nearly twice as often as boys. Joint involvement is almost always asymmetrical. The joints affected most commonly are the knee joints, followed in frequency by the ankle (and subtalar) joints (Fig. 13.3.1), wrists and elbows. Onset usually is with pain, loss of function and swelling of the involved joint(s).

The diagnosis of oligoarthritis is initially one of exclusion. The child presenting with an acute monoarthritis must initially be evaluated carefully for infective or other causes (Ch. 12.2). Hip disease is rare in this early-onset form of oligoarthritis, and a child presenting with isolated hip involvement as the initial manifestation of an arthritis must be investigated carefully for disorders such as septic arthritis or osteomyelitis and, in the appropriate age groups, avascular necrosis of the femoral head (Perthes disease) and slipped femoral capital epiphysis (Ch. 8.1).

There is little or no systemic disturbance in oligoarthritis. Radiographs of involved joints show soft tissue swelling and sometimes effusions and widening of the joint space but erosions are not present. Epiphyseal overgrowth and lengthening of the involved limb is common as a result of the increased blood supply in the presence of chronic inflammation, particularly if untreated. Rheumatoid factor is not present but approximately 70% of all children with oligoarthritis have a positive serological test for ANA. This group is at higher risk of anterior uveitis (see below). Approximately 25% of patients with

Clinical example

Tianna was a 2-year-old girl who had 8 weeks of a painful left knee that was stiff in the mornings and became progressively more swollen. She had been admitted under orthopaedic care, had arthroscopic drainage of the knee joint and was being treated with antibiotics with little improvement in her knee. The synovial fluid showed over 20 000 white blood cells but was negative on culture. The histopathology report of a synovial biopsy stated that the synovium looked injected and thickened.

On further review by a paediatric rheumatologist it was noted that the knee had an effusion and synovial thickening and minor flexion deformity with significant quadriceps wasting. Tianna also had mild (asymptomatic) swelling of her left ankle. Investigations revealed an ESR of 41 and a positive antinuclear antibody titre of 1:160. Ophthalmology review revealed evidence of cells and flare in the anterior chamber of Tianna's left eye consistent with chronic iridocyclitis. Her diagnosis was juvenile idiopathic arthritis of the oligoarthritis type, and an associated uveitis.

Tianna was commenced on a non-steroidal anti-inflammatory agent but after mild improvement in 2 weeks it was elected to reaspirate and inject the knee and ankle with long-acting corticosteroid (triamcinolone). Within 3 weeks all signs of her arthritis had resolved and her range of motion was near normal after several sessions of physiotherapy. Her eye disease was treated with topical steroids and mydriatics for 6 weeks and responded rapidly, although it recurred several times during the next 2 years. Her arthritis recurred twice in the following few years, requiring further corticosteroid injections with further excellent response. By 10 years of age Tianna's arthritis and uveitis had been in remission off all treatment for over 2 years.

oligoarthritis will pursue a progressive course after the first 6 months, which is termed *extended oligoarthritis*.

Polyarthritis

Polyarthritis accounts for about 25% of all JIA cases. By definition, five or more joints are involved in the first 6 months of disease, and usually many more. Girls are affected almost twice as often as boys and, although the presentation may be at any age in childhood, onset is more common between the ages of 2 and 4 years.

Young children with polyarthritis usually have asymmetrical large joint involvement, with any of the large joints being susceptible. Asymmetrical small joint involvement is also common. Hip disease may occur, particularly later in the disease course. The degree of disability with polyarthritis can be considerable. Joint deformities are common, includ-

ing asymmetric overgrowth (particularly knees) and undergrowth (temporomandibular joint and mandible) and destruction and fusion in some (especially the wrist and cervical spine). Considerable muscle wasting occurs with prolonged active disease, adding to levels of disability.

Rheumatoid factor is absent in most such children with polyarthritis. A small subgroup are rheumatoid-factor-positive, often with a symmetrical small and large joint arthritis (see below). Tests for ANA are positive in 30–40% of children, again sometimes associated with a risk of uveitis. X-rays show similar changes to those in oligoarthritis, although over time significant joint damage, evidenced by joint space loss, erosions and joint destruction, may occur.

Systemic arthritis

Systemic arthritis (formerly called 'Still disease') may have its onset at any age in childhood and has also been described as a rare occurrence in adults. Extra-articular manifestations are the predominant features at onset, and affected children may not develop evidence of joint disease for many months, making diagnosis difficult.

Systemic arthritis affects both sexes equally and accounts for about 10% of cases of chronic arthritis in childhood. The initial presentation is with a daily recurrent (quotidian) fever, usually above 39°C, returning to or below 37°C between spikes (Fig. 13.3.2A) The fever spikes may occur once or twice daily. At the time of the fever, affected children are very irritable and movement appears painful. Individual joints may have no or minimal evidence of inflammation in the early phases of the illness. Spikes of fever are usually associated with a classical rash, which consists of small, salmon pink macules (Fig. 13.3.2B). The macules usually are less than 5 mm in diameter and appear and fade rapidly. The rash is commonly seen on the upper trunk and the upper aspects of the arms and thighs. It may be induced by a warm bath or by scratching or rubbing the skin (Koebner phenomenon). Notably, in some individuals the rash may be more urticarial and papular (particularly in darker-skinned children).

Generalized lymphadenopathy is frequent and there may be significant hepatosplenomegaly. Serositis occurs, with abdominal pain (peritonitis), pleuritis and pericarditis. Pericardial effusions may be detected by cardiac ultrasound and may be subclinical.

Diagnosis is often difficult in the early stages of disease because of the absence of apparent joint involvement. Many of the features of the presentation mimic an infective process and investigations undertaken are those for fever of unknown origin, including serial blood, urine and other cultures.

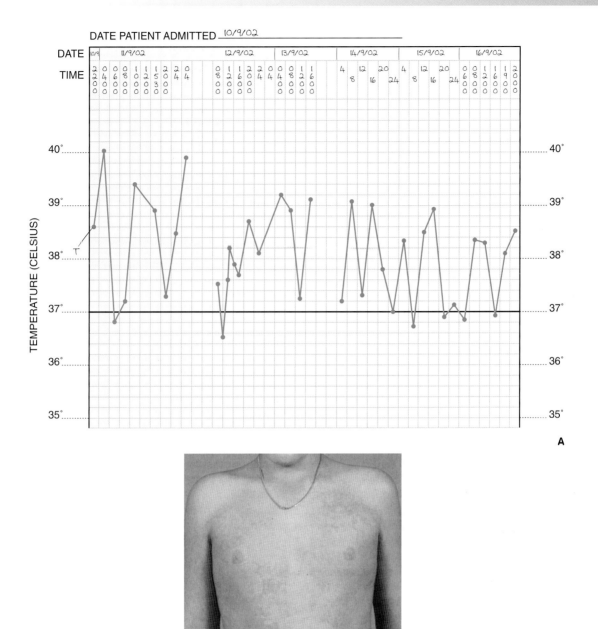

Fig. 13.3.2 **A** The typical fever chart of systemic-onset JIA, with high spiking fever 1–2 times daily, returning to baseline. **B** Typical rash of systemic-onset type JIA in a 10-year-old boy, which is widespread, macular and salmon pink in colour.

Marked elevation of white cell counts, platelets and the ESR are typical. Some malignancies (such as lymphomas and neuroblastomas) can present with similar features. Most children require admission to hospital for observation and extensive investigation.

In many cases, the diagnosis is confirmed only later in the course of the disorder when other causes have been excluded and arthritis becomes evident.

Joint involvement can be in large and small joints. In approximately half of cases the arthritis will respond relatively well to treatment and eventually remit within a few years with relatively little damage. In others the course is of a relentless polyarthritis (often with persistent fever and rash for the initial years), which is resistant to most treatment. Mortality occasionally occurs in this group from infections or a complication known as macrophage activation syndrome.

Clinical example

Andrew presented to the emergency department with chest pain and difficulty breathing. He had been unwell for 4 weeks with a daily high spiking fever and a widespread rash that was much worse with the fever or if he scratched himself. He had been given several courses of antibiotics by his GP. Examination revealed an unwell, dyspnoeic boy with a temperature of 39.5° and a widespread erythematous macular rash that faded at times of defervescence of his temperature. He had widespread lymphadenopathy and mild hepatosplenomegaly. Cardiovascular examination revealed poorly heard heart sounds.

Investigations revealed an ESR of 131 and a haemoglobin of 89 g/l, a white cell count of 29 000 and a platelet count of 829 000. Blood cultures were negative on multiple occasions. A chest X-ray revealed a large heart and the echocardiogram revealed a moderate pericardial effusion. Andrew had a moderate response to NSAIDs while in hospital over several weeks but during this time he developed a widespread polyarthritis of both small and large joints. He was ANA- and rheumatoid-factor-negative. A diagnosis was made of JIA of the systemic arthritis type. He was given pulse methylprednisolone therapy daily for 3 days followed by oral steroids, with dramatic improvement in his fever, rash and joint swelling. His pericarditis had resolved within a week. Attempted tapering of Andrew's steroids after discharge led to breakthrough fever and worsening of his arthritis. He was started on methotrexate (20 mg/m²) and subsequently was able to reduce his oral steroids to a small dose.

Six months later Andrew's polyarthritis worsened again and he responded only briefly to pulse methylprednisolone infusions. He was then started on the biological agent etanercept (anti-TNF) subcutaneously twice weekly, with dramatic and sustained improvement in his arthritis during the following 6 months. The etanercept therapy was continued in conjunction with methotrexate for several years.

Other forms of juvenile idiopathic arthritis

Rheumatoid-factor-positive polyarthritis

Some children, particularly girls, may present in later childhood or in adolescence with an arthritis associated with persistently positive blood tests for rheumatoid factor. The arthritis is usually symmetrical and involves predominantly small joints and then in time large joints equally. There may be erosions on X-ray of involved joints early in disease. This disorder is considered to be the same as early-onset adult-type rheumatoid arthritis and may have a poor outlook in terms of eventual joint deformity and function, with relative resistance to treatment.

Extended oligoarthritis

A small number of children with onset of arthritis as an oligoarthritis later have involvement of more than four joints. The arthritis may involve the temporomandibular joints, cervical spine and many other joints, often in an asymmetrical pattern. It may be very destructive in some patients.

Psoriatic arthritis

Some children with oligoarthritis or polyarthritis have features suggestive of an association with psoriasis, although the skin rash of psoriasis may not appear for many years. Dactylitis (sausage-like swelling of one or more fingers or toes) may be seen (Fig. 13.3.3A), and nail abnormalities (pitting or onycholysis) or the presence of a family history of psoriasis may provide clues to the likelihood of psoriasis being linked to the arthritis. Psoriasis of the skin, when seen, may be subtle, e.g. umbilical, in the scalp (Fig. 13.3.3B) or behind the ears. The severe form, arthritis mutilans, is very rare in childhood.

Enthesitis-related arthritis

This form of arthritis was formerly known as juvenile spondyloarthropathy or HLA-B27-associated arthritis. Enthesitis means inflammation of tendon insertions and fascia, and is thought to be present in almost all patients (though subclinical in many). The most common entheses involved include the Achilles tendon (Fig. 13.3.4A), patellar tendon and plantar fascia insertions. Most patients tend to be older boys (>6 years) who present with lower limb asymmetrical arthritis (similar to the oligoarthritis pattern) with a predilection for the tarsus and great toe and later hip involvement. In some patients it may be associated with the later development of axial disease, with sacroiliac and lumbar spine inflammation (Fig. 13.3.4B) and occasionally true ankylosing spondylitis (<10%). Children with enthesitis-related arthritis are usually but not always B27-positive. Many early-onset cases may remit as they get older. Some children may present with enthesitis-related arthritis associated with occult or unrecognized inflammatory bowel disease.

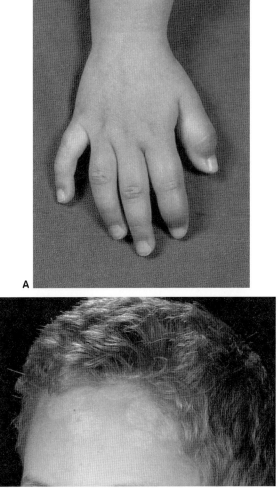

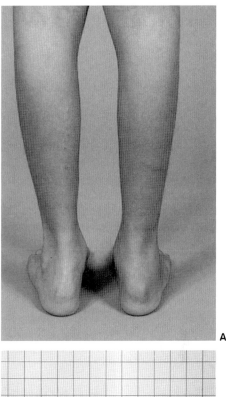

Fig. 13.3.3 **A** Dactylitis of the thumb and index finger of a 4-year-old boy with psoriatic arthritis. **B** Psoriatic plaques on the scalp of the same boy.

Arthritis in association with other connective tissue disorders

Persisting arthritis occasionally may be seen in some of the other connective tissue disorders such as systemic SLE, juvenile dermatomyositis, sarcoidosis and scleroderma (both localized and systemic).

Eye disease in juvenile arthritis

Inflammatory disease of the uveal tract of the eye (uveitis or iridocyclitis) is a very important associated abnormality in children with almost all forms of chronic arthritis. The highest risk group is those who are female with an early-onset oligoarthritis, especially those who are ANA positive, of whom many will develop uveitis in one or both eyes at some stage during the course of the disease. However,

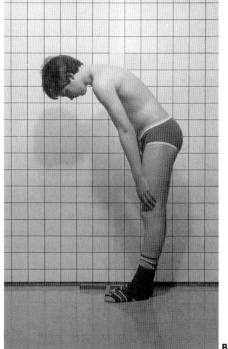

Fig. 13.3.4 **A** Enthesitis of the right Achilles tendon insertion in a 13-year-old boy with enthesitis-related arthritis (juvenile spondyloarthropathy). **B** Limited forward bending and flattened lumbar spine, typical of the inflammatory spinal involvement, that occurred early in the disease course of the same boy.

inflammatory changes in the eyes may occur occasionally in ANA-negative children with arthritis, and in children with polyarthritis, systemic arthritis and psoriatic arthritis.

The inflammatory changes of anterior uveitis are usually entirely asymptomatic and young children are unlikely to verbalize the experience of visual abnormalities. Therefore, regular examination of the eyes by an ophthalmologist using a slit lamp is essential. This needs to be performed at 2–6-monthly intervals depending on the risk level (e.g. less frequent assessment is needed in systemic arthritis). The degree of inflammation in the eye does not relate to the severity or duration of the arthritis: some children may have minimal joint involvement and have severe blinding uveitis. Treatment is with mydriatics and topical steroid preparations, and occasionally disease-modifying agents such as methotrexate. Untreated eye disease may lead to severe impairment of vision due to cataract formation and the development of adhesions of the iris (synechiae). Glaucoma may also occur. An acute symptomatic form of iritis may occur in the enthesitis-related arthritis form of JIA (spondyloarthropathy syndromes). This acute uveitis usually remits rapidly with treatment. A granulomatous panuveitis or posterior uveitis may occur in paediatric sarcoidosis.

Investigation of chronic arthritis in childhood

Useful initial investigations are listed in Table 13.3.2. A microcytic anaemia may be present secondary to the chronic inflammatory state, particularly with more extensive forms of arthritis. The ESR is usually elevated but may be normal, especially in oligoarthritis and ERA. The ANA pattern, when positive, is usually homogeneous. Rheumatoid factor (IgM antibody against IgG) is persistently positive in significant titres only rarely, usually indicating rheumatoid factor positive polyarthritis. It may be useful to look for the presence of the HLA B27 antigen if an enthesitis-related arthritis is suspected or there is an asymmetric lower limb arthritis in older boys. The B27 antigen is demonstrable by genotyping in approximately 8% of the normal Caucasian population but is present in at least 90% of those with ankylosing spondylitis and up to 75% of children with ERA.

Radiology

Radiographs of involved joints in the early stages usually show no abnormalities or only soft tissue changes. Changes seen later in the course of the disorder may include bone overgrowth, progressive joint damage and ultimately joint ankylosis. Ankylosis may be seen in the cervical spine particularly. In very severe disease, and in rheumatoid-factor-positive disease, there may be discrete joint erosions, but these are a relatively unusual finding. Radiographs also are important in excluding some other disorders that may mimic idiopathic arthritis, e.g. bone or synovial tumours, unsuspected fractures and radiopaque foreign bodies. Magnetic resonance imaging (MRI) has increasing use in difficult diagnostic situations or in assessing deep joints such as the hip (Fig. 13.3.5). When performed with gadolinium, MRI can exquisitely show the presence and burden of synovitis in the examined joint. High-frequency ultrasound shows promise in assessing synovial pathology, although it is very operator-dependent.

Management of idiopathic arthritis

Management of JIA has been revolutionized in the last few decades with vastly improved drug regimes and the presence of multidisciplinary centres with allied health professionals.

Maintenance of joint function

Joint function is maintained by physiotherapy, and joint splinting when necessary. When a joint is acutely inflamed and painful, rest is necessary to relieve pain. However, gentle passive movement is still important to maintain the full range of joint movement. As inflammation improves, an active exercise programme is introduced as soon as it is tolerated to further improve the range of joint movement and to strengthen muscles around the involved joint. This is done with the guidance of an experienced physiotherapist. Hydrotherapy is an important adjunct to therapy and usually involves a regular exercise programme in a heated pool.

Table 13.3.2   Initial investigations in suspected juvenile arthritis

- Full blood count (CBC)
- Erythrocyte sedimentation rate and/or C-reactive protein
- Rheumatoid factor
- Antinuclear antibody
- HLA B27 (older children, especially males)
- Liver function and renal function tests in those who are systemically unwell
- Radiography of major involved joints (may X-ray contralateral joints for comparison)
- Ophthalmological assessment using a slit lamp
- Magnetic resonance imaging of joint if unusual or uncertain history or haemarthrosis found at aspiration – especially useful for assessing hips and spine

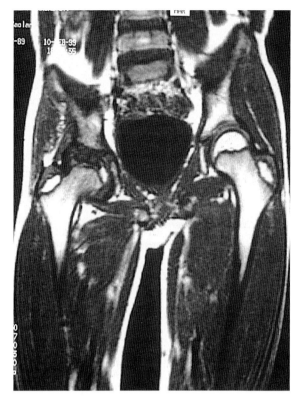

Fig. 13.3.5 MRI of an actively inflamed and damaged right hip joint in a 12-year-old girl.

Splinting is used to maintain involved joints in a good functional position when at rest. This is used most commonly as knee extension splints in bed at night. Other joints where splints are used frequently are the ankle and the wrist.

Relief of pain

Persisting pain in the involved joints is a major burden for many children. Pain in the joints of the lower limbs interferes with walking. Pain in any joint can lead to poor sleeping, irritability and a decreased appetite. Inability to do simple activities because of specific joint pain has a marked effect on the child and family. For example, children with painful wrists and fingers may no longer be able to dress themselves or feed themselves. Resting of joints in a functional position may assist in pain control. Warmth may relieve the discomfort of stiff joints, whereas the hot and acutely inflamed joint may be made more comfortable with ice packs. Simple analgesics such as paracetamol are important. The non-steroidal anti-inflammatory agents (NSAIDs) can help with pain control by relieving inflammation, although they do not have primary analgesic activity. Emotional pain and distress is important to identify and is easy to confuse with physiological or pathological pain, but usually understood by simple observation of the child. More importantly, perhaps, intensive medical therapy with treatments detailed below (such as joint injections and disease-modifying antirheumatic drugs (DMARDs) have raised the bar in terms of what is acceptable in ongoing chronic inflammation and hence pain.

Specific drug therapy

Non-steroidal anti-inflammatory drugs
The NSAIDs form the cornerstone of initial therapy for JIA because of their rapid, though often modest, effect on inflammation. An important consideration in young children is that the NSAID should be available in syrup form so that it can be taken easily and so that the dose can be titrated accurately. Naproxen is available in many countries in syrup form (125 mg/5 ml), as is ibuprofen. Piroxicam is available in a dispersible tablet form. All NSAID medications can cause gastrointestinal irritation, vomiting or bleeding, although these effects seem to be less common in children than in adults. Some children experience poor concentration and sleep disturbance. NSAIDs should be taken with meals. It may be 6 weeks or more before a full anti-inflammatory effect is seen.

Renal dysfunction has been reported only rarely in children receiving NSAIDs. Some children may develop a scarring, porphyria-like rash, particularly on sun-exposed areas of the skin: the forehead, bridge of the nose, cheeks and dorsum of the hands. This rash is seen particularly with naproxen in fair-skinned children. The newer, so-called 'gastroprotective' COX-2-selective agents have been used in some instances, but cardiovascular concerns with one agent (rofecoxib) led to discontinuation. Celecoxib is still used on occasion (off-licence) in older children. Subsequent studies suggest that most if not all NSAIDs carry an increased cardiovascular risk if used in the longer term, at least in older adults with co-morbidity. Whether this has relevance for children is uncertain.

Joint aspiration and injection
This procedure has supplanted chronic NSAID use in many centres. Instillation of the long-acting tri-amcinolone drugs into inflamed joints, particularly weightbearing joints and wrists, has demonstrated profound benefits in many studies, with resolution of joint inflammation for long periods. Young children usually require a general anaesthetic (as do older children if multiple joints or deep joints such as hip or subtalar are to be injected). In other circumstances, somewhat older children may manage with

nitrous oxide or conscious sedation. Considerably older children are injected under local anaesthetic cover as for adults. Complications are rare but include steroid atrophy of nearby soft tissues, which can be profound and long-lasting in children. Infections subsequent to injection are exceedingly rare.

Methotrexate

In children in whom joint inflammation is not controlled adequately with joint injections and/or NSAID medications, methotrexate therapy, given as a single weekly dose, has been shown in randomized controlled trials to be of major benefit in doses of up to 15–20 mg/m^2. This should be undertaken only under the supervision of a paediatric rheumatology service. The dose can be increased in several steps to ensure tolerance, with careful monitoring of hepatic and haematological function. It may be several months before improvement in joint inflammation and function is apparent. Methotrexate is considered the gold standard with the best evidence for efficacy of all available DMARDs. It is also the most widely studied, and tends to have good levels of tolerance in children. Efficacy and compliance may be improved with subcutaneous administration in some children.

Leflunomide

Leflunomide is a further second-line agent used frequently in adult arthritis for which there is some preliminary evidence of efficacy in childhood. It is not recommended for use in young children but may have a place in treatment in adolescents with active arthritis who are unable to tolerate methotrexate.

Sulfasalazine

Sulfasalazine may be of benefit in some children, particularly in those with enthesitis-related arthritis (spondyloarthropathy) or with arthritis associated with inflammatory bowel disease. It may also be used in polyarthritis but usually as an adjunct to methotrexate.

Corticosteroids

As with their efficacy in the joint injections, intravenous (so called pulse therapy) and oral steroids still have a role to play in treatment of arthritis. With severe disease, particularly systemic onset (with fever rash, hepatosplenomegaly, etc.), such therapy is mandated for rapid control of inflammation. It is also very useful for severe polyarthritis at the start of treatment for rapid effect. Oral steroids have a role as a short course in similar patients or perhaps during major flares. At all times attempts to reduce such doses should be made over time and steroid-sparing/disease-modifying agents such as methotrexate should be used instead. Corticosteroid eye drops are an important part of therapy for uveitis, along with mydriatics and occasional depot steroids, but in time, because of complications, DMARDs such as methotrexate are gaining favour to also control eye disease.

Biological therapies

The so-called biological agents are designed using molecular genetics and the knowledge of important cytokine actions in inflammation. Anti-tumour-necrosis-factor (TNF) therapies (etanercept, infliximab) are now being used for some children with severe arthritis not controlled by other agents, usually in combination with methotrexate. Initial studies, particularly with etanercept, suggest profound benefit and remission induction in numbers of patients who were previously resistant to treatment. Newer biological agents such as adalumimab (anti-TNF) and anakinra (anti-IL1-receptor antagonist) have been licensed for use in rheumatoid arthritis and early data suggest that they may have efficacy in some subsets of JIA. A specific anti-IL6 antibody has been trialled in systemic-onset JIA with great promise in this most resistant from of JIA.

Experimental therapies

The use of thalidomide in a few studies suggests possible efficacy. The use of autologous stem cell transplantation has also been reported in over 50 children with the most severe unremitting arthritis, with remission induction in many but also associated with several deaths. Time will show whether autologous stem cell transplantation becomes safe enough to be used more routinely.

> ### ▶ **Practical points**
>
> - In a swollen joint with marked pain, limitation of motion, or associated fever, septic arthritis should be considered and should be ruled out by aspiration and culture
> - Swelling of a joint or joints, lasting longer than 6 weeks, and with other causes excluded, is highly likely to be a form of juvenile arthritis
> - All children diagnosed or suspected as having JIA should be seen by an ophthalmologist to detect uveitis. The risk is highest in young females with oligoarthritis and a positive ANA
> - Chronic arthritis of the lower limbs in an older boy who is HLA-B27-positive, associated with painful/swollen entheses, is likely to be enthesitis-related arthritis
> - For any joint with persistent chronic synovitis unresponsive to NSAIDs, injection with a long-acting steroid is usually very efficacious
> - For any polyarthritis unresponsive to simple therapies, use of a disease-modifying drug such as methotrexate is mandated

Prevention and management of disability

Because drug treatment may take considerable time to suppress inflammatory arthritis and may never do so completely, the mainstay of treatment of chronic arthritis in children includes the physiotherapy programme to maintain joint function. The programme needs to be tailored to the needs of each joint and to be appropriate to the level of activity and needs of the child and his or her family. Home exercise programmes and guidance with sporting activities are essential. Appropriate seating at home and at school, encouragement and assistance with activities of daily living and information for other caregivers, for example schoolteachers, are all important.

Surgical intervention is needed rarely in childhood but is appropriate when joints have become severely deformed and when joint replacement is necessary, e.g. for severe and long-standing hip disease. Many whose disease has 'burned out' in childhood may eventually require surgery for accelerated degenerative disease.

In children with severe disease and with significant disability, psychological support is also needed. Many children, particularly adolescents, who face challenges of altered body image and threats to their independence, benefit from appropriate counselling. Parents often require supportive therapy particularly soon after diagnosis. Social work involvement is often required for children with severe arthritis. For example, disabled parking access, health-care cards and disability support allowances are an important part of assistance for parents to provide the extra care needed. Patient travel allowances and specific pharmaceutical benefits for children with chronic diseases and high drug costs are also available. Parent and patient support groups (such as the Arthritis Foundation) are valued greatly by families with affected children.

Management of associated abnormalities

The management of uveitis has been described above. Growth may be impaired in any chronic inflammatory state, and nutritional assessment and advice is important. Growth hormone has been used in selected patients to help restore growth velocity, particularly during less active phases of disease. Osteoporosis is a well recognized complication of severe juvenile arthritis and is exacerbated by steroid use. Attention to calcium and vitamin D intake is important and on occasions the use of bisphosphonates may be considered for those who are at great fracture risk.

Outcome of juvenile arthritis

In spite of the significant joint disease seen during the active phases of arthritis, the long-term outcome is good when appropriate therapy is provided. Approximately 70% of affected children will have minor or no residual joint dysfunction 15 years after onset. The best outlook is for those with oligoarticular disease with onset in early childhood. Long-term disability is seen most frequently in those with severe polyarticular-onset disease and in those whose systemic disease progresses rapidly to widespread and progressive polyarticular involvement. However, the physical function and level of future education and employment may be impaired in adults who have had more moderate disease if multidisciplinary input is not provided. Severe impairment of vision with synechiae and cataract formation may occur with aggressive or late-diagnosed uveitis.

Other disorders associated with arthritis in childhood

Reactive arthritis conditions occur when, after (or during) a specific infection elsewhere in the body, a non-septic inflammation of joint(s) occurs for some period of time (usually less than 6 weeks). Transient synovitis of the hip or 'irritable hip' is considered a form of reactive arthritis that occurs in early childhood and is self-limiting. Post-streptococcal reactive arthritis and post-mycoplasma reactive arthritis are increasingly recognized clinical entities, along with reactive arthritis induced by *Salmonella*, *Yersinia* and *Campylobacter* gastrointestinal infection. Usually, reactive arthritis has an oligoarthritis pattern, which may be severe in terms of pain, occasionally migrates, but lasts for a few weeks only. Treatment with NSAIDs is usually effective but occasionally a short course of steroids is beneficial. The Reiter triad of conjunctivitis, urethritis and arthritis is rare in childhood.

Some viral infections may be associated with arthralgia or arthritis. These include rubella, Ross River virus, Epstein–Barr virus and hepatitis virus infections. Some bacterial infections may cause a persistent arthritis: tuberculosis is still an important cause of chronic joint infection in some countries and may also be associated with a reactive arthritis (Poncet disease).

Lyme disease is rare in Australia but is an important cause of arthritis in some parts of the world. Infection with tick-borne *Borrelia* species leads to a rash known as erythema chronicum migrans, neurological signs and a relapsing arthritis, usually of one or more large joints. It is responsive to penicillin.

Rheumatic fever (Ch. 15.2) and Henoch–Schönlein purpura (Chs 16.2, 18.2) have an associated arthritis which is transient in nature. Haemophilia

(Ch. 16.2) with recurrent intra-articular joint bleeding leads to chronic synovitis and destructive changes in joints often indistinguishable from inflammatory arthritis, particularly in the knee and the ankle.

Miscellaneous disorders that may present as joint pain or dysfunction in childhood

Other conditions that may present with joint pain or dysfunction are listed in Table 13.3.3.

Systemic lupus erythematosus

Systemic lupus erythematosus is a chronic multisystem disorder of unknown aetiology. Polyclonal activation of B cells is associated with excessive antibody formation, and disease results from immune complex deposition. Autoantibodies are seen in serum and in tissue biopsy samples but their role in the manifestations of disease remains speculative. The disorder is relatively uncommon in childhood but 10–20% of all SLE has its onset at less than 18 years of age. Presentation under the age of 4–5 years is very rare. Girls are affected more commonly than boys, although the female:male ratio is lower in childhood than in adult life. Although SLE is often a mild and slowly progressive disorder when it has its onset in adult life, in childhood it is often severe and may present very acutely. There is a high incidence of severe renal involvement and significant levels of morbidity and mortality.

Table 13.3.3 Miscellaneous conditions that may be associated with joint pain or dysfunction in childhood

- Legg–Calvé–Perthes disease
- Slipped upper femoral epiphysis
- Transient synovitis (e.g. irritable hip)
- Chronic recurrent multifocal osteomyelitis
- Foreign body synovitis (e.g. plant thorn synovitis)
- Chondromalacia patellae and anterior knee pain syndromes
- Unrecognized trauma
- Some metabolic and inherited disorders and syndromes
- Malignancy, including acute lymphoblastic leukaemia
- Dysplastic bone/cartilage disorders
- Hypermobility conditions
- 'Overuse' conditions, especially in elite child athletes and gymnasts
- Reflex sympathetic dystrophy (complex regional pain syndrome II)
- Chronic pain and fatigue syndromes ('fibromyalgia')
- Conversion symptoms and hysterical gait abnormalities

Clinical features

The onset of SLE is often associated with non-specific symptoms of lethargy, low-grade fever, loss of appetite and oral ulceration. Raynaud's phenomenon may be present and patchy alopecia may occur. By the time of presentation a rash is usually present. This is characteristically a photosensitive vasculitis rash with scaling and erythema over the malar area of the face (Fig. 13.3.6A). Often there are also vasculitic lesions on the extremities such as the pulp of the digits (Fig. 13.3.6B), extensor surfaces of the arms and legs, and the palate. Purpura or ecchymoses may be present as a result of thrombocytopenia or associated coagulopathy.

Arthralgia and joint symptoms are common but resolve rapidly when treatment is commenced. Myositis is not uncommon, contributing to weakness. Renal involvement causes microscopic hematuria and proteinuria. Some children will present with macroscopic hematuria and proteinuria in a mixed nephritic–nephrotic picture, or with hypertension. Autoimmune hepatitis may occur with elevation of transaminases.

Many children with SLE will have neurological manifestations such as severe headache, mood disorder and cognitive dysfunction. Seizures, psychosis, chorea, polyneuropathy or transverse myelitis are less common but associated with poorer disease outcome. Lung and cardiac abnormalities may also occur.

Laboratory findings

Common laboratory findings are:

- elevated ESR
- leucopenia (specifically lymphopenia)
- Coombs-positive haemolytic anaemia or anaemia of chronic disease
- thrombocytopenia
- low C3 and/or C4
- microscopic haematuria, proteinuria, cellular casts and altered renal function.

Important diagnostic immunologic findings in SLE are the presence of autoantibodies. ANA is universally present, often in very high titre. The ANA may be directed against specific identifiable extractable nuclear antigens (ENA) such as anti-Sm (Smith), anti-Ro (SSA) and anti-La (SSB). Antibody to double-stranded (native) DNA is typical. High concentrations are almost specific for SLE and are associated with more severe renal disease and central nervous system disease. Anticardiolipin antibody may be present and is often associated with the lupus anticoagulant phenomenon. The associated risk of thrombosis with such antibodies seems to be rarer in by biopsy is important for guiding therapy and determining outcomes. Diffuse proliferative glomerulonephritis (grade IV), the most severe form, is the commonest finding in children with kidney disease.

Management

It is often necessary to use high dose prednisolone initially in SLE in childhood to control the disease process rapidly after diagnosis. Doses of 2 mg/kg/day may be needed, sometimes in split daily doses. In very severe disease, pulses of intravenous methylprednisolone at a dose of 25–30 mg/kg up to a maximum of 1 g per dose may be required for up to 3 consecutive days. The doses of steroids required often lead to significant side effects, including increased susceptibility to infection. SLE itself increases susceptibility to infection and thus infection is an important cause of morbidity and mortality. Treatment of SLE requires careful and expert supervision often by multiple specialists.

Steroid-sparing or disease-modifying immuno-suppressive agents should be used in most patients. Hydroxychloroquine is used for mild (especially skin) disease, and methotrexate is useful if arthritis is dominant. Azathioprine is used in moderate disease and cyclophosphamide is probably mandated for severe renal involvement or any major central nervous system involvement. Mycophenolate mofetil can also be used in these instances, although the evidence for its overall benefit in children and young people is still accumulating. Plasmaphaeresis is probably of little use but more recently autologous stem cell transplantation has been successful in inducing remission in some severe, treatment-resistant cases, as has the use of the biological agent rituximab. This anti-B-cell (CD20) antibody may be especially useful for severe haematological manifestations.

As for juvenile arthritis, multidisciplinary team involvement of multiple medical specialists, dietitians, psychologists and physiotherapists is essential for optimal outcome. Most children and young people with SLE will require steroid use for some or all of their disease and good dietary management including calcium and vitamin D is essential. Most patients will develop significant dyslipidaemia and are at risk of atherosclerotic complications in adult life, which thus needs to be monitored and treated.

The outcome for children with SLE has improved markedly in recent decades with more intensive and successful therapies. With careful therapy, renal function is usually maintained. There must always be a high index of suspicion for infection in any febrile patient. Side effects of steroid therapy, including avascular necrosis of the femoral heads, decreased spinal mineralization and growth suppression,

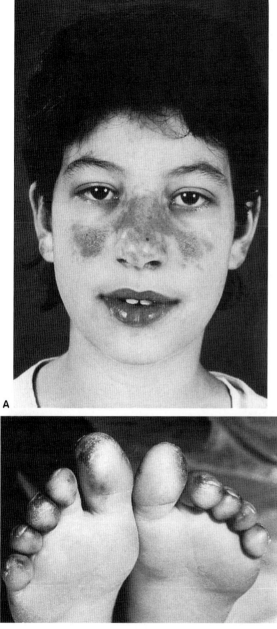

Fig. 13.3.6 **A** Systemic lupus erythematosus: facial rash in a girl with active lupus vasculitis. There are also vasculitic lesions on both ears. **B** Systemic lupus erythematosus: vasculitic lesions on the toes of a 9-year-old girl with active disease. She also had a diffuse proliferative glomerulonephritis and anaemia in association with thrombocytopenia.

children than in adults but may be a severe complication.

Biopsy of involved tissues such as skin and kidney shows evidence of characteristic inflammation and immunoglobulin and complement deposition in blood vessels and tissues. The staging of renal disease remain difficult areas of management. For many children, however, the aim should be a near normal life expectancy and preservation of fertility, with minimal disease and minimal treatment morbidity.

Neonatal lupus syndrome

Some infants born to mothers with serological evidence of SLE-type antibodies will have transient manifestations of SLE. The mothers rarely have a diagnosed rheumatic disorder (such as SLE or Sjögren disease) but may go on to do so in later life. The neonatal manifestations are due to transplacental passage of maternal IgG autoantibody, particularly anti-Ro and anti-La antibody. The most common abnormality is a discoid lupus-like skin rash, mild thrombocytopenia and transaminitis, which gradually improve as maternally acquired antibody titres decrease. Usually no treatment is required. The most important complication is congenital heart block, which seems to occur in isolation from the other manifestations, may lead to fetal or neonatal death, persists throughout life and usually requires placement of a cardiac pacemaker.

Sjögren disease

Sjögren syndrome is very rare in childhood, presenting with constitutional symptoms, rash, recurrent or chronic parotitis and conjunctivitis. Xerostomia and the sicca complex are rarely seen in childhood but other organ vasculitis may be seen. Serology is similar to SLE with a prominence of anti-Ro and anti-La antibodies.

Juvenile dermatomyositis

Dermatomyositis in children can occur at any age, but is seen most commonly between the ages of 4 and 10 years. Weakness and pain in the proximal muscle groups of the limbs is a major component of the disorder and a presenting feature may be a gait abnormality or even an inability to walk. Weakness of muscles may progress to involve the trunk and respiratory muscles in severe disease. In some children onset may be rapid and life-threatening; in others progression may be insidious.

The typical rash of dermatomyositis is a heliotrope (purplish) discoloration, and a rash on the eyelids with an associated erythematous facial rash and oedema is common (Fig. 13.3.7A). A scaly erythematous rash over the dorsum of the small joints of the hands (Gottron's papules) and elbows and knees are common and typical. Occasional other patterns such

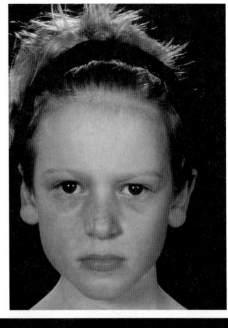

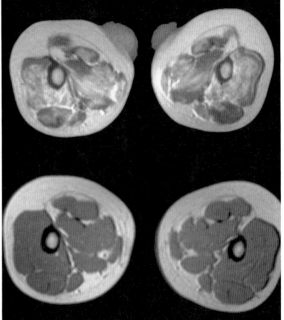

Fig. 13.3.7 **A** Facial erythema and eyelid rash in a boy with juvenile dermatomyositis. **B** MRI images of the mid-thigh in the same boy, with upper images showing widespread signal increase in the muscles and images below showing improvement after therapy.

as a 'shawl' distribution, 'V' neck or photosensitive distribution rash may be seen. In some, the rash may be ulcerative, usually associated with severe treatment resistant disease.

Muscle enzymes in serum are usually elevated (CK, ALT, AST, aldolase). Electromyography will show typical myositis changes and imaging-guided muscle biopsy often shows typical changes. MRI shows characteristic signal changes in the involved muscles (Fig. 13.3.7B) and along with the clinical findings often negates the need for biopsy and electromyography. Treatment is initially with corticosteroids in high dose (oral or i.v. form) and with very gradual reduction. In most children, early commencement on a drug such as methotrexate or ciclo-

---

Clinical example

Joshua was aged 6 years and developed a scaly erythematous rash over his face after sun exposure that persisted for several months despite topical allergy treatments. He became very fatigued, often sleeping on return from school for several hours. He had stopped playing sport and riding his bike, and complained of painful legs. Over several weeks his rash worsened and spread to his elbows, knees and the back of his hands. When seen by his GP, Joshua had difficulty getting up on to the examination couch.

Examination revealed a boy who had lost some weight. He had a scaly red rash over the small joints of his hands and knees and elbows. He had a macular erythematous rash on his face and his eyelids had a violaceous hue. He had evidence of marked muscle weakness in his proximal leg muscles, shoulders and trunk, was unable to get up from lying unaided and was unable to raise his arms above his head for more than a few seconds.

Investigations revealed a normal blood count, an ESR of 25, normal renal function and LFTs showing an AST of 145 and ALT 109 with a normal bilirubin and albumin. Subsequently he was shown to have a creatine kinase of 2988, an LDH of 1468 and an aldolase of 108. He was admitted to hospital and a diagnosis of inflammatory myositis was made. A subsequent MRI of his thighs showed typical widespread but patchy signal changes in the muscle and fascial tissues. A biopsy of the lateral thigh confirmed the inflammatory nature of his myositis. His specific diagnosis was juvenile dermatomyositis based on the clinical picture and investigations. By this stage, Joshua was having difficulty walking any distance and getting up out of a chair, with considerable muscle pain evolving.

Treatment was commenced with pulse intravenous methylprednisolone for 3 days followed by 1 mg/kg oral steroids. At the same time Joshua was started on oral methotrexate 20 mg/m². He also started a graduated physiotherapy programme in the hydrotherapy pool. During the first week he gradually improved and after a second course of intravenous methylprednisolone he was able to be discharged with marked improvement in his muscle rash and muscle strength. He was able to walk and started to be able to use the stairs. Over the subsequent 3 months his steroids were slowly weaned and he had progressive improvements in his muscle strength and was able to start some junior soccer training. His parents had noticed several small lumps on Joshua's knees and inner thighs, which proved to be calcinosis on X-ray.

---

sporin is used for more optimal disease control and for a steroid-sparing effect, although some will require steroids for many years. Few children are able to have treatment withdrawn in less than 2 years.

Some children have persistent chronic disease activity or multiple relapses despite intensive therapy. Other treatments used or added in these situations are azathioprine and cyclophosphamide (particularly in ulcerative disease). Complications include muscle wasting, joint contractures, a form of progressive chronic arthritis, calcinosis of areas of skin and subcutaneous tissue, and rarely a lipodystrophy syndrome. However, many children have a very good outcome after a number of years with appropriate intensive multidisciplinary treatment.

Scleroderma disorders

The major feature of scleroderma is induration or sclerosis of skin and subcutaneous tissue and subsequent atrophy of sweat sebaceous glands and underlying muscle and bone. This may occur in several forms. Systemic sclerosis occurs in a diffuse or limited form (the latter being known formerly as CREST syndrome). It is very rare in childhood and when seen is in adolescents. A typical widespread, symmetrical, waxy, tightened, indurated skin with atrophy of muscles is seen, and is associated with anti-PMScL antibody in some. The associated vasculopathy causes serious renal and cardiopulmonary disease, and major gut involvement with reflux and malabsorption is seen. Treatment remains difficult, with methotrexate and cyclophosphamide perhaps offering some benefit. Symptomatic treatment with antihypertensives (such as ACE inhibitors) and pulmonary vasodilators contribute to management and reduction in early mortality. Autologous stem cell transplantation has also been used successfully in a number of cases.

Localized scleroderma, though uncommon, is seen 10–20 times more frequently than systemic sclerosis in childhood. It occurs as either morphea (isolated patches) or linear scleroderma or combinations of the two lesions, and may be very widespread. The involved skin becomes shiny and thickened, deeply tethered, and has patches of depigmentation and also often areas of excess pigmentation. Major joint contractures occur when it crosses joints and there may be failure of limb growth. A form occurring on the head (known as *en coup de sabre*) may be severe enough to cause hemifacial atrophy (Parry–Romberg syndrome), occasionally with uveitis and central nervous system involvement. There are usually no associated systemic features. Evidence now indicates that early treatment with steroids and maintenance with methotrexate for more severe lesions over a number of years may benefit many patients. Topical treatments have been largely unsuccessful, and cosmetic and corrective surgery may be required.

Overlap syndromes

Some children appear to have features of several of the disorders described above, or some features without having any complete disorder. One specific type of 'overlap syndrome' disorder is called mixed connective tissue disease (MCTD), in which there is Raynaud's phenomenon, skin nodules, arthralgia or arthritis, sclerodactyly and sometimes myositis. Patients with MCTD characteristically have a speckled-pattern high-titre ANA with specificity for U1RNP. Some children with MCTD later develop major manifestations of SLE or scleroderma. Other children develop what is termed *undifferentiated connective tissue disease*, where they may have a positive ANA and phenomena such as Raynaud's and mild small vessel vasculitis. They may rarely develop more major features of a more formally recognizable connective tissue disorder in later life.

Chronic recurrent multifocal osteomyelitis

Chronic recurrent multifocal osteomyelitis is a condition that usually presents in children aged over 2 years with painful bony swelling or apparent arthritis if near a joint, or occasionally as atypical pain in a limb or the back. Radiology reveals characteristic lesions with bone lysis and new bone formation, and typical sites include the medial clavicle (Fig. 13.3.8A, B), distal tibia or femur, vertebrae or cranium. Lesions may occur singly or may be multiple. Multiple lesions may be associated with some constitutional symptoms and elevation of inflammatory markers. Some may get more widespread synovitis, acne pustulosis, hyperostosis and osteitis of bones (so called SAPHO syndrome). Biopsies of the lesions reveal chronic inflammation and no evidence of malignancy (such as Langerhans cells), and are always negative on culture.

Many affected children will have received several courses of antibiotics from initial practitioners with little evidence of efficacy. It is no longer considered an infectious entity and is now recognized as a chronic inflammatory disorder. In general the condition waxes and wanes over several years but may 'burn out' after 5–6 years in many. Severe bony destruction and altered limb growth may mandate

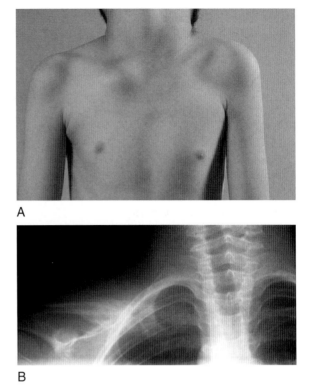

A

B

Fig. 13.3.8 **A** 7 year old boy with a swollen right medial clavicle due to chronic recurrent multifocal osteomyelitis. **B** radiograph of the same lesion showing both osteolysis and new bone formation or hyperostosis.

aggressive treatment. Initial treatment is with NSAIDs but courses of steroids and/or DMARDs (such as methotrexate) may be required.

Vasculitis syndromes

Table 13.3.4 provides a classification of primary vasculitic disorders in childhood according to the predominant vessels involved. The commonest are Henoch–Schönlein purpura (Chs 16.2, 18.2) and Kawasaki disease.

Kawasaki disease

Kawasaki disease has been described worldwide but is more common in children of Japanese descent. It is seen most often between the ages of 1 and 4 years. Diagnostic or classification criteria have been developed. They are a fever of more than 38.5°C for 5 or more days in the absence of evidence of a streptococcal (or other specific) infection with at least four of the following five manifestations:

- bilateral non-purulent conjunctival injection
- oral mucosal changes (erythema or dry cracked lips or strawberry tongue)

Table 13.3.4 Primary vasculitic disorders in childhood based on predominant size of vessel involved
Small vessel vasculitis
• Henoch–Schönlein purpura
• Infantile haemorrhagic oedema
• Hypersensitivity angiitis
• Hypocomplementaemic (urticarial) vasculitis
Medium vessel vasculitis
• Polyarteritis nodosa
• Cutaneous polyarteritis
• Microscopic polyangiitis, isolated (renal/lung 'PAN')
• Kawasaki disease
• Wegener disease (granulomatous)
• Churg–Strauss disease
• Primary angiitis of the central nervous system
• Moya moya disease
Large vessel vasculitis
• Takayasu's arteritis
Other
• Sarcoidosis
• Behçet disease
• Mucha–Haberman
• Cogan syndrome

- cervical lymphadenopathy with one node 1.5 cm or more in diameter
- changes in the extremities (swelling of hands or feet, or erythema of palms or soles, or membrane-like peeling of the skin)
- a generalized rash, which often is morbilliform in appearance.

Other clinical features include arthritis, cholecystitis, orchitis and occasionally central nervous system disease.

The diagnosis is often particularly difficult in young infants, where clinical findings can be subtle or missed, and may be made without fulfilling all the above criteria (atypical Kawasaki) and treated presumptively. A major complication of this disorder, reflecting its vasculitic nature, is a propensity to develop proximal arterial aneurysms. This is seen in the coronary arteries particularly and is found in approximately 20% of untreated patients on echocardiography. The incidence of coronary artery aneurysm formation can be reduced greatly by treatment with intravenous immunoglobulin (IVIG) during the early phase of the acute illness. Steroids may play a role in those who are resistant to IVIG. Aspirin is used in the early phase to prevent thrombosis. Atherosclerosis and ischaemic heart disease may follow later in life.

All the other vasculitis disorders are rare in childhood, often presenting with constitutional symptoms, fever, weight loss and rash (Fig. 13.3.9). The disorders often evolve later into more organ-specific features, such as nephritis and hypertension in polyarteritis nodosa, or respiratory symptoms in Wegener granulomatosis. Biopsy of affected tissues or angiography is usually required to establish the diagnosis. Therapy usually involves corticosteroids and often immunosuppressive or cytotoxic medications for long periods, with significant risk of morbidity and mortality.

Clinical example

David was 2 years old and had been well previously when he developed a high fever. He became very irritable, refused to eat and developed marked swelling of his cervical nodes, particularly on the right side. His mouth and throat were reddened and he was thought to have a viral infection. Two days later, he had marked conjunctival reddening, a measles-like rash on his trunk and swelling of his hands and feet. His lips had become more inflamed and cracked. A diagnosis of Kawasaki disease was made on the basis of the clinical features. David was admitted to hospital and was given 2 g/kg of intravenous immunoglobulin. The fever, rash and irritability resolved rapidly. Echocardiograms were performed on admission, at 6 weeks and at 3 months, but no coronary artery aneurysms were seen. Low-dose aspirin (5 mg/kg per day) was given as a single daily dose until the echocardiogram at 3 months after onset was shown to be normal.

Practical points

- When more than one system appears to be involved in an inflammatory disorder, suspect a connective tissue disorder or vasculitis
- Autoantibodies such as ANA may be useful in a child suspected of a connective tissue disorder and are more specific if found in high titre or with specific antibodies such as dsDNA or extractable nuclear antigens such as anti-Ro, anti-La, anti-Sm, etc.
- In children with an acute illness comprising high fever, rash, lymphadenopathy and oral mucosal changes, Kawasaki disease should be considered and echocardiography and IVIG treatment considered
- When steroid therapy is required the minimal effective dose should be used and steroid-sparing agents should be introduced as soon as practical if prolonged use is expected
- All children who require any prolonged steroid therapy should have calcium and vitamin D supplementation and bone mineral density studies to help prevent pathological osteoporosis.

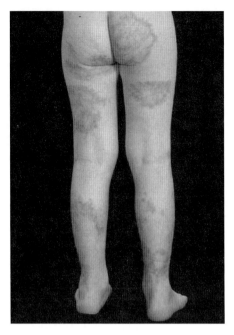

Fig. 13.3.9 Vasculitic rash on the buttocks and legs of a 5-year-old boy with polyarteritis nodosa also affecting his renal and hepatic vessels.

Non-inflammatory musculoskeletal disorders

General practitioners and paediatricians see many children with joint symptoms, the majority of whom will not have an inflammatory arthritis or connective tissue disorder. The history for these children is often shorter or more episodic and usually the joint discomfort is associated with activities relieved by rest. These symptoms are mechanical in origin and are related to underlying factors such as ligamentous laxity (hypermobility), overuse, poor fitness or specific inherited physiques (such as pes planus or genu valgus).

Hypermobility disorders

Marked ligamentous (and soft tissue) laxity is often seen in specific genetic disorders such as Ehlers–Danlos syndrome and Marfan syndrome, but also occurs in Down syndrome and Stickler disease. Far commoner is so called benign joint hypermobility, where inherited ligamentous laxity is associated with musculoskeletal symptoms such as 'growing pains', recurrent lower limb arthralgia, painful flat feet, anterior knee pain syndrome and adolescent mechanical back pain. Bursitis and tendonitis can also be seen, particularly in older children. Mechanical spinal pain disorders in adolescence are becoming more common and appear to be associated with increasing sedentariness and obesity. It is possible that these may predispose to premature degenerative spinal disease and osteoarthritis in later life.

Chronic pain disorders

In some children, musculoskeletal symptoms develop in the absence of any definable organic pathology. Fibromyalgia or chronic widespread pain disorder is a symptom complex of chronic muscle and joint pain, marked sleep disturbance and the presence of typical tender or trigger points in the musculature. Another form of chronic pain disorder is more localized and is called reflex sympathetic dystrophy or chronic regional pain syndrome. This takes the form of a limb or joint that becomes painful after minor injury and is immobilized with avoidance of movement. Subsequent sensory and vasomotor disturbance may follow with discoloration, altered sweating and eventually atrophy of tissue if untreated. Patients are typical preadolescent or early-adolescent females who are often highly disabled by their symptoms, with cessation of physical activities and school absence.

These disorders are considered by most practitioners to have a major psychogenic component but physical deconditioning and tissue changes may become significant and physical treatment of this is an important part of rehabilitation. Psychological therapies are usually required but children have a much better outcome overall than adults.

PART 14

RESPIRATORY DISORDERS

Acute upper respiratory tract infections in childhood

C. Mellis

Upper respiratory tract infections (URTIs) are the scourge of young children and their parents. In the first 5 years of life children average six to eight episodes a year. The timing and frequency of these infections depends largely on the level of exposure; therefore they occur earlier and more often in those with older siblings and those who attend day care (Fig. 14.1.1). By far the majority of URTIs are viral in origin, of mild severity and of short duration (5–7 days). These illnesses are self-limiting and require no specific pharmacological intervention (Tables 14.1.1, 14.1.2). The age of the child is the major predictor of type, severity and extent of a viral respiratory tract infection (Table 14.1.2).

Nevertheless, these recurring URTIs of early childhood are important, particularly when they occur repeatedly during the winter months. Local complications of viral URTIs do occur in a significant percentage, especially acute otitis media and acute sinusitis (Fig. 14.1.2). Progression of the infection into the lower respiratory tract is a risk, particularly with some of the more potent respiratory viruses such as parainfluenza (the usual cause of viral 'croup'), respiratory syncytial virus (RSV – the usual cause of acute viral bronchiolitis), influenza virus and the recently recognized human metapneumovirus (HMP – which is closely related to RSV). The proportion who develop these lower respiratory tract complications depends largely upon the child's age and the specific infecting virus, plus other host and environmental factors (Fig. 14.1.3).

Additional issues with URTIs are: the clinical problem of differentiating common viral pharyngitis from uncommon streptococcal pharyngitis; viral URTIs can lead to significant systemic illnesses (such as Henoch–Schönlein purpura); and common respiratory viruses are by far the most common trigger of severe acute exacerbations of asthma in young children.

A difficulty with URTIs is the arbitrary definitions used to describe them, such as rhinitis, rhinosinusitis, pharyngitis, tonsillitis, stomatitis and otitis media. There is clearly substantial overlap with these syndromes, as the viral infection will frequently cross anatomical boundaries. Indeed, viral inflammation of the respiratory tract is usually diffuse rather than focal, while bacterial infections of the respiratory tract (such as streptococcal tonsillitis) are generally more anatomically localized.

The most common form of URTI is the 'common cold', which is also known as viral nasopharyngitis, acute coryzal illness or viral catarrh, but overall it is probably best described as an uncomplicated viral URTI.

Common cold (uncomplicated viral URTI)

This is defined as an acute illness where the major symptoms are:

- nasal (snuffliness, sneezing and rhinorrhoea)
- sore throat
- conjunctival irritation (red, watery eyes).

The symptoms are mild, fever is often minimal or absent and all symptoms resolve between 5 and 7 days.

The usual pathogen responsible for an uncomplicated viral URTI is rhinovirus, which has over 100 types. However, there are a large number of other respiratory viruses that can produce this syndrome (Table 14.1.1). These viruses are highly infectious and spread via both droplets (particularly by sneezing) and nasal secretions on hands and fomites (clothing, handkerchiefs, toys, cot sides). Viral shedding is maximal in the 7 days after inoculation and most have a short incubation period (2–3 days). Therefore, close proximity such as household contacts with older school-age siblings, day care attendance, overcrowding, lower socioeconomic status and poor personal hygiene are all associated with high rates of URTI (Fig. 14.1.3).

Local ENT complications of the common cold include otitis media and acute rhinosinusitis (Fig. 14.1.2), and a small proportion progress to involve the lower respiratory tract.

Pharyngitis (oropharyngitis/tonsillitis)

Pharyngitis is a clinical syndrome in which the major complaint is acute sore throat and/or discomfort on swallowing (dysphagia). The illness is generally mild and self-limiting, with three-quarters of patients free of pain within 2–3 days of onset, whether due to a respiratory virus or to beta-haemolytic streptococ-cus. However, there are a number of specific, recognizable syndromes of oropharyngitis/tonsillitis.

Ulcerative pharyngotonsillitis

This is usually due to an adenovirus infection and typically occurs in infants and toddlers. It produces an isolated exudative tonsillitis resembling strep-tococcal tonsillitis or Epstein–Barr pharyngitis. Adenoviruses (types 3, 4, 7, 14 and 21) also produce the very specific 'pharyngoconjunctival fever'. The enteroviruses (Coxsackie virus and echovirus) and herpes simplex virus can also produce ulcerative pharyngotonsillitis. Other respiratory viruses (including RSV and parainfluenza) usually cause a more diffuse nasopharyngitis rather than this focal tonsillar inflammation.

Epstein–Barr virus pharyngitis/tonsillitis

Although this typically occurs in older, school-age children it can cause an exudative tonsillitis in the very young. The tonsillitis is associated with a membrane and marked cervical lymphadenopathy may be associated with generalized symptoms, including fever, lethargy, anorexia and headache (this generalized illness is referred to as infectious mononucleosis, or 'glandular fever').

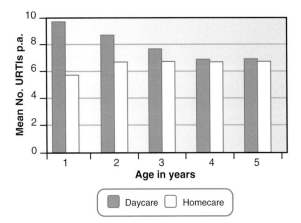

Fig. 14.1.1 Number of respiratory tract infections per year in infants and preschoolers (day care versus home care). From data in Isaacs D, Moxon E R 1996.

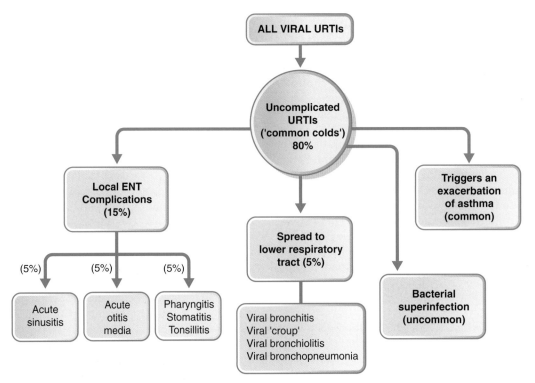

Fig. 14.1.2 Complications of viral upper respiratory tract infections.

Table 14.1.1 Infecting agents in upper respiratory tract infections

	Usual	Common	Uncommon
Common cold	Rhinoviruses	Coronaviruses Enteroviruses	Adenovirus Influenza A and B Respiratory syncytial virus (RSV)* Human metapneumovirus Parainfluenza[†]
Pharyngitis	Adenovirus[a]	Epstein–Barr virus[b] *Streptococcus*[d]	Herpes simplex[c] Coxsackie/echo[e,f] Parainfluenza Influenza A and B Coronaviruses

* School age children (infants and preschoolers commonly develop lower respiratory tract infection with RSV). [†] Parainfluenza, especially type 1, is the major cause of 'croup' in preschool children.
a–f, see text for details – a, ulcerative pharyngotonsillitis; b, Epstein–Barr viral pharyngitis; c herpes stomatitis; d, streptococcal tonsillitis; e, herpangina; f, hand, foot and mouth disease.

Table 14.1.2 Age of child and type of respiratory tract infection

Age	Type of infection
Newborn	Risk of acute, more generalized systemic illness with respiratory viruses (looks 'septic')
Infant	High risk of lower respiratory tract involvement with respiratory viruses (particularly acute viral bronchiolitis with respiratory syncytial virus and human metapneumovirus)
Toddler/preschooler	High risk of viral laryngotracheobronchitis ('croup') with respiratory viruses (especially parainfluenza viruses) Very frequent viral respiratory tract infections, mostly confined to upper respiratory tract
School age (5–15 years)	Lower rates of viral respiratory tract infections Suspect bacterial tonsillitis (streptococcal) Suspect Epstein–Barr viral pharyngitis/tonsillitis Suspect *Mycoplasma pneumoniae* if lower respiratory tract involvement (bronchitis and bronchopneumonia)

Primary herpes simplex stomatitis

This is due to infection with herpes simplex virus (HSV) types 1 and 2. The peak incidence is in children aged 1–3 years and it typically causes multiple discrete ulcers on the *anterior* regions of the oropharynx – tongue, gums and palate. It is generally accompanied by vesicles on the lips or circumoral region, significant fever and lymphadenopathy (especially submental and anterior cervical lymph glands). The ulcers generally persist for 5–7 days and can cause considerable pain, feeding difficulty and irritability. Asymptomatic oral shedding of HSV is common and can transmit the virus. Infection may be widespread in children with eczema and severe in those who are immunocompromised.

The usual treatment is orally or rectally administered analgesia, such as paracetamol. Local anaesthetic gels are commonly tried but are often ineffective because they sting when the child already has a painful mouth. There have also been adverse effects reported – including aspiration from pharyngeal numbness and seizures from excessive absorption.

Acyclovir is generally administered only in immunocompromised children. While there is a study showing benefit from acyclovir in HSV stomatitis in normal hosts, it is only effective if given within 72 hours of onset, which is often before the peak of the number of ulcers and commonest timing of presentation. Acyclovir is expensive and has to be given 5 times a day orally to a child with a very sore mouth. The risk of persisting HSV infection and recurrent

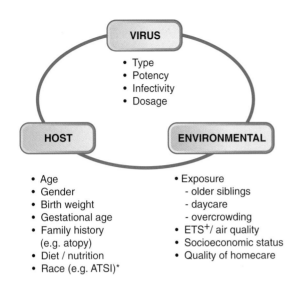

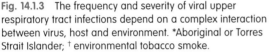

Fig. 14.1.3 The frequency and severity of viral upper respiratory tract infections depend on a complex interaction between virus, host and environment. *Aboriginal or Torres Strait Islander; [†] environmental tobacco smoke.

cold sores after treatment of primary stomatitis has not been studied but in primary genital herpes infections treatment has been associated with earlier and more severe recurrences when treatment groups were compared with placebo groups.

The virus may result in persistent dormant infection in the oral region, with recrudescent orolabial infections ('cold sores'). These episodes may be triggered by the fever of future intercurrent viral infections, stress, menstruation and exposure to cold or ultraviolet radiation.

Herpangina

This typically occurs in preschool children and is due to one of the enteroviruses (Coxsackie virus or echovirus). It results in a number of discrete mouth ulcers, localized to the *posterior* portion of the oropharynx – tonsillar pillars, pharyngeal wall, uvula and palate. This distribution contrasts with the anterior ulcers due to herpes simplex virus.

Hand, foot and mouth disease

This illness of young children is due to enteroviruses and results in lesions similar to those of HSV. The usual symptoms are sore throat and refusal to eat and drink. These symptoms are often accompanied by a vesicular or macular papular rash on the hands, feet, buttocks or trunk. The mouth ulcers are generally on the tongue, palate and buccal mucosa. The illness classically occurs in mini-epidemics, making clinical recognition relatively simple.

Acute bacterial tonsillitis ('streptococcal pharyngitis')

Group A beta-haemolytic streptococcus is the usual bacterial cause of acute pharyngitis (Table 14.1.3) and is the only common form of pharyngitis for which antibiotics have a role. While it is important to distinguish viral pharyngitis from streptococcal pharyngitis, unfortunately this is not easy on clinical grounds; however, if three or more of the following characteristics are present then it is more likely that the child has a streptococcal infection:

- fever
- tonsillar exudate

Clinical example

At the age of 18 months, Jennifer developed a high fever and became very irritable. She cried loudly when given cordial to drink and spat it out. She could not swallow her saliva and was dribbling constantly. Her mouth looked red and inflamed, and her mother took her immediately to see her GP.

Jennifer was difficult to examine but her mouth seemed very painful. She had submental and cervical lymphadenopathy. With gentle persuasion, her GP encouraged her to open her mouth. The gingivae and anterior oropharynx were bright red, and there were many small ulcers on her gums and on the tongue and hard palate, many of which were covered by a grey-white exudate.

Jennifer had an acute gingivostomatitis, almost certainly due to herpes simplex virus. She was given small frequent sips of water and milk to maintain her hydration. She could not take paracetamol because she had difficulty swallowing in the first 24 hours, and it was difficult to apply a topical analgesic gel because of pain. The first night, a paracetamol suppository was used to provide some analgesia. The ulcers healed after 4 days and did not leave any scars.

Table 14.1.3   Clinical features of group A beta-haemolytic streptococcal tonsillitis

History
- Age 5–15 years
- Abrupt onset
- Severe sore throat (pain and difficulty swallowing)
- Systemic symptoms
  - headache
  - abdominal pain/nausea/vomiting
- No cough or coryzal/nasal symptoms

Examination
- Tonsillar exudate, purulent and patchy (rather than a membrane); marked inflammation of throat and tonsils
- Enlarged, tender bilateral anterior cervical lymph nodes
- No nasal discharge

- tender, enlarged anterior cervical lymph nodes
- absence of cough and/or coryzal symptoms.

While this clinical dilemma can be overcome by use of rapid laboratory (antigen detection) tests, a throat culture remains the gold standard for confirming the presence of streptococcal pharyngitis and rational use of antibiotics.

While it would appear logical to give antibiotics in the presence of streptococcal pharyngitis, current evidence casts doubts on efficacy. A Cochrane review of randomized control trials concluded that antibiotics confer little benefit (in terms of pain relief) in the treatment of sore throat, irrespective of whether the infection is due to a virus or streptococcus. However, in children known to be at high risk of complications of streptococcal infection (poststreptococcal glomerulonephritis and/or rheumatic fever), the threshold for giving antibiotics should be considerably lower. Populations at particular risk include Aboriginal and Torres Strait Islanders, Maori and Pacific Islander children.

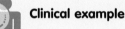

Clinical example

Adam who was not Aboriginal, Torres Strait Islander, Maori or Pacific Islander and was 3 years old, presented with fever, sore throat and difficulty swallowing during the previous 24 hours. When first seen he had an axillary temperature of 38.2°C and both tonsils were swollen and inflamed, with a visible yellow exudate scattered over both tonsils. There was bilateral enlargement of the lymph nodes in the anterior cervical chain. A clinical diagnosis of acute streptococcal tonsillitis was made, a throat swab was taken for culture and oral penicillin was considered but not prescribed at this time as Adam was at low risk of suppurative or rheumatic complications of streptococcal infection. He represented several days later because of ongoing fever and the development of a clear nasal discharge and watery eyes. He had a mild dry cough but was now drinking well and not complaining of a sore throat. His throat culture was sterile. The illness was almost certainly due to a respiratory virus (such as parainfluenza or adenovirus). Several days later Adam's mother rang to say that he was now virtually back to his normal self. This case clearly demonstrates the major clinical difficulty in distinguishing a bacterial from a viral tonsillitis/pharyngitis.

Acute sinusitis (rhinosinusitis)

Bacterial infection of the paranasal sinuses occurs in approximately 5–10% of viral URTIs and generally involves the maxillary sinuses. The usual manifestation is a profuse, mucopurulent nasal discharge with nasal obstruction. Uncomplicated acute viral rhinosinusitis normally resolves without specific treatment in 7–10 days. Thus, if the child has a purulent nasal discharge continuing beyond 10 days, the possibility of secondary bacterial sinusitis needs to be considered.

Although a Cochrane review of five randomized control trials involving over 400 children found that 10 days of antibiotics would reduce the probability of persistence of nasal discharge in the short to medium term, the benefits are modest and no long-term benefits have been documented. Despite this, current American Academy of Pediatrics Clinical Practice Guidelines (2001) recommend antibiotics for acute bacterial sinusitis to achieve a more rapid clinical cure. However, this controversial recommendation is restricted to those children diagnosed with 'persistent' or 'severe' sinusitis. Because complications of acute bacterial sinusitis can be serious, the sicker the child (high fever, toxic or constitutionally ill), or the more prolonged the symptoms (>10–14 days) the more prudent it is to prescribe antibiotics. The usual organisms responsible for acute bacterial sinusitis are *Streptococcus pneumoniae*, non-typeable *Haemophilus influenzae* and *Moraxella catarrhalis*. Amoxicillin plus clavulanic acid (co-amoxiclav) is therefore generally considered the antibiotic of choice.

Acute otitis media

See also Chapter 22.1.

This local complication of viral URTIs is characterized by earache, fever, reduced hearing and non-specific discomfort and irritability in the very young child. Examination shows a red tympanic membrane, loss of the normal anatomical landmarks on the tympanic membrane, the presence of a middle ear effusion and the eardrum may be visibly bulging. However, because not all of these signs may be easily observed, the diagnosis of acute otitis media is often made with a degree of uncertainty, particularly in infants and very young children.

Acute otitis media is the most frequent complication of viral URTI, particularly in the very young (6 months to 2 years of age). Virtually all children will have at least one episode of otitis media and some are particularly prone to this complication. Viral inflammation of the nasopharynx disrupts the function of the eustachian tubes, impairing ventilation, thus rendering the middle ear liable to infection. The microbiology of otitis media has been accurately documented in a recent large study from Finland. In this study, middle ear fluid was obtained (by myringotomy) in over 90% of 2500 episodes of clinical acute otitis media during the first 2 years of life. A bacterial pathogen, particularly pneumococcus,

M. catarrhalis and *H. influenzae*, was cultured in over 80%.

Although this suggests that young children with acute otitis media should be treated with an antibiotic, such as amoxicillin plus clavulanic acid (co-amoxiclav), the evidence is unimpressive. A Cochrane review of seven randomized control trials (over 2000 children) found no reduction in earache at 24 hours between antibiotics and placebo, and only a 6% absolute reduction in pain at 2–7 days. The authors found that approximately 80% of all children with acute otitis media, irrespective of treatment, will be pain-free by 2–7 days. Thus, the benefit of antibiotics is small and is possibly outweighed by the 5% risk of adverse effects (rash, diarrhoea and/or vomiting). Consequently, simple oral or topical analgesics (anaesthetic ear drops) may be the best option. However, as with streptococcal pharyngitis, in patients at increased risk of suppurative complications of otitis media (particularly Aboriginals, Torres Strait Islanders, Maoris and Pacific Islanders) the threshold for prescribing antibiotics should be substantially lower.

The duration of antibiotic administration has also been addressed in a Cochrane review, which concluded that 5 days of antibiotics is adequate treatment for uncomplicated ear infections in children. This review considered those randomized control trials that compared short-course antibiotics (<7 days) to longer courses (≥ 7 days) and found no difference in outcome.

Streptococcus pneumoniae is the most common reported bacterial cause of acute otitis media (between one-third and one-half of all cases) and initial trials of multivalent conjugate vaccines against the serotypes responsible for otitis media have been shown to be effective.

The recent (2004) American Academy of Pediatrics Clinical Practice Guideline for diagnosis and management of acute otitis media is an excellent summary of the published data about this condition.

Approach to management of respiratory tract infections

Uncomplicated viral URTIs (common cold)

It should be evident that antibiotics are not indicated in this condition. A Cochrane review has demonstrated that antibiotics offer no advantage over placebo; further, antibiotics were associated with a 6% rate of adverse events (rashes and gastrointestinal symptoms).

Numerous potential therapies for the common cold have been the subject of Cochrane reviews. These include antihistamines, nasal decongestants, vitamin C, zinc, *Echinacea* and heated, humidified air.

Antihistamines as monotherapy do not alleviate nasal congestion, rhinorrhoea nor sneezing. While combinations of antihistamines and nasal decongestants are not effective in preschool children, in older children they are of benefit as regards both nasal symptoms and general recovery. However, the clinical relevance of these beneficial effects is unclear and need to be balanced against potential side effects. For example, in the most recent randomized controlled trial, almost 50% of the children receiving the 'antihistamine and nasal decongestant' combination were asleep within 2 hours of the medication, compared to 27% in the placebo. Obviously, from the parents' viewpoint this 'adverse' event would be seen as desirable. Nevertheless, antihistamines have been associated with paradoxical excitability, hallucinations, agitation and seizures. Furthermore, 10% of all poison centre calls are related to overdose with various cough and cold medications.

When used as prophylaxis, vitamin C failed to reduce the rate of common colds; and when introduced at the onset of colds (as therapy) vitamin C did not show any benefit. The evidence for zinc lozenges for treating colds is inconclusive, although the reviewers felt that this deserved further study. *Echinacea* has been popularized over recent years for both preventing and treating the common cold. Cochrane reviewers concluded that, although the majority of available studies reported positive results, the quality of the trials was poor and the results were inconclusive, because of the heterogeneity of both the preparations used and the outcome measures employed. Obviously, further high-quality multicentre randomized control trials are indicated to address this question appropriately. Conflicting results have been published about heated, humidified air and Cochrane reviewers recommend a multicentre randomized control trial using a standardized outcome measure.

Reduce exposure

Reducing exposure to respiratory viruses is extremely difficult. In day-care settings, cohorting of children into smaller and age-specific groups is of benefit. While the cohorting, or exclusion, of children suffering from URTIs may help, unfortunately person-to-person spread often occurs before the child has obvious symptoms of an URTI.

Simple measures such as handwashing by both staff and children, improving ventilation and reducing overcrowding are all of value (Table 14.1.4).

Reduced exposure to environmental tobacco smoke

While the evidence relating to respiratory infections and passive smoking relates predominantly to lower

Table 14.1.4 Prevention of upper respiratory tract infections
Reduction of exposure in day care   • Cohorting (both age and symptomatic of respiratory tract infection)   • Reducing overcrowding   • Improving ventilation   • Individual use of personal items (e.g. toothbrushes and facecloths)   • Strict handwashing by both staff and children
Education of parents about spread of respiratory viruses and appropriate care   • Similar issues to those outlined above for day care   • Education concerning no antibiotics for URTIs   • Symptomatic treatment should be minimal (e.g. oral analgesics)

Reduced exposure to environmental tobacco smoke, especially in homes and cars
 Vaccination
 • Influenza vaccine
  • to prevent serious influenza A and B infections in young children
  • to reduce the pool of infection to protect the elderly community
 • Pneumococcal conjugate vaccine (to reduce rates of acute otitis media)

respiratory infections, there is also evidence that URTIs in young children are increased in those exposed to environmental tobacco smoke.

Immunization

The effect of immunization against the serotypes responsible for pneumococcal otitis media has now been demonstrated, although further trials are essential.

The use of influenza A and B vaccine in infants and young children remains controversial. Recent American studies found that, during years when influenza viruses predominate, the rates of hospitalization with acute respiratory disease in children under 2 years of age (without specific risk factors) were as high as 2% per annum. Consequently, it has been suggested that routine influenza immunization be considered in all young children. A recent Japanese study found that routine immunization of schoolchildren caused a major reduction in mortality from influenza in the elderly. This confirms that children are the major disseminators of influenza, and routine annual influenza immunization for children could become policy in the near future.

In children over the age of 1 year, it is possible to use neuraminidase inhibitors, which are potent, safe agents effective against both influenza A and B virus.

A recent Cochrane review concluded that both inhaled zanamivir and oral oseltamivir were effective in shortening illness duration (by 1.0–1.5 days) and hastening return to normal activity in previously healthy children with influenza. Efficacy in 'at risk' children remains to be proved. Emergence of drug-resistant strains of viruses has not been a significant problem.

Summary

The vast majority of respiratory tract infections in young children are uncomplicated 'common colds' that require no specific treatment. Although local ENT complications are not uncommon, antibiotic treatment for acute sinusitis and acute otitis media offers very limited benefit but does cause adverse effects (particularly rashes and gastrointestinal symptoms). A very small proportion of URTIs are bacterial. Streptococcal tonsillitis resolves quickly without complication in the majority of children without antibiotics. When treating populations known to be at high risk of suppurative complications, high rates of poststreptococcal glomerulonephritis or rheumatic fever, there must be a substantially lower threshold for antibiotic treatment.

The age of the child, the specific infective agent and other host and environmental factors have a major bearing on the nature of the respiratory infections, including the timing, frequency, severity and likelihood of either local or distant complications.

Practical points

- Young children experience six to eight viral URTIs per year. A large variety of respiratory viruses can cause URTIs in young children
- The vast majority (approx. 80%) of respiratory tract infections in young children are mild, self-limiting viral URTIs ('common colds') that require no treatment
- The child's age and the specific type of virus are the most powerful predictors of the type of respiratory infection the child will experience
- Local ENT complications of viral URTIs (e.g. acute sinusitis, acute otitis media, pharyngitis) occur in approximately 15% of URTIs. Although these may benefit from symptomatic therapy (such as analgesics), antibiotics are not generally necessary
- A very small proportion of URTIs are bacterial (and may have a slight benefit from antibiotics). The most common is streptococcal pharyngitis ('tonsillitis'), especially in school-age children
- Both spread of the viral infection into the lower respiratory tract and secondary bacterial infection are uncommon complications

Stridor and croup

P. D. Sly

Stridor and croup are both disorders that have obstruction of the middle airways as an underlying cause of the symptoms with which they present.

Stridor

Physiological principles

Stridor is defined in *Dorland's Illustrated Medical Dictionary* (28th edition) as 'a harsh, high-pitched respiratory sound such as the inspiratory sound often heard in acute laryngeal obstruction'. While this definition is strictly correct, it is not all that helpful and gives no information about how and why stridor comes about. Stridor is a harsh, high pitched noise heard predominantly during inspiration. Consideration of the physiological principles underlying this fact gives some clue as to the site of the lesion causing the stridor. The presence of an added respiratory sound implies an obstruction to the free flow of gas through the airway tree. This obstruction is usually known as flow limitation. Flow limitation in a compliant tube, such as the airways, is accompanied by fluttering of the walls, which occurs to conserve energy when driving pressure exceeds the pressure required to produce the maximal flow. The fluttering of the walls produces a respiratory noise. When this phenomenon occurs during inspiration, the resultant noise is known as stridor, and when it occurs during expiration, the noise is known as wheeze.

During breathing, there are pressure gradients between the airway opening and the alveoli. Inspiration occurs when alveolar pressure is lowered below atmospheric pressure and air flows in to equalize the pressures. At the onset of expiration, alveolar pressure exceeds atmospheric pressure and air flows out. There are also pressure gradients across the airway wall and these tend to alter airway calibre. The pressure around the extrathoracic airways, that is, those above the thoracic inlet, is atmospheric, while the pressure around the intrathoracic airways essentially is equal to the pleural pressure. As illustrated in Figure 14.2.1, the pressure gradients across the airway wall during inspiration means that there is a net force tending to narrow the extrathoracic airways

and to dilate the intrathoracic airways (Fig. 14.2.1A). During expiration, the direction of the forces is opposite, resulting in a tendency to narrow intrathoracic airways and dilate extrathoracic airways (Fig. 14.2.1B).

As stridor is an inspiratory noise, the predominant site of obstruction (the site responsible for the flow limitation) is generally in the extrathoracic airways. Stridor with an expiratory component, that is, where the noise can also be heard at the beginning of expiration, can result from either a severe obstruction producing flow limitation during expiration as well, or from a lesion that extends into the intrathoracic airways.

Differential diagnosis

When considering the differential diagnosis, several factors need to be taken into consideration. These include:

- *Age of onset.* A stridor present from the first few days of life suggests a congenital or structural cause
- *Speed of onset of symptoms.* Infective causes such as croup tend to come on quickly; however, most cases of congenital or structural stridor commonly first present following a viral upper respiratory illness
- *Progression of stridor.* Stridor increasing in severity over weeks to months suggests a progressive lesion, such as subglottic haemangioma
- *Effect of body position.* Stridor that is worse when lying supine is seen commonly with laryngomalacia
- *Presence of an expiratory component.* This suggests a more severe obstruction that limits flow during expiration as well as during inspiration
- *Quality of voice.* While the voice is frequently normal, a hoarse voice would suggest a vocal cord lesion
- *Other medical conditions that could contribute to the pathogenesis or presentation:* febrile illness, ex-premature infant, gastro-oesophageal reflux, cutaneous haemangiomas, Möbius syndrome (a very rare syndrome characterized by congenital palsy of the external rectus and facial muscles, usually bilateral, associated with paralysis of the sixth and seventh nerves)

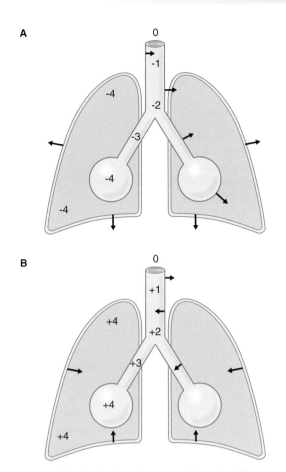

Fig. 14.2.1 The distribution of pressures throughout the respiratory system during (**A**) inspiration and (**B**) expiration. Atmospheric pressure is shown as zero. During inspiration, the expansion of the thorax results in pleural pressure falling below atmospheric. This relatively negative pressure is transmitted to the alveoli and a pressure gradient is established between the airway opening and the alveoli. Gas flows into the lungs along this pressure gradient. The pressure outside the airways is essentially pleural pressure and results in net forces that tend to expand intrathoracic airways and to collapse the extrathoracic trachea. As shown in B, the pressure gradients are opposite during expiration.

Classification

1. Acute stridor

a. Common causes:
   • laryngotracheobronchitis (croup)
b. Rare causes (in developed countries):
   • laryngeal trauma
   • acute angioneurotic oedema
   • retropharyngeal abscess
   • peritonsillar abscess (quinsy)
   • acute epiglottitis (typically a low-pitched rumbling noise coming from the supraglottic area)
   • diphtheria

2. Persistent stridor

a. Common causes:
   • laryngomalacia (infantile larynx)
   • congenital subglottic stenosis
   • acquired subglottic stenosis in a premature infant who required intubation
b. Uncommon causes:
   • subglottic haemangioma
   • vocal cord palsy (unilateral or bilateral)
   • laryngeal webs
   • cysts of the posterior tongue or aryepiglottic folds
   • subglottic mucus retention cysts in a premature infant who required intubation
   • vascular ring (note that this usually presents with a predominantly expiratory noise)
c. Rare causes:
   • laryngocele
   • laryngeal cleft
   • tracheal stenosis (note that this usually presents with a predominantly expiratory noise).

Characteristics of the more important causes of stridor

Laryngomalacia

Laryngomalacia, which is sometimes known as infantile larynx, is the most common cause of persistent stridor. It is not well named, as the larynx and vocal cords are actually normal. The supraglottic tissues appear as if they are too large for the size of the glottis and narrow the glottic aperture during inspiration instead of the more normal widening during inspiration. This can occur in a number of ways, the most common being:

• a long, curled (sometimes called omega-shaped) epiglottis collapsing during inspiration so that the lateral walls touch, restricting the free passage of air
• floppy arytenoid processes prolapsing into the glottic aperture during inspiration
• a long epiglottis collapsing against the posterior pharyngeal wall during inspiration.

In more severe cases combinations of these mechanisms may be responsible for the inspiratory obstruction.

Laryngomalacia classically produces a cog-wheel stridor, with no expiratory component. The cog-wheel nature to the stridor is likely to come from vibrations of the supraglottic tissues as the degree of obstruction varies during the inspiratory effort. The stridor may be worse when the infant is lying supine, although this feature is not always seen. More severe obstruction may be associated with suprasternal and sternal retraction during inspiration.

Laryngomalacia is usually a benign condition that does not require any treatment, except to reassure the parents that this is the case. Severe laryngomalacia may be associated with failure to thrive and gastro-oesophageal reflux. The importance of parental reassurance should not be underestimated, as the stridor is likely to last for 2–3 years. Frequently, parents find the most distressing part of having a child with laryngomalacia are the looks from people when they take the child out in public and the well intentioned advice received from relatives.

Clinical example

Tran was a 3-month-old infant who had been referred to the respiratory medicine clinic for assessment of persistent stridor. She was born at term following an uneventful antenatal course and normal vaginal delivery. The stridor was not present at birth and was noticed for the first time at the age of 2 months when she caught a cold from her older brother. Her mother was extremely concerned that something was seriously wrong with her baby as several relatives had told her it is not normal for a baby to make this type of noise.

Since that time the stridor had been present on most days but was less commonly heard when Tran was sleeping. Her mother was concerned that the stridor was becoming louder and, on questioning, reported that sometimes an expiratory component could be heard. The stridor was typically worse when Tran was crying or when lying supine for nappy changes.

Examination revealed a female infant who looked scrawny. Her height was on the 50% percentile but her weight was just below the 10% percentile. She had two typical strawberry naevi on her trunk. While being held in her mother's arms, a cog-wheel stridor with no expiratory component could be clearly heard. When she was lying supine, the stridor was associated with a soft but definite expiratory component and mild suprasternal retraction.

Discussion points
- What is the most likely diagnosis?
- What investigations are warranted?

A flexible bronchoscopy was performed under general anaesthesia and revealed laryngomalacia, with a tightly coiled epiglottis and prolapsing arytenoid processes. The subglottic area and lower airways were normal.

Discussion points
- Is any treatment warranted?
- Is the fact that Tran's weight percentile is lower than her height percentile of concern?
- Is the laryngomalacia likely to be responsible for her relative failure to thrive (lower weight percentile than height percentile)?
- How could this come about?

The bronchoscopic findings are diagnostic of laryngomalacia and one can be confident that the symptoms will resolve spontaneously with time. The relative failure to thrive may be related to the increased work of breathing required to overcome the obstruction. However, a dietary assessment is warranted before attributing the failure to thrive to this mechanism. As the obstruction decreases with time, Tran's work of breathing will also decrease and the failure to thrive should resolve.

Subglottic stenosis

Subglottic stenosis refers to a narrowing in the upper part of the trachea, immediately below the glottis. This narrowing may be congenital or acquired. Congenital subglottic stenosis occurs typically at the level of, and involves, the cricoid cartilage. The tracheal epithelium typically appears normal but the cross-sectional area of the lumen is reduced and typically does not vary with respiration. Acquired subglottic stenosis usually results from trauma and is most commonly seen in premature infants who required intubation. Older infants and children who require prolonged intubation are also at risk. Here the tracheal epithelium is more likely to be replaced by scar tissue.

Subglottic stenosis may present soon after birth or the presentation may be delayed. The stenosis, either congenital or acquired, is usually not progressive but the degree of obstruction may increase, e.g. as the child's activity levels increase or at times of respiratory infection. The typical presentation is with stridor, particularly at times of respiratory infection. If the obstruction is severe enough, the stridor may have an expiratory component and be associated with suprasternal and sternal retractions.

Many cases of subglottic stenosis do not require treatment and most will improve with growth. Laser and dilatation treatments are generally disappointing. More severe obstruction may require surgery, usually involving a procedure in which the cricoid cartilage is split and reconstructed.

Subglottic haemangioma

The subglottic area can also be narrowed by a haemangioma occurring in this area. These are typical haemangiomas occurring in the submucosal layer of the tracheal wall. As with other haemangiomas, they enlarge during the first year of life and typically present with increasing stridor and inspiratory obstruction. The stridor is rarely present at birth and most come to attention around 4–6 months of age. As the obstruction becomes worse, the stridor develops an expiratory component and is associated with sternal and suprasternal retractions. Approximately 50% of subglottic haemangiomas are associated with cutaneous haemangiomas, although the converse association is much less frequent.

The earlier a subglottic haemangioma presents, the more likely that surgical treatment will be necessary. Tracheostomy remains the definitive treatment, although some cases do respond to medical treatment with corticosteroids or interferon.

Investigations

The most important investigations in elucidating the cause of a stridor are a thorough history and physical examination. As discussed above, the characteristics of the stridor, the time of onset, the progression and whether or not an expiratory component is present will clarify the cause of the stridor on many occasions.

The definitive investigation for stridor is a bronchoscopy, preferably performed with a flexible, fibreoptic bronchoscope. Laryngoscopy is not sufficient as the subglottic area and lower trachea cannot be safely and adequately assessed. Frequently the trachea can be visualized on penetrated radiographs of the chest and lateral neck; however, these X-rays rarely replace the need for bronchoscopy.

Croup (laryngotracheobronchitis)

Croup is usually considered to exist in two forms:

• acute viral croup
• recurrent (or spasmodic) croup.

While these two conditions have a number of similarities, they are likely to be distinct entities. They have in common that they involve the larynx, trachea and bronchi and present with a typically barking cough. The cough is so typical it is usually referred to as a 'croupy' cough.

Acute viral croup

Acute viral croup is typically a disease of toddlers, being rare in the first 6 months of life and reaching a peak incidence of 5 cases per 100 children per year during the second year of life. Boys are affected more commonly than girls. Most children who get acute viral croup will only ever have one or two episodes. These episodes typically begin with the symptoms of an upper respiratory infection and progress to typical croup over 1–2 days. The most common viruses isolated from children with croup are parainfluenza virus type 1 (up to 50% in some series), parainfluenza virus type 3 (up to 20%) and respiratory syncytial virus (approximately 10%).

Clinical manifestations

As mentioned above, croup usually begins with signs and symptoms of an upper respiratory infection, including fever and rhinitis. A cough may be present. The typical barking, croupy cough usually begins during the night or the early hours of the morning. As the disease progresses, stridor may be heard on exertion initially. If the subglottic obstruction progresses further, stridor may be heard at rest and an expiratory component may be heard. The typical cough continues to be heard.

If the degree of obstruction continues to worsen, the stridor may become more difficult to hear and the child may become distressed and restless. Cough may be absent at this stage. The lack of stridor comes about because the amount of air moving through the obstructed airway is not sufficient to generate the noise (see above). The distress and restlessness are most likely to be due to hypoxia and signal impending complete respiratory obstruction.

Clinical example

Jane was a 4-year-old girl who was brought to the emergency department by her mother, who reported increased wheezing over the past day, associated with a cold. Jane had a history of troublesome episodes of asthma for the past 3 years. She was reasonably well between episodes but, since starting preschool, her mother had noticed that Jane wheezed when running and appeared to tire more easily. Jane's mother reported that the wheeze was not really helped by bronchodilators and that inhaled steroids did not help prevent the attacks. On examination, Jane had an expiratory wheeze but had a prominent inspiratory component to her wheeze. She was not particularly distressed and her oxygen saturation was normal.

Discussion points
• What is the most likely diagnosis?
• What investigations are warranted?
 A chest X-ray showed an odd appearance to the upper mediastinum but was otherwise normal. Closer examination revealed a right-sided aortic arch and the ED consultant diagnosed the problem as being due to a vascular ring.

Discussion points
A vascular ring causes an obstruction to the intrathoracic portion of the trachea. Using the distribution of pressures throughout the respiratory system shown in Figure 14.2.1, explain the physical signs Jane presented with.

Practical points

• A careful history of the age of onset, features of preceding viral infection, nature and respiratory timing of the stridor are important for diagnosis.
• Many children with stridor will need no investigations.
• Persistent stridor with an expiratory component always warrants further investigation.

The viral illness generally lasts 7–10 days, but the typical croupy cough usually only occurs on the first 2–3 nights.

Investigations

Most children with croup do not warrant any investigations. Viral diagnosis on nasal secretions, usually obtained by per nasal aspiration, can be helpful from an epidemiological point of view but will not alter management. Chest X-rays are not helpful for children with typical croup.

Children less than 6 months old who present with croup or those whose croup runs an atypical course warrant investigation. The most useful investigations are likely to be a lateral neck X-ray and flexible bronchoscopy.

Management

The majority of children with croup do not require any treatment. Symptomatic treatment for fever and cold symptoms may be warranted. Children with a croupy cough and stridor on exertion (but not at rest) can usually be managed with supportive treatment only. There is a widespread belief that exposing these children to steam, especially by steaming up the home bathroom, helps relieve stridor. There is no evidence to support this treatment. The only benefit that is likely to come from sitting with the child in a steamy bathroom is from sitting quietly with the child and not from the steam.

Children with stridor at rest warrant medical assessment. The most useful treatment for croup that has reached this severity is corticosteroids. These can be give orally in syrup form or inhaled (nebulizer or metered dose inhaler and spacer). The mechanism of action is not known but is likely to be via a topical action. A single dose of steroids decreases the risk of hospitalization dramatically.

More severe obstruction can be relieved by nebulized adrenaline (epinephrine). Traditionally this has been given as a 50:50 mix of the L- and D-isoforms (known as racemic adrenaline), but the L-isoform (as found in standard ampoules of intravenous adrenaline) is as effective and is now commonly used. This relieves obstruction by causing a topical vasoconstriction, which wears off in 1–4 hours, depending on the severity of the underlying obstruction.

Severe obstruction may require intubation or even tracheostomy, although the need for these types of treatment has become much less with the widespread use of oral corticosteroids in the emergency departments of paediatric hospitals in Australia.

Practical points

- Use of corticosteroids can favourably modify the course of acute viral croup
- Severe croup can lead to complete airway obstruction and death

---

Recurrent (spasmodic) croup

Some children suffer recurrent episodes of croup, frequently without the preceding viral prodrome usually seen in acute viral croup. Typically these children are well when they go to bed and wake in the early hours of the morning with a barking cough and stridor. Fever is unusual in this form of croup. The same viruses as found in acute viral croup may be found in the upper airways of children with spasmodic croup, although the relationship between the viruses and the symptoms is less clear. Frequently children with recurrent croup have a family history of atopy and asthma or have asthma themselves. This, together with the uncertain relationship between the clinical symptoms and the presence of a virus, have led to the concept that spasmodic croup maybe a manifestation of upper airway hyperresponsiveness. There are no direct data to support or refute this hypothesis.

Spasmodic croup may be severe enough to require treatment with oral corticosteroids, nebulized adrenaline or even intubation; however, the episodes are frequently short lived and often settle by the time the child presents to the emergency department.

While controlled trials have not been carried out, there is a substantial body of anecdotal evidence that frequent bouts of recurrent croup can be prevented by maintenance therapy with inhaled corticosteroids via a spacer.

Asthma 14.3

R. Henry

Asthma is the most common chronic illness in children. It is the major acute illness requiring admission to hospital in most developed countries, including Australia and New Zealand, and is the major chronic condition associated with absence from school. Despite its frequency, there is no definition of asthma that encapsulates its features and is of practical value in making the diagnosis in an individual child.

For the clinician, asthma is recurrent episodes of wheeze, cough and breathlessness. This is an oversimplification, because it is possible to have asthma without the triad of wheeze, cough and breathlessness. Furthermore, a minority of children with these symptoms will have other conditions.

For the physiologist, asthma is a condition associated with airway hyperreactivity (loosely referred to as 'twitchy airways') and with reversible airways obstruction. Objective measurement of airway hyperresponsiveness can be obtained by measuring lung function such as peak expiratory flow (PEF) or forced expiratory volume in 1 second (FEV_1) in a bronchial challenge test. Airway hyperreactivity is defined as a significant fall (usually about 15–20%) in lung function after inhalation of chemicals (such as methacholine, histamine or mannitol), after inhalation of hypertonic saline, after cold, dry air or following exercise. Airway hyperreactivity and reversible (or variable) airways obstruction also may be demonstrated by an increase in PEF or FEV_1 of more than 10% following a bronchodilator, or by fluctuations in PEF measurements obtained on a regular basis at home. There are limitations to this physiological definition of asthma. These include the fact that most children are unable to cooperate with challenge tests to measure airway hyperresponsiveness (AHR) until they are 5 or 6 years old, and that there is an imperfect correlation between children with AHR and clinical features of asthma.

For the pathologist, the definition of asthma relates to mucosal oedema, mucous hypersecretion and smooth muscle spasm in the small airways. Airway inflammation is prominent. A limitation of this definition is that airway specimens have been difficult to obtain before death. In recent years non-invasive methods, such as induction of sputum with hypertonic saline or measurement of exhaled nitric oxide (NO), or invasive methods, such as bronchoalveolar lavage (BAL) at bronchoscopy, have enabled research into airway inflammation.

For the immunologist, the focus for asthma is on the atopic state. In an allergic response, degranulation of mast cells occurs, with the release of chemical mediators into the airways and a resultant asthmatic response. Our understanding of the cytokines that are important in asthma remains incomplete. Indeed, the mast cell, the eosinophil and the neutrophil all seem to have important roles in the pathogenesis of asthma.

What causes asthma?

The causes of asthma may be thought of at a number of different levels (Table 14.3.1). Genetic factors are important in predisposition. If one identical twin has asthma, the other twin has a 60% chance of developing asthma. Genetic markers for asthma have been reported on many different chromosomes, including 5, 6, 7, 11 and 12. It may be that there is genetic heterogeneity or that different components of heredity are being described, such as inheritance of atopy in contrast to inheritance of airway hyperresponsiveness. Even when an individual is born with a genetic predisposition to asthma, environmental stimuli are necessary to induce (or sensitize to) the asthmatic state. Identification of inducers of asthma is difficult but they may include allergens and cigarette smoke (particularly in the early months of life). One explanation for the observed increase in asthma incidence is the 'hygiene hypothesis'. The hypothesis is that early exposure to infection stimulates a T helper 1 (Th1) lymphocyte response, whereas absence of infection stimulates a Th2 lymphocyte response, with production of IgE. If there are few infections in early life, the Th2 response may persist for longer in childhood. In developed countries with advantaged living standards, the frequency of infections in early life, particularly severe infections, is less than in disadvantaged countries. This is an explanation for the observations that asthma is more common in developed than developing countries, and that older siblings and attendance at day care are protective against asthma.

Table 14.3.1 Causes of asthma
Predisposing • Genetic: ? chromosomes 5, 6, 7, 11, 12
Inducers (sensitizers) • Hygiene hypothesis • Allergens • Cigarette smoke • Other irritants, such as ozone • Occupational (rare in children)
Triggers • Infections, e.g. viral, *Mycoplasma*, pertussis • Exercise, especially in cold, dry air • Allergens, e.g. house dust mite, pollen, animal dander, foods • Environment, e.g. cigarette smoke, ozone, SO_2 • Emotional, such as laughing • Chemicals, e.g. salicylates, metabisulphite
Sustainers (maintainers) • Allergens • Viruses • Environmental irritants

Once asthma has developed, a variety of triggers may precipitate individual attacks. Viral respiratory infections are by far the most important, with at least 80% of admissions to hospital with asthma being associated with viral infections. Other triggers are listed in Table 14.3.1. Once asthma is established, ongoing environmental factors are necessary to sustain (or maintain) the asthmatic state. Allergens, viruses and non-specific irritants have all been shown to increase airway hyperresponsiveness.

Diagnosis

The diagnosis of asthma is easy to make in the child who has:

• recurrent episodes of wheeze
• breathlessness
• cough

and who is

• completely well between attacks.

Other clinical presentations may be less classical, such as:

• nocturnal cough
• persistent cough in association with acute respiratory infections
• a history of 'rattly breathing' in the absence of a definite history of wheeze.

In each of these scenarios asthma is possible, although unlikely. One approach is a therapeutic trial of asthma medications, such as a bronchodilator at the time of symptoms. In other cases, investigations may be necessary to support the diagnosis of asthma or to suggest another diagnosis. Useful tests may be:

• chest X-ray (abnormalities will suggest another diagnosis)
• measurement of FEV_1 before and after a bronchodilator (reversible airways obstruction would confirm asthma)
• a bronchial provocation test (a significant fall in FEV_1 or PEF after inhalation of hypertonic saline would support asthma)
• allergen skin prick tests (demonstration of atopy would support asthma).

Investigations

The majority of children with asthma, especially those with infrequent episodic symptoms, do not require any investigations. As indicated above, tests such as a chest X-ray or tests of airway hyperresponsiveness have more of a role in making the diagnosis or suggesting another cause than in assessing the asthma.

Lung function

Spirometry to measure FEV_1 and forced vital capacity before and after a bronchodilator may help assess severity and response to therapy. Between exacerbations, children with episodic disease will have normal lung function and no further improvement after bronchodilators. Children with persistent symptoms may show airways obstruction with improvement after inhalation of a bronchodilator. Fixed airways obstruction suggests either severe asthma or an alternative diagnosis such as cystic fibrosis.

Portable peak flow meters can be used at home on a regular basis to measure PEF. Children with well controlled disease will have normal values with little variability between readings. Poorly controlled asthma is associated with both decreased PEF and wide fluctuations in PEF over days or weeks. In most cases regular PEF measurement will be unnecessary.

Allergy tests

The role of allergen skin prick testing in asthma is controversial. Some paediatricians believe that allergen testing does not result in information that is of any clinical relevance; others believe it is an essential part of assessment of the child with asthma. Most children with asthma are atopic but allergen avoidance measures have not been shown to have a major role in management (Ch. 13.1).

Pattern of asthma

There is a wide spectrum of severity of asthma. This is relevant in terms of management and prognosis. Some children have episodic symptoms, with extended periods when they are totally symptom-free. Others have persistent asthma, with symptoms present on most days. One way to classify the spectrum of severity of asthma is:

- *infrequent episodic*
- *frequent episodic*
- *persistent asthma.*

The distinctions between these three categories are somewhat arbitrary. Children with infrequent episodic symptoms may be typified as those who have up to five exacerbations of asthma a year and are well clinically and have normal lung function in the symptom-free intervals. About 75% of children with asthma have infrequent episodic disease. About 20% of children with asthma have frequent episodic asthma. They may have six or more attacks per year but are well between exacerbations. Those with persistent asthma (about 5%) will have symptoms on most days.

Questions that are particularly helpful in clarifying the pattern of asthma include:

- are there nocturnal symptoms?
- are there symptoms on waking in the morning?
- is there normal exercise tolerance?
- how much school is missed because of asthma?
- how frequent is the use of bronchodilator medication?
- how frequent are asthma symptoms?

Management

Drugs used to treat asthma

There are two main strategies in the drug treatment of asthma. The first is the use of *reliever* medications to reverse acute airway obstruction. The main drugs are:

- bronchodilators (beta-2 sympathomimetic agents, anticholinergic agents and theophyllines)
- corticosteroids.

The second is preventing symptoms by decreasing airway inflammation and bronchial hyperreactivity. The main *preventer* medications are:

- corticosteroids (inhaled and oral)
- sodium cromoglycate and nedocromil sodium (inhaled non-steroidal)
- leukotriene antagonists (oral non-steroidal).

Symptom controllers (long-acting beta-2 sympathomimetic agents) are used in combination with inhaled corticosteroids to augment asthma preventer therapy.

Beta-2 sympathomimetics (beta-2 agonists) are the most widely used reliever medications. They are available as metered-dose aerosol inhalers, powder inhaler devices, nebulizer solutions, oral and injectable preparations. The preferred route of administration is by inhalation. Most children can use a powder inhaler device effectively from 5–6 years of age and a standard metered dose aerosol from 7–8 years. Spacer attachments, with a flexible facemask or with a one-way mouthpiece, will allow younger children to use a metered aerosol and are standard in acute attacks of asthma. The beta-2 agonists can be nebulized with a compressed air pump or using oxygen as the driving gas but this mode of drug delivery is only required for acute severe exacerbations.

Beta-2 agonists can be used immediately prior to exercise to help prevent exercise-triggered asthma.

Ipratropium bromide is an anticholinergic agent that is available as a nebulizer solution or as a metered aerosol. Its main use is in combination with beta-2 agonists in acute severe asthma.

Theophyllines are available as oral, rectal and intravenous preparations. Intravenous aminophylline used to be a first-line therapy in acute asthma but has been replaced by beta-2 agonists, the early use of oral corticosteroids and ipratropium bromide. The absorption of the rectal form is erratic and this preparation is not recommended. Long-acting oral preparations have been popular, especially to control nocturnal symptoms, but the emphasis on preventive therapy has led to decreased use.

Sodium cromoglycate is available as dry powder inhaler, metered aerosol or nebulizer solution, while nedocromil sodium is available as a metered aerosol. For both, the main target population is children with frequent episodic asthma in whom the aim is to prevent asthma symptoms. They are used on a regular basis over a number of months. In addition, either may be taken immediately before exercise to block asthma provoked by exercise.

Montelukast sodium is a leukotriene receptor antagonist and is available in oral form. It is an option as a preventer in frequent episodic asthma.

Corticosteroids are available as oral or injectable forms, metered-dose aerosols, dry powder inhaler devices and nebulized preparations. Oral corticosteroids are required by a minority of children for the treatment of acute exacerbations and by a small proportion of children with persistent asthma to optimize control. Inhaled corticosteroids are effective preventers. They are the therapy of choice for persistent asthma and one of the options with frequent episodic asthma. The use of spacer devices, especially in children receiving higher doses of inhaled corticosteroids (more than 200 µg of fluticasone propionate daily) is recommended to minimize the possibility of side effects from oropharyngeal deposition.

Clinical example

John was a 12-year-old boy who presented with a history of breathlessness and chest pain that occurred towards the end of an 800 m run. Neither cough nor wheeze was present. He had received bronchodilators and sodium cromoglycate before exercise without benefit. A trial of inhaled corticosteroids for 6 weeks had also been ineffective. His parents were both keen athletes and hoped that John would become a champion athlete.

Physical examination was normal. FEV_1 was normal and a hypertonic saline challenge test was negative, with no evidence of airway hyperresponsiveness. He was nonatopic on allergen skin tests. After an explanation to John and his parents that he did not have asthma, John indicated that he was not interested in competitive athletics. He was discharged on no treatment. One year later he was completely well. He could play regular sport with no difficulties. The tests used were helpful in confirming that John did not have asthma.

Clinical example

Jill was a 4-year-old who had persistent asthma. She had been admitted to hospital at the age of 3 months with bronchiolitis. Since then she had 6–8 episodes of wheezing each year, usually triggered by colds. Even at her best, she tended to wheeze after a few minutes of exercise and had about two nights each week when her sleep was disturbed by cough and wheeze. Her treatment had been with a beta agonist as required. This relieved her symptoms but she tended to have it most days. Jill was started on inhaled steroids administered via a spacer device. Within 2 weeks, there was dramatic improvement, with cessation of nocturnal symptoms and marked improvement in exercise tolerance. Her dose of inhaled steroids was decreased, with continued benefit. Over the next 6 months she did not require beta agonists more than once a month.

Acute exacerbations of asthma

The focus of management of acute attacks of asthma is assessment of severity of the episode and treatment to restore baseline lung function. The initial assessment attempts to identify those whose asthma is mild and will be managed at home, those who may require admission to hospital and those who will definitely require admission and may need management in an intensive care unit.

- *Mild asthma* usually involves coughing, a soft wheeze, minor difficulty in breathing, no difficulty in speaking in sentences, initial PEF at least 60% of predicted and oxygen saturation (S_aO_2) of at least 94%
- *Moderate asthma* involves persistent cough, loud wheeze, obvious difficulty in breathing with use of accessory muscles, able to speak in phrases, PEF 40–60% of predicted and S_aO_2 91–93%
- *Severe asthma* involves a very distressed and anxious child, gasping for breath, unable to speak more than a few words in one breath, pale and sweaty, possibly cyanosed, palpable pulsus paradoxus and poor air entry with a silent chest. The PEF will be less than 40% of predicted and S_aO_2 90% or less.

One protocol for the management of acute asthma would be to begin with a beta-2 agonist agent such as salbutamol or terbutaline. In mild and moderate cases this may be given by inhalation using a metered-dose aerosol and spacer device. In severe asthma it is delivered via a nebulizer, with oxygen as the driving gas.

If the bronchodilator does not provide relief for at least 3–4 hours, further beta agonist may be given together with oral corticosteroids. Children who are expected to require inhaled beta agonist more frequently than 3–4 hourly should be managed in hospital. When there is an inadequate response to therapy with beta agonists, oxygen and corticosteroids, inhaled ipratropium bromide has been shown to have a small additive effect.

Intravenous aminophylline is an effective bronchodilator but until recently there was little evidence that it had an effect additive to that achieved with maximal doses of beta agonists. Many paediatric units have not used aminophylline for asthma for many years but it has had a resurgence of use in intensive care units with the sickest children with asthma.

The resolution of an acute attack of asthma is not the end of treatment and should be used as an opportunity to consider the background control and management of the child's asthma.

Episodic and persistent asthma

Drug therapy for infrequent episodic asthma is a beta agonist as required. A 35-year follow up of

Table 14.3.2 Asthma management
Assess severity
• History
• Lung function
Aim for optimal control of symptoms and normal life style
Drugs
• Beta-2 sympathomimetics
• Sodium cromoglycate and nedocromil sodium
• Leukotriene antagonists
• Inhaled corticosteroids
• Oral corticosteroids
• Ipratropium bromide
• Theophyllines
• Long-acting beta agonists
Control trigger factors if possible
Review regularly
• Check inhaler technique
• Consider compliance
• Consider decreasing dose of medications
• Education of child and parents
• Address family concerns and expectations
• Crisis plan
• Monitor symptoms and lung function

Melbourne schoolchildren showed that those with infrequent episodic asthma who were not treated with preventer medication had an excellent prognosis, with no evidence of long-term abnormalities in lung function. Children with frequent episodic asthma should receive preventer medication. Current guidelines are either montelukast, sodium cromoglycate (or nedrocromil) or inhaled steroids. Inhaled corticosteroids are the preventers of choice in persistent asthma.

The management of asthma is more than drug treatment. Some of the issues are shown in Table 14.3.2. The child and family need education about asthma and its management. Avoidable factors such as cigarette smoke should be eliminated from the child's environment. Allergen avoidance measures have a role for some children but the clinician needs to be wary about creating false expectations that allergen avoidance is likely to have a major beneficial impact for most children. Explanation of the difference between reliever and preventer therapy is vital (many patients find it useful to remember that most reliever medications are blue, metered-dose inhalers). Demonstration of correct inhaler technique and reinforcing the need for good compliance are essential. An appropriate *crisis management plan* should be developed by the doctor and implemented by the family. In particular a *written action plan* should be provided, together with arrangements for follow-up.

Clinical example

Amy was a 4-year-old girl who had had four admissions to hospital with asthma in the past year. She had also had disturbed sleep due to wheeze three or four times a week. After a few minutes exercise she had to stop because of wheeze and breathlessness. She had been treated with salbutamol on an 'as necessary' basis. On average she had salbutamol at least once a day. You decide to start her on inhaled corticosteroids on a regular basis.

Write an asthma management plan for Amy's parents, including day-to-day management and how to treat an acute exacerbation.

Prognosis

Approximately 60% of those children with infrequent episodic asthma will cease wheezing by early adult life, but only 20% of those with frequent episodic asthma and less than 5% of those with persistent asthma become wheeze free in adult life. Nevertheless, with appropriate therapy asthma can be controlled. For children with frequent episodic and persistent asthma the price of a normal life will be taking regular preventive medication and avoiding smoking.

Practical points

- Diagnosis is usually based on history
- Assess background severity
- Decide whether to start a preventer
- Provide a written asthma action plan
- Review response to therapy
- Check the basics such as inhaler technique, adherence to therapy, avoidance of cigarette smoke

Wheezing disorders other than asthma

R. Henry

The child who wheezes

Although asthma is by far the most common cause of a recurrent wheeze, the term 'wheeze' should not be used interchangeably with asthma, as there are many other possible causes. It is difficult to describe a sound and this makes a definition of wheeze imprecise. Wheeze is typically a high-pitched, musical whistle heard during expiration. The term wheeze refers to the noise heard either with or without a stethoscope.

In the normal situation, a child's breathing is inaudible without a stethoscope because the velocity of airflow in the airways is too low to produce a sound. When the airways narrow, turbulence occurs. Wheeze may occur when the velocity of airflow increases as a consequence of the airways narrowing. In diseases such as asthma and bronchiolitis, the pathology is in the small airways. This sometimes leads to the erroneous assumption that the wheeze is due to air whistling through narrowed small airways. Theoretically, the velocity of airflow in the smaller airways is far too low to cause a wheeze, even when there is significant narrowing. The wheeze is generated in the trachea and major bronchi, which are made narrower by secondary compression during expiration. The physiological explanation is that the small airways obstruction leads to a forced expiration with positive (rather than the usual negative) intrapleural pressure. This positive intrapleural pressure exceeds the pressure within the lumen of the trachea and other large airways, resulting in compression of these airways during expiration and producing a wheeze in these dynamically narrowed larger airways. Examples are demonstrated in Figures 14.4.1 and 14.4.2.

Although obstruction in the small airways is the usual reason for wheeze generated in the large airways, obstructive lesions in the trachea or main bronchi can also cause wheeze. In this case, the wheeze may be generated by the increase in velocity of airflow at the level of the obstruction. Thus, foreign bodies in the intrathoracic part of the large airways or large airway compression from tuberculous lymph notes may manifest themselves as wheeze.

Since wheeze can develop because of narrowing of either the small or large airways, there are many potential causes. One way of classifying the likely causes of wheeze in an individual child is to consider wheeze in different age categories.

Wheezing in infants, toddlers and the preschool child

Table 14.4.1 lists potential causes of wheezing in younger children.

Obstruction of small airways

Acute viral bronchiolitis

This is the most common cause of wheeze in the first year of life and is usually due to respiratory syncytial virus (RSV). The clinical features of acute viral bronchiolitis are described in detail in Chapter 14.5.

Transient infant wheeze versus asthma

The natural history of wheezing in the first 6 years of life has been studied to try to assess the factors that determine whether children wheeze and whether they outgrow the symptoms. One cohort study found that about 50% of children had no wheezing in the first 6 years of life; 20% had at least one lower respiratory tract illness with wheezing during the first 3 years of life but no wheezing by 6 years (transient infant wheezing); about 15% had persistent wheezing; and 15% developed wheezing after the age of 3 years.

Children with transient infant wheeze appear to have airways that are of relatively small calibre and may be floppy. Maternal smoking is a risk factor but neither a personal nor family history of atopy is more common than in children who do not wheeze. Transient infant wheezing is a benign condition.

Children who continue to wheeze at 6 years of age are more likely to have had wheezing without colds, to be atopic, to have a first degree relative with asthma, to be male and to have a mother who smokes.

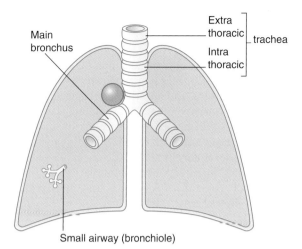

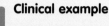

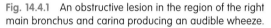

Fig. 14.4.1 An obstructive lesion in the region of the right main bronchus and carina producing an audible wheeze.

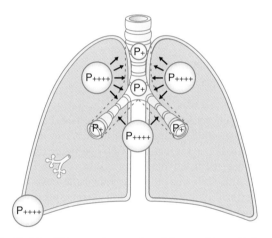

Fig. 14.4.2 Widespread narrowing of the small bronchioles – e.g. in viral bronchiolitis.

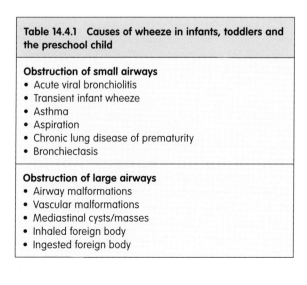

Table 14.4.1 Causes of wheeze in infants, toddlers and the preschool child

Obstruction of small airways
- Acute viral bronchiolitis
- Transient infant wheeze
- Asthma
- Aspiration
- Chronic lung disease of prematurity
- Bronchiectasis

Obstruction of large airways
- Airway malformations
- Vascular malformations
- Mediastinal cysts/masses
- Inhaled foreign body
- Ingested foreign body

It is often difficult to distinguish infants with wheezing who have or will develop asthma from those with a transient problem. For this reason the appropriate management of individual infants with wheeze may require the input of a consultant paediatrician.

> ### Clinical example
>
> Edward was 10 months old when he was referred to a paediatrician because of an 8-month history of wheeze. His mother reported that he wheezed all the time. She was embarrassed to take him out in public because people would stop her and tell her to take Edward to see a doctor. She indicated that he did not ever seem to be in discomfort with his wheeze. Neither cough nor breathlessness had been present. He had been treated with inhaled corticosteroids and salbutamol for 3 months, both without apparent clinical benefit. There was no family history of asthma. Edward was thriving, with a weight of 10.5 kg. He was smiling and playing contentedly, but had a loud wheeze. The diagnosis of transient infant wheeze was suspected. The nature of this entity was explained to his mother and his medications were ceased. During the next 12 months his wheezing resolved gradually.

Aspiration bronchitis/bronchiolitis/pneumonia

This possibility should always be considered in small infants with recurrent or persistent lower respiratory symptoms, including cough and wheeze. Aspiration is usually due to gastro-oesophageal reflex or incoordinate swallowing, or a combination of the two. Incoordinate swallowing will lead to aspiration occurring during feeds, whereas there will be a delay between feeding and coughing with reflux. Some children have incoordinate swallowing due to delayed maturation of the normal mechanisms for swallowing, while others have problems secondary to disease of the central nervous system (such as cerebral palsy). Less commonly, aspiration may be due to an anatomical communication such as a tracheo-oesophageal fistula.

Chronic lung disease of prematurity (bronchopulmonary dysplasia)

The preterm infant who develops hyaline membrane disease and requires ventilation and high concentrations of supplemental oxygen may develop chronic lung disease (Ch. 11.3). This is thought to result from the interaction of immaturity of the lung, oxygen toxicity, mechanical ventilation and possibly repeated aspiration. This is now a common condition seen in tertiary referral paediatric centres, and persistent cough and wheeze for the first year or two of life is common. When these children develop acute viral bronchiolitis, it is likely to be a particularly severe disease.

Suppurative lung disease

Familial reasons for suppurative lung disease (bronchiectasis) are important. Cystic fibrosis occurs in 1 in 2500 live births in the Caucasian population (Ch. 14.6). Infants with cystic fibrosis may have lower respiratory tract symptoms such as cough, wheeze and manifestations of repeated lower respiratory infections. The wheeze in this situation is usually due to bronchiolitis, sometimes viral and sometimes bacterial.

Other familial forms of suppurative lung disease that may present in infancy with cough and wheeze include immunodeficiences such as X-linked hypogammaglobulinaemia (Ch. 13.2) and primary ciliary dyskinesia (immotile cilia syndrome).

Acquired bronchiectasis may occur after bronchiolitis or pneumonia. Well recognized causes include adenovirus infection (especially types 7 and 21) and measles (Ch. 12.1). Ongoing aspiration may also lead to bronchiectasis. Often the aetiology is unknown.

Obstruction of large airways

Congenital airway malformations

Tracheomalacia/bronchomalacia
This is a primary malformation of either tracheal or bronchial cartilage resulting in excessive floppiness of the central airways. This causes wheeze and a brassy cough, likened to the 'bark' of a seal. Children who have had a repaired tracheo-oesophageal fistula (TOF) have tracheomalacia. Their cough is referred to as a 'TOF cough'. Tracheomalacia may be complicated by sudden, very severe obstructive episodes known as 'dying spells'. These are due to transient total apposition of the anterior and posterior tracheal walls.

Congenital lobar emphysema
This is a result of a congenital deficiency of cartilage in a lobar bronchus, which causes obstruction to the bronchus, overdistension of that lobe and subsequent displacement of the adjacent lung and mediastinum. Generally, these infants present in the neonatal period with respiratory distress accompanied by wheeze and overdistension of the chest. Treatment is surgical removal of the affected lobe, and the long-term prognosis is excellent.

Subglottic/tracheal haemangioma
These lesions are absent at birth (as are haemangiomas of the skin) but appear during the first few months of life. The symptoms of expiratory wheeze, inspiratory stridor and respiratory distress typically occur between the ages of 6 weeks and 6 months. The actual noise produced depends upon the anatomical site of the mass. Laryngeal or subglottic lesions cause inspiratory stridor; and intrathoracic tracheal lesions cause expiratory wheeze. Approximately half of these infants will also have cutaneous haemangiomas in the head and neck region. The diagnosis can only be made reliably by bronchoscopy under general anaesthesia. Spontaneous resolution of the haemangioma may take a few years and intervention (such as laser therapy) may be necessary. (See also Ch. 21.1).

Congenital tracheal/bronchial stenosis
This may occur anywhere in the central tracheobronchial tree, resulting in varying degrees of obstruction. Normally, these infants will present with breathlessness, expiratory wheeze and/or inspiratory stridor, depending upon the site and extent of the narrowing.

Vascular malformations

Vascular ring
The true vascular ring is usually due to a double aortic arch malformation. This results in early onset of wheeze and stridor, cough and recurring lower respiratory tract infections. Classically the diagnosis has been made on barium swallow, which demonstrates an abnormal indentation of the oesophagus posteriorly plus an indentation of the anterior wall of the tracheal air column on lateral views. Diagnosis is confirmed at bronchoscopy and surgical excision of the smaller arch is indicated after delineation of the anatomy by angiography. Other vascular malformations that may cause symptoms include innominate artery compression of the trachea (often associated with localized tracheomalacia), aberrant subclavian artery and rare forms of pulmonary artery sling. Other investigations may supplement or replace some of the above, such as echocardiography and computed tomography scanning.

Large left to right cardiac shunt
External compression of the bronchi can occur in the presence of enlarged, hypertensive pulmonary arteries, particularly when there is associated left atrial enlargement. The left atrium lies immediately adjacent to the tracheal bifurcation and infants with this combination seem particularly prone to bronchial compression, e.g. ventricular septal defect and persistent ductus arteriosus. Clinically, this obstruction results in overdistension of one or both lung fields with associated wheeze and breathlessness.

Mediastinal cysts and tumours

Cystic hygroma/lymphangioma

Usually these contain elements of both cystic hygroma (cavernous lymphangioma) and capillary lymphangioma within the same lesion. Although the majority of these are in the neck, they can involve the mediastinum, where they tend to be more cystic and can cause compression of the central airways. In this site surgical removal may be indicated.

Bronchogenic cysts

These are usually adjacent to the lower trachea, carina or main bronchi. Although embryological in origin, they can present quite late in childhood, or even in adult life; however, if large, they will present with wheeze and breathlessness, and an obvious middle mediastinal mass will be noted on chest X-ray. Treatment is surgical excision.

Oesopageal duplication cysts, neurenteric and gastroenteric cysts

These are usually in the posterior mediastinum and therefore are less likely to impinge upon the airway; however, duplication cysts may be in the middle mediastinum and may result in wheeze and respiratory difficulty. Treatment is by surgical excision.

Teratomas

These are the most common of the germ cell tumours and, while most are in the sacrococcygeal region, 10–15% are found in the anterior mediastinum and frequently cause compression of adjacent structures, particularly the trachea or main bronchi. These tumours may be benign (dermoid cysts) or malignant. Malignancy can be determined only after histological evaluation; excision is mandatory.

Mediastinal lymphadenopathy

Extrinsic compression of the main bronchi may occur that is due to enlarged hilar lymph nodes secondary to primary tuberculosis. Classic features are recent weight loss, cough, fever, wheeze and breathlessness. The chest X-ray will show hilar lymphadenopathy, narrowing of the adjacent mainstem bronchus and frequently a parenchymal lesion, representing the primary complex (Fig. 14.4.3). Other causes of enlarged hilar lymph nodes in this age group include lymphoma.

Inhaled foreign body

The majority of children presenting with an inhaled foreign body are toddlers and preschool children. The most common foreign bodies are nuts (especially peanuts) but other food material and small objects (e.g. plastic toys, grass seeds, leaves) can be inhaled into the airways. Only one-third of children

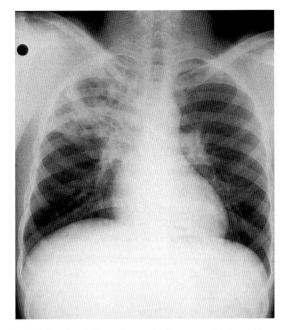

Fig. 14.4.3 Chest X-ray demonstrating consolidation of the right upper lobe; this child had a strongly positive Mantoux test. Diagnosis – primary pulmonary tuberculosis.

present with the classic diagnostic triad of choking, asymmetrical air entry and abnormal chest X-ray. Many children present with acute onset of wheeze, accompanied by cough and breathlessness. Chest X-rays may show air trapping from a ball valve

Clinical example

Pablo, a 3-year-old boy, had no past history of chest problems. Ten days previously he had been to a friend's birthday party and was observed to have a choking episode while laughing. Shortly beforehand he had been seen emptying a bowl full of salted peanuts into his mouth. During the choking episode he was blue around the lips and he coughed uncontrollably for 2–3 minutes. Following this episode, he appeared to be normal and continued playing at the party. Since the party, however, his mother had noted a troublesome cough and a soft, but persistent, wheeze. On examination, the only abnormal finding was localized expiratory wheezing and softer inspiratory breath sounds over the right chest, both front and back. A chest X-ray (inspiratory film) was normal; an expiratory film showed right-sided hyperinflation and mediastinal shift to the left. Because of the history and physical signs, a foreign body inhalation was suspected and Pablo was admitted to hospital for a bronchoscopy. Two large fragments of peanut were removed from the right main bronchus. There were no abnormal chest findings following this procedure, and at follow-up 2 weeks later he was perfectly well.

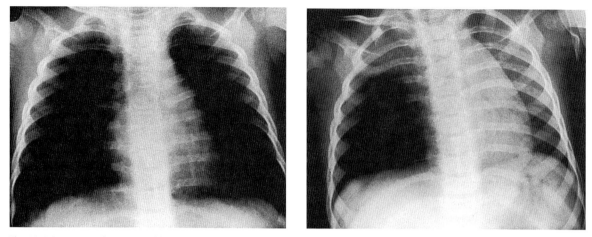

Fig. 14.4.4 X-rays of a 3-year-old child with acute wheeze during inspiration (left) and expiration (right). The inspiratory film is normal. The expiratory film shows marked trapping in the right lower zone, consistent with a ball valve (partial obstruction) in the right main bronchus. At bronchoscopy, a peanut was removed from the right main bronchus.

obstruction, particularly if both inspiratory and expiratory views are taken (Fig. 14.4.4). Other X-ray findings include atelectasis and radiopaque foreign bodies; however, about one-third of children with an inhaled foreign body have a perfectly normal chest X-ray. Similarly, although there may be diminished breath sounds over one side of the chest, or localized high pitched expiratory wheeze, physical signs may be absent. If a foreign body is suspected, then bronchoscopy should be considered.

Ingested foreign body

Quite large foreign bodies (coins, toys, bones) may be swallowed and may fail to pass through the relatively narrow upper oesophagus. If these foreign bodies are large (Fig. 14.4.5) or irregularly shaped, they may cause significant obstruction to the adjacent extrathoracic trachea. In most cases this will produce inspiratory stridor, but expiratory wheeze may also be audible. These children will have difficulty swallowing of recent onset, plus persisting fever and malaise as a consequence of inflammation of the oesophagus from the large foreign body. Radiopaque foreign bodies will be visible on X-ray providing the upper portion of the airways is present on the chest film. Management is by removal of the foreign body by oesphagoscopy under general anaesthesia.

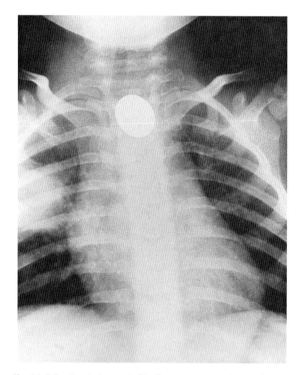

Fig. 14.4.5 A coin impacted in the upper oesophagus has distorted the adjacent trachea causing wheeze and consolidation – collapse of the right upper lobe.

Wheeze in school aged children/adolescents

Causes of wheezing in older children are listed in Table 14.4.2.

Obstruction of small airways

As well as the conditions mentioned previously, *Mycoplasma pneumoniae* is a common cause of wheezing in school-age children. This organism is an important trigger for asthma and will often be seen as one of the causes of an exacerbation of asthma. Other children, without a history of previous wheezing, may develop symptoms with *Mycoplasma* infec-

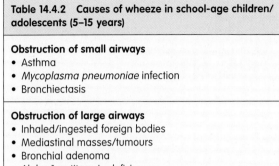

Table 14.4.2   Causes of wheeze in school-age children/adolescents (5–15 years)

Obstruction of small airways
- Asthma
- *Mycoplasma pneumoniae* infection
- Bronchiectasis

Obstruction of large airways
- Inhaled/ingested foreign bodies
- Mediastinal masses/tumours
- Bronchial adenoma
- Alpha-1-antitrypsin deficiency
- Hysterical wheeze/stridor

tions. Suggestive clinical features include protracted cough and fever, combined with widespread crackles on chest auscultation and extensive radiological changes (especially parahilar and peribronchial) in a child who looks well. An oral macrolide (erythromycin or roxithromycin) is the appropriate antibiotic.

Obstruction of large airways

Bronchial adenomas

These are rare and usually present with wheeze and breathlessness due to the mechanical effects of the tumour. A persistent irritating cough and failure to respond to asthma therapy are typical.

Alpha-1-antitrypsin deficiency

Most children and adolescents will present with neonatal hepatitis or a known family history of this disorder. Respiratory symptoms usually develop in the third or fourth decade but cough, wheeze and breathlessness may begin in childhood.

Hysterical wheeze/stridor

This problem is sometimes seen, particularly in young females. It is more common for there to be inspiratory stridor rather than wheeze. The noise is generated by the vocal cords, which are held in apposition during exhalation, and by dynamic compression of central airways due to the violent expiratory effort. Usually there is considerable emotional turmoil involving the child and family, and the possibility of sexual abuse needs to be considered. Exercise-induced vocal cord dysfunction is a similar entity that occurs on exercise in high-achieving athletic teenagers (more commonly female). It can be mistaken for exercise-induced asthma.

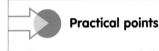

Practical points

- There are many causes of wheezing in childhood other than asthma
- The causes of non-asthma wheezing are different in different age groups
- Many of the disorders are only seen in children
- The role of the general practitioner is to recognize that the diagnosis is probably not asthma
- Referral is needed to consider appropriate investigations

Lower respiratory tract infections and abnormalities in childhood

P. N. Le Souëf

Lower respiratory tract infection

Most respiratory tract infections involve both the upper and lower airway. For respiratory tract infections that appear to involve mainly the upper airway, a degree of involvement of the lower airway is usually present to some degree. A lower respiratory tract infection can be considered to be present when significant symptoms or signs arise from the intrathoracic airway. In developing countries, acute lower respiratory infections remain the greatest cause of mortality in children under the age of 5 years.

Pneumonia

Pneumonia is a common cause of morbidity and mortality in children and is characterized by infection, inflammation and consolidation of the lung. There are many different causes of pneumonia, the most common being:

- viral infections
- bacterial infections
- atypical infections
- aspiration.

Symptoms of acute infective pneumonia include dyspnoea, fever and malaise. Cough may be dry or moist but is not always present. Pleuritic chest pain is often present. If the pneumonia involves the apices, neck pain may be present and can be confused with the neck stiffness of meningism. If the diaphragmatic pleural surface is involved, pain can be referred to the abdomen or shoulder tip.

Signs include tachypnoea and respiratory distress, dullness to percussion and, on auscultation, localized crackles and bronchial breathing. Of these signs, tachypnoea is the most consistent and reliable, and pneumonia should be suspected in any child with an unexplained tachypnoea. However, none of these symptoms or signs is specific for pneumonia and the clinical diagnosis should be suspected when the history and examination are consistent. Signs of complications of pneumonia include those related to:

- pleural effusion – shifting of mediastinum or trachea, dullness to percussion (stony dullness with large effusions), reduced or absent breath sounds, and bronchial breathing above the effusion
- pneumothorax – uncommon, shifting of mediastinum or trachea, reduced breath sounds.

Investigations

Chest radiography is the most reliable investigation. If the chest radiograph is normal, pneumonia can be considered to be not present at that time, but, if the X-ray is taken very early in the disease process, this does not preclude radiological changes developing later. In general, patchy or peripheral consolidation may be more in keeping with a viral infection, lobar opacification is suggestive of bacterial pneumonia, and a more central peribronchial infiltrate may indicate *Mycoplasma* infection, but the specificity of these changes is relatively poor. Importantly, all these radiological features can be found with asthma. Repeat X-ray to establish resolution of the pneumonia is important to reduce the risk of missing an unrecognized, underlying or unresolved pathology but preferably this should be done after at least 4–6 weeks, as the abnormalities may not have resolved prior to that time necessitating a further X-ray.

Blood culture may be performed if clinically indicated. Bacteraemia is not common in the majority of bacterial pneumonias.

Polymerase chain reaction (PCR) or *antigen examination of a nasal aspirate* can detect the presence of causative respiratory viruses, but positive results for PCR in particular are common in normal individuals.

Sputum is often difficult to obtain and of limited usefulness because of contamination by upper airway bacteria.

Bacterial antigen detection in the peripheral blood is of also of limited use.

Immune function: In recurrent or atypical pneumonia, consideration should be given to the possibility of immunodeficiency. Initial examinations may include assessment of serum immunoglobulins and tests for human immunodeficiency virus (HIV).

Pneumococcal pneumonia

Streptococcus pneumoniae is the most common cause of bacterial pneumonia in children at any age. Pneumococcal pneumonia is most common in children under 3 years of age. Risk factors include male gender, indigenous race and preterm delivery. It is partially a vaccine-preventable illness, and the recent introduction of conjugate pneumococcal vaccine into the routine childhood immunization schedule should be beneficial.

Pneumococcal pneumonia may be preceded by symptoms suggestive of a mild upper respiratory infection and typical symptoms and signs of pneumonia may then appear. While these can be non-specific with this form of pneumonia, symptoms are more likely to include fever, tachypnoea and pleuritic chest pain and cough can be absent, and signs are more likely to include nasal flaring, grunting, reduced movement of the chest wall on the affected side, dullness to percussion, reduced breath sounds and bronchial breathing over the area involved. Dullness to percussion may indicate the presence of an empyema. If the upper lobes are involved, neck stiffness may be present and the child may be misdiagnosed as having meningitis.

Chest X-ray findings vary widely but the most common finding is lobar involvement (Fig. 14.5.1), and a well defined round opacification or patchy

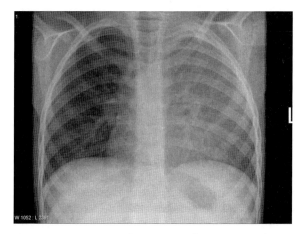

Fig. 14.5.1 Pneumococcal pneumonia showing consolidation throughout the left upper lobe.

changes are not uncommon. Empyema, abscesses and pneumatoceles are less common than in staphylococcal pneumonia. An increased white cell count in peripheral blood is common and blood culture may be positive.

The diagnosis should be made as early as possible and treatment commenced as soon as possible with penicillin and a third-generation cephalosporin. The response to treatment is usually rapid and complete recovery can be expected.

Clinical example

Ben, a 3 year-old boy, presented with a 4-day history of cough, and fever. He was noted to be mildly unwell and to have a respiratory rate of 50 breaths per minute and bronchial breathing over the left base posteriorly. A chest X-ray showed opacification confined to the left lower lobe. Ben was treated with parenteral then oral penicillin and was afebrile within 8 hours. The bronchial breathing had disappeared the next day and he was back to normal health within a week. A repeat X-ray 1 month later was normal.

Staphylococcal pneumonia

When *Staphylococcus aureus* causes pneumonia, it is usually a more severe form. It is more common in younger children, especially those under 2 years of age, and an important risk factor is a socially disadvantaged or indigenous background.

Compared with other forms of pneumonia, the child with staphylococcal pneumonia usually appears more unwell, with a high fever, and is more likely to have pallor, tachypnoea and respiratory distress. The onset is usually acute and the course more rapid. Chest signs are non-specific, but the chest X-ray is more likely to show severe involvement. Early in the course of the illness, staphylococcal pneumonia may have radiological features that are similar to other forms of bacterial pneumonia, including lobar consolidation, patchy shadowing and a small pleural effusion. However, within days, more serious findings may be evident, including widespread opacifications, large pleural effusions and displaced intrathoracic structures. More specific to staphylococcal pneumonia are abscesses, either single or multiple, and large or encysted pleural effusions with thick walls. Air leaks are common and highly specific for staphylococcal pneumonia; they include pneumothorax, pneumomediastinum, pneumopericardium and, in particular, pneumatoceles (Fig. 14.5.2A). However, these are not pathognomonic of this condition, as air leaks including pneumatoceles

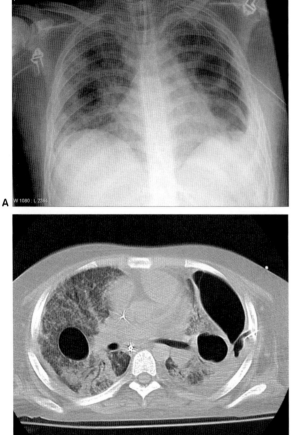

Fig. 14.5.2 Chest X-ray (**A**) and single slice from a thoracic CT scan (**B**) in an immunocompromised 15-year-old with staphylococcal pneumonia and bronchopleural fistulae. There is diffuse air space opacification with several pneumatoceles and a left-sided pneumothorax.

can be found in other bacterial pneumonias, including those caused by *Escherichia coli*, *Klebsiella* sp., *Pseudomonas* sp., group A streptococci and pneumococci. For staphylococcal pneumonia, computed tomographic (CT) scans of the chest (Fig. 14.5.2B) are often useful in defining the nature and extent of these complications.

Investigations

Blood cultures may be positive in the acute phase of the illness. Pleural effusions should be aspirated to assist with diagnosis but the fluid from an empyema may be sterile if sufficient antibiotic treatment has been given.

Management

Infants in whom staphylococcal pneumonia is suspected should be hospitalized to allow adequate observation during the acute phase of the illness, as deterioration can be rapid and air leaks can occur and require immediate treatment. Broad-spectrum antibiotics should be used until an accurate diagnosis can be made. The combination of a beta-lactamase-resistant penicillin such as flucloxacillin and a third-generation cephalosporin, both given intravenously, is useful, as it combines direct treatment of staphylococci as well as coverage of other common respiratory pathogens. In children under 2 years of age with clinically significant pneumonia, flucloxacillin should be included in the treatment regimen because of the much higher prevalence of staphylococcal pneumonia in this age group. In some communities, resistance to beta-lactamase-resistant penicillins (so called methicillin- or multiresistant *Staphylococcus aureus* (MRSA)) may occur, so other drugs such as clindamycin should be considered. Nosocomial staphylococcal infections are more likely to show multiple drug resistance than community-acquired MRSA infections. The duration of antibiotic treatment needs to be extended to around 6 weeks to reduce the risk of relapses.

Surgical intervention

Surgery may be undertaken early in the course of the illness to assist in diagnosis or to reduce the mechanical effects of large effusions. Video-assisted thoracoscopic surgery (VATS) is likely to be a better option than open thoracotomy, as it is less invasive and postoperative hospital stay is generally shorter with VATS. However, use of VATS depends on the availability of a surgeon who has been appropriately trained and has the necessary skill for this approach. Whether or not surgery reduces the total duration of illness is less clear, although the decision to drain an effusion is often taken with the expectation that drainage will reduce the space-occupying and pressure effects of a large effusion as well as reducing the recovery time.

Long-term outcome

Clinical recovery from staphylococcal pneumonia is usually good with a very high likelihood of a complete return to normality. Radiological recovery is usually also complete, as children examined radiologically some years after recovery generally show no evidence of previous problems, despite extensive, serious abnormalities in chest X-rays at the time of the illness.

Haemophilus influenzae type b pneumonia

Pneumonia due to *H. influenzae* is now relatively uncommon because of immunization against this organism. *H. influenzae* is found in the upper respiratory tract of the majority of normal, non-immunized children, and less commonly in those who have been immunized. Three-quarters of invasive infections occur in children aged under 2 years. Other risks factors for *H. influenzae* infection include indigenous

Clinical example

Jasmine, a 9-month-old girl, was brought to the local doctor by her mother. She had been unwell for 24 hours, with increasing fever, lethargy and difficulty feeding. The doctor noticed that she was pale, listless and tachypnoeic and scattered coarse inspiratory and expiratory crackles were heard on auscultation of her chest. She was transferred by ambulance to hospital where a chest X-ray showed opacification in the right upper and left lower lobes. She was treated with oxygen and intravenous flucloxacillin and cefotaxime. Blood culture was positive for *S. aureus* and treatment with flucloxacillin was continued for 6 weeks. She slowly improved and she was fully recovered when seen after the antibiotic treatment had been completed.

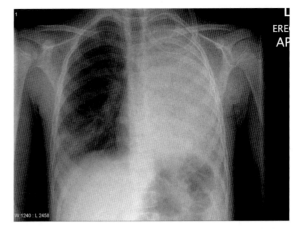

Fig. 14.5.3 *Mycoplasma* pneumonia in a 7-year-old girl presenting with cough and fever. There is extensive consolidation in the left lung with air bronchogram formation and focal consolidation in the lateral basal segment of the right lower lobe.

race, lower socioeconomic group, male gender and immunodeficiency.

The signs and symptoms of *H. influenzae* pneumonia are not distinguishable from those found in other pneumonias. Similarly, the radiological features are not specific to this organism. For children who are ill, treatment with a parenteral third generation cephalosporin is recommended, and for children who are less unwell, oral amoxicillin/clavulanic acid is appropriate. Other children in the family do not require prophylactic treatment if they are adequately immunized.

Mycoplasma pneumoniae

Mycoplasma pneumoniae is a frequent causative organism of pneumonia in children; it is uncommon in infancy. The clinical course is often protracted and characterized by the gradual development of fever, malaise, upper respiratory symptoms and cough. Signs can include widespread sparse fine crackles or coarse crackles. In children with a tendency to asthma, wheeze is commonly present. The chest X-ray often shows changes that are more striking than expected for the degree of clinical illness. The findings themselves are usually non-specific but can include perihilar opacification, and consolidation of one or more lobes (Fig. 14.5.3). The diagnosis is supported by positive serology. Co-infection with *S. pneumoniae* is not uncommon. Treatment with a macrolide (e.g. roxithromycin, erythromycin) is indicated but the response to treatment may be restricted to a reduction in general symptoms, as the clinical course of the pneumonia itself may not be affected by treatment.

Other causes of bacterial pneumonia

Other bacteria that can cause pneumonia in the community include:

- *Group A beta-haemolytic streptococci* (*S. pyogenes*). This organism is not a common cause of pneumonia, although it is a common cause of bacterial pharyngitis. When it does cause pneumonia, this is less likely to be in children under the age of 5 years and, compared with other causes of bacterial pneumonia, tends to be more rapidly progressive, severe and poorly responsive to antibiotic therapy. Fever, chest pain and haemoptysis are more common than in other forms of pneumonia, and a higher percentage of cases will have large pleural effusions and empyema. Treatment is with high-dose intravenous penicillin G
- *Group B beta-haemolytic streptococci*. This organism is a common and important cause of neonatal pneumonia, which occurs within hours of birth, has a rapidly progressive course, can mimic respiratory distress of prematurity and has a high mortality. After the neonatal period, it rarely causes pneumonia and, when it does, the disease course is usually less acute
- *Klebsiella pneumoniae*. This organism typically causes pneumonia in neonates and immunocompromised host. In children, it is a rare cause of pneumonia and when *Klebsiella* infection is present, bacteraemia is more common than pneumonia.. The clinical picture of *Klebsiella* pneumonia initially is not distinguishable from other forms of pneumonia but the complications of lung abscess and pneumatocele may occur and, without appropriate treatment, the mortality is high. Recommended treatment depends on individual resistance patterns but is likely to include an aminoglycoside and/or a third-generation cephalosporin

- *Other bacterial organisms* that can cause pneumonia in children include anthrax, *Bordetella pertussis*, *Brucella*, *Burkholderia cepacia*, *Citrobacter* sp., *Corynebacterium* sp., *E. coli*, *Listeria monocytogenes*, *Mycobacterium* sp., *Neisseria meningitidis*, *Pasteurella* sp., *Proteus* sp., *Pseudomonas aeruginosa*, *Salmonella* sp. and *Yersinia* sp.

Viral pneumonia

Viruses are common causes of pneumonia in children of all ages and the spectrum of disease varies widely. Risk factors for viral pneumonia include:

- *Age.* Children under 5 years of age are at greatest risk of viral pneumonia, but the risk remains high throughout the first decade of life
- *Season.* Peak seasonal incidence is in winter
- *Passive smoke exposure.* Maternal smoking increases the risk, especially in the first year of life
- *Poor socioeconomic status.* A risk factor in both the developing and the developed worlds
- *Pre-existing chronic problems.* The risk is increased in chronic chest problems such as cystic fibrosis, chronic postneonatal lung disease, congenital heart disease and HIV infection.

The most important causative viruses are parainfluenza viruses, influenza viruses, respiratory syncytial virus (RSV) and adenoviruses. Human metapneumovirus (HMV) has recently been recognized to be an important pathogen that causes similar clinical patterns of disease to RSV. All of these viruses can cause other respiratory illnesses apart from pneumonia, including acute upper respiratory tract infection, acute laryngotracheitis, bronchitis and bronchiolitis. Symptoms of these illnesses can co-exist with those of pneumonia. Rhinoviruses, cytomegalovirus and measles can also cause pneumonia. In recent years, rhinovirus has been identified as the most common cause of exacerbations of acute asthma in both children and adults, so that care is needed to avoid misdiagnosing pneumonia in children with X-ray changes due to rhinovirus-induced asthma. The radiological features of viral pneumonias are non-specific, but patchy, widespread infiltrates are more characteristic than lobar involvement (Fig. 14.5.4). Treatment with antiviral agents is rarely indicated in normal children, but supportive measures are commonly required.

Fungal pneumonia

Fungal causes of pneumonia or pneumonia-like illnesses occur most commonly in immunocompromised children and include *Actinomyces*, *Aspergillus*, *Candida*, *Cryptococcus*, *Histoplasma* and *Nocardia* spp.

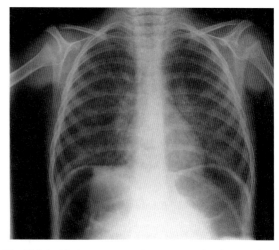

Fig. 14.5.4 Viral pneumonia showing typical widespread diffuse opacification.

Clinical example

Dana, an 8 year old girl, was brought to her general practitioner with a 3-day history of fever, increasing dry cough and loss of appetite. Her 12-year-old brother had also been unwell with a cough and a fever. On examination, her doctor noted a temperature of 37.8°C, a respiratory rate of 28 breaths per minute, mild soft tissue recession, and the presence of sparse, coarse crackles bilaterally on auscultation. A chest X-ray showed scattered areas of patchy opacification. She was diagnosed as having viral pneumonia, treated symptomatically and recovered uneventfully over the next few days.

Protozoal pneumonia

Protozoa that are causes of pneumonia or pneumonia-like illnesses also occur most commonly in immunocompromised children and include *Cryptosporidium* spp., *Pneumocystis jiroveci* (formerly *carinii*) and *Toxoplasma* spp.

Acute viral bronchiolitis

This is the most common significant respiratory infection in the first year of life and approximately 2% of children are admitted with bronchiolitis during infancy. It is less common but not rare after 1 year of age. In most locations, bronchiolitis occurs in winter epidemics but, in climates with more precipitation in summer than winter, this situation can be reversed. Important risk factors include maternal smoking, congenital heart disease, chronic lung disease of prematurity, immunodeficiency and cystic fibrosis.

> **Practical points**
>
> **Pneumonia**
> - *Tachypnoea*: the most useful clinical sign
> - *Pneumococcal pneumonia*: the most common cause of bacterial pneumonia at all ages including the first year of life.
> - *Staphylococcal pneumonia*: uncommon, but when it does occur, it most commonly occurs in the first year or two of life
> - *Follow-up X-ray*: taken to ensure that there is no significant underlying pathology
> - *Follow-up X-ray timing*: leave for at least 4 to 6 weeks to allow enough time for complete clearing of the abnormalities

Recent evidence suggests that for bronchiolitis in the community, rhinovirus is the most common causative organism rather than respiratory syncytial virus (RSV). For children admitted to hospital, RSV is the most common causative organism. Bronchiolitis can also be caused by parainfluenza 1–3, influenza A and B, adenovirus and HMV. It is rarely due to bacteria and secondary infection with bacteria is also rare.

Clinical features are usually sufficient to allow a clinical diagnosis to be made and consist of an illness with a gradual onset over several hours to a day or two, low-grade or no fever, expiratory wheeze, dry cough, tachypnoea, hyperinflation of the chest and fine inspiratory crackles. Respiratory distress can vary from minimal to severe. Bronchiolitis usually lasts for 2–3 days but more severe episodes last longer. If the condition has not resolved within 2 weeks, an underlying risk factor is likely to be present. The principal differential diagnosis is early-onset asthma. The presence of inspiratory fine crackles is more indicative of bronchiolitis than asthma, but the two conditions can be similar clinically and precipitated by the same viruses, so that in some cases there is no reasonable way to separate these two diagnoses.

A nasal aspirate should be taken for diagnosis in cases severe enough to require hospital admission. The main radiological feature in most cases is hyperinflation but non-specific widespread opacification can be found in more severe cases. Oxygen saturation should be measured to assess severity and to determine the need for supplementary oxygen therapy.

Treatment consists of providing support in the form of oxygen to keep arterial saturation at a level of 94% or above and fluid and nutritional maintenance. Great care needs to be taken with administering fluids by nasogastric tube, as infants with severe respiratory distress are at high risk of aspiration if they vomit, as they are less able to defend their airway. Hence, more severe cases should receive maintenance fluids intravenously. Pharmacological therapy is not indicated in most patients even if the condition is severe. Bronchodilators have not been shown to be effective and may increase requirement for supplementary oxygen. Specific anti-viral therapies such as anti RSV immunoglobulin or palivizumab are poorly effective and expensive, although they may reduce cause a modest reduction in the need and length of hospitalization.

Long-term sequelae of bronchiolitis are probably few. Follow-up studies show that infants who have had bronchiolitis are more likely to wheeze in the future and develop asthma, but this appears to be more of a reflection to their pre-existing predisposition to respiratory disease, including bronchiolitis, rather than problems caused by bronchiolitis.

> **Practical points**
>
> **Bronchiolitis**
> - Most common cause of wheeze in early life
> - Rhinovirus the most common cause of mild bronchiolitis, RSV the most common cause of severe bronchiolitis
> - Clinical features: low-grade fever, cough, wheeze, hyperinflation, fine inspiratory crackles
> - Treatment: supportive only – oxygenation, hydration, nutrition

Pertussis (whooping cough)

This is caused by the bacterium *Bordetella pertussis*. It can affect patients of any age but infants, particularly those aged less than 6 months, are at greatest risk of complications (e.g. apnoea, severe pneumonia, encephalopathy) and death.

Its incidence and severity is greatly reduced by pertussis vaccine. A major value in immunization is the increased herd immunity which reduces transmission to young babies from older siblings and adults.

Infected subjects are most infectious in the prodromal phase where coryza is more prominent than cough, and continue to be infectious for up to 3 weeks.

Clinical features

There is a prodromal phase with nasal discharge and an unremarkable cough, which lasts a few days, before the phase of pronounced coughing begins. There may be prolonged paroxysms of coughing often accompanied by vomiting and terminated by a characteristic inspiratory 'whoop'. Young infants also commonly have apnoea and may develop severe pneumonia and encephalopathy, which can be fatal.

Investigations

A nasopharyngeal aspirate for immunofluorescence and culture is the investigation of choice. Serology is available but can be difficult to interpret and rarely affects clinical management.

Management

Infants less than 6 months of age are more likely to require hospital admission for supportive therapy.

Macrolide antibiotics (e.g. erythromycin, clarithromycin, azithromycin) reduce the period of infectivity and can alter the course of the illness, but only if commenced before the paroxysmal phase. Thus, they are indicated in those seen very early in the course of the illness or those with severe symptoms.

Household contacts are usually also treated to reduce spread of infection. Infected individuals should be excluded from school, creche, etc., until they have had at least 5 days of antibiotics or have had the illness for at least 21 days. Pertussis is a notifiable disease in most states of Australia.

Pulmonary tuberculosis

Tuberculosis is caused by infection with *Mycobacterium tuberculosis*. Pulmonary tuberculosis remains an important cause of morbidity and mortality in children worldwide. The tubercle bacillus was discovered by Koch in 1822, and in the 20th century the spread of the disease was reduced in developed countries by effective public health and therapeutic approaches. However, late in the century the incidence began to increase because of the dismantling of control measures and in the 21st century the incidence of the disease is likely to increase further because of the presence of large numbers of people with HIV infection.

Children usually acquire the infective agent from an adult or adolescent rather than from other children. Tuberculosis in children is most common under 5 years of age, with a lower incidence between 5 and 15 years. Other risk factors are low socioeconomic conditions and an indigenous racial background. The organism is transmitted mainly by inhalation in the indoor environment and only a small percentage of those infected will develop disease.

Signs of pulmonary tuberculosis do not appear for weeks, months or years after infection. The initial lesion is often subpleural, occurring with an associated lymph node response that comprises a primary. The disease does not progress further in most patients but, when it does, effusions may occur, lymph nodes may enlarge and obstruct major airways, and the lung may be damaged by extensive caseation. The disease may then disseminate and produce miliary, meningeal or renal tuberculosis.

Early in the course of the disease there are often few symptoms or signs of pulmonary disease, but non-specific symptoms, including weight loss, malaise and fever may be found. Most patients will eventually develop a cough and, if there is airway compression, wheeze may result.

Diagnosis is established by:

- suggestive chest X-ray findings
- a positive tuberculin skin test (>15 mm skin induration from 5TU of PPD-S is taken as evidence of disease; 10–15 mm suggests that infection has occurred but disease may not be present; false negatives can occur in early or severe disease)
- culture of the organism from early morning gastric lavage
- light microscopic identification of bacilli from sputum, bronchoalveolar lavage fluid or pleural fluid.

Treatment has traditionally been with triple therapy which consists of 6 months treatment. Rifampicin, isoniazid and pyrazinamide are given for 2 months, then rifampicin and isoniazid for a further 4 months. A positive skin test without any evidence of pulmonary disease is treated with isoniazid alone for 6–9 months.

Atypical mycobacterial infection

Atypical mycobacteria (*Mycobacterium avium, intracellulare, scrofulaceum*) can, on rare occasions, cause pulmonary disease in immunocompetent children, particularly in Australia. Pulmonary lymphadenopathy can be so marked as to obstruct airways. Diagnosis is made by specific skin testing and by identification of bacilli from fluid or tissue. Response to treatment is slow and therapy may need to be continued for 12–24 months but prognosis for full recovery appears to be excellent.

Congenital disorders of the lower respiratory tract

Congenital lung abnormalities

Congenital anomalies of the lung are rare but they may present well into childhood and their symptoms can be non-specific; most can be detected on chest X-ray:

- *Lung cysts* can vary from being simple and solitary to multiple and complex. Cysts can become infected if they communicate with the airway. They can also cause symptoms if they become enlarged and compress surrounding structures
- *Cystic adenomatoid malformation* consists of multiple cysts and abnormal proliferation of lung elements. It can present at birth and if, sufficient lung is involved, cause chronic respiratory insufficiency. Surgery may be needed to remove troublesome cysts
- *Congenital lobar emphysema* is characterized by overinflation of a lung lobe and commonly presents before 6 months of age with respiratory distress or tachypnoea. Surgical intervention may be required if the emphysematous lobe causes significant compression of neighbouring lung
- *Sequestration* of the lung refers to an abnormality of the lung where a part of the lung is discontinuous with the rest of the lung and can be intra pulmonary or extrapulmonary. The former is much more common and more likely to become infected and require surgical removal. The latter is most frequently left-sided, with an aberrant systemic blood supply and asymptomatic.

Congenital chest wall abnormalities

- *Pectus excavatum* is a midline concave depression of the lower sternum. It is very common, not usually associated with any underlying respiratory abnormality and usually does not affect rib cage or lung function
- *Thoracic dystrophies* are characterized by impaired development of the chest wall and are associated with pulmonary hypoplasia
- *Scoliosis* can cause a restrictive functional defect in chest wall function if the angle of the curve is great enough
- *Congenital diaphragmatic hernia* can present with early onset respiratory distress and can be misdiagnosed if the gut above the level of the diaphragm on the chest X-ray is misinterpreted as opacified or cystic lung.

Congenital lower airway abnormalities

- *Tracheomalacia and bronchomalacia* (Ch. 14.4).
- *Oesophageal atresia and tracheo-oesophageal fistula* (Ch. 11.5).
- *Bronchogenic cysts* (Ch. 14.4).

14.6 An approach to chronic cough and cystic fibrosis in children

A. B. Chang, S. M. Sawyer

Cough is the most common symptom of respiratory disease, particularly in childhood, and it is one of the most common reasons for parents to seek medical attention for young children. The presence of cough can indicate the entire spectrum of cardiorespiratory childhood illness, ranging from a symptom of the 'common cold' to a symptom of severe, life-limiting disorders such as cystic fibrosis. Most cough in children is acute and resolves promptly. Prolonged or chronic cough is defined as cough lasting longer than 4 weeks. It is abnormal and deserves careful consideration of the cause.

Pathophysiology

Cough is generally considered a reflex but as it is subject to cognition and can be voluntarily generated there are non-reflex elements to cough. Cough is made up of three phases (inspiratory, compressive and expiratory) and serves as a vital defensive mechanism for lung health. The forceful expiration provided by coughing occurs after a build-up of pressure in the thorax (up to 300 mmHg) by contraction of expiratory muscles against a closed glottis. This leads to expulsion of air at high velocity, which sweeps material within the airways towards the mouth. Inspiration of a variable volume of air occurs when cough is stimulated. Successive coughs may or may not be preceded by inspiration.

Cough is an important component of normal respiratory function through two mechanisms. Firstly, mechanical stimulation of the larynx causes immediate expiratory efforts through the expiratory reflex, a primary defensive mechanism that is stimulated when foreign objects (such as food or fluid) are inhaled. Secondly, cough enhances mucociliary clearance. The absence of a forceful cough (e.g. generalized muscular weakness) has important clinical repercussions, such as difficulty clearing secretions, atelectasis, lobar collapse and recurrent pneumonia.

Issues to keep in mind when the presenting symptom is cough are:

- cough, especially nocturnal cough, is unreliably reported when compared to objective measures of cough
- cough usually resolves spontaneously (called the period effect), which makes evaluation of therapeutic interventions difficult
- many cough treatments are not based on the results of randomized controlled trials
- as the aetiology and management of cough in childhood is quite different from adults, extrapolation of information from the adult cough literature to children can be harmful.

 Practical points

- Children with chronic cough should:
  - be carefully evaluated especially for symptoms and signs of an underlying respiratory or systemic disease
  - have spirometry (if age-appropriate) and chest radiograph performed
  - be re-evaluated as minimal airway secretions may be present in dry cough and hence wet cough may initially present as dry cough
  - be assessed for a history of environmental exposures in particularly tobacco smoke exposure should be sought and intervention initiated if appropriate
  - be reviewed to ensure there is resolution of the cough
- Chronic cough can be classified based on the likelihood of an underlying disease or process; specific cough and non-specific cough (an overlap is present)

Approach to diagnosis and management

Figure 14.6.1 outlines a schematic approach to the diagnosis and management of chronic cough. The key questions are presented in Table 14.6.1. Initial categorization of cough into acute cough, subacute cough and chronic cough according to duration is helpful. There is, however, no strict definition of chronic cough. Most acute cough arises from respiratory viruses and settles within 2 weeks. Subacute

506

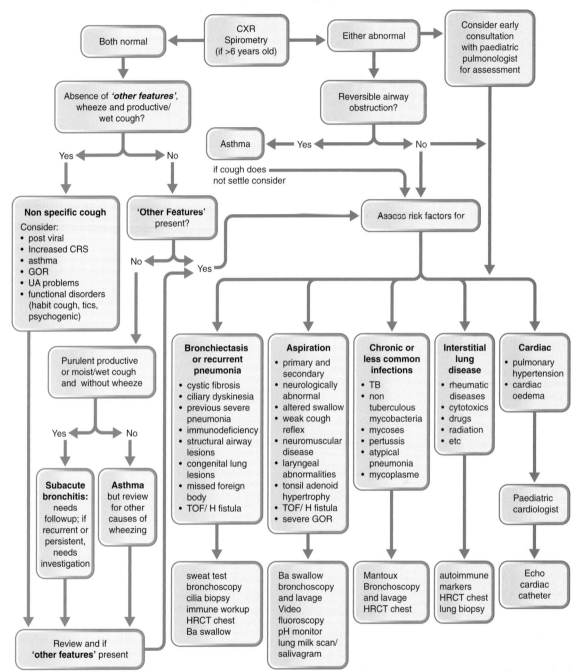

Fig. 14.6.1 Guide for approaching a child with a persistent cough. Symptoms and signs vary according to age and illness severity. ARI, acute respiratory infection; CRS, cough receptor sensitivity; CXR, chest X-ray; FTT, failure to thrive; GOR, gastro-oesophageal reflux; HRCT, high-resolution computed tomography of the chest; LTB, laryngotracheobronchitis; TEF, tracheo-oesophageal fistula; TB, tuberculosis; UA, upper airway. Adapted with permission from Chang AB, Asher MI 2001 A review of cough in children. Journal of Asthma 38: 299–399.

Table 14.6.1 Key questions to consider

- Is the cough representative of an underlying respiratory disorder?
- Are any of the symptoms and signs in Table 14.6.2 present?
- Are exacerbating environmental factors present (passive or active tobacco smoking, other lung toxicants)?
- Should the child be referred promptly?

Table 14.6.2 Symptoms and signs alerting to the presence of an underlying disorder

- Auscultatory findings
- Cough characteristics e.g. cough with choking, cough quality (Table 14.6.3), cough starting from birth
- Cardiac abnormalities (including murmurs)
- Chest pain
- Chest wall deformity (Fig. 14.6.3)
- Chronic dyspnoea
- Daily moist or productive cough
- Digital clubbing (Fig. 14.6.4)
- Exertional dyspnoea
- Failure to thrive
- Feeding difficulties
- Haemoptysis
- Immune deficiency
- Neurodevelopmental abnormality
- Sinopulmonary infections

Table 14.6.3 Classical recognizable cough in children

Barking or brassy cough	Croup, tracheomalacia, habit cough
Honking	Psychogenic
Paroxysmal	Pertussis and parapertussis
Staccato	*Chlamydia* in infants
Cough productive of casts	Plastic bronchitis

cough in children is a chest radiograph and lung spirometry (if over 6 years old). Diagnoses to be considered include bronchiectasis, cystic fibrosis, asthma, retained foreign body, aspiration lung disease, atypical respiratory infections, cardiac anomalies and interstitial lung disease. If basic investigations are not helpful, referral to a general or respiratory paediatrician is indicated rather than further investigations.

Clinical example

Adrienne, a 13-year-old girl, was referred to a respiratory physician for a chronic cough. She had been managed incorrectly as an asthmatic for more than 10 years. On specific questioning, Adrienne indicated that she had been coughing for as long as she could remember and she indicated that her cough was worse in the mornings and she often expectorated sputum. Her cough had been stable and she had not noticed any exertional dyspnoea. She had no growth failure and did not have digital clubbing.

Given that she had some features of bronchiectasis, a high resolution computed tomography (CT) scan of Adrienne's chest was performed and it revealed focal changes in the right basal segment (Fig. 14.6.2). Her immunoglobulin profile was normal and she was Mantoux- and sweat-test-negative. On flexible bronchoscopy. a retained foreign body (piece of shell) was visualized and removed from the right medial segment of her right lower lobe. The foreign body had caused prolonged partial bronchial obstruction and was the aetiology for Adrienne's localized bronchiectasis.

It is important to define the aetiology of any child's chronic cough. This child had features, listed in Table 14.6.3, that indicated that she had specific cough and further investigations were indicated. In children it is best for investigations to be performed in a children's facility.

Management of non-specific cough

The majority of children with non-specific cough have postviral cough and/or increased cough receptor sensitivity. There is no serious underlying cause of non-specific cough and reassurance is a large part of management. Understanding and listening to parental concerns and expectations is important. There is no evidence that 'over the counter' (nonprescription) medications reduce cough in young children.

Identification of exposure to environmental tobacco smoke (ETS) in children and active smoking in adolescents is an important part of respiratory history taking. Environmental tobacco smoke exposure can cause non-specific cough and exacerbate a variety of respiratory disorders including otitis media, asthma and pneumonia. Non-specific cough is a

cough commonly lasts 2–4 weeks, while chronic cough is cough lasting longer than 4 weeks.

The key point in the assessment of chronic cough is whether it is specific or non-specific, according to the presence or absence of particular features (Table 14.6.2). Children younger than 6 years do not generally expectorate sputum. Thus the productive cough of older children and adults manifests as a moist or 'rattly' cough in younger children. The presence of any of these symptoms or signs raises the possibility of an underlying disorder. Certain cough characteristics are associated with particular types of illness (Table 14.6.3).

The choice of investigation depends on the clinical findings. However, minimum investigation of chronic

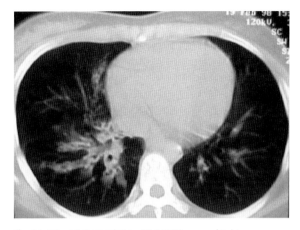

Fig. 14.6.2 High-resolution CT (HRCT) scan of Adrienne, as described in the clinical example. 13-year-old girl with a moist cough for more than 10 years. She had been incorrectly managed as an asthmatic for 10 years until referred for another opinion. The HRCT scan shows focal bronchiectasis of the right basal segment. Flexible bronchoscopy was undertaken. A foreign body (a piece of shell) was removed from the right basal medial bronchus.

reason to encourage parents to stop smoking. If smoking cessation cannot be achieved, aim to reduce smoking in enclosed spaces such as the house and car.

Habit cough is a cause of non-specific cough, especially in older children and younger adolescents. The age of diagnosis is broad but is commonly from 4–15 years. Severe cases are more common in adolescents than in children. The cough is classically 'honking'. It is generally absent in sleep and is worse at times where attention is focussed on the cough. Habit cough generally settles promptly once parents are aware that there is no underlying respiratory problem. Mental health expertise is required for those with more severe or prolonged symptoms, especially if there are other features of somatization or concerns of underlying psychopathology.

Cough, asthma and allergy

There is little doubt that children with asthma can present with cough. However, most children with chronic cough do not have asthma. Furthermore, while nocturnal cough is a feature of children with asthma, nocturnal cough alone is uncommonly due to asthma. In a randomized placebo-controlled trial of inhaled salbutamol or corticosteroids in children with recurrent cough, the presence of airway hyper-responsiveness did not predict the efficacy of these medications for cough. If asthma 'preventer' medication is used, it should be introduced on a trial basis with early review (2–4 weeks) and cessation of medication if the cough does not respond to asthma 'preventer' therapy. Failure to do so will result in

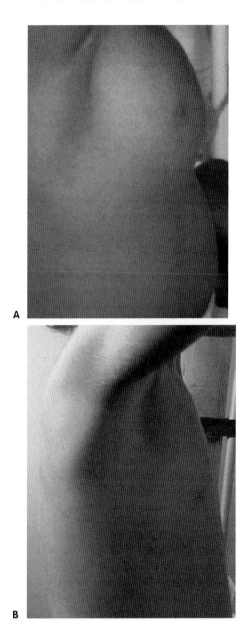

A

B

Fig. 14.6.3 **A** Severe pectus carinatum. This can be present in children with any chronic lung disease. Gross pectus carinatum as shown in this picture is now rarely seen. **B** Normal-shaped chest.

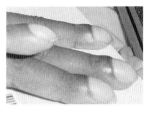

Fig. 14.6.4 Digital clubbing in a boy with bronchiectasis. Digital clubbing is non-specific and may or may not be present in children with suppurative lung disease.

509

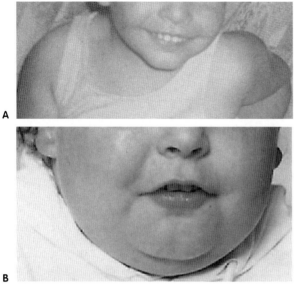

A

B

Fig. 14.6.5A, B This previously normal child had a chronic dry cough, which was incorrectly treated with escalating doses of inhaled corticosteroids. Two years later, he was cushingoid in appearance without any change in his cough. Children with isolated cough should not be treated with increasing doses of asthma therapy.

Clinical example

Gino was first seen by a paediatric respiratory physician when aged 8 years. He had been receiving 2000 μg/d of inhaled corticosteroids for the last 6 years for a chronic dry cough and had been managed as an 'asthmatic': his medications were escalated when his cough did not respond to the steroids. When seen, his chest X-ray and spirometry were normal, he was cushingoid and earlier pictures of him showed a normal-sized 3-year-old boy (Fig. 14.6.5). His 6-year-old brother's body habitus was also normal. Gino had been exposed to tobacco smoke and had an element of habitual cough. His asthma medications were subsequently withdrawn and his cough eventually subsided when he was no longer exposed to tobacco smoke and received appropriate counselling.

This example illustrates the importance of obtaining a history of smoke exposure. Also, it is crucial not to 'overdiagnose' asthma on the basis of the presence of isolated cough. In children, when cough is representative of asthma, the cough should subside within 2 weeks of appropriate asthma treatment. If the cough does not subside, the asthma therapy should be withdrawn and not escalated.

escalation of medication dose with the risk of significant side effects.

A longitudinal population study of cough in infants and children revealed that recurrent cough (rather than chronic cough) presenting in the first year of life resolves over time in the majority of children. The group of children with recurrent cough without wheeze had neither airway hyperresponsiveness nor atopy and differed significantly from those with classical asthma, with or without cough, in the persistence of symptoms over time. It is believed that these infants may have more narrow airways and that airway growth leads to symptomatic improvement. This group of infants is clinically hard to differentiate from those who continue to have recurrent cough from asthma, making predictions of future illness difficult in infancy.

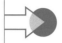

Practical points

- Over-the-counter (OTC) or prescription medications are ineffective for chronic non-specific cough and should not be used for the symptomatic relief of cough
- Treatment for chronic cough should be aetiologically based. Medications are largely unhelpful for non-specific cough. If medication trials are undertaken, a response should not be assumed to be related to the medication tried, especially for asthma medications. A diagnosis of asthma should not be made based on a single episode in the absence of other symptoms of asthma
- Chronic suppurative lung disease or bronchiectasis should be suspected in children with chronic wet cough that does not resolve on oral antibiotics or that recurs. These children should be investigated for an underlying cause such as cystic fibrosis, primary ciliary dyskinesia, immune deficiency and aspirated foreign body
- Children with chronic suppurative lung diseases should be managed by a multidisciplinary team. The medical elements include airway clearance techniques, attention to nutrition and early intervention for pulmonary exacerbations and other complications

Cough, gastro-oesophageal reflux and aspiration lung disease

Gastro-oesophageal reflux (GOR) can be associated with cough. However, while GOR can cause cough, cough can also cause GOR and causative links are hard to identify. The view that GOR is a frequent cause of cough is now challenged. GOR is neither a specific nor frequent cause of chronic cough in children. As cough is very common in children and respiratory symptoms may exacerbate GOR, it is difficult to delineate cause and effect. Infants regularly regurgitate, yet few if any well infants cough with these episodes.

Aspiration lung disease can result from severe GOR and from laryngopalatal discoordination or discoordinated swallowing. These children present with chronic cough but usually in the context of severe developmental or neurological disturbance. The investigatory evidence for aspiration lung disease can be difficult. Ambulatory oesophageal pH studies can identify gastro-oesophageal reflux. However, a positive result does not confirm that aspiration has occurred. Similarly primary aspiration (from swallowing discoordination) is also difficult to confirm as current standard tests like nuclear medicine milk scan or a barium swallow provide only a 'single moment' test which may not be representative of the child's routine feeding pattern.

Cough, sinusitis and postnasal drip

Although it is widely stated that sinusitis/postnasal drip is a common cause of cough there is little supportive evidence. There are no cough receptors in the pharynx or postnasal space. Although sinusitis is common in childhood, it is not associated with asthma or cough once allergic rhinitis, a common association, is treated. The relationship between nasal secretions and cough is more likely linked by common aetiology (infection and/or inflammation causing both) or due to throat clearing of secretions reaching the larynx.

Bronchiectasis

Bronchiectasis can be the end result of a number of different respiratory disorders. In contrast to data in the 1960s, bronchiectasis is now an uncommon disorder in non-indigenous Australian children. Bronchiectasis can be diffuse or focal. Diffuse disease usually develops secondary to an underlying disorder such as cystic fibrosis, immunodeficiency or primary ciliary dyskinesia, although it can be idiopathic. Focal bronchiectasis more commonly reflects airway narrowing, either congenital (e.g. bronchial stenosis) or acquired (e.g. retained foreign body). In indigenous Australians, bronchiectasis is not uncommon and is thought to result from earlier childhood respiratory infections (postinfectious bronchiolitis obliterans). Congenital forms of bronchiectasis (e.g. Williams–Campbell syndrome) are rare.

The spectrum of bronchiectasis varies from mild to severe. Symptoms and signs reflect the extent of the disease. Children with bronchiectasis have a chronic moist or productive cough and are typically clubbed but not necessarily so. The cough is characteristically worse in the mornings. Physical findings are non-specific: clubbing, chest wall abnormality (hyperinflation or pectus carinatum (uncommon)), coarse crepitations and localized wheeze. All these

Clinical example

Deanna was hospitalized on several occasions for pneumonia. The first occurred at 2 months of age. She was first referred for further assessment at 2.5 years of age and had a prolonged moist cough. She had a hyperinflated chest wall, early digital clubbing and growth failure. Her weight was below the 3rd percentile and her height was at the 3rd percentile. Her chest high-resolution CT showed postinfectious bronchiolitis obliterans and bronchiectasis. Other investigations were normal.

Deanna was admitted for a prolonged course of intravenous antibiotics, and her parents were taught home physiotherapy. Following discharge, Deanna remained on maintenance co-trimoxazole. Her daily moist cough disappeared when her bronchiectasis was aggressively treated with antibiotics and physiotherapy.

may or may not be present and absence of these signs does not imply absence of disease.

Plain radiography will show suggestive features in severe disease (dilated and thickened bronchi may appear as 'tram tracks') but is insensitive in mild disease. Confirmation is by high-resolution computed tomography (CT) scan of the chest (routine CT scan provides insufficient detail).

A child with suspected bronchiectasis should be referred for investigation for a specific cause and specific treatment will be instituted when indicated, e.g. cystic fibrosis, immunodeficiency. The general approach to managing children with bronchiectasis is similar to that outlined under 'key elements of respiratory management' described for cystic fibrosis below. In addition, children aged more than 2 years should receive a pneumococcal 23 valent vaccine once every 5 years and influenza vaccine yearly. Pooled immunoglobulin replacement is indicated for those with identified immunodeficiency syndromes. Surgery is very rarely indicated, and only for those with focal disease.

Primary ciliary dyskinesia

Primary ciliary dyskinesia (PCD) syndromes encompass several congenital disorders, all of which affect the ciliary function of several organs, including the upper and lower respiratory tracts and genitourinary tract. The term includes Kartagener syndrome (situs invertus associated with bronchiectasis), immotile cilia syndrome, ciliary dysmotility and primary orientation defects of ciliary components. Primary ciliary dyskinesia has a prevalence of 1:20 000, is mostly autosomal recessive in inheritance and is probably genetically heterogenous.

Cilial ultrastructure consists of a $9 + 2$ arrangement: the axoneme consists of nine peripheral microtubular doublets surrounding a central pair of microtubules. Abnormalities in cilial function are due to alteration of its ultrastructure or its function, the ciliary beat frequency. Secondary abnormalities in both ultrastructure and function can also occur as a result of infection, smoking or pollutants. Cilial dysfunction markedly reduces mucociliary clearance and results in recurrent infections of both the upper and lower respiratory tract (middle ear infections, pneumonia, bronchitis, bronchiectasis). In the genitourinary tract, ciliary dysfunction can lead to infertility in males and ectopic pregnancies in females. Increasingly, structural ciliary abnormalities have been found to be associated with other organ diseases such as the eye (retinitis pigmentosa), the ear (hearing loss) and kidneys (cystic diseases of the kidney).

The severity of pulmonary manifestations of PCD varies widely. Presentation can be early in life with neonatal respiratory illness. In infants and older children, the diagnosis should be considered in those with chronic cough, bronchiectasis, recurrent pneumonia, atypical asthma, recurrent rhinosinusitis and chronic secretory otitis media. Specific investigations for PCD include assessment of mucociliary clearance, measurement of ciliary beat frequency and electronic microscopic identification of cilial ultrastructure.

Cystic fibrosis

Cystic fibrosis is the most common life-threatening autosomal recessive disorder in Australians, affecting approximately 1 in every 2500 births. It is caused by a defect in the cystic fibrosis transmembrane conductance regulator gene (*CFTR*). The *CFTR* gene encodes a protein for a cyclic adenosine monophosphate (cAMP)-regulated chloride channel present on many epithelial cells, including those of the conducting airways, gut and genital tract. The commonest mutation, Δ508, accounts for approximately 70% of mutant alleles and more than 1300 mutations have been described.

Diagnosis

All infants in Australia are now screened at birth for cystic fibrosis. A two-stage screening procedure is widely used. Initially, immunoreactive trypsin (IRT) is measured in Guthrie blood spot samples. Samples with an IRT level above the 99th percentile are then tested for the common mutation (additional mutations are tested in some states).

Most Australian children with cystic fibrosis are identified by neonatal screening, with the diagnosis confirmed with a sweat test (pilocarpine iontophoresis) at 6–10 weeks. However, newborn screening does not detect all children with the condition. A sweat test should be arranged if there are phenotypic features suggestive of cystic fibrosis. An elevated sweat chloride (>60 mmol/l) and sweat sodium is diagnostic (some centres use a lower cutoff). To minimize the multiple errors that can occur (especially false negatives), sweat testing should be undertaken in a laboratory that routinely does sweat tests. A diagnostic complication is that, very infrequently, patients have been identified with an abnormal cystic fibrosis genotype yet have a normal sweat test result. A borderline sweat test result is more commonly seen in those with retained pancreatic function.

Between 15% and 20% of Australian infants with cystic fibrosis present before the results of screening are known with meconium ileus, a form of neonatal intestinal obstruction. Antenatal diagnosis for cystic fibrosis is available when both parents are known carriers of the cystic fibrosis gene because they have had a previous child with cystic fibrosis or a family history of the disorder. Community screening is not currently undertaken in Australia.

Clinical features

Cystic fibrosis affects multiple organ systems, causing a range of clinical problems of varying severity (Table 14.6.4). It is a severe disorder, although the occasional child has mild disease. Rarely, it is so mild that it is not diagnosed until adult life, following a presentation of *Pseudomonas* pneumonia or male infertility.

Cystic fibrosis has a major impact on the lungs, where the altered physicochemical properties of the airway epithelium result in abnormally viscid mucus and bacterial colonization of the respiratory tract. The lungs of a child with cystic fibrosis are normal at birth but with time, chronic airway infection develops that causes progressive obstructive lung disease. Clinically, chronic productive cough develops as bronchiectasis progresses and lung function deteriorates. Clubbing is a feature in later stages of the disease.

Malabsorption is present in approximately 90% of children with cystic fibrosis from failure of the exocrine pancreas. Additionally, there are various degrees of gastric and duodenal hyperacidity, impaired bile salt activity and mucosal dysfunction. Stools are abnormal, being typically frequent and bulky. Growth failure may result from many reasons, including inadequate energy intake, malabsorption and chronic bacterial infection. Long-term retention

Table 14.6.4 Common manifestations of cystic fibrosis disease
Respiratory system • Chronic productive or moist cough • Features of bronchiectasis • Clubbing
ENT • Nasal polyps • Sinusitis
Gastrointestinal system • Meconium ileus • Features of malabsorption • Distal intestinal obstruction syndrome • Liver disease • Endocrine pancreatic insufficiency (diabetes mellitus)
Reproductive • Male infertility
General • Growth delay
Metabolic • Salt depletion
Others • Osteoporosis • Urinary incontinence

ments has contributed to these improved health outcomes, including a stronger focus on nutrition and the development of more specific and potent antibiotics. However, a key intervention has been the development of specialized cystic fibrosis centres, characterized by a multidisciplinary team of health professionals including respiratory physicians, gastroenterologists, physiotherapists, nutritionists, nurses, surgeons, social workers and mental health therapists. The goal of treatment is to maintain as high a quality of life as possible for as long as possible in order to slow the relentless progression of lung disease that occurs in cystic fibrosis.

The key elements of respiratory management consists of:

- prompt use of antibiotics to delay the onset of bacterial colonization
- aggressive treatment of recurrent respiratory infections
- promotion of mucociliary clearance by daily physiotherapy
- minimization of other causes of lung damage (e.g. smoking, aspiration)
- promotion of normal growth through high-energy diet and pancreatic supplementation
- identification and treatment of complications as they arise (asthma like disease, allergic bronchopulmonary aspergillosis (ABPA), haemoptysis, pneumothorax, etc.).

of pancreatic function is associated with better survival.

As survival of patients with cystic fibrosis improves, the range of cystic-fibrosis-related diseases and effects becomes more important. This includes altered growth and nutrition, diabetes mellitus and liver disease (both seen in approximately 15–20% of adolescents and adults), arthropathy and arthritis, and osteoporosis. Men are generally infertile as a result of bilateral absence of the vas deferens. Women are fertile, although pregnancy presents a range of health risks to both the fetus and the mother. Women have increased rates of vaginal yeast infections and stress incontinence.

Principles of management of a child with cystic fibrosis

The median age of survival has dramatically improved as a range of clinical improvements has developed over time. Three decades ago, the median survival was less than 10 years. The current median survival is to the mid-30s in years, although there is a marked gender differential, with males surviving significantly longer than females. A range of improve-

Respiratory infections should be treated aggressively, as recurrent infection and the accompanying inflammation promote loss of lung function. The most common respiratory bacteria are *Staphylococcus aureus* and *Haemophilus influenzae* in the early years, followed by *Pseudomonas aeruginosa* and *Burkholderia cepacia*. With increasing use of antibiotics, a plethora of other microorganisms are now increasingly isolated, ranging from fungi (*Aspergillus* species, *Acedosporium prolificans*) and other bacteria (*Stenotrophomonas maltophilia*) to non-tuberculous mycobacteria, *Nocardia*, *Ralstonia* and *Pandoraea* species. Children colonized with certain types of microorganism (such as *B. cepacia*) should also be separated from non-colonized children. Most clinics currently cohort children who have similar organisms in their airways (sputum or bronchoalveolar lavage) to prevent cross-colonization.

Gastroenterological and nutritional management of cystic fibrosis consists of:

- pancreatic enzyme replacement (lipase, protease, amylase) at each meal
- high energy diet
- vitamin supplementation with vitamin A, D, E and K, and salt tablets

- early identification of liver disease
- early identification of distal intestinal obstruction syndrome.

Cystic fibrosis is a lifelong chronic condition. As children grow and mature into adolescents and young adults, the psychosocial aspects of the disease take on different dimensions for individuals, siblings and parents. In adolescence, attention to body image issues and feelings of difference due to chronic disease can help maintain young people's adherence with the health-care regimen. Declining health despite good adherence can be especially demoralizing, however.

Lung and liver transplantation are increasingly undertaken to treat end-stage lung and liver disease respectively. Gene therapy is still in the experimental phase.

Summary

Cough is the commonest manifestation of respiratory problems in children. Although it can be a distressing symptom, its presence is vital for respiratory health. A chest radiograph and spirometry are the minimal investigations in a child with a chronic cough (>4 weeks). When cough is associated with other symptoms (specific cough), investigations and/or referral are required to identify the cause. Nonspecific cough is largely managed expectantly, trying to explore parent anxieties, minimize investigations and environmental triggers such as tobacco smoke. There is little evidence that the common causes of persistent, isolated cough in adults (asthma, gastro-oesophageal reflux, sinusitis and nasal disease) cause chronic cough in children and adolescents.

PART 15

CARDIAC DISORDERS

Assessment of the infant and child with suspected heart disease

J. Wilkinson

Cardiac abnormalities or disease affect approximately 1% of children in the developed world and 2–3% in developing countries, the difference largely being related to rheumatic heart disease in such areas. (See also Chapter 15.2.)

The prevalence of congenital malformations of the heart is approximately 8 in 1000 newborn infants. Acquired heart disease in developed countries includes:

- myocarditis
- septic pericarditis
- cardiomyopathies
- Kawasaki disease.

Transient involvement of the heart may occur in viral illnesses such as mumps and measles but this seldom leads to long-term problems. Acute myocarditis may follow viral infections (especially Coxsackie B) and often appears to be immunologically mediated. Coronary arteritis with the formation of multiple coronary aneurysms is an important feature of Kawasaki disease (Ch. 13.3).

Manifestations

Heart disease may manifest itself with symptoms, due either to congestive heart failure or to cyanosis. Many patients are asymptomatic and their heart defect comes to light with the discovery of a heart murmur at a routine examination.

Evaluation in symptomatic patients

A careful note needs to be made of the onset of symptoms. In babies, breathlessness, feeding difficulties, inability to complete feeds and poor weight gain are important (Fig. 15.1.1). Is cyanosis persistent or intermittent? Its relationship to feeding, crying or other activities or precipitating factors should be sought. Normal infants and children may manifest peripheral cyanosis when cold (often noted after a bath) or when running a fever; cyanosis may also be associated with breath-holding in children with normal hearts. Particular attention should be paid to the palpation of peripheral pulses and auscultation.

Pulses

Examination of pulses should include both left and right arms and femoral pulses, best felt simultaneously to make comparison easy. Reduced lower limb pulses suggest coarctation but apparently normal lower limb pulses do not exclude this diagnosis, especially in the newborn period. Bounding pulses may be associated with persistent ductus. Pulses (especially lower limb pulses) may be difficult to feel in the first few days of life, even in normal babies, and this requires practice. The pulse rate in children varies markedly with activity and the resting rate is the only rate that needs to be noted (Table 15.1.1).

Blood pressure

Measurement of blood pressure should be a routine part of examination in children. Use of an appropriate cuff is vital. The balloon should be of sufficient length to encircle at least two-thirds of the arm, centred over the artery and wide enough to cover two-thirds of the distance from the antecubital fossa to the acromion of the scapula. In practice, the largest cuff that can be fitted to the upper arm without covering the antecubital fossa is appropriate. Blood pressure should normally be recorded by auscultation of Korotkoff sounds, as in adults, although palpation (of the brachial or radial pulse) may be employed to assess systolic pressure in young children and infants if auscultation proves to be difficult. Significant errors in blood pressure are more likely to result from the use of a cuff that is too small than one that is overlarge.

For measurement of leg pressure a cuff may be placed on the thigh. Again, the balloon should encircle at least two-thirds of the limb and be centred over the artery. An adult arm cuff may be large enough

Table 15.1.1 Approximate normal upper limit for pulse, respiratory rate and systolic blood pressure, at rest; resting measurements consistently above these values should arouse suspicion

Age group	Pulse rate (beats/min)	Respiratory rate (breaths/min)	Systolic BP (mmHg)
0–8 weeks	160	50	70
Older infant (2–12 months)	145	40	85
Toddler (1–3 years)	130	30	100
Older child (4–7 years)	115	20	115

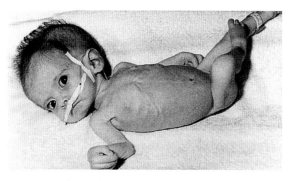

Fig. 15.1.1 Infant with evidence of severe failure to thrive, dyspnoea and feeding difficulties (note nasogastric tube) due to a large ventricular septal defect.

for young children but larger children or adolescents will require a 'thigh cuff', which is larger than an adult arm cuff.

Normal blood pressure varies at different ages (Table 15.1.1).

Palpation of the cardiac impulse

Location of the apex beat and documentation of any abnormal/forceful impulse is important, as is palpation for thrills.

Auscultatory findings

Splitting of the second sound should be noted (Fig. 15.1.2). Splitting is normally only audible during inspiration. A wide split is present when splitting is heard during both phases of respiration. Fixed splitting, a feature of atrial septal defect, implies both wide splitting and absence of variation between inspiration and expiration (Fig. 15.1.3).

Accentuation of the pulmonary component of the second sound tends to be associated with a loud second sound, which may be palpable, often with no definite splitting, and implies the presence of pulmonary hypertension. However, it should be noted that

the normal aortic closure sound may be loud in children with a thin chest wall and is sometimes palpable at the upper left sternal border. The presence of an ejection click (Fig. 15.1.2) is a useful ancillary auscultatory finding. Such sounds are heard shortly after the first heart sound and tend to be high-frequency and discrete in character. If heard at the apex, it usually implies a bicuspid aortic valve or aortic stenosis. When originating from the pulmonary valve, it is heard at the left sternal edge and varies with respiration, being louder on expiration. This finding is characteristic of pulmonary valve stenosis.

Murmurs

When a heart murmur is heard, a process of 'murmur analysis' needs to be applied. This involves:

- timing
- localization
- amplitude (grading)
- characterization
- radiation.

Timing
Murmurs may be systolic (limited to systole), diastolic (limited to diastole) or continuous (extending from systole into diastole). Note that continuous murmurs are not necessarily present throughout the cardiac cycle. Murmurs should be timed against the carotid pulse or apical impulse. Distal pulses, such as the radial pulse, can produce incorrect assessment of timing.

Localization
The point of maximum intensity of the murmur should be identified.

Amplitude
Murmurs may be graded according to the scale in Table 15.1.2.

Characterization
Ejection murmurs (Fig. 15.1.4) are systolic and are crescendo–decrescendo in character, starting shortly

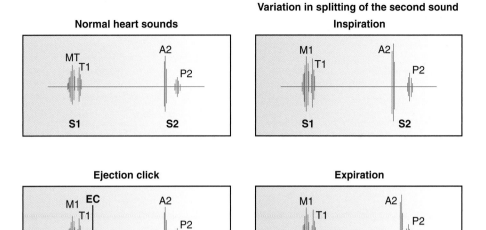

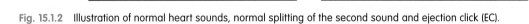

Fig. 15.1.2 Illustration of normal heart sounds, normal splitting of the second sound and ejection click (EC).

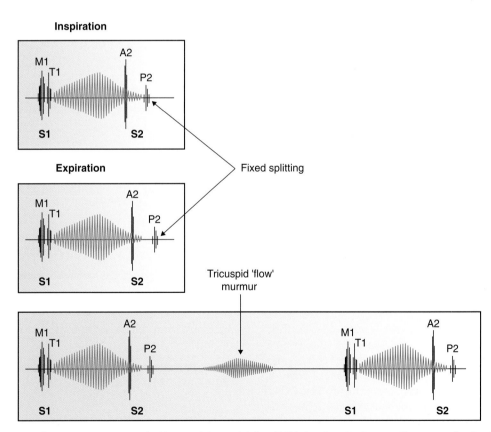

Fig. 15.1.3 Auscultatory signs associated with an atrial septal defect (ASD) showing ejection systolic murmur, fixed splitting of S_2 and tricuspid flow murmur (Ch. 15.2).

Table 15.1.2   Grading of murmurs

Grade	Amplitude	Thrill	Comments
1	Very soft	Absent	Scarcely audible
2	Soft	Absent	Easily audible
3	Loud	Absent	Very easily audible
4	Loud	Faint/localized	Very easily audible
5	Very loud	Easily felt/widespread	Very easily audible
6	Very loud	Easily felt/widespread	Heard with stethoscope off chest wall

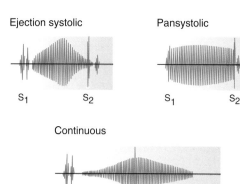

Ejection systolic   Pansystolic

S_1 S_2 S_1 S_2

Continuous

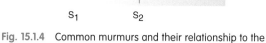

S_1 S_2

Fig. 15.1.4   Common murmurs and their relationship to the heart sounds S_1 and S_2.

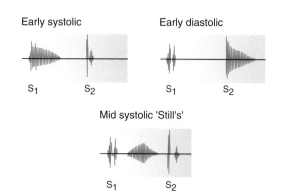

Early systolic   Early diastolic

S_1 S_2 S_1 S_2

Mid systolic 'Still's'

S_1 S_2

Fig. 15.1.5   Other murmurs: early systolic, early diastolic and Still's murmur.

after the first sound. Good examples are the murmurs of pulmonary or aortic valve stenosis.

Pansystolic murmurs (Fig. 15.1.4) are murmurs which commence at the first sound and continue to the second sound. They may be due to atrioventricular valve incompetence (e.g. mitral incompetence) or a ventricular septal defect (VSD).

Diastolic murmurs may be *early diastolic* (Fig. 15.1.5) (commencing at the second sound) or *mid diastolic* (Fig. 15.1.3). The former reflect either aortic or pulmonary incompetence, whereas mid-diastolic murmurs are due to turbulence during ventricular filling and reflect stenosis of or increased flow through the mitral (or tricuspid) valve.

Other characteristic murmurs include *early* (Fig. 15.1.5) and *late systolic* murmurs (reflecting a tiny muscular VSD or mitral valve prolapse, respectively) and the *late diastolic* murmur associated with atrial contraction in patients with mitral stenosis.

Characterization of murmurs also includes assessment of the pitch of the murmur and its quality, e.g. 'harsh', 'musical' or 'vibratory'.

Radiation
A murmur that is easily audible/loud away from the precordial area (e.g. the neck or axilla) is said to 'radiate' towards the area in question.

Innocent murmurs

There are four characteristic types of innocent murmur:

- Still's murmur
- pulmonary flow murmur
- carotid bruit
- venous hum.

Still's murmur
This is a short mid-systolic murmur best heard at the left sternal border or between the apex and left sternal edge. This murmur is sometimes referred to as 'Still's' murmur (Fig. 15.1.5) or a 'vibratory' murmur. The murmur is of medium frequency and

has a vibratory or slightly musical quality. It tends to become softer if the patient stands and is louder when the patient is squatting or lying supine.

Pulmonary flow murmur

This is a soft, blowing ejection murmur, maximal in the pulmonary area. Murmurs of this kind are frequently heard in early infancy and may radiate softly to the axillae, when they may be labelled as innocent with a high degree of confidence, and are less common later in childhood. In older children, distinction from an atrial septal defect or mild pulmonary stenosis can be difficult, and usually requires an electrocardiogram (ECG) and X-ray and in many cases an echocardiogram.

Carotid bruit

This medium-frequency, rough ejection systolic murmur heard over the carotid artery (right or left or bilateral) at the root of the neck is very common in children, being usually softer or inaudible below the clavicle.

Venous hum

A high-pitched, blowing, rather variable, continuous murmur, heard over the sternoclavicular junctions or over the neck and changing with the position of the head, is frequently heard in children. This murmur almost always disappears completely when the patient lies flat and may be eliminated by gentle compression of the neck veins.

It should be appreciated that innocent murmurs may be heard in around 50% of normal school-age children and adolescents. In early infancy, the frequency of soft murmurs is probably around 80%. Because of the very high frequency of soft heart murmurs, it is essential that all doctors involved in caring for infants and children become familiar with the common innocent murmurs and should be able to recognize them with confidence and be able to exclude organic heart disease (Fig. 15.1.6). Simple ancillary investigations (e.g. ECG, chest X-ray) may be helpful. Echocardiography is not usually necessary. Where doubt exists, patients should be referred for formal cardiological assessment.

Cyanosis

The distinction between peripheral and central cyanosis is important. The terms are often thought to describe the site at which cyanosis is seen, whereas they reflect the site of origin of cyanosis. Peripheral cyanosis, originating in areas of poor tissue perfusion, is not seen in areas of good perfusion. By contrast, central cyanosis is generalized. Examination of the tongue and mucous membranes will usually exclude central cyanosis. In the presence of central cyanosis the arterial PO_2 will be depressed, with the rare exception of cyanosis associated with methae-moglobinaemia. Where doubt exists about the presence of cyanosis the use of pulse oximetry is frequently very helpful.

Manifestations of heart failure

Cardiac failure in infancy tends to be dominated by pulmonary congestion, which leads to dyspnoea/tachypnoea.

Dyspnoea contributes to feeding difficulties, reduced intake and increased metabolic rate. Failure to thrive often results. Chronic dyspnoea may lead to the appearance of Harrison's sulci, which are deformations of the ribcage at the site of the diaphragmatic attachments. Crepitations at the lung bases are usually a manifestation of superimposed infection rather than heart failure in infants.

Systemic venous congestion is manifest by liver enlargement and/or oedema. Liver engorgement results in an enlarged, abnormally firm liver with its edge palpable 2.5–5 cm below the costal margin. In infants, oedema is often diffuse and difficult to detect. It is often best seen around the face and eyes (periorbital oedema). Elevated jugular venous pressure cannot be assessed easily in infancy.

Other evidence of cardiac failure may include persistent tachycardia, a chronic dry cough and profuse sweating, especially of the forehead and scalp.

Investigations

Chest X-ray

The chest X-ray provides information about heart size, shape and lung vascularity. The heart is enlarged when, on a posteroanterior chest film, the cardiothoracic ratio exceeds 0.5 in an adult or 0.55 in a child. In infancy the cardiothoracic ratio may be as large as 0.6 (Fig. 15.1.7). If vascular shadows in the hilum are increased, this implies high pulmonary flow (pulmonary plethora; Fig. 15.1.7) or pulmonary venous congestion. Diminished vascular marking, with abnormally dark lung fields (pulmonary oligaemia), is associated with the decreased pulmonary flow occurring in some forms of cyanotic heart disease, e.g. tetralogy of Fallot. Individual cardiac chamber size is often difficult to assess on plain chest X-rays, although variations in cardiac contour may provide useful clues.

Electrocardiogram

The ECG provides information about heart rate and rhythm and about atrial or ventricular hypertrophy or hypoplasia.

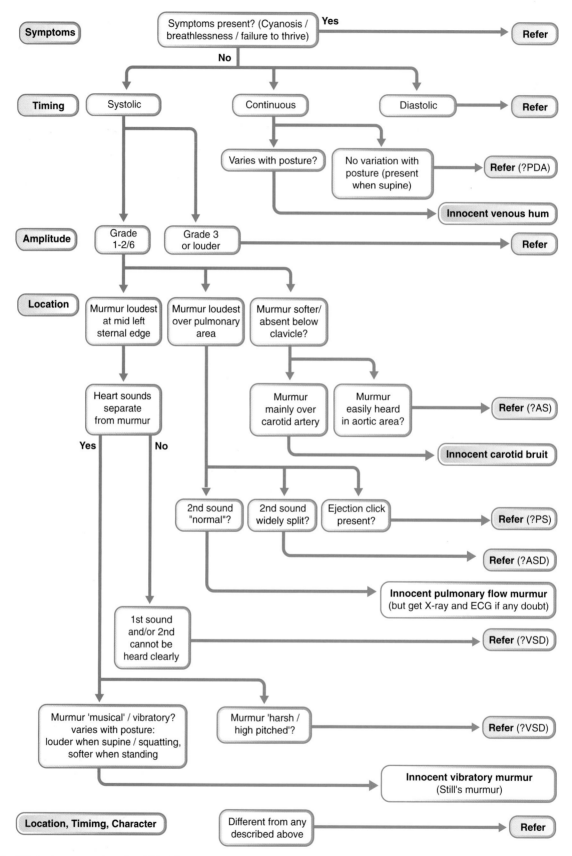

Fig. 15.1.6   An approach to the child with a murmur.

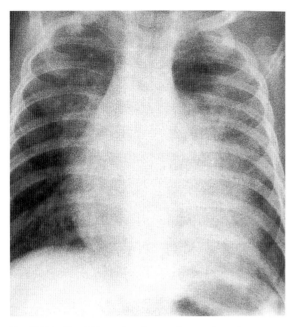

Fig. 15.1.7   Chest X-ray showing cardiomegaly and pulmonary plethora in a child with a large ventricular septal defect (Ch. 15.2).

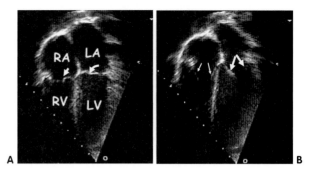

Fig. 15.1.8   Echocardiogram: 'four chambers view'. **A** Four chambers with the mitral valve (curved arrow) and tricuspid valve (straight arrow) closed during ventricular systole. **B** Same anatomy during diastole with the mitral (large arrows) and tricuspid (small arrows) valves open. The atrial and ventricular septa can be seen separating the left heart chambers (LA and LV) from the right sided chambers (RA and RV).

Cardiac catheterization

Cardiac catheterization allows measurement of intracardiac pressures and shunts. It also allows for angiographic demonstration of abnormal anatomy. As much of this can be obtained using echocardiography, the requirement for catheterization has diminished substantially. It may also be used for therapeutic purposes, such as balloon dilation of valves (valvuloplasty) for pulmonary or aortic valve stenosis, or placement of an occlusion 'device' to close a persistent ductus arteriosus, atrial septal defect or ventricular septal defect.

In the vast majority of cases, a diagnosis can be made and treatment instituted on the basis of non invasive investigations without cardiac catheterization. However, catheterization may be necessary for planning surgical treatment, especially in more complicated heart defects.

In the newborn infant, right ventricular forces tend to dominate, whereas by the end of the first year of life left ventricular forces predominate. This evolution reflects changes in ventricular wall thickness, and evaluation of ventricular hypertrophy needs to take into account the normal values for children of each age group. Additionally, normal values for heart rate, PR interval, QRS duration, QT interval and T wave axis vary at different ages.

Echocardiography

Current echocardiographic instruments allow the sectional anatomy of the heart, as it beats in 'real time', to be displayed on a television monitor. This is referred to as cross sectional echocardiography (Fig. 15.1.8).

Doppler echocardiography allows quantitation of the direction and flow velocity at individual sites. This can provide useful quantitative information about the presence and severity of valvar stenoses, regurgitation and septal defects.

Colour flow Doppler is a modality in which the lines of information are split, with Doppler sampling at different sites being displayed as colour on the television monitor. Computerized image processing generally allows good quality imaging along with colour flow maps, which provides a visual display of flow in the areas being examined.

Treatment

Cardiac failure

The development of heart failure in infancy should be regarded as an emergency requiring urgent hospitalization, usually at a major cardiac centre. The transportation of such infants can present a major challenge and may well be best achieved by arranging for the patient to be accompanied by well trained medical and/or nursing personnel with appropriate resuscitation equipment.

Circulatory support

Intravenous dobutamine or dopamine may be life saving. Digoxin should usually be avoided in such cases as renal impairment leads to rapid accumulation and toxicity.

Prostaglandin

In infants developing symptoms in the newborn period, due to congenital heart disease, a 'ductus dependent congenital defect' is often responsible. Infants with such defects (coarctation of the aorta, pulmonary atresia, transposition) may benefit from infusion of prostaglandin E_1 to reopen/maintain patency of the ductus.

Respiratory support

In the presence of severe cardiac and/or respiratory failure, positive pressure ventilation may be helpful in allowing stabilization of the child's condition.

Correction of acidosis

Where respiratory or metabolic acidosis are present, these should be corrected by ventilatory support and/or circulatory support (inotropes/volume expansion).

Diuretics

Frusemide (furosemide) is usually the diuretic of choice. This may be given parenterally initially. If diuretics are required for more than a limited period, potassium depletion may develop and potassium supplements or co-administration of a potassium-sparing diuretic such as spironolactone (Aldactone) should be considered.

Oxygen

Oxygen should be administered if significant hypoxia is detectable, although in the presence of significant cyanotic congenital heart disease the administration of oxygen will seldom produce much improvement in oxygenation.

Feeding

Gavage feeding via nasogastric tube may be helpful if the infant is too breathless to feed adequately. Introduction of high-calorie feeds may be helpful. Infants with heart failure tend to tolerate small frequent feeds better than larger feeds. In the presence of more severe congestive failure feed volume should be reduced to 120 ml/kg/24 h (or less) to avoid fluid overload.

Clinical example

Stacey, aged 6, presented with fever, cough and breathing difficulty. She had been known to have a heart murmur since infancy, which was labelled as being 'innocent' by her paediatrician. Examination showed her to be febrile with a temperature of 39.6°C, a red throat and crepitations over the lungs, with widespread rhonchi. A grade 2/6 murmur was audible at the upper sternal edge that extended from systole into early diastole. Her chest X-ray showed a normal cardiac contour with patchy opacity in the right lower zone. The ECG was normal. An echocardiogram showed a small patent ductus arteriosus with no chamber enlargement.

Stacey had pneumonia following a viral respiratory infection. Her murmur was 'continuous', although only audible during systole and early diastole. It could easily be mistaken for a purely systolic murmur unless careful attention was paid to assessing the timing. For this reason (being judged to be a soft systolic murmur) it had been incorrectly labelled as innocent. The persistent ductus was an incidental finding and the normal heart size on X-ray, normal ECG and absence of chamber enlargement demonstrated by the echocardiogram all indicated that the shunt was small and hence not likely to be contributing to her current symptoms. Her pneumonia was treated with appropriate antibiotics and the PDA was reassessed and treated (probably with a catheter procedure to implant a coil or occlusion device) after she had recovered from her current illness.

Clinical example

Ryan was a 2-month-old infant with recent onset of episodic cyanosis when distressed. He had been noted to have a heart murmur a few days ago but had been feeding well and gaining weight normally. His mother thought that his colour was normal most of the time but when he cried his lips and fingers became purple. His chest X-ray was normal but the electrocardiogram indicated right ventricular hypertrophy. Pulse oximetry showed a saturation of 92% while he was asleep, but when upset the saturation was 65%.

This baby was likely to have a cyanotic heart defect, as evidenced by his low saturations on pulse oximetry – both at rest and more so when crying. Minor desaturation (with saturations above 85%) may be difficult to detect clinically and Ryan might appear to be pink when he was comfortable. However, when distressed his oxygen demands would increase and he would become more obviously hypoxic, with reduced saturations and clinically apparent cyanosis. An echocardiogram was organized to establish the nature of his heart defect – the commonest problem to present like this being Fallot's tetralogy (Ch. 15.2).

Practical points

- Most heart disease in childhood is congenital, but various acquired disorders are important
- Clinical assessment, including auscultation, remains vital and should not be omitted – even though investigations such as echocardiography are usually necessary
- Cardiac catheterization is seldom required to establish the diagnosis but is frequently used for therapeutic (interventional) procedures
- Many serious heart defects, which lead to symptoms in the early days/weeks of life, are 'ductus-dependent'. Use of prostaglandin E_1 infusion to reopen the ductus may be life-saving

Surgery

In many cases, surgical treatment offers the best means of alleviating the problem that has produced heart failure, and medical treatment should only be pursued in an effort to achieve stabilization of the infant's condition and allow a diagnosis to be reached so that planning of surgical management may proceed.

15.2 Common heart defects and diseases in infancy and childhood

J. Wilkinson

Congenital malformations affecting the heart and/or great vessels occur in a little under 1% of newborn infants. Eight defects are relatively frequent and together make up approximately 80% of all congenital heart disease (Table 15.2.1). The remaining 20% of defects comprise a large number of abnormalities, some being quite rare and/or complex malformations.

Presenting features

The major presenting features are:

- the presence of an abnormal murmur
- development of symptoms or signs of congestive heart failure
- central cyanosis
- any combination of the above.

Acyanotic defects

These comprise approximately 75% of all congenital heart defects and can be subdivided into (1) those that are associated with an isolated left-to-right shunt and (2) those that are not associated with any shunting, in which no septal defect is present.

Defects with a left-to-right shunt are:

- ventricular septal defect (VSD)
- persistent ductus arteriosus (PDA)
- atrial septal defect (ASD)
- atrioventricular septal defect (AVSD).

Ventricular septal defect

These comprise around 30% of all cardiac defects. They vary from tiny defects, of pinhole size, to huge defects. Small defects are more common than large ones and are usually asymptomatic. Defects are frequently situated in the region of the membranous septum but VSDs involving the muscular septum are also common (Fig. 15.2.1). Very tiny muscular defects may be demonstrated by echocardiography in infants with no clinical signs to suggest a septal defect.

With a small VSD, there is usually a loud, harsh, high-pitched systolic murmur audible at the left sternal border, frequently associated with a thrill. The heart sounds otherwise may be normal and there are often no other abnormal findings. The murmur is most often 'pansystolic' in timing, but this is not invariably so. Alternatively there may be an early systolic (decrescendo) murmur, which is often well localized at the mid left sternal border and reflects a very small muscular defect that is functionally closing with each systolic contraction.

With a larger VSD, signs of cardiac failure may be present and the physical signs are different. These may include a parasternal heave, a displaced apex and the systolic murmur may be softer and less harsh. An additional diastolic murmur may be heard at the apex, due to increased flow through the mitral valve. Infants with a large VSD often thrive poorly, suffer dyspnoea with feeds and are prone to recurrent chest infections. Tachypnoea, dyspnoea, sweating and hepatomegaly are frequent findings.

With small defects, the chest X-ray and electrocardiogram (ECG) are frequently normal. With larger defects, the X-ray shows cardiomegaly and increased pulmonary vascular markings (pulmonary plethora) (see Fig. 15.1.7). The ECG often shows biventricular hypertrophy. The site and size of the defect can be documented well with echocardiography.

The natural history of a VSD varies. Small defects frequently undergo spontaneous closure, which may occur in 50% or more. Some moderate defects may also diminish in size and the shunt becomes minor. Important complications include progressive aortic incompetence, when one leaflet of the aortic valve is sucked into (prolapses) into an adjacent VSD, or the development of infundibular pulmonary stenosis. Small isolated defects may be left alone if the evidence shows no significant haemodynamic disturbance and the patient remains symptom-free.

Large VSDs are associated with a variable degree of pulmonary hypertension, which is related to transmission of systemic pressure through the defect into the right ventricle. In the presence of a large (non-restrictive) defect, pulmonary artery systolic pressure may be 'systemic' (similar to that in the

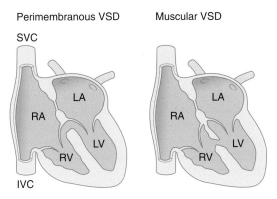

Perimembranous VSD   Muscular VSD

Fig. 15.2.1 Sites of ventricular septal defect (VSD). In the left panel, the defect is close to the membranous part of the ventricular septum (perimembranous VSD). In the right panel, the defect is in the muscular septum.

Table 15.2.1 Relative frequency of common congenital heart defects	
Defect	Approximate frequency (%)
Ventricular septal defect (VSD)	30
Persistent arterial duct (ductus arteriosus; PDA)	12
Atrial septal defect (ASD)	8
Pulmonary stenosis	8
Aortic stenosis	5
Coarctation of the aorta	5
Tetralogy of Fallot	5
Transposition of the great arteries	5

aorta). Pulmonary 'hypertension' is present from birth and may lead to the development of pulmonary vascular obliterative disease. Progression of pulmonary vascular damage, with increasing vascular resistance in the pulmonary circulation, will eventually result in reversal of the shunt, with the appearance of cyanosis (Eisenmenger syndrome), developing in adolescence or early adult life.

Early surgical repair (before age 6 months) of a VSD is indicated if congestive heart failure appears in infancy, or if pulmonary hypertension is present. Surgery can be carried out at any age from the newborn period. However, many infants with a large VSD do not become symptomatic until they are several weeks old. Repair at a later age may be indicated if the defect fails to close and continues to cause a significant shunt, or if complications such as aortic valve prolapse develop. In practice only around 25% of children with a VSD will need surgery for it. Non-surgical closure, with a catheter device, is feasible in selected patients but is not yet regarded as the first choice option for 'repair' of VSD.

Persistent ductus arteriosus

Failure of the ductus arteriosus to close in the newborn period may be due to severe prematurity or to a congenital abnormality. The clinical findings depend on the size of the ductus. Patients with a small PDA frequently remain asymptomatic and the only abnormal finding may be a continuous murmur audible at the upper left sternal border (in or above the pulmonary area). Such murmurs may be present throughout the cardiac cycle ('machinery murmur') but sometimes disappear during diastole and may be sufficiently short to be mistaken for a purely systolic murmur, especially if the ductus is large and there is associated pulmonary hypertension.

In the presence of a large ductus, collapsing pulses are frequently apparent. The apex may be displaced and forceful and an apical mid-diastolic murmur may be heard (due to increased blood flow across the mitral valve).

Symptoms such as failure to thrive, dyspnoea and recurrent chest infections are similar to those of a large VSD.

The presence of cardiomegaly and pulmonary plethora on the chest X-ray indicates a large shunt and left ventricular hypertrophy may be seen on the ECG. The diagnosis can be confirmed by echocardiography.

In symptomatic premature infants, medical treatment with indomethacin, which inhibits prostaglandin synthesis, may be effective in promoting ductal constriction. Unfortunately, drug treatment is not effective in mature infants and in such patients intervention to close the ductus is indicated. This should be carried out at an early stage in symptomatic patients (including premature infants if indomethacin is ineffective) but may be delayed until the second year of life or subsequently in asymptomatic patients with a small ductus. When the ductus is small, intervention is indicated to eliminate the risk of infective endocarditis rather than to treat cardiac failure or pulmonary hypertension. The preferred method of closure is device occlusion, via a cardiac catheter, either by introduction of one or more spring coils or by placement of an occlusion device via a cardiac catheter. The alternative of surgical ligation is preferred for premature infants and some patients with very large PDAs.

Atrial septal defect

Defects of the atrial septum are usually situated in the region of the fossa ovale and are termed 'secundum' ASD (Fig. 15.2.2). Unlike small VSDs and PDAs (which tend to be associated with loud murmurs), small ASDs may go completely undetected. With larger defects, a significant shunt is present, but this is not associated with pulmonary hypertension (with rare exceptions) and seldom leads to symptoms during infancy. Isolated ASDs hardly ever lead to Eisenmenger syndrome.

The characteristic findings in children with an ASD are related to the increased blood flow through the right side of the heart. An ejection systolic murmur, due to high pulmonary flow, is present in the pulmonary area but not usually louder than grade 2/6 and not harsh in character, and a soft mid-diastolic murmur may be heard at the lower end of the sternum, secondary to increased tricuspid flow. A parasternal heave related to a dilated right ventricle may be palpable. The aortic and pulmonary components of the second heart sound are widely separated and frequently remain equally separated during both phases of respiration (fixed splitting) (see Fig. 15.1.3).

While most children are free of any major symptoms, their growth is often mildly impaired compared with siblings, and exercise tolerance may be slightly reduced. If they reach adult life without surgery, they may develop atrial flutter or fibrillation in middle adult life and frequently become increasingly handicapped by exertional dyspnoea and effort intolerance at the age of 40–50 years, even if arrhythmias are not a problem.

The chest X-ray characteristically shows an increase in transverse cardiac diameter with pulmonary plethora. The electrocardiogram tends to show features of partial right bundle branch block. The diagnosis may be confirmed by echocardiography.

Closure should be recommended in cases where there is evidence of a significant shunt. In most cases a transcatheter procedure is performed with placement of an 'occluder' device, which is an appropriate non-surgical option for many patients with central defects of small to moderate size with good margins but is not applicable for very large defects or those with poorly formed margins. Surgical repair may be required for defects that are unsuitable for 'device closure'. This can usually be achieved by direct suture but may require insertion of a patch.

Atrioventricular septal defect

This category of defect, which accounts for approximately 3% of all congenital cardiac defects, includes a group of ASDs low in the atrial septum that abut on the atrioventricular valves and may involve the upper part of the ventricular septum. When the ventricular septum is intact (partial AVSD), only an atrial communication is present. This is referred to as an 'ostium primum' ASD (Fig. 15.2.2) and is almost invariably associated with leaflet abnormalities (a 'cleft') of the mitral valve, which is usually incompetent.

Children with this type of defect may, if mitral incompetence is severe, become symptomatic in infancy or early childhood. In the absence of significant mitral regurgitation, however, the features resemble those of a secundum ASD.

When a significant VSD coexists (complete AVSD – 'common atrioventricular canal'; Fig. 15.2.3), the presentation resembles that of an isolated large VSD with difficulty feeding and failure to thrive.

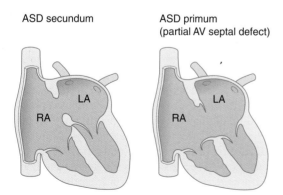

Fig. 15.2.2 Common types of atrial septal defect (ASD). Secundum defects are in the fossa ovale (mid-atrial septum). Primum defects are low in the atrial septum and abut on the atrioventricular valves, which are abnormal and often incompetent.

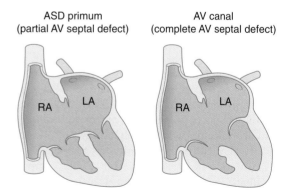

Fig. 15.2.3 Atrioventricular (AV) septal defect. The complete form is associated with a common AV valve and the septal defect allows communication between all four cardiac chambers.

This defect is commonly associated with Down syndrome.

The chest X-ray usually shows quite marked cardiomegaly and pulmonary plethora, especially in the complete form of the defect. The ECG characteristically shows left axis deviation accompanied by partial right bundle branch block. The presence of left axis deviation distinguishes 'primum' ASDs from 'secundum' defects. Echocardiography confirms the diagnosis and will differentiate partial from complete atrioventricular defects.

Surgical repair is almost always required. When pulmonary hypertension is present this is generally recommended in the early months of life (3–4 months) in order to obviate the risk of pulmonary vascular disease. In patients with an isolated ostium primum ASD, when pulmonary hypertension is absent, surgery may be delayed until the age of 2–4 years. Operation involves placement of a patch to close the ASD and repair of the mitral valve cleft to eliminate mitral incompetence, if present.

The following defects have no shunt, and are obstructive lesions:

- pulmonary stenosis
- aortic stenosis
- coarctation of the aorta.

Pulmonary stenosis

Pulmonary stenosis, usually valvar in site, is the commonest of the pure obstructive malformations. The pulmonary valve is abnormal, with thickened leaflets and partially fused commissures. In some cases the valve may be bicuspid.

Other sites of pulmonary stenosis, occurring as isolated abnormalities, are less frequent. These include muscular subpulmonary obstruction involving the right ventricular outflow tract (infundibular stenosis) and supravalvular or branch pulmonary stenosis.

Most patients are asymptomatic in infancy and childhood. An ejection systolic murmur, best heard in the pulmonary area and radiating through to the back, is the characteristic finding. The murmur is usually not associated with a thrill. The pulmonary component of the second sound is often abnormally soft or inaudible, although in mild cases it may be heard and the degree of splitting is often increased. An early ejection sound (ejection click) is usually audible at the left sternal border (Fig. 15.2.4) with valvar stenosis. Characteristically the click is louder during expiration and fades on inspiration.

The chest X-ray usually demonstrates a normal heart size but the main pulmonary artery is often unusually prominent (poststenotic dilatation). This produces an abnormal convexity on the upper left

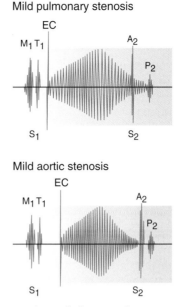

Fig. 15.2.4   Auscultatory findings in pulmonary and aortic stenosis. The ejection click (EC) is earlier in pulmonary stenosis and the second sound is widely split. In aortic stenosis the click is best heard at the apex.

heart border just below the aortic knuckle. The ECG may be normal with mild obstruction but shows right ventricular hypertrophy in more severe cases.

Mild pulmonary stenosis is generally a benign condition and is often non-progressive. More severe pulmonary stenosis leads eventually to effort intolerance, angina on exertion and cardiac failure. 'Critical' (very severe) pulmonary stenosis may present in early infancy with cyanosis due to right-to-left shunting through the foramen ovale or an associated ASD.

The diagnosis may be confirmed by echocardiography. Treatment involves a catheter technique involving inflation of a balloon in the valve orifice to separate the fused commissures (balloon pulmonary valvotomy or valvuloplasty). This procedure is simple and effective in most cases, requires only a very short hospital stay and saves the patient an open heart operation. If this is not effective, then surgical valvotomy may be performed.

Aortic stenosis

As in pulmonary stenosis, the valve is abnormal with thickened leaflets and fused commissures. In most cases the valve is bicuspid. Subaortic stenosis with a fibrous stricture or with muscular obstruction (hypertrophic subaortic stenosis) also occurs but is less common. Stenosis in the ascending aorta, above the aortic valve, also may be encountered (supra-aortic stenosis).

Except in very severe cases, affected children are symptom-free in infancy and early childhood and present with the chance finding of an ejection systolic murmur over the precordium and in the aortic area. Characteristically, with valvar stenosis the murmur is best heard to the right of the sternum and radiates to the carotids. A thrill is commonly present over the carotids and may also be felt in the aortic area. An ejection click is usually heard with valvar stenosis (Fig. 15.2.4) and is often most easily audible at the apex or lower left sternal border. In more severe cases a forceful apical impulse due to left ventricular hypertrophy may be apparent. In subaortic stenosis the murmur is best heard at the left sternal edge and a click is not heard. Conversely, the murmur of supravalvar stenosis is often best heard over the carotid artery.

The natural history of aortic stenosis is generally one of gradual progression. Symptoms include dizziness and syncope on exertion, angina pectoris, effort intolerance and sudden death. In a small minority of cases, with 'critical' stenosis, severe congestive heart failure may appear in early infancy.

In mild and even moderate aortic stenosis, the chest X-ray and ECG may show little abnormality. In more severe cases the ECG tends to show left ventricular hypertrophy but this is often late in appearing. Echocardiography allows assessment of the site and severity of the obstruction.

Treatment should be recommended if significant stenosis is present, even in the absence of symptoms. Balloon aortic valvotomy is feasible as an alternative to surgery and is currently the preferred treatment option for most cases, but may lead to worsening aortic incompetence. Operation involves aortic valvotomy on heart–lung bypass.

Coarctation of the aorta

In this condition a discrete stricture is present in the distal part of the aortic arch. The maximal site of obstruction is usually opposite to, or just proximal to, the aortic end of the ductus arteriosus or ligamentum arteriosum (Fig. 15.2.5).

Coarctation of the aorta is often associated with other cardiac defects, including aortic stenosis, ventricular septal defect and mitral valve abnormalities. A bicuspid aortic valve is present in 40% of cases even in the absence of other malformations.

Coarctation usually leads to the development of severe cardiac failure in the newborn period, with oliguria and acidosis, often in the second or third week of life. Alternatively, in around 30% of cases, presentation may be delayed until late in childhood or even adolescence or adult life.

The characteristic physical findings are of diminished or absent femoral pulses. Simultaneous palpa-

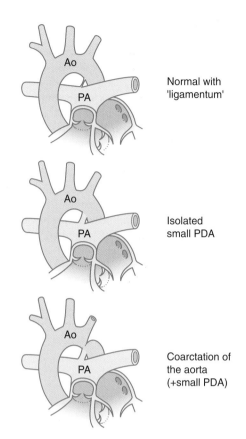

Fig. 15.2.5 Aorta and pulmonary artery showing persistent ductus and site of coarctation (often associated with persistent ductus arteriosus, PDA).

tion of the right brachial pulse and a femoral pulse frequently shows quite obvious delay in the appearance of the latter. Upper limb blood pressure is often elevated, sometimes severely so, and there is a marked discrepancy between arm and leg blood pressure, usually greater than 20 mmHg.

The chest X-ray and ECG findings vary according to the age of presentation. In symptomatic infants cardiomegaly and pulmonary congestion are usually seen on the chest X-ray, and the ECG shows right ventricular hypertrophy. In later childhood the X-ray may show an abnormal appearance of the aortic knuckle and rib notching due to the presence of enlarged intercostal arteries, which act as collateral routes for flow of blood into the lower systemic segment. This is seldom seen before the age of 8 years. The ECG may show left ventricular hypertrophy.

In infancy the onset of congestive heart failure is often related to closure of the ductus arteriosus. Before closure of the ductus, the pulmonary artery pressure is usually sufficient to allow adequate flow of blood into the descending aorta via the ductus, but after the ductus starts to close the flow of blood in the lower part of the circulation becomes inadequate. For this reason infusion of prostaglandin E_1 intravenously may palliate symptoms by causing the ductus to reopen. Other medical measures may help to ameliorate heart failure and improve the condition of the infant before operation. Early surgery, as soon as the diagnosis is established, is always indicated in symptomatic cases. Patients who remain free of symptoms should be assessed carefully for the development of hypertension and, if this is present, surgery should be carried out during early childhood. In other patients intervention may be deferred until later in childhood. In selected cases, with a localized coarctation shelf, balloon angioplasty (or placement of a stent) may be employed as an alternative to surgical repair. Patients who have required surgical relief of coarctation (especially those operated in early infancy) and those who have had balloon angioplasty may develop restenosis at the coarctation site, although this is less common with newer surgical techniques. Such re-stenosis is frequently treated with further balloon angioplasty or stent implantation.

Unoperated patients with coarctation (i.e. those who escape detection during childhood) are at a high risk from serious complications or death during adolescence or early adult life. Complications include left ventricular failure, aortic dissection and subarachnoid haemorrhage due to ruptured berry aneurysm.

Hypoplastic left heart syndrome

A small subgroup of infants with both severe aortic stenosis and coarctation may present with associated hypoplasia of the left ventricle. In some cases the aortic valve and/or mitral valve are atretic (Fig. 15.2.6).

Such infants present with severe cardiac failure or shock in the early days of life. All peripheral pulses are diminished or absent and manifestations of cardiac failure are severe.

The condition is invariably lethal without surgery. Medical treatment, including infusion of prostaglandin and other measures, may lead to improvement. Palliative surgery (the Norwood procedure) is possible and can produce long-term survival. Heart transplantation, even in the newborn period, is offered to some infants, mainly in a small number of centres in the USA.

Cyanotic defects

The presence of cyanosis in a child with congenital heart disease indicates that deoxygenated blood

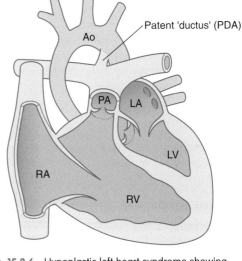

Fig. 15.2.6 Hypoplastic left heart syndrome showing hypoplasia of: left ventricle, mitral valve, aortic valve, ascending aorta. The ductus provides the only effective route through which the systemic circulation can be maintained from the right ventricle with right-to-left shunting across the duct.

from the systemic venous system is being directed back into the systemic circulation without transiting the pulmonary vascular bed. Cyanotic defects account for approximately 25% of all congenital heart malformations. Such defects are almost always associated with the presence of a septal defect, coupled with additional abnormalities that alter the pressure relationship between the two sides of the heart so that, instead of pure left-to-right shunting, right-to-left or bidirectional shunting occurs, producing cyanosis.

Three major subgroups exist. In the first group (exemplified by tetralogy of Fallot) pulmonary blood flow is reduced as a result of a combination of obstruction to normal flow into the lung circulation and a septal defect behind the obstruction through which blood may shunt from right to left. In tetralogy of Fallot the shunt is almost completely right to left, whereas in some other defects associated with low pulmonary flow the physiology is more complex, with right-to-left shunting at one level and left-to-right shunting at another, e.g. tricuspid atresia and pulmonary atresia.

In the second group of cyanotic defects bidirectional shunting is associated with very large communications between the left and right sides of the heart with free mixing of blood, e.g. 'single ventricle', and truncus arteriosus. In such defects pulmonary blood flow is usually high and pulmonary hypertension is a feature. Cyanosis is generally mild and may pass unnoticed.

A third group of cyanotic defects, best exemplified by transposition of the great arteries, may be considered as a 'plumbing problem'. In transposition, the aorta and pulmonary artery are connected to the wrong side of the heart and as a result systemic venous blood is directed straight through into the systemic circulation again (see below).

Tetralogy of Fallot

Of the four components that comprise Fallot's tetralogy (VSD, pulmonary stenosis, right ventricular hypertrophy, overriding aorta) the important ones are pulmonary stenosis and the VSD (Fig. 15.2.7). The presence of severe pulmonary stenosis, which characteristically is associated with infundibular muscular obstruction coupled frequently with valvar hypoplasia and commissural fusion, leads to elevation of right ventricular pressure. In most patients, the systolic pressure in the left and right ventricles is equal but the increased resistance to ejection into the pulmonary circulation, due to the stenosis, produces right-to-left shunting into the aorta.

Clinical features

Cyanosis is not usually obvious in the newborn period but appears later in infancy in most affected children. Oxygen saturations (with pulse oximetry) may be normal or mildly depressed in the early weeks of life. A harsh ejection systolic murmur is audible at the left sternal edge and/or in the pulmonary area (infundibular stenosis) and radiates through to the back. The second heart sound is often quite loud but single because the pulmonary closure sound is inaudible (Fig. 15.2.8).

Cyanosis appears gradually during the first 6–12 months of life or rarely later, and is characteristically more obvious on crying or on exertion. A characteristic feature is the development of intermittent episodes of severe cyanosis ('hypoxic spells'), which may appear spontaneously but are quite commonly precipitated by stress or exercise. Such spells are characterized by marked pallor or cyanosis with dyspnoea and distress. Loss of consciousness may occur. Hypoxic spells are associated with increased right-to-left shunting and a sharp reduction in pulmonary flow. In the past these have been attributed to infundibular 'spasm', although in practice the physiology is more complex and spasm does not occur. First aid treatment of these spells, which are potentially dangerous, involves soothing and pacifying the distressed infant with a view to trying to induce sleep. In severe cases intramuscular morphine may be helpful. Older infants and children have reduced exercise tolerance and often adopt a squatting posture at intervals during exertion. This manoeuvre, in which the child squats down on the haunches with knees up to the chest, increases systemic venous return and systemic vascular resistance. The latter reduces right-to-left shunting and the increased venous return produces a significant transient rise in pulmonary blood flow with improved oxygenation.

Course and prognosis

Cyanosis generally progresses gradually, with diminishing exercise tolerance, finger clubbing and in severe cases growth retardation. Development of cardiac failure is unusual but the severe cyanosis leads to compensatory polycythaemia and cerebral thromboembolic complications, e.g. stroke, may occur. Infective endocarditis and cerebral abscess also are important complications.

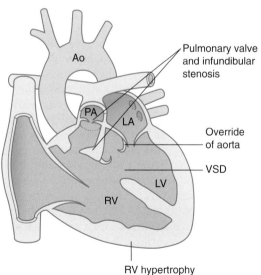

Fig. 15.2.7 Fallot's tetralogy, showing infundibular and valvar pulmonary stenosis and hypoplasia of the branch pulmonary arteries, all of which are frequent.

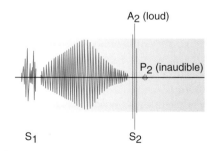

Fig. 15.2.8 Auscultatory signs in Fallot's tetralogy. The systolic murmur is 'ejection', due to the pulmonary stenosis. The aortic closure sound is accentuated and pulmonary closure is so soft as to be inaudible. The second sound appears to be 'single'.

Investigations

The chest X-ray shows the heart size to be normal with an uptilted apex and concave pulmonary segment associated with reduced lung vascularity (oligaemia). In severe cases the cardiac contour may resemble the shape of a wooden clog – *coeur en sabot* – often referred to as 'boot-shaped'. The ECG usually shows right ventricular hypertrophy. Echocardiography is diagnostic.

Differential diagnosis

In infancy, before the onset of cyanosis, the murmur often is mistaken for that of a small VSD. Other cyanotic defects, such as tricuspid atresia, may be differentiated by ancillary investigations, such as ECG and echocardiogram.

Treatment

Total correction involving repair of the VSD and relief of the infundibular and pulmonary valve stenosis can be carried out even in early infancy if the anatomy is suitable. However, many affected children have quite marked hypoplasia of the branch pulmonary arteries and this may make it desirable to delay repair and to carry out a palliative shunt operation first. This involves creating a communication between the aorta and a pulmonary artery to increase pulmonary blood flow, allowing better growth of the branch pulmonary arteries. Currently, most surgeons use a prosthetic tube graft (Gore-Tex) to create an anastomosis between a subclavian artery and the ipsilateral pulmonary artery branch.

Infants who are having significant hypoxic spells can be treated medically in the short term with beta-adrenergic blocking drugs, for example, propranolol, to prevent spells while the child is awaiting surgery.

Transposition of the great arteries

In this condition the aorta and pulmonary arteries arise from the incorrect ventricles. This is described as 'ventriculoarterial discordance' (Fig. 15.2.9). Systemic venous blood is directed through the right side of the heart back into the aorta and pulmonary venous blood through the left side of the heart back into the pulmonary circulation. Survival is dependent on transfer of blood across from each circuit into the other via a foramen ovale, ductus arteriosus or a septal defect. Affected infants generally survive for several days or even weeks because of shunting through the foramen ovale and/or ductus arteriosus, but few live longer than a month without help, unless they have a coexisting septal defect, e.g. a VSD.

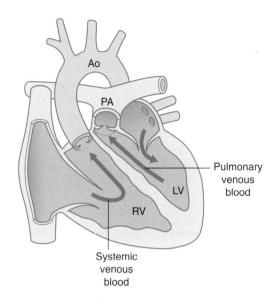

Fig. 15.2.9 Transposition of the great arteries. Systemic venous blood is ejected from the right ventricle to the aorta, while pulmonary venous blood passes from the left ventricle to the pulmonary artery.

Clinical features

Cyanosis is present from the early hours of life and usually progresses gradually over the next few days. Metabolic acidosis also may develop, because of the tissue hypoxia, if the situation persists untreated. Apart from the cyanosis the infant may appear completely normal. Palpation reveals a forceful right ventricular impulse at the left sternal edge, but on auscultation there is frequently no murmur audible.

Investigations

The chest X-ray shows a normal-sized or mildly enlarged heart with a contour that sometimes resembles 'an egg on its side'. Pulmonary vascular markings are usually increased. The ECG shows normal ventricular complexes but may manifest T-wave abnormalities. The diagnosis may be established rapidly by echocardiography.

Treatment

Balloon atrial septostomy
Cardiac catheterization is performed as an emergency procedure and a catheter with an inflatable balloon at the tip is passed into the left atrium via the foramen ovale. After inflation of the balloon the catheter is withdrawn with force into the right atrium, producing a tear in the atrial septum and hence creating an atrial septal defect. This allows more effective shunting with amelioration of the cyanosis and hypoxia.

Surgery

After successful balloon septostomy most infants will manage comfortably for many days or weeks. Surgical correction involves transferring the pulmonary artery and the aorta back to their appropriate ventricles. It is also necessary to transfer the tiny coronary arteries across from the aortic root (above the right ventricle) to the new aortic origin from the left ventricle. The operation needs to be performed in early infancy, usually the first 2–3 weeks of life, before the left ventricle has become acclimatized to feeding the low-pressure pulmonary circulation and no longer has sufficient muscle mass to support the systemic circulation.

Tricuspid atresia

In this malformation the tricuspid valve is blocked completely and there is no communication between the right atrium and ventricle. Systemic venous blood passes via the foramen ovale or an ASD into the left side of the heart, and at ventricular or arterial level a left-to-right shunt exists (via a VSD or PDA). This allows blood to perfuse the pulmonary circulation, usually in reduced amounts.

Clinical features

Cyanosis develops early. A systolic murmur is audible along the left sternal border.

Diagnosis

The diagnosis may be suspected on the characteristic ECG pattern of left axis deviation, right atrial hypertrophy, left ventricular hypertrophy and right ventricular hypoplasia. Echocardiography confirms the diagnosis.

Treatment

A palliative shunt operation may be performed in infancy (see above under Tetralogy of Fallot). Later in childhood reconstructive cardiac surgery is usually feasible and involves the creation of an anastomosis/connection between the systemic veins (superior and inferior vena cava) and the pulmonary arteries, allowing systemic venous blood to pass directly into the pulmonary circulation (Fontan operation).

Pulmonary atresia

In this condition the origin of the pulmonary artery from the right ventricle is completely obstructed or absent. Blood in the right side of the heart passes via an ASD, foramen ovale or VSD into the left ventricle and aorta. The pulmonary circulation depends on collateral flow from the aorta via a PDA or other collateral channels.

Clinical features

Cyanosis develops early and many infants have an easily audible continuous murmur due to the associated PDA or other collaterals feeding the pulmonary circulation from the aorta.

Diagnosis

The diagnosis is usually confirmed by echocardiography, although it may be suspected strongly on clinical grounds coupled with ECG and X-ray findings.

Treatment

Initial medical therapy may involve prostaglandin infusion to maintain patency of the ductus. Early surgical treatment usually involves a systemic-to-pulmonary shunt procedure. At a later stage, which depends on the associated defects, surgical correction may be performed by opening up a way through from the right ventricle into the pulmonary arteries, often by insertion of a 'valved conduit'.

Persistent truncus arteriosus ('truncus')

This defect is associated with the presence of a single artery, which branches shortly after arising from the heart to give rise to the pulmonary artery and aorta. The truncal valve usually sits astride a large VSD and receives blood from both right and left ventricles.

Clinical features

Cyanosis is usually mild or absent and congestive heart failure often appears in the newborn period. Most infants will have a systolic murmur and in some cases a diastolic murmur may be heard that is due to incompetence of the abnormal truncal valve.

Diagnosis

The diagnosis can be made by echocardiography. Chest X-ray and ECG findings are usually non-specific.

Treatment

The only effective treatment is surgical correction, which needs to be carried out in early infancy. The pulmonary artery is separated from the truncus and, after closure of the VSD leaving the aorta arising from the left ventricle, a valved conduit is placed to connect the right ventricle to the pulmonary arteries.

Clinical example

Aaron was 6 months old and had gained weight poorly since birth. Birth weight was 2.8 kg and his present weight was 4.1 kg. Several doctors had examined him but had failed to find a cause for his poor weight gain.

Examination showed a thin infant who is tachypnoeic with a respiratory rate of 60 per minute. All pulses were easily palpable and large-volume (bounding). The cardiac impulse was forceful, with the apex displaced towards the anterior axillary line. Auscultation revealed a grade 2/6 ejection systolic murmur of non-specific character audible over the precordium and in the pulmonary area. A soft diastolic murmur was also heard at the apex.

A chest X-ray showed a large heart and plethoric lungs. An ECG showed left ventricular hypertrophy.

The fact that the murmur had not been heard before suggested that it might have been soft or dismissed as being innocent. The signs suggested a significant VSD or patent ductus arteriosus with pulmonary hypertension. It was not possible to make a definite diagnosis without echocardiography, which needed to be organized as soon as possible. The X-ray and ECG abnormalities indicated a major haemodynamic disturbance and the defect was likely to be large. Aaron's failure to thrive was likely to be the consequence of the cardiac abnormality.

The diagnosis, confirmed by echocardiography, was a large patent ductus arteriosus. The absence of a continuous murmur was due to the presence of severe pulmonary hypertension.

Acquired heart disease in children

There are several forms of acquired heart disease in children.

Kawasaki disease

This condition is described elsewhere (Ch. 13.3). It may lead to the development of coronary artery aneurysms, with risk of myocardial ischaemia or infarction.

Myocarditis

This condition follows a viral infection, although the aetiological mechanism may well be, in part, immunologically mediated. The disease quite frequently follows Coxsackie B infection, but may be associated with a wide variety of other viruses. The ausculta-

tory signs are non-specific, with soft heart sounds, a gallop rhythm but no murmur in most cases. Congestive heart failure may develop rapidly or insidiously and the condition is accompanied by ECG, X-ray and echocardiographic evidence of myocardial damage, ventricular dilatation and depressed myocardial function. In the past, the condition was frequently fatal, although some patients recovered. Use of immunoglobulin or immunosuppressive drug therapy (e.g. steroids, azathioprine, cyclosporin) may improve the prospects for recovery.

Cardiomyopathy

This term encompasses a group of conditions with heart muscle disease and myocardial dysfunction, often associated with progressive effort intolerance, arrhythmias and/or heart failure. The condition may result from an earlier episode of myocarditis but in most cases the aetiology is unknown and no specific treatment is available. In those patients where the condition progresses to end-stage heart failure, cardiac transplantation offers the only prospect of survival.

Rheumatic heart disease

Rheumatic heart disease is now very uncommon in the developed world. The condition follows acute rheumatic fever, although a clear history of rheumatic fever may be absent in some cases. It is probably the result of an abnormal immune response on the part of the host to certain streptococcal antigens, which results in an autoimmune disorder affecting the heart, synovial membranes and other tissues.

The main cardiac sequelae of rheumatic fever are the development of damage to heart valves, resulting in the development of mitral stenosis and/or incompetence and aortic stenosis/incompetence. Other valves are occasionally affected.

Clinical manifestations

Rheumatic fever follows a streptococcal infection, usually tonsillitis.

Major criteria for diagnosis include:

- migratory polyarthritis mainly affecting large joints
- evidence of carditis with tachycardia, cardiac enlargement, the development of new murmurs and, in severe cases, cardiac failure
- choreiform limb movements: Sydenham chorea
- a transient demarcated skin rash on the trunk: erythema marginatum
- the development of nodules over bony prominences.

535

Minor criteria are:

- fever
- arthralgia
- previous history of rheumatic fever
- raised erythrocyte sedimentation rate (ESR) or C reactive protein
- prolonged PR interval on ECG.

All patients with suspected rheumatic fever should have throat cultures and be tested for evidence of streptococcal antibodies (ASO titre, anti-DNAase titre).

Diagnosis

The diagnosis cannot usually be regarded as established unless evidence of a recent streptococcal infection is demonstrable, i.e. a positive throat culture or positive antibody titres. If such evidence is found, however, the presence of two minor criteria and one major criterion as listed above, or the presence of two or more major criteria, may be regarded as indicative of the presence of rheumatic fever.

Treatment

Treatment involves bed rest and administration of aspirin in full anti-inflammatory doses. Steroids may also be administered in the presence of more severe carditis and will usually reduce the duration of the acute episode, although they probably do not affect the development of chronic valve disease.

Infective endocarditis

The presence of structural cardiac abnormalities associated with turbulent blood flow within the heart or major arteries predisposes to seeding of bacteria into endothelial erosions associated with jet lesions. Once infection becomes established, vegetations develop in the affected area and progressive destruction of adjacent structures follows. The development of a transient bacteraemia is usually the precursor of such infection, although the source of the bacteraemia is often not clear.

Symptoms include fever, rigors, anorexia and weight loss. Physical signs may include evidence of anaemia, sometimes with petechial haemorrhages, splinter haemorrhages in the nailbeds, splenomegaly and finger clubbing. In many cases the manifestations are relatively subtle and a high index of suspicion is required if the diagnosis is to be reached. Any child with known structural heart disease, whether operated or not, is at risk (with the exception of a PDA or a secundum ASD that has been closed surgically or with a device more than 6 months previously). Should such a patient become chronically unwell or have pro-

longed unexplained fever, s/he should be investigated with a view to excluding infective endocarditis. Investigations should include a full blood count and ESR, multiple blood cultures and careful echocardiography, including, if necessary, transoesophageal echocardiography to identify vegetations.

Occasionally, infective endocarditis may develop in a patient with no previously known cardiac defect.

The responsible organism is most commonly *Streptococcus viridans* or *Staphylococcus* (both *aureus* and *albus*). Other organisms include enterococci, *Escherichia coli* and fungi, especially *Candida albicans*.

Treatment involves intravenous antibiotic therapy, usually for a period of 6 weeks. Bactericidal drugs should be used and the choice of antibiotic(s) should be made on the basis of sensitivity testing of the infecting organism from cultures. Rarely, where severe valve damage develops during the acute illness, or with large vegetations in the heart, surgery may be required to remove vegetations and/or repair or replace damaged valves.

Prophylaxis against endocarditis should be advised in all patients who are considered to be at risk and should be administered on occasions when a bacteraemia is likely to result from surgical or dental procedures. Such procedures include dental extractions and other dental procedures involving significant gingival trauma, other oropharyngeal instrumentation and surgery on the bowel and genitourinary tract. Effective cover can usually be achieved with amoxicillin (with an aminoglycoside, in addition, to cover procedures on the genitourinary or gastrointestinal tract). In the main a single dose of antibiotic, administered an hour prior to the procedure (oral dose) or at induction of anaesthesia (intravenous dose), is adequate as the bacteraemia induced by such procedures is very transient.

Cardiac arrhythmias

Phasic variation in heart rate (*sinus arrhythmia*) is a normal phenomenon in children. It is usually related to respiration, although not invariably so.

Paroxysmal supraventricular tachycardia

This condition is characterized by the sudden onset of very rapid tachycardia, usually with a rate of 200–300 beats per minute. Affected infants usually become pale and appear mildly distressed with tachypnoea and poor feeding. Heart failure may develop and the appearance of supraventricular tachycardia in an infant requires urgent treatment. Older children are often aware of their rapid heart rate and adult observers may notice pulsation in the neck.

The acute episode may sometimes be terminated by vagal manoeuvres, such as the application of ice packs to the face or the Valsalva manoeuvre. Intravenous adenosine will usually terminate the episode, or alternatively a DC shock may be applied.

The ECG between episodes will often show evidence of pre-excitation with Wolff–Parkinson–White syndrome.

Some patients have recurring attacks over many years and need chronic antiarrhythmic drug treatment or definitive intervention to ablate the substrate of the arrhythmia, although this is seldom needed in early childhood.

Heart block

Congenital heart block is an uncommon problem in the newborn period. It may present with fetal bradycardia, which can be misinterpreted as indicating fetal distress. Among affected infants, 50% have no structural cardiac abnormality but a range of congenital anomalies may be associated with heart block. Infants with otherwise normal hearts may develop heart block due to the presence of maternal autoimmune antibodies, which should be looked for in the mother of all affected children. Some mothers will have evidence of systemic lupus erythematosus or other collagen disease. Others are asymptomatic but have autoimmune antibodies, which are probably responsible for damage to the conduction system of the fetus.

The heart rate is usually in the range of 40–70 beats per minute. Infants with heart rates above 55 beats per minute are often asymptomatic and will tolerate the bradycardia well. Slower heart rates and/or the presence of associated structural cardiac defects often lead to the development of heart failure and the need for implantation of a permanent pacemaker.

Ventricular arrhythmias

Sustained ventricular arrhythmias are uncommon during childhood; however, the presence of ventricular premature beats may be detected as irregularities in the pulse on routine examination or on a chance ECG. The presence of such premature beats in an otherwise normal child with no other evidence of heart disease may be regarded as benign, and even when premature beats occur frequently they very rarely lead to any symptoms or require treatment.

Long QT syndrome

A small number of families or individual children manifest electrocardiographic evidence of prolonged repolarization with increase in the corrected QT interval on the ECG. Such patients are vulnerable to development of paroxysmal ventricular tachycardia or ventricular fibrillation, usually associated with a sudden emotion (e.g. fright) or with exertion. Any patient developing dizziness or syncope on exertion should, therefore, be assessed with a view to excluding this condition, which often is familial and may lead to sudden death.

Treatment may involve antiarrhythmic medication, implantation of a pacemaker or surgical stellate ganglionectomy.

 Practical points

- VSD is the commonest congenital heart defect
- Minor heart defects (small VSD/PDA; mild pulmonary or aortic stenosis) may be well tolerated with no symptoms but carry a risk of infective endocarditis
- Necessity for treatment depends on careful assessment of the severity of disturbance to cardiac function and risk of complications (including endocarditis). Some defects (e.g. small VSD; mild pulmonary stenosis) pose little threat and do not need intervention
- Treatment for congenital heart defects was, in the past, usually surgical. In the current era many heart defects can be managed with catheter interventions – but choice of surgery versus catheter procedures still requires careful assessment of the risks and benefits of the different options

PART 16

HAEMATOLOGICAL DISORDERS AND MALIGNANCIES

Anaemias of childhood 16.1

P. Monagle

Definition

Anaemia is a common medical condition throughout all ages of childhood. However, the common causes vary with age. Anaemia refers to a reduction in haemoglobin (and hence red cell mass) below that which is considered normal for the patient in question. Normative haemoglobin data differs with age and, in teenage years, gender. Clinicians need to ensure that, when considering a diagnosis of anaemia, correct age-specific and, where applicable, sex-specific reference ranges are used. These reference ranges may vary according to the laboratory analyser in use. Thus each laboratory should report their own specific age-related reference ranges. An example of the age-related variation is shown by the reference ranges in Table 16.1.1. The majority of reference ranges in clinical use reflect 95% confidence intervals, so that 2.5% of individuals who are in fact 'normal' would be expected to consistently have haemoglobin levels just below the lower limit of the reported reference range.

Physiology

The prime function of haemoglobin is tissue oxygen delivery. Hence anaemia threatens this critical bodily function. Acutely, severe anaemia can lead to hypoxic tissue injury, and chronic anaemia can lead to growth failure and organ dysfunction as a result of chronic hypoxia or failure of compensatory mechanisms. The physiology of tissue oxygen delivery is critical to understand, as it enables the clinician to understand the concepts of relative anaemia and to determine appropriate treatment of the anaemic patient.

> Tissue oxygen delivery (ml/min)
> = cardiac output (l/min) × haemoglobin (gm/l)
> × haemoglobin saturation (%) × 1.34 (ml/g),

where 1.34 is a constant and represents the amount of oxygen carried by 1 g of normal haemoglobin.

The key issues in this basic physiological equation are that:

- the parameters are multiplied, such that small decreases in cardiac output *and* haemoglobin *and* haemoglobin saturation lead to an overall large decrease in tissue oxygen delivery. Thus patients with cardiac disease may tolerate less reduction in

haemoglobin before developing tissue hypoxia, and hence often have considerable urgency in treating their anaemia. No single haemoglobin (Hb) level can be used as a indication for transfusion therapy as these other factors need to be considered

- in the presence of anaemia, cardiac output must be increased to maintain tissue oxygen delivery (Hb saturation cannot be increased above 100%). Failure of this compensatory mechanism or limitation of cardiac output by another disease will result in tissue hypoxia. Cardiac output is determined by cardiac stroke volume and heart rate. Therefore, heart rate is an important measure of the stress the anaemia is placing on the patient's cardiac reserve. All anaemic patients should have their vital signs, especially heart rate and respiratory rate, assessed as part of their initial medical evaluation, and these parameters should be used to monitor progress and response to therapy

- Hb saturation is normally close to 100% in children without cyanotic congenital heart disease or significant lung pathology. Thus, in otherwise well children with severe anaemia, or children in whom the Hb saturation is measured as 99–100%, inspired oxygen therapy makes little if any contribution to improving tissue oxygenation. Recovery of red cell mass (and hence Hb) is the most effective therapy

- in children with cyanotic congenital heart disease or pulmonary pathology, the natural compensation for reduced Hb saturation is to increase Hb concentration. Hence, if a child with cyanotic congential heart disease who usually has a relatively increased Hb was to develop a 'relative anaemia', they might develop symptoms of anaemia at Hb levels that would be considered normal in most children. Treatment of 'relative anaemia', if required, is based on the same principles as treatment of 'true anaemia'.

Clinical presentations

Children with anaemia most often present with pallor (reflecting the reduced Hb) or signs of reduced exercise tolerance (reflecting inability to increase tissue oxygen delivery to meet the demands of exercise). Reduced exercise tolerance manifests differently according to age. In infants, poor feeding is

Table 16.1.1 Normal haemoglobin values for age

Age	Hb (g/l)
Birth	135–200
1 month	100–180
2 months	90–140
6 months	95–135
1 year	105–135
2–6 years	110–145
6–12 years	115–155
>12 years (female)	120–160
>12 years (male)	130–180

often described. In older children, shortness of breath on exertion or generalized lethargy are more common. Alternatively, incidental finding of anaemia when full blood examination has been performed for another indication is also very common.

Once the presence of anaemia is confirmed, thorough history taking and examination of the patient is required. Patient age and the duration of symptoms is important as a first step in determining the likely aetiology of the anaemia.

In addition, during the history and examination, other key considerations are:

- is there evidence of cardiac decompensation or other adverse events as a result of the anaemia? This clearly makes appropriate therapy a matter of urgency
- are there clues to the aetiology of the anaemia?
- is there evidence of multilineage cytopenias (neutropenia and thrombocytopenia)?
- is there evidence of an associated, perhaps causative, disease?

Information that assists in answering these questions is shown in Table 16.1.2.

Table 16.1.2 Relevant information required on history and examination for patients with anaemia

Critical question	Information obtained on history and examination
Cardiac decompensation	Exercise tolerance Heart rate and respiratory rate Signs of congestive heart failure Altered conscious state, irritability, restlessness
Aetiology	Duration of symptoms (bone marrow failure and haematinic deficiency usually have a longer duration of symptoms) Family history (hereditary spherocytosis, G6PD deficiency, haemoglobinopathies and others are inherited causes of anaemia. Maternal history, e.g. veganism, may be associated with B_{12} deficiency in infants) Birth and neonatal history (blood loss at birth, birth asphyxia and maternal blood group compatibility are all important in assessing neonatal anaemia. Jaundice at birth may give a clue to an episodic haemolytic disorder in older children) Presence or absence of jaundice (haemolysis) Drug exposure: as a cause of haemolysis, or bone marrow suppression Blood loss: trauma, recent surgery, iatrogenic in neonates, epistaxis, menstrual loss Dietary history: iron deficiency can be predicted in infants less than 12 months of age fed cow's milk, or in toddlers who have failed to transfer to solid foods adequately
Multilineage cytopenias	Bruising or bleeding, especially petechiae (thrombocytopenia) Infection, mouth ulceration (neutropenia)
Associated disease	Gastrointestinal symptoms (e.g. coeliac disease, inflammatory bowel disease) Joint or bone pain (e.g. leukaemia, sickle cell disease, arthritis) Renal disease Malignancy Infection: as a primary cause (e.g. malaria), a precipitant of acute deterioration in a more chronic anaemia, or a trigger to acute haemolysis Neurological disorders, developmental delay/regression, failure to thrive may reflect functional B_{12} deficiency in infants. Pica may be associated with iron deficiency Eating disorders in older children Bleeding disorders

Initial investigations

Progressive selective investigation, guided by the history, the clinical findings and the result of the blood count, is recommended. The first investigation will be a blood count, which automatically includes red cell indices (full blood examination (FBE) or complete blood count (CBC)), reticulocyte count and examination of the blood film. These initial investigations will usually allow classification of the anaemia. The presence or absence of polychromasia on the blood film, and the reticulocyte count, enable the anaemia to be classified as regenerative or are-generative. This is a most important initial decision to be made. The red cell indices, in particular the mean corpuscular volume (MCV), and the blood film, enable the anaemia to be classified by red cell size into microcytic, normocytic and macrocytic. Finally the blood film enables any specific red cell morphology to be determined and confirms the platelet and leukocyte parameters. At this stage a probable aetiology is likely and thus the direction of further investigations can be determined.

In the interpretation of these initial tests, there are a number of important considerations. First, sample integrity is vital, and preanalytical variables such as a clotted or inadequately mixed specimen can cause significant erroneous results. If the results do not match the clinical findings, repeat testing should always be considered. Second, MCV also varies with age. MCV is highest in the neonate (98–118 fl), falls to its lowest value between 6 and 24 months of age (79–86 fl), then increases progressively throughout childhood (75–92 fl). A low MCV indicates microcytosis and a high MCV indicates macrocytosis. Reticulocyte counts may be expressed as a percentage of the total red cell count (3–7% in the neonate, thereafter 0–1%), or more usually as an absolute count (normally $20–100 \times 10^9/l$). If expressed as a percentage, the reticulocyte count can be misleading, so an absolute count is preferable. An increased reticulocyte count indicates active regeneration of red cells, seen after blood loss, haemolysis or in response to correct haematinic therapy. Blood loss and previous hematinic therapy can usually be excluded on history, so that an increased reticulocyte count is often suggestive of haemolysis. A low reticulocyte response in the presence of anaemia indicates a lack of marrow response, because of a deficiency of the necessary iron or vitamins or inappropriate therapy for the anaemia, or inability to respond, such as marrow aplasia or infiltration.

Examination of the blood film

This is as important as the evaluation of the red cell indices, leukocyte count and platelets. The presence of abnormal red cell size, shape, inclusions, Hb content, and evidence of regeneration will usually suggest the cause of the anaemia and direct the next stage of investigation. The presence of abnormal leukocytes or abnormal platelet numbers may suggest a specific diagnosis such as leukaemia. Examples of a normal blood film and blood films in some conditions associated with anaemia are shown in Figure 16.1.1. Further investigations are suggested by the algorithms in Figures 16.1.2 and 16.1.3.

Practical points

Determining the urgency of investigation of anaemia

- Mild anaemia (Hb > 8 g/l) may still require urgent investigation and management, depending on the cause. Hence, until the cause of anaemia has been determined in a broad sense, discharge from emergency department/hospital should not be considered
- Acute regenerative anaemia (blood loss or haemolysis) has the capacity to rapidly develop severe anaemia. Blood loss is usually obvious, so haemolysis must be excluded or the rate of haemolysis (multiple Hb levels over a number of hours) understood before a patient can safely leave hospital. Thus a FBE, reticulocyte count, blood film examination and serum bilirubin are almost always indicated in initial investigations
- Megaloblastic anaemia in infancy, irrespective of the level of anaemia, requires urgent investigation because of the potential for rapid neurological deterioration. Hence the MCV is a crucial piece of information in the initial FBE, as is the blood film examination. A history of failure to thrive and neurological impairment in infancy should lead to consideration of megaloblastosis, as anaemia is often not the presenting symptom. An FBE with careful consideration of the red cell parameters is always warranted in this circumstance
- Anaemia as part of a multilineage failure may have a degree of urgency because of the potential for febrile neutropenia or thrombocytopenic haemorrhage

---

Specific disease entities

Disorders of stem cell proliferation

Pluripotential stem cell failure (aplastic anaemia)

Normal marrow function is dependent on stem cell renewal and maturation of all cell lines. Failure of stem cell proliferation and differentiation results in aplastic anaemia. Both genetically determined and acquired forms occur (Table 16.1.3).

Fanconi anaemia
Fanconi anaemia, the commonest of the genetic forms of aplastic anaemia, is recessively inherited and is characterized by a variable phenotype,

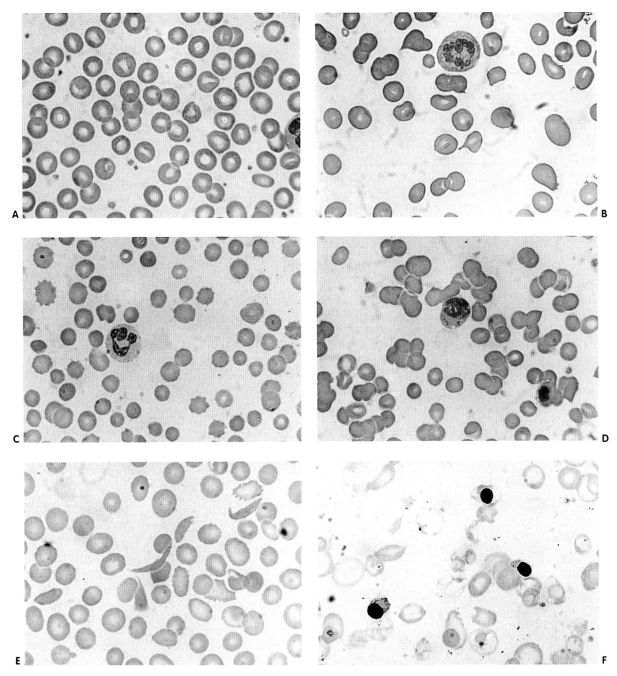

Fig. 16.1.1 Blood films. **A** Normal. **B** Macrocytosis – note hypersegmented polymorph. **C** Spherocytes in hereditary spherocytosis. **D** Autoimmune haemolytic anaemia showing red cell agglutination. **E** Sickle cell disease. **F** Thalassaemia major showing hypochromic microcytes and macrocytes, with nucleated red cells.

progressive marrow failure and an increased risk of malignancy. There appear to be multiple gene defects in this condition which explains the diversity of clinical manifestations.

Approximately 75% of children have congenital abnormalities, with a wide range of defects. The commonest are café au lait spots, short stature, microcephaly and skeletal anomalies, with thumb and radial hypoplasia or aplasia being most characteristic. Renal anomalies, stenosis of auditory canals, micro-ophthalmia, hypogenitalism and a variety of anomalies of the gastrointestinal tract may also occur. The child shown in Figure 16.1.4 shows many features of this disorder.

The diagnosis may be suspected at birth if there are congenital abnormalities. Haematological

Table 16.1.3   Causes of anaemia due to defective stem cell proliferation

Pathological process	Aetiology	Disease entity	Usual age of presentation
Pluripotential stem cell failure	Congenital	Fanconi anaemia	Variable, majority <10 years
	Acquired Drugs Infection Idiopathic	Aplastic anaemia	Any age
Erythroid stem cell failure	Congenital Acquired	Blackfan–Diamond syndrome	Neonate–6 months <5 years
	Idiopathic	Transient erythroblastopenia of childhood	
	Erythropoietin deficiency	Chronic renal failure Hypothyroidism	
	Unknown	Chronic infection Chronic inflammatory disease	
Bone marrow replacement	Malignant transformation of progenitors	Leukaemia	Infant–adult
	Marrow infiltration	Disseminated malignancy	
	Abnormal accumulation of metabolic substrates	Lipid 'storage' disease	

abnormalities are rare at birth. Pancytopenia develops gradually, usually by the age of 10 years. Onset is earlier in boys than girls. Macrocytosis is followed by thrombocytopenia, neutropenia, then anaemia. Bone marrow aspirate and trephine show hypoplasia or aplasia.

In contrast, infants with the thrombocytopenia–absent radii (TAR) syndrome are severely thrombocytopenic at birth and have radial anomalies without thumb abnormalities.

The diagnosis of Fanconi anaemia is established by special chromosome studies of lymphocytes. Chromosomes from patients with Fanconi anaemia show markedly increased spontaneous and alkylating agent (cells incubated with mitomycin C or diepoxybutane) induced chromosomal breaks, gaps, rearrangements, exchanges and endoreduplication. Antenatal diagnosis is possible.

Androgen therapy may produce long remissions of the anaemia but has little effect on thrombocytopenia and neutropenia. Its use is associated with masculinization and therefore is undesirable in young children, particularly girls. Granulocyte–macrophage colony-stimulating factor has been used with some success. Bone marrow transplantation offers the only possibility of cure of the aplasia. Supportive care with transfusions and antibiotics is required for patients without a marrow donor but death from infection, bleeding or the development of leukaemia usually occurs within a decade of diagnosis.

Clinical example

John, aged 5 years, presented with pallor and bruising of several months duration. He had a past history of tracheo-oesophageal fistula and had always been small, with his height and weight on the 3rd centile for age. His teacher had expressed concern about his hearing. On examination he was pale and had multiple bruises and several café au lait spots. He had a convergent squint and his external auditory canals were narrow. There was no hepatosplenomegaly or lymphadenopathy. A blood test showed a macrocytic anaemia with an Hb of 80 g/l and a white cell count of 1.4×10^9/l with neutrophils 0.7×10^9/l. The platelet count was 25×10^9/l. A bone marrow aspirate showed hypocellular fragments, and trephine biopsy confirmed marrow aplasia. Cytogenetic studies on peripheral blood lymphocytes confirmed that John had Fanconi anaemia by showing an increased rate of spontaneous and mitomycin-C-induced chromosome breaks. His sister was found to be HLA-identical with normal cytogenetic studies, and plans were made for elective bone marrow transplantation within the next few months.

Acquired aplastic anaemia

A number of agents may cause marrow failure, either in a dose-dependent fashion (irradiation and cytotoxic drugs) or in an idiosyncratic fashion. Some viral infections are associated with marrow suppression. No cause is identified in about 50% of children

Further Investigation of aregenerative anaemias

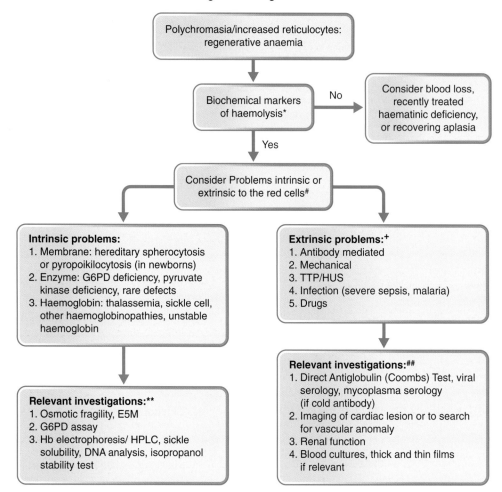

Reasonable first line investigation screen in haemolytic patients includes FBE, reticulocyte count, serum bilirubin, E5M, G6PD assay, Hb HPLC, DAT, renal function, and in neonates urine and blood culture.

BEWARE: Severe intravascular haemolysis (G6PD, some antibodies, microangiopathic (TTP/HUS, mechanical, sepsis)) may release free Hb which falsely elevates the measured haemoglobin. Always check that the red cell count is proportional to the measured Hb. Methaemoglobinaemia in severe G6PD haemolysis may increase tissue hypoxia for any given measured haemoglobin. All acute haemolytic anaemias have the potential for life threatening haemolysis to develop within hours and as such should be treated with extreme caution. In general, admission to hospital, close monitoring of vital signs and FBE until the tempo of the haemolysis is established is recommended. Folate deficiency in haemolysis may reduce the ability of the bone marrow to respond and worsen the anemia as well as causing diagnostic confusion

* Biochemical markers of haemolysis: in most cases the presence of an elevated unconjugated serum bilrubin is sufficient. Haptoglobins and LDH are frequently non contributory in small children.

\# Blood film may be diagnostic. Eg G6PD- blister and bite cells, spherocytosis (in neonates reflects etiher HS, ABO incompatability or severe sepsis), sickle cells

** Osmotic fragility requires a large blood sample (up to20 mls) and is not performed in many routine laboratories. The test is time-consuming and unsuitable for use in small children because of the volume of blood required. E5M requires less than 0.5 ml and is now offered by some laboratories instead of osmotic fragility. G6PD assay may be elevated in the presence of a reticulocytosis so borderline results should be repeated after the acute event and at least 3 months post transfusion if the clinical and blood film findings are suggestive.. Most laboratoriess perform HPLC to detect abnormal haemoglobins and use electrophoresis to identify abnormal bands. DNA testing should not be ordered acutely, but as a confirmatory test electively. HPLC and sickle solubility are most useful initial tests.

\+ Antibody mediated haemolysis may be warm (usually IgG, spherocytes on film) or cold (usually IgM, +/_ complement fixation, agglutination on film). Haemolysis due to mechanical, TTP/HUS or severe sepsis (DIC) are usually characteristically microangiopathic in blood film morphology

\#\# The Direct Antiglobulin (Coomb's) Test (DAT) is crucial to perform in all haemolysing children as IgG mediated haemolysis can be life threatening, and so the diagnosis should not be missed.

Fig. 16.1.2 Further investigation and initial management of a regenerative anaemia. * Biochemical markers of haemolysis: in most cases the presence of an elevated unconjugated serum bilirubin is sufficient. Haptoglobins and lactate dehydrogenase are frequently non-contributory in small children. † Blood film may be diagnostic, e.g. G6PD – blister and bite cells, spherocytosis (in neonates reflects either hereditary spherocytosis, ABO incompatibility or severe sepsis), sickle cells. ‡ Antibody-mediated haemolysis may be warm (usually IgG, spherocytes on film) or cold (usually IgM ± complement fixation, agglutination on film). Haemolysis due to mechanical damage, thrombotic thrombocytopenic purpura (TTP)/haemolytic–uraemic syndrome or severe sepsis (DIC) is usually characteristically microangiopathic in blood film morphology. § Osmotic fragility requires a large blood sample (up to 20 ml) and is not performed in many routine laboratories. The test is time-consuming and unsuitable for use in small children because of the volume of blood required. E5M requires less than 0.5 ml and is now offered by some laboratories instead of osmotic fragility. G6PD assay may be elevated in the presence of a reticulocytosis so borderline results should be repeated after the acute event and at least 3 months post-transfusion if the clinical and blood film findings are suggestive. Most laboratories perform HPLC to detect abnormal haemoglobins and use electrophoresis to identify abnormal bands. DNA testing should not be ordered acutely but as a confirmatory test electively. HPLC and sickle solubility are the most useful initial tests. ¶ It is crucial to perform the direct antiglobulin (Coombs) test (DAT) in all haemolysing children as IgG-mediated haemolysis can be life-threatening and so the diagnosis should not be missed. HPLC, high performance liquid chromatography; HUS, haemolytic–uraemic syndrome; TTP, thrombotic thrombocytopenic purpura.

with marrow failure. Fanconi anaemia must be excluded by cytogenetic studies, as not all affected individuals have congenital abnormalities.

Common causes are:

- drugs: chloramphenicol, anticonvulsants, non-steroidal anti-inflammatory agents and cytotoxic drugs
- chemicals: benzene, organic solvents, insecticides
- viral hepatitis: usually non-A, non-B, non-C hepatitis, less commonly Epstein–Barr virus, cytomegalovirus, parvovirus or human immunodeficiency virus (HIV)
- preleukaemic: acute lymphoblastic leukaemia occasionally has a transient period of aplasia before the onset of the disease
- paroxysmal nocturnal haemoglobinuria.

Presentation is with the gradual onset of pallor, lethargy and bruising. There may be a history of recent infection. Physical examination reveals little other than pallor, bruising, petechiae and oral mucosal bleeding. Importantly there is no enlargement of liver, spleen or lymph nodes but there may be fever and focal infection associated with the neutropenia.

The blood shows a pancytopenia with a normocytic anaemia without regeneration. Bone marrow aspirate and trephine biopsies reveal absent or decreased haemopoiesis.

Initial management depends on the severity and clinical manifestations of the aplasia. Potentially causative agents must be removed. Infections are treated vigorously. Supportive red cell and platelet transfusions are given as required. The general principles of transfusion therapy in aplastic anaemia are to avoid HLA sensitization by using leukocyte-depleted cellular products, and to minimize alloimmunization by minimizing donor exposure through the appropriate selection of blood products. Early

referral to a tertiary centre is vital. Although a small number of children will recover within a few weeks, bone marrow transplantation from an HLA-compatible sibling is generally regarded as the treatment of choice for severe aplastic anaemia, particularly in the under-5-years age group. Only 30% of children will have a matched sibling donor. For the remainder, antithymocyte globulin, together with granulocyte colony-stimulating factor and ciclosporin, produces improvement or complete recovery in about two-thirds of children. Onset of response may not occur for 2–3 months after initiation of therapy and supportive care during this time is vital. For those failing to respond, unrelated donor transplantation is an option and a donor search should be initiated early.

Red cell aplasia (erythroid stem cell failure)

Isolated aplasia of red cells results in a normocytic normochromic anaemia without reticulocytosis. The platelets and white blood cells are normal. Congenital and acquired forms occur.

Congenital red cell aplasia (Diamond–Blackfan syndrome). This disorder is almost certainly heterogenous, with sporadic, dominant and recessive forms occurring. The defect has not been determined but the disorder is possibly due to a defect in the erythroid progenitor cell.

Normocytic anaemia may be present at birth and usually is evident by 2–3 months of age. However, diagnosis beyond 1 year of age is reported. Early treatment with steroids results in a reticulocytosis and increase in Hb in about two-thirds of patients. In steroid responders, long-term low-dose steroids are recommended before total weaning is attempted. Some steroid-responsive patients are successfully weaned off steroids but many remain steroid-dependent. Those failing to respond to steroids or

Further Investigation of aregenerative anaemias

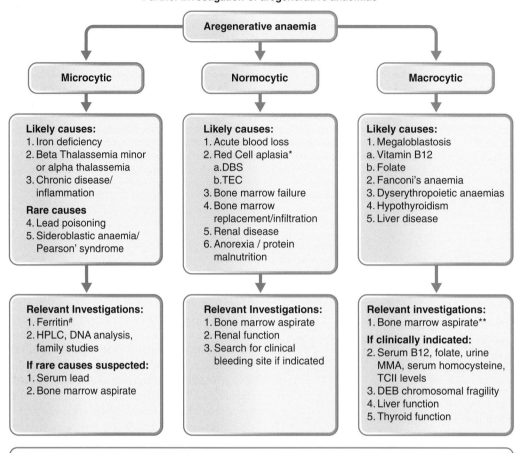

Aregenerative anaemia

Microcytic

Likely causes:
1. Iron deficiency
2. Beta Thalassemia minor or alpha thalassemia
3. Chronic disease/ inflammation

Rare causes
4. Lead poisoning
5. Sideroblastic anaemia/ Pearson' syndrome

Relevant Investigations:
1. Ferritin#
2. HPLC, DNA analysis, family studies

If rare causes suspected:
1. Serum lead
2. Bone marrow aspirate

Normocytic

Likely causes:
1. Acute blood loss
2. Red Cell aplasia*
   a.DBS
   b.TEC
3. Bone marrow failure
4. Bone marrow replacement/infiltration
5. Renal disease
6. Anorexia / protein malnutrition

Relevant Investigations:
1. Bone marrow aspirate
2. Renal function
3. Search for clinical bleeding site if indicated

Macrocytic

Likely causes:
1. Megaloblastosis
   a. Vitamin B12
   b. Folate
2. Fanconi's anaemia
3. Dyserythropoietic anaemias
4. Hypothyroidism
5. Liver disease

Relevant investigations:
1. Bone marrow aspirate**

If clinically indicated:
2. Serum B12, folate, urine MMA, serum homocysteine, TCII levels
3. DEB chromosomal fragility
4. Liver function
5. Thyroid function

BEWARE: Megaloblastic anaemia in infancy (<2 years) is often accompanied by severe failure to thrive and neurodevelopmental regression. Often these patients deteriorate very rapidly once they have finally reached medical attention, and investigation is a matter of urgency so that replacement therapy can be commenced ASAP and long term neurological sequelae minimized. The bone marrow aspirate confirms megaloblastic tissue quickly, such that treatment can be commenced pending further investigations of child and if a breast fed infant, investigation of the mother for Vitamin B12 or folate deficiency.

---

*Red cell aplasia may be isolated or part of broader marrow dysfunction. The differential between transient erythroblastopenia of childhood (TEC) and Diamond Blackfan Syndrome (DBS) is often difficult, even with thorough investigations.

Investigation of iron deficiency in children needs to be appropriate. In children with classic history of cow's milk intake before 12 months, or inadequate transition to solids, no investigations may be required after the blood film diagnosis, and treatment should be commenced. In otherwise normal children, ferritin is the most useful investigation and other iron studies are rarely contributory. Ferritin is an acute phase protein, so testing may need to be delayed if an acute febrile illness is coexistent. Full iron studies may be of value in children with complex medical problems.

** In the absence of clear renal, liver or thyroid disease, bone marrow aspirate is indicated for most significant normocytic or macrocytic anaemias. Bone marrow aspirates must always be examined in conjunction with the peripheral blood smear, and ancillary investigations. Hence consultation with a haematologist early in the investigation of such patients is often worthwhile. With the exception of megaloblastic anaemia, where bone marrow examination is often an emergency procedure to allow commencement of replacement therapy immediately, BMA can often be performed electively, and should never delay transfusion of a borderline or decompensating patient. In cases of suspected aplasia, bone marrow trephine may assist in assessing marrow cellularity.

Fig. 16.1.3   Further investigation of a regenerative anaemia. *Red cell aplasia may be isolated or part of broader marrow dysfunction. The differential between transient erythroblastopenia of childhood (TEC) and Diamond–Blackfan syndrome (DBS) is often difficult, even with thorough investigation. † Investigation of iron deficiency in children needs to be appropriate. In children with a classic history of cow's milk intake before 12 months, or inadequate transition to solids, no investigations may be required after the blood film diagnosis, and treatment should be commenced. In otherwise normal children, ferritin is the most useful investigation and other iron studies are rarely contributory. Ferritin is an acute-phase protein, so testing may need to be delayed if an acute febrile illness is coexistent. Full iron studies may be of value in children with complex medical problems. ‡ In the absence of clear renal, liver or thyroid disease, bone marrow aspirate is indicated for most significant normocytic or macrocytic anaemias. Bone marrow aspirates must always be examined in conjunction with the peripheral blood smear, and ancillary investigations. Hence consultation with a haematologist early in the investigation of such patients is often worthwhile. With the exception of megaloblastic anaemia, where bone marrow examination is often an emergency procedure to allow commencement of replacement therapy immediately, BMA can often be performed electively, and should never delay transfusion of a borderline or decompensating patient. In cases of suspected aplasia, bone marrow trephine may assist in assessing marrow cellularity. DEB, diepoxybutane; HPLC, MMA, methlymalonic acid; TCII, transcobalamin II.

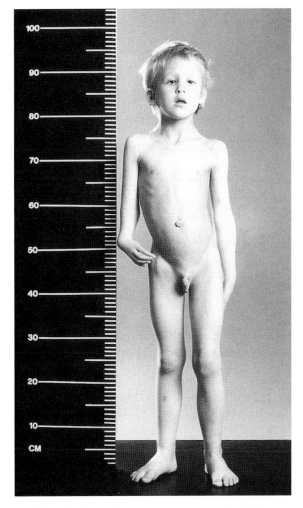

Fig. 16.1.4   Child with Fanconi anaemia. Note short stature, absent right radius and thumb, micro-ophthalmia and the presence of a hearing aid.

requiring large doses will need regular blood transfusion and chelation therapy. Bone marrow transplantation has corrected the condition in steroid-resistant patients.

Acquired red cell aplasia. Pure red cell aplasia (PRCA) is primarily a disease of adults but cases have been documented in teenagers. A large number of disorders, including thymoma, malignancy, autoimmune disease, viral infection and drug administration, have been implicated. Therapy is directed primarily toward the cause but may include immunosuppression, plasmaphaeresis, thymectomy and splenectomy.

Transient erythroblastopenia of childhood (TEC). This self-limiting, aregenerative anaemia occurs typically in children between 1 and 3 years of age. The aetiology remains unclear but antibodies directed against early red cell precursors have been documented in some children. Parvovirus B19 has not been consistently isolated.

The typical presentation is with pallor of gradual onset in an otherwise well child. The only abnormal clinical finding is pallor. The anaemia may be marked, without evidence of regeneration. A bone marrow aspirate will generally show absent or diminished erythropoiesis but if spontaneous recovery is already occurring at the time of presentation there may be many early erythroid progenitors present.

As the onset of the anaemia is gradual, most children will have compensated well and tolerate quite marked degrees of anaemia. If, however, there is no evidence of recovery occurring by the time the Hb falls to levels below 50 g/l, transfusion is likely to be required. Folic acid supplements should be given during the recovery phase. Spontaneous recovery usually occurs within 1–2 months and it is unusual for more than one transfusion to be required. Steroids have no role in the management of this disorder.

In some cases the distinction between DBS and TEC is extremely difficult. Neither the clinical scenario nor the bone marrow findings are absolutely diagnostic. In such cases, transfusion therapy without steroids may be useful initially to enable the patient every opportunity to recover. If steroids are introduced early, on the presumption of DBS, and recovery occurs, one is reluctant to cease steroid therapy quickly for fear of relapse and a spontaneously recovering TEC could potentially receive unnecessary steroids for a prolonged period.

Transient erythroid aplasia in chronic haemolytic anaemias. An aplastic crisis may occur in patients with one of the chronic haemolytic anaemias, such as sickle cell disease, hereditary spherocytosis and autoimmune haemolytic anaemia. Infection with human parvovirus B19 has been documented as the usual cause. Folic acid deficiency may be a further precipitating factor.

Because of the shortened red cell survival, there is a precipitous fall in Hb when erythroid proliferation ceases. Pallor and lethargy develop relatively quickly. The absence of jaundice, lack of increase in the degree of splenomegaly and absence of a reticulocyte response enables one to distinguish an aplastic crisis from increased haemolysis. Blood transfusion is likely to be required. Spontaneous recovery usually begins within 10–14 days.

Marrow replacement

Infiltration with neoplasia, particularly leukaemia, is the commonest cause of marrow failure in childhood. Several other childhood malignancies (neuroblastoma, non-Hodgkin lymphoma, Ewing sarcoma and rhabdomyosarcoma) metastasize to the bone marrow. Progressive pancytopenia with a normocytic anaemia and an associated shift to the left in the erythroid and myeloid series develops. Nucleated red cells and immature granulocytes (left shift) may be seen in the peripheral blood (leukoerythroblastic blood picture). Replacement of marrow with storage cells (e.g. Gaucher disease), fibrous tissue (myelofibrosis) or bone (osteopetrosis) will have a similar result. Careful examination of the blood film looking for leukaemic blasts, and a bone marrow examination that will identify abnormal cells, are required in any child with pancytopenia.

Dyserythropoietic/ineffective erythropoiesis

Congenital dyserythropoietic anaemias

This group of rare hereditary disorders of erythropoiesis is characterized by ineffective erythropoiesis resulting in shortened red cell survival with associated jaundice, a variable degree of anaemia, with normocytic to macrocytic red cell morphology, and anisopoikilocytosis and fragmentation in some types (Table 16.1.4). Bone marrow findings are characterized by erythroid hyperplasia, multinuclearity and internuclear bridging. The aetiology is unknown. Some patients in whom haemolysis is severe require regular transfusions.

Megaloblastic anaemia

Megaloblastic anaemias in childhood are rare but prompt diagnosis of the cause, especially in infants, is important to prevent potentially irreversible neurological damage, which may result from deficiencies of vitamin B_{12} or its transport protein transcobalamin II.

Vitamin B_{12} deficiency

Because the daily requirement for vitamin B_{12} is low and body stores are generally high, dietary deficiency of vitamin B_{12} is rare, occurring only after prolonged inadequate intake, as may occur in vegans. Breastfed infants of vitamin-B_{12}-deficient mothers are at risk and may present with anaemia in the first year of life. The commonest causes of maternal deficiency are undiagnosed pernicious anaemia and veganism. In infants with megaloblastosis it is important to determine whether maternal deficiency or transcobalamin II deficiency is the cause. Maternal deficiency requires short-term parenteral therapy of the infant; however, transcobalamin II deficiency requires long-term high-dose parenteral B_{12} injections. The majority of older children with vitamin B_{12} deficiency have a malabsorptive problem, either specific to vitamin B_{12}, as in pernicious anaemia, or secondary to inflammation or loss of the ileum, the portion of the small bowel in which vitamin B_{12} absorption occurs.

Vitamin B_{12} deficiency results in an anaemia with oval macrocytosis, hypersegmentation of neutrophils and thrombocytopenia. Bone marrow examination shows erythroid hyperplasia with megaloblastosis characterized by abnormally large erythroid and myeloid progenitors, in which nuclear maturation is delayed as compared to cytoplasmic maturation. Intramedullary destruction of erythroid precursors leads to a mild unconjugated hyperbilirubinaemia. Elevated serum homocysteine and urinary methyl malonic acid are useful to confirm the presence of intracellular vitamin B_{12} deficiency.

Therapy depends on the cause of the vitamin B_{12} deficiency. Dietary deficiency is treated by an initial dose of parenteral vitamin B_{12}, followed by dietary correction. Abnormalities of absorption, whether due to pernicious anaemia, ileal malabsorption or resection, require long-term intramuscular injection of the vitamin (hydroxycobalamin) at 1–3-month intervals according to the severity of the malabsorption.

Table 16.1.4 Anaemias that are due to ineffective erythropoiesis and dyserythropoiesis

Pathological process	Aetiology	Disease entity	Usual age of presentation
Impaired DNA synthesis	Unknown Vitamin B$_{12}$ deficiency Congenital Acquired	Congenital dyserythropoietic anaemia Transcobalamin II deficiency Congenital pernicious anaemia Maternal B$_{12}$ deficiency Juvenile pernicious anaemia Ileal resection Regional ileitis Blind loop syndrome	Infancy to adulthood (megaloblastosis) Neonates–3 months <3 years 3–12 months <10 years Any age
	Folate deficiency Congenital Acquired	Rare metabolic abnormalities Dietary deficiency Malabsorption (coeliac disease) Increased utilization (haemolysis)	Infancy Any age

Defective haem synthesis (microcytosis)	Iron deficiency	Dietary deficiency
		Malabsorption
		Blood loss
		  Occult
		  Overt
			Infancy, adolescence
			Any age

Reduced/absent globin chain synthesis	Gene deletion/mutation	Beta-thalassaemia major HbH disease (alpha-thalassaemia) Thalassaemia traits	6 months–5 years Any age
Abnormal globin chain production	Gene mutation/amino acid substitution	Haemoglobinopathies Sickle cell disease	Any age 1–4 years

Folate deficiency

Daily folate requirements are low but body stores are small. Folate is heat-labile and, although ubiquitous in food, is often destroyed by cooking.

Extra folate is required at times of rapid growth, during pregnancy and in patients with haemolytic anaemia. Deficiency is most likely to occur under these circumstances. Dietary deficiency most commonly occurs in infants fed exclusively on goat's milk, which is deficient in the vitamin. Malabsorption occurs in generalized malabsorptive syndromes such as coeliac disease and Crohn disease.

Some anticonvulsant drugs, e.g. phenytoin, may interfere with folate absorption, and megaloblastic changes are common among patients taking these drugs.

Inherited disorders of folate metabolism are rare and may present diagnostic difficulty.

Folate deficiency presents with a macrocytic anaemia without neurological abnormality. Oral administration of folic acid is effective in reversing deficiencies. Doses required are small, as 0.1 mg daily produces an optimal haematological response. In patients with increased requirements or malabsorption, higher doses of 0.5–5 mg daily are given. It is essential to exclude coexistent vitamin B$_{12}$ deficiency before treatment as the haematological picture may improve initially with folate therapy but progression of the neurological effects of vitamin B$_{12}$ deficiency will still occur.

Defective haem synthesis

Iron deficiency

Iron deficiency is the commonest cause of anaemia in childhood, being particularly common in the first 2 years of life when iron requirements are increased because of rapid growth and dietary intake is often inadequate. Early adolescence is another risk period for development of iron deficiency because of rapid growth.

Low-birth-weight infants and infants having exchange transfusions or frequent blood sampling have low total body iron stores and are at high risk of early development of iron deficiency anaemia, as iron stores and dietary intake are inadequate to keep up with rapid postnatal growth. Breast milk and cow's milk have a similar iron content but iron bioavailability from breast milk is approximately 50%, compared with 10% from cow's milk. Breastfed term babies therefore are rarely iron-deficient in the first 6 months of life but iron concentrations in breast milk decline postnatally and the iron content of breast milk is insufficient to meet the needs of the infant over the age of 6 months.

Oral iron supplementation (2 mg/kg/d) is given to low birth weight infants, generally from approximately 3 months of age. Iron-containing foods should be introduced by 6 months of age to all term babies. Most infant formulae are iron-fortified. Infants weaned early on to cow's milk (before 12 months of age), particularly those in whom milk continues to be the major component of the diet without the appropriate introduction of mixed solid feeding, are the group presenting most commonly with gross iron deficiency. In some, iron deficiency is exacerbated by the development of cow's milk protein enteropathy, leading to peripheral oedema secondary to hypoalbuminaemia in addition to anaemia.

Older children with diets poor in iron-containing foods (red meat, white meats, legumes, green vegetables, egg yolk) are also at risk. Blood loss must always be considered in an iron-deficient child or adolescent without an appropriate dietary history. Menorrhagia is an important cause of iron deficiency in adolescent girls. Occult blood loss is usually gastrointestinal in origin, from such diverse causes as cow's milk enteropathy, polyps, haemangiomas, Meckel's diverticulum and hereditary telangiectasia, but repeated epistaxes and chronic blood loss from the renal tract must be excluded.

Iron malabsorption is uncommon and is usually associated with malabsorption syndromes such as coeliac disease or chronic inflammatory bowel disease.

Iron deficiency initially leads to depletion of marrow iron stores without any haematological abnormality. When iron stores are exhausted, serum iron concentration and transferrin binding falls and there is reduced intracellular iron availability for haem synthesis, with a consequent reduction in Hb production, leading to microcytosis and the development of anaemia.

Symptoms of early iron deficiency with no or minimal anaemia may include poor attention span and irritability. As anaemia develops, cognitive deficits may increase and lethargy and pallor become apparent. Some chronically iron-deficient children exhibit pica (the ingestion of non-food items such as dirt and clay, and chewing of ice).

Examination reveals pallor, most easily detected in the palmar creases and conjunctivae. Signs of cardiac decompensation will occasionally be present if the anaemia is severe. Mild splenomegaly is found occasionally but is more common in thalassaemia minor, from which iron deficiency must be distinguished.

Therapy of iron deficiency involves correction of the underlying cause and replenishment of iron stores. Improvement in the dietary intake of iron-containing foods is the most important strategy in the majority of iron-deficient children. Reduction in the total milk content of the diet may be necessary to allow the child to develop an appropriate appetite. If a source of blood loss is identified, appropriate therapy is undertaken and iron supplements are given until the deficiency is corrected.

Therapeutic iron is optimally given orally in two to three divided doses daily in a dose of 6 mg/kg per day of elemental iron. Absorption is enhanced when iron is taken with vitamin C and between meals but the side effects of abdominal discomfort are reduced when iron is taken with food. Ferrous sulphate is cheaper and better absorbed than ferrous gluconate but the gluconate is better tolerated. A reticulocyte response to iron should be seen within 7–10 days but iron therapy should continue for 3 months to replenish

Clinical example

Tan, a 15-month-old boy, had been breastfed for 10 months and then was given cow's milk. He had occasional solid foods only, and rarely had any foods with a significant iron content. He had become irritable, seemed to be low in energy and slept more than his parents thought was usual. When he was seen by his doctor because of an upper respiratory tract infection, he was noted to have pale conjunctivae and pale palmar creases.

Tan's Hb was 51 g/l, his MCV was 51 fl, and his mean corpuscular haemoglobin concentration (MCHC) was 15 pg. The total WBC was normal and his platelet count was $432 \times 10^9/l$. The blood film showed microcytic and hypochromic red cells; there was no reticulocytosis and no basophilic stippling. The serum ferritin was 4 µg/l (normal range 16–300).

Tan's anaemia had all the features of an iron-deficiency anaemia due to a deficient iron intake in his diet. A dietitian assisted in instructing his mother in ways to improve his diet by including foods such as red and white meats, green vegetables, legumes and egg yolks. Tan was given ferrous gluconate mixture at a dose of 6 mg/kg of expected weight per day, to be taken as two doses daily. His parents were asked to give this with orange juice to improve absorption. They were warned that the mixture could make Tan's stools a grey-black colour but that this was not of concern. They were asked to brush his teeth after each dose to prevent any minor staining. They were warned of the toxic effects of iron if taken in overdose accidentally by an inquisitive toddler; the mixture was provided in limited amounts only in a bottle with a safety top, and they were asked to keep it in a secure place, preferably a locked cupboard.

The iron mixture was continued for 3 months. Tan's reticulocyte count rose in a few days, and his Hb began to rise in 10 days. By 6 weeks of therapy his Hb was normal; the iron mixture was continued for another 6 weeks to ensure that his iron stores were replenished.

iron stores. The stools are grey-black in individuals on iron.

It is rarely necessary to use the parenteral route for iron administration but, in occasional children with poor absorption or poor compliance, intravenous infusions of iron may be required.

Haemoglobinopathies

Haemoglobin is a compound protein made up of two pairs of globin chains with a haem molecule inserted into each. One of these globin chains is designated as the alpha chain, the other variably being termed beta, delta, epsilon (ε), gamma and zeta (ζ). Zeta and epsilon chains are expressed only in early embryonic life, with zeta chain production switching to alpha chain production and gamma chain production replacing epsilon chain synthesis in the early weeks of gestation. In the perinatal period there is a further switch from gamma to beta chain production. The predominant fetal haemoglobin is HbF ($\alpha_2\gamma_2$). In children beyond 6 months of age and adults, the major haemoglobins are HbA ($\alpha_2\beta_2$) and HbA2 ($\alpha_2\delta_2$). A number of abnormalities of globin chain production or point mutations within globin genes may result in significant disease.

Thalassaemias

These are genetic disorders characterized by reduced or absent production of one or more of the globin chains of haemoglobin.

The thalassaemias are found commonly in people originating from the Mediterranean region, the Middle East, the Indian subcontinent, south Asia and Africa. The inheritance is in a mendelian recessive manner.

Beta thalassaemia

Beta thalassaemia occurs as a result of point mutations or deletions within one or both of the two beta globin genes, resulting in reduced or absent production of beta globin chains. The heterozygous state is termed thalassaemia minor and the homozygous state thalassaemia major.

Beta thalassaemia minor. Affected individuals are usually asymptomatic, with mild anaemia detected either during investigation of another illness or as a result of family screening. Mild pallor and splenomegaly may be noted but the examination is often unremarkable. There is a mild microcytic hypochromic anaemia with occasional target cells. The differential diagnosis is iron deficiency, although both may coexist. The HbA$_2$ level is elevated. If present, iron deficiency may mask the thalassaemia minor, preventing diagnosis until the iron deficiency is corrected.

Beta thalassaemia major (Cooley anaemia). This is caused by the inheritance of two abnormal beta genes. At birth the haemoglobin is normal but, as the γ–β switch occurs, there are no (β^0) or insufficient (β^+) beta chains to balance alpha chains. Excess alpha chains precipitate, causing shortened red cell survival with destruction within the bone marrow (ineffective erythropoiesis) and spleen. HbA production is inadequate to compensate for the gradual fall in HbF as gamma chain production switches to inadequate beta chain production.

Children with thalassaemia major usually present between 3 months and 1 year of life with pallor and hepatosplenomegaly. There may be mild jaundice. Occasionally presentation is delayed to 4–5 years, with these children having increased skin pigmentation, frontal bossing and malar prominence due to chronic marrow expansion. The Hb may be very low, with blood examination revealing hypochromia, red cell stippling, microcytosis, macrocytes, target cells and nucleated red cells (Fig. 16.1.1F). An elevated HbF level (usually 50–100%) confirms the diagnosis. Globin chain synthesis studies can differentiate between β^+ and β^0 thalassaemia.

Without treatment, the severe chronic anaemia leads to growth retardation, poor musculoskeletal development and increased iron absorption, resulting in skin pigmentation. Extramedullary haemopoiesis in liver and spleen together with hypersplenism result in organ enlargement and abdominal distension. Marrow expansion produces the characteristic facial appearance with frontal bossing, maxillary hypertrophy with exposure of the upper teeth, prominence of the malar eminences and a flattened nasal bridge. Skull X-rays show expansion of the diploic space, and the subperiosteal bone has a typical 'hair on end' appearance. There is cortical thinning of long bones and fractures may occur. Death usually occurs within 10 years from cardiac failure, cardiac arrhythmias or infection.

Current treatment is with regular transfusion at 3–4-weekly intervals, aiming to suppress endogenous haemopoiesis (preventing marrow expansion) and to keep the Hb level above 100 g/l. Regular transfusion results in iron loading and chelation therapy must accompany transfusion support to prevent the toxic effects of iron on the myocardium, liver, pancreas and gonads (cardiac arrhythmias, cardiac failure, diabetes mellitus, hepatic fibrosis, infertility). The chelator desferrioxamine is currently given by subcutaneous infusion via a syringe pump over 10 hours nightly, usually after approximately 5 years of age. Compliance, particularly during adolescence, is often a problem. Many centres now transfuse by erythrocytaphaeresis to reduce iron loading. All patients receive folic acid supplements and hepatitis

B vaccination and are encouraged to participate in all normal activities. Splenectomy, preceded by appropriate vaccinations, is occasionally required.

Bone marrow transplantation from matched siblings is producing high cure rates provided it is carried out before hepatic dysfunction develops, but long-term results are still to be evaluated.

With improvements in therapy some patients are now surviving into the fifth decade. A proportion of adults have preservation of gonadal function and have had children.

Haemoglobin E/β thalassaemia. Haemoglobin E ($\beta^{26Glu-Ly}$) occurs extensively throughout south-east Asia. Neither the heterozygous nor the homozygous state produces clinical abnormalities. The doubly heterozygous state of HbE with beta thalassaemia results in a clinical condition similar to thalassaemia major. Diagnosis is confirmed by blood examination and haemoglobin electrophoresis. Clinical presentation and management are similar to a moderately severe beta thalassaemia.

Alpha thalassaemia

There are four alpha globin genes and alpha thalassaemia results from the loss of one or more of these. The loss of one gene produces neither haematological nor clinical abnormality (silent carrier). Loss of two genes results in hypochromia and microcytosis, but no anaemia, and is known as alpha thalassaemia trait. Alpha thalassaemia occurs with a very high incidence in Asian populations and is assuming increasing importance in our community.

Haemoglobin H disease. The loss of three alpha genes results in the formation of excess beta chains, which form an unstable tetramer (β_4), accounting for 30–40% of the total haemoglobin. The clinical picture is similar to beta thalassaemia intermedia, with pallor, jaundice and moderate hepatosplenomegaly. There is a moderate anaemia (Hb 80–100 g/l) and persistent reticulocytosis. The anaemia is aggravated by infections, pregnancy and oxidant drugs (e.g. phenacetin or primaquine), which should be avoided. No specific treatment is necessary other than folic acid supplements.

Haemoglobin Barts (hydrops fetalis syndrome). All four alpha genes are deleted and no alpha chains are produced. The haemoglobins present are HbBarts (γ_4) 70%, HbH (β_4) 0–20% and HbPortland ($\zeta_2\gamma_2$). Severe fetal anaemia develops, resulting in cardiac failure, hepatosplenomegaly and generalized oedema. The infants are generally stillborn or die shortly after birth. In utero transfusions may result in a liveborn infant, and exchange transfusion followed by ongoing transfusion support has led to the survival of a few patients. Bone marrow transplantation should cure these patients.

Sickle cell disease

Haemoglobin S (HbS) results from a single amino acid substitution in the beta globin chain ($\beta^{6Glu-Val}$). Under hypoxic conditions, deoxyhaemoglobin S polymerizes into fibre bundles, which distort the cell into a sickle shape. Sickling may be reversible on reoxygenation or may become irreversible. The sickle cell gene occurs in people from Africa, the Middle East and the Mediterranean region, as well as in the African-American population.

The heterozygous carrier (*sickle trait*) is asymptomatic, with normal Hb and red cell morphology. Haemoglobin electrophoresis reveals an HbA of approximately 60% and an HbS level of 30–40%.

In the homozygous state (*sickle cell anaemia*) there is a normochromic normocytic haemolytic anaemia with target cells, sickle cells, nucleated red cells, fragments and spherocytes (Fig. 16.1.1E). The diagnosis is confirmed by finding an elevated HbS (60–90%) on electrophoresis with approximately 2% HbA$_2$, the remainder being HbF. The higher the level of HbF the less severe the symptoms of the disease.

The doubly heterozygous *sickle trait–beta thalassaemia* is expressed with clinical features very similar to those of homozygous sickle cell disease. In contrast to sickle cell anaemia, the red cells are microcytic and hypochromic and target cells are present. Sickling can be demonstrated and both HbS and HbA$_2$ are elevated. Examination of the parents' blood confirms sickle cell trait in one and thalassaemia minor in the other. The management of this condition is similar to that for sickle cell anaemia.

The clinical course of the patient with sickle cell disease, or doubly heterozygous sickle/thalassaemia, is characterized by 'crises' as a result of sickling of red cells that obstruct the lumen of capillaries and small venules, causing infarction of surrounding tissues. Haemolytic 'crises' may also occur during infective illness.

Presentation is usually between the ages of 6 months and 4 years with pallor, jaundice, abdominal or limb pain and/or swelling of the hands and feet. Haemolytic crises are characterized by increased pallor and jaundice, infarctive 'crises' with acute pain, generally of limbs or back, and aplastic crises with an aregenerative anaemia. Splenic sequestration crises occur in young children predominantly under the age of 5 years. In this potentially life-threatening complication, red cells are trapped in splenic sinusoids, resulting in hypovolaemia, a rapid increase in splenic size and profound anaemia. Patients with sickle cell disease have an increased risk of infection, particularly pneumococcal infection. Functional asplenia secondary to repeated splenic infarction occurs in most patients.

The emphasis in management is on avoidance of environmental factors known to precipitate a crisis. The following protective measures are recommended:

- good nutrition with regular folic acid supplements
- penicillin prophylaxis from infancy, with prompt treatment of infections
- appropriate immunization schedule
- maintenance of adequate hydration, particularly during hot weather
- prevention of vascular stasis. This may occur with tight clothing, the use of tourniquets applied during an operative procedure, and exposure to cold.

Vaso-occlusive crises require prompt control of pain, the maintenance of hydration and treatment of underlying infection. Severe crises (pulmonary syndrome or cerebral infarction) require blood transfusion to reduce the HbS concentration. Occasionally exchange transfusion may be required.

Patients with splenic sequestration require prompt restoration of intravascular volume and correction of acidosis.

Patients with frequent crises may be managed with hydroxycarbamide (hydroxyurea), which increases the proportion of HbF and reduces the number of sickle crisis. Hydroxycarbamide is not usually commenced until at least 3 years of age, but usually 5 years. In more severe cases, regular blood transfusions to suppress endogenous HbS production are required. These patients also require iron chelation. Successful bone marrow transplantation has been reported.

Genetic counselling

Current DNA techniques allow prenatal diagnosis of the thalassaemias and sickle cell disease. With increased community awareness and education, many couples who carry either a thalassaemia or sickle trait are now seeking antenatal counselling and prenatal diagnosis. This will have significant effects on the incidence of newly diagnosed homozygotes in the future.

Anaemia due to increased red cell destruction (haemolysis)

Anaemia secondary to haemolysis (Table 16.1.5) occurs when bone marrow replacement does not keep pace with the rate of destruction.

Haemolysis may be intravascular or may occur by phagocytosis within the spleen or liver. Intravascular haemolysis occurs in some autoimmune haemolytic anaemias, acute haemolysis in G6PD deficiency,

Table 16.1.5 Anaemias due to increased red cell destruction			
Pathological process	Aetiology	Disease entity	Usual age of presentation
Oxidative cell damage	Enzyme defects of the glycolytic pathway	G6PD deficiency Pyruvate kinase deficiency	Neonate–10 years Neonate–adult
Membrane abnormality (decreased red cell deformability)	Congenital – splenic destruction	Hereditary spherocytosis Hereditary elliptocytosis	Neonate–adult
Antibody-mediated membrane damage	Fetomaternal Rh and ABO incompatibility Autoantibodies ± complement reacting with red cell membrane Infection Drugs Autoimmune disease	Haemolytic disease of newborn Autoimmune haemolytic anaemia	In utero–24 hours Any age
Toxic membrane damage	Infection Heavy metals	*Clostridium perfringens* Wilson disease	Any age Late childhood–adult
Mechanical membrane damage	Membrane damage	Disseminated intravascular coagulopathy Haemolytic–uraemic syndrome Cardiac prosthesis	Any age Childhood

and acute transfusion reactions. Free haemoglobin is released and combines with haptoglobin. The complex is cleared by the reticuloendothelial system of the liver and spleen. If the free plasma haemoglobin concentration exceeds the haptoglobin binding capacity, haemoglobinuria occurs. The colour of the urine may vary from pink through brown to almost black, depending on the amount of free haemoglobin excreted.

If haemolysis occurs predominantly in the reticuloendothelial system (autoimmune haemolytic anaemia, membrane abnormalities), there is little free haemoglobin in plasma. Haemoglobin is converted to bilirubin within phagocytes, transported to the liver bound to albumin, then conjugated and excreted into the bile. Jaundice is variable, depending on the rate of haemolysis and hepatic conjugation. To compensate for the reduced red cell survival, the bone marrow increases its output of red cells, releasing immature reticulocytes and, in acute severe haemolysis, nucleated red cells into the peripheral blood.

Intracellular enzyme defects

Mature red cells lack a nucleus and intracellular organelles necessary for synthesis of proteins and generation of adenosine triphosphate (ATP) via oxidative pathways. Energy production for maintenance of the integrity of the red cell is via one of the two glycolytic metabolic pathways within it. About 95% of glucose metabolism is via the anaerobic Embden–Myerhof pathway and 5% through the hexose monophosphate shunt (pentose phosphate pathway). Enzyme defects in either pathway result in oxidative damage and haemolysis. Deficiencies or abnormalities of G6PD, the first enzyme in the hexose monophosphate shunt, are extremely common worldwide. All the documented enzyme deficiencies of the Embden–Myerhof pathway resulting in haemolytic anaemias are rare. Examples are pyruvate kinase deficiency and glucose phosphate isomerase deficiency.

G6PD deficiency

This X-linked enzyme deficiency is the commonest inherited disorder of the red cell. It is fully expressed in hemizygous males and in homozygous females. Heterozygous females show a variable level of enzyme activity due to variation in X chromosome inactivation. There are over 200 variant enzymes and the clinical expression of the disorder is variable, with four major clinical syndromes. Neonatal jaundice is common in the Chinese and Mediterranean variants; favism (acute haemolysis after ingestion of broad beans or inhalation of pollen) is a feature of the Mediterranean variant; while oxidative-stress-induced haemolysis (drugs, infection), although common to all variants, is the predominant feature in affected individuals of African descent. Individuals of northern European descent have chronic moderate haemolysis, while other variants only experience haemolysis with appropriate stress. Patients typically present severely anaemic with dark urine, having been well until 1–2 days prior to presentation. The precipitating factor is usually identifiable on history. Because of the rapidity of the fall in haemoglobin there often is profound lethargy and restlessness at presentation.

Examination of the blood film shows polychromasia and anisocytosis, and typically 'blister' cells. The diagnosis is established by enzyme assay in mature red cells. Enzyme levels are higher in reticulocytes in some variants and a normal enzyme level at the time of an acute haemolytic episode does not exclude the diagnosis. Management is to avoid precipitating factors. Patients having acute crises may require blood transfusion, although a brisk reticulocyte response may result in rapid spontaneous recovery.

Clinical example

Thomas was an 8-year-old boy from Hong Kong. He presented with the onset of pallor over 24 hours and was passing very dark urine. He had recently been treated for tonsillitis. He had no past history of serious illness. On examination, apart from marked pallor, splenomegaly was present. His urine contained haemoglobin. Blood tests revealed a haemoglobin of 40 g/l with an elevated reticulocyte response. Blister cells were evident on the blood film. The G6PD assay was borderline normal and assays on the parents showed that Thomas's mother was heterozygous for G6PD deficiency. One month after this episode, Thomas was shown to have a severe deficiency of G6PD activity. The earlier borderline result was caused by the presence of many young red cells with high G6PD activity.

Intrinsic membrane defects

Abnormalities of the red cell membrane result in alterations of cell shape, usually due to changes in transmembrane electrolyte flux. Changes in cell shape cause decreased deformability, splenic trapping and destruction within the spleen, resulting in chronic haemolytic anaemia. The commonest membrane abnormality is hereditary spherocytosis, a dominantly inherited condition.

Hereditary spherocytosis

There is a marked variability in the severity of haemolysis in this condition. Neonatal jaundice is common. Some children present with anaemia in infancy while others remain asymptomatic until a haemolytic or aplastic crisis occurs in association with a viral infection. Hypersplenism or gallstones may result in the presentation of a previously asymptomatic patient with well compensated haemolysis. A positive family history is often obtained. Examination reveals pallor, often mild jaundice and a variable degree of splenomegaly. The diagnosis is suggested by the presence of spherocytes in the peripheral blood (Fig. 16.1.1C). The best test currently to confirm the diagnosis is the E5M test. In this test, the dye eosin-5-maleimide reacts covalently with Lys-430 on the extracellular loop of band 3 protein. Reduced E5M staining is seen in patients with hereditary spherocytosis, Congenital dyserythropoietic anaemia type II and south-east Asian ovalocytosis and cryohydrocytosis.

Folic acid supplements should be given. Blood transfusion may be required for anaemia resulting from inadequately compensated haemolysis and for aplastic crises, during which the haemoglobin may fall precipitously. Aplastic crises usually are associated with parvovirus B19 infection. Haemolysis is abolished by splenectomy. Overwhelming postsplenectomy infection may occur, particularly in children less than 5 years of age. Pneumococcal, meningococcal and *Haemophilus influenzae* b immunizations should be given presplenectomy, and penicillin prophylaxis should be continued indefinitely postsplenectomy.

Decisions about splenectomy should be based on the following:

- degree of haemolysis and anaemia
- age
- size of spleen
- presence of gallstones.

Clinical example

Angela was 9 years of age. In the neonatal period she required exchange transfusion for severe jaundice. She had always been pale and had a small appetite. With upper respiratory tract infections, her pallor increased and jaundice had appeared. At 2 years of age hereditary spherocytosis was diagnosed and folic acid supplements were commenced. Angela's father also had this condition. She presented with abdominal pain, pallor, icterus and splenomegaly of 6 cm. Ultrasound examination confirmed the presence of gallstones. Following pneumococcal and *Haemophilus influenzae* b vaccination, splenectomy and cholecystectomy with removal of gallstones was undertaken. Prophylactic penicillin was commenced after the surgery and would continue indefinitely.

Extrinsic membrane damage

Acquired membrane damage leading to haemolysis can result from antibody–antigen reactions, mechanical insults (e.g. intravascular prosthetic patches), burns, toxins (e.g. copper) and infective agents (e.g. *Clostridium perfringens*).

Antibody-mediated haemolysis

The binding of immunoglobulin or complement, or a combination of the two, to the red cell membrane may result in premature cell destruction or immune haemolysis. The antibody involved may be IgG (warm antibody) or IgM (cold antibody). Immune haemolytic anaemias may be classified as follows:

Isoimmune haemolysis in the newborn
- Rhesus incompatibility (mother Rh −ve; baby Rh +ve)
- ABO incompatibility (mother group O: baby group A or B).

Autoimmune haemolysis in children
- *Idiopathic.* In many instances of IgG warm-antibody-mediated haemolysis, no definite aetiological agent is identified
- *Postinfectious.* Many common infectious diseases, such as measles (IgG), infectious mononucleosis (IgM) and mycoplasmal infection (IgM) may be associated with acute haemolysis
- *Drug related.* This is very uncommon in children. Some drugs, e.g. α-methyl dopa, stimulate the production of antibodies that are directed against red cell antigens but not against the drug. A second mechanism involves a drug, such as penicillin, binding to the red cell membrane, with antibody to the drug being formed and attaching to the drug. The antibody-coated red cells then undergo destruction in the spleen. The third mechanism of drug-related haemolysis involves the deposition of antibody–antigen complexes on the red cell surface with activation of complement and brisk intravascular haemolysis
- *Associated with connective tissue disease or malignancy.* This is rare in childhood but may be associated with systemic lupus erythematosus in adolescence.

Presentation of a child with immune-mediated haemolysis is usually acute with rapid onset of pallor, severe anaemia and dark urine. Jaundice may be present. Life-threatening anaemia may develop rapidly, with vasoconstriction, cardiac failure and hypoxia. Modest splenomegaly is often present.

The peripheral blood shows a predominantly normocytic anaemia with spherocytes, fragmented red cells and rouleaux formation (Fig. 16.1.1D). In cold agglutinin disease, agglutination is seen on the blood film. As a compensating reticulocytosis develops, polychromasia and macrocytosis are seen. A positive direct antiglobulin test (DAT) confirms the diagnosis. The specificity of the positive DAT classifies the type of antibody involved. The commonest are warm IgG antibodies, but cold IgM antibodies are found in association with mycoplasmal infection and infectious mononucleosis.

Urgent blood transfusion may be required. In some cases the presence of strong autoantibody in recipient plasma makes the provision of compatible blood and the exclusion of underlying alloantibodies difficult. Transfused cells may be haemolysed rapidly and careful observation is required. Repeated transfusions may be necessary. Adequate hydration must be maintained to avoid renal tubular damage from haemoglobinuria. Where a warm antibody is identified, steroid therapy is instituted and maintained until the Hb stabilizes, then tapered gradually. Haemolysis is usually self-limiting over the course of days to weeks. Occasional patients may have severe ongoing haemolysis, or frequent relapses. Plasma exchange, exchange transfusion or high-dose immunoglobulin may be useful but, if these measures fail, splenectomy may be life-saving.

Blood loss

Blood loss, if acute, results in vasoconstriction, then tachycardia and finally hypotension. The haemoglobin, if measured very early in the course of a bleeding episode, will be normal or only slightly reduced. When there has been time for haemodilution to occur, the haemoglobin falls. A compensatory reticulocytosis occurs after approximately 48 hours. Chronic blood loss results in iron-deficiency anaemia.

Blood transfusion therapy

The majority of children with anaemia do not require transfusion therapy. The critical questions that must be addressed in deciding whether to transfuse are:

- Has the patient evidence of cardiovascular decompensation?
- Is the anaemia likely to be progressive and at what rate?
- What is the likely timing of spontaneous recovery?
- Are there alternative therapies that are likely to succeed?

Major acute blood loss due to trauma, acute haemolytic anaemias and chemotherapy-induced anaemia are the most likely causes of acute anaemia to require transfusion. The exact transfusion trigger will be a function of the physiological considerations discussed previously in this chapter. Major haemoglobinopathy and bone marrow failure syndromes may require chronic transfusion programmes. Nutritional anaemia rarely requires transfusion therapy in the absence of cardiovascular instability.

There are specific indications for exchange transfusion in neonates and, for example, older children with sickle cell disease.

Risks of blood transfusion therapy

Parents worry about viral infections from blood transfusion, although this remains an extremely low risk. If the clinician has used the principles above to determine the need for transfusion, then the risks of not transfusing usually far outweigh the risks of transfusion. In terms of viral safety Australia has one of the safest blood supplies in the world. Factors contributing to this are that every blood donor is a volunteer (unpaid) and must meet strict selection criteria, including answering a comprehensive questionnaire about their health and lifestyle and undergoing a personal interview by trained staff at which they sign a declaration. Every blood donation is screened for syphilis, hepatitis B and C, HIV and human T-cell leukaemia/lymphoma virus (HTLV). Two types of test for hepatitis C and HIV are now performed – antibody testing and nucleic acid testing (detects viral materials directly and therefore infection at an earlier stage). Only blood that is negative for all these tests is released for use.

Current risks of transfusion transmitted infection

Australian Red Cross Blood Service (ARCBS) uses sophisticated mathematical models to calculate the current infection risks for blood transfusions in Australia, which are shown in Table 16.1.6. These risks are very small compared to the risks of everyday living. The chance of being killed in a road accident in Australia is about 1 in 10 000.

Non-viral risks associated with blood and blood products

ABO incompatibility remains one of the most common fatal complications of blood transfusion and most cases are due to avoidable errors (most commonly associated with patient/sample identification). Table 16.1.7 gives estimates of risk based on reports from a number of countries, which are subject to the problem of underestimation due to lack of reporting and recognition of transfusion reactions (hence the broad ranges). The transfusion of autologous blood is not without risk and the same indications apply as for the use of homologous blood.

Practical points

Deciding if a patient needs a red cell transfusion
- The actual haemoglobin level, while important, does not alone determine the need for a transfusion
- Consider the cause and time-course of the anaemia. Haematinic deficiencies rarely need transfusion. Acute blood loss (especially if ongoing) and acute haemolysis frequently need transfusion
- Coexistent disease is important in determining the likely ability of the patient to cope with a degree of anaemia. Cardiac and lung function, as well as haemoglobin level, are important determinants of oxygen delivery. The ability to maintain oxygen delivery is the key question when considering most acute red cell transfusion questions
- Reduced oxygen saturation measured by pulse oximetry may reflect lung disease, cyanotic heart disease or abnormal Hb with reduced oxygen affinity (e.g. methaemoglobin) and may reduce the transfusion threshold. In the absence of adequate cardiac output or Hb, normal pulse oximetry does not equate to adequate tissue oxygen delivery
- Clinical signs of cardiac stress (increased heart rate) or hypoxia (restlessness, altered conscious state/behaviour) are critical indicators of the need for urgent transfusion. In children, hypotension is a late sign in acute blood loss. These factors should be monitored closely in anaemic patients. In a child with cardiovascular decompensation from anaemia, do not delay urgent transfusion therapy in favour of thorough investigation. A live child who remains a diagnostic dilemma is better than a dead child in whom you know the diagnosis

Table 16.1.6 Risks based on ARCBS data 1 July 2000 to 30 June 2003

Infection	Residual risk with tested blood per unit transfused
HIV	1 in 7 299 000
Hepatitis C	1 in 3 636 000
Hepatitis B	1 in 1 339 000
HTLV	Considerably less than 1 in 1 000 000
Syphilis	Considerably less than 1 in 1 000 000
Variant CJD	Unknown: possible and cannot be excluded

CJD, Creutzfeldt–Jakob disease; HIV, human immunodeficiency virus; HTLV, human T-cell leukaemia/lymphoma virus.

Table 16.1.7 Non-viral serious risks of blood transfusion (per unit transfused unless specified)

	Morbidity	Mortality
Bacterial sepsis		
Red cells	1 in 40 000 to 500 000	1 in 4 000 000–8 000 000
Platelets	1 in 10 000 to 100 000	1 in 50 000–500 000
Haemolytic reactions		
Acute	1 in 12 000 to 38 000	1 in 600 000–1 500 000
Delayed	1 in 1 000 to 12 000	1 in 2 500 000
Anaphylaxis – IgA deficiency	1 in 20 000 to 50 000	
Fluid overload/cardiac failure	1 in 100–700 per patient	
TRALI*	1 in 5000–100 000	1 in 5 million
TA-GVHD†	Rare	90% cases fatal

* Transfusion-related acute lung injury (TRALI) is characterized by acute respiratory distress (within hours of transfusion) with non-cardiogenic pulmonary oedema. Full recovery in 48 hours is usual if the patient is well resuscitated/supported. TRALI is likely to be significantly under-reported. † Transfusion-associated graft versus host disease (TA-GVHD) is due to viable engraftment of T lymphocytes and usually affects severely immunocompromised patients or recipients who share an HLA haplotype with a specific donor. Gamma-irradiation of blood products for specific at-risk groups of patients (refer to hospital guidelines) prevents this rare but usually fatal event.

16.2 Abnormal bleeding and clotting

B. Saxon

Bleeding disorders range from those that are severe and potentially life-threatening through to mild disorders that may be difficult to distinguish from normal.

Abnormal bleeding is the result of a disorder of one of the following:

- the blood vessel or its supporting tissue
- the platelets
- the coagulation mechanism.

Clinical approach to diagnosis

As a general rule, history taking, physical examination and a small number of relatively simple laboratory tests will find most causes of abnormal bleeding. The history, with particular reference to the past and family history, will usually provide the most valuable information.

Practical points

Bleeding disorder assessment
- History to determine normal from abnormal is the most valuable tool
- Simple coagulation tests such as platelet count, activated partial thromboplastin time (aPTT), prothrombin time (PT/INR) and fibrinogen will confirm the majority of diagnoses
- Mucosal bleeding needs assessment for von Willebrand disorder
- Assessment of other family members is often required

History

What is abnormal?

The main question to answer in the history is whether the bleeding symptoms are within or outside normal limits. Isolated bruises over the shins are common, while spontaneous petechiae are abnormal. Finger-induced epistaxis is common and not indicative of a bleeding disorder; however, recurrent nose bleeds lasting more than 10 minutes or leading to anaemia are often related to a bleeding disorder. Table 16.2.1 gives some clinical guidance.

When did the bleeding start?

Prenatal and neonatal
- congenital infection may result in a bleeding disorder
- mucosal bleeding occurs with haemorrhagic disease of the newborn
- umbilical stump bleeding is associated with factor XIII deficiency and dysfibrinogenaemias
- intracranial haemorrhage may occur with factor deficiencies and with neonatal alloimmune thrombocytopenia
- prolonged bleeding following circumcision is suggestive of haemophilia and may be the presenting feature of haemorrhagic disease of the newborn

Early childhood
- often implies a congenital defect
- bruising, muscle and joint bleeding is strongly suggestive of haemophilia
- petechiae and mucosal bleeding suggests a platelet problem or von Willebrand disorder

Sudden onset
- usually an acute problem such as immune thrombocytopenic purpura
- non-accidental injury may have a haemorrhagic presentation with inadequate explanations for each specific bruise, which may have an unusual distribution (Ch. 3.9). Skeletal trauma and other stigmata of non-accidental injury may be present

Where is the bleeding?

Specific bleeding sites have characteristic associations:

- *Joint bleeding*: haemophilia A and B
- *Nasal mucosa*: local irritation; von Willebrand disorder and platelet dysfunction
- *Gums, periosteum, skin*: scurvy
- *Gastrointestinal*: haemorrhagic disease of the newborn in babies; liver disease in older children

Table 16.2.1   What symptoms and signs may be related to a bleeding disorder?

Site	Within normal limits	May be abnormal and due to a number of causes	Usually due to a bleeding disorder
Nose	Finger-induced	Unilateral	Recurrent, requiring medical intervention or causing anaemia
Oral	Blood on brush	Gum ooze < 30 min	Gum ooze > 30 min
Gut	Rectal fissure, blood in nappy	Haematemesis, melaena	
Menstrual loss	4–7 days	'Same as Mum'	Loss leading to anaemia or transfusion
Skin	Shins don't count	Bony prominences	Spontaneous bruising over soft areas, laceration bleeding >30 min
Joints and muscles		Trauma induced	Spontaneous
Intracranial		Neonatal, trauma-induced	Spontaneous

- *Retro-orbital*: haematological malignancy or disseminated solid tumour.

Other aspects of history

Family history
Haemophilia A and B are X-linked; most von Willebrand disorder subtypes and haemorrhagic hereditary telangiectasia are recessive and several platelet function disorders are dominantly inherited. Clinical penetrance in haemophilia carriers and von Willebrand disorder may be variable.

Past history
Easy bruising, bruising at abnormal sites, prolonged bleeding following trivial trauma or bleeding following surgery and dental extractions are all indications for investigation.

Associated diseases
In the presence of disorders such as systemic lupus erythematosus, liver disease, extrahepatic portal hypertension, gross splenomegaly, giant haemangiomas, reticuloendothelial malignancies and leukaemia, bleeding is anticipated and is readily explicable.

Drug ingestion
Drugs may produce abnormal bleeding through:

- *depression of clotting factors*: anticoagulants, liver toxins
- *bone marrow depression*: chloramphenicol, cytoxic agents, radiation
- *antigen–antibody reactions with platelet membranes*: quinine group of drugs
- *direct inhibition of enzymes in platelets*: aspirin effects on platelet cyclooxygenase.

Physical examination

The following should be noted on physical examination.

The type of skin bleeding

Petechiae alone strongly suggest a platelet or vessel problem, while ecchymoses alone suggest a factor deficiency. Combined petechiae and ecchymoses suggest a severe disorder, often of platelet origin.

The site of the bleeding

Confirmation of history, defining the number of all different bleeding sites and assessment of severity of bleed and functional implications are all important aspects for both diagnosis and management.

Splenomegaly

Hypersplenism occurs when a large spleen removes platelets from the circulation, which leads to bleeding. The problem is the underlying cause of the splenomegaly. Hepatomegaly, splenomegaly, lymphadenopathy and/or anaemia, in association with bleeding, strongly suggest leukaemia.

Miscellaneous

Bleeding in association with eczema is a feature of Wiskott–Aldrich syndrome; telangiectasia and mucosal bleeding are typical of hereditary haemorrhagic telangiectasia. Hyperelastic skin, hyperextensible joints and bruising are associated with Ehlers–Danlos syndrome.

561

Table 16.2.2 Interpretation of initial blood tests in children with abnormal bleeding

Test	Result	More common causes	Less common causes
Blood count	Isolated thrombocytopenia	ITP NAIT	Congenital anomaly Early SAA
	Pancytopenia	Leukaemia SAA	Myelodysplasia Osteopetrosis
	High white cell count and thrombocytopenia	Leukaemia Infections	Myeloproliferative disorders
Blood film	Thrombocytopenia and red cell fragmentation	Microangiopathic anaemia, e.g. HUS	
	Small platelets		Wiscott–Aldrich syndrome
	Giant platelets		Bernard–Soulier syndrome
Prothrombin time (PT/INR)	Isolated prolongation	Vitamin K deficiency Warfarin therapy	Congenital factor VII deficiency
	Prolonged PT and aPTT	DIC Septicaemia Liver disease	Factor X, factor V, prothrombin or fibrinogen deficiency
aPTT	Isolated prolongation	Unfractionated heparin therapy Haemophilia A or B 'Lupus anticoagulant'	Factor XI deficiency Contact system* deficiency
All tests	Normal	Non-accidental injury	

* Contact system refers to factor XII, prekallikrein and high-molecular-weight kininogen.
aPTT, activated partial thromboplastin time; DIC, disseminated intravascular coagulation; HUS, haemolytic–uraemic syndrome; INR, international normalized ratio; ITP, immune thrombocytopenic purpura; NAIT, neonatal alloimmune thrombocytopenia; SAA, severe aplastic anaemia.

Investigation of bleeding in childhood

The tests in Table 16.2.2 are the most important.

Other tests

Measurement of von Willebrand factor level (antigen), activity (ristocetin cofactor and/or collagen binding assay) and factor VIII level are required to diagnose von Willebrand disorder. The bleeding time has lost favour because of its scarring potential but is characteristically prolonged in thrombocytopenia (normal 2–7 min), von Willebrand disorder and platelet function disorders and will be normal in other coagulation disorders.

Disorders of bleeding due to vascular defects

The commonest vascular defects seen in childhood are:

- anaphylactoid purpura
- infective states
- nutritional deficiency.

Anaphylactoid purpura (Henoch–Schönlein purpura)

The aetiology of this disorder is still not clear. It is readily recognized by the characteristic distribution of the rash over the buttocks, legs and backs of the elbows (Fig. 16.2.1). Frequently, it is accompanied by abdominal pain, melaena, joint swellings and occasionally a glomerulonephritis. In anaphylactoid purpura the bleeding time, international normalized ratio (INR), activated partial thromboplastin time (aPTT) and platelet counts are normal; the Hess test is positive in only 25% of cases. Thus, diagnosis must be made on the clinical picture alone. The outlook is excellent, except for an occasional child who develops a progressive renal lesion (Ch. 18.1). No specific therapy exists, although in children with severe abdominal pain corticosteroids may be helpful.

Infective states

The purpura associated with such disorders as meningococcaemia, other septicaemias and dengue haemorrhagic fever are the result of a severe angiitis

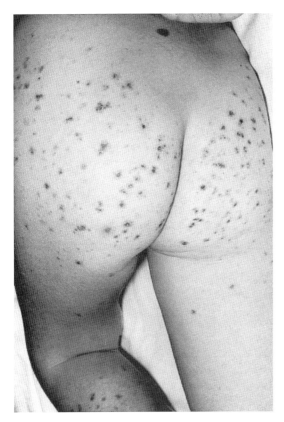

Fig. 16.2.1 Anaphylactoid purpura. The rash is typically distributed over the buttocks and backs of the legs.

caused by antigen–antibody complexes. Severe bleeding, which may accompany these states, is the result of activation of the coagulation mechanism producing disseminated intravascular coagulation. Management involves that of the infection and of the associated vascular collapse.

Nutritional deficiency

Scurvy is uncommon and occurs in the artificially fed infant with inadequate vitamin C supplementation. The child is often pale, with skin bruises; is immobile in the frog position because of painful subperiosteal haemorrhages; and has gingival bleeding. A wrist X-ray will demonstrate the characteristic dense lines in the metaphyses of the radius and ulna and the 'eggshell'-like epiphyses. Treatment with vitamin C (100–200 mg/d) reverses the clinical features within a week.

Purpura fulminans

This is a life-threatening and rare form of non-thrombocytopenic purpura that may follow such infections as scarlet fever, varicella, measles and some other viral infections. Typically there are rapidly spreading skin haemorrhages involving the buttocks and lower extremities. Congenital deficiencies of either protein C or protein S are the cause of neonatal purpura fulminans.

Miscellaneous

Bleeding from vascular wall defects is a feature of a group of rare disorders. These include hereditary haemorrhagic telangiectasia, polyarteritis nodosa, other vasculitides and uraemia. Anoxia, and thus damage to the capillary wall, may cause purpura in the asphyxiated newborn. The bleeding that accompanies Cushing syndrome, Ehlers–Danlos syndrome and cutis laxa is the result of defects in vascular supporting issue.

Bleeding due to platelet disorders

Bleeding disorders resulting from platelet abnormalities are usually due to thrombocytopenia but may be due to qualitative platelet defects. The various types of inherited and acquired thrombocytopenia are listed in Table 16.2.3.

Immune thrombocytopenic purpura

Immune thrombocytopenic purpura is the most common acquired bleeding disorder in children. It may be acute or chronic (defined as lasting longer than 6 months), episodic or continuous. Common to all clinical variations is the marked reduction in platelet life span due to immune-mediated splenic sequestration.

Features of typical acute immune thrombocytopenic purpura:

- 80–90% of paediatric immune thrombocytopenic purpura cases
- preceding viral illness is common
- peak age 2–5 years
- abrupt onset of bleeding
- mucosal and skin bleeding
- petechiae common
- otherwise normal examination, i.e. no lymphadenopathy or hepatosplenomegaly
- platelet count usually $<20 \times 10^9/l$
- normal red cell and white cell parameters.

There is no need for other investigations if these 'typical' features are present.

Differential diagnosis is predominantly that of evolving aplastic anaemia.

Chronic immune thrombocytopenic purpura occurs in 10–20% of cases and often has an insidious onset in children aged over 7 years; it affects girls

Table 16.2.3   Inherited and acquired thrombocytopenias

	Disorder	Key information
Inherited		
With platelet dysfunction	Bernard–Soulier syndrome	GpIb–V–IX adhesion re ceptor defect – inability to bind with vWF
	Wiscott–Aldrich syndrome	Small platelets, eczema, infections, X-linked, *WASP* mutations
	X linked thrombocytopenia	Small platelets, X-linked, *WASP* mutations
	Grey platelet syndrome	Granule defect, bone marrow fibrosis
Without platelet dysfunction	May–Hegglin anomaly	Large platelets, Dohle bodies in neutrophils
	Alport syndrome	Large platelets, nephritis, deafness, cataracts, several variants
	Thrombocytopenia with absent radii (TAR)	Decreased megakaryocytes, typical bone anomalies
	Mediterranean macrothrombocytopenia	Large platelets, autosomal dominant
	Fanconi anaemia	Thrombocytopenia often precedes other cytopenias
Acquired		
Neonatal	Immune thrombocytopenia	Neonatal alloimmune or maternal autoimmune
	Intrauterine infection	TORCH
	Pre-eclampsia	
	Birth asphyxia	
	Giant haemangioma	'Kasabach–Merritt syndrome' features platelet consumption
Any age	Immune thrombocytopenia (ITP)	The most common acquired thrombocytopenia
	Autoimmune disorders	Antiphospholipid antibodies may be present
	Disseminated intravascular coagulation	Sepsis or other cause evident. Low coagulation factors
	Haemolytic–uraemic syndrome	Microangiopathic haemolysis, usually normal INR and aPTT
	Bone marrow infiltration	Leukaemia, lymphoma, disseminated solid tumours, HLH
	Bone marrow failure	Severe aplastic anaemia
	Drug induced	Cytotoxic therapy, chloramphenicol
	Hypersplenism	Platelets trapped in spleen, as in portal hypertension

HLH, haemophagocytic lymphohistiocytosis; TORCH, *t*oxoplasmosis, *o*ther (e.g. HIV and parvovirus B19), *r*ubella, *c*ytomegalovirus, *h*erpes simplex; vWF, von Willebrand factor.

more commonly than boys. *Recurrent immune thrombocytopenic purpura* is rare and is characterized by thrombocytopenia at more than 3-month intervals.

Treatment approaches to *immune thrombocytopenic purpura* are shown in Table 16.2.4.

Bleeding due to qualitative platelet defects

The child with a functional platelet defect will have a normal platelet count but abnormal platelet function tests. These tests analyse aggregation of platelets in response to several stimuli. The more common disorders in this group are the 'aspirin-like' syndrome and platelet storage pool disorders. The most severe disorder is Glanzmann disease. Before undertaking

Clinical example

Chloe presented at the age of 4 years, 2 weeks after a viral upper respiratory infection, with a 3-day history of a petechial rash on her face and gum bleeding with toothbrushing. Examination revealed several fresh skin bruises along with the petechiae. There was no hepatosplenomegaly and the only palpable lymph nodes were slightly tender, 2 cm diameter tonsillar nodes. The only abnormality on full blood examination was a platelet count of 9×10^9/l. Chloe was treated with prednisolone 4 mg/kg daily in three divided doses for 4 days as an outpatient, with alternate daily platelet counts. On the second day of treatment her platelet count was 65×10^9/l and the count became normal within 5 days. She had no further episodes of thrombocytopenia.

Table 16.2.4 Treatment options for acute immune thrombocytopenic purpura with either bleeding problems or if the platelet count is less than $10 \times 10^9/l$

Treatment option	Advantages	Disadvantages	Time course to resolution
First-line therapy			
Conservative	No drug side effects	Longest time to platelet $>20 \times 10^9/l$ <1% risk of ICH while awaiting platelet recovery	75% remission in 4–6 weeks 15% take 4–6 months
Corticosteroids (standard dose*)	No blood product exposure	Steroid side effects‡ common	1 week
Corticosteroids (high dose†)	No blood product exposure Rapid rise in platelets	Steroid side effects‡ less common	Platelets $>20 \times 10^9/l$: 2 days Platelets $>50 \times 10^9/l$: 3–4 days
Intravenous gammaglobulin (IVIG)§	Rapid rise in platelets	Pooled blood product with two viral inactivation steps	Platelets $>20 \times 10^9/l$: 1–2 days Platelets $>50 \times 10^9/l$: 3 days
Second-line therapy			
Anti-Rh(D) antibody		Only useful in Rhesus-positive children Similar efficacy to IVIG and steroids	
Splenectomy	Most useful in children >5 years old with chronic ITP	Immunizations for meningococcus, *Haemophilus influenzae* and pneumococcus are mandatory Lifelong antibiotic prophylaxis	Rapid in the majority

* Standard dose: prednisolone 2 mg/kg body weight daily for 21 days. † High dose: prednisolone 4 mg/kg body weight daily for 4 days. ‡ Steroid side effects include gastric irritation, transient diabetes and other metabolic derangements, immune suppression, cushingoid body fat distribution, growth delay, osteopenia and rarely avascular necrosis of the femoral head. § IVIG (e.g. Intragam P, Sandoglobulin) 0.8 g/kg body weight, repeat within 1–7 days if platelets remain $<10 \times 10^9/l$ or any platelet count with problematic bleeding. IVIG side effects include flu-like symptoms and rarely transient aseptic meningitis. Blood products may theoretically transmit viral and prion particles.
ICH, intracranial haemorrhage; ITP, immune thrombocytopenic purpura.

 Practical points

Acute bleeding history
- Differentiate 'wet' purpura (mucosal bleeding) from 'dry' purpura (skin bleeding) as some authorities claim increased likelihood of intracranial bleeding in the presence of wet purpura
- Always examine the fundi for bleeding changes
- Splenomegaly, lymphadenopathy or hepatomegaly indicate a systemic illness, e.g. Epstein–Barr virus infection, leukaemia
- Anaemia and reticulocyte response aid determination of severity and duration of bleeding

platelet function studies one must ensure that there has been no ingestion of aspirin for at least 7 days.

Bleeding due to coagulation disorders

Physiology of coagulation

Following the formation of a platelet plug at the site of vessel injury, fibrin is laid down and is cross-linked to form a protein mesh. This process (coagulation) is usually initiated by factor VIIa binding to exposed tissue factor (Fig. 16.2.2) This complex activates factors IX and X. Activated factor X recruits a cofactor, factor Va, to activate prothrombin (factor II). This process takes place on a phospholipid surface such as a platelet. Thrombin is a

Practical points

Understanding coagulation
- The aPTT and PT/INR are screening tests which represent how various 'factors' interact in the test tube. Useful tests to determine which factor may be low
- In vivo coagulation does not occur as a 'cascade', rather a series of positive feedback reactions starting with tissue factor and factor VII and culminating in a thrombin burst
- Clotting occurs at the site of injury by thrombin cleaving fibrinogen to fibrin
- Thrombin inhibits coagulation by binding with thrombomodulin on normal blood vessels

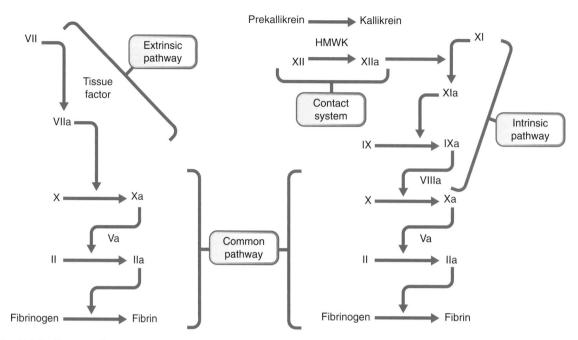

Fig. 16.2.2   The coagulation system as measured by initial blood tests: prothrombin time (INR; left) and aPTT (right). HMWK, high-molecular-weight kininogen; 'a' indicates activated factor. This figure does not represent in vivo coagulation, rather the coagulation factors (in test tubes) that influence the prothrombin time and aPTT.

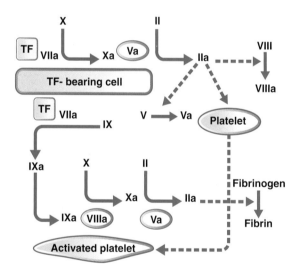

Fig. 16.2.3   Initiation of coagulation and the production of a fibrin clot. TF, tissue factor.

Clinical example

Albert was born at term, received intramuscular vitamin K and developed a large bruise in his thigh. No circumcision was performed. He always seemed to have fingerprint bruises under his arms from being picked up. When he began sitting unaided he developed buttock bruising and when he began walking he presented to the accident and emergency department with a swollen, hot right ankle. The joint had virtually no movement and an ultrasound confirmed a fluid-filled joint. The history was highly suggestive of haemophilia. The INR was normal, the aPTT was 90 seconds and the factor VIII level was less than 1%. Haemophilia A was diagnosed and prophylaxis with 25 U/kg recombinant factor VIII three times per week was commenced. At the age of 4 years Albert fell from a chair on to his occiput after missing a dose of prophylaxis. Within 2 hours he had a falling level of consciousness and respiratory depression. A computed tomography scan diagnosed a subdural haematoma. Treatment with high-dose factor VIII and neurosurgical intervention led to an uneventful recovery.

powerful procoagulant, activating factors V, VIII and XI and cleaving fibrinogen to form fibrin. The activation of 'upstream' coagulation factor causes more thrombin generation (Fig. 16.2.3). Fortunately, thrombin also activates key inhibitors of coagulation to prevent excessive clot formation. Clearly a defect in any major protein could lead to significant bleeding problems.

Haemophilia

Prevalence

- Haemophilia A (factor VIII deficiency): 5–10 males per 100 000
- Haemophilia B (Christmas disease, factor IX deficiency): 0.5–1 per 100 000.

- Factor XI deficiency (haemophilia C): rare
- other factor deficiencies: exceedingly rare

Genetics

Haemophilia A and B are both X-linked. Up to one-third of all new cases of haemophilia are due to new mutations. Female carriers sometimes have low levels of factor VIII or IX and may have a bleeding disorder.

Severity

Defined by plasma factor level and correlates with clinical severity:

- *severe*: <2%, frequent spontaneous deep tissue bleeding
- *moderate*: 2–5%, infrequent spontaneous bleeding
- *mild*: 6–30%, bleeding with trauma and surgery, not spontaneously.

Clinical manifestations

Neonatal
A positive family history or known carrier status allows for definitive diagnosis in the newborn period. Cord blood genetics are most reliable. Some laboratories will perform factor VIII or factor IX assays on cord blood but technical difficulties may arise and results should be interpreted with caution. There is prolonged bleeding following circumcision. Intracranial haemorrhage is suspicious of a bleeding disorder in the term neonate.

Early childhood
Skin and soft tissue bleeds are common in the first year and beyond. Haemarthroses usually only occur once the child is walking. The ankles are common bleeding sites in young children; elbow and knee bleeding (Fig. 16.2.4) occur more commonly in older children.

Specific bleeds
Bleeding into the forearm may occlude the neurovascular bundle and cause a Volkmann ischaemic contracture. Bleeding into the posterior pharyngeal wall may interfere with respiration and cause dysphagia. Iliopsoas bleeding may be complicated by femoral nerve compression. Intracranial vascular accident is the cause of death in 7% of patients with haemophiliacs. Haematuria is common in adolescents and is seldom serious.

Chronic illness
There is synovial hypertrophy and arthritis. HIV/AIDS occurred in more than 50% of patients receiv-

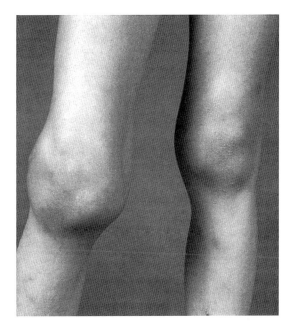

Fig. 16.2.4 Haemarthrosis of the right knee in a boy with haemophilia.

ing blood products in the years 1980–1985. Hepatitis C infection is also common prior to viral identification, screening and viral inactivation of plasma products. Variant Creutzfeldt–Jakob disease (vCJD) is a prion disease. It has been shown to be transmissible in blood products and is not removed by current viral inactivation processes. Fortunately there have been no cases of vCJD described in patients with haemophilia. Psychosocial problems arise as a result of chronic illness, lifestyle restrictions and the need for injections.

Complications

Inhibitors are anti-factor-VIII or anti-factor-IX antibodies, which prevent regular doses of factor concentrate from working. Central lines may be required to ensure venous access in young children. These may be complicated by infection or large vein thrombosis.

Management

Correct or prevent the bleeding tendency
- mild and moderate haemophilia A often responds to desmopressin acetate infusions to elevate plasma factor VIII
- 1 unit of factor VIII/kg body weight given intravenously increases the factor VIII by approximately 2%
- life-threatening bleeds require plasma factor levels of more than 80%

- most other bleeds require plasma factor levels of 30–60%
- prophylactic infusions of 25–40 U/kg three times a week 'converts' severe disease into moderate disease, thereby decreasing the risk of spontaneous bleeding.

Choice of product
- most developed countries, including Australia, now offer recombinant product to all haemophilia patients
- plasma-derived factor products are still available. These are screened for HIV and hepatitis B and C and then undergo two viral inactivation steps in the processing.

Orthopaedic
- rest, immobilization, ice, compression and elevation (RICE) are usually sufficient to control pain
- splinting followed by exercises when pain has settled preserves function.

Haemophilia centres
- focus of education and training for patient and family
- multidisciplinary group with expertise in haemophilia management.

Inhibitors
- occur in up to 30% of patients
- at least half of these are low-titre inhibitors, which can be treated by high-dose factor VIII
- high titre inhibitors require 'immune tolerance' therapy for eradication of inhibitor, and infusions of the factor VIII and IX bypass agent, recombinant factor VIIa, to treat bleeds.

Clinical example

Vanessa was a 13-year-old girl with menorrhagia since menarche. She had always had 'easy bruising' and required a transfusion after tonsillectomy due to excessive bleeding. She often bled from her gums after brushing her teeth. Her older sister and her mother both had heavy periods but neither had had severe postsurgical bleeding. Platelet count, INR and aPTT were all normal. von Willebrand antigen was 30%, activity (ristocetin cofactor) 25% and factor VIII 35%. She was diagnosed with mild von Willebrand disorder.

Von Willebrand disorder

This disorder has the following features:

- quantitative (types 1 and 3) or qualitative (type 2) defect in von Willebrand factor (vWF), a molecule which assists platelet adhesion to the subendothelium

- Common: 125 per million population
- Type 1 is inherited as autosomal dominant, is mild and is the most common
- Types 2 and 3 are rare
- Mucosal bleeding, excessive bruising and postoperative or post-traumatic bleeding
- Prolonged bleeding time but normal INR and aPTT, unless severe disease is present
- Abnormal vWF antigen and activity (ristocetin cofactor)
- Treatment for type 1 vWF is DDAVP which releases stored vWF/factor VIII
- DDAVP may be repeated once stores have reaccumulated, usually after 12–24 hours
- Plasma derived factor VIII products often contain vWF and may be used in those unresponsive to DDAVP
- Cryoprecipitate should be avoided due to lack of viral inactivation.

Haemorrhagic disease of the newborn

Haemorrhagic disease of the newborn fortunately is now rare, since the introduction of routine vitamin K administration for all babies at the time of delivery. Features of haemorrhagic disease of the newborn:

- Coagulation factors requiring vitamin K for post-transcriptional modification:
  - factor II (prothrombin)
  - factor VII
  - factor IX
  - factor X
  - protein C and S
  These fall in neonates as a result of nutritional deficiency
- Bleeding is usually from the gastrointestinal tract or following circumcision
- Occurs early, often day 2–3
- Prophylactic vitamin K eliminates this disease
- Vitamin K 1 mg given by the intramuscular route stops bleeding rapidly.

Clotting due to coagulation disorders

Physiology of anticoagulation

The formation of a fibrin clot is tightly regulated in its local environment by anticoagulants. Local thrombin binds thrombomodulin located on normal endothelium which activates protein C. Activated protein C (APC) with the cofactor, protein S, inhibits

Table 16.2.5 Major causes of thrombosis in childhood

Cause	Clinical features	Diagnostic tests	Treatment
Venous access device	Blocked access/emboli, limb swelling	Echocardiography and contrast radiography	Heparin. Removal of device
Phospholipid antibodies	Superficial/deep vein thrombosis	Prolonged INR/aPTT, not corrected by normal plasma	Often no therapy, may require corticosteroids or heparin
Protein C and S homozygous	Purpura fulminans	Very low protein C or S	Protein C replacement + heparin
Protein C and S heterozygous	Superficial/deep vein thrombosis; rare cerebral, mesenteric and renal vein thrombosis	Low protein C or S	Heparin followed by long term warfarin
Factor V mutation, (Arg506 to Gln), 'FV Leiden'	Early onset vascular disease in family	Activated protein C resistance test	Heparin and long term warfarin
Antithrombin deficiency	Venous thrombosis in adolescence	Decreased level of antithrombin	Antithrombin replacement, heparin and warfarin
Dysfibrinogenaemia	Rare thrombosis in childhood	Prolonged thrombin time and snake venom times	Replacement therapy
Homocysteinaemia	Arterial and venous thrombosis	Biochemical tests	Diet and short-term anticoagulants

factors Va and VIIIa by cleaving the molecules. A mutation of factor V at one cleavage point prevents the APC inhibitory effect and is termed APC resistance. The mutation is called factor V Leiden. The other key coagulation inhibitor is antithrombin, a direct inhibitor of thrombin and also factors Xa, IXa, XIa and XIIa. Heparins potentiate the effect of antithrombin greatly. The largest risk factor for paediatric thrombosis is not a protein deficiency but the presence of a central venous catheter.

Table 16.2.5 lists the causes and features of thrombosis in childhood.

Childhood cancers

T. A. O'Brien

The last 30 years have seen dramatic improvements in the treatment of childhood cancer. Survival rates have climbed from below 30% to more than 80%. This improvement is largely due to the use of clinical cancer trials conducted through collaborative national and international childhood cancer study groups and underpins the need for a cohesive approach to the treatment of rare diseases. Prompt referral to a paediatric oncology centre for diagnostic workup and management is critical for all children with a suspected malignancy. A multidisciplinary team approach utilizing skills of specialist medical, nursing and allied health practitioners is the gold standard in delivery of excellence in care to children with cancer.

Reflecting improved cure rates, it is projected that by 2010, one in every 250 adults will be a survivor of childhood cancer. This has lead to widespread study of potential late effects of cancer treatments in childhood. Despite these remarkable improvements, it is sobering to acknowledge that 20–25% of children diagnosed with cancer are not cured with current therapies. Childhood cancer remains the leading cause of disease-related mortality among children. This clearly dictates the need for ongoing research to improve survival outcomes.

There are four principal therapeutic modalities used in the treatment of childhood cancers; surgery, radiotherapy, chemotherapy and biological therapies. These are used as single agents or in combination depending on tumour type and stage.

Incidence and distribution of childhood cancers

Approximately 1 in 600 children will be diagnosed with cancer before the age of 15 years.

The distribution of cancer types in children aged 0–14 years is shown in Table 16.3.1. Acute leukaemia (acute lymphoblastic (ALL) or acute myeloblastic leukaemia (AML)) accounts for close to one-third of all childhood cancer. Primary brain or central nervous system (CNS) tumours are the most common solid cancer, followed by lymphoma, neuroblastoma, Wilms tumour, bone tumours and soft tissue sarcomas.

Aetiology of childhood cancer

When confronted with a diagnosis of childhood cancer, parents often ask 'Why did this happen to my child?' or 'Did this happen because of something I have done or passed on to my child?'. With the exception of several known predisposing genetic syndromes (Table 16.3.2) the proportion of paediatric cancers that have a clearly hereditary component is small. Similarly, despite extensive epidemiological studies, few environmental agents have been consistently linked with childhood malignancy. Broadly speaking, it is hypothesized that cancer initiation results from a series of genetic mutations resulting in the inability of a cell to respond normally to intracellular and/or extracellular signals that control cell proliferation, differentiation or death (apoptosis). Examples include mutations involving tumour suppressor genes (e.g. *RB1*, *p53* or *WT1*) or activation of cellular proto-oncogenes (e.g. *myc* or *abl*). The number of required genetic alterations may differ depending on the type of malignancy from as few as one to a complex cascade arising directly or indirectly from inherited gene mutations, environmental, chemical or radiation-induced DNA damage or random errors in DNA synthesis.

Acute leukaemia

While the cause of leukaemia remains unknown, the prevailing theory for leukemic development is that a mutant stem cell, capable of indefinite renewal, gives rise to abnormal proliferation of lymphoblasts (ALL) or myeloblasts (AML) in the bone marrow. These cells occupy the marrow space, leading to reduced numbers of normal haematopoietic cells, resulting ultimately in pancytopenia. Secondary involvement of the reticuloendothelial system (leading to lymphadenopathy and hepatosplenomegaly), bone, joints and rarely CNS, testes and skin can occur. A two-step pathogenesis for ALL (Greaves' hypothesis) has been suggested, with the initial event, occurring during fetal life, driving clonal expansion and a second trigger occurring during childhood, possibly resulting from viral stimuli of cellular proliferation.

Table 16.3.1 Frequency of malignancy in childhood

Malignant disease	Frequency (%)
Leukaemia	35
Primary central nervous system tumours	20
Lymphoma: non-Hodgkin and Hodgkin	10
Wilms tumour	6–8
Neuroblastoma	6–8
Rhabdomyosarcoma, soft tissue sarcoma	5
Sarcoma of bone: Ewing and osteosarcoma	4
Histiocytosis	5
Teratoma	2
Retinoblastoma	1
Hepatic	1
Others	5

Table 16.3.2 Inherited/genetic syndromes associated with increased risk of childhood malignancy

Cancer	Associated syndrome
Leukemia	Trisomy 21, Bloom syndrome, Fanconi anaemia, ataxia telangiectasia, neurofibromatosis, Kostmann syndrome, Klinefelter syndrome, Li–Fraumeni syndrome, Diamond–Blackfan anaemia, Noonan syndrome
CNS Tumours	Neurofibromatosis, tuberous sclerosis, Li–Fraumeni syndrome, von Hippel–Lindau syndrome
Lymphoma	Immunodeficiency disorders
Wilms tumour	Denys–Drash syndrome, Beckwith–Weidermann syndrome, WAGR syndrome
Rhabdomyosarcoma	Li–Fraumeni syndrome

This theory stems from evidence that a significant proportion of children presenting with ALL have molecular evidence of leukaemic clones identified retrospectively at birth on newborn screening cards.

ALL accounts for 80% of all childhood leukaemia, with AML accounting for the majority of the remainder. In ALL, presentation peaks at age 2–5 years, whereas there is no peak in AML. Chronic leukaemia, including chronic myeloid leukaemia (CML) and juvenile myelomonocytic leukaemia (JMML), is rare, accounting for fewer than 5% of cases.

Leukaemia can be further classified on the basis of morphological characteristics, immunobiology and cytogenetic or molecular markers. Immunophenotype as determined by flow cytometric detection of cell surface antigens is commonly used to differentiate distinct ALL categories into:

- precursor B-cell ALL (early pre-B, pre-B, transitional pre-B) – 80–85%
- mature B-cell ALL – 2–3%
- T-cell ALL – 10–15%.

In AML, characteristic morphological and cytochemical features include the presence of Auer rods as well as positive staining for myeloperoxidase and monocyte-associated esterases. Classification into one of eight morphological subclasses using the French/American/British (FAB) system is possible. In addition to morphology and immunophenotype, genetic features of leukaemic cells can provide diagnostic and prognostic information. In ALL, for example, the number of chromosomes per leukaemic cell influences prognosis, with more favourable survival in patients with hyperdiploid leukaemic cells (>50 chromosomes per cell). Specific chromosomal translocations can also be identified, e.g. t(8;14) in B-cell ALL and the unfavourable t(9;22) or the *BCR-abl* gene (Philadelphia chromosome) identified in CML and 5% of paediatric patients with ALL. In AML, characteristic translocations are seen within FAB morphological subgroups: for example, M3 or acute promyelocytic leukaemia (APML) is identified by the translocation t(15;17), and t(8;21) is a favourable cytogenetic abnormality seen in FAB M1 and M2.

Acute lymphoblastic leukaemia

The clinical presentation of ALL can be quite variable; however, most children will present with a 3–4-week prodrome that may include pallor, increased bruising or bleeding, lethargy, anorexia, recurrent infection or fevers, anorexia, bone pain or reluctance to walk. Physical examination may show:

- pallor (80%)
- petechiae (50%)
- lymphadenopathy (35%)
- hepatomegaly or splenomegaly (50–60%)
- rarely, skin infiltration (chloroma) and testicular infiltration (usually presents as a painless swelling).

The peripheral blood film can be normal but will usually demonstrate the presence of leukaemic blasts with or without anaemia and thrombocytopenia. The white blood cell count (WCC) is frequently elevated at diagnosis (leucocytosis), with a presenting WCC below $10 \times 10^9/l$ in 25%, $10–50 \times 10^9/l$ in 50% and above $50 \times 10^9/l$ in 25% of patients. A bone marrow aspirate and biopsy (trephine) are the gold standard diagnostic tests and will show replacement of normal haematopoiesis by leukaemic cells. A lumbar puncture is also done during the staging work-up with approximately 5–10% of patients showing leukaemic spread to the cerebrospinal fluid (CSF). T-cell leukaemia, more common in older boys, presents with a mediastinal mass in 50% that can result in life-threatening airway compression and obstruction of the superior vena cava. 30% of patients with T-cell ALL present with a leucocyte count greater than $100 \times 10^9/l$ and there is a higher incidence of CNS disease.

Table 16.3.3 shows prognostic risk factors for ALL. Clinical features such as age and WCC at diagnosis are becoming less significant with the advent of newer molecular methodologies. Furthermore, the response to treatment is becoming a critical determinant in prognosis. For example, reduction of initial blast count following steroid therapy is an important prognostic factor, as is detection of minimal residual disease (MRD) by molecular methods after exposure to chemotherapy.

Current combination chemotherapy protocols for ALL result in cure of 80% of patients. Much of the required therapy can be given on an outpatient or day-stay basis. Treatment consists of phases of therapy including induction, consolidation, CNS directed therapy, re-induction and continuation or maintenance therapy. By the end of the first month of therapy (induction) with 3–4-drug combination chemotherapy (vincristine, asparaginase, prednisone, daunorubicin), remission will be achieved in more than 95% of patients. Further combination therapy is required to prevent relapse. The optimal total duration of therapy is not known – most centres elect to treat for 2–3 years. CNS-targeted therapy using high-dose intravenous and intrathecal methotrexate has allowed for cranial irradiation to be generally avoided except in patients with overt CNS disease at diagnosis, sparing potential deleterious effects on cognition and growth.

Clinical example

Sally was a 3-year-old girl who presented with a 2–3-week history of intermittent fever, lethargy and poor appetite. Reluctance to walk and increased bruising were also noted for 1–2 days prior to presentation. Examination confirmed a pale child with truncal petechiae, limb bruising, cervical lymphadenopathy, splenomegaly and hepatomegaly. What was the differential diagnosis?

The presence of fever suggested infection, pallor suggested anaemia and petechiae and bruising suggested thrombocytopenia. A blood count would confirm this. Lymphadenopathy and hepatosplenomegaly were consistent with infection (e.g. infectious mononucleosis, cytomegalovirus) or leukemic infiltration. Reluctance to walk, fever and mild anaemia may be consistent with a primary joint problem such as juvenile rheumatoid arthritis or osteomyelitis but were not consistent with lymphadenopathy, hepatosplenomegaly and thrombocytopenia. A blood count and film were warranted and a bone marrow aspirate was needed to confirm the diagnosis of acute leukaemia. Other paediatric malignancies that may present with bone marrow involvement should be considered, including lymphoma, neuroblastoma, rhabdomyosarcoma and Ewing sarcoma.

Table 16.3.3 Risk group classification for acute lymphoblastic leukaemia		
Risk group	Clinical features	Molecular/genetic features
Low risk	Age 2–10 years, WCC $<50 \times 10^9/l$ Not T-cell phenotype No central nervous system or testicular disease Rapid response to induction therapy	DNA index >1.16 Absence of: $t(9;22)$ BCR–abl $t(4;11)$ MLL/AF$_4$ $t(1;19)$ MLL rearrangement $t(12;21)$ TEL/AML1
High risk and very high risk	Induction failure Age < 12 months Poor prednisone response High MRD levels	$t(9;22)$, $t(4;11)$ MLL rearrangements

Acute myeloid leukaemia

AML accounts for 20% of acute leukaemia. Presenting symptoms and signs are similar to ALL and can include pallor, bleeding, fever, anorexia, malaise and bone pain. Certain subtypes of AML have more distinctive presenting clinical features. Acute promyelocytic leukaemia (APML) can present with serious haemorrhage or disseminated intravascular coagulation, whereas acute monoblastic or myelomonoblastic leukaemia may present with skin infiltration (chloroma) or gum hypertrophy. CNS leukaemia is diagnosed in 5–15% of patients. Like ALL, the differential diagnosis can include infection, juvenile rheumatoid arthritis, idiopathic thrombocytic purpura, aplastic anaemia and osteomyelitis.

In contrast to ALL, therapy for AML is of shorter duration and more intensive, often requiring frequent hospital admissions with aggressive supportive care, including blood products and antimicrobials during lengthy periods of marrow suppression. Overall, the outlook for patients with AML is less optimistic, with survival rates reported of 50–70%.

Clinical example

Angela was a 10-year-old girl who presented with a 1-week history of lethargy, poor appetite, recurrent epistaxis and gum bleeding on brushing her teeth. Examination revealed anaemia, gum hypertrophy, bruising on the lower limbs and trunk, hepatosplenomegaly and inguinal lymphadenopathy. A full blood count confirmed anaemia and thrombocytopenia with a haemoglobin of 8.2 g/l and platelets $12 \times 10^9/l$. Leukocytosis was noted, with a white cell count of $120 \times 10^9/l$ with circulating blast cells. Coagulation profile was prolonged, consistent with mild disseminated intravascular coagulation. Bone marrow aspirate confirmed the diagnosis of acute monocytic leukaemia. Lumbar puncture was performed to exclude CNS spread. A double-lumen central line was inserted following attention to thrombocytopenia and coagulation abnormalities, and combination chemotherapy was commenced as soon as practical. Tumour lysis syndrome or uric-acid-induced nephropathy can be an early complication of leukaemia therapy as tumour cells die, releasing uric acid, potassium and phosphate with consequent life-threatening electrolyte abnormalities and renal impairment. Vigorous hydration with intravenous fluid, forced diuresis and allopurinol are standard. Dialysis is occasionally required.

Haematopoietic stem cell transplant

For most patients with high-risk, relapsed or refractory leukaemia, haematopoietic stem cell transplantation is the treatment of choice. Stem cells can be sourced from the bone marrow, from peripheral blood or from the umbilical cord of a newborn infant. Siblings have a 25% chance of being an identical match. Those lacking a sibling donor are reliant on volunteer bone marrow and cord blood donors sourced through international donor registries. Umbilical cord blood transplants are used with increased frequency because of the advantages of speed of availability and greater likelihood of matching.

Brain and central nervous system tumours

Brain tumours or tumours of the CNS are the most common solid cancer, representing approximately 20% of all childhood malignancies. Brain tumours as a group are heterogeneous with regard to clinical presentation, location, histological type and natural history. 95% of CNS tumours occur within the brain, often in specific sites for different age groups. Posterior fossa tumours are more common in childhood, except during the first year of life, and in adolescence, where supratentorial sites predominate. The most common histological subtypes are:

- astrocytomas (50%)
- primitive neuroectodermal tumours (21%)
- gliomas (15–20%)
- ependymomas (9%).

Table 16.3.4 shows a working classification of CNS tumours. Early symptoms and signs of CNS tumours may be few and difficult to elicit (Table 16.3.5). Evidence of raised intracranial pressure is the most common because posterior fossa and deep midline tumours usually obstruct CSF pathways. Treatment of brain tumours depends on tumour type and location and can include surgery, chemotherapy and radiation therapy. A number of factors impact on outcome and survival, including age, tumour location and operability, histological subtype and

---

Table 16.3.4 Central nervous system tumours

1. Supratentorial
   a. *Hemisphere*: astrocytoma; glioblastoma; primitive neuroectodermal tumour
   b. *Midline*: craniopharyngioma; optic nerve glioma; pineal
2. Infratentorial
   a. *Cerebellar and fourth ventricle*: astrocytoma; medulloblastoma; ependymoma
   b. *Brain stem*: brain-stem glioma
3. Spinal cord
   Astrocytoma; ependymoma

Table 16.3.5	Signs and symptoms of brain and central; nervous system tumours
Raised intracranial pressure	Headache, often on waking Vomiting Papilloedema Tense fontanelle and increased head circumference in infants indicating hydrocephalus Drowsiness, bradycardia and hypertension (late signs)
Posterior fossa signs	Truncal ataxia due to central cerebellar tumours Coordination difficulties and tremor due to lateral lesions Cranial nerve palsies, suggesting a brain-stem lesion Defective upward gaze with tumours of the pineal region Deep midline tumours around the third ventricle Impaired visual acuity and visual field defects due to craniopharyngioma or optic nerve glioma Diabetes insipidus and growth failure Severe wasting and anorexia due to the diencephalic syndrome of a hypothalamic tumour
Seizures	Uncommon as sole presenting symptom Consider tumour with focal seizures or progressively more difficult to control seizures

presence or absence of neuraxis dissemination. Survival has improved considerably over time for some types of tumour, notably medulloblastoma. For other tumour subtypes, however, such as brain-stem gliomas, outcome remains poor. Additionally, increasing attention is being paid to the longer-term toxicity of treatment. This is particularly true of radiation therapy, which, where possible, is spared in younger children because of the potential impact on cognition and growth.

Lymphoma

Lymphomas, accounting for approximately 10% of childhood cancers, are the third most common form of malignancy in childhood. There are two basic types: non-Hodgkin lymphoma (NHL) and Hodgkin disease. Both are more common in boys than in girls. Although lymphadenopathy attributable to an infectious aetiology is more common in childhood, any child with persistent adenopathy (>2–3 weeks) should be considered for a biopsy. Site of adenopathy (e.g. supraclavicular) or character (firm, >1–2 cm) may indicate the need for earlier biopsy.

Non-Hodgkin lymphoma

Childhood NHL has quite different features from its adult counterpart. Childhood NHL is more often disseminated, diffuse not nodular, high-grade immature T- or B-cell lineage with frequent spread to extranodal sites, marrow and CNS. In contrast, NHL occurring in adulthood is usually a low-grade malignancy with predominantly nodal involvement. Clinical and pathological staging is achieved with organ imaging (computed tomography (CT) of chest/abdomen/pelvis, positron emission tomography (PET) scan or gallium scan), lymph node biopsy/resection, bone marrow aspirate and biopsy (trephine) and CSF examination. When more than 25% of bone marrow is involved, disease is classified as T- or B-cell ALL. NHL in childhood can be classified as:

- lymphoblastic NHL – diffuse, poorly differentiated, primarily T-cell lineage
- small non-cleaved (undifferentiated) Burkitt or non-Burkitt subtypes, primarily of B-cell origin. A t(8;14) translocation is characteristic of Burkitt lymphoma
- large cell lymphoma – can be cleaved or non-cleaved and of B-cell or T-cell origin.

A mediastinal primary of T-cell immunophenotype accounts for 25% of NHL and often presents with acute superior vena caval and/or airway obstruction (a medical emergency) producing stridor and cough, usually with an associated pleural effusion and characteristically occurring in preteen or early teenage males. Diagnosis, immunophenotyping and cytogenetics may be made on pleural aspirate, suprasternal or supraclavicular node biopsy, or rarely on direct biopsy of the mediastinal mass. Abdominal lymphoma accounts for 35–40%, is of B-cell immunophenotype and characteristically presents as either local tumour causing intussusception and readily removable, or massive diffuse abdominal disease, often with ascites. The later is often associated with uric-acid-induced nephropathy or tumour lysis syndrome. Release of uric acid, potassium and phosphate from rapidly growing tumours, particularly following commencement of chemotherapy, can result in significant renal impairment and life-threatening electrolyte disturbances (hyperkalaemia, hyperphosphataemia, hypocalcaemia).

Following pathological diagnosis and staging, multiagent chemotherapy is initiated; the intensity and duration depends upon stage and immunophenotype. Stages I and II have a more than 90% cure rate and stages III and IV a 70–80% cure rate.

Clinical example

Luke was a 12-year-old boy with a short history of cough, wheeze and sudden onset of faint stridor. Examination revealed supraclavicular adenopathy, a mass palpable in the suprasternal notch, decreased air entry and dullness to percussion note at the right base. Luke's face was suffused with venous distension.
  Symptoms and signs suggested superior vena caval syndrome with airway obstruction. This constituted an oncological emergency. Chest X-ray confirmed a large mediastinal mass and a right pleural effusion. Urgent diagnosis and commencement of therapy (steroids) was required to prevent complete airway obstruction. Thoracentesis and cytological analysis confirmed that the diagnosis was T-cell lymphoblastic lymphoma. Precautionary admission to the intensive care unit was recommended. Full staging workup required chest/abdo/pelvis CT, nuclear medicine PET or gallium scan, bone marrow biopsies and lumbar puncture. Although uncommon, the diagnosis of an obstructive mediastinal mass should be entertained in children/adolescents with onset of wheezing, particularly when there is no prior history of asthma.

Hodgkin disease

Hodgkin disease, more common in boys than girls, is rare before the age of 5 years, with a progressively increasing incidence in adolescents. A viral aetiology is suspected, with the genome of Epstein–Barr virus identified in some Hodgkin cells; however, the significance of this is not clear. A painless progressive swelling of lymph nodes (above the diaphragm in two-thirds of patients) is the most common clinical presentation. Dissemination to spleen, liver, lungs, bones and bone marrow can occur. Constitutional symptoms, including weight loss, night sweats, rash and fever, occur in one-third of patients. Open biopsy confirms the diagnosis and pathological staging with CT chest/abdo/pelvis, gallium or PET scan and marrow aspirate and trephine completes the workup. Chemotherapy is the mainstay of treatment, with radiotherapy having a supplemental role in patients with massive mediastinal involvement. Cure rates are excellent, with survival greater than 90%. Emphasis on cure without cost has become paramount in this disease, with a shift to therapy combi-

nations that allow for preservation of fertility, reduction in rates of secondary cancers (associated with the use of radiation and etoposide) and reduced longer-term organ morbidity (e.g. lung toxicity with bleomycin, cardiomyopathy with anthracyclines) without compromising cure rates.

Neuroblastoma

Accounting for about 8–10% of childhood cancers, neuroblastoma is the most common extracranial solid tumour in childhood. Most cases occur in children under the age of 5 years, with a median age at presentation of 23 months. Neuroblastoma along with ganglioneuroblastoma and ganglioneuroma derive from primitive neural crest cells. Variations in the location, degree of differentiation, clinical and biological behaviour of these tumours are diverse. Spontaneous regression and differentiation into benign neoplasms is seen at one end the spectrum and highly aggressive tumours resistant to intensive chemotherapy at the other. Metastatic neuroblastoma in children older than 1 year has a poor prognosis. Unfortunately, over 75% of patients present with metastatic disease at the time of diagnosis.

The clinical manifestations of neuroblastoma are variable and depend on primary site and the extent of disease. The classic presentation is of a 3–4-year-old, pale, irritable child reluctant to walk, with periorbital ecchymoses. Primary tumours can commonly arise in the abdomen (70%), in the adrenal gland or abdominal paravertebral sympathetic chain. Disease arising in the thorax (25%) or pelvis (5%) occurs less commonly. Various paraneoplastic syndromes, including hypertension, secretory diarrhoea and opsomyoclonus, have been reported at presentation. The latter, occurring in 5% of patients with neuroblastoma, is a syndrome of myoclonic, irregular, jerking random eye move-ments that can be associated with cerebellar ataxia. Common sites for metastatic disease are bone, lymph nodes and bone marrow. Neuroblastoma can present in the newborn or early neonatal period. Infants <12 months with Stage IVs disease (localized primary tumour with metastatic disease to skin, liver or bone marrow, but not bone cortex) generally have excellent survival, with tumours spontaneously regressing without the need for treatment.

Biopsy is required for histological diagnosis. Staging investigations include CT/magnetic resonance imaging (MRI) scan of the primary tumour, bilateral bone marrow aspirate and trephine (core) biopsies, bone scan and meta-iodobenzylguanidine (MIBG) scan. MIBG is a radiolabelled compound taken up by cells of the sympathetic nervous system that demonstrates catecholamine synthesis.

Approximately 90–95% of neuroblastomas show uptake of MIBG. Measurement of urinary catecholamines is also a valuable test both at diagnosis and to assess disease responsiveness, with 90–95% of patients with neuroblastoma excreting elevated levels of vanillylmandelic acid, homovanillic acid and other catecholamines. Serum levels of lactate dehydrogenase, ferritin and neuron-specific enolase are also elevated in neuroblastoma.

Diagnosis is confirmed by histology following biopsy of tumour. Neuroblastoma is one of the 'small, round, blue cell' cancers of childhood that also include Ewing sarcoma, NHL, rhabdomyosarcomas and primitive neuroectodermal tumours. Pathological grading systems, including the Shimada criteria and the International Neuroblastoma Pathology Classification, help in defining the patient with a poor prognosis. The N-*myc* oncogene is present in increased numbers of copies in about 30% of neuroblastomas and correlates with poor survival.

Treatment depends on staging and includes surgical resection only in stage I and II disease, chemotherapy and surgery in stage III disease and intensive chemotherapy, surgical resection, tumour bed irradiation and autologous bone marrow transplantation in stage IV patients, as well as a subset of patients with high-risk stage III disease. Long-term survival in stage IV patients remains poor at 30–50%. Novel cytotoxic agents, targetted radionucleotide therapy and immune-mediated therapy are all currently being investigated in clinical trials.

Wilms tumour (nephroblastoma)

Wilms tumours account for 6% of childhood malignancies and represent the vast majority of primary renal cancers in childhood. Over 90% of children diagnosed with Wilms tumour are under 5 years of age.

Clinical presentation, differential diagnosis, staging and treatment of Wilms tumour

- Clinical presentation is most commonly with abdominal swelling or an asymptomatic abdominal mass
- Malaise, abdominal pain, gross or microscopic haematuria, fever, anorexia or hypertension occur in approximately 25% of patients
- 8–10% of patients with Wilms tumour will have an acquired von Willebrand factor abnormality with prolonged coagulation studies at diagnosis
- Differential diagnosis includes polycystic kidney disease, hydronephrosis, hepatoblastoma and neuroblastoma
- Common sites of blood-borne metastases are liver and lung. Extension to regional lymph nodes, hepatic adhesion and tumour invasion of the renal vein and inferior vena cava which can extend up to the right atrium can occur rarely
- Investigations usually include a contrast-enhanced CT scan of abdomen ± lungs, chest X-ray and abdominal ultrasound, with Doppler if tumour extension or involvement of the inferior vena cava is suspected
- Through collaborative multimodal clinical trials, survival of Wilms tumour patients exceeds 90% overall. Surgery can be performed up front or delayed until after response to chemotherapy. The frequency and intensity of chemotherapy depends on stage and histological subtype (favourable versus unfavourable or anaplastic). Radiotherapy is used in patients with stage III and IV disease. Cure rates exceed 90% for stage I–III and 85–90% for stage IV disease.

> ### Clinical example
>
> Brigitte, aged 4 years, was brought into the Emergency Department with a short history of abdominal pain, fever, general malaise and weight loss. On examination, she appeared to be an irritable child with tachycardia and mild hypertension. She had a distended abdomen with a large, poorly defined, palpable, hard mass in the periumbilical area. A plain X-ray showed calcification within the mass. A large primary adrenal mass was confirmed on CT imaging. Open biopsy confirms neuroblastoma and the remaining staging examination (bone marrow biopsy, nuclear medicine bone scan and MIBG scan) demonstrated metastatic disease to the bone marrow and bone cortex of three vertebrae. Differential diagnosis of an abdominal mass in childhood includes neuroblastoma, Wilms tumour, lymphoma, rhabdomyosarcoma and germ cell tumours.

Rhabdomyosarcoma and soft tissue sarcoma

Soft tissue sarcomas make up 5% of paediatric cancer; about 50% of these are rhabdomyosarcomas. Rhabdomyosarcomas occur in early childhood with a median age at diagnosis of 5 years. There is a recognized association between rhabdomyosarcoma and familial syndromes, including neurofibromatosis and Li–Fraumeni syndrome. Li–Fraumeni syndrome includes clusters of soft tissue sarcomas, adrenocortical carcinoma and early-onset breast cancer and results from germline mutations in the *p53* tumour suppressor gene. Rhabdomyosarcomas are included in the small, round, blue cell tumours of childhood and are thought to arise from mesenchymal cells committed to muscle differentiation. There are two major histological subtypes of rhabdomyosarcoma: embryonal (80%) and the more aggressive alveolar (20%).

Clinical presentation varies widely depending on the site of the primary disease, which can include:

- orbit, head and neck including parameningeal (40%)
- extremities (20%)
- genitourinary (20–25%)
- trunk (10–15%).

Approximately half of all patients will have unresectable tumours at diagnosis. Less than 25% of patients will have metastatic disease at diagnosis involving lung, bone marrow, bone or lymph nodes. MRI of primary tumour is the investigation of choice for children with rhabdomyosarcomas. Technetium-99m bone scan, CT of the lung and bone marrow biopsy are required to assess for metastatic disease. Therapy for rhabdomyosarcomas depends on the location and stage of disease and is often multimodal, involving surgery, adjuvant chemotherapy and radiotherapy. Prognostic variables include metastatic disease at diagnosis, site of disease, surgical resectability, histological subtype and age. Early-stage disease is curable in more than 85% of patients. Patients with more aggressive disease have a poorer prognosis, ranging from 30–50% depending on risk factors.

Osteosarcoma and Ewing sarcoma

Primary bone tumours in childhood occur less frequently than bony metastases to the skeleton. Bone tumours are the sixth most common tumour type in childhood, increasing to the third most frequent tumour type in adolescence and young adults. Osteosarcoma is more common than Ewing sarcoma.

Osteosarcoma

The peak incidence of osteosarcoma occurs in the second decade of life during the adolescent growth spurt, and the condition occurs more commonly in males. For the most part, the aetiology of osteosarcoma is not clear. There is a known association with exposure to ionizing radiation, although this accounts for only a small proportion of patients diagnosed with osteosarcoma. Mutations in two recessive oncogenes, *RB* (the retinoblastoma susceptibility locus) and *p53*, have been postulated to play a role in tumorigenesis in osteosarcoma. The commonest mode of presentation is with bone pain, with associated swelling and decrease in activity.

The following are important to note:

- approximately 60% of osteosarcoma arise around the knee, in the metaphysis of the femur or tibia
- metastatic disease can occur to lungs and less commonly to bones
- diagnostic workup should include a plain X-ray and MRI ± CT of primary lesion, CT of the lung and bone scan to identify potential disease spread

- surgical biopsy is needed for definitive histological diagnosis. Treatment consists of chemotherapy followed by surgical resection of tumour. The traditional surgical approach to achieve local control of osteosarcoma of the extremity is amputation; however, modern techniques allow for limb-salvage surgery in the majority of patients
- cure rates for patients with non-metastatic disease at diagnosis are over 70%. Histological response of tumour following chemotherapy is a predictor of outcome, with patients with a good response (defined as >90% necrosis) having a long-term survival rate in excess of 80%, compared with poor or standard responders with a survival rate of 40–60%. The survival outcome for patients with metastatic disease at diagnosis remains poor, at less than 50%.

Clinical example

Peter, aged 13, had a 4-month history of pain around the knee. In the last 2 weeks this had become severe and he was able to walk short distances only. Peter recalled a minor injury playing sport at the onset of his symptoms 4 months ago. Examination demonstrated swelling on the medial aspect of the proximal tibia with a diffuse, firm, non-tender mass present. The most likely diagnosis was a bone or soft tissue sarcoma. Plain X-ray of the tibia confirmed a soft tissue mass and destructive bony lesion with 'sunburst' appearance reflecting periosteal elevation in the metaphyseal region. CT and MRI scan were required to delineate anatomy, followed by biopsy, which confirmed osteosarcoma. Staging with CT lung and bone scan to determine extent of the disease were required. Prognosis and the therapy required depend on staging. A history of trivial injury is often associated with bone tumours but there is sparse evidence to suggest a causal relationship and more probably the injury serves as a trigger to seek medical attention.

Ewing sarcoma

Ewing sarcoma accounts for 10–15% of primary malignant bone tumours in childhood and adolescence. Most originate in the bone, although they can occasionally arise in soft tissue (extraosseous Ewing). The primary site of disease in Ewing sarcoma is either in the extremities (53%) or the axial skeleton (47%). The most common sites are:

- pelvis (25%)
- chest wall (20%)
- femur (15%)
- tibia (9%)
- vertebra (8%)
- fibula (7%)
- humerus (5%).

Unlike osteosarcomas, which typically arise from the metaphysis, Ewing tumours of the long bone more commonly originate from the diaphysis. Pain (96%) and a palpable mass (61%) are the most common presenting features. About 15% of patients have a pathological fracture at time of diagnosis. Approximately 25% of patients have a evidence of metastatic disease at diagnosis. Common sites of spread are lung, bone and bone marrow.

Diagnostic tests include plain X-ray of the lesion in two planes, with MRI as the gold standard for local staging. A CT scan of the primary lesion may also be required, particularly to demonstrate cortical fractures. A bone scan, bilateral bone marrow aspirates and biopsies and CT of the chest are performed at diagnosis to define the metastatic spread of disease. The typical X-ray appearance of Ewing sarcoma shows a poorly defined, destructive or 'moth-eaten' pattern, often accompanied by a multi-laminated 'onion skin' periosteal reaction with elevation (Codman's triangle). A tumour biopsy is required in all patients to confirm the histological diagnosis. The differential diagnosis includes non-malignant pathology (osteomyelitis, eosinophilic granuloma) and malignant pathology (osteosarcoma, lymphoma, neuroblastoma, spindle cell sarcoma). Molecular testing will identify a translocation involving t(11;22) or *EWS* (Ewing sarcoma gene) in over 90% of Ewing tumours.

Treatment consists of a combination of surgery, radiation and combination multiagent chemotherapy. Several prognostic factors have been identified, including tumour site, tumour size, histological grade, response to therapy and the presence or absence of overt metastatic disease at diagnosis. With current therapies, 60–70% of patients with localized disease will be cured. Survival for patients with metastatic disease remains poor, at less than 50%, underpinning the need for ongoing investigation into novel agents.

Rare tumours

A detailed review of all childhood malignancy is beyond the scope of this chapter. The reader is referred to more extensive paediatric oncology material for a review on retinoblastoma, hepatoblastoma, germ cell tumours, histiocytic disorders, nasopharyngeal carcinomas and other malignant diseases occurring in childhood.

Late effects of cancer therapy

It is projected that by 2010 1 in 250 persons aged 15–45 years will be a survivor of childhood cancer.

Although there has been considerable effort to reduce the toxicity of treatment protocols without compromising cure, based on current data, approximately 50% of long-term survivors of childhood cancer will have or develop disabilities that impact on quality of life. Clearly, the potential for the long-term toxicity of treatments should be discussed up front at the time of initial diagnosis, prior to treatment. Late effects depend on prior treatment exposure and can include growth failure, skeletal abnormalities, endocrinopathies, dental anomalies, learning disabilities, cardiopulmonary disease, hearing loss, infertility and second malignancy. Systematic surveillance and management of late effects of therapy is now the focus of many childhood cancer units and cooperative study groups.

Palliative care

Cancer is the most common cause of non-accidental death in childhood, with approximately 20–25% of children diagnosed with a malignancy dying of their disease. Optimal palliation requires open and ongoing communication between all members of the health-care team, the child and family. Management of symptoms, including pain, dyspnoea, nausea/vomiting and bowel abnormalities, is important, as is optimization of psychological, social and spiritual needs. Open discussion regarding the desired place of death (e.g. home, hospital or hospice) should take place in advance. A child's understanding of death will vary depending on age and the individual but many studies suggest that children as young as 6 have an understanding of death and should be given the opportunity to talk openly about their illness. Following the death of a child, one of the essential roles of the treating team is to provide bereavement support for parents and siblings.

> **Practical points**
>
> **Childhood cancer**
> - Childhood cancer is rare, with excellent survival rates for most cancer types
> - A multidisciplinary team approach delivers best therapy to children with cancer
> - Acute leukaemia and brain tumours account for a significant proportion of all childhood cancer
> - Treatment depends on cancer type and stage and can include surgery, radiation, chemotherapy and immunotherapies
> - The long-term consequences of therapy must be considered, including the impact on growth, fertility, learning and development as well as late organ toxicity and second cancers

PART 17

SEIZURE DISORDERS AND DISORDERS OF THE NERVOUS SYSTEM

Seizures and epilepsies 17.1

A. S. Harvey

Few events are more alarming to parents than their child having a breath-holding attack, febrile convulsion or first epileptic seizure. Seizures of some type occur in up to 5% of children but fortunately most are single episodes of a non-serious nature.

Terminology and classification

An epileptic seizure is a neurological event in which there is a sustained and abnormal, hypersynchronous discharge from neurons in the cerebral cortex, either localized or widespread, usually associated with electrical, metabolic and clinical alterations. Epilepsy is classically defined as the group of conditions where a person has recurrent, unprovoked epileptic seizures. This definition excludes single seizures; febrile and other provoked seizures, seizures in newborns, seizures in the context of acute neurological insults, and non-epileptic attacks such as faints and breath-holding spells.

The International League Against Epilepsy classification of seizures, based on clinical and electroencephalography (EEG) features (1981), recognizes two major categories: focal (partial) seizures and generalized seizures. Focal seizures originate in a localized part (hence, partial) of the cerebrum, usually on one side, whereas generalized seizures commence synchronously in both cerebral hemispheres. Several, pathophysiologically-distinct generalized seizures types are recognized by different clinical and EEG patterns, the most common being generalized tonic–clonic, absence and myoclonic seizures (Table 17.1.1). Focal seizures have similar pathophysiological features and are distinguished by the part of the brain involved and the resultant clinical manifestations.

The epilepsies or *epileptic syndromes,* the conditions that predispose to epileptic seizures, are best conceptualized in terms of the underlying aetiology and their predominant seizure types (Table 17.1.2). Idiopathic (primary) epilepsies are seizure disorders with no identifiable cause other than a presumed genetic predisposition to seizures. These epilepsies usually manifest with characteristic focal or generalized seizures, predictable age at seizure onset, stereo-typic EEG patterns, absence of other neurological problems, good response to treatment and favourable neurological outcome. The idiopathic generalized epilepsies are being gradually understood as abnormalities of neuronal ion channels. The cause of idiopathic partial epilepsies is not fully understood, although delay in cerebral maturation is postulated. Symptomatic (secondary) epilepsies are seizure disorders due to known or presumed (cryptogenic) underlying cerebral abnormalities such as cortical tumours, malformations, injuries or metabolic disturbances. These epilepsies tend to have variable seizure and EEG manifestations depending on the nature, location, extent and timing of the underlying cerebral abnormality. Symptomatic epilepsies usually have a poor prognosis for seizure control and are often associated with other neurological problems such as learning difficulties, intellectual disability, behavioural problems and hemiplegia, again depending on the nature and extent of the underlying cerebral abnormality.

These terminologies and classifications are imprecise and sometimes confusing, especially when terms are used to describe types of seizures and syndromes, e.g. febrile seizures, infantile spasms. Furthermore, there is much overlap of categories, with some patients having epilepsies with focal and generalized seizures, idiopathic epilepsies occurring in children with pre-existing developmental disabilities, and seizures arising as a result of an underlying cerebral abnormality and a genetic predisposition.

Prospective studies of new-onset epileptic seizures in childhood reveal that approximately 50% of patients with a first seizure have a recurrence. Epilepsy as classically defined occurs with an annual incidence of about 60–80 in 100 000 and a prevalence of about 5 in 1000 in childhood, the incidence and prevalence being highest in infancy. Studies of new-onset epilepsy in childhood indicate a greater proportion with focal seizures than generalized and undetermined seizures, and about equal proportions of idiopathic, symptomatic and undetermined/cryptogenic aetiologies. Prospective studies of treated and untreated new-onset epilepsy reveal that about 80% of children go into remission, some with subsequent seizure relapses, and about 20% of children have treatment-resistant epilepsy.

Table 17.1.1   Classification of epileptic seizure type, based on clinical and EEG features

Focal (partial)
- Simple partial – consciousness preserved
- Complex partial – consciousness impaired
- Partial seizures with secondary generalization

Generalized
- Tonic–clonic
- Absence
- Myoclonic
- Clonic
- Tonic (epileptic spasms are series of brief tonic seizures)
- Atonic

Table 17.1.2   Common types of epilepsy in childhood, grouped by age

Infancy
- Benign familial/non-familial neonatal convulsions*
- Febrile seizures (*not classically considered epilepsy*)
- Infantile epileptic encephalopathy with epileptic spasms (West syndrome)[†]
- Severe myoclonic epilepsy of infancy (Dravet syndrome)
- Benign familial/non-familial infantile convulsions*
- Symptomatic focal epilepsies of infancy – commonly hemispheric and multilobar[†]

Childhood
- Typical childhood absence epilepsy *
- Benign focal (rolandic) epilepsy of childhood with centrotemporal spikes*
- Benign occipital epilepsy *
- Primary generalized epilepsy with tonic–clonic seizures*
- Childhood epileptic encephalopathy with tonic seizures (Lennox–Gastaut syndrome)[†]
- Symptomatic focal epilepsies – commonly temporal lobe epilepsy and frontal lobe epilepsy[†]

Adolescence
- Primary generalized epilepsy with tonic–clonic seizures*
- Juvenile absence epilepsy*
- Juvenile myoclonic epilepsy*
- Symptomatic focal epilepsies – commonly temporal lobe epilepsy and frontal lobe epilepsy[†]

* classical idiopathic epilepsy syndromes, [†] classical symptomatic epilepsy syndromes.

Common epilepsies of infancy, childhood and adolescence

Febrile seizures

Fever and seizures may coexist with infections of the central nervous system (not epilepsy) and with non-specific febrile illnesses in children with epilepsy. However, fever and seizures most often occur together as a manifestation of the syndrome of *febrile seizures,* a condition in which some infants and young children have a presumed genetic predisposition to fit in the presence of fever. Although not considered part of the classical definition of epilepsy, the syndrome of febrile seizures does have several features in common with the idiopathic epilepsies, including an age-limited predisposition to seizures, a family history of seizures in more than 30% of children, an evolution to idiopathic generalized or partial epilepsy in a minority, and mutations in neuronal ion channel genes in some rare instances. Febrile seizures are the focus of ongoing epilepsy genetic research and are no longer considered just a non-specific susceptibility to seizure with fever in infants.

Simple febrile seizures are defined as a brief, generalized tonic and/or clonic seizures in which there is neither clinical nor laboratory evidence of central nervous system infection, the temperature is 38°C or higher and the child has no history of previous afebrile seizures, neurological deficits or developmental delay to suggest an underlying neurological problem. Most febrile seizures are associated with upper respiratory or urinary tract infections or viral exanthemas and occur once at the beginning of the illness. Complicated febrile seizures are those that are prolonged, focal or multiple.

Febrile seizures occur in approximately 3% of the population, commencing between the ages of 5 months and 5 years, with most manifesting in the first 2 years of life. In approximately one-third of children febrile seizures are recurrent, the risk increasing to 50% if onset is in infancy or there is a family history of febrile seizures. Only 3% of children with febrile seizures go on to have later afebrile seizures, i.e. epilepsy, the risk being increased further if there is evidence of abnormal development or neurological problems, if the child has a family history of epilepsy or if the seizures are complicated. When epilepsy follows febrile seizures it is invariably a later manifestation of the same underlying seizure predisposition, i.e. idiopathic epilepsy. Very rarely, later epileptic seizures may be the result of brain injury from prolonged and focal febrile seizures. Febrile seizures are not associated with any increased mortality or later intellectual impairment.

Treatment

The cause of the febrile illness is investigated and treated on its own merits. There is no role for EEG or brain imaging in febrile seizures. There is debate about the role of antipyretics and gentle cooling. Seizures have usually ceased before medical help is obtained; however, if a febrile seizure continues after

3–5 minutes, it should be terminated urgently, usually with rectal or intravenous diazepam. Meningitis or encephalitis should be considered if the child has a history of vomiting, is younger than 6 months, has repeated seizures following presentation, has been treated with antibiotics, has not recovered promptly from the seizure or seems more ill than would be expected following a simple febrile seizure.

Antiepileptic medication does not diminish the likelihood of later epilepsy. Given the benign nature of the seizures and the potential adverse effects of antiepileptic medication, treatment is rarely prescribed for the syndrome of febrile seizures. Parents and carers need explanation and reassurance about the likelihood of further febrile seizures, the infrequency of later epilepsy, the rarity of neurological problems and the management of subsequent febrile illnesses and seizures. Some children with a history of recurrent or prolonged febrile seizures may be prescribed prophylactic oral diazepam or emergency rectal diazepam, respectively, although these remain controversial issues.

Infantile spasms

The syndrome of *infantile spasms* is the most common symptomatic generalized epilepsy syndrome in childhood. Onset of epileptic spasms is usually between 3 and 8 months of age and males are affected twice as commonly as females. Flexor or salaam spasms are the most common and consist of sudden drawing up of the legs, hunching forward of the neck and shoulders and flinging out of the arms; opisthotonic or extensor spasms are less common. Epileptic spasms are essentially brief tonic seizures and they typically occur in series over a minute or more, usually many times a day. The EEG usually shows a diffusely disorganized pattern with high-voltage, multifocal epileptic activity, called hypsarrhythmia (Fig. 17.1.1). Development may be delayed prior to the onset of spasms, or there may be loss of visual attention and arrest of developmental progress at seizure onset. The term *West syndrome* is often used synonymously with infantile spasms but classically refers to the triad of epileptic spasms, developmental delay and hypsarrhythmia. Differential diagnosis includes a variety of normal or benign infant behaviours, such as sleep jerks, colic, shuddering attacks, benign myoclonus of infancy and gastro-oesophageal reflux, as well as other less sinister myoclonic epilepsies of infancy.

Infantile spasms are an age-dependent manifestation of a severe, localized or diffuse, acquired or developmental, disturbance in the immature central nervous system. An underlying cause is identified in about two-thirds of infants, including prenatal/perinatal stroke or infection, focal or diffuse brain malformations, tuberous sclerosis and metabolic disorders such as pyridoxine (vitamin B_6) deficiency or phenylketonuria. In these symptomatic cases, the outcome for seizures and development is usually poor. In the cryptogenic cases where no cause is apparent from history, examination, brain imaging and metabolic screening, outcome is more variable; if there is a prior history of developmental delay and spasms are not quickly controlled with treatment, outcome is again poor. Overall, 70–80% children with infantile spasms develop some degree of

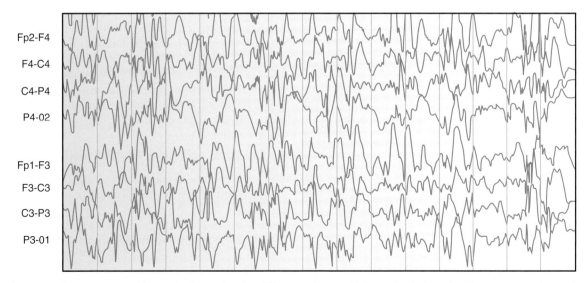

Fig. 17.1.1 The EEG pattern of hypsarrhythmia, showing diffuse, continuous, high-amplitude, irregular sharp waves, spikes and slow waves on a disorganized background, typical of that seen in infantile spasms.

intellectual disability and 30–50% develop a chronic, focal or generalized epilepsy. In many children with a symptomatic generalized epilepsy following infantile spasms, the electroclinical picture is that of the *Lennox–Gastaut syndrome* with refractory tonic and other seizures, generalized slow spike wave and paroxysmal fast activity on EEG, and severe intellectual disability. The neurological sequelae of infantile spasms seem to be the result of both the underlying cerebral or metabolic abnormality and the deleterious effects of frequent seizures and EEG disturbance on the developing brain.

Treatment

The syndrome of infantile spasms needs urgent diagnosis, investigation and treatment. Treatment choices include corticosteroids (e.g. intramuscular adrenocorticotrophic hormone (ACTH), oral prednisolone), vigabatrin and benzodiazepines (e.g. nitrazepam, clonazepam). Pyridoxine should always be given as a trial, prior to commencement of antiepileptic drugs or steroids, to exclude pyridoxine dependency syndrome. In infants with unilateral strokes or malformations and drug-resistant seizures, epilepsy surgery may be considered. The aims of all treatments are to stop seizures, suppress the epileptic EEG disturbances and maximize neurological development.

Clinical example

Baby Jonathan presented at the age of 5 months with episodes of stiffening and drawing up of his legs, thought to be colic. The attacks lasted only seconds but occurred in clusters up to 10 times each day. During the attacks, his eyes rolled up, he appeared unaware and he would cry briefly. Jonathan's parents were also concerned that he seemed irritable, was not fixing on their faces and was no longer smiling. The pregnancy, birth and early developmental milestones had been unremarkable. On examination, Jonathan fixed and followed poorly and had poor head control. Examination revealed several depigmented patches of skin on the legs and trunk. A cluster of typical bilateral infantile spasms occurred during the assessment, with head and eye deviation to the right side. An EEG that day showed a modified hypsarrhythmic pattern, confirming West syndrome with infantile spasms, and vigabatrin was started promptly. An MRI the week following showed cortical tubers and periventricular nodules, confirming the underlying diagnosis of tuberous sclerosis. Spasms ceased after the second day of vigabatrin and there was some improvement in visual attention the week following. However, Jonathan's motor development was slow over subsequent months and smiling was sporadic. EEG continued to show prominent multifocal epileptic activity, although reduced.

Absence epilepsies

Absence epilepsies are idiopathic generalized epilepsies that manifest in otherwise normal children with predominantly absence seizures. Absence seizures are manifest by sudden cessation of activity with staring, usually lasting only 5–15 seconds. Blinking, upward deviation of the eyes, slight mouthing movements and some fidgeting hand movements (automatisms) may occur. The child is unresponsive, does not fall, is rarely incontinent and returns promptly to normal activity at the offset of the absence, with no memory of the seizure. The EEG shows generalized spike-wave activity during the seizure (Fig. 17.1.2). Usually, many attacks occur in a day. Absence seizures can generally be precipitated in the clinic room and during EEG recordings with forced hyperventilation. Differential diagnosis of absence seizures includes daydreaming and complex partial seizures.

Absence seizures usually commence after the age of 4 years and there are two common types described. In *typical childhood absence epilepsy* (so called petit mal epilepsy), absences usually begin before the age of 7 years, tonic–clonic seizures are rare, the EEG shows runs of regular 3 Hz spike-wave activity and prognosis for seizure remission is good. In *juvenile absence epilepsy,* onset of absences is later, sometimes in the teen years, the EEG shows faster and more irregular spike-wave activity, there may be associated tonic–clonic seizures, and prognosis for seizure remission is poorer. Intellectual development is usually normal in absence epilepsies.

Treatment

EEG is needed to confirm absence seizures and characterize the epilepsy syndrome; brain imaging is unnecessary. Sodium valproate, ethosuximide and lamotrigine are the medications used commonly to treat absence seizures. Treatment is usually for 2 years in typical childhood absence epilepsy, with an expectation of seizure remission, and through puberty into the teen years in juvenile absence epilepsy. Rare refractory cases may respond to treatment with a ketogenic diet.

Benign focal epilepsies of childhood

The benign or idiopathic focal (partial) epilepsies of childhood are some of the most common epileptic syndromes in children. They occur in otherwise normal preschool and primary-school-age children and typically manifest with infrequent sleep-related focal seizures and prominent focal epileptiform patterns on routine EEG, these remitting in the second decade. The two most common varieties are *benign rolandic epilepsy (benign epilepsy with centrotemporal*

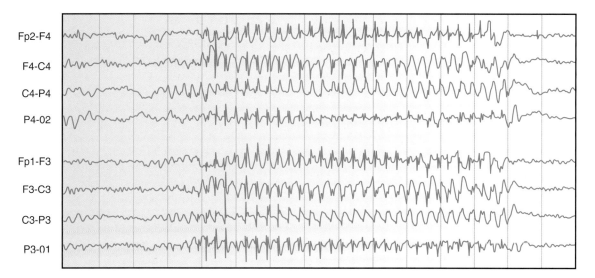

Fig. 17.1.2 The EEG of typical absence epilepsy during an absence seizure, showing a paroxysm of generalized 3 Hz spike-wave activity.

Clinical example

Nadine, a 6-year-old girl, was noted by her parents to frequently 'blank out' while sitting at the dinner table and most recently, to stop walking and talking while shopping with her mother. These episodes were occurring several times a day and seemed to last only a few seconds. Her class teacher had not noticed any problems. Hyperventilation in the clinic room provoked a typical absence episode lasting 12 seconds, during which Nadine was seen to stop hyperventilating, be unresponsive, fidget with her shirt and have slight bobbing of her eyes. Typical childhood absence epilepsy was confirmed with an EEG, which showed 3 Hz generalized spike-wave activity during spontaneous and hyperventilation-induced absence seizures. Sodium valproate was introduced slowly over 3 weeks with no absences noted after the second week of treatment and none precipitated with hyperventilation when reviewed. Slight irritability and moodiness were reported by Nadine's parents as potential side effects of treatment.

spikes), in which the seizure and EEG focus is low in the central sulcus (rolandic) region on one or both sides, and *benign occipital epilepsy,* in which the seizure and EEG focus is in the occipital lobe on one or both sides. The aetiology and pathogenesis of the idiopathic focal epilepsies is unclear in that they are not due to underlying structural brain lesions and they share only limited genetic associations with the idiopathic generalized epilepsies. The EEG abnormalities of the benign focal epilepsies can be found in children with no history of seizures, sometimes leading to diagnostic errors.

In *benign rolandic epilepsy,* seizure onset is usually between 5 and 10 years of age and there is a male predominance. Focal seizures may be simple partial with tingling or twitching of the mouth and preserved consciousness, often with associated drooling of saliva, choking noises and inability to speak. Seizures may progress to jerking of one side of the body, with or without impairment of consciousness. Some children have secondarily generalized seizures in which the focal onset is not recalled or witnessed. Attacks are most commonly from sleep. EEG recordings that include sleep reveal very frequent focal epileptiform activity over the centrotemporal regions on one or both sides (Fig. 17.1.3). In *benign occipital epilepsy*, the presentation is usually before the age of 6 years and there is a female predominance. Seizures are characteristically from sleep with complex partial or secondarily generalized attacks beginning with staring, vomiting, head rotation, eye deviation and hemiclonic jerking. Seizures can sometimes be prolonged and raise concern about encephalitis. Daytime attacks may occur with episodic visual distortions or hallucinations and migraine-like headaches. Again, EEG recordings that include sleep reveal characteristic focal epileptiform activity over the occipital region. In typical cases of benign focal epilepsy, brain imaging is unnecessary.

Treatment

Seizures tend to be infrequent in the benign focal epilepsies, many children having only one or two seizures before they ultimately remit. Because of this, and the tendency for nocturnal occurrence, treatment with antiepileptic medications is not

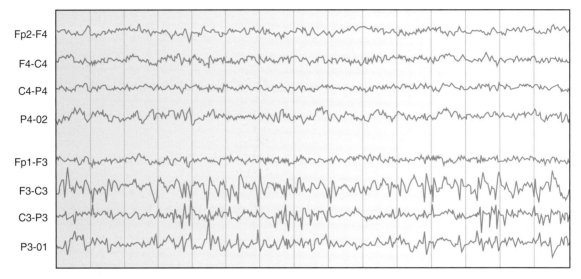

Fig. 17.1.3 The EEG of benign focal epilepsy of childhood with centrotemporal spikes (benign rolandic epilepsy) showing focal epileptiform activity in the left central region (lower three channels).

always necessary. If warranted, treatment with sodium valproate or low dose carbamazepine for 1–2 years is usually adequate. Prognosis is excellent, with absence of cognitive and behavioural problems, and remission of seizures by the teen years, hence the term 'benign'. In rare instances, these epilepsies may

manifest in an atypical way with more problematic seizures, continuous bilateral EEG disturbances and deleterious effects on language and motor development; this tends to occur in children with pre-existing neurological problems.

Primary generalized epilepsies with tonic–clonic seizures

The primary or idiopathic generalized epilepsies with tonic–clonic seizures are a somewhat heterogenous group of seizure disorders occurring in otherwise normal children and adolescents, sometimes with additional absence and myoclonic seizures. Generalized tonic–clonic seizures typically begin with loss of consciousness, stiffening (tonic), temporary cessation of breathing and falling if standing, then progress to a phase with generalized, rhythmic jerking (clonic), which is initially rapid but gradually slows. Tonic–clonic seizures invariably cease spontaneously, usually within a few minutes, and are followed by a postictal period with depressed consciousness and headache, during which the person usually sleeps. There are no warning symptoms (auras), no significant focal features to the seizure and no memory of the actual seizure. Generalized tonic–clonic seizures often occur during intercurrent febrile illnesses in young children and either during sleep or following periods of sleep deprivation or stress in older children and adolescents.

Generalized tonic–clonic seizures may begin at any age but onset around puberty is common. Sometimes there is a history of prior febrile seizures or absence seizures; in these cases, the later occurrence of tonic–clonic seizures usually represents an age-

Clinical example

Michael, a developmentally normal 8-year-old boy, presented to the emergency department of a regional hospital after being heard fitting in his motel bed at 5 am while holidaying with his family. The seizure was brief, seemingly generalized tonic–clonic, associated with prominent gurgling noises and followed by a 10–15-minute period during which his speech was slurred and his face drooped on one side. The parents recalled hearing similar noises from Michael's bedroom once or twice previously and occasionally finding his pillow wet with saliva in the morning. Michael described waking from his sleep in this seizure, having an fuzzy feeling in his mouth and being unable to call out to his parents, who were sleeping in the same room. An EEG arranged subsequently showed very frequent left central and temporal epileptiform discharges that became almost continuous in sleep. A diagnosis of benign rolandic epilepsy was made. Computed tomography (CT) of the brain, which was performed in the regional hospital, was normal. Following much parental counselling and reassurance about the benign nature of this type of epilepsy, it was decided to not perform a magnetic resonance imaging (MRI) scan and to defer treatment with antiepileptic medication. General safety and lifestyle advice was given about seizures, although it was appreciated that seizure occurrence in the day was unlikely.

dependent, evolving expression of the same underlying, genetically determined seizure tendency. As for other idiopathic epilepsies, there is no demonstrable cerebral or metabolic abnormality, usually normal intellect and sometimes a family history of seizures. The routine EEG shows characteristic generalized spike-wave and polyspike-wave discharges. *Juvenile myoclonic epilepsy* is a type of primary generalized epilepsy typically beginning in the teen years with generalized tonic–clonic seizures, early morning myoclonic jerks and sometimes brief absence seizures, seizures often being precipitated by sleep deprivation. The EEG in this syndrome shows 4–7 Hz generalized polyspike-wave activity. *Photosensitive epilepsy* with generalized tonic–clonic seizures is another type of idiopathic generalized epilepsy, where the seizures and EEG abnormalities are almost exclusively related to flashing light stimulation.

The differential diagnosis of generalized tonic–clonic seizures includes focal seizures with secondary generalization, convulsive syncope and psychogenic seizures. A preceding aura, focal or asymmetric features to the seizure, transient postical weakness of a limb (Todd's paresis), focal neurological deficits on examination, or a history of a prior cerebral trauma or infection should suggest a focal basis for an apparently generalized tonic–clonic seizure. Seizures of brief duration with rapid recovery and seizures occurring in typical vasovagal settings (see below) should suggest a syncopal rather than an epileptic basis. Psychogenic seizures are highly variable in their manifestations and can occur in patients with epilepsy, making their diagnosis sometimes difficult.

Treatment

Sodium valproate is the drug of choice for generalized tonic–clonic seizures, especially when there is documented generalized spike-wave on EEG or there is a history to suggest additional absence or myoclonic seizures. Carbamazepine is sometimes used for generalized tonic–clonic seizures when other features of primary generalized epilepsy are lacking, there being a risk of exacerbating absence and myoclonic seizures in predisposed patients. Lamotrigine, phenytoin, oxcarbazepine, topiramate and benzodiazepines are also effective for generalized tonic–clonic seizures. Seizure control is usually possible with medication and lifestyle adjustments (e.g. avoiding sleep deprivation). Many children and adolescents with primary generalized epilepsy and isolated tonic–clonic seizures outgrow their need for medication but adolescents with juvenile myoclonic epilepsy specifically usually require treatment into adult life.

Clinical example

Stephanie, a 13-year-old girl with a history of a single febrile seizure in infancy, presented to a regional hospital emergency department after having a generalized tonic–clonic seizure at school camp. The seizure occurred in the shower at 7 am, the morning after girls in Stephanie's cabin had stayed awake until 4 am. Stephanie was heard to fall in the shower and was found by a friend convulsing on the shower floor. She sustained a forehead bruise and hot water scalding on her back. There was no history of staring episodes or isolated jerking of the limbs. Stephanie recalled that on one occasion she had had to walk away from a computer game that her brother was playing because she felt sick and her head started jerking. There was no family history of epilepsy. Subsequent EEG recording showed frequent bursts of generalized fast spike-wave activity at rest and during photic stimulation. A diagnosis of primary generalized epilepsy with tonic–clonic seizures and associated photosensitivity was made. Long discussions were held with Stephanie and her parents over the initial and subsequent consultations, highlighting safety and lifestyle factors. Sodium valproate was commenced after discussion of the high likelihood of further seizures. The potential for weight gain and mild hair loss as side effects of treatment was also discussed, these concerning Stephanie more than the risk of further seizures. The family was given a guarded prognosis for seizure remission in the later teen years and regular review was arranged.

Temporal and frontal lobe epilepsies

Temporal lobe epilepsy (TLE) and *frontal lobe epilepsy* (FLE) are focal epilepsies in which seizures arise in the temporal or frontal lobes on one or both sides. TLE and FLE are generally considered symptomatic focal epilepsies in which an underlying scar, tumour, cyst or malformation is either known or suspected to be the basis of the recurring focal seizures. Symptomatic focal epilepsies can arise in any part of the brain, and in infants and young children they can often be due to multilobar or hemispheric lesions. TLE and FLE are the most common varieties of symptomatic focal epilepsy in children and adults, presumably because they make up the largest brain surface area of the brain. Seizures may commence at any age but often not until later childhood or adolescence, even when due to congenital malformations.

Focal seizures may be simple partial with preserved consciousness, complex partial with impaired consciousness, or secondarily generalized, the exact clinical manifestations of the seizures depending on the location of seizure onset and propagation. Some patients with complex partial and secondarily generalized seizures have prior warning symptoms, or auras, these being the simple partial phase of an evolving focal seizure.

Seizures in *temporal lobe epilepsy* are usually complex partial in type, characteristically manifest by motionless staring, fearful or bewildered facial expression, unresponsiveness, fidgeting hand movements (automatisms) and postictal amnesia and confusion. In some patients there may be head turning or stiffening or jerking of the limbs on one side during the seizure. Autonomic disturbances such as facial flushing or pallor, lip smacking, salivation, chewing, swallowing and sometimes vomiting are common; apnoea may be the predominant manifestation of complex partial seizures in infancy. Warning of an impending seizure (aura) is often present but may not be described at the time or recalled in a young or developmentally delayed child; fear, unusual smells or tastes, abdominal discomfort and dizzy or dreamy states are the usual descriptions. Complex partial seizures may secondarily generalize. Complex partial seizures last longer than absence seizures, generally 30–60 seconds, and are followed by postictal confusion and sleepiness. They are usually infrequent and commonly occur in clusters over several days, alternating with seizure-free periods.

Seizures in *frontal lobe epilepsy* often occur from sleep are brief in duration and commonly manifest with prominent motor features such as unilateral or bilateral stiffening or jerking, asymmetric tonic posturing with head deviation to one side, loud vocalization and hyperkinetic behaviours (automatisms) such as tapping, cycling and running. Seizures may occur on a multiple nightly basis. Secondary generalization is common.

The routine EEG in symptomatic focal epilepsy may be normal, show non-specific abnormalities or show localized epileptic patterns over the affected brain region. Video-EEG monitoring with recording of seizures is sometimes necessary to confirm the diagnosis and localize the seizures. The differential diagnosis of TLE, with episodes of staring and confused behaviour, includes daydreaming, absence seizures, behavioural outbursts, migraine and psychogenic seizures. The differential diagnosis of FLE, with nocturnal convulsive or thrashing seizures, includes parasomnias and primary generalized epilepsy. Benign focal epilepsies can usually be distinguished from TLE and FLE by their characteristic rolandic or occipital seizure and EEG manifestations, occurring at typical ages in otherwise normal children. Brain imaging with MRI is needed to search for an underlying cerebral lesion in all patients with focal seizures not due an idiopathic epilepsy syndrome, although causative lesions are not always found.

Treatment

Carbamazepine is the drug of first choice for seizures in all symptomatic focal epilepsies, including TLE and FLE. Seizures may be resistant to treatment and, over time, the patient may be tried on other medications (Table 17.1.3). Cognitive, physical and behavioural problems may be present in some children with TLE and FLE, as non-seizure manifestations of the underlying temporal or frontal lobe disturbance or lesion. These comorbidities may require specific assessment and intervention in their own right. Spontaneous seizure remission occurs in some patients, mainly when a lesion is not identified on MRI. In children with uncontrolled seizures that impact significantly on the life of the child and family, or are exerting detrimental effects on neurological development, resection of the responsible lesion or affected lobe(s) may be considered.

Table 17.1.3 Antiepileptic medications most effective in different seizure types	
Seizure type	Antiepileptic medication
Focal (simple, complex and secondarily generalized)	Carbamazepine, oxcarbazepine, lamotrigine, sodium valproate, topiramate, levetiracetam, phenytoin, gabapentin, benzodiazepines
Generalized tonic–clonic (primary)	Sodium valproate, lamotrigine, topiramate, carbamazepine, phenytoin, oxcarbazepine, benzodiazepines, levetiracetam
Absence	Sodium valproate, ethosuximide, lamotrigine
Myoclonic, atonic, tonic	Sodium valproate, lamotrigine, benzodiazepines, topiramate
Neonatal seizures	Phenobarbital, phenytoin, clonazepam
Infantile spasms	Vigabatrin, prednisolone/ACTH, benzodiazepines

Clinical example

Steven, a 9-year-old boy with a history of learning problems and aggressive outbursts, was referred for management of refractory seizures. Seizures began at age 5 years, occurred in clusters each week and were characterized by a scared feeling in the abdomen followed by cessation of activity, loss of responsiveness, stiffening of the right hand and rocking movements. Twice during illnesses, these seizures secondarily generalized. None of the three antiepileptic medications used over the years had controlled Steven's seizures. An MRI showed a lesion of benign appearance in the uncus of the left temporal lobe, thought to be a developmental tumour. Video-EEG recording of seizures showed electrical onset in the left temporal lobe region. Cognitive testing showed normal intellect but decreased verbal abilities. Left temporal lesionectomy was performed and the histopathology revealed a ganglioglioma. After a 2-year period free of seizures, Steven was gradually weaned off his medication. Learning and behavioural difficulties persisted but were better managed with understanding of their cause, abolition of seizures and institution of specific behavioural and educational strategies.

Non-epileptic episodic disorders

Not all episodes of neurological dysfunction in infancy and childhood are epileptic. Sleep disorders, movement disorders, circulatory disturbances, migraine and some normal behaviours may mimic epileptic seizures (Table 17.1.4). Disorders frequently misdiagnosed as seizures are breath-holding attacks in infancy and syncope in older children and adolescents, because of their paroxysmal nature with loss of consciousness and sometimes associated convulsive movements. In such attacks, the neurological manifestations are secondary to transient cerebral ischaemia and not to any intrinsic cerebral dysfunction.

Table 17.1.4 Differential diagnosis of epileptic seizures

- Normal behaviours, e.g. sleep jerks, day dreaming, masturbation
- Parasomnias, e.g. night terrors, sleep walking
- Breath holding spells
- Syncope e.g. vasovagal, cardiac arrhythmia/outflow obstruction
- Migraine and migraine variants, e.g. benign paroxysmal vertigo/torticollis
- Movement disorders, e.g. tics, tremor, clonus, shuddering attacks
- Non-neurological, e.g. gastroesophageal reflux, hypoglycaemia
- Psychiatric, e.g. rage attacks, psychogenic seizures

Breath-holding attacks

Attacks usually commence in the first or second year of life and are reported in up to 4% of children. Crucial to the diagnosis is recognition that attacks are precipitated by either physical trauma, such as a knock or a fall, or emotional trauma such as fright, anger or frustration, the precipitants not always being significant and noticed. Attacks usually commence with crying, but this may be brief or absent. Apnoea and bradycardia then occur, either suddenly or gradually, with cyanosis or pallor following. The attack may then terminate without loss of consciousness, or progress, with the child becoming unconscious, limp and sometimes briefly stiffening or jerking in response to the cerebral ischaemia. Recovery is usually rapid, although some children are drowsy and lethargic after an attack with convulsive features. Attacks usually cease by the third or fourth year of life.

The pathophysiology of breath-holding attacks is not well understood but affected children probably have an age-related dysfunction in cardiorespiratory reflexes. Iron-deficiency anaemia is an exacerbating factor in some children with frequent attacks or prominent convulsive features. Breath-holding attacks are not a cause of death, epilepsy, intellectual disability or cerebral damage and families should be reassured about their benign nature.

Syncope

Syncope, or fainting, is not uncommon in childhood. As in adults, it is the result of decreased cardiac output and cerebral perfusion leading to loss of consciousness and falling. Brief tonic stiffening, clonic jerking or incontinence can accompany the loss of consciousness and lead to misdiagnosis as an epileptic seizure. Recovery is usually prompt following syncope. Light-headedness, dizziness, visual loss and auditory or sensory changes may be recalled prior to loss of consciousness, being manifestations of focal cortical ischaemia. Sweating and tachycardia during recovery are common, as a result of reflex sympathetic drive. However, a more important clue to the diagnosis than the recalled or observed clinical features is the situation in which the episode occurred. Syncope should be suspected as the basis of loss of consciousness or convulsing when attacks occur contemporaneously with vomiting illnesses, prolonged standing (e.g. classroom, church), hairbrushing, injury, venepuncture, other medical procedures and veterinary procedures. Syncope without an obvious orthostatic or noxious precipitant, or syncope during exercise or while in water, should prompt concern about a primary cardiac cause, such as prolonged QTc syndrome or left ventricular outflow obstruction. No investigations, other than perhaps an ECG, are needed in syncope and most patients and families need only explanation and reassurance. Patients' recognition of precipitating situations and presyncopal symptoms is helpful in taking evasive action.

Assessment of children with seizures

Three important and successive steps in the assessment of a child with suspected seizures are to:

- distinguish epileptic seizures from non-epileptic attacks
- determine the type(s) of seizure the child is having, most importantly whether they are generalized or focal, and determine if unrecognized minor seizures are occurring
- determine the type of epilepsy in the child having recurrent seizures, or at least try and determine whether the epilepsy is likely to be idiopathic or symptomatic.

The diagnosis of epileptic seizures should be made on clinical grounds with investigations used to confirm the diagnosis, help characterize the seizure disorder and determine the underlying cause. Good detailed history from the patient and observers, sometimes combined with home video recordings of attacks are the basis of making a correct diagnosis. Children with epilepsy should be examined for dysmorphic features, neurocutaneous stigmata, focal neurological deficits, signs of raised intracranial pressure and markers of systemic disease.

Metabolic disturbance, especially hypoglycaemia and hypocalcaemia, should always be considered, especially in infants with seizures and children with no identifiable cause for their epilepsy. Pyridoxine deficiency, although very rare, should be considered in refractory infant-onset epilepsy.

EEG is invaluable in the characterization of seizures and epilepsies, and should generally be requested in all children with definite afebrile seizures, although this last point is somewhat controversial. EEG is of no value in the investigation of infants and young children with febrile seizures. In epilepsy, the EEG helps distinguishing focal from generalized seizures and aids diagnosis of specific epilepsy syndromes, especially idiopathic epilepsies. In this way, the EEG may assist in making the correct choice of antiepileptic medication and determining the need for brain imaging. It is important to note that the interictal EEG is normal in many patients with epilepsy, particularly symptomatic focal epilepsies. Conversely, epileptiform abnormalities, particularly

centrotemporal spikes and brief generalized spike-wave bursts in drowsiness, are seen in up to 4–5% children without seizures, more frequently in children with underlying neurological and developmental problems. EEG should therefore not be done to exclude epilepsy in a child with undiagnosed attacks. In children with undiagnosed recurrent attacks, or children with epileptic seizures of uncertain type, simultaneous video-EEG monitoring may be needed.

Brain imaging, usually with MRI, is indicated when one suspects an underlying cerebral abnormality, i.e. symptomatic epilepsy. Thus, imaging should be done in children with focal seizures or significant focal EEG abnormalities, except when they are characteristic of a benign focal (rolandic or occipital) epilepsy. Imaging should also be performed in children with focal or generalized seizures who have significant developmental delay, abnormal neurological findings on examination, a history of a prior neurological insult, or poorly controlled seizures. Brain imaging is unnecessary in typical cases of idiopathic focal and generalized epilepsy.

 Practical points

Diagnosis
- A detailed description of the attacks and the situations in which they occurred, sometimes supplemented with a home video recording, are the keys to correct diagnosis of epileptic and non-epileptic events
- The differential diagnosis of episodic staring includes daydreaming or inattention, absence seizures and complex partial seizures
- The differential diagnosis of collapse and convulsing includes syncope, generalized tonic–clonic seizures, focal seizures with secondary generalization and psychogenic attacks
- Seizures in the classroom, church, bathroom, medical surgery or veterinary surgery should be considered to be syncopal attacks until proved otherwise
- EEG is helpful in characterizing seizures and epilepsies but should not be done to clarify the nature of undiagnosed events. Further history, home video-recording or video-EEG monitoring may be needed for undiagnosed episodic phenomena
- Idiopathic focal and generalized epilepsies usually have prominent and characteristic epileptic patterns on routine EEG, such that their absence should prompt consideration of non-epileptic attacks or a symptomatic epilepsy requiring imaging
- Imaging is performed when the seizures, EEG, history or examination suggest an underlying cerebral abnormality. Imaging is not performed in idiopathic focal or generalized epilepsies
- Learning and behavioural problems in a child with epilepsy are often the result of the underlying neurological problem rather than being secondary to seizures or medications

General principles of treatment of seizures in children

Explanation and reassurance, provision of information about the child's specific seizure disorder, first aid advice about how to manage future seizures, discussion of potential seizure precipitants, consideration of lifestyle modification and safety advice regarding bathing, swimming, heights and driving are all important aspects of seizure management. The decision to treat a child with antiepileptic medication and the choice and duration of treatment depend on the type of epilepsy and several patient and family factors. Antiepileptic medications reduce the likelihood of seizures but do not alter the course of epilepsy: that is, seizures do not remit any sooner on treatment. The appropriate antiepileptic drug is usually indicated by the seizure type (Table 17.1.3), treatment being generally initiated after specialist assessment.

Seizures can usually be controlled with one medication at an optimal dose, especially in idiopathic epilepsies. Children vary greatly in their dosage requirements and tolerance of antiepileptic drugs, patient age and associated disabilities being the main determinants. Except in status epilepticus and other situations with frequent or severe seizures, antiepileptic medications are usually commenced singly and in low dosage, and then increased gradually to a dose where seizure control is obtained, side effects appear or maximum dosage and serum levels are achieved. The duration of therapy depends on the type of epilepsy and its natural history, the degree of seizure control and the patient's lifestyle. Several years of freedom from seizures are desirable before antiepileptic drugs are ceased, and this is best done slowly over a period of months. Antiepileptic drug interactions are common, both pharmacokinetic and pharmacodynamic, some being advantageous (e.g. sodium valproate and lamotrigine) and others leading to side effects (e.g. barbiturates and benzodiazepines).

Almost all antiepileptic drugs produce side effects such as drowsiness and unsteadiness if given in excess (Table 17.1.5). These effects are common when medications are commenced and the dose is increased but they often wear off after the maintenance dose is reached. Some antiepileptic medications have side effects of an idiosyncratic type, such as rash or behaviour disturbance.

Use of serum levels for monitoring some antiepileptic medications is particularly useful if seizure control is inadequate, side effects attributable to toxicity are suspected or compliance is uncertain. Blood level monitoring is of particular value in young infants, in children with intellectual disability and in patients with impaired consciousness, i.e. patients who are not able to describe side effects. Barbiturate and phenytoin levels correlate well with both seizure control and side effects, a weaker correlation being present with carbamazepine. However, there is little role for blood level monitoring with the other antiepileptic medications, including sodium valproate and the benzodiazepines.

In addition to regular prescription of antiepileptic medication to prevent seizures, some parents and carers are instructed in the use of rectally administered diazepam or buccally administered midazolam to treat prolonged or recurring seizures, in children with a tendency to prolonged or clustering seizures.

For children with uncontrolled epilepsy, in whom seizures continue despite correct diagnosis

Table 17.1.5 Side effects of antiepileptic medications	
Medication	Side effects
Toxicity	
Common to most antiepileptic medications	Drowsiness, ataxia, tremor, nystagmus, dysarthria, confusion, nausea, vomiting, sleepiness or insomnia
Idiosyncratic	
Carbamazepine	Rash, leukopenia, hyponatraemia, irritability, weight gain
Clonazepam	Behaviour disturbance, increased bronchial and salivary secretions
Lamotrigine	Rash, severe hypersensitivity syndrome
Levetiracetam	Behaviour disturbance
Oxcarbazepine	Hyponatraemia
Phenytoin	Rash, serum-sickness-type illness
Phenobarbitone	Rash, behaviour disturbance
Sodium valproate	Weight gain, alopecia, pancreatitis, hepatic failure (rare)
Topiramate	Kidney stones, weight loss, speech disturbance
Vigabatrin	Peripheral vision impairment, behaviour disturbance, weight gain

and correct prescription of antiepileptic medications, specialized treatments such as epilepsy surgery, a ketogenic diet and vagal nerve stimulation may be considered. Surgical treatment is reserved for children with well characterized and refractory focal epilepsy in whom seizures are impacting greatly on quality of life. Surgery is most effective when the seizure focus is discrete, away from critical functional cortex and associated with a lesion on MRI. Epilepsy surgery is only carried out after detailed evaluation in a centre with special experience in paediatric epileptology. A ketogenic diet, with high fat and low carbohydrate and protein intake, is sometimes effective in refractory epilepsy, especially in younger children, uncontrolled absence and myoclonic epilepsies. Vagal nerve stimulation, a form of chronic brain stimulation for the treatment of refractory epilepsy, is being increasingly utilized in children with uncontrolled seizures where drugs and surgery are ineffective.

When treating epilepsy it is necessary to consider the whole child and family in their environment, and not only the seizures. Problems pertaining to education and vocation, problems related to adjustment to the diagnosis, and associated psychological and behavioural problems may be more difficult to manage than the actual seizures. Disentangling the effects of seizures, medications, underlying lesions, pre-existing states, family dynamics and psychosocial factors can often be difficult and require specialist involvement.

Practical points

Treatment
- Explanation, reassurance, lifestyle modification and first-aid advice are important aspects of epilepsy management
- For febrile seizures, reinforce that febrile seizure recurrence is common, epilepsy development is uncommon and neurodevelopmental sequelae are rare
- In a child with epilepsy, the decision to treat, the choice of medication and the duration of therapy are determined by the type of seizure and epilepsy
- As a general rule in antiepileptic drug therapy, 'start low and go slow' and withdraw medications slowly
- Antiepileptic drug level monitoring is important with phenobarbital and phenytoin, often helpful with carbamazepine but of limited value with sodium valproate and other drugs
- If seizures continue despite treatment with antiepileptic medication, consider whether the diagnosis of epilepsy and the seizure/syndrome type are correct, whether the choice of medication is appropriate, and whether medication is being given and taken in appropriate doses

Cerebral palsy and neurodegenerative disorders

17.2

D. Reddihough, K. Collins

Cerebral palsy

Cerebral palsy is the term used for a persistent but not unchanging disorder of movement and posture due to a defect or lesion of the developing brain. It is generally applied to children with permanent motor impairment due to non-progressive brain disorders occurring before the age of 5 years. There are many different causes, a wide range of manifestations of the motor disorder and various associated problems.

Cerebral palsy is not a single disorder but a group of disorders with diverse implications for children and their families.

For some young people with mild cerebral palsy, the only motor deficit may be a minimal hemiplegia, causing clumsiness with certain movements. In other children with severe cerebral palsy, the motor deficit may be spastic quadriplegia with little or no independent movement. Because each child with cerebral palsy is different, individual assessment and treatment are essential.

Prevalence

Cerebral palsy is the most common physical disability in childhood. Studies from several parts of the world, including Western Australia, Sweden and the UK, have shown that the prevalence of cerebral palsy is between 2.0 and 2.5 per 1000 live births. The overall prevalence of cerebral palsy has remained fairly stable since 1970 (Fig. 17.2.1).

Aetiology

The cause of cerebral palsy is unknown in many children. There is a significant association with prematurity and low birth weight but *it is important to remember that most low-birth-weight infants do not develop cerebral palsy.*

In a significant proportion of children who have cerebral palsy, there appears to have been no single event but rather a sequence of events responsible for the motor damage. This has led to the concept of 'causal pathways', a sequence of interdependent events that culminate in disease. It is likely that interdependent events are responsible for many cases of cerebral palsy.

Historical aspects

There has been a fundamental change in our understanding of aetiological factors during the past 20 years. Before this time, most cases of cerebral palsy were thought to be caused by lack of oxygen either during labour or during the perinatal period and it was expected that improvement in obstetrics and neonatal care would result in lower rates of cerebral palsy. Subsequently, there was an increased use of interventions such as caesarean section and electronic fetal monitoring but, despite a decline in stillbirth and neonatal deaths, the cerebral palsy rate remained constant.

In the past, cerebral palsy was attributed to minor obstetric and neonatal events, often incorrectly. Current research suggests that about 8–10% of cases are associated with perinatal asphyxia, the preferred term to describe a situation in which there have been perinatal events likely to reduce oxygen supply, evidenced by significant acidosis, followed by a failure of function in at least two organs (usually the brain and kidney). It is important to remember that perinatal asphyxia may not necessarily be the primary cause of the cerebral palsy and is generally not preventable. Because it is often impossible to ascribe clinical signs and symptoms to an event during birth, the term 'birth asphyxia' should be avoided.

Current knowledge about aetiology

It is helpful to consider the timing of the brain insult:

- prenatal events are thought to be responsible for approximately 75% of all cases of cerebral palsy
- perinatal events contribute 10–15%
- postnatal causes account for about 10% of all cases.

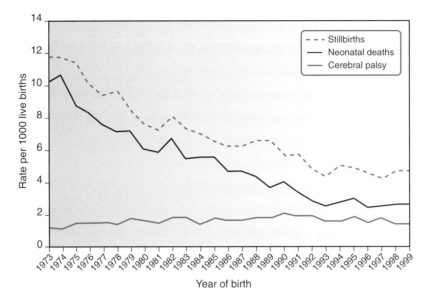

Fig. 17.2.1 Cerebral palsy, stillbirth and neonatal death rates per 1000 births in Victoria using published and unpublished data from the Victorian Cerebral Palsy Register and the Victorian Perinatal Data Collection Unit. Reid S, Lanigan A, Reddihough DS. Report of the Victorian Cerebral Palsy Register, 2005.

A prenatal cause is assumed in the absence of clear evidence for a perinatal or postnatal cause.

Prenatal causes

Malformations. Disturbances of brain development result in a variety of abnormalities, including malformations of cortical development. These typically arise at about 12–20 weeks gestation and may be identified by brain imaging, particularly magnetic resonance imaging (MRI). While genetic causes are being increasingly recognized, the basis for these malformations often remains unexplained.

Vascular. Brain imaging provides evidence of previous vascular events such as middle cerebral artery occlusion (Fig. 17.2.2).

Infective. Maternal infections during the first and second trimesters of pregnancy, including the **TORCH** group of organisms (*t*oxoplasmosis, *r*ubella, *c*ytomegalovirus and *h*erpes simplex virus), may cause cerebral palsy. It has also been suggested that maternal infections in the perinatal period may form part of the causal pathway to cerebral palsy in some children.

Genetic. There are some uncommon genetic syndromes associated with cerebral palsy.

Metabolic. Iodine deficiency in early pregnancy is an important cause of cerebral palsy in many parts of the world. Maternal thyroid disease has also been implicated.

Toxic. There have been reported cases associated with lead and methylmercury ingestion.

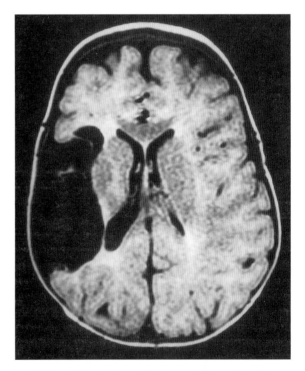

Fig. 17.2.2 MRI brain scan of a 2-year-old boy with left spastic hemiparesis, showing loss of brain tissue in right frontal and parietal lobes, consistent with an old (prenatal) right middle cerebral artery territory infarct.

Perinatal causes

Problems during labour and delivery. Obstetric emergencies such as obstructed labour, antepartum haemorrhage or cord prolapse may compromise the fetus.

Neonatal problems. Conditions such as severe hypoglycaemia or untreated jaundice may be responsible.

Premature and low-birth-weight infants. Premature and low-birth-weight infants differ from those born at term in their higher risk of cerebral palsy. The rate of cerebral palsy in children born before 33 weeks is up to 30 times higher than in those born at term. Some premature infants develop brain damage from complications of their immaturity, such as intraventricular haemorrhage, while others are damaged earlier in pregnancy. Intrauterine growth retardation is associated with cerebral palsy in both term and preterm infants. Periventricular leukomalacia is a common radiological finding in premature children with cerebral palsy. It is caused by an ischaemic process, usually occurring between 28 and 34 weeks of gestation, in the watershed zone that exists in the periventricular white matter of the immature brain. Periventricular leukomalacia may also be found in infants born at term, suggesting that the insult occurred early in the third trimester even though the pregnancy progressed to term.

Multiple pregnancy. Multiple births are associated with preterm delivery, poor intrauterine growth, birth defects and intrapartum complications and with an increased risk of both mortality and cerebral palsy. The increased risk to twins of cerebral palsy is not entirely explained by their increased risk of prematurity and low birth weight. Intrauterine death of a co-twin is a factor unique to multiple pregnancies and is associated with a sixfold increase in the rate of cerebral palsy per twin confinement, or an 11-fold increase in rate per child.

Postnatal cerebral palsy

Infection and injuries are responsible for most cases of postnatal cerebral palsy in developed countries:

- the introduction of vaccines against *Haemophilus influenzae* type b, meningococcus and pneumococcus should have a significant effect on the occurrence of bacterial meningitis in young children but other organisms remain
- injuries are an important group as there are clear prospects for prevention. Injuries may be accidental (e.g. motor vehicle accidents and near-drowning episodes) or due to physical abuse. Important preventive measures include improved road safety and mandatory fencing around home swimming pools.

Other causes of postnatal cerebral palsy include apparent life-threatening events and cerebrovascular accidents. Meningitis, septicaemia and infections such as malaria are important causes of cerebral palsy in developing countries.

Clinical example

Caitlin's mother went into labour at 33 weeks' gestation after an uneventful pregnancy. The delivery was rapid and Caitlin's Apgar scores were 6 at 1 minute and 8 at 5 minutes. Her parents remembered some panic in the labour ward and felt that more could have been done to slow the labour. Caitlin developed hyaline membrane disease and mild jaundice. In the early neonatal period she had difficulty sucking, which was attributed to her prematurity. She was slow in her motor development and did not sit until the age of 15 months. A diagnosis of cerebral palsy was made at that time.

When Caitlin was 2 years old, her parents requested an opinion as to whether subsequent children were likely to have cerebral palsy, believing that her prematurity and problems at birth were responsible for her condition. MRI of the brain demonstrated a brain malformation with bilateral clefts in the cerebral cortex, dating the problems to early pregnancy rather than the perinatal period.

Practical points

- Cerebral palsy is a diverse disorder with multiple risk factors and aetiologies
- Perinatal asphyxia is responsible for only a small proportion of cases (approximately 8–10%)
- It is important to establish the cause of cerebral palsy if at all possible. It is helpful for families and essential for genetic counselling
- When determining aetiology, distinguish risk factors from causes
- Many cases of cerebral palsy relate to events long before birth
- Take a careful history and examination to determine possible factors
- Brain imaging should be undertaken to establish timing and possible cause

Classification

There are three major ways in which cerebral palsy is classified – by type, by topographical distribution and by the severity of the motor disorder.

Type of motor disorder

Cerebral palsy is a disorder of movement (difficulties with voluntary movement and/or abnormal movements), posture and muscle tone. Children with cerebral palsy may present with various types of movement disorder.

Spastic cerebral palsy (70%)

This is the most common type. Spasticity involves increased muscle tone with characteristic clasp knife quality. Children with spasticity often have underlying weakness. In spastic cerebral palsy, there is damage to the motor cortex or corticospinal tracts, in contrast to dyskinetic and ataxic cerebral palsy, which are associated with abnormalities of the basal ganglia and cerebellum, respectively.

Dyskinetic cerebral palsy (10–15%)

This refers to a group of cerebral palsies with involuntary movements and is characterized by abnormalities of tone involving the whole body. Several terms are used within this group:

- *Dystonia* is a syndrome of sustained muscle contractions, frequently causing twisting and repetitive movements or abnormal postures
- *Athetosis* refers to slow writhing movements involving the distal parts of the limbs
- *Chorea* is the term for rapid jerky movements.

Ataxic cerebral palsy (less than 5%)

Children have a fine tremor, more noticeable when movements are initiated, as well as poor balance and hypotonia. Ataxia is associated with other neurological conditions that must be excluded before this diagnosis is made. Some children have a mixed motor disorder.

The topographical distribution

The terms diplegia, hemiplegia and quadriplegia are used and generally apply to children with spastic cerebral palsy as the other types usually involve four limbs:

- the term *diplegia* is used where the predominant problem is in the lower limbs. There is usually some upper limb involvement, which may be subtle. The majority of these children have normal intelligence. Spastic diplegia is the pattern most commonly seen in premature infants who have the radiological finding of periventricular leukomalacia
- children with *spastic hemiplegia* usually have normal intelligence, frequently have epilepsy (50–70%), may have sensory impairments in the upper limb and may have visual deficits (homonymous hemianopsia)
- children with *spastic quadriplegia* frequently have problems such as intellectual disability, epilepsy and visual difficulties. There is often poor trunk control and oromotor difficulties in addition to four limb involvement.

Severity of the motor disorder

The gross motor function classification system (GMFCS), provides information about the movement problems of children with cerebral palsy based on their motor abilities and their need for walking frames, wheelchairs and other mobility devices. There are five levels: children in levels I and II walk independently, children in level III generally need walking frames or elbow crutches and children in levels IV and V use wheelchairs. This classification system does not consider cognitive and other deficits, which may have a profound effect on the eventual outcome.

Using the GMFCS, growth motor development curves have been constructed that provide some guide to prognosis for motor development.

▶ **Practical points**

- Cerebral palsy can be classified according to motor type, distribution and severity (the latter using the GMFCS)
- New methods of classifying severity provide information about motor prognosis
- Co-morbidities such as epilepsy are more common in certain types of cerebral palsy

---

Presentation

The diagnosis of cerebral palsy is not always easy, particularly in children born prematurely. Signs may evolve during the first year of life. For example, spasticity is not usually present in the early weeks of life, involuntary movements are generally not seen in the first year of life and, conversely, abnormal neurological signs may disappear. Cerebral palsy may present as:

- follow-up of 'at risk' infants, such as those born prematurely or those with a history of neonatal encephalopathy
- delayed motor milestones, particularly delay in learning to sit, stand and walk
- development of asymmetric movement patterns, e.g. strong preference for one hand in the early months of life
- abnormalities of muscle tone, particularly spasticity or hypotonia. the latter in isolation should always be treated with caution as it may be an early sign of global developmental delay rather than cerebral palsy
- management problems, e.g. severe feeding difficulties or abnormalities of behaviour such as unexplained irritability. These problems should be

interpreted carefully, as many other conditions can present with these features.

Examination involves a search for abnormalities in muscle tone, posture and deep tendon reflexes, along with persistence of primitive reflexes. It is important to exclude other conditions that may present with motor delay, including neuromuscular, neurodegenerative and metabolic disorders. It is generally recommended that MRI be part of the investigation of the child with cerebral palsy, particularly where the cause or causes are uncertain or unknown.

Practical points

- Observation of the child often provides more information than 'hands on' examination. It will provide information about the presence or absence of age appropriate motor skills and their quality

Associated disorders

- Visual problems occur in about 40% of children with cerebral palsy and include strabismus, refractive errors, visual field defects and cortical visual impairment
- Hearing deficits occur in 3–10% of children with cerebral palsy. High-frequency hearing loss may be found in children with congenital rubella or other viral syndromes
- Speech and language problems: receptive and expressive language delays and articulation problems occur
- Epilepsy occurs in up to 50% of children with cerebral palsy, most commonly in those with severe motor problems
- Cognitive impairments: while intellectual disabilities and learning problems are common, there is a wide range of intellectual ability in children with cerebral palsy and children with severe physical disabilities may have normal intelligence. Perceptual difficulties are also frequent.

Some children with cerebral palsy have only a motor disorder.

Management

A team approach is essential, involving a range of health professionals and teachers, with input from the family of paramount importance. Management of the child with cerebral palsy involves:

- management of the associated disabilities, health problems and consequences of the motor disorder
- assessment of the child's capabilities and referral to appropriate services for the child and family.

Management of the associated disabilities, health problems and consequences of the motor disorder

Associated disabilities
- All children require a **hearing** and **visual** assessment
- Assessment and advice about **epilepsy** and prescription of anticonvulsants when appropriate
- Children may benefit from formal **cognitive assessment** and may need help with their educational programme. Assessment of cognitive abilities can be difficult when children have severe physical disabilities

Health problems
- **Growth** should be monitored and dietary advice sought to ensure that nutrient and calorie intake is adequate. Failure to thrive and undernutrition are frequent problems, caused by eating difficulties due to oromotor dysfunction. Nasogastric or gastrostomy feeds should be considered if there is difficulty in achieving satisfactory weight gains or if the length of time taken to feed the child interferes with other activities. Conversely, **obesity** is a significant problem and may interfere with progress in motor skills
- Investigation and management of **gastro-oesophageal reflux,** which occurs commonly in cerebral palsy. It can result in oesophagitis or gastritis, causing pain and poor appetite, and, if severe, aspiration can result
- Dietary and laxative advice regarding the frequent problem of **constipation.** Immobility, low-fibre diet and poor fluid intake are contributory factors
- Lung disease. Some children with severe cerebral palsy develop chronic **lung disease** due to aspiration from oromotor dysfunction or severe gastro-oesophageal reflux occurring over a period of time. The presence of coughing or choking during meal times, or wheeze during or after meals, may signal the possibility of aspiration but it may also occur without clinical symptoms or signs. There is no 'gold standard' test for aspiration but barium videofluoroscopy may be helpful. Alternative feeding regimens, such as the use of a gastrostomy, should be considered if aspiration is present
- Many children with cerebral palsy, particularly those born prematurely, have **hydrocephalus** requiring **ventriculoperitoneal shunts**
- **Dental health.** Children are at risk of dental problems and should be regularly monitored
- **Osteoporosis.** Pathological fractures may occur in children with severe cerebral palsy
- Most importantly, **emotional problems** can be overlooked and may be responsible for suboptimal performance, either with academic tasks or in the self-care area

Consequences of the motor disorder
- Management of **drooling** (poor saliva control). Speech pathologists can assist with behavioural approaches and methods to improve oromotor control. Medication (anticholinergics) and surgery are helpful in some children
- **Incontinence.** Children may be late in achieving bowel and bladder control due to cognitive deficits or lack of opportunity to access toileting facilities because of physical disability and/or inability to communicate. Sometimes children have detrusor overactivity causing urgency, frequency and incontinence
- **The testes** may be in the normal position at birth but may ascend with time (secondary to chronic spasm of the cremaster muscle), requiring the same treatment as in other boys with this problem (usually **scrotal orchidopexy**)
- **Orthopaedic problems.** Children may develop contractures that require orthopaedic intervention. Surgery is mainly undertaken on the lower limb but is occasionally helpful in the upper limb. Physiotherapists are essential in the postoperative rehabilitation phase
  - *The hip.* Non-walkers and those partially ambulant (GMFCS levels III–V) are at risk of hip subluxation and dislocation. Early detection is vital and hip X-rays should be performed at yearly intervals. If there is evidence of subluxation or dislocation, children should be referred for an orthopaedic opinion. Dislocation causes pain and difficulty with perineal hygiene. Ambulant children rarely develop hip problems
  - *The knee.* Flexion contractures at the knee may require hamstring surgery
  - *The ankle.* Equinus deformity at the ankle is the commonest orthopaedic problem in children with cerebral palsy. Toe-walking is treated conservatively in young children with orthoses, inhibitory casts and botulinum toxin A therapy. Older children benefit from surgery for a definitive correction of the deformity
  - *Multilevel surgery.* Sometimes children require surgery at several different levels (e.g. hip, knee and ankle). This involves a single hospitalization and is called 'single event multilevel surgery'. It is of most benefit to children who walk independently or with the assistance of crutches. The usual age is between 8 and 12 years. The aims of surgery are to correct deformities and to improve both the appearance and efficiency of walking. An accurate assessment of the walking problems is undertaken in a gait laboratory. A carefully planned intensive rehabilitation physiotherapy programme lasting up to 1 year is required to maximize the benefits
  - *The upper limb.* Procedures can be offered following careful assessment

- *Scoliosis.* Correction is sometimes necessary
- **Spasticity management** is aimed at improving function, comfort and care and requires a team approach. Options include:
  - *Oral medications,* e.g. diazepam, dantrolene sodium and baclofen. These medications may not be effective or may cause unwanted effects
  - *Inhibitory casts* aim to increase joint range and facilitate improved quality of movement. The main application is below-knee casts for equinus but occasionally casts are used in the upper limb
  - *Botulinum toxin A* is injected into muscles and reduces localized spasticity
  - *Intrathecal baclofen* is administered by a pump implanted under the skin. This treatment is suitable for a small number of children with severe generalized spasticity and may enhance quality of life
  - *Selective dorsal rhizotomy* is a neurosurgical procedure whereby specific posterior spinal roots are sectioned to reduce spasticity. It is used mostly in young children aged 3–7 years with spastic diplegia. Randomized trials have provided evidence of some benefits in carefully selected cases. An intensive rehabilitation period is required.

Clinical example

Tom was born at 26 weeks' gestation. He had many neonatal problems, including a grade IV intraventricular haemorrhage. The parents were informed that some degree of cerebral palsy was likely. At 4 months corrected age, Tom's mother noted that his right hand was fisted. The diagnosis of cerebral palsy was confirmed and a physiotherapy programme was commenced.

When he began to walk independently at 24 months corrected age, Tom's gait was noted to be asymmetrical, with a tendency to walk on his toes on the right side. This problem was more apparent by 30 months and he fell more than would be expected for his age. Inhibitory casts were applied for 4 weeks and he was fitted with an ankle–foot orthosis (AFO). His walking pattern was much improved after this treatment but after a further 10 months the problem had recurred. This time Tom appeared not only to walk in equinus but was also flexed at the knee. Hamstrings as well as calf muscles were tight. Botulinum toxin A injections were given to both muscle groups with an excellent result. A new AFO was given as Tom had grown considerably over this time. When Tom was 5 years old, he required further botulinum toxin A injections. At 6 years of age, surgery was undertaken by the same orthopaedic surgeon who had been monitoring him since the age of 24 months. Now he is 10 years old and no treatment is currently planned, although the family has been advised that further surgery may be required following his adolescent growth spurt.

Assessment of the child's capabilities and referral to appropriate services for the child and family

The role of the team

Careful assessment in conjunction with a multidisciplinary team is essential to enable children to achieve their optimal physical potential and independence:

- *Physiotherapists* give practical advice to parents on positioning, handling and play to minimize the effects of abnormal muscle tone and encourage the development of movement skills. They also give advice regarding the use of orthoses, special seating, wheelchairs and other mobility aids
- *Occupational therapists* help parents to develop their child's upper limb and self-care skills, and also recommend suitable toys, equipment and home adaptations
- *Speech pathologists* assist in the development of communication skills, including advising about augmentative communication systems for children with limited verbal skills. They provide guidance about feeding difficulties and saliva control problems
- *Orthotists, medical social workers, psychologists, special education teachers* and *nurses* are helpful.

Therapy approaches

Therapy to address movement problems and to optimize children's progress in all areas of development is incorporated into early intervention and school programmes. The two most commonly used approaches by therapists in Australia are:

- *Neurodevelopmental Therapy (NDT).* This is a therapeutic approach to the assessment and management of movement problems with the goal of maximizing the child's functional ability. This therapy was developed by Dr and Mrs Bobath and hence is sometimes known as 'Bobath therapy'. Family members receive education in NDT principles so that they can implement the programme at home, preschool and school
- *programmes based on the principles of Conductive Education.* Conductive education is a Hungarian system for educating children and adults with movement disorders. It provides an integrated group programme where children and parents learn to develop skills in all areas of life, e.g. daily living, physical, social, emotional, cognitive and communication skills.

Assistive technology

Appropriate equipment tailored for the individual child can enhance communication, mobility, learning and socialization. Examples include powered wheelchairs, electronic communication devices and computers for educational and recreational purposes.

Trends in service provision

Services are best provided within local communities. Therapists and special education teachers work with children at home and later in child-care centres, kindergartens and schools. Most children attend mainstream preschools and schools but others benefit from attendance at centre-based early intervention programmes and special schools. It is essential that parents are made aware of all available options.

Alternative therapies

There are many non-mainstream (or 'alternative') treatments available. Sometimes great claims, usually not justified, are made for alternative approaches. Families can be reassured that any new treatment that is of value will be assessed and incorporated into mainstream practice. There is no evidence to suggest that alternative methods are superior to conventional treatments and some may do harm. It is important that professionals are aware of alternative approaches and are prepared to critically examine their claims.

Working with families

Care of the child with cerebral palsy involves developing a trusting and cooperative relationship with the parents. The child is part of a family unit and concerns in parents or siblings must be addressed. As with all children, a supportive home environment builds self-esteem and confidence. Parents may need practical support, such as provision of respite care, and may be helped by meeting other families in similar circumstances or by attending parent support groups. Provision of information about financial allowances is an important aspect of care.

Life expectancy

Children with mild and moderate cerebral palsy have a normal life span. Those with severe motor impairment, particularly those who are wheelchair dependent and require tube feeding, have a reduced life expectancy. Chronic lung disease is the most common cause of morbidity and mortality in this group.

Practical points

- In the child with cerebral palsy, the associated disorders and health problems may require more attention than the motor disorder itself
- Optimal management of the child with cerebral palsy involves the collaborative efforts of a team

Neurodegenerative disorders

This section addresses the problem of the child who presents because of concern about regression in development that has been normal previously, or with apparent worsening of a pre-existing neurological disorder. In infants and young children, concern may arise because of loss of gross and fine motor, personal social and language skills. Declining school performance may lead to referral of the older child.

An approach to this problem will be outlined, with examples of the many disorders that may present in this way. Some of these disorders are mentioned in Chapter 10.5. The suggested Further reading associate with this chapter provide a more detailed account of the wide range of neurodegenerative conditions. The diagnostic process is presented here as a series of questions.

Is there evidence of regression or lack of progress in any area of development?

This is sought in a sequential history of progress in each area of development, supplemented by questions such as 'How is your child's speech now, com-

pared with this time last year? Is there any area where your child has gone backward or shown no progress at all?'

A clear ongoing loss of former skills, as shown in the latter part of curve C in Figure 17.2.3, raises obvious concern about a progressive disorder, but this may be less certain during the earlier 'plateau' phase before actual regression appears.

This is to be distinguished from the pattern of abnormally slow, but consistent, progress shown in curve A. This is often found in children with an intellectual disability or cerebral palsy, who may be seen to fall behind other children in abilities while in fact continuing to acquire new skills, but at a slower pace because of a static brain disorder arising in the prenatal or perinatal period.

A variation on this pattern, seen in curve B, occurs in the child whose initially normal progress is interrupted by an acute injury or illness (e.g. meningitis or encephalitis) causing brain damage with later slower development.

Could the apparently progressive symptoms be due to a static disorder complicated by other factors?

Such factors are often amenable to treatment and include:

- frequent seizures, especially subtle myoclonic and atonic episodes, which may severely impair alertness and coordination
- drug toxicity, particularly from antiepileptic drugs
- psychological or emotional factors, including depression, withdrawal and psychosis; a particular problem is the tendency for children with autism to show arrest or regression in social and language skills during the second year of life
- joint deformities due to soft tissue contractures in spastic 'cerebral palsy', leading to worsening of postural stability and gait.

If this is a progressive disorder, what is its distribution in terms of brain anatomy?

Important anatomical patterns to consider are as follows.

One lesion

Progressive hemiparesis, perhaps associated with focal seizures, suggests a cerebral hemisphere tumour, while spinal cord tumours may produce progressive weakness and spasticity affecting the lower limbs, either alone or with variable upper limb

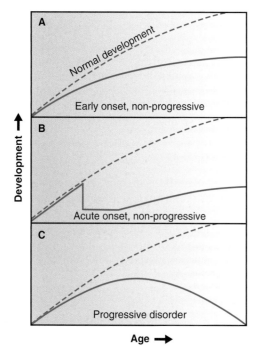

Fig. 17.2.3 Curves demonstrating the course of development over time in a child with static (A and B) and progressive neurological disease (C) compared with expected normal development. The actual age scale will vary and a different curve may apply to each aspect of development in each child or disease process.

involvement, thus imitating diplegic cerebral palsy. This clinical pattern, sometimes with associated ataxia, is also seen in slowly progressive hydrocephalus, even in the absence of a cerebral neoplasm. The triad of cranial nerve palsies, corticospinal tract signs and ataxia suggests a brain-stem glioma. Most other childhood tumours of the nervous system raise clear concern because of symptoms of raised intracranial pressure, but the insidious visual loss associated with optic nerve glioma and craniopharyngioma is often not recognized as a progressive problem until late in its course.

One functional system or group of systems

The prototype of 'system degenerations' is Friedreich ataxia. In this disorder, abnormalities of spinocerebellar, corticospinal and sensory tracts arise in the second decade of life. In other cerebellar ataxia syndromes there is involvement not only of neural pathways but of other body organs, as with ataxia telangiectasia, in which chromosomal breaks, immunological defects and skin lesions occur. A system disorder involving basal ganglia or extrapyramidal motor function may be inferred from the signs of dystonia, rigidity and choreoathetosis. An important example in this category is Wilson disease, which is treatable with penicillamine. Peripheral neuromuscular diseases, which also may be regarded as system disorders, are discussed separately in Chapter 17.3.

A multifocal process, with several discrete lesions in the brain

This is exemplified by recurrent cerebral infarctions associated with cyanotic congenital heart disease. In the absence of cardiac disease, repeated cerebral vascular occlusions are suggestive of moya-moya disease, a well recognized but poorly understood syndrome. Angiography here shows progressive occlusion of the major cerebral arteries, with a curious network of fine collateral vessels in the basal ganglia.

Among a group of disorders known collectively as mitochondrial encephalomyelopathies, one form (MELAS) may present with repeated stroke-like episodes and multifocal brain lesions, associated with abnormal mitochondria in muscle, increased lactate levels in blood and cerebrospinal fluid, and deletions of the nuclear or mitochondrial DNA controlling mitochondrial enzyme activity.

Homocystinuria, an inborn error of amino acid metabolism, may present with recurrent cerebral venous or arterial thromboses. While multiple sclerosis is a major cause of multifocal lesions in young adults, it seldom begins in childhood.

A diffuse degenerative disorder of the nervous system

Diseases causing widespread loss of neurological function are generally separated into those that begin by affecting predominantly cortical grey matter, or nerve cell bodies, and those in which white matter, or nerve sheath myelin, is primarily involved. While this distinction is of clinical value, many disorders are not easily classified in this way.

Diffuse disorders of grey matter
These tend to cause seizures (often myoclonic) and early loss of intellectual function, with progressive impairment of language, comprehension and memory. In addition, involvement of nerve cells in the retina leads to a variable pattern of visual loss. This clinical syndrome is seen in several of the lipid storage disorders, of which Tay–Sachs disease is the best known. Subacute sclerosing panencephalitis is an infrequent complication of measles and evolves as a sequence of behavioural change, intellectual decline, myoclonic jerks and later rigidity.

Diffuse disorders of white matter
By involving corticospinal tracts, these tend to present with early motor impairment and spasticity, and may masquerade initially as 'cerebral palsy'. Impaired vision, when present, reflects optic pathways disease. Peripheral nerve myelin also may be involved, with clinical effects, as in Krabbe disease and metachromatic leukodystrophy, both of which are lipid storage disorders.

The above three questions can generally be answered after a careful clinical history and examination, but the remaining steps in diagnosis require knowledge of a growing number of recognized but rare diseases. In practice, this will involve specialist consultation.

Which disorders are known to occur in children of this age, and to produce the other clinical features present in this child?

Individual neurodegenerative diseases tend to have a characteristic age of onset. It is useful to consider broad age ranges (early infancy, late infancy and later childhood) in narrowing the diagnostic field. Next, by matching possible diagnoses against associated clinical findings, such as enlargement of liver and spleen, ocular abnormalities or unusual facial features, the physician may further refine the search and select the most relevant diagnostic tests.

A diagnosis is often reached merely by answering these questions. If not, it is useful next to turn from clinical features to pathophysiology.

Clinical example

Vincent, aged 6 years, was referred to a paediatric neurologist because the teachers at his special school were concerned about his deterioration over several months, with loss of speech and comprehension of language, impaired coordination and increasingly hyperactive, aggressive behaviour. He had been diagnosed as having developmental delay at the age of 3 because of limited speech and overactive behaviour. On examination, in addition to the developmental and behavioural findings, he had slightly coarse facial features with thickened eyebrows, a palpably enlarged liver and a mild thoracic kyphosis. These features raised the clinical suspicion that he had Sanfilippo disease, one of a group of disorders in which a deficiency of lysosomal enzymes leads to an accumulation of mucopolysaccharides in the tissues and excretion in the urine. The diagnosis was confirmed on specific blood and urine tests. Much professional support was needed by Vincent's parents, confronted with the prospect of their son's progressive dementia and immobility, as well as the autosomal recessive inheritance of his condition.

Are any other, less evident diagnoses suggested by a systematic review of known mechanisms of disease?

The previous selective clinical correlations can be investigated further by considering in turn the major categories of:

- disease process, including metabolic errors, neurocutaneous disorders, slow virus infections and chronic intoxications
- biochemical substrates, such as lipids, vitamins and minerals
- cellular organelles, including lysosomes, peroxisomes and mitochondria, with their respective disorders.

This search may yield a further short list of possible diagnoses known to the clinician but not considered, usually because of limited recent experience with them.

Are there any treatable disorders among the diagnoses being considered in this child?

This important question may alter the priority of investigation, as a potentially treatable disorder, however unlikely, must be rigorously excluded at an early stage. The major groups to recognize are:

- neoplasms and other space occupying lesions involving the brain, and especially the spinal cord or optic nerves, where they are often not suspected until late, after irreversible damage
- subacute and chronic infections of the nervous system, such as tuberculous and cryptococcal meningitis and HIV infection
- intoxications: lead poisoning, glue sniffing, prescribed medications and, occasionally, chronic drug administration by a disturbed parent
- inborn errors of metabolism. The use of a modified diet in phenylketonuria is well known but may also be of value in rarer disorders. Removal of toxic agents, e.g. copper chelation in Wilson disease, may be possible. In seizures due to pyridoxine dependency and in other vitamin dependency syndromes, large doses of vitamins may effectively compensate for the metabolic defect
- deficiency states, especially of vitamins required for normal growth and function of the nervous system.

Effective treatment is not yet available for most degenerative neurological disorders of childhood but accurate diagnosis remains the basis for genetic counselling and for offering a realistic prognosis. A specific diagnosis or 'answer' is of great value to parents in coping with the distress of having a disabled child.

Neuromuscular disorders 17.3

A. J. Kornberg

Neuromuscular disease in childhood has until recently received little attention. This is not surprising, given that many of the conditions were difficult to diagnose without sophisticated investigations and they were generally untreatable. However, this group of disorders cannot be ignored because of the significant morbidity and mortality associated with them, the genetic implications and the arrival of potential therapies. The establishment of an early diagnosis is important in the rational management of these disorders as it allows prognostic and genetic information to be provided. Accurate diagnosis in this wide array of disorders is dependent on a careful clinical assessment followed by confirmatory and appropriate investigations. While recent advances have unravelled the molecular biology of many neuromuscular conditions, the clinical assessment of patients remains the cornerstone of diagnosis and management. If clinical assessment is found wanting, the use of even the best technology may not supply the required diagnostic information.

The management of peripheral neuromuscular disease requires recognition, diagnosis, therapy and counselling.

Recognition that a child's presenting symptoms or signs may be due to peripheral neuromuscular disease

Please listen to the patient, he's trying to tell you what disease he has.

Michael H. Brooke, *The Clinician's View of Neuromuscular Disease*

Although the hallmark of neuromuscular disease is weakness, parents do not come into the consulting room saying 'I'm worried because my child is weak'. The physician needs to recognize that the presenting symptoms or signs relate to the peripheral neuromuscular system before the diagnostic process begins. The failure of recognition results in diagnostic delay, with frequent presentations to a doctor, be it the family doctor or other specialist. While this failure does not usually affect the ultimate prognosis, it adds considerably to patient and parental frustration. The main tragedy occurs when opportunities for preventive strategies are missed and a second affected child is born in the immediate or even extended family.

Common presenting complaints of neuromuscular disease include:

- difficulty walking and running
- poor at sports
- clumsy or poorly coordinated
- not able to keep up with peers
- frequent falls
- tires easily.

Another trap in the recognition of neuromuscular disease in childhood is that classical neurological signs, readily demonstrated at the end of a disease process in adult patients, are expected to be present in children at the beginning of the disease process. For example, in Charcot–Marie–Tooth disease, adult patients will have gross pes cavus, areflexia and the so-called 'inverted champagne bottle legs'. In children, the early features are commonly an abnormal walk or run, clumsiness and frequent falls, with foot deformity as a presenting symptom in a minority. In addition, although areflexia is the rule in adult patients, about 10% of children with Charcot–Marie–Tooth disease have normal reflexes at presentation. Not understanding the age-dependent symptoms and signs of various neuromuscular disorders will lead to the failure of recognition of a neuromuscular disease in childhood.

Other modes of presentation include a family history of neuromuscular disease; weakness, hypotonia, respiratory or feeding difficulty in the neonatal period; delayed motor milestones; abnormal gait (particularly toe walking) and orthopaedic abnormality, such as foot deformity or scoliosis. Some patients present with non-neuromuscular problems, such as intellectual disability or delayed language development, as, for example, in Duchenne muscular dystrophy.

Diagnosis of neuromuscular disease based on anatomical, electrophysiological, biochemical, histopathological or DNA identification

After recognizing that the symptoms are due to neuromuscular disease, the differential diagnosis is

603

usually based on a logical anatomical approach. Although this may appear to be simplistic, as some disorders may affect more than one anatomical area or be multisystem, this approach will provide a broad differential diagnosis that may lead to a definitive diagnosis.

The anatomical localization is based on the clinical findings listed in Table 17.3.1 and includes disorders affecting the:

- anterior horn cell
- anterior and posterior nerve roots
- peripheral nerve (motor, sensory, autonomic)
- neuromuscular junction
- muscle.

The use of a time frame of symptoms, such as acute, subacute or chronic, may also provide an important filter for the differential diagnosis.

The definitive diagnosis rests on a combination of:

- clinical history and examination
- family history
- serum enzymes, particularly creatine kinase (CK)
- electrophysiology (e.g. nerve conduction studies, electromyography, repetitive nerve stimulation)
- histology of muscle and/or nerve
- metabolic studies (e.g. muscle glycogen, carnitine assay, mitochondrial studies)
- DNA studies.

With only a few exceptions, electrophysiological, biopsy and/or DNA studies should be undertaken, as the implications of a neuromuscular disease diagnosis are so great for the child and immediate family, and sometimes the extended family.

Anterior horn cell disorders

Acute

Poliomyelitis

This disorder is rare in developed countries. It should still be considered where there is acute onset of lower motor neurone flaccid paralysis of a single limb, or with patchy asymmetrical distribution, particularly if associated with fever, vomiting, neck or spine stiffness and muscle pain or spasm. Sensory abnormalities are absent.

Hopkins syndrome

A clinical syndrome of asthma with flaccid paralysis of a limb resembling poliomyelitis has been recognized (Hopkins syndrome). Anterior horn cell dysfunction has been identified with magnetic resonance imaging through the clinically affected segments of the spinal cord. Coxsackie virus and echovirus infections have occasionally produced weakness thought to be of anterior horn cell origin.

Chronic

In childhood the chronic disorders, characterized pathologically by degeneration of anterior horn cells and associated clinically with progressive muscle weakness, are called the spinal muscular atrophies (SMAs). The important clinical syndromes and their classification are listed in Table 17.3.2.

Table 17.3.1 Clinical clues helpful in establishing the site of the lesion in neuromuscular disease				
Clinical feature	Anterior horn cell	Peripheral nerve	Neuromuscular junction	Muscle
Weakness	Proximal	Distal	Cranial/proximal	Proximal
Hypotonia	++	+	+/−	++
Hyporeflexia	+/−	Early	+/−	Late
Fasciculations	+++	+	−	−
Sensory abnormalities	−	+/−	−	−
Myotonia	−	−	−	+/−
Autonomic dysfunction	−	+/−	−	−
Muscle enlargement	−	−	−	+/−

Table 17.3.2 Clinical classification of childhood-onset proximal spinal muscle atrophy

Designation	Symptom onset (months)	Course	Death (years)
I (severe)	0–6	Never sits without support	<2
II (intermediate)	<18	Never stands without aid	>2
III (mild)	>18	Stands alone	Adult

Spinal muscular atrophy type I (Werdnig–Hoffmann disease)

This autosomal recessive disorder occurs in approximately 1 in 25 000 live births, making it one of the commonest fatal autosomal recessive disorders in humans. The earliest symptom may be decreased fetal movements in late pregnancy. Presentation is invariably before 6 months of age and is either at birth, with hypotonia, weakness, joint deformity and respiratory difficulty, or more commonly later with marked hypotonia and limb weakness, poor feeding, poor cough and cry. The onset is sometimes relatively rapid and when first seen the child is usually severely weak (Fig. 17.3.1). Weakness, although generalized, is maximal proximally in the shoulder and hip girdle muscles. Intercostal muscle weakness leads to chest deformity, a poor cough and a weak cry. The respiratory pattern becomes diaphragmatic. Deep tendon reflexes are absent. Fasciculations of the tongue are an important clinical clue, but this can be an exceedingly difficult sign to be certain about and one can only be confident if the baby is relaxed and there are no 'voluntary' movements of the tongue. Facial weakness is only mild and extraocular movements remain full, giving the baby an alert appearance. Death, usually from pneumonia and respiratory failure, occurs by 18 months of age in 95% of patients, with those with onset in the first 2 months of life having the shortest survival.

The genetic abnormality has been mapped to chromosome 5q13.3 and involves several different genes (*SMN* and *NAIP*). Prenatal diagnosis is available.

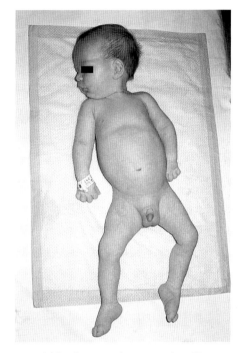

Fig. 17.3.1 Child with SMA I, showing profound hypotonia and weakness.

Studies of various therapeutic strategies are being trialled. Most of the therapeutic strategies are designed to upregulate SMN via a variety of mechanisms.

Spinal muscular atrophy type II (chronic childhood spinal muscular atrophy)

Clinical onset is almost invariably before 3 years of age, with SMA type II at least as common as Werdnig–Hoffmann disease. About one half of children affected by this disorder never walk, and only 5% are still walking by 20 years of age. Survival varies from 18 months through to adult life. Prompt treatment of chest infections will prolong survival.

The clinical picture is one of severe generalized weakness and wasting, with proximal predominance. Deep tendon reflexes are decreased or absent and often there are fasciculations of the tongue. The

Practical points

- A positive diagnosis of fasciculations of the tongue should not be made unless the tongue has no voluntary movement, i.e. is not protruded, and the child is not crying or actively moving the tongue
- The presence of deep tendon reflexes makes it extremely unlikely that the child has type I SMA and an alternative diagnosis should be considered

facial muscles may be mildly weak but eye movements remain normal and the patient is usually normal intellectually. Some patients have a fine, rapid tremor of the hands. Major management problems include the prevention of orthopaedic deformity, especially scoliosis, and the management of the respiratory complications of muscle weakness. The genetic abnormality is allelic to that for SMA type I.

Spinal muscular atrophy type III (Kugelberg–Welander syndrome)

Patients with late onset and a moderately benign clinical course are classified as SMA type III (Kugelberg–Welander syndrome). Most have onset in the first two decades, with only a few in the third decade, and survival is usually for many decades. While many remain ambulant over many years, particularly those with later onset, some do lose the ability to walk during childhood years. The genetic abnormality is allelic to that for SMA types I and II.

Peripheral nerve disorders

A number of peripheral neuropathies occur in childhood, with various time courses (acute, subacute or chronic). They may be inherited or acquired; they may involve motor, sensory or autonomic fibres, or commonly mixtures of all three. Pathologically, they may be associated with combinations of demyelination and axonal degeneration. Some central nervous system degenerative disorders, such as Krabbe disease and metachromatic leukodystrophy, may also have a peripheral neuropathy component. The commonest disorders in childhood are Guillain–Barré syndrome and peroneal muscular atrophy or Charcot–Marie–Tooth disease. Chronic inflammatory demyelinating peripheral neuropathy (CIDP), while uncommon, is important because it is responsive to immunotherapies.

Acute neuropathies

Guillain–Barré syndrome

Guillain–Barré syndrome (GBS) is the most common acute neuropathy in clinical practice and can occur at any age, although it is rare in infancy. An infection, commonly of the upper respiratory tract or gastrointestinal tract (*Campylobacter jejuni*), precedes the neurological syndrome in at least 50% of cases. Typical GBS is a monophasic illness with symmetrical, ascending weakness involving proximal and distal muscles. Paraesthesia and muscle pain may be presenting complaints but sensory impairment is usually minimal. Severe back pain and stiffness may occur, especially in young children. Tendon reflexes are lost early in the course of the illness. Cranial nerve involvement, particularly the facial nerve, is relatively common. Autonomic involvement can cause wide fluctuations of the blood pressure as well as cardiac arrhythmias and bladder dysfunction. Respiratory failure occurs in about 30% of patients and in addition may be associated with pharyngeal dysfunction. GBS typically progresses over a period of less than 4 weeks, with most patients reaching their maximal deficit within 2 weeks of onset. Artificial ventilation for periods of up to 8 weeks may occasionally be required. Recovery continues over weeks to many months, with most children returning to normal function. Some more severely affected children may have residual weakness, particularly with dorsiflexion. Fatigue is common during the recovery period.

Diagnosis is based on the clinical features, with elevation of the cerebrospinal fluid (CSF) protein with only a few, if any, cells. A nerve conduction study may be useful in difficult diagnostic situations. Intravenous gammaglobulin or plasmaphaeresis, if used early, may hasten recovery. Supportive therapy is very important.

Management of GBS requires special expertise in medical and nursing care and children should be referred to centres used to dealing with this condition. Monitor blood pressure and cardiac rhythm, as autonomic dysfunction is one of the potentially serious complications. In severely affected individuals who are ventilated and with little movement, it may appear that the patient is unresponsive. The patient can see, hear and think. It is important to explain what is happening at all times and reassure them that they will get better.

Chronic neuropathies

Chronic inflammatory demyelinating peripheral neuropathy

This condition is rare but treatable and is thought to be an autoimmune disorder. It usually presents as a subacute or chronic neuropathy. The course can be monophasic but is usually relapsing and remitting over many weeks or months duration. Acute presentations can occur and may cause confusion with Guillain–Barré syndrome. Symptoms and signs of weakness, often most prominent proximally, bring the child to medical attention. The diagnosis is confirmed by nerve conduction studies, elevated CSF protein and, if there is diagnostic doubt, pathological abnormalities in a nerve biopsy.

Intravenous immunoglobulin, corticosteroids, other immunosuppressive agents and plasmaphaeresis have all been used with varying degrees of success. Many children regain normal strength, although some are left with muscle weakness.

Peroneal muscular atrophy (Charcot–Marie–Tooth; hereditary motor and sensory neuropathy) syndrome

Peroneal muscular atrophy (PMA) is the commonest chronic inherited neuropathy in childhood. Various forms of it are known and are based on electrophysiological and DNA studies. Most families show autosomal dominant inheritance, but autosomal recessive and X-linked forms can occur. Approximately 60% have onset of symptoms in the first decade of life.

Pes cavus, loss of foot dorsiflexion and eversion, hyporeflexia and sensory loss are typical clinical features in childhood. However, relatively asymptomatic children may present because of a family history, while others present with gait disturbance, particularly toe walking, frequent falling or poor coordination. Weakness and wasting in the legs may progress slowly and distal weakness in the arms is sometimes seen. Thickened peripheral nerves can occasionally be palpated.

The diagnosis can be confirmed by a nerve conduction study but readily available DNA studies are the usual first step in diagnosis. The DNA studies show a duplicated region on chromosome 17p (*PMP-22* gene). Parents of children with suspected PMA should be examined.

No cure is available but ankle–foot orthoses or orthopaedic procedures to correct foot deformity are often required and helpful. Progression is only relatively slow, with patients leading a fairly full life.

Children with neuromuscular disease often do not have all the clinical features seen in adults and sometimes it is the family history that gives the vital clue.

Clinical example

Claudine, a 5-year-old girl, was seen by her paediatrician because of frequent falling. He found mild ataxia of gait and areflexia but no other abnormality. There was an extensive family history (autosomal dominant inheritance pattern) of a chronic neuropathy consistent with peroneal muscular atrophy. Claudine's mother was asymptomatic.

Examination of Claudine's mother revealed minor sensory loss in the feet and hyporeflexia. Both mother and child had DNA evidence of the *PMP-22* gene duplication, confirming the diagnosis of peroneal muscular atrophy.

The clinical severity of PMA varies considerably and some adults can be asymptomatic. Careful clinical examination of a parent and further diagnostic studies sometimes unmask the apparent missing link. The absence of foot deformity or sensory disturbance in a child does not exclude PMA.

Neuromuscular junction disorders

Acute

Infant botulism

Infant botulism results from the production of *Clostridium botulinum* exotoxin in the gastrointestinal tract. It differs from botulism associated with food poisoning, in which there is ingestion of preformed toxin from contaminated food. In infant botulism, botulinum spores are ingested, with honey implicated in some cases. The disease usually occurs in infants under 9 months of age.

Constipation for days or weeks typically precedes the onset of symptoms of floppiness, weakness and ptosis, which occur over hours or 1–2 days at most. Feeding and swallowing difficulty, a poor cough, weak cry, hyporeflexia and respiratory insufficiency are typical. Extraocular movements may be impaired and dilated; sluggishly reacting pupils are often seen and can be helpful diagnostically. Deterioration may be rapid, with many patients requiring artificial ventilation for up to 2 months while the neuromuscular junctions regrow.

Diagnosis is clinical, supported by isolation of the organism and its toxin from faeces. Treatment is supportive. Botulinum antitoxin has been used but has not been shown to be helpful. Human intravenous botulism immune globulin (BabyBIG) may have a place in therapy if the child is treated early. The prognosis is excellent, with full recovery unless complications from cerebral hypoxia intervene. Prompt recognition and transfer to a facility capable of long-term ventilatory support is essential.

Chronic

Autoimmune myasthenia gravis

Myasthenia gravis in most children has an autoimmune basis, with antibody directed against neuromuscular junction postsynaptic acetylcholine receptors. Onset occurs at any time from the second year of life onwards. Symptoms are present for less than 1 month in the majority of patients and many have an episode of respiratory failure if untreated. Symptoms and signs are similar to those in adults, although relatively more prepubertal patients have only ocular problems. Ptosis, eye movement disorder, diplopia, difficulty chewing and swallowing, and slurred speech with or without predominantly proximal limb muscle weakness of recent onset should raise the suspicion of myasthenia gravis. Fatigability, the hallmark of myasthenia, is usually prominent, but this is not invariable.

Suspicion of myasthenia gravis should trigger an urgent diagnostic assessment. Diagnosis is based on clinical observation of fatigability, often best seen in the upper eyelid, response to intravenous or intramuscular anticholinesterase agents such as edrophonium or neostigmine, repetitive nerve stimulation and assay of acetylcholine receptor antibodies. Symptomatic relief may be obtained by oral administration of an anticholinesterase, commonly pyridostigmine. Corticosteroids, thymectomy, intravenous immunoglobulin and plasmaphaeresis have a role in selected circumstances. Although myasthenia gravis is a serious long-term and potentially fatal disorder, the disease remits in some children.

Transient neonatal myasthenia gravis

Transient neonatal myasthenia gravis occurs in about 10% of offspring of mothers with myasthenia gravis. It is due to placental transfer of antiacetylcholine receptor antibodies from a myasthenic mother to her fetus during pregnancy. This was one of the reasons why a humoral mechanism for myasthenia gravis was considered highly likely, prior to proof of this mechanism by passive transfer of myasthenia from human to mouse accomplished in the mid-1970s.

Onset of symptoms is not immediately after birth but is usually in the first 96 hours; feeding difficulty, respiratory difficulty and weakness or hypotonia are the main features. Myasthenic symptoms in the mother may be minimal. Appropriate supportive measures and anticholinesterase medication are used until the syndrome resolves over the ensuing weeks. This correlates with the expected diminution of passively transferred IgG antiacetylcholine antibodies that had been transferred from mother to infant. The infant returns to normal and does not subsequently have myasthenia gravis.

Congenital myasthenic syndromes

Congenital myasthenic syndromes are not one disease but many different rare genetic–biochemical disorders of the neuromuscular junction encompassing both the pre- and postsynaptic regions. They are not autoimmune disorders. Detailed electrophysiological and morphological testing, available in only a few laboratories, is usually required to diagnose and characterize these disorders definitively. Hypotonia, limb weakness, facial weakness, ptosis, ophthalmoplegia and apnoeic episodes, particularly with infections, may be seen but the emphasis varies with the particular syndrome. Some show improvement with time despite life-threatening episodic apnoea in infancy, while others have more persistent problems. Individuals do not have acetylcholine receptor antibodies. Some respond to anti-anticholinesterase preparations while others do not or worsen. As these are not autoimmune disorders, immunomodulatory therapies normally used in myasthenia gravis are without benefit.

Muscle disorders

Acute myopathies

Myopathic disorders with acute onset of weakness are uncommon. Snake bite or drugs may rarely trigger rhabdomyolysis or acute muscle breakdown. The dominantly inherited, sometimes fatal, syndrome of malignant hyperthermia during anaesthesia causes muscle necrosis and myoglobinuria. This disorder is associated with central core disease (see below). Rhabdomyolysis with myoglobinuria appears occasionally after an upper respiratory tract infection or after exercise and is probably related to an underlying metabolic disorder of muscle.

Chronic myopathies

Congenital myopathies

The congenital myopathies are a group of inherited disorders clinically relatively non-specific but with specific or distinctive findings on morphological analysis of the muscle biopsy. Advances in histochemical and electron microscopy techniques over the last 30–40 years have enabled characterization of patients into well-defined myopathies, whereas previously they were given non-specific diagnoses such as 'floppy infant syndrome'. The identification of these disorders allows important genetic and prognostic information to be given to the family.

These myopathies, usually inherited, are characterized by onset of weakness and hypotonia at or shortly after birth, or occasionally later in childhood or adulthood. Weakness may be mild or severe and is usually only slowly progressive. Pathologically there are structural changes in individual muscle fibres or variations in the number or size of the muscle fibre types.

Some of the well recognized disorders are central core myopathy (Fig. 17.3.2) and nemaline myopathy.

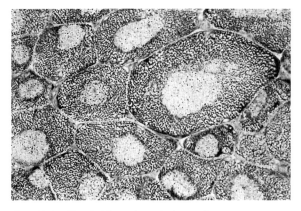

Fig. 17.3.2 Muscle biopsy in central core disease.

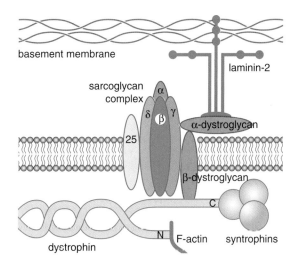

Fig. 17.3.4 Subsarcolemmal cytoskeleton.

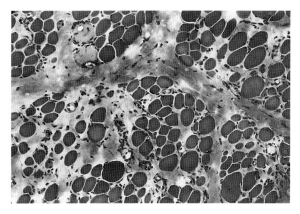

Fig. 17.3.3 Dystrophic muscle biopsy.

Practical points

- In a family exhibiting autosomal dominant inheritance of a muscle disorder consistent with a congenital myopathy, central core disease should be considered a possibility and precautions taken against malignant hyperthermia if an anaesthetic is given (e.g. for a muscle biopsy)

Progressive muscular dystrophies

The muscular dystrophies are a group of inherited disorders of muscle characterized by weakness presenting from birth to late adulthood, with the common feature being the pathological appearance of dystrophic muscle (Fig. 17.3.3). These disorders primarily affect skeletal muscle but other tissues may be involved; for example, congenital muscular dystrophy may be associated with white matter abnormalities in the brain. The dystrophies are the commonest serious muscle diseases and as a group place a significant burden on the patient, the family and the community in medical, social and economic terms.

The various forms of muscular dystrophy share a common pathogenesis of muscle plasma membrane instability secondary to the lack of, or abnormality of, proteins and glycoproteins linking the subsarcolemmal cytoskeleton to the extracellular matrix (Fig. 17.3.4). Not all dystrophies have had the absent or abnormal protein characterized. Absence or dysfunction of these structural proteins makes the muscle fibre more prone to damage.

Many of the muscular dystrophies share common clinical features, although the severity varies. The age of onset, pattern of weakness, family history and relatively specific findings on examination are important in diagnosing the type of muscular dystrophy. Some of the muscular dystrophies are named because of their pattern of weakness but these labels will probably change with the identification of specific protein defects.

The clinical features of some muscular dystrophies are described below.

Duchenne muscular dystrophy

Duchenne muscular dystrophy (DMD) is the most common muscular dystrophy, occurring in 1 in 3500 live male births. It is an X-linked disorder and occurs nearly exclusively in males. It is a disease of devastating proportions as it is progressive, it has significant genetic implications, there are no curative treatments available and it has serious medical complications. It causes death in the second or third decade and ranks high on the list of devastating diseases as judged by its effect on the person, the family and the requirements for community resources.

DMD is caused by a mutation at the Xp21 chromosome site. This causes a lack of dystrophin, a muscle protein that is thought to be important in the stability of the muscle membrane. Two-thirds of patients have a family history of muscular dystrophy or are isolated cases with an unsuspecting female carrier in the family, while one-third appear to arise as spontaneous mutations.

Development in the first year of life is usually normal. The first symptoms are usually recognized from 18 months to 4 years of age, with delayed walking being the most common presenting complaint. Approximately 50% of children with DMD do not walk before 18 months of age. Abnormal walking or running, toe walking, difficulty in climbing, difficulty in getting up from the floor or chair, and frequent falls are other prominent early features. A significant percentage of children will also have developmental problems other than motor delay, such as intellectual impairment or delayed language development. The intellectual impairment and language delay are non-progressive and mean IQ is approximately 85. While many are intellectually normal, some children are moderately intellectually disabled. The dual problems of motor and intellectual disabilities are severely incapacitating socially and educationally.

Proximal muscle weakness accounts for the motor difficulties. This can be demonstrated on formal testing or alternatively by functional testing, such as getting the child to rise from the floor. Typically, with this action the Gowers sign is exhibited (Fig. 17.3.5). A Gowers sign is not specific for DMD and is seen in other disorders with proximal muscle weakness. Enlargement (pseudohypertrophy) and firmness of the calf, quadriceps and triceps muscles is commonly seen (Fig. 17.3.6).

Some variability in course is exhibited from child to child, although the following generalizations encompass most children with DMD. Between the ages of 4 and 6 years there is an apparent improvement in mobility, with the children typically performing new motor activities. This is because normal muscle development (and regeneration) outstrips the degenerative process. After this period of improvement, relentless decline in function occurs, with increasing proximal and distal weakness in the limbs. Trunk muscles are also weakened. This leads to a worsening waddling gait, increasing lumbar lordosis and increasing equinovarus foot deformities.

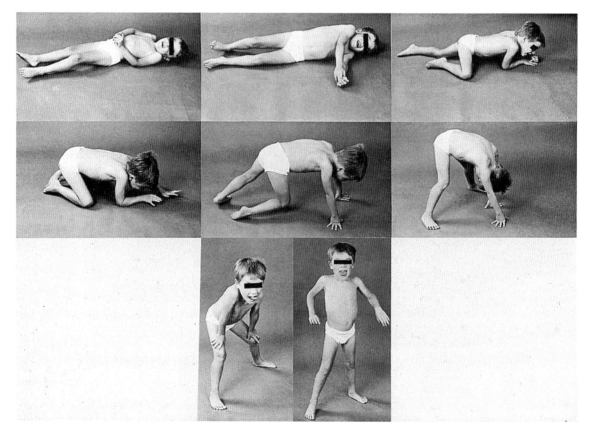

Fig. 17.3.5 The Gowers sign in a patient with Duchenne muscular dystrophy, illustrating the sequence of manoeuvres required to rise from the supine position. (With permission from Williams 1982.)

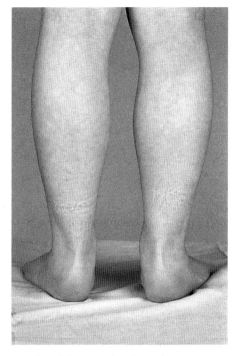

Fig. 17.3.6 Pseudohypertrophy of muscles.

Independent mobility is lost, usually between 8 and 13 years of age, with the child becoming wheelchair-bound, after which scoliosis generally develops. During the second decade of life there is a gradual decline in pulmonary function, related to the scoliosis and progressive muscle weakness. Death is usually due to respiratory complications, although cardiac failure secondary to a cardiomyopathy can occur. Cardiac arrhythmias may be a terminal event.

The diagnosis of DMD should be based on the family history (if any), clinical features, serum CK, DNA deletion testing and muscle biopsy. Pathological confirmation of the diagnosis is essential except where the diagnosis has been confirmed in another family member or by a DNA deletion. The CK is a reliable screening test and is invariably grossly elevated in a child with DMD, even from the neonatal period. Conversely, a normal CK test after the neonatal period excludes the later development of DMD.

Effective genetic counselling can be offered only if the first case in the family is diagnosed before other affected males are born. The early diagnosis of DMD can be facilitated by using the following criteria for ordering serum creatine kinase estimations in males:

- known or suspected family history of dystrophy
- male not walking before 18 months of age without obvious cause

- unexplained gait disturbance (particularly toe walking)
- unexplained mental retardation
- unexplained language delay.

Detection and counselling of female carriers is a most important aspect of family management. The male offspring of a known carrier have a 50% risk of having DMD, while 50% of female offspring will be carriers. Females may still be carriers even though there is no other family history. Only 60% of known carriers have an elevated CK level and hence a normal level does not exclude the carrier state. DNA technology can now be applied to offer antenatal diagnosis by detecting deletions from the X chromosome or by linkage analysis.

Currently there is no cure for muscular dystrophy. Corticosteroids may provide symptomatic improvement in strength, with the prolongation of ambulation. The prolongation of ambulation decreases the complications associated with being wheelchair-bound.

Management involves a very positive approach to satisfying the emotional, social and educational needs of the child and his family, together with judicious use of physiotherapy, orthotic devices and surgery for orthopaedic deformity.

Practical points

- The commonest reason for the late diagnosis of Duchenne muscular dystrophy is not thinking of the diagnosis in a young male with delayed motor, mental or language development

Becker muscular dystrophy

Becker muscular dystrophy is a disorder allelic to DMD but much less common. It is less severe than DMD and has a variable age of presentation.

Facioscapulohumeral syndrome

Facioscapulohumeral (FSH) muscular dystrophy is a relatively common autosomal dominant disorder that predominantly affects the shoulder girdle, in particular the periscapular, humeral and facial muscles. It is a relatively mild disorder with very slow progression. Onset is commonly in adolescence or early adult life, although occasionally it may be very early childhood.

In a typical case, facial muscle weakness is one of the first symptoms. Patients have difficulty closing the eyes, blowing out the cheeks, whistling or sucking through a straw. The shoulder girdle weakness usually begins at the same time as the facial weakness is noted and can be quite asymmetric. Symptoms include difficulty lifting the arms above the head. There is obvious winging of the scapulae in adult patients but this may not be so obvious in children. On abduction of the shoulders, the scapulae move upwards and give the shoulders a characteristic appearance. Foot drop is not uncommon. An infantile form has been described that presents with more severe weakness. The infantile form of FSH dystrophy is associated with deafness and visual loss.

The locus for autosomal dominant FSH has been mapped to the distal arm of chromosome 4.

Sensorineural hearing loss and Coats disease, a proliferative retinopathy, are associated with early-onset FSH dystrophy. Aggressive treatment of these associated disorders is important.

Myotonic disorders

These are a clinically heterogeneous group, with myotonia being the characteristic clinical feature. Myotonia is the inability of muscles to relax after voluntary contraction or stimulation. Myotonia can be detected during attempted relaxation of a voluntary contraction, such as after shaking hands or eyelid closure, by percussion of a muscle or by electromyography. Older children may describe myotonia as stiffness or cramping.

Many of these disorders have been shown to be due to defects of muscle ion channels. In some instances different mutations within the one gene can cause myotonia and/or periodic paralysis.

Myotonia congenita (Thomsen disease)

Autosomal dominant and autosomal recessive forms occur. Onset is in infancy or early childhood with symptoms due to myotonia, such as stiffness, difficulty initiating rapid movements and sometimes feeding difficulties. Muscle hypertrophy is common. The myotonia decreases with continued activity and may be aggravated by cold. Improvement occurs with increasing age. Symptomatic relief of myotonia with quinine or mexiletine may be useful.

Myotonic dystrophy (Steinert disease)

Myotonic dystrophy is an autosomal dominant disorder but an affected parent may be relatively asymptomatic and not diagnosed until detailed examination and investigation is undertaken. The disease is due to an excessive number of repeats of the sequence CTG on the long arm of chromosome 19 and this can be used for diagnostic testing in difficult cases and for antenatal diagnosis. The spectrum of clinical severity in myotonic dystrophy is extremely broad, requiring genetic testing to help clarify the diagnosis in minimally affected patients.

Juvenile type
The clinical features are similar to those seen in adults, with distal muscle weakness, wasting and myotonia, an expressionless face due to facial muscle weakness, and ptosis. Cataracts, frontal alopecia, testicular atrophy, cardiopulmonary insufficiency and dementia may occur in adult life.

Congenital type
A syndrome of hypotonia, weakness, arthrogryposis, feeding difficulty, respiratory difficulty and marked facial weakness all present at birth, along with other dysmorphic features, has been recognized. Invariably, the mother has myotonic dystrophy. Intellectual disability is common if the child survives the neonatal period.

Clinical example

Mrs McGill, aged 25 years, had myotonic dystrophy, as did her father, sister and brother. She had a son and twin daughters who were normal at birth and who remained asymptomatic. Her next child, Tessa, was 4 weeks premature and at birth was very hypotonic, had some respiratory difficulty and required gavage feeding. There was marked bilateral facial weakness, talipes equinovarus and mild flexion deformity at the knees. The respiratory and feeding difficulties gradually resolved, but the facial muscle weakness remained and Tessa later showed delay in motor and language milestones. There was no clinical myotonia when she was seen at 3 years of age.

Tessa had typical features of the congenital form of myotonic dystrophy, which typically occurs if it is the mother who is the affected parent. Some babies are stillborn, while others do not survive the neonatal period. Tessa was only moderately affected and will survive into adult life, but will almost certainly require special schooling. The dominant inheritance is clear from the family history. Mrs McGill and her husband wanted to know if the other children might develop the disease. Although they were asymptomatic at the time, there was still a chance that they had inherited the abnormal gene. DNA testing for the triplet expansion on chromosome 19 could be used to allow antenatal diagnosis.

Practical points

• Facial diplegia with respiratory difficulty or pharyngeal incoordination in a neonate should raise the suspicion of congenital myotonic dystrophy

Inflammatory myopathy

Acute viral myositis

Acute viral myositis is a clinically recognizable syndrome of acute onset of pain and tenderness of the gastrocnemius and soleus muscles several days after an upper respiratory tract infection, often with influenza B virus. Recovery occurs in a few days.

Chronic inflammatory myopathy

This may occur as 'idiopathic' disorders, such as dermatomyositis or polymyositis, or as part of a recognized collagen vascular disease.

Metabolic myopathies

A large number of individually uncommon metabolic disorders may produce episodic, acute or chronic muscle weakness, hypotonia, stiffness or cramping, exercise intolerance or myoglobinuria. Symptoms are sometimes accentuated or precipitated by exercise, rest after exercise, fasting or excessive carbohydrate intake.

The underlying metabolic defects usually are in glycogen metabolism (e.g. Pompe disease), lipid metabolism (e.g. carnitine deficiency, carnitine palmitoyltransferase deficiency), potassium metabolism (e.g. the periodic paralyses associated with hyper-, hypo- or normokalaemia) or a variety of mitochondrial functions (e.g. myopathies with cytochrome oxidase deficiency and Kearns–Sayre syndrome of progressive external ophthalmoplegia).

Knowledge of the underlying metabolic causes of many of these disorders is increasing and the hope is that, once the underlying pathophysiological processes are elucidated, more specific and effective therapies will become available.

The 'floppy' infant syndrome

Hypotonia, or floppiness, is a common observation in infancy and has many different causes. Normal muscle tone depends not only on the peripheral neuromuscular system but also on spinal cord and higher centres. Indeed, disorders affecting the central nervous system are more frequently the cause of the floppy infant syndrome than peripheral neuromuscular causes. Muscle tone is assessed by observation of posture, assessment of the resistance of joints to passive movements and of range of movement.

When an infant or young child is found to be significantly hypotonic, an important question is whether the hypotonia is 'central' or 'peripheral' in origin. Hypotonia of peripheral neuromuscular origin usually is associated with significant weakness (e.g. Werdnig–Hoffmann disease), while central hypotonia is usually not associated with significant weakness (e.g. Down syndrome or Prader–Willi syndrome). In practice, the differentiation in early childhood can sometimes be quite difficult. Apart from the absence of significant weakness, clues to a central cause of hypotonia may be:

- a history of adverse perinatal events
- abnormal behaviour in the neonatal period
- delayed mental development
- seizures
- abnormality of head size or shape
- the presence of normal or brisk deep tendon reflexes.

Hypotonia of peripheral neuromuscular origin is usually, but not invariably, accompanied by hyporeflexia in an alert baby with normal mental development.

Acknowledgements

I would like to thank Dr Lloyd K. Shield, who has been my mentor and the person who kindled my interest in neuromuscular disease. Dr Shield's previous contributions to this textbook form the major part of this chapter.

Large heads

A large head may be due to enlargement of the brain substance or the fluid-filled spaces of the brain. The more common causes include:

- a large cerebrum
- an oversized, overweight brain (as in megalencephaly)
- a dilated cerebrum (as in hydrocephalus)
- a tiny cerebrum (as with large chronic subdural hygromas)
- no cerebrum (as in hydranencephaly).

The two major categories of aetiology responsible for megalencephaly are anatomical and metabolic. A large head with normal-sized ventricles and normal neurodevelopmental examination may be related to familial factors, as in benign familial anatomical megalencephaly or macrocephaly. However, the large dolichocephalic head in cerebral gigantism will have large ventricles but normal ventricular pressure and associated limited intellect, poor coordination and coarse facial features.

Head enlargement in metabolic megalencephaly is a late manifestation of many cerebral degenerative disorders such as lysosomal storage diseases. Megalencephaly occurs in a wide variety of clinical disorders and syndromes, can be unilateral or bilateral, and is associated with a wide spectrum of developmental symptoms and signs. An acute increase in intracranial pressure should prompt consideration of the possibility of drug intoxication (tetracycline, vitamin A, nalidixic acid), lead encephalopathy, subdural haematoma and Reye syndrome.

Hydranencephaly is a condition of uncertain aetiology. The cerebral cortex is represented by a thin membrane composed of glial cells, with islands of cerebral cortex sometimes scattered in this tissue. The third ventricle, basal ganglia, brain stem and cerebellum are present but may reveal morphological abnormalities. The head size is usually normal at birth but increases rapidly within a few weeks of life.

Neurological function initially may be normal, shortly after gross neurological abnormality is evident (rigid muscle tone, tremors, and persistent and exaggerated primitive reflexes). Optic atrophy is common and the head transilluminates readily. The child sleeps excessively, is irritable, feeds poorly and has unstable thermoregulation. Electroencephalography reveals a flat tracing or a few low voltages over islands of cerebral cortex.

Hydrocephalus

Hydrocephalus (Greek: *hydro* meaning 'water', and *cephale,* 'head') refers to a group of conditions characterized by:

- an increase in cerebrospinal fluid (CSF) volume
- ventricular dilatation
- elevation of intraventricular pressure.

Hydrocephalus occurs when there is an imbalance between the formation and absorption of CSF. Impaired absorption is almost always due to some degree of obstruction along the CSF pathways. If the passage of CSF is obstructed within the ventricular system, the resultant hydrocephalus is labelled *non-communicating,* while if obstruction exists in the surface pathways, the hydrocephalus is described as being *communicating.* The rate of this volume change varies from patient to patient and depends in large part on the degree of obstruction. The lesions that commonly produce hydrocephalus are listed in Table 17.4.1.

In supratentorial lesions, CSF obstruction is a late event, so that neurological or endocrinological abnormalities often precede symptoms of raised intracranial pressure. Less commonly, cerebral tuberculoma, torular meningitis or an aneurysm of the vein of Galen may simulate intracranial neoplasms. The latter should be suspected if, in addition to hydrocephalus, a loud intracranial bruit, high output failure and vascular naevi are also present in the same patient.

Table 17.4.1 Lesions producing hydrocephalus

Non-communicating
Aqueduct stenosis or atresia
- Commonest site of intraventricular obstruction in infants with congenital hydrocephalus
- May occur as an isolated anomaly or be associated with myelomeningocele and the Arnold–Chiari malformation
- Histologically, subependymal gliosis around the aqueduct is demonstrable
- May be slowly progressive in some, not being clinically apparent for several years before obstructive symptoms appear

Sporadic
Familial
- Inherited as a sex-linked trait; features include a short flexed thumb, mental retardation and other cerebral abnormalities

Obstruction at the fourth ventricle
- Dandy–Walker syndrome
  - Cystic dilatation of the fourth ventricle, with cerebellar hypoplasia; other structural brain anomalies may also occur
  - Associated with atresia of the exit foramina of the fourth ventricle
  - Hydrocephalus may be present at birth or may develop subsequently
  - Diagnosis is suggested in typical cases by the shape of the skull and the presence of cerebellar signs
- Arachnoiditis

Obstruction due to intracranial mass lesions
- Should always be considered in any child where head enlargement develops in late infancy or childhood
- Neoplasm, cysts
  - Childhood tumours usually arise in the posterior cranial fossa and include medulloblastoma, astrocytoma and ependymoma
  - Intracranial pressure develops early, because of their close proximity to the fourth ventricle
  - Ataxia, incoordination, nystagmus and papilloedema are suggestive of the diagnosis
  - Differential diagnosis includes craniopharyngioma, gliomas, pinealomas and arachnoid cysts
- Haematoma
- Galenic vein aneurysm

Ventricular inflammations (rare)

Communicating
Arnold–Chiari malformation
With myelomeningocele (Type 2) (Fig 17.4.5)
Without myelomeningocele (Type 1)
- Consists of:
  - downward displacement and elongation of the hind brain
  - herniation of the medulla, cerebellar vermis and inferior part of the fourth ventricle into the upper cervical canal
- CSF flow is impaired, usually within the subarachnoid space
- Hydrocephalus usually develops in early infancy
- Frequently associated with cranium bifidum, myelomeningocele and hydromyelia

Encephalocele
Meningeal adhesions
Postinflammatory
Posthaemorrhagic
- May be secondary to neonatal meningitis (post inflammatory adhesions), or intraventricular or subarachnoid haemorrhage
- Hydrocephalus is common, and is usually communicating
- Neurological deficit, developmental delay and seizures are usually the result of the infective process, but the hydrocephalus, if not relieved, will aggravate the brain injury

Choroid plexus papilloma
- A rare cause of hydrocephalus.
- Hydrocephalus is produced by excessive fluid secreted by the tumour, sometimes with obstruction to CSF flow
- Recurrent haemorrhage from the tumour may play a role
- Total excision of the tumour usually leads to a resolution of the hydrocephalic process

Clinical example

Ivan, a 5-year-old boy, presented with a 2-month history of early morning headache and vomiting. This was associated with a decline in his school performance and he was noted to be increasingly unsteady on his feet. The significant findings on examination included a wide-based, unsteady gait, horizontal nystagmus and severe bilateral papilloedema. A computed tomography (CT) scan revealed the presence of a large mass in the cerebellar vermis, which was distorting the fourth ventricle.

Ivan underwent a craniotomy and the tumour arising in the cerebellar vermis was excised. Following operation the symptoms of raised intracranial pressure subsided and serial CT scans showed a resolution of the dilated lateral and third ventricles.

With this patient, excision of the obstructing mass was an effective form of treatment for a significant degree of non-communicating hydrocephalus. The presenting symptoms were in part due to raised intracranial pressure and in part due to interference with cerebellar function.

Approach to clinical diagnosis

The clinical appraisal of the hydrocephalic child involves:

- the establishment of the diagnosis
- elucidation of the aetiology
- assessment of neurological and mental function
- a search for other associated malformations.

It is essential to determine the age and rapidity of onset of hydrocephalus and its rate of progression. In most clinical situations, the child presents with a large head, which may already be apparent at birth or at a few months of age. Despite the obviously large head, many babies thrive and may develop normally, apart from poor head control. Other infants with hydrocephalus, however, feed poorly, are irritable, vomit excessively and fail to gain weight. In infants with congenital hydrocephalus, the birth weight, nature of delivery and neonatal course should be noted. In addition, enquiry as to whether there has been a similar illness in an older sibling or possible intrauterine infection is relevant.

Hydrocephalus that develops in an older and previously normal child suggests the possibility of a posterior fossa neoplasm. Because ventricular dilatation is generally subacute in children with cerebellar tumours, symptoms of raised intracranial pressure are often associated with changes in behaviour, a clumsy gait, abnormal articulation, tremors and incoordination. If elevation of ventricular pressure occurs abruptly, attacks of nausea, vomiting, head retraction and extensor spasms are prominent.

In very ill children, symptoms of a primary illness, such as cranial infection and haemorrhage, may obscure symptoms of intracranial hypertension. It is important in all cases to ascertain any neurological symptoms, determine the time of onset of head enlargement and assess the developmental progress of the child.

In children with myelomeningocele and shunted hydrocephalus, raised intracranial pressure is usually secondary to a blocked shunt. Children may present with features typical of a blocked shunt (irritability, headache, somnolence, vomiting, loss of consciousness) but may also present with atypical features such as seizures or unusual behaviours. Diagnosis requires exclusion of other underlying causes, and a high index of suspicion prompting the clinician to question shunt dysfunction.

Clinical example

William was an 11-year-old boy with spina bifida and shunted hydrocephalus. During the course of the clinical consultation as part of long-term follow-up of his condition, he complained that he had been experiencing some facial pain on the right side of his face for the past 3 days. He had a decreased appetite and his mother noted that he had been confused about his daily routine, which surprised her.

On examination, William had a flaccid lower limb paralysis and was wheelchair-mobile. He had mild hyperreflexia in his upper limbs and nystagmus of gaze, both long-standing problems associated with his condition. His shunt appeared to empty, but was slow to refill. His fundi did not show evidence of papilloedema. There was no history of recent trauma or infection to explain his facial pain, and it was decided that he should have a CT scan to exclude hydrocephalus as a cause. This revealed enlarged ventricles and William was taken to theatre that day by the neurosurgical team to revise his shunt.

In this situation, the classical signs of raised intracranial pressure were not present and diagnosis of shunt dysfunction required a high index of suspicion. This boy might well have progressed to developing further signs later but by then the risk of an adverse outcome would probably have increased.

Physical examination

Classically, hydrocephalus is recognized by a progressive increase in occipitofrontal head circumference out of proportion to other bodily dimensions. A single head circumference measurement that greatly exceeds the 97th percentile strongly suggests the existence of hydrocephalus. Where head enlargement is equivocal, and neurological abnormality is absent, serial head measurements will often indicate the need for further diagnostic studies. It must be emphasized that, once enlargement of the skull is clinically obvious, the ventricles are already grossly dilated and the cerebral cortex is thinned.

Clinical signs that frequently precede obvious enlargement of the head include:

- a large and bulging fontanelle
- thinning of the bones of the calvarium
- widening of the coronal, sagittal and lambdoidal sutures.

With advancing hydrocephalus:

- the scalp thins and becomes shiny and pale
- there is upward retraction of the eyelids
- the eyes are fixed in a downward gaze (the 'setting sun' sign)
- hair appears sparse
- superficial scalp veins become distended
- the brow overhangs the small, triangular face.

Despite the enormous head size, papilloedema is uncommon in congenital hydrocephalus. The shape of the skull should be noted. A large protruding occiput is typical of a Dandy–Walker cyst, while an asymmetrical head may be due to unilateral obstruction at the foramen of Monro. In addition, auscultation for cranial bruit should be performed over the eyeballs and over the calvarium.

Many mildly affected hydrocephalic children have remarkably normal development and minimal neurological deficit. Gross abnormalities in a child with mild hydrocephalus are usually related to the underlying disorder that caused the hydrocephalus. However, prolonged stretching and compression of neural structures will lead ultimately to profound neurological injury. Where the increase in intracranial pressure is rapid and there has been no compensatory increase in head size, the highly irritable child frequently gives a short, high-pitched 'cerebral cry'. During these screaming episodes, decerebrate posturing may be evident. In the older child with 'arrested' hydrocephalus, it is important to evaluate the mental and psychological status. These children are frequently talkative, jovial and euphoric ('cocktail party syndrome') but their capacity for concentration, language comprehension and abstract thinking is often lacking. Manifestations of long-standing hydrocephalus include a variety of endocrinological and metabolic disorders such as precocious puberty, diabetes insipidus and abnormal thermoregulation. Various anomalies, particularly neural tube defects, skeletal defects and cutaneous naevi, are known to coexist with obstructive hydrocephalus.

Investigations

The child's assessment, based on the history and examination, will often enable a diagnosis of hydrocephalus to be made with some degree of certainty. However, in all cases, investigations are required to confirm the diagnosis, determine the extent of the disorder and if possible define the aetiology. Investigations are also of assistance in deciding the need or otherwise for active treatment and also as a means of assessing the success or otherwise of treatment. The plain skull X-ray may be a useful initial investigation.

Ultrasound

The widespread use of ultrasound scanning (Fig. 17.4.1) has in recent times greatly facilitated the assessment of infants with suspected hydrocephalus. Real-time ultrasound imaging through the open fontanelle provides a clear demonstration of the ventricles and may define other structural anomalies well. This non-invasive risk-free investigation can be undertaken with little or no sedation and can be repeated as often as required. When the fontanelle closes, satisfactory imaging can no longer be obtained. Ultrasound examination during pregnancy can indicate whether the fetus has hydrocephalus.

Computed tomography

In the older child, and occasionally in infants where more detail is required, computed tomography (CT) scanning (Fig. 17.4.2) is the investigation of choice.

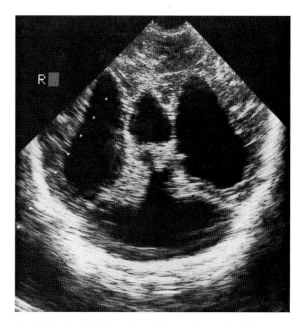

Fig. 17.4.1 Frontal view of a real-time ultrasound study showing markedly dilated lateral ventricles on either side of a large posterior fossa cyst in a patient with Dandy–Walker malformation.

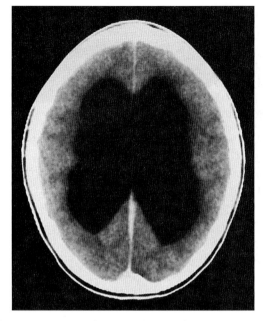

Fig. 17.4.2 Computed tomography scan demonstrating gross ventricular dilatation in hydrocephalus.

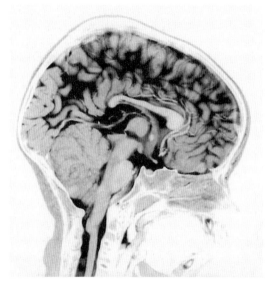

Fig. 17.4.3 Magnetic resonance image of a child with a spina bifida showing the Arnold–Chiari malformation. Note the herniation of the cerebellum into the upper cervical canal.

This technique provides excellent detail of the intracranial anatomy and the images may be enhanced by the injection of contrast material. Many children can have CT scans without sedation while others will require sedation or occasionally a general anaesthetic. The radiation involved in a single scan is of an acceptable degree but a limitation should be placed on repeated studies.

Magnetic resonance imaging
Magnetic resonance imaging (MRI) (Fig. 17.4.3) is rarely undertaken as a primary investigation but may be of value in defining the cause of the condition. Small tumours in the region of the aqueduct causing obstruction to CSF flow may not be visualized by a CT scan but are clearly defined by an MRI study. Special techniques can visualize CSF flow patterns.

Treatment

The indications for treatment are based on a clear understanding of the natural history of the disorder. Three patterns may be described:

- the process continues, followed by neurological deterioration
- the process progresses to a point, then stabilizes ('compensated hydrocephalus')
- the process is temporary.

In the majority of patients, the ventricles will continue to enlarge and the overlying brain will become

stretched, compressed and thinned. If the process starts in infancy before the skull bones have developed significant attachment to each other, massive head enlargement will result and under these circumstances significant brain injury will result. This type of progression will be detected by the presence and persistence of signs of raised pressure, an excessive rate of head growth and, less commonly, by the finding of neurological abnormality and developmental delay. Serial imaging will confirm progression of ventricular dilatation. In this group treatment is essential if brain injury is to be avoided or minimized.

In a lesser number of patients limited enlargement of the ventricles will occur and then cease. The term 'arrested hydrocephalus' has been applied to this group. The ventricles remain somewhat larger than normal but there are no clear signs of raised intracranial pressure and brain function appears normal. The head may be large but the rate of growth will either be normal or only slightly excessive and serial images will show no significant alternation in ventricle size. With this pattern, decisions regarding treatment are less well defined. If the degree of dilatation is mild to moderate there is no good evidence that treatment will influence the outcome favourably. Under these circumstances, frequent assessment is required to ensure that stability is maintained.

With the widespread use of head imaging techniques, it has become apparent that hydrocephalus may be a temporary state in certain circumstances. Posthaemorrhagic hydrocephalus in the low-birth-weight infant is often of this type, as is the disorder complicating certain forms of meningitis. In these patients it appears likely that the CSF pathways have regained their patency. These patients are usually defined by repeating imaging. Such studies would show reduction in size of ventricles to normal and this satisfactory state would be associated with the disappearance of all physical signs of progressive hydrocephalus. Obviously, no long-term treatment is required in this group but intermittent removal of CSF by either a lumbar puncture or a ventricular puncture may help to resolve the process and prevent any excess ventricular dilatation during the period before effective CSF flow is established via normal pathways. On occasions, a reservoir may be inserted into a lateral ventricle to facilitate such intermittent removal. In addition, drugs that reduce CSF production, such as acetazolamide and isosorbide, have been used with the same intent.

Operative treatment

The definitive treatment of hydrocephalus is a surgical procedure. The usual method of treatment is by a shunt that diverts the CSF to some other site in the body. In some cases of non-communicating hydrocephalus, ventriculostomy may successfully re-establish normal CSF pathways.

Ventriculoperitoneal shunt. This is the operation performed most frequently in paediatric patients with hydrocephalus. A Silastic catheter is placed in a lateral ventricle through a burr hole and the other end of the tube is passed subcutaneously to the abdomen and then placed in the peritoneal cavity. A valve is interposed and an adequate length of tube is placed in the peritoneal cavity to allow for growth. The peritoneum absorbs CSF effectively.

Ventriculoatrial shunt. In this procedure the lower end of the shunt is passed via a neck vein to the right atrium. The catheter is so designed so that CSF can pass from the catheter tip but blood cannot flow back into the lumen. The turbulent blood flow in the atrium prevents thrombus formation around the catheter. This operation is not undertaken often in childhood as maintenance may involve the lengthening of the atrial catheter on several occasions.

Complications of ventricular shunts

The operation is generally well tolerated with infrequent early difficulties. Common complications include meningitis, ventriculitis, and shunt obstruction.

The most common presentation of a child with a blocked shunt is that of a vague illness. Irritability and vomiting are frequent and headache may be present. The symptoms are very similar to those of many childhood illnesses and difficulties are often experienced in trying to decide whether the symptoms are a consequence of shunt malfunction or an unrelated illness. Definite signs of raised intracranial pressure, if present, are of great assistance but are often not ascertained readily. Palpation of the shunt mechanism may also frequently be inconclusive.

The treatment of shunt obstruction is usually a simple procedure and involves the replacement of the defective component. However, a small number of patients suffer from repeated episodes of obstruction and management can be difficult and may involve many variations of shunt equipment and surgical technique.

Clinical example

Sara, a 6-year-old child with a past history of having had a ventriculoperitoneal shunt inserted in infancy for congenital hydrocephalus, presented at the outpatient clinic for review having missed a previous planned attendance. Her mother stated that Sara was generally well but was concerned by her visual function. Sara insisted on sitting immediately adjacent to the television set and had been moved to the front of her class to enable her to see the blackboard.

When examined, Sara appeared to be generally well but head measurement indicated an excessive rate of growth. Her visual acuity was markedly diminished in each eye and funduscopy revealed severe secondary optic atrophy. On palpation the shunt tubing was disconnected and an immediate CT scan showed very large ventricles. The shunt was revised immediately but unfortunately there was no improvement in Sara's poor vision.

The shunt had obviously been malfunctioning for a prolonged period of time and had resulted in chronic raised intracranial pressure. Sara had not complained of any symptoms but the presence of intracranial pressure produced marked optic atrophy over this interval of time. If Sara had attended for the planned reviews, the abnormality might well have been recognized and corrected before visual deterioration resulted.

Neural tube defects

The term neural tube defect (NTD) refers to a group of malformations involving the brain and/or spinal cord in association with varying degrees of absence or malformation of the overlying tissues: meninges, bone, muscle and skin. *Myelomeningocele* (*myelo* meaning 'cord'; *meninges,* coverings of the spinal cord; *cele,* 'sac') involves all the tissue layers including the skin and bone and is an outpouching of the spinal cord through the posterior bony vertebral column that has failed to form. *Meningocele* is an outpouching of the meninges or coverings of the spinal cord only, and not the cord itself. The term *spina bifida* refers to the normal bony projection over the spine being divided or 'bifid'. *Spina bifida occulta* is the failure of the formation of the posterior elements of the vertebrae but without any out pouching of the meninges or spinal cord. It occurs in 5–10% of the population and is most often asymptomatic. X-rays of the spine documenting the incomplete vertebral arch confirm the diagnosis. Accompanying associated features may include dermal hyperpigmentation, a fatty swelling, a tuft of hair or a dermal sinus on the back. *Spina bifida cystica* refers to myelomeningocele and meningocele. Myelomeningocele is the much more serious and much commoner type of spina bifida cystica. *Spinal dysraphism,* which includes spina bifida occulta, meningocele and myelomeningocele, is part of the family of neural tube defects that encompasses abnormalities of the cranium and its contents (anencephaly, encephalocele and cranial meningocele) as well as abnormalities of the spine.

Incidence

The incidence has varied in different countries, the highest rates being recorded in the past in Northern Ireland, the west of Scotland and south Wales. In South Australia, the total incidence of neural tube defects during 1966–1991 was 2.01 per 1000 births and the incidence of myelomeningocele was 0.97 per 1000 births, with no upward or downward trend. Despite the total incidence remaining stable, prenatal diagnosis and termination of pregnancy resulted in an 84% fall in the birth prevalence of all neural tube defects during the years studied. Screening by serum alpha-fetoprotein measurements or mid trimester ultrasonography, or both, detected over four-fifths of cases in 1986–1991 in South Australia.

Recurrence risks in families have been documented extensively. Recurrence risk statistics suggest a polygenic or environmental aetiology. The risk of recurrence following the birth of the first child with a neural tube defect is approximately 4–8%, or 1 in 25. The risk increases to at least 10% after the birth of two affected children.

Neural tube defects are found commonly in spontaneous first trimester miscarriages. Neural tube defects are more common in females and in lower socioeconomic groups and the incidence varies with different ethnic groups.

Embryology and pathogenesis

The neural tube is the embryological structure from which the brain and spinal cord develop. The human neural tube closes just before the 30th day post fertilization and thus any influence affecting the closure of the neural tube must be present before this early stage of pregnancy. The typical motor, sensory and sphincter dysfunctions of spina bifida and myelodysplasia are the most evident clinical manifestations but represent only one aspect of this complex teratological anomaly. There is a high incidence of gross and microscopic brain-stem, cerebellar and cerebral malformations. The aetiology of neural tube defects is still debated. Polygenic inheritance and environmental and teratogenic factors have been implicated. It has been unequivocally demonstrated that vitamin supplementation with folic acid reduces the incidence of recurrence in high-risk populations. Dietary factors may therefore play a major part in low-risk populations. Many other potential aetiological causes have been examined also during the last 20 years.

Antenatal diagnosis, antenatal counselling and fetal surgery

The presence of abnormally high levels of alpha-fetoprotein in the amniotic fluid has a high correlation with myelomeningocele. Alpha-fetoprotein is a component of fetal CSF and it probably leaks into the amniotic fluid from the open neural tube defect. Closed lesions often do not cause increased alpha-fetoprotein. The false-positive rate for the determination of myelomeningocele is less than 0.5% and the false-negative rate is 2%. Alpha-fetoprotein is synthesized by the yolk sac, hepatic cells and gastrointestinal tract of the fetus and is normally excreted in the amniotic fluid in fetal urine. The detection rate for open neural tube defects using maternal serum screening is approximately 80%, with a low false-positive rate. Ultrasonography can detect or confirm the extent of the neural tube defect.

Offering counselling for the family with an antenatal diagnosis of a neural tube defect is important, especially as the family will probably consider their options about whether to continue with the pregnancy or elect for termination. Great care should be taken about the information conveyed. Preferably, it should be given by a specialist experienced in caring for children with a neural tube defect, in an appropriate environment and with time available to answer the family's questions about all the facets of raising a child with this diagnosis. The antenatal scan can offer some guidance but it must be remembered that ultrasound scan findings cannot predict all aspects of functioning (physical and cognitive) accurately. In addition, families can be offered further counselling through community-based organizations (e.g. the Spina Bifida and Hydrocephalus Association). All families should be made aware of preventative measures (periconceptional folate) and offered genetic counselling if they wish to have other children in the future.

Fetal surgery (for closure of the myelomeningocele lesion) at 20–30 weeks gestation, after which the fetus is returned to the uterus, has been developed with the hope of preventing significant complications in the affected child. Early studies have demonstrated good cosmetic closure of the lesion but the complication rate (primarily due to the fetus being delivered prematurely) was found to be high. There is currently a randomized control trial being undertaken in the USA. The primary outcome is a significant reduction of the development of hydrocephalus in the treatment group. Until the results of this important trial are completed, however, this mode of treatment cannot be recommended.

Clinical features

Neural tube defects may be classified as in Table 17.4.2.

Management of myelomeningocele

A team approach that includes the parents is essential for the proper management of myelomeningocele. An important factor, which compounds the disability, is that the defect is apparent at birth. Information given to the parents and the manner in which it is conveyed will influence their reaction at this most vulnerable time and will affect the future of the child and the family. Medical specialists in this team include the neurosurgeon, orthopaedic surgeon and urologist. The medical team leader is most appropriately a paediatrician or paediatric rehabilitation specialist with special skills in the field of child development and rehabilitation. The medical team leader will coordinate care but, importantly, will also manage and advise on the multiple problems experienced by the children and their families. These include disability issues, school integration, interventions to improve functional outcome and various activities to support the parents and child through the many problems, both physical and psychological, that invariably arise. The physiotherapist, occupational therapist, orthotist, psychologist and medical social worker, together with trained hospital and community-based nursing staff and teachers, are important members of this team. The team has three major goals:

- to promote good health in the short and long term
- to promote maximum function in the child so that, as nearly as possible, normal developmental sequences and timing can be followed to enable maximal independence for the child and family
- to promote good family functioning.

Table 17.4.2   Classification of neural tube defects
Anencephaly • At birth, presents as an opened, malformed skull and brain • Most babies are stillborn • No effective treatment is possible • Death usually occurs within hours or days
Cranium bifidum **Cranial meningocele** • The underlying brain is normal • A meningeal sac protrudes through a skull defect
Encephalocele • A midline sac protrudes that may contain brain • Hydrocephalus is common

Spina bifida occulta
• One or more vertebral arches are incomplete posteriorly but the overlying skin is intact
• Diagnosed incidentally, e.g. as the result of an X-ray of the spinal column during other investigations
• Spinal cord usually normal; however, a number of abnormalities of the spinal cord have been described
• Ectodermal abnormalities may be associated:
  • a dermal pit
  • a depression with a tuft of hair
  • a fatty swelling (Fig. 17.4.4)
• The ectodermal component
  • may communicate with the dura
  • may pose some risk of intraspinal infection (if associated with a dural sinus)
• The fatty swelling may be a lipomeningocele
• The ectodermal component, if present, warrants full neurological examination

Spina bifida cystica
Myelomeningocele (Figs 17.4.5, 17.4.6), in which vertebral column skin, meninges and spinal cord are involved
Meningocele (Fig. 17.4.7), where the spinal cord is not involved
• Almost always obvious at birth (most frequently, a midline sac protrudes through a spinal defect (Fig. 17.4.4))
• May occur anywhere along the length of the spinal column
• The lumbar and lumbosacral regions are the most frequent anatomical levels
• Abnormal spinal cord tissue and nerve roots may be readily apparent macroscopically
• There may be spinal abnormalities such as kyphosis at the site of the lesion
• Functional deficits include:
  • paraplegia, with motor and sensory impairment
  • hydrocephalus
  • variable intellectual impairment
  • neuropathic sphincter dysfunction

Sacral agenesis

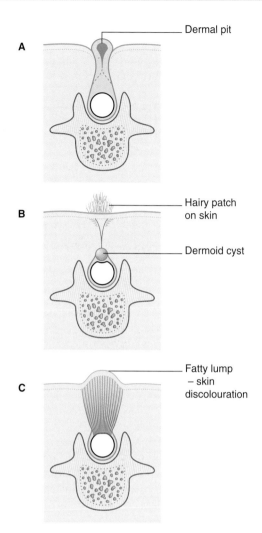

Fig. 17.4.4 Schematic representation of spina bifida occulta.
A. Dermal sinus. B. Intraspinal cyst pressing on the cord.
C. Lipomatous mass infiltrating the cord elements.

Specific problems in the management of the newborn with spina bifida

It is possible to predict with considerable accuracy the potential for future impairment in a number of areas. These include ambulation and subsequent mobility, probable bowel and bladder function, and hydrocephalus, with its probable sequelae. It is much more difficult to predict the effects that these impairments will have on the lifestyle of the individual and family. Also, it is possible to recognize early those lesions that are inoperable because of massive bony deformity and extensive skin loss, which would prevent closure of the defect. The specific problems are as follows:

1. children with high lesions (thoracic and thoracolumbar), significant hydrocephalus at birth, major kyphosis or other significant problems (either congenital or acquired) have a significantly

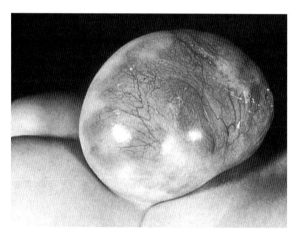

Fig. 17.4.5 A lumbosacral myelomeningocele.

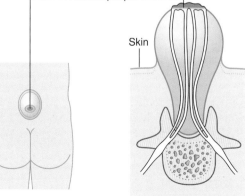

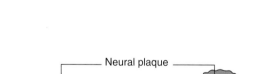

Transverse section

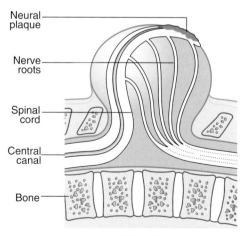

Longitudinal section

Fig. 17.4.6 Myelomeningocele: diagrammatic representation.

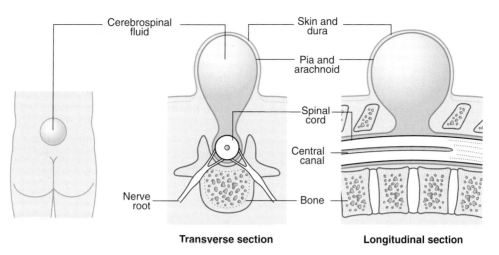

Fig. 17.4.7 Meningocele: diagrammatic representation.

increased mortality in early life and substantial morbidity if they survive. In these circumstances, in discussion with the family, supportive care only may be recommended. If the infant survives the perinatal period, elective surgical care may be indicated. In the absence of such adverse factors, in discussion with the family, early surgical repair/removal of the lesion usually is recommended.

2. careful serial evaluation of head circumference and ventricular size by ultrasound or CT scan will indicate if hydrocephalus is developing. Once it is established that progressive hydrocephalus is present, a shunt procedure is recommended.

3. baseline orthopaedic, urology and neurosurgery assessments provide the basis for ongoing discussions with the family and management of the condition. Occasionally, active urological intervention is required for urinary retention.

4. it is critical to begin to establish an empathetic, therapeutic relationship with the parents in the newborn period that forms the foundation for ongoing support throughout childhood.

Ongoing management issues

Management of physical disability and mobility

Physiotherapists play an essential role in reducing deformities and encouraging mobility. Foot deformities are common at birth as a result of unopposed muscular activity in utero. Splinting and passive stretching are the mainstays of treatment in early life. Persistent foot deformities may require corrective orthopaedic surgery. Surgery also may be needed for dislocated hips, particularly if the child is likely to walk. At times, three-dimensional gait analysis (3DGA) is beneficial for surgical decision making and can assist in planning for this intervention.

The outlook for walking depends on the level of the spinal cord lesion, intelligence and motivation. Most children with a lesion at L4 or lower will walk, with or without splints and crutches. Children with higher lesions may walk with orthotics in early childhood but most will choose wheelchair mobility by mid to late childhood.

Spinal deformities

A significant percentage of children will develop scoliosis and many of these will require spinal instrumentation. Spinal jackets are not well tolerated and have a very limited role in the management of paralytic scoliosis.

Neuropathic fracture

Fractures of the lower limbs, due to osteopenia, are common in children with myelomeningocele. Fractures may occur with minimal trauma. Encouraging children to walk, or stand in a standing frame on a regular basis may improve the mineralization of long bones and lessen the likelihood of further fractures. However, nutrition, calcium and vitamin D from sunlight may also be important factors in management.

Sensory deficit and skin care

Pressure ulcers or burns in anaesthetic areas are common. Parents are encouraged to check anaesthetic areas daily for the presence of pressure sores. Early recognition and treatment is essential to prevent long periods of morbidity and hospitalization.

Neuropathic bladder

Almost all children with myelomeningocele have a neuropathic bladder. Failure to empty the bladder may lead to recurrent urinary tract infections, vesicoureteric reflux, renal calculi and hydronephrosis. Hypertension and renal failure may be seen in a small number of cases. Management of the neuropathic bladder is by clean intermittent catheterization performed four or five times daily by the parents, and later by the child. This is usually commenced at around 3–4 years of age, or earlier if repeated urinary infections occur. Prophylactic antibiotics may be required for recurrent urinary infections. Bladder augmentation and/or artificial sphincter operations may be indicated if the clinical situation dictates. The use of anticholinergic medications and of oxybutynin to increase bladder capacity may be tried. Regular assessment of renal function is essential throughout the person's life.

Neuropathic bowel

Most children have limited or absent rectal sensation and have little or no bowel control. Constipation with megacolon, faecal impaction and overflow incontinence is the major risk in spina bifida. Faecal softeners may be needed in infancy. Some children can attain continence simply by regular toileting, while others may need high-fibre diets, faecal softeners, suppositories or microenemas. Aperients are avoided whenever possible. Refractory cases may require regular bowel washouts.

Sexual function

Many people with spina bifida achieve a satisfactory sexual relationship. In females, pregnancy has been achieved in many individuals and is generally a positive experience. Predictably, there are a number of potential difficulties with pregnancy and confinement. Urinary tract infections, worsening pressure sores and spinal problems are particularly common. In males, the situation is more complex. Difficulties range from impotence to retrograde ejaculation and infertility. Sexual counselling is important in adolescence.

Tethered spinal cord

Following repair of a myelomeningocele, the lower end of the spinal cord may become tethered to the site of repair. As the child grows, this may cause progressive neurological deterioration in motor or sensory function, or in bladder control. Regular monitoring of the neurological state is essential particularly during the rapidly growing phase. MRI scans are performed to demonstrate the tethering process. If the neurological deterioration is significant, consideration should be given to neurosurgical release of the tethered cord.

Arnold–Chiari malformation

This has been described earlier (Fig. 17.4.3). It is present in a significant number of children with myelomeningocele and is elegantly demonstrated by MRI scan. Symptoms are variable: they may be quite minor, e.g. strabismus or mild difficulties with chewing and swallowing, or they may be severe, with laryngeal stridor and apnoeic spells. Life-threatening episodes may necessitate neurosurgical intervention to decompress the posterior fossa.

Education

Children with myelomeningocele often have specific learning problems, requiring assistance at school. Overall intelligence is generally in the low average range, with a wide range of abilities. Verbal IQ is usually considerably higher than performance IQ, and many children have apparently very good expressive language but with a paucity of meaning and content of speech (often referred to as 'cocktail party syndrome'). Difficulties with mathematical concepts are very common, as are problems with abstract reasoning. Many children have a poor attention span, with distractibility. Problems with fine motor control and visual perceptual difficulties are frequently present. Most children with spina bifida attend normal schools, with varying levels of assistance for physical and cognitive/learning difficulties from support teachers. Schools may require modification to provide access and suitable toilet arrangements.

Social and emotional adjustment and transition to adulthood

A child with a chronic disability places severe strains on the emotional and financial resources of a family. Members of the team must be alert to signs of distress and be ready to provide the necessary support. During the teenage years, the usual problems of adolescence are superimposed on the difficulties associated with the disability, and these young people need sensitive counselling. For the families, parent groups provide valuable practical and emotional support.

There are now increasing numbers of young adults with spina bifida. A coordinated approach to management is still desirable but more difficult to attain, because of the wish of the young people to be independent and to break away from what they perceive as overprotection by the medical fraternity. Nevertheless, problems continue to occur, particularly pressure ulcers, shunt and urinary complications. In South Australia, the Spina Bifida and Hydrocephalus Association employs community nurses, who maintain close contact with all the adults with spina bifida and refer problems to appropriate agencies. This service has been invaluable in maintaining physical and emotional wellbeing and ongoing health education, and has helped to avoid hospital admissions among the group.

Prevention of neural tube defects

Neural tube defects (spina bifida, anencephaly and encephalocele) result from defective closure of the neural tube in early pregnancy. The human neural tube closes just before the 30th day post-fertilization and thus any influence affecting the closure of the neural tube must be present before this early stage of pregnancy. Primary prevention of this group of conditions may now be feasible. Research has suggested a relationship between maternal diet and the birth of an affected infant. Medical evidence has confirmed that folic acid (a water-soluble vitamin found in many fruits, leafy green vegetables, wholegrain breads, cereals and legumes) may prevent the majority of neural tube defects.

A randomized controlled clinical trial carried out by the Medical Research Council of the UK demonstrated a 72% reduction in risk of recurrence by periconceptional (i.e. before and after conception) folic acid supplementation of 4 mg daily. Other epidemiological research, including work done in Australia, suggests that primary occurrences of neural tube defect births may also be prevented by folic acid, either as a supplement or in the diet, and this has been confirmed in a randomized controlled trial from Hungary, which found that a daily multivitamin supplement containing 0.8 mg folic acid was effective in reducing the occurrence of neural tube defects in first births.

The National Health and Medical Research Council of Australia has recommended the following

- *All women planning a pregnancy or likely to become pregnant* should be offered advice about folate in the diet and encouraged to increase their dietary intake of folate-rich foods, particularly in the month before and in the first 3 months of pregnancy

In addition:
- *Low-risk women* (no family history of neural tube defects, not on anticonvulsants) should be offered periconceptional folic acid supplementation (0.5 mg daily). Generally, periconceptional supplementation with other vitamins is not necessary. When supplements are used, the potential risks of vitamin overdose should be considered. In particular, large therapeutic doses of vitamin A may predispose to birth defects

- *Women with a close family history of neural tube defects* (e.g. they or their partner has spina bifida, they have already had an affected child, they have a sibling or other close relative with a neural tube defect):
  - should be referred for genetic counselling
  - should be advised to take periconceptional folic acid supplementation 5 mg daily (the 4 mg formulation is not available in Australia)
  - should continue to be offered prenatal diagnosis with alpha-fetoprotein estimation and tertiary level ultrasound, by an operator experienced in anatomical scans, at 16–18 weeks gestation. Although the risk of recurrence is reduced significantly if folic acid supplementation is used appropriately, there is a residual risk of about 1% in women taking supplements who have had a previously affected infant
- *Women on anticonvulsant drugs* should take folic acid supplementation only under the supervision of and with close monitoring by their physician
  - because of the increased risk of neural tube defects in the offspring of women taking some anticonvulsants (notably sodium valproate), these women also should be counselled and offered prenatal diagnosis

Fortification of staple foods with folic acid
- Fortification of staple foods, such as bread and cereals, with folic acid should be introduced in Australia. After mandatory wheat flour fortifications in the US, there has been a 30% reduction of neural defects, with 1000 fewer cases every year. Each case of spina bifida prevented saves an estimated US$ 500 000 in lifetime costs. In Canada and Chile substantially further reductions (50% and 70% respectively) have been proven with even higher amounts of folic acid added to flour than in the US. More than 40 countries around the world have now made it mandatory.

Folic acid fortification of flour is cheap, less than 0.1% of the cost of flour.

Education, research and monitoring
- There should be education programmes, for health professionals and the public, on how to achieve adequate folate intake with diet and supplementation to prevent neural tube defects
- There should be continued research into the mechanisms of action of folic acid and the minimum dose of folic acid required for prevention
- Close monitoring of both the prevalence of neural tube defects (including terminations of pregnancy) and the increase in folate intake should be undertaken to evaluate the effectiveness of any health promotion campaigns

• Further research should be monitored, and these recommendations reviewed in the light of any developments.

In Australia, health promotion campaigns have been undertaken to inform health professionals and women about folate and the prevention of neural tube defects. For example, folic acid (folate) in fruit and vegetables is easily destroyed by cooking and prolonged storage. It is wise to eat fruit and vegetables that are fresh and either raw or lightly cooked. For good health and enough folate per day, one would need to aim for at least two servings of fruit, five servings of vegetables and seven servings of bread and cereals every day. The safety of increased folate ingestion before and during early pregnancy appears to be confirmed. Furthermore, an intake of folate from fortified food is unlikely to be high enough to constitute a hazard for those people with untreated vitamin B_{12} deficiency.

Children with headaches 17.5

I. Wilkinson

Headache occurs in most children at some time. In a number of these, frequent headaches are a disabling problem. In one study in primary schools in Australia, 23% of parents believed that their children suffered from 'frequent headaches'.

Many processes result in headache. These will be considered in two major classes: 'cranial' headaches, where the cause of pain is a process directly involving the brain and associated structures, including meninges, cerebral blood vessels and scalp; and 'extracranial' headaches, where the primary cause is remote from the brain.

The actual mechanisms of headache are multiple but it should be recognized that the brain itself is insensitive to pain. Some neurosurgical operations for intractable epilepsy are actually performed on the brain with the patient awake.

Structures that are sensitive to pain include:

- blood vessels
- meninges
- cranial nerves 5, 7, 9 and 10.

Pain is also generated from integumentary structures surrounding the skull, including:

- skin
- muscle
- periosteum
- blood vessels.

This chapter will deal particularly with recurrent or chronic headaches and not with those that accompany acute events such as trauma, intracranial bleeds or infections of the nervous system.

Cranial causes

Migraine and stress or tension types are the most common of chronic or recurrent headaches with origins in and around the brain. The migraine subset is numerically the biggest in Australian children. Stress and tension components often interact with a predisposition to migraine. Pure stress and tension headaches are less common than in adults. Often headaches in children that are classified as 'stress' or 'tension' start out as migraine headaches but, as a consequence of recurrent pain, disability and fear

of the next headache, develop strong features suggesting that stress or tension is the primary cause.

Of the different headache types in children, migraine, because of its great prevalence and associated morbidity, will receive most attention in this discussion.

Migraine

Epidemiological features

Migraine is:

- the commonest cause of recurrent headaches
- increasing prevalence. In a 1974 Finnish study using rigid criteria, 1.9% of children suffered from migraine headaches. In 1992 the study was repeated with the same criteria and the prevalence had increased to 5.7%. Other studies suggest up to 10% incidence
- leading cause of referrals to a child neurologist
- more common in males before puberty but in females after puberty

Clinical manifestations

Childhood migraines result from the same biological process as those in adults but clinical manifestations may be quite different. Some of these differences relate to the difficulty a child has in describing or explaining the features; for example, young children may not be able to describe throbbing, or lateralization, or sensory associations. Nevertheless, there are some features, such as dizziness and vomiting, that are clearly more common in children.

'Classical' migraine (which is a relatively uncommon type of migraine even in adults) includes aura, or transitory neurological dysfunction, especially of the visual system, and may involve sophisticated hallucinations such as fortification spectra, which often precede the onset of headache and then disappear as the headache commences. This classic sequence may occur in older children and adolescents but often instead there is a description of sensory hallucination that occurs with, or during, the headache. This may be a visual disturbance described in unsophisticated terms, such as 'flashing lights', 'seeing things double' or 'blurry, like looking through a curtain', or something more complex and bizarre-sounding and often very frightening. Such hallucinations include the appearance that objects are too big or too small, or that things moving in the environment appear to be going too fast or too slow. It is suggested that Lewis Carroll drew on personal migraine experiences when describing Alice's distorted body perception after she ate the magic substance.

Such hallucinations can involve the auditory process, e.g. things sounding too loud or someone speaking too fast. At times, the aura for a child defies description but may involve a sense of unreality or depersonalization.

What can make the migraine process more difficult to unravel in a child is the not uncommon situation where the actual sensory hallucination is not accompanied (during that event) by a headache. This is referred to as migraine dissociée and there is frequently more alarm and distress for a child or parent than when there is an accompanying headache.

Other variations from adult migraine involve the location of the pain. Whereas in adult migraine attacks the pain can often be lateralized (a true 'hemicrania' – one origin of the word migraine), this is frequently not the case in young children, who will simply point to their forehead (without lateralization) as being the location. As the child grows older a description of pain that is unilateral and sometimes located in one or other temple becomes more common. The pain is more often in the frontal half of the head and pain that is only located posteriorly raises the possibility of more sinister causes of headache.

A description of the quality of the pain in migraine in children is often difficult for them. The pain tends to more of an aching type 'like a tummy ache' rather than sharp 'like a needle'. A combination of the two may be described. Further, in adults with pure migraine attacks it is frequent for the pain to be described as throbbing, implying involvement of vascular structures. Children with migraine may well experience throbbing pain but may not be able to describe it as such, although, as the child becomes older, he or she may describe it as 'beating like a drum' or 'like a hammer'.

Although many adults do not acknowledge headaches as being migraine unless they are severe and resulting in cessation of usual activities, in children there can be a great range in the severity of migraine events, from the situation where the child is able to continue in school or at play, to the level where all activity must cease and the child retreats to bed in misery.

Adults with migraine attacks may not change greatly in external appearance but children are often extremely pale.

Nausea and vomiting may occur in association with adult migraine and not uncommonly continue throughout and exacerbate the headache, resulting in treatment with an antiemetic. During the attack, abdominal pain, nausea and vomiting are extremely common in children but the sequence may be that a single vomit, often followed by a sleep, seems to terminate the attack.

Formulating rigid diagnostic criteria for childhood migraine has proved very controversial and strict requirements for certain features to be present in combination before a diagnosis can be made may be counterproductive in clinical practice. In practice, children with headaches with some of the previously mentioned features, occurring intermittently and with symptom-free periods, who are normal to neurological examination, may be considered to suffer from migraine.

The single feature that has caused most disagreement between those studying children with headaches and those studying adults is a requirement for the headache to be of a certain duration. A diagnosis of migraine had originally required, by International Headache Society criteria, a duration of at least 4 hours. Eventually it was conceded that childhood migraine attacks may last as little as 1 hour.

Classic teaching about headaches due to tumours and other situations of raised intracranial pressure has been that they are present upon awakening, or actively cause the patient to waken. Although in reality this is not always the case, a contrast remains with childhood migraine, where the onset is more commonly later in the day, perhaps approaching midday or during the afternoon or evening.

Childhood migraine is a very cyclical condition. Patients may have a bout of recurrent headaches that lasts weeks or months, followed by a period of remission that may last a year or more, to be followed by another bout. Hot weather may be a factor in relapses.

Types of migraine

In the International Headache Society classification (2004) there are six categories and 17 subcategories of migraine. Precise classification is necessary in migraine research but is not always so important in clinical diagnosis and management, and there is often overlap between different types in children. To categorize according to the presence or absence of 'aura' in children can be very difficult. The 'aura', in children who can describe it, may often occur during the headache and not precede it, and frequently involves some sense of disequilibrium, perhaps true vertigo. Visual auras are often basic, such as blurring or double vision, and unsophisticated.

There are some conditions that are considered to be part of the migraine phenomenon, although appearing to have little relationship with adult migraine types:

- in early childhood, usually before the age of 5 years, some may experience recurrent episodes with sudden onset of true vertigo. These are extremely distressing and cause the child to seek a cuddle, or lie on the ground to relieve the feeling of spinning. These events last a few minutes, sometimes hours, and may be associated with pallor, nausea and vomiting. In some studies up to 80% of these children who are described as having benign paroxysmal vertigo subsequently develop migraine headaches
- unexplained attacks of vomiting, without associated headache, may also be precursors of migraine. These attacks can be very puzzling diagnostically and often very debilitating, possibly recurring after a predictable interval and sometimes requiring intravenous fluids and hospitalization. With the passage of time, headaches may become more of a feature of these attacks, which are labelled cyclical vomiting
- recurring episodes of unexplained abdominal pain defying diagnosis despite multiple investigations can also be very debilitating. There may be a family history of migraine and as time goes by the child's abdominal pain may become associated with and eventually replaced by migraine headaches.

The most recent International Headache Society Classification (2004) now includes a section 'Childhood periodic syndromes that are common precursors of migraine', incorporating (1) cyclical vomiting, (2) abdominal migraine and (3) benign paroxysmal vertigo.

In infancy, paroxysmal torticollis, where the head becomes tilted strongly to one or either side for periods of hours or days, may be a precursor of migraine, although simultaneous headache may not be apparent. A similar process involving the trunk has been described. These infants have been demonstrated to be at greater risk of later developing migraine headaches.

Hemiplegic migraine may present with unilateral weakness, or unilateral sensory disturbance, and this often precedes the actual headache.

Expressive or receptive language difficulties also may be a presenting feature of some attacks, with the headache not occurring till an hour or so later.

In acute confusional migraine the patient is quite disoriented and distressed, with short-term memory loss. This condition raises concerns about more sinister neurological processes, or drug intoxication, perhaps leading to invasive investigations. Again, the headache may not become apparent until later.

Aetiology

The basic mechanisms causing migraine in adults have been investigated extensively and there has been controversy, contradiction and revision of theories as to causation. It is beyond the scope of this text to detail all the theories, but historically the two main schools have postulated either:

- an initial central process involving neuronal pathways or
- a peripheral process involving blood vessels.

Current thinking suggests a very complex multifactorial mechanism, perhaps centred on the brain stem, where there is sensitization of nociceptor sites and central pain facilitation and receipt of various trigger inputs. There is also sensitivity of the cerebral cortex, leading to auras, and neurogenic inflammation and dilatation of blood vessels in pain-sensitive structures.

At a chemical level both noradrenergic and serotonergic transmitter pathways are implicated, and this has relevance for drug therapy.

Genetic factors play a major role in childhood migraine. As many as 90% of children with migraine have a first-degree relative with the condition. In some types, such as hemiplegic migraine, genetic loci have been found on particular chromosomes. In more common types of migraine it has been variously proposed that inheritance may be autosomal dominant, recessive, sex-linked or polygenic.

Given that some children are at risk genetically of developing migraine, it is clear that there may be provoking factors for individual attacks. These include head injuries, not necessarily severe ones. The head injury may be the commencing point for recurrent bouts of migraine headache, and this may have legal ramifications. Other provoking factors are:

- intercurrent systemic infections, particularly with fever
- strenuous physical exercise
- hot weather
- dehydration
- worry and stress, either domestic, social or educational in origin. While these factors remain, they may greatly complicate treatment. The distinction from 'stress' or 'tension' headaches without an underlying migraine basis may be very difficult
- foodstuffs. This is a very controversial area, with evidence for and against. Citrus fruit, cheese, chocolate and processed meat have been implicated
- food additives, such as monosodium glutamate, sodium nitrite, benzoic acid, tartrazine.

Treatment

Treatment can be divided into the following tiers:
- avoidance of triggers
- non-specific analgesia for attacks
- specific antimigraine medication for attacks
- prophylactic medication
- non-medication treatments.

Avoiding specific triggers in childhood migraine can be difficult. In many they do not exist. In Australia, hot weather and exercise are common precipitants that are part of a normal childhood lifestyle. Ensuring adequate hydration in the above situations may be helpful.

The role of restrictive diets is controversial. If it is evident that certain foodstuffs or drinks regularly provoke attacks then they should be avoided. Placing children on very limited diets is not only unpleasant and difficult to enforce but may even have nutritional consequences.

The use of non-specific analgesics in attacks is the simplest means of treatment. The most commonly used is paracetamol, best given in an initial dose of 20 mg/kg. Unfortunately, children may not seek medication, or as a result of being at school may not be able to access medication, until the attack is advanced. The paracetamol may not be effective at this time, or may be vomited. There may be a role for rectal paracetamol in this latter situation.

A recent study has indicated that ibuprofen in a dose of 10 mg/kg may be more effective then paracetamol. Other non-steroidal anti-inflammatory drugs (NSAIDs) may be helpful.

In recent years aspirin has been avoided in childhood because of concerns about its relationship with Reye syndrome, a rare but severe acute encephalopathy with potentially fatal outcome. Nevertheless, aspirin in doses of 15 mg/kg may be employed in older children with recurrent headaches.

The use of codeine and powerful narcotics in childhood headache is not usually necessary and is potentially hazardous, although restricted infrequent use of combinations of paracetamol and codeine in older children may be necessary and effective.

Ergotamine has long been a useful antimigraine drug in adults, particularly at the beginning of the attack. Although some studies have shown efficacy of oral dihydroergotamine in children, ergotamines have had limited use because children often delay seeking treatment and also because they may pro-duce side effects such as vomiting and abdominal discomfort.

Triptans are a new generation of serotonin-active drugs that abort migraine attacks. There have now been controlled trials in children supporting their use, but triptans have not yet been accepted for childhood use in some countries. Nasal sumatriptan has been shown to be effective but administration by the oral route has not been successful. Subcutaneous sumatriptan may be effective but is unpleasant to administer. Other triptans have generally not been proved to be effective.

Prophylactic medications may be considered for frequent disabling attacks. What constitutes 'frequent' is arbitrary but more than two severe attacks per month may justify treatment. Controlled trials of prophylaxis in childhood migraine are confounded by the cyclical nature of childhood migraine and the tendency to remit spontaneously, as well as the high placebo response rate.

A 2004 Cochrane data base study confirmed the paucity of evidence for successful treatment of childhood migraine and concluded that only one study each for propranolol and flunarizine was identified showing efficacy as prophylaxis for paediatric migraine. Nevertheless, the following medications are commonly used in clinical practice:

- cyproheptadine, an antihistamine with serotonin-blocking and calcium-channel-blocking properties. Side effects include drowsiness (which may be minimized with a single night-time dose regimen) and increased appetite. Effective doses range from 0.1–0.3 mg/kg per day, given either once or twice daily
- propranolol, a beta-adrenergic blocking drug, also blocks release of serotonin from platelets. It is contraindicated in asthma. Doses range from 0.5–2.0 mg/kg per day in two or three equal doses. Propranolol and similar drugs have been proven in adults but trials in children have produced conflicting results
- pizotifen, with antiserotonin and antihistamine properties, has side effects of increased appetite, weight gain and drowsiness. The latter may be avoided by a single night-time dose. Doses are limited by the single-size pill format (0.5 mg) but range from one to three at night
- flunarizine, a calcium-channel blocker, has been widely used in children in Europe but has restricted availability in Australia
- clonidine, a vasoactive drug, has been trialled in a range of conditions in children but lacks good evidence for use in migraine and has significant potential side effects
- amitriptyline, originally marketed as an antidepressant, has been used for migraine prophylaxis in children. It may be particularly useful where there are stress and depressive features, but care must be taken to avoid provoking cardiac arrhythmias.

Because of the high remission rates in children, prophylactic medications should not be used continuously for more than 6 months without attempting to wean patients from them.

Not surprisingly, given that there has been a swing towards accepting primary brain-stem and other neurological mechanisms as a major mechanism in the aetiology of migraine, anticonvulsant drugs are now being employed in prophylaxis. Studies of valproate, lamotrigine topiramate, gabapentin and levetiracetam in adults and to a limited extent in children have been promising but at this time they have not gained approval in Australia. Riboflavine (vitamin B_2) has been shown to be effective in one study in adults, and there is a trial of this under way in Australian children.

Non-medication treatments may at times be successful but again there is a paucity of controlled trials in children. Biofeedback and relaxation techniques have been used, particularly in Europe and North America. Acupuncture has proved to be successful in adults but is a potentially painful procedure. Homeopathic formulations are enjoying increased popularity in many conditions but lack evidence in childhood migraine. Chiropractic treatments are controversial, lack controlled trials and may be dangerous in young children.

Although discussion in this section has focused on migraine, the non-specific medications and treatments cited may be useful in all headache types.

Prognosis

Childhood migraine is often cyclical, with bad bouts followed by prolonged remissions, sometimes followed by relapses in later childhood or adult life. Various studies have indicated an overall 30–40% 10-year remission rate. It is not uncommon when taking a family history to find that parents, when pressed, remember childhood migraines long since in remission. Similarly, in apparent adult-onset migraine, a long forgotten history of severe childhood headaches may eventually be recalled.

Other children, like adults, will have a history of infrequent migraines throughout their developing years.

Clinical example

Jason, who was 8 years old, presented in March with headaches that had occurred about twice a week for the previous 3 months, although he had had some following soccer last winter. They commenced after lunch at school, were frontal and throbbing, and Jason looked very pale. Paracetamol sometimes helped him but often he would vomit, go to sleep and then awake without headache and eat his evening meal.

His mother had a history of migraine. Neurological examination in Jason was normal. After daily treatment with cyproheptadine for 2 weeks his headaches ceased.

The history is consistent with childhood migraine.

Stress and tension headaches

There is a broad spectrum of headache types in some way associated with emotional factors, perhaps more frequently seen in older children and adolescents. At one end is a small group where the symptoms of headaches may be used in a conscious and malingering way to avoid a situation. Examples include:

- the child who consistently develops a severe headache on a Monday morning in a setting of school difficulties
- the child who develops a severe headache when an unwelcome visit to a disliked non-custodial parent is planned.

Further along the spectrum is the situation where the child is being exposed to a great deal of stress, often multifactorial, and this apparently constitutes the sole underlying aetiological basis for headaches. High parental expectations may be major factors here. It is a reality of modern urban life that children may be involved in a demanding combination of schooling, additional tutoring, competitive sport, training in the performing arts and so on to the point where their life allows for little relaxation or personal time.

In situations such as this, a pattern of headache may develop. The nature of this headache may differ from that of migraine. In migraine the headache does not usually occur daily, and indeed daily headaches by many definitions are not migraine. In addition, the quality of the headache may differ; for example, they:

- may occur at all times and throughout the day
- cannot be localized or described in other than vague terms
- lack an association with pallor, nausea, vomiting, or disturbance of vision or balance.

For the clinician it may be frustratingly difficult to come to grips with the nature of these headaches.

Somewhere along this spectrum is the child who has a primary psychiatric disorder and in whom the symptom of headache may be part of a conversion reaction or a major psychosis.

Perhaps the more common situation is where the child with a past history of intermittent headaches sounding just like migraine, and a family history of this, experiences a crescendo effect, in which the headaches become daily, unremitting but not always severe. Although daily headaches may be indicative of a more sinister process, such as raised intracranial pressure, this is not necessarily the case. In this group where the crescendo effect is seen, it may be that the exposure to frequent pain and the expectation of further severe pain results in secondary stress and anxiety, which in turn provokes further headaches, becoming a vicious circle.

The sequence whereby individual stress events provoke a severe migraine attack is perhaps less frequently seen in children than in adults, but can still occur. Sometimes it is the 'let down' phenomenon following a period of stress that provokes a headache.

In childhood headaches associated with emotional aetiologies there is usually no abnormality on neurological examination. The facial appearance can range from complete indifference through to intense anxiety.

Radiological investigations rarely contribute in any positive sense but sometimes the performance of a normal brain scan in an extremely anxious patient may be the only way to allay anxiety and enable successful treatment. On the other hand, where there is a conversion reaction it may produce a reinforcement that there really is an organic problem.

Treatment is often difficult. Where there appears to be an original underlying basis of migraine, treatment with adequate doses of analgesia, possibly NSAIDs, may be able to break the cycle. It may be prudent to commence migraine prophylaxis as well.

Where the headache appears to be further along the spectrum towards psychiatric disorders, then consultation with a child psychiatrist is strongly advised.

As mentioned earlier, the tricyclic antidepressants may have a separate specific analgesic effect and can be particularly useful where an element of depression is a factor. Although monoamine oxidase inhibitors can also be useful in treating migraines in adults, the use of these in children may present dangers because of dietary interactions.

Caution must be exercised in drug treatment in this group of headaches, as it is common for such patients to finish up on combinations of medications in large doses and they may become dependent on these medications.

Several non-pharmacological therapies may have a role. These include:

• muscle relaxation
• stress avoidance
• biofeedback
• hypnosis
• acupuncture.

These therapies are used quite widely in Europe and North America but are often resource-intensive.

Headaches due to raised intracranial pressure

The possibility of childhood headaches being caused by raised intracranial pressure, especially due to tumours, is often a cause for great concern in the treating physician as well as the child and family. In reality, only a very small number of childhood headaches are due to raised pressure. Even when there is pressure, the ability of the child's skull to expand may mitigate some of the effects.

Although headaches due to raised intracranial pressure have classically been described as worse in the morning upon awakening, or causing the patient to awaken, and associated with vomiting, this is not always the case.

Raised intracranial pressure can be a result of abnormal fluid collections, solid masses or vascular malformations. Interference with fluid dynamics without discrete collections can result in the condition of benign intracranial hypertension.

Fluid can collect abnormally either within ventricles, within the substance of the brain or over the surfaces:

• build up of fluid within the ventricles is referred to as hydrocephalus (Ch. 17.4). This often presents in infancy, and the ability of the skull to expand, coupled with the inability of the child to report the pain, may be the reason that headache is not a presenting feature. In older children, the onset of hydrocephalus is often associated with a mass lesion obstructing the intracerebral cerebrospinal fluid pathways, and this may result in major headaches
• intracranial abscesses are uncommon in children in Western society. Children with cystic fibrosis or cyanotic heart disease are at increased risk. Abscesses can develop by spread from infections of the paranasal sinuses. Headaches resulting from abscesses are often associated with systemic manifestations such as fever, and tend to build up in severity over days or weeks
• arachnoid cysts occur in a number of different locations, often adjacent to the surface of the brain. They result from fluid collecting within a split arachnoid membrane and may be asymptomatic, but can produce headaches
• fluid, including blood, can collect in the subdural or extradural spaces, often as a result of trauma. Accompanying headaches are often crescendo in frequency and severity, and may be associated with focal signs
• headaches due to tumours are most often due to mass effect, or obstruction of cerebrospinal fluid pathways, and are less likely to be due to direct local involvement of pain-sensitive structures. Intracranial tumours in children are usually primary and are most frequently found in the posterior fossa, where they readily obstruct fluid pathways. It is not uncommon that there is a substantial delay in detection of the tumour in such headaches

- aneurysms are uncommon in children but arteriovenous malformations or cavernous angiomas are found at this age. These may produce headache due to their size or obstruction of fluid pathways.

The signs associated with raised pressure often involve the eyes.

Papilloedema may take days to develop, even in the presence of grossly elevated pressure. Abnormalities of ocular movements, particularly failure of abduction with resultant paralytic convergent strabismus, or failure of upward gaze, can occur. Sluggish pupillary light reflexes may be found. Deep tendon reflexes are often brisk. There may be neck stiffness. Bradycardia and systemic hypertension are later effects.

Treatment of such headaches usually involves surgical approaches, either directly to the mass or to drain fluid from the ventricles or brain surface via a shunt. Oedema surrounding a mass may be treated with corticosteroids or osmotic diuretics, but these are temporary measures only.

Benign intracranial hypertension

This condition, also known as 'pseudotumour cerebri' because the clinical feature can mimic a tumour, occurs in children and adults. It results from a build-up in intracranial pressure, without a space occupying lesion, probably due to an imbalance between production and resorption of cerebrospinal fluid. It is potentially serious as it can eventually result in visual loss. There is often an association with adolescent females, who may be overweight but otherwise apparently healthy. This may have a hormonal basis.

Other proposed causes in individual cases include:

- recurrent middle ear infections, sometimes associated with mastoiditis, where the draining cerebral venous sinuses near the ear become obstructed
- head trauma
- oral contraceptives
- the use or withdrawal of corticosteroids
- excessive amounts of vitamin A
- tetracyclines
- growth hormone treatment.

In some cases a specific cause is not found and the entity of 'benign intracranial hypertension' should probably be divided into idiopathic and symptomatic categories.

The clinical features include:

- headache, which tends to be daily, often worse in the morning but not necessarily severe

- abnormalities of the eyes, most commonly papilloedema (which may be asymptomatic) and lateral rectus palsies due to pressure on the abducens nerves
- nausea and vomiting
- raised pressure at lumbar puncture, to figures of 20–40 cmH$_2$O or more
- normal laboratory findings in cerebrospinal fluid.

In the presence of papilloedema or other eye signs it is prudent to perform a structural study (computed tomography (CT) or magnetic resonance imaging (MRI)) before performing the lumbar puncture. A magnetic resonance venogram may be helpful in demonstrating obstructed venous sinuses.

Cerebral images are usually otherwise quite normal, without a space-occupying lesion or dilatation of the ventricles. Even in the presence of a normal scan, it is reasonable to examine the cerebrospinal fluid for malignant cells, as in rare cases undifferentiated tumours can present with raised intracranial pressure in the presence of apparently normal scans.

Treatment is varied but includes:

- repeated lumbar punctures to remove fluid; this is quite traumatic and not always effective
- acetazolamide, which potentially reduces production of cerebrospinal fluid by interfering with the carbonic anhydrase enzymes, or more powerful diuretics, such as furosemide, if acetazolamide fails
- steroids
- shunting procedures to remove fluid from the cranial cavity; these should be reserved for drug-resistant cases

---

Clinical example

Lisa, 14 years old, developed daily headaches. These were often present by the time she had breakfast and were distressing, but she could get to school most days. The pain continued throughout the day and was all over her head. She had noticed some visual difficulty. The problem started after she was placed on an oral contraceptive for dysmenorrhoea.

On examination, Lisa was obese. There was papilloedema but no other neurological abnormality. Her blood pressure was normal. Cranial tomography was normal and a lumbar puncture resulted in the fluid pressure rising out of the top of the tube. The fluid was normal in the laboratory.

Lisa responded to cessation of the contraceptive and treatment with 250 mg acetazolamide each morning.

The history is consistent with benign intracranial hypertension.

- decompression procedures on the optic nerves
- anticoagulation if there are thrombosed draining venous sinuses.

Patients must be seen by an ophthalmologist, to monitor visual function, as prolonged papilloedema can lead to optic nerve damage.

The prognosis for benign intracranial hypertension is generally good. The process, particularly where no underlying cause is demonstrated, often remits spontaneously.

Seizure-related headaches

In adults, severe headaches are common following a major seizure. In young children, postictal headaches tend to be less debilitating. Children may describe a headache during an actual epileptic event, while conscious. This is often associated with focal discharges, possibly from the temporal lobe, and may be only a brief event, not always associated with other clinical features. Electrical discharges in the occipital region may give visual hallucinations, vomiting and headaches not always associated with motor convulsions. This condition may be familial and often difficult to diagnose.

Extracranial causes

Headache is a frequent associate of systemic illness, without there being a primary pathological process in the nervous system:

- the most frequent association is with systemic febrile illnesses not directly involving the nervous system
- connective tissue disease, especially 'mixed connective tissue disease', may lead to vascular-type headaches
- systemic hypertension is much less common in children, and hypertensive encephalopathy is not seen frequently. Nevertheless, in persistent severe hypertension in children a major encephalopathy may develop, with headache, seizures and altered consciousness. Acute glomerulonephritis may present in this way
- metabolic pathway disturbances such as urea cycle defects can produce headaches, especially during biochemical decompensation
- hypoglycaemia is a potent trigger for migraine but can also result in non-specific headaches and may be a result of poor diabetic control
- hunger without demonstrable hypoglycaemia may also provoke headaches
- although controversial, allergic disorders may be associated with migraines and other headaches

- obstructive sleep apnoea and other sleep disorders may produce a clinical picture of daytime headaches and somnolence.

In these situations treatment of the underlying cause is preferable to symptomatic relief.

Overrated causes of childhood headaches

Children with recurrent headaches are frequently initially referred to optometrists or ophthalmologists. The basis for these headaches is often migraine.

Glaucoma (rarely seen in children) and iritis may product aching in and around the orbit. Convergence insufficiency and other ocular muscle imbalances are common findings in children. Headaches may be attributed to these problems but the evidence is not convincing.

Minor refractive errors detected on examination, but with doubtful clinical relevance, may be blamed incorrectly as a cause of childhood headache. Spectacles or ocular movement exercises may result in apparent temporary relief of the headaches, but not infrequently they return.

Acute sinusitis is a potential cause of headache in children, often associated with other features such as fever, purulent nasal or postnasal discharge, local tenderness and puffiness around the eyes. The pain can be widespread in the skull and the location can be confusing. This is a potentially dangerous condition, occasionally leading to intracranial abscesses.

More frequently seen is the situation where recurrent frontal migraine headaches are attributed to chronic sinusitis and referral for a radiographic series is the first investigation. These are frequently negative. With the increasing availability of CT and MRI performed for other reasons, it is not uncommon that asymptomatic fluid collections are detected in paranasal sinuses, usually with no clinical consequences.

The frontal and other sinuses are not formed in early childhood and may be not be capable of harbouring infections until the end of the first decade.

Headaches found in adults but not children

- Giant cell or temporal arteritis is a potentially serious cause of headaches in the elderly and can lead to visual impairment or cerebrovascular accidents if not treated. Fortunately, it is not a condition of childhood

• Acute angle closure glaucoma is another cause of pain in the ocular region. It is uncommon for this to occur in isolation in childhood

• Cluster headaches are a condition of adult life and can result in some of the most severe headaches known. They can be very resistant to treatment. Although there are isolated reports, they are fortunately rarely seen in childhood

• Headaches due to arthritic changes in the neck, often chronic disabling headaches, generally relate to long-standing degenerative processes and are not common in children

Investigations

Childhood headaches are frequently overinvestigated. In general, blood investigations have little yield. Plain radiographs of the skull may demonstrate signs of chronically raised pressure, or sinusitis, but are of little use in most situations.

CT is necessary only rarely but is most useful in hydrocephalus, other fluid collections and tumours, although it is not ideal for visualization of the middle or posterior fossae and is associated with significant radiation exposure and risk of subsequent malignancy. MRI is more likely to detect tumours and masses, particularly in the middle and posterior fossa. Magnetic resonance arteriography or venography is quite sensitive for detecting vascular abnormalities and is relatively non-invasive. Lumbar puncture is the diagnostic test for benign intracranial hypertension.

Specialist consultation is frequently more rewarding and less expensive then laboratory investigation.

PART 18

URINARY TRACT DISORDERS AND HYPERTENSION

Urinary tract infections and malformations

C. Jones

Urinary tract infections

Urinary tract infection is the second most common bacterial infection affecting children. Urinary tract infection can cause septicaemia or chronic ill health with failure to thrive and is often an indication of an underlying urinary tract malformation.

Epidemiology

Epidemiologic studies have shown that 2% of boys and 8% of girls have had a urinary tract infection by the age of 7 years; 75% of urinary tract infections occur under the age of 1 year in males and 50% under the age of 1 year in females. The prevalence of urinary tract infection in febrile infants under the age of 3 months presenting to emergency departments is 20–30% and boys outnumber girls. After the age of 3 months the prevalence of urinary tract infection in febrile children falls to around 8% in females and 2% in male children. The incidence of urinary tract infection in uncircumcised boys is 4–10 times that in circumcised boys in the first 3 months of life. Common clinical patterns of urinary tract infection are described in Table 18.1.1.

Diagnosis

The frequency of symptoms of urinary tract infection in a recent series of 304 children less than 5 years of age presenting to a Sydney hospital emergency department is listed in Table 18.1.2. The presentation varies with age because of the developmental status of the child. While a wide range of symptoms can occur, an infant will probably have an acute illness with fever and vomiting or a chronic illness with failure to thrive, reflecting the systemic response to infection at this age. The preschool child, who has usually achieved continence, will often show wetting or frequency, complain of generalized abdominal pain and sometimes indicate dysuria. The teenage girl will usually present with symptoms of cystitis (fever, frequency, dysuria, strangury and accurately localized pain) or pyelonephritis (fever, often with rigor, and loin pain and tenderness). At any age, symptoms of fever, vomiting and systemic unwellness occur with pyelonephritis.

Urinalysis and microscopy

The finding of a positive urinary dipstick test for leukocyte esterase is sensitive for urinary infection (approximately 80% of urine infections detected) and urinary nitrite testing is specific (97% of positive tests indicate infection). Taking the prevalence rates for urine infection at different ages (see Epidemiology) into account, a positive testing for both nitrites and leukocyte esterase in a child under 3 months of age predicts a 90% chance of a urine infection, but negative tests are found in 10% of infants with infection. This is not good enough for clinical purposes as the diagnosis of urine infection would be missed in a significant number of ill infants. In a child aged 3 years or more, or in a circumcised male, the prevalence of urine infection is much lower and the finding of negative tests (leukocyte esterase and nitrites) is reassuring as there is then only a 1% chance of urine infection. Thus, negative tests are quite useful in this older age group in excluding urinary infection and at least justifying withholding antibiotic treatment until the results of urine culture are available. Microscopy will usually reveal leukocytes and non-glomerular red cells (red cells that appear normally haemoglobinized and of uniform size and shape under phase-contrast microscopy) in freshly examined urine. The presence or absence of bacteria on microscopy can be unreliable: the presence of bacteria on microscopy of a fresh, well collected specimen (e.g. by suprapubic aspirate of urine (SPA)) can be sensitive and specific for urinary tract infection, particularly if the white cell count is high (>10 white cells/μl). The finding of epithelial squamous cells indicates a poorly collected sample and the absence of leukocyturia in a sample with mixed growth or low colony count on culture may indicate a contaminated sample.

Urinary nitrite tests are frequently used in monitoring the urine of children prone to recurrent urinary tract infection (for example, continent children with vesicoureteric reflux). Nitrite testing of early morning urine on a weekly basis has been reported to detect urinary tract infection in asymptomatic children, enabling treatment to be initiated earlier than would otherwise occur.

Table 18.1.1 Common clinical patterns of urinary tract infection

Age	Infancy	Toddler and young child	Adolescent
Presentation	Males more common than females, especially under 3 months High fever Systemically unwell Commonly recurs	Common for females, uncommon for males Mild fever, wetting, dysuria and smelly urine Frequent recurrences	Common for females, rare for males Pyelonephritis or cystitis
Precipitating factors	*Males:* High-grade VUR (often associated with significant congenital renal malformation), physiological phimosis *Females:* Low-grade VUR, usually associated with no or minor renal malformation *Both:* Immature voiding pattern with high voiding pressure and detrusor hyperactivity	Low-grade VUR – ? associated with development of acquired renal injury Dysfunctional elimination symptoms Detrusor dyssynergia Infrequent voiding Constipation Vulvovaginitis	Often history of VUR Sexual activity Vulvovaginitis
Prevention of recurrence	Prophylactic antibiotic	Treatment of precipitating factors identified	Counselling Adjustment of sexual habit (void post-intercourse, antibiotic at time of sexual activity)

VUR, vesicoureteric reflux.

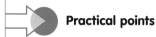

Practical points

Dipstick testing
- Positive leukocyte esterase is a reasonably sensitive test but is not at all specific for urinary tract infection (UTI)
- Positive nitrites is less sensitive but quite specific for UTI
- Negative testing for leukocyte esterase and nitrites does *not* exclude UTI, especially in babies. 10% of babies with UTI will have negative dipstick testing
- Always send urine for culture if UTI is suspected
- Negative dipstick testing may reasonably be used in making the decision to withhold antibiotics from children over 3 years of age while awaiting urine culture results

Urine culture

The urine culture is the gold standard for diagnosis, but management decisions often have to be made before the results are available.

The five common forms of urine collection are compared in Table 18.1.3.

Microbiology
Escherichia coli accounts for 80–90% of pathogens isolated. *Proteus* species are the cause of infection in 30% of males over 1 year of age. Coagulase-negative

Staphylococcus species are common in teenagers and *Klebsiella* is frequent in the neonatal period. *Pseudomonas* species are frequently isolated in children with more complicated anatomical malformations and in those children who have had surgical procedures, especially where foreign materials (e.g. urinary stents) have been left in situ. The enterococcus causes around 5% of urinary tract infections and is the most common organism found that is resistant to gentamicin. Approximately 5% of children will have two organisms isolated.

Initial treatment

Once the urine culture has been obtained a decision on acute treatment must be made. Intravenous therapy is required where the child is systemically unwell (dehydrated, signs of septic shock such as hypotension, tachycardia and decreased conscious state), where there is vomiting, so that oral medications will not be retained, and, in general, in the infant under the age of 6 months. In the child in whom an infection is likely on the basis of urinalysis and presentation, and the child is reasonably well (generally older and not vomiting), oral antibiotics may be commenced, with review once the culture is through in 24–48 hours. In the child in whom a urinary infection is a possibility and the child is not

Table 18.1.2   Frequency of symptoms in children under 5 years with symptomatic urinary tract infections

Symptom	%
History of fever	79.6
Axillary temperature >37.5°C	59.5
Irritability	52.3
Anorexia	48.7
Malaise/lethargy	44.4
Vomiting	41.8
Diarrhoea	20.7
Dysuria	14.8
Offensive urine	13.2
Abdominal pain	13.2
Family member with past history of UTI*	11.2
Previous unexplained febrile episodes	10.5
Frequency	9.5
Urinary incontinence†	6.6
Macroscopic haematuria	6.6
Febrile convulsion	4.6

* First-degree relative. † Defined as a noticeable increase in the frequency of daytime wetting.
Source: from Craig et al, 1998.

unwell then the results of the culture are obtained before starting treatment. The intravenous antibiotics and oral antibiotics used acutely are listed in Table 18.1.4. Intravenous antibiotics are usually ceased within 2–3 days once culture results have been obtained and the child has improved clinically. Acute treatment is completed with oral antibiotics, usually of 5 days duration.

Prophylactic antibiotics

After acute treatment the child may be placed on prophylactic antibiotics given once each night. The antibiotics usually used for prophylaxis are listed in Table 18.1.4. These antibiotics are excreted in the urine, achieve high urinary concentrations and are well tolerated over long periods of time without inducing excessive microbiological changes in the gut (leading to the emergence of resistant organisms or candidiasis). They are usually given until the results of imaging tests are available, and perhaps for prolonged periods with the aim of reducing the risk of further UTI. This is an area of medical controversy and further research into the benefits of prophylactic antibiotics is currently underway.

Investigations

The investigation necessary after a first urinary tract infection is an area of medical controversy. After several decades where the trend was to perform several detailed investigations, many centres are now more conservative and reserve more invasive investigations, and those involving irradiation, for special situations.

Investigations are aimed at excluding obstructive urinary tract lesions and determining whether there are significant underlying urinary tract malformations. Nearly all centres perform a renal ultrasound. This enables the presence, site, size and shape of the kidneys to be determined. In the age group under 5 years, only 15% of abnormalities found on DMSA scan ('scars/dysplasia') will be seen on ultrasound examination. The ureters are not visualized unless enlarged. The finding of hydronephrosis or hydroureter leads to further nuclear medical imaging (discussed below) to diagnose obstructive lesions of the urinary tract. An idea of bladder function can be determined by measuring the postvoid residual volume (normally <20 ml in children under 7 years).

The radiological examination of the urethra and bladder, using a micturating cystourethrogram (MCU), is performed in some centres as a routine on infants (less than 1 year of age) and selectively at older ages where visualization of the bladder surface and urethra is required. This investigation is performed less frequently than in the past because the demonstration of vesicoureteric reflux (VUR, see below) does not alter management at many centres. The patient and parental acceptability of the test is poor and against the ethos of development of 'pain- and anxiety-free' paediatric procedures. I generally have MCU tests performed under general anaesthesia.

Nuclear medicine investigations with technetium-99m-labelled radioisotopes are useful for a number of purposes. These investigations carry radiation toxicity of less than one-tenth of a routine chest X-ray.

The *DTPA* radionuclide is injected intravenously, is filtered by the glomerulus and then is neither secreted nor absorbed by the tubule of the kidney. Like creatinine or insulin, it can be used to obtain an accurate measure of the glomerular filtration rate.

641

Table 18.1.3 Comparison of methods of urine collection

Urine collection method	Advantages	Disadvantages	Recommended use
Paediatric bag	Widespread use in primary care paediatrics Considered convenient Avoids invasive procedure	Contamination with skin flora common so that only results of <10^8 cfu/l (excluding infection) are useful Should not be used where immediate antibiotic treatment is required	Collection of urine from infant or toddler at low risk for UTI (not febrile and no known urological abnormality) for urinalysis: if +ve for leukocytes or nitrites, another urine collection method should be used for culture
Clean catch	Non-invasive Good correlation with SPA/MSU/CSU results	Perceived to be difficult to collect (majority can be collected within 1 h)	Method of choice in infants and toddlers >10^8 cfu/l indicates infection, although presence of squamous epithelia and lack of pyuria indicates contamination
Midstream urine collection (MSU)	Non-invasive Widespread patient acceptance	Poor technique (failure to withdraw foreskin or wash labia) results in contamination Difficult with phimosis or for obese females	Method of choice in toilet trained child >10^8 cfu/l indicates infection, although presence of squamous epithelia and lack of pyuria indicates contamination
Catheter sample (CSU)	Usually results in collection of sample of urine, reasonable for diagnosis especially if 1st drops of urine discarded	Invasive – poor acceptance by parents and can establish fear in child of future clinic visits Difficult with phimosis	Second choice to SPA in infants and toddlers with high risk of UTI (febrile and proven urological abnormalities) where treatment is required before culture available >10^6 cfu/l may indicate infection, although presence of squamous epithelia and lack of pyuria indicates contamination
Suprapubic aspirate of urine (SPA)	Gold standard as avoids contamination. Less invasive than CSU collection	'Dry tap' relatively common (ultrasound confirmation of full bladder can minimize this)	Method of choice in infants and toddler at high risk of UTI Useful in obese females with recurrent contaminated MSUs Any growth significant

cfu, colony-forming unit on bacterial culture.

Table 18.1.4   Antibiotic treatment of urinary tract infection

Antibiotic	Dose	Organisms sensitive* (%)
Acute **Intravenous** (sick, <6 months old, pyelonephritis) 1. Benzyl penicillin *and*	50 mg/kg (max. dose 2 g) 6 h	Covers enterococcus

2. Gentamicin	8 mg/kg day 1, then 6 mg/kg/day for <10 years,
	    7 mg/kg day 1, then 5 mg/kg/day for >10 years
	    (max. dose 360 mg)
	Monitoring: trough level <1 mg/l taken
	    on 3rd day and serum creatinine 3rd day
		95+

Oral Trimethoprlm *or*	4 mg/kg (max. dose 150 mg) 12 h	85+
Co-trimoxazole	(40/200 mg/5 ml) 0.5 ml/kg (max. dose 20 ml) 12 h	85+
or Cephalexin	15 mg/kg (max. dose 500 mg) 8 h	95
or Augmentin†	10–25 mg/kg/8 h	95
Prophylactic Co-trimoxazole	(40/200 mg/5 ml) 0.25 ml/kg/night	85+
Nitrofurantoin	1–2 mg/kg/night	85+
Cefalexin‡	5 mg/kg/night	95+

* Percentage of bacteria causing urinary tract infection diagnosed in the emergency department of major Australian hospitals that are sensitive to antibiotics. † Amoxicillin alone only covers 60% of organisms encountered, so Augmentin is preferred.
‡ The suspension forms of the cephalosporins and penicillins lose activity after a few weeks.

The *Mag 3* scan has largely replaced the DTPA scan because, in addition to some glomerular filtration, the isotope is mainly secreted by the proximal tubular cells into the urine so that the signal to background ratio is higher than in the DTPA scan. This is particularly useful in children with renal impairment or infants in the first 3 months of life when the glomerular filtration rate is low. Both of these investigations are useful for diagnosing the presence of obstruction to urinary flow from the kidneys to the bladder, for determining the 'split' of kidney function (between the right and left kidneys), and for estimating overall renal function.

The *DMSA* radionuclide is filtered by the glomerulus and taken up by the proximal tubular cells. Scanning takes place when it has been taken up by these cells, which are in the renal cortex. Lack of uptake gives a defect on the scan and this can be due to either transient impairment of the tubular cell function (e.g. following acute inflammation with pyelonephritis for a period of up to 3–4 months) or absence of kidney tissue (renal 'scarring/dysplasia').

Delayed uptake of any of these three radionuclides may occur in conditions where perfusion to the kidney is abnormal (e.g. renal artery stenosis in a unilateral case or dehydration in a bilateral case).

The ongoing management depends on the results of investigations. A flow diagram of possibilities is shown in Figure 18.1.1.

Urinary tract infection and normal renal ultrasound

If the child is afebrile and asymptomatic, I do not perform another urine culture at the end of treatment. In the case of an infant, prophylactic antibiotics are continued for 6–12 months. In the case of an older child with recurrent infections and normal baseline investigations, the ultrasound would be repeated and an examination for precipitating factors (see Table 18.1.1) such as constipation or a functional voiding disorder (daytime wetting) would be undertaken. Sexual activity should be considered in teenagers.

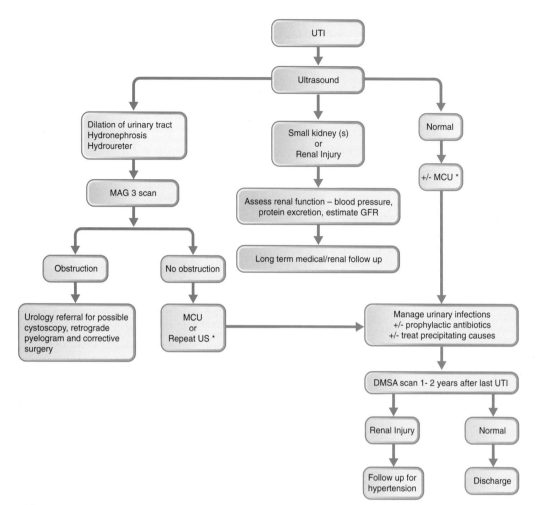

Fig. 18.1.1 A flow diagram of ongoing management following a proven urinary tract infection. A normal ultrasound does not exclude scarring. This age is chosen for convenience. Boys uncommonly get recurrent infections after 1 year; girls commonly have recurrent infection until about 3 years. Follow-up includes a yearly blood pressure check. The finding of a normal DMSA scan normalizes the risk of developing hypertension. MCU, micturating cystourethrogram; U/S, ultrasound; VUR, vesicoureteric reflux.

Clinical example

Johnnie had a birth weight of 3.3 kg. He was breastfed and weighed 5.1 kg at 2 months of age. For the next month he put on no weight and his mother noted that he was irritable, fed poorly and had the occasional vomit. The family doctor took a bag sample of urine and found more than 10^8/l colony forming units (cfu) of an organism growing on culture the next day. The doctor arranged for a suprapubic aspirate of urine to be performed at the emergency department. This was done after a bladder scan showed a moderately full bladder. The child was admitted to hospital and received treatment with gentamicin and penicillin given intravenously for 48 hours before an *E. coli* sensitive to co-trimoxazole was identified.

The infant was discharged to complete 3 days of oral co-trimoxazole therapy and then to commence night-time co-trimoxazole prophylactic antibiotic treatment. An MCU and renal ultrasound were performed in the next few days.

The ultrasound showed right-sided hydronephrosis and hydroureter with a normal left kidney. The MCU showed a mild trabeculated bladder with right-sided vesicoureteric reflux; the urethra was abnormal in appearance with dilation of the posterior urethra suggesting a diagnosis of posterior urethral valves (Fig. 18.1.2). Prophylactic antibiotic treatment was continued and the child was referred to a paediatric urologist for cystoscopy and evaluation of the urethra.

Clinical example

Amy, a 14-year-old girl, presented to her local doctor on three occasions over 6 months with culture-proven urinary tract infections. There was no family history of urine infections, Amy had never had a urinary tract infection before, and there was no evidence of a wetting disorder. Further history revealed the onset of sexual activity at about the same time as the urinary tract infections started.

Amy was counselled regarding contraception and sexually transmitted diseases and she and her parents were offered counselling regarding her sexual activity. She was advised to have a 300 ml glass of water with a citravescent sachet immediately prior to or just after sexual intercourse. However, 1 month later Amy re-presented with another urinary tract infection. She was then advised to take nitrofurantoin (100 mg capsule immediately after sexual intercourse). She was seen for review 3 and 6 months after this treatment, reported no further symptoms and remained compliant with the treatment. As she was frequently changing sexual partners she was advised to continue on the treatment.

Asymptomatic infection

Up to 4% of adolescent girls have asymptomatic bacteriuria. A number of these children will have vesicoureteric reflux or reflux-associated nephropathy (see below). There is no evidence that treatment of asymptomatic bacteriuria is beneficial, and colonization frequently recurs after treatment, sometimes precipitating symptomatic infection caused by a more pathogenic organism.

Practical points

Management of urinary tract infection in infancy
- Suspect in febrile infant with vomiting or failure to thrive
- Urine sample:
  - Acutely unwell: SPA 1st choice (or CSU)
  - Not unwell: clean catch
- Unwell: commence treatment with intravenous gentamicin and intravenous penicillin initially, changing to oral antibiotic to finish course when improved
- Prophylactic antibiotic until renal ultrasound evaluated
- Long-term follow-up essential unless DMSA scan normal

Management of recurrent urinary tract infection in childhood
- Characterize symptoms as pyelonephritis or cystitis
- Identify precipitating factors: wetting, vulvovaginitis, phimosis or balanitis, constipation
- Bladder abnormality
- Individualize therapy to minimize development of symptomatic urine infection
- Longer term follow-up essential unless DMSA normal

Abnormalities of the urinary tract

Vesicoureteric reflux

This is a disorder in which urine passes in a retrograde direction from the bladder through the vesicoureteric junction into the ureter. It is a common disorder, affecting 40% of children under 1 year of age who are investigated for a first urinary tract infection. The diagnosis is made by MCU or by an indirect MCU done without urinary catheterization.

Vesicoureteric reflux (VUR) is a familial trait affecting between 30% and 50% of first-degree relatives of index cases. This developmental abnormality is characterized by the distal end of the ureter running less obliquely through the wall of the bladder and having less muscle around it. In some cases, it is associated with renal malformation (variously referred to as renal scarring, dysplasia, reflux-associated nephropathy), excessive dilatation and tortuosity of the ureter, occurrence on the contralateral side and abnormalities of bladder function including premature detrusor contractions (causing urgency symptoms and wetting) and poor bladder emptying. Higher grades of VUR are associated with higher recurrence rates of UTI.

The treatment of VUR has been controversial. Controlled trials (Table 18.1.5) have shown no advantage of either anti-reflux surgery or antibiotic prophylaxis in preventing urinary infections, hypertension, renal injury or renal failure. In fact, it is not clear whether these treatments are better than no treatment or episodic treatment of urine infection alone. Much of the renal injury leading to renal failure in a small number of patients with VUR is congenital and the significance of acquired injury is

---

Table 18.1.5 Management of vesicoureteric reflux: evidence and controversies

Evidence-based analysis of surgical versus antibiotic treatment of VUR shows

- No difference in overall rate of urinary tract infection (but reduced rate of pyelonephritis with surgery)
- No difference in occurrence of 'new scarring' or extension of 'old scarring'
- No difference in incidence of renal failure
- No difference in incidence of hypertension

Continuing controversies:

- Whether VUR surgery or antibiotics make any difference to development of acquired renal injury
- The frequency of acquired or congenital renal injury as a cause of reflux nephropathy
- The effectiveness of prophylactic antibiotic therapy
- The significance of smaller renal scars

debated. Thus, the aim of treatment of VUR is prevention of symptomatic UTI, not prevention of renal injury. Attention to reducing and treatment precipitating factors for UTI, the use of antibiotic treatment in a prophylactic or episodic manner and the selective use of antireflux surgery for patients with intractable symptoms form the basis of treatment.

VUR often resolves spontaneously (of a cohort of children with reflux, 20% will have resolution occurring spontaneously each 3-year period, with less severe degrees of reflux resolving earlier than more severe degrees). Resolution of reflux is often not associated with resolution of urine infection, which can be expected to occur periodically throughout life in affected females, particularly with sexual activity and pregnancy.

Reflux-associated nephropathy

Once thought to be due to the combination of VUR and infection, this abnormality of the kidney is most often congenital in origin. It is found in approximately 10% of children with VUR. The importance of this lesion lies in the possibility of development of hypertension, which is rare in early childhood but occurs in up to 15% of cases by the age of 20 years. Bilateral extensive reflux associated nephropathy is a cause of renal failure occurring from mid childhood.

Posterior urethral valves

This abnormality is also referred to as congenital obstructive posterior urethral membranes (COPUMs). It affects males and causes obstruction to urine flow at the level of the posterior urethra. The bladder is often thick-walled and trabeculated; there may be associated VUR with tortuous and dilated ureters draining grossly hydronephrotic kidneys. Antenatal ultrasound demonstrating hydronephrosis and megacystis is a common presentation, as is urinary infection in early infancy, but some children present later with dribbling and wetting.

Diagnosis is made on the urethrogram phase of the MCU (Fig. 18.1.2) and confirmation is obtained by cystoscopy. Treatment involves complex surgical procedures performed in the setting of a team approach to the patient, involving medical staff and continence physiotherapists. Preparation for end stage renal failure treatment is often necessary.

Bladder abnormalities

Bladder malfunction is strongly associated with urinary tract infections and often overlooked in clinical management. Table 18.1.6 describes common bladder abnormalities and their management.

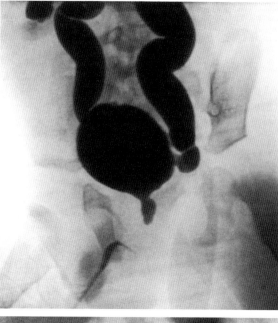

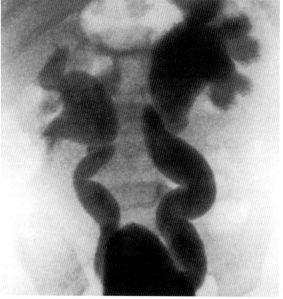

Fig. 18.1.2 **A.** The MCU (from the clinical example) showing a dilated posterior urethra, mildly irregular appearance of the edge of the bladder ('trabeculation') and bilateral vesicoureteric reflux into dilated tortuous ureters. **B.** Hydronephrosis with 'clubbing' of the calyces.

Duplication

A kidney is said to be duplex if two separate collecting systems are identified. The ureters may join before entry into the bladder or they may have separate openings into the bladder. The upper pole ureter enters the urinary tract more distal to the lower pole ureter and may enter the urethra, giving rise to incontinence, or may be obstructed at its lower end

Table 18.1.6   Common bladder abnormalities

Bladder abnormality causes	Urodynamic assessment	Symptoms	Treatment

Small bladder
  Primary
  Posterior urethral valves
  Bladder extrophy
  Neurogenic
	Low volume
	High pressure
		Day and night wetting
		UTI
		Hydroureter
			Frequent voiding
			Bladder augmentation

Large bladder
  Primary
  Neurogenic
  Vesicoureteric reflux
	Large volume
	Low pressure
	High residual volume
		Infrequent voiding
		UTI
		Wetting
			Frequent voiding
			Drainage by vesicostomy,
			  CIC or catheterizable conduits

Detrusor dyssynergia
  syndrome
  Primary
  Vesicoureteric reflux
	Premature detrusor
	  contractions
		Urge symptoms
		Wetting
		UTI
			Anticholinergic drugs
			Frequent voiding
			Usually resolves

Neurogenic
  Cord injury*
  'Non-neurogenic'†
	All of the above found	Wetting with 'overflow'
		UTI
		Obstructive nephropathy
			Bladder drainage by vesicostomy,
			  CIC or catheterizable conduit
			Bladder augmentation

* Cord injury may be clinical apparent (spina bifida) or determined by US in a neonate when the cord can be imaged or MRI at later ages. † Non-urogenic neurogenic bladder is a term used for the clinical and investigational features of a neurogenic bladder but do not have demonstrable spinal pathology.
CIC, clean intermittent catheterization; UTI, urinary tract infection.

(ureterocele), in which case the upper pole of the kidney will be abnormal. The lower pole ureter often has vesicoureteric reflux.

Other causes of urinary obstruction

Pelviureteric junction obstruction. This is now most commonly diagnosed following the evaluation of hydronephrosis detected on antenatal scanning of the fetus. At least nine out of 10 such cases will resolve spontaneously over the first year of life. Periodic renal ultrasound observation, sometimes supplemented by diuretic renography using DPTA or Mag 3, or magnetic resonance imaging (MRI), is used to follow these infants. Pelviureteric junction obstruction may present in later childhood with renal colic and these cases usually require surgery.

Vesicoureteric junction obstruction. This often presents following investigation of urinary tract infection, with the ultrasound showing a dilated ureter and MRI showing delayed passage of urine from the ureter to the bladder with a widened ureteric image. Treatment is reimplantation of the ureter.

Renal calculi. These may present following urinary tract infection, in which case the calculus is usually a triple phosphate (magnesium, calcium and ammonium) stone and the infecting organisms often urea-splitting (such as *Proteus mirabilis*), or renal colic. Other stones occasionally encountered are composed of cystine (autosomal recessive cystinuria), calcium oxalate and uncommonly uric acid.

Table 18.1.7   Antenatal renal abnormalities: postnatal diagnoses

Diagnosis	%
Non-refluxing non-obstructive hydronephrosis	55
Vesicoureteric reflux	15
Pelviureteric junction obstruction	5
Multicystic kidney	5
Vesicoureteric junction abnormalities	5
Duplex	5
Agenesis	5
Posterior urethral valves	2

Table 18.1.8 Forms and presentation of cystic renal disease

Cystic renal disease	Incidence	Genetics	Clinical features
Autosomal dominant polycystic kidney disease	1–2 in 1000 M = F	Three gene defects cause it; 50% risk in subsequent children	Usually discovered because of family history Uncommon cause of hypertension oroin/abdominal discomfort in childhood Progresses to renal failure later in life
Autosomal recessive kidney disease	1–2 in 10 000 births M = F	One gene defect identified; 25% risk in subsequent pregnancies	Often present in infancy with enlarged kidneys, polycystic and oligohydramnios, which in turn is associated with pulmonary hypoplasia. Later may get hypertension, renal impairment Associated with hepatic fibrosis causing portal hypertension in mid childhood
Cystic renal dysplasia	Common	Polygenic; low recurrence risk	Often asymptomatic. Associated with vesicoureteric reflux. May be bilateral
Multicystic dysplastic kidney	Relatively uncommon	Unknown; low recurrence risk	Enlarged completely cystic non-functioning kidney without blood flow. Contralateral kidney usually normal but may be associated with vesicoureteric reflux or pelviureteric junction obstruction

Antenatal renal abnormalities

The advent of almost routine antenatal scanning at 18 weeks gestation has led to the detection of approximately 1 in 200 infants having an increased renal pelvis diameter (>4 mm at 18 weeks). The postnatal diagnoses are shown in Table 18.1.7.

Management

The antenatal ultrasound should be repeated in the third trimester of pregnancy. The presence of bilateral severe hydronephrosis with an enlarged bladder in the male infant suggests the diagnosis of posterior urethral valves. The presence of oligohydramnios suggests reduced urine output and this is associated with the development of pulmonary hypoplasia.

After birth, the infant should be placed on prophylactic trimethoprim until the diagnosis is determined. If the child is unwell or if significant severe abnormalities are suspected, imaging of the kidneys and urinary tract should be performed immediately. In contrast, if the baby is well and without severe urinary tract dilatation, a postnatal ultrasound is undertaken towards the end of the first week of life when the baby is well hydrated. Further investigations, usually looking for reflux or obstruction, are performed, depending upon the results of this ultrasound.

Cystic renal disease

Common forms of cystic renal disease and the modes of presentation are listed in Table 18.1.8.

Glomerular disease, renal failure and hypertension

S. J. McTaggart

Glomerular disease presents with various clinical manifestations that include:

- isolated urinary abnormalities, e.g. recurrent haematuria, proteinuria
- acute glomerulonephritis (nephritic syndrome)
- nephrotic syndrome
- chronic renal failure.

Isolated urinary abnormalities

Benign microscopic haematuria

Asymptomatic isolated microscopic haematuria is common, with screening studies in children of all ages showing a prevalence of 0.5–2%. However, persistent microscopic haematuria is less common (<0.5%) indicating that investigation of isolated microscopic haematuria should only be instigated once persistence has been established in at least 3 different specimens taken over a period of 2–3 weeks. Persistent microscopic haematuria is usually benign providing there is no infection or proteinuria, renal function is normal and no structural abnormality is present on ultrasonography. Renal biopsy sometimes shows thinning of basement membrane on electron microscopy (thin basement membrane disease). Often, inheritance is in an autosomal dominant fashion.

IgA nephropathy

This glomerulopathy is present in 50% of children who have recurrent episodes of macroscopic haematuria. The episodes of haematuria often occur simultaneously with intercurrent viral infections and may be associated with flank pain. Other presentations include abnormal urinalysis on medical examination and, rarely, an acute glomerulonephritis with renal failure. The histology of focal proliferative glomerulonephritis with IgA in the mesangium is similar to that of Henoch–Schönlein purpura (Fig. 18.2.1). While the prognosis for most children with IgA nephropathy is good, long-term studies show that about 10% progress to chronic renal failure by 15 years after onset of disease.

Alport syndrome

This is a familial disorder in production of type IV collagen and is inherited as an X-linked dominant (85% of cases), autosomal dominant or autosomal recessive condition. In the X-linked form, males are affected more severely than females. In males this disorder presents in the first 10 years of life with haematuria and proteinuria. Renal histology shows a proliferative glomerulonephritis, with typical changes in the basement membrane of splitting of the internal elastic lamina found on electron microscopy. Renal failure develops in the teenage years. High-tone nerve deafness and eye abnormalities are the other features of the syndrome.

Postural proteinuria

Intermittent or orthostatic proteinuria occurs in 10% of children and is more common in adolescents. Testing with Albustix or protein:creatinine ratio shows a normal amount of urinary protein in the early morning and increased protein during the day. The 24-hour protein estimation can sometimes be as high as 500 mg/d. This phenomenon is benign but proteinuria in an overnight urine specimen will usually require biopsy to determine the cause.

Glomerulonephritis

Most forms of glomerulonephritis result from an immunologically mediated injury involving either deposition of circulating immune complexes in the glomerulus or a specific antibody to the glomerular basement membrane.

The clinical features of acute glomerulonephritis are:

- haematuria
- proteinuria
- acute fluid overload – oedema, pulmonary oedema, congestive cardiac failure
- hypertension
- renal impairment – oliguria, elevated plasma creatinine.

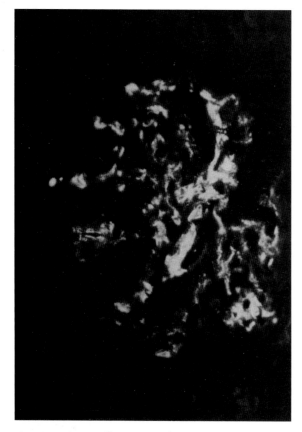

Fig. 18.2.1 Immunofluorescence shows mesangial IgA deposits (×600).

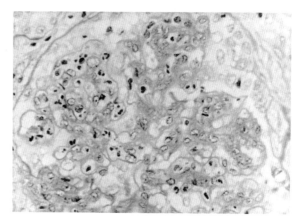

Fig. 18.2.2 Mesangial proliferation and neutrophil infiltration in post-streptococcal glomerulonephritis (periodic acid–Schiff ×800).

Table 18.2.1 Causes of acute nephritis

- Postinfectious glomerulonephritis
- Henoch–Schönlein purpura
- IgA nephropathy
- Lupus erythematosus
- Membranoproliferative glomerulonephritis
- Vasculitis

Acute presentation with these clinical features is seen most commonly in poststreptococcal glomerulonephritis. Other forms of glomerulonephritis (Table 18.2.1) in childhood may have a less severe onset.

Poststreptococcal glomerulonephritis

This disorder follows 7–14 days after group A haemolytic streptococcal throat infection and 3–6 weeks after streptococcal skin infection. It is hypothesized that streptococcal antigens deposit in glomeruli with activation of the complement system. The pathological appearance consists of proliferation of mesangial and endothelial cells with neutrophil infiltration (Fig. 18.2.2). Crescents may be present. Immunofluorescence shows IgG and C3 and electron-dense deposits are demonstrated by electron microscopy.

The usual presentation is a child, usually of school age, with macroscopic haematuria, acute fluid overload and hypertension. Lassitude, fever and loin pain also may be present. Physical examination may reveal hypertension, papilloedema, facial and leg oedema. On laboratory investigation urinalysis shows red blood cell casts and dysmorphic red cells. Serum urea, creatinine and potassium concentrations are often elevated. Mild normocytic normochromic anaemia is common and indicates haemodilution due to fluid overload.

The antistreptolysin O titre (ASOT) and antistreptococcal DNAase B are elevated in 90% of cases. Activation of the classical complement pathway leads to low serum levels of C3, which generally return to normal within 6–12 weeks. Complement C4 may be low in the early stages of the disease.

Careful management of the acute renal failure, and especially of the hypertension, is the basis of treatment in this condition. Salt and water accumulation, with suppression of plasma renin, is the major cause of hypertension. Mild hypertension is best managed with furosemide 2–4 mg/kg per day and fluid restriction. Moderate to severe hypertension requires management with oral nifedipine or prazosin, while parenteral hydralazine or nitroprusside are rarely required. Beta blockers should be avoided in the presence of pulmonary oedema. Bed rest is necessary only when the blood pressure is elevated. A course of oral penicillin for 10 days eradicates any existing streptococcal infection but does not alter the natural history of this condition. When renal insufficiency is present the diet consists of restricted protein (1 g/kg/d) and low salt and potassium intake.

The major *complications* of acute post-streptococcal glomerulonephritis are hypertensive encephalopathy, left ventricular failure and acute renal failure. Hypertensive convulsions are often associated with papilloedema and a temporary cortical blindness and require emergency treatment to lower blood pressure.

Acute heart failure is related to hypertension and fluid overload. Severe fluid restriction, high dose furosemide administration and adequate control of hypertension are then necessary.

The period of oliguria lasts up to 10 days and dialysis is indicated in cases where the blood urea rises above 50–60 mmol/l, or when hyperkalaemia or pulmonary oedema are not controlled by intravenous furosemide and fluid restriction. Dialysis should be performed only in a centre with the appropriate expertise. The long-term prognosis is excellent, with only 1% developing chronic renal failure. Microscopic haematuria may continue for 2 years but proteinuria should clear within 6 months. Renal biopsy is not indicated unless there is uncertainty of diagnosis with the initial investigations or the period of oliguria lasts longer than 3 weeks.

Other infectious agents including viral and bacterial organisms rarely can produce an illness similar to poststreptococcal nephritis. These organisms include staphylococci and pneumococcus, Echo, Coxsackie and Epstein–Barr viruses.

Henoch–Schönlein purpura

This disease is a vasculitic illness predominantly involving small vessels in the skin, large joints and gastrointestinal tract (Ch. 16.2). The illness is preceded by upper respiratory tract infection in 30–50% of patients. These children present with a petechial or purpuric rash, abdominal pain and arthritis. A mild nephritis is seen in 50–70% of cases, manifest usually by microscopic haematuria and proteinuria. Rarely, blood pressure and serum creatinine are elevated. Renal histology shows a proliferative glomerulonephritis with IgA in the mesangium. The prognosis is good, with fewer than 5% developing chronic renal failure.

Lupus erythematosus

Systemic lupus erythematosus (SLE) in childhood is seen more in females in the later childhood years. Facial rash, arthritis and fever are common presenting symptoms. Renal biopsy is indicated if haematuria and proteinuria are present. Serum C3 complement is usually low. This disorder is discussed further in

Chapter 13.3. The type of glomerular disease in SLE can vary from a mild focal proliferative glomerulonephritis to a diffuse crescentic glomerulonephritis with associated membranous features. The treatment includes prednisolone, azathioprine, cyclophosphamide and mycophenolate. The amount of immunosuppression is dependent on the severity of renal impairment, proteinuria and type of renal histology.

Nephrotic syndrome

Nephrotic syndrome is defined as:

- oedema
- proteinuria
- hypoalbuminaemia and
- hyperlipidaemia.

The annual incidence in children is approximately 2–4 in 100 000. The major conditions associated with a primary nephrotic syndrome are listed in Table 18.2.2.

Minimal change nephrotic syndrome

Evidence now suggests that the aetiology of minimal change nephrotic syndrome is caused by an alteration in the glomerular anionic status. Sensitized lymphocytes secrete a number of lymphokines that alter the normal, negatively charged sialoproteins on the glomerular basement membrane. Loss of membrane negative charge allows anionic proteins to leak across the basement membrane into Bowman's space. Light microscopy shows normal glomeruli but in some cases a mild increase in mesangial cells and mesangial matrix may occur. Immunofluorescence is negative and electron microscopy shows fusion of foot processes.

Generalized oedema is the usual presenting symptom (Fig. 18.2.3). Minimal change nephrotic syndrome comprises 80% of cases of nephrotic syndrome in childhood and is more frequent in males than females, the majority presenting between the ages of 1 and 4 years. Renal biopsy is not initially

---

Table 18.2.2   Classification of primary nephrotic syndrome

- Minimal change disease
- Focal segmental glomerulosclerosis
- Membranoproliferative glomerulonephritis
- Membranous glomerulopathy
- Congenital nephrotic syndrome

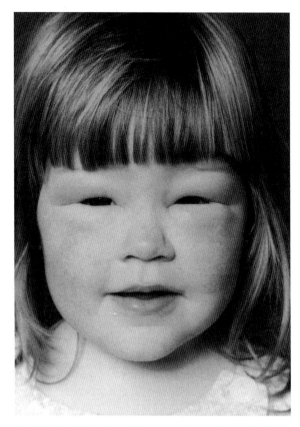

Fig. 18.2.3 Child with facial oedema due to the nephrotic syndrome.

Table 18.2.3 Clinical features of minimal change nephrotic syndrome

- Age 1–10 years
- Blood pressure normal
- Renal function normal
- Microscopic haematuria 30%
- Complements normal
- Selective index – low-molecular-weight protein urine loss

---

indicated if clinical features suggest minimal change (Table 18.2.3).

Unless large pleural effusions, gross ascites or severe genital oedema are present, strict bed rest is not necessary and the child should be allowed normal ward activity. A low-salt diet is encouraged. Fluid intake is generally not restricted because of the risk of hypovolaemia but mild fluid restriction may be beneficial in some children with significant oedema. Prednisolone 2 mg/kg per day or 60 mg/m² per day induces a remission in 90% of cases. The prednisolone dose is then reduced over 6 months, with later doses being given on alternate days to reduce side

effects. If remission, as defined by complete loss of proteinuria, has not occurred by 4 weeks, the nephrotic syndrome is steroid-resistant and a renal biopsy is then indicated to exclude other pathology, particularly focal segmental glomerulosclerosis.

Approximately 70% of children have relapses, which are more likely to occur in association with viral upper respiratory tract infections. Frequent relapses (≥4/year) may be prevented by regular prednisolone 5–15 mg given on alternate days. A course of cyclophosphamide is indicated when steroid side effects become significant. Of children given cyclophosphamide, 50% have no further relapses while most of the remainder have substantially fewer episodes of nephrotic relapse. Cyclosporin reduces the frequency of relapses and preliminary studies suggest that mycophenolate may have a similar effect. Neither drug gives long-lasting remission, with relapse common after withdrawal of treatment,

The major complications of the nephrotic syndrome are infections, hypovolaemia and thromboembolism. *Infections* such as peritonitis and septicaemia can be caused by both Gram-positive and Gram-negative organisms. The susceptibility to infections is related to loss of opsonins and immunoglobulins in the urine. If the patient develops a serious infection, the initial antibiotic treatment should cover both Gram-positive and Gram-negative organisms until cultures and sensitivity results are available. *Hypovolaemia* is due to loss of plasma water into the tissues with a consequent fall in the circulating blood volume. It occurs in 5% of cases and should be suspected if a child develops oliguria (<100 ml/day), poor peripheral perfusion, abdominal pain, tachycardia or postural hypotension. This

---

Clinical example

Sasha, a girl aged 5 years, presented with nephrotic syndrome at 2 years. At presentation serum albumin was 18 g/l and 24 hour urine protein 1.5 g/l. Microurine showed 30 rbc/mm³. Blood pressure and complement were normal. Prednisolone 60 mg/m² per day induced remission in 10 days. In the next 2 years Sasha had six relapses with upper respiratory tract infections and was then managed with prophylactic prednisolone. In the last 6 months she had two further relapses while still on maintenance prednisolone. She was now cushingoid and her height percentile had fallen from the 25th to below the 10th percentile. She commenced a 10-week course of cyclophosphamide (2.5 mg/kg/d).

Sasha had steroid-dependent nephrotic syndrome with significant steroid side effects requiring a change in therapy.

complication is confirmed by a high haematocrit and a low urine sodium (<10 mmol/l). The preferred treatment is intravenous 20% albumin (1 g/kg over 3–6 h), which may need to be repeated, according to response. Intravenous furosemide (2 mg/kg) is given in the middle and at the end of the infusion to promote a diuresis.

A hypercoagulable state exists for a number of reasons. These include haemoconcentration and loss of antithrombin III in the urine. Renal vein thrombosis and pulmonary embolism are relatively rare occurrences that require prompt treatment with anticoagulants. The avoidance of bed rest and the treatment of hypovolaemia probably account for the decreasing incidence of these complications.

Approximately 90% of children with relapsing nephrotic syndrome cease relapsing by 16 years of age. Even those children who continue to relapse into adult life usually remain steroid-sensitive. It is very rare for a child with a steroid-sensitive minimal change lesion nephrotic syndrome to progress to chronic renal failure. The 20-year mortality has now decreased from 60% to less than 5% since the introduction of antibiotics and corticosteroids. The morbidity and mortality should continue to decrease with adequate management of complications and avoidance of excess immunosuppression.

Focal segmental glomerulosclerosis

This glomerulopathy comprises 5–10% of children with nephrotic syndrome. The presentation is often similar to a minimal change lesion but with steroid resistance. Renal biopsy (Fig. 18.2.4) shows segmental sclerosis or hyalinosis with other glomeruli completely sclerosed or normal. Immunofluorescence shows IgM and IgG in the affected segmental lesions. Mutations in podocin, a podocyte structural protein,

are found in 10–30% of sporadic cases of steroid-resistant focal segmental glomerulosclerosis.

The majority of children with this lesion are resistant to steroids, cyclophosphamide and cyclosporin. Those children who remain nephrotic require treatment with diuretics (furosemide, spironolactone), mild fluid restriction and a low-salt diet. Approximately 60% progress to end-stage renal failure over 10 years. This glomerulopathy has a 30% recurrence risk in a transplanted kidney and in some cases plasmaphaeresis is beneficial.

Congenital nephrotic syndrome

Nephrotic syndrome in the first 3 months of life is most common in Finland, where the pathology is described as microcystic disease. Other types with minimal lesion histology, diffuse mesangial sclerosis or congenital syphilis are seen occasionally. The Finnish types are now seen in descendants of other European communities and the condition is inherited in an autosomal recessive fashion. The gene is localized to chromosome 19q13.1 and encodes a transmembrane protein called nephrin, which is expressed in the slit diaphragm between glomerular podocytes. Oedema is noted in the first weeks of life, with placentomegaly and prematurity being common precursors. There is no specific treatment, but transplantation can be performed. Proteinuria may occasionally recur following transplantation as a result of the formation of antinephrin antibodies.

Acute and chronic renal failure

The causes of acute renal failure are listed in Table 18.2.4.

Haemolytic–uraemic syndrome

Haemolytic–uraemic syndrome (HUS) is the most common cause of acute intrinsic renal failure in childhood and is characterized by the triad of:

- microangiopathic haemolytic anaemia
- thrombocytopenia
- acute renal insufficiency.

It has been broadly classified into two groups: the typical or epidemic form, also known as diarrhoea-associated (D+) HUS; the atypical or sporadic form, diarrhoea-negative (D−) HUS.

This disorder is more common under the age of 3 years. Usually it follows a mild gastroenteritis, but the diarrhoea is often blood-stained. Over the next few days, the child becomes pale, oliguric and unwell. Examination of the blood film shows fragmented red

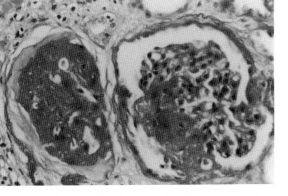

Fig. 18.2.4 Segmental and global sclerosis (periodic acid–Schiff ×500).

Table 18.2.4 Causes of acute renal failure		
Prerenal	Renal	Post-renal
Hypovolaemia 　Gastroenteritis 　Haemorrhage 　Hypoalbuminaemia	Kidney disease 　Glomerulonephritis 　Haemolytic–uraemic syndrome 　Interstitial nephritis	Posterior urethral valves Neurogenic bladder Ureterocele Calculi
Peripheral vasodilation 　Sepsis	Myoglobinuria, haemoglobinuria Nephrotoxic drugs	Tumours Uric acid (tumour lysis 　syndrome)
Decreased cardiac output 　Congestive cardiac failure		

blood cells and thrombocytopenia. Urinalysis reveals haematuria and proteinuria. The serum creatinine is usually elevated and hypertension is often severe.

Pathogenesis is related to verocytotoxin production by *Escherichia coli,* usually serotype O157 : H7, although other serotypes are also involved. The toxin crosses the damaged gut mucosa and adheres to endothelial cells in arterioles, with consequent swelling and widening of the subendothelial space with fibrin deposition. Atypical cases may follow pneumococcal pneumonia in which neuraminidase causes T-cell activation.

Dialysis is often necessary in the management of acute renal failure. Management is complex and should only be undertaken by an expert in paediatric renal disease; 90% of children make a complete recovery. Bad prognostic signs are oliguria lasting more than 2 weeks, cerebral involvement and age of onset over 5 years.

Chronic renal failure

The incidence of chronic renal failure in children is 2–4 per million total population per year. The commonest causes include:

- chronic glomerulonephritis
- reflux nephropathy
- obstructive uropathy
- medullary cystic disease.

The principles of management are as follows:

- control of hypertension
- adequate nutrition. Growth becomes impaired when the glomerular filtration rate is less than 25% of normal/1.73 m^2. With this degree of renal impairment, hyperfiltration can produce further sclerosis of the remaining functioning glomeruli. A low protein diet (0.8–1.5 g/kg/d) with low phosphate and adequate calorie intake may delay the progression of renal failure. Salt and fluid intake will vary with the type of renal disease

- prevention of renal osteodystrophy. Hyperphosphataemia should be vigorously treated with a low-phosphate diet and dietary phosphate binders (calcium carbonate or aluminium hydroxide) in an attempt to prevent secondary hyperparathyroidism. Vitamin D supplementation with calcitriol (1,25-dihydroxycholecalciferol) is given in early renal failure to prevent rickets
- administration of alkali to control acidosis (2–3 mmol/kg/d)
- anaemia is corrected by erythropoietin. This is administered subcutaneously once each week. Iron supplementation is necessary
- growth retardation is improved by growth hormone. Resistance to growth hormone is caused by low free insulin-like growth factor-1 levels.

Dialysis and transplantation are now standard for young children with end-stage renal failure. Under 1 year of age there are considerable technical, ethical

Clinical example

Thomas, aged 30 months, had chronic renal failure from birth from urethral valves and dysplastic kidneys. He had a poor appetite and required nasogastric feeding from 3 months. X-ray of the wrist at 18 months showed rickets requiring treatment with calcitriol. At 24 months he developed anaemia (Hb 9.5 g/l) and commenced weekly subcutaneous darbepoietin. Thomas had grown 2 cm in the last 12 months. Investigations showed Hb 11.3 g/l, serum sodium 136 mmol/l, potassium 4.5 mmol/l, urea 42 mmol/l, creatinine 0.65 mmol/l, calcium 2.4 mmol/l, phosphate 2.4 mmol/l, alkaline phosphatase 850 U/l. Parathormone was elevated.

Thomas had now reached end-stage renal failure and will commence peritoneal dialysis. Growth hormone was indicated for growth failure. He continued calcium carbonate at meal times in addition to calcitriol for renal osteodystrophy and erythropoietin for anaemia.

Practical points

Glomerular disease
- Microscopic haematuria without proteinuria is rarely associated with significant renal disease
- Non-postural proteinuria is a more important diagnostic and prognostic finding and requires specialist assessment
- Children with typical features of nephrotic syndrome that respond to prednisolone treatment do not require a renal biopsy
- Children with frequently-relapsing (2 relapses within 6 months of initial episode or ≥4/year) or steroid-dependent (relapse on prednisolone) nephrotic syndrome require specialist referral
- Control of hypertension and fluid overload is the key to management of acute post-streptococcal glomerular nephritis

and psychological problems. Young children tolerate peritoneal dialysis better than haemodialysis and the use of automated machines for overnight dialysis facilitates attendance at school. Both cadaver and live related transplants are performed in children, with good results. Approximately 80% of children survive for at least 10–15 years after entering dialysis/transplant programmes.

Hypertension

The recording of blood pressure should be part of the normal examination in children older than 3 years age. The blood pressure cuff bladder length should cover 80–100% of the circumference of the upper arm, as a smaller cuff will often lead to a falsely high reading. The child should be still and not crying. Using sphygmomanometry, the diastolic component is best recorded by the disappearance of Korotkoff sounds but if difficulties arise in obtaining an accurate recording a machine using oscillometric techniques can be used.

Normal blood pressure for children varies with gender, age and height (Fig. 18.2.5). A child should not be regarded as being hypertensive unless three recordings give levels above the 95th percentile for age and height. In borderline hypertension oscillometric 24-hour ambulatory blood pressure recordings are useful to distinguish persistent blood pressure elevation from 'white coat hypertension'.

The major causes of hypertension are given in Table 18.2.5. Renal disease accounts for approximately 80% of cases prior to adolescence.

The investigation of hypertension should commence with a good history and examination. The history should specifically include enquiries about urinary tract infections, neonatal umbilical artery

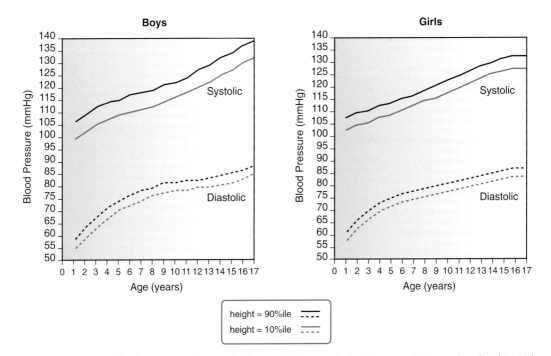

Fig. 18.2.5   95th percentile blood pressure in boys and girls aged 1–17 years, by height percentile (upper line, height = 90th percentile; lower line, height = 10th percentile).

catheterization, medication use and hypertension or early stroke in any relatives. Symptoms may relate to the underlying cause (polyuria and polydipsia in chronic renal failure) or the hypertension itself (headaches, irritability). Physical examination may assist in making a specific diagnosis (palpable renal mass, neurocutaneous pigmentation, delayed femoral pulses, renal artery bruits) or may suggest essential hypertension (obesity). The initial evaluation of hypertensive children is summarized in Table 18.2.6.

Treatment of hypertension depends on the severity, presence of symptoms and underlying cause. Children with a hypertensive emergency usually present with signs and symptoms involving the:

- nervous system – encephalopathy, facial palsy, retinopathy

- heart – left ventricular hypertrophy or congestive cardiac failure
- kidneys – raised serum creatinine, proteinuria.

An acute hypertensive emergency requires immediate intervention with intravenous drugs (Table 18.2.7), which can produce a controlled reduction in blood pressure. The aim is to decrease blood pressure by 25% over the first 8 hours, with gradual normalization over the subsequent 24–48 hours. Severe hypertension without imminent serious clinical sequelae is managed as a hypertensive urgency and blood pressure may be gradually reduced over 24–48 hours.

In essential hypertension, advice on a low-salt diet, weight reduction and exercise may assist reduction in blood pressure. Intervention techniques such as transluminal angioplasty for renal artery stenosis, resection of coarctation of the aorta and

---

Table 18.2.5   Causes of hypertension – REDCAT

R Renal parenchymal disease
- Acute glomerulonephritis
- Chronic glomerulonephritis
- Reflux nephropathy
- Obstructive uropathy
- Haemolytic uraemic syndrome
- Polycystic kidneys
  Renovascular (renal artery stenosis, renal vein thrombosis)
E Essential
D Drugs (corticosteroids, ciclosporin)
C Coarctation of aorta
A Adrenogenital syndrome, hyperaldosteronism
T Tumours (Wilms, phaeochromocytoma, neuroblastoma)

Table 18.2.7   Drug therapy of severe hypertension

Hypertensive emergency	
Sodium nitroprusside	0.5–10 µg/kg/min i.v. infusion
Labetalol	0.5–3 mg/kg/h i.v.
Hydralazine	0.1–0.5 mg/kg i.v. or i.m. every 4–6 h
Diazoxide	1–3 mg/kg stat i.v. then every 6 h
Hypertensive urgency	
Nifedipine	0.5–1 mg/kg oral 12 h
Minoxidil	0.1–0.5 mg/kg oral 12 h

Table 18.2.6   Evaluation of hypertension

Investigations	Potential diagnosis
Initial screening	
Creatinine and serum biochemistry	Acute or chronic renal failure
	Hyperaldosteronism (hypokalaemia)
Urinalysis and urine culture	Acute or chronic glomerulonephritis (haematuria, proteinuria), urinary tract infection
Renal ultrasound with Doppler	Reflux nephropathy, cystic disorders, tumours, renal artery stenosis
DMSA/micturating cystourethrogram	Reflux nephropathy
Mag3 or DTPA renal scan	Obstructive nephropathy
Echocardiogram	Aortic coarctation, assessment of end-organ damage
Second line	
Complement, antistreptolysin O titre and anti-DNAase B	Post-streptococcal glomerulonephritis
Renal angiogram/renal vein renin sampling	Renal artery stenosis
Plasma renin/aldosterone	Adrenal disorders, renal artery stenosis
Catecholamines/MIBG scan	Phaeochromocytoma
Renal biopsy	Acute or chronic glomerulonephritis

nephrectomy for a small scarred kidney may cure a small percentage of children.

The drug treatment of chronic hypertension is similar to that of adult patients; drugs used include:

- angiotensin converting enzyme inhibitors (captopril, perindopril)
- angiotensin receptor blockers (irbesartan, losartan)
- calcium channel inhibitors (nifedipine, amlodipine)
- beta-adrenergic blockers (atenolol, metoprolol)
- vasodilators (hydralazine, prazosin)
- diuretics (hydrochlorothiazide, furosemide).

Clinical example

Sally, aged 6 years, had a blood pressure recording of 140/100 mmHg at the time of tonsillectomy. Urine analysis, renal function and renal ultrasound were normal; an echocardiogram showed left ventricular hypertrophy; a Mag 3 scan showed that the left kidney contributed 44% and the right kidney 56% of total function; a renal angiogram showed a midaortic syndrome with bilateral renal artery stenosis from fibromuscular hyperplasia.

Sally's blood pressure was controlled with metoprolol 7.5 mg daily and amlodipine 5 mg daily. Left balloon angioplasty to 3–4 mm has been performed and she is awaiting a similar procedure on the right renal artery.

Practical points

Hypertension
- Hypertension is defined as repeated systolic blood pressure and/or diastolic blood pressure measurements ≥ 95th percentile for gender, age and height. Some hypertensive children may have a normal blood pressure at presentation if they are in cardiac failure
- 'White coat' hypertension is common in children and can be excluded by 24-hour ambulatory blood pressure monitoring
- All hypertensive children should be evaluated for target organ damage and have investigations to identify secondary causes of hypertension
- Intravenous treatment to achieve a slow, controlled reduction of blood pressure is indicated for hypertensive emergencies
- The goal for antihypertensive treatment is reduction of blood pressure to ≤95th percentile

PART 19

ENDOCRINE DISORDERS

Growth and variations in growth

J. Batch

Growth is the process in our lives that is unique to paediatric and adolescent medicine and distinguishes the health of children and young people from all other branches of clinical medicine. Growth is a multifactorial process and is influenced by the interplay of genetic, nutritional, hormonal, psychosocial and other factors, including the general health of a child. As such, growth mirrors the psychosocial and physical wellbeing of a child and adolescent.

The study of normal and abnormal growth is facilitated by a knowledge of the effects of physiological and pathological processes on growth and development at the different stages of life. The three major determinants of growth are:

- genetic factors
- nutritional factors
- hormonal factors.

Genetic factors

The genetic background of individuals is the basis for the major determinant of growth potential: tall parents tend to have tall children, while short parents have short children. Although children's heights at maturity resemble those of their parents, little is known about the exact location of the individual height controlling genes, how many genes are involved or how they direct cellular growth. Major genetic disturbances such as occur with chromosomal abnormalities are often reflected in growth patterns. For example, with loss of a sex chromosome in 45,XO Turner syndrome as shown in Figure 19.1.1 (see also Ch. 10.3), adult stature is severely compromised. Other less severe chromosomal abnormalities also may result in abnormalities in stature.

Many inherited genetic conditions can also result in growth disturbance. The most striking of these are the skeletal dysplasias, which often follow an autosomal dominant mode of inheritance. The classic example of a skeletal dysplasia is achondroplasia, which is described in Chapter 10.3. Chromosomes may also influence tall stature, as seen in the case of an individual with an extra sex chromosome, for example Klinefelter syndrome XXY, which frequently leads to an adult height above that anticipated from the family pattern.

Nutritional factors

Nutrition is the second most important factor determining normal growth in childhood and adolescence. In a global sense, malnutrition is the world's primary cause of poor growth. Both undernutrition and overnutrition may have long-lasting effects on growth patterns. Undernutrition, particularly if it occurs in utero or at significant postnatal periods, may affect both the weight and height growth patterns and also the development of body organs. In utero, undernutrition has also been associated with increased long-term risks of cardiovascular morbidity and mortality in children who are born small for dates. Undernutrition later in life is complicated by the interaction between the quality and the quantity of the diet and the duration of dietary inadequacy.

Emotional deprivation also has a profound influence on the growth process and may interact with provision of food. Furthermore, the mechanism of poor growth in many chronic illnesses of childhood is at least in part due to undernutrition or to nutritional influences on the balance of hormones and growth factors. Overnutrition may lead to obesity with advanced linear growth and early pubertal maturation. Overnutrition at a time when linear growth is declining in late adolescence may lead to lifelong obesity with the attendant risks of hypertension, insulin resistance and the development of type 2 diabetes.

Hormonal factors

Those of significance in growth are:

- growth hormone
- thyroid hormone
- testosterone and adrenal androgens
- oestrogens.

Growth hormone–insulin-like growth factor I axis

The major hormonal influence involved in growth regulation at all ages is the growth hormone–insulin-like growth factor 1 axis (GH–IGF-I). Growth

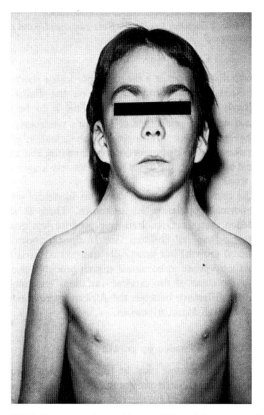

Fig. 19.1.1 Turner syndrome. Note webbing of the neck and the broadly spaced nipples.

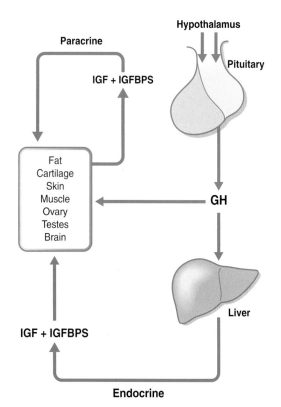

Fig. 19.1.2 A model showing the factors regulating pituitary growth hormone (GH) release and its targets in specific tissues as well as the liver, inducing release of insulin-like growth factor I (IGF-I) and its binding proteins (IGFBPs).

hormone is secreted by the anterior pituitary gland in a pulsatile pattern. Major peaks of secretion occur particularly at night. Growth hormone is bound to a specific growth hormone binding protein and subsequently acts on a broad range of tissues via cell surface receptors, resulting in a range of metabolic and growth-related effects. Many of these effects are mediated via IGF-I, which is produced by the liver and many other tissues (Fig. 19.1.2). The secreted IGF-I then acts either locally on adjacent tissues (paracrine action) or via endocrine mechanisms (i.e. via the circulation). IGF-I levels are age-dependent, being low in the fetus, rising through infancy and childhood, peaking during puberty and then falling to adult levels. IGF-I is very sensitive to nutritional status and in itself is of limited diagnostic value in the assessment of short stature. It circulates bound to one of its major binding proteins (IGFBPs).

Thyroid hormone

Thyroxine is very important for postnatal growth. Children with untreated hypothyroidism show profound both mental and growth retardation, with very delayed bony development. In many developed countries, neonatal thyroid screening programmes have been set up and treatment of congenital hypothyroidism ensures normal growth and intellectual development.

Testosterone and adrenal androgens

These hormones are anabolic and growth promoting. In males, testosterone and growth hormone act synergistically to promote the adolescent growth spurt. Excess androgens in childhood due to exogenous treatment, arising from adrenal enzyme disorders (congenital adrenal hyperplasia), precocious puberty or tumours will rapidly cause bone age advancement and may limit the potential for final height.

Oestrogens

Oestrogens in small doses may synergize with growth hormone to cause growth promotion. In higher doses, oestrogens will inhibit growth and promote early fusion of the bony epiphyses.

Phases of growth

There are three main phases of growth: fetal and childhood growth, and the pubertal growth spurt.

Fetal growth

Fetal growth is the most rapid phase of growth. Fetal growth is characterized by rapid differentiation of body organs, while late fetal growth involves continued rapid enlargement in tissues and organs and growth in length. The most rapid linear growth velocity of all ages occurs in the weeks before birth. Factors controlling fetal growth include placental supply of nutrients and oxygen and a range of local growth factors including insulin-like growth factors (IGFs). Pituitary growth hormone probably plays a relatively small part in this phase of growth, while thyroxine is involved in brain and bone growth in the fetus. Pituitary gonadotrophins (luteinizing hormone (LH), follicle stimulating hormone (FSH)) regulate testicular testosterone synthesis in the male fetus, which is essential for normal growth of the male phallus. Thus a male infant with hypopituitarism may have a micropenis at birth.

Childhood growth

During the first years of life, linear growth velocity is still very rapid (on average 8–12 cm/year) but it plateaus through childhood to an average of approximately 5 cm/year. The growth velocity immediately before the prepubertal growth spurt may be lower than this and represents a transient phase of poor growth. If the onset of the pubertal growth spurt is delayed then this phase of poor growth may be prolonged. During the childhood growth phase the limbs grow faster than the trunk, so that the ratio of the upper to lower body segments (divided at the pubic symphysis) diminishes from approximately 1.7:1 during infancy to 1:1 by age 10. It may fall to around 0.8 by mid puberty. The span:height ratio remains unchanged at approximately 1:1.

Factors controlling this phase of growth include genetic determinants, nutrition, absence of chronic disease and hormones, the most important of which are growth hormone and thyroxine.

Pubertal growth spurt

Puberty is associated with the onset of sex hormone production in boys and girls under the influence of pulsatile release of gonadotrophins (FSH/LH) from the pituitary gland. The earliest sign of puberty in boys, usually occurring at an average age of 11 years, is testicular enlargement (volume greater than 3–4 ml measured with an orchidometer). Penile and scrotal growth follow, with development of pubic and axillary hair in response to testosterone synthesis. In girls, ovarian oestrogen secretion leads to the earliest pubertal sign of breast development at an average age of 10.5–11 years, followed by pubic and axillary hair growth in response to adrenal and ovarian androgens. In boys, testosterone also leads to muscle growth, while in girls, oestrogens cause pelvic broadening and fat redistribution, leading to a female body shape. In both sexes, the onset of puberty is followed by a peak linear growth velocity, at an average age of 12.5 years in girls and 14.5 years in boys.

The hormonal events of puberty include an increase in the amplitude of growth hormone pulses, probably due to sex hormone effects. IGF-I levels rise during puberty in association with the high growth hormone levels. The sex hormones (testosterone or oestrogens) also appear to have direct effects at the skeletal growth plate, ultimately leading to fusion of the bony epiphyses and cessation of growth at an average age of 15 years in girls and 17 years in boys. The pubertal growth spurt may be influenced by genetic factors and also may be affected adversely by poor nutrition or chronic disease, both of which can cause pubertal delay.

> **Practical points**
>
> **Puberty**
> - The earliest sign of puberty in females is breast budding at an average age of 10.5–11.0 years
> - The earliest sign of puberty in males is testicular enlargement, at an average age of 11 years
> - The pubertal growth spurt occurs at an average age of 12.5 years in females, and 14.5 years in males
> - The growth spurt in puberty is the most rapid phase of postnatal growth

---

Assessment of growth

Percentile charts

Any health professional who deals with children must have a working knowledge of normal variations in growth and development and must be able to use a percentile chart. The childhood and pubertal growth patterns can be appreciated by examining growth charts, including linear height and weight charts (Fig. 19.1.3) as well as height velocity charts, indicating annual rate of growth (Fig. 19.1.4).

These charts demonstrate the range of normal growth, expressed either as percentiles or as standard deviations (SD) from the mean for age. The

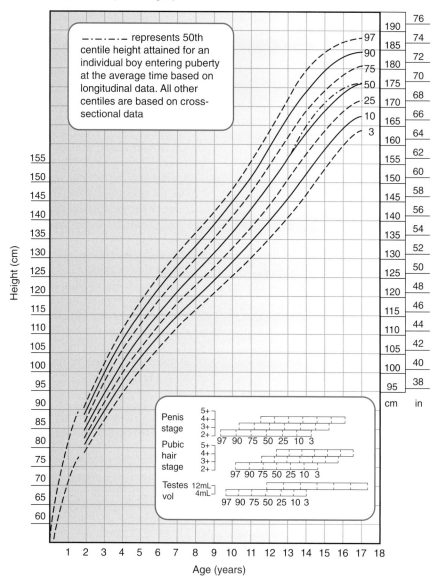

Boys: 2 to 18 years height percentile

–·–·–·– represents 50th centile height attained for an individual boy entering puberty at the average time based on longitudinal data. All other centiles are based on cross-sectional data

Fig. 19.1.3 Male height centile chart. A similar chart is available for females.

percentile curves are derived from the overall distribution (bell-shaped curve) of the data. The median or mid point is the 50th percentile and the normal range of average height or weight on the charts falls between the 3rd and 97th percentiles (Fig. 19.1.3). The median or 50th percentile indicates that 50% of the measurements of a normal group of children are above and 50% are below that point. The 50th centile 'final' height value for males is 177 cm and for females is 164 cm. The range between the 3rd and 97th (or approximately –2 SD to +2 SD) includes 94% of all normal children. It must be realized that there will be three normal children in every 100 who will be at or below the 3rd centile and three in every 100 who will be at or above the 97th centile.

Assessment of growth velocity (Fig. 19.1.4) is of far greater clinical significance than single measurements of height, and should be based on sequential measurements taken at 3-monthly intervals during a period of 6–12 months. When measured over this time period, a normal child will tend to follow the same height percentile. A child with an organic or endocrine disease will tend to deviate away from the percentile line and may move downwards across percentile lines. Thus serial measurement of children is the key to the assessment of their growth status.

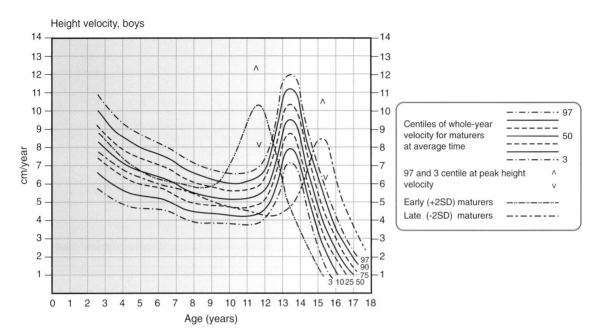

Fig. 19.1.4 Male height velocity centile chart. A similar chart is available for females.

> **Practical points**

Growth
- There is a wide variation of normal growth
- 3% of normal children will be above the 97th percentile or below the 3rd percentile
- Assessment of growth velocity (growth over time) is of more value than a single growth measurement
- The average growth rate during childhood is 5 cm/year

Bone age

Bone age is an index of physiological maturity, indicating the state of bony epiphysial maturation. A bone age is obtained by performing an X-ray of the left wrist and hand and is interpreted according to an atlas of age- and sex-specific standards. The bone age indicates the average age of children at a similar stage of bony maturation and is a guide to the remaining growth potential of the child. In normal children the bone age can be delayed up to 2 years behind the chronological age but it is rarely advanced a year beyond the chronological age.

Height age

Height age is the age at which a child's current height would represent the 50th percentile. This means that the height age indicates the average age of children of a similar height.

Midparental height

The midparental height (MPH), also known as the target height, allows the height of any individual child to be considered in relation to the heights of his/her biological parents. The midparental height can be calculated using the following formulae:

For boys: MPH = (father's height + (mother's height + 13))/2, ± 7.5 cm

For girls: MPH = (mother's height + (father's height − 13))/2, ± 6 cm.

A child should not be assumed to be short 'because s/he has a short family' unless the actual height of the child has been plotted on the growth chart and found to be consistent with the midparental height outlined above.

Short stature

The management of a child with short stature requires consideration of a number of issues. It is important to realize that the majority of short children will have no pathology but will either be following a familial pattern or have a variant of normal growth. The main causes of short stature in order of frequency of diagnosis are summarized in Table 19.1.1. As can be seen from the table, endocrine causes of short stature are the least common.

Table 19.1.1   Causes of short stature

- Genetic/familial short stature
- Constitutional delay
- Intrauterine growth retardation
- Chronic illness – malnutrition
- Skeletal dysplasia
- Iatrogenic (steroids/irradiation)
- Chromosomal abnormality/syndrome
- Psychosocial
- Endocrine

Table 19.1.2   The relationship between chronological age, bone age and height age for common growth problems

Growth problem	Chronological age (CA) (years)	Height age (HA)	Bone age (BA)
Genetic short stature	10	HA < CA	BA = CA
Constitutional delay	10	HA < CA	BA < CA
			BA = HA
Delayed puberty	15	HA < CA	BA < CA
Precocious puberty	6	HA > CA	BA > CA

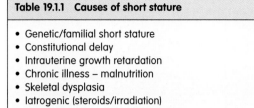 **Practical points**

Short stature
- The majority of short children are normal and healthy
- The most common causes of short stature are familial short stature and constitutional delay of growth
- Chronic disease is a major cause of short stature and is characterized by a fall off in both height and weight velocity

Variations from normal

Familial (genetic) short stature

Important features of familial short stature are as follows:

- these children will be growing on the 3rd centile or below, but the rate of growth is parallel to the 3rd centile
- the growth rate (growth velocity) is usually normal.
- the adult height percentiles of both parents should be plotted on the child's growth chart to assess whether the child's height is appropriate for the heights of the parents
- pubertal development usually occurs at the appropriate time
- markers of physical maturation such as bone age tend to be consistent with chronological age.

Constitutional delay in growth and pubertal development

Constitutional delay in growth and pubertal development is a very common variation of growth and leads to short stature during childhood with a height prognosis consistent with the midparental height expectation. Important features are:

- affects boys far more commonly than girls
- often there is a family history of a parent being short as a child, with delayed puberty and eventual catch-up with peers
- these children are the so called 'slow growers and late bloomers'. The typical growth pattern shows a

growth rate that is mostly normal except for a period of 6–12 months in the first 2 years of life, when the growth rate falls transiently
- the nadir in the growth velocity prior to puberty may be exaggerated, with the delayed appearance of pubertal development
- markers of physical maturation such as bone age are delayed and are consistent with the height age, indicating a true constitutional delay in growth
- the delay in puberty and associated delay in closure of bony epiphyses means that both the pubertal growth spurt and the completion of growth will be slowed according to the delay in bone age
- these children (most often boys) tend to grow into their late teenage years or early twenties.

The remaining causes of short stature are all pathological causes. The differences in growth patterns between genetic short stature, constitutional delay and pathological short stature are summarized in Figure 19.1.5. The relationship between chronological age, bone age and height age for common growth abnormalities is summarized in Table 19.1.2.

Pathological causes

Intrauterine growth retardation

This results in growth-retarded babies of appropriate gestational age. Major causes include a variety of genetic disorders primarily affecting the fetus. An abnormal intrauterine environment due to maternal illness, placental insufficiency or intrauterine infection may also lead to poor fetal growth. If the insult to the fetus occurs early in gestation, cell number is reduced and the potential for catch up is diminished.

Chronic disease

Chronic disease is a major cause of growth failure:

- usually the growth failure is associated with a similar fall off in weight velocity

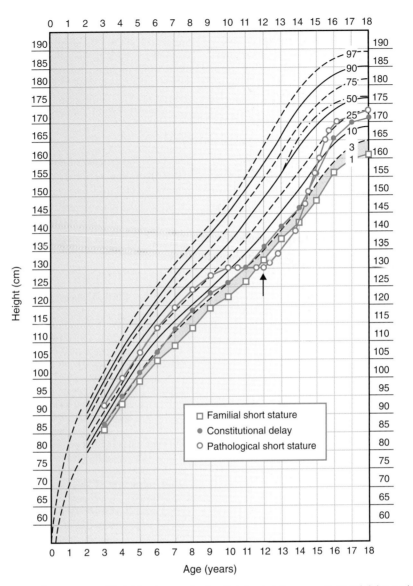

Fig. 19.1.5 The typical growth patterns and height outcomes for familial short stature, constitutional delay and pathological short stature are illustrated on the percentile chart. The arrow indicates detection of the cause of the pathological growth pattern and commencement of appropriate therapy, thus allowing catch-up growth.

- Chronic infections may also present as failure to grow and gain weight
- A hormone or endocrine problem is unlikely to be the cause of poor growth if both the weight and height are affected
- Nutritional insufficiency may contribute to the growth failure of chronic disease due to inadequate or inappropriate intake, poor absorption or impaired or excessive tissue utilization.

Skeletal disorders

Skeletal disorders are usually familial, involving intrinsic cartilage or bone defects. Examples include achondroplasia (the classic dwarf), other milder bony dysplasias (particularly hypochondroplasia) and the mucopolysaccharidoses. The major distinctive features of all of these disorders is body segment disproportion, i.e. increased upper to lower body segment ratios. The limbs are usually short, leading to a reduced span:height ratio. Weight gain is usually normal. These disorders in their mild form are relatively common and often overlooked. More information is given in Chapter 10.3.

Iatrogenic

Iatrogenic causes include corticosteroid excess, seen in children with steroid-treated chronic illnesses, such as severe asthma, juvenile arthritis and nephrotic syndrome. Marked growth failure is associated with weight gain. Irradiation to the head and spine may result in hypothalamic–pituitary dysfunction and poor spinal growth, which may lead to poor growth of the trunk with increased span:height ratio and a reduced upper to lower body segment ratio.

Chromosomal abnormalities and syndromes

Turner syndrome and its variants are the most common chromosomal cause of short stature. This condition must be excluded in any girl with short stature, as the typical phenotypic features may not be seen, particularly in the mosaic forms of Turner syndrome. The most common associated abnormality is ovarian dysgenesis resulting in failed pubertal development in 95% of cases. Other commonly seen features include a webbed neck (Fig. 19.1.1), small ears, increased carrying angle, coarctation of the aorta, horseshoe kidney, dysplastic nails and recurrent otitis media. All or none of these dysmorphic and clinical features may be present. The full range of features is summarized in Table 19.1.3.

Table 19.1.3   Features of Turner syndrome
General
• Short stature
• Developed puberty
• Amenorrhoea
Lymphatic abnormalities
• Neck webbing
• Low posterior hairline
• Lymphoedema
• Nail convexity/dysplasia
Skeletal abnormalities
• Micrognathia
• High arch palate
• Short fourth/fifth metacarpals
• Increased carrying angles
• Madelung deformity
• Kyphoscoliosis
• Broad chest
• Abnormal upper/lower body segment ratio
Metabolic
• Thyroiditis
• Carbohydrate intolerance
Miscellaneous
• Recurrent middle ear infections
• Decreased hearing
• Cardiac: coarctation or aortic stenosis (bicuspid aortic valve)
• Renal anomaly
• Naevi

Other chromosomal disorders are less common causes of short stature. Common dysmorphic syndromes presenting with short stature include Noonan syndrome, intrauterine growth retardation (Russell–Silver dwarfism) and Aarskog syndrome. Further details of these conditions are found in Chapter 10.3.

Psychosocial

Psychosocial causes of short stature cover the spectrum from severe deprivation to overt abuse, and may be associated with nutritional deficiencies. Fall off in weight gain is usually as striking as failure of linear growth. Short stature due solely to psychosocial deprivation is uncommon.

Clinical example

Tahlia's parents were concerned about her growth. Tahlia was aged 7 years and had an average birth weight and length but, since she had gone to school, her mother had noticed that she was one of the smaller girls in her class, and she did not seem to be growing as fast as the other children. Tahlia had several urinary tract infections as a toddler, and an ultrasound done after these had shown that she had a single horseshoe kidney. She also had recurrent middle ear infections, and her general practitioner noted that she had a heart murmur. An echocardiogram by a paediatric cardiologist showed that Tahlia had a bicuspid aortic valve. Tahlia had no other medical problems.

Tahlia's height at 7 years of age was 6 cm below the 3rd percentile and well below her midparental height range. Unfortunately despite having seen several doctors over the years, no past height measurements had been recorded. Tahlia's growth progress was monitored during a 6-month interval, during which time she only grew 1.6 cm (annualized growth velocity = 3.2 cm). Her position on the growth chart moved further away from the 3rd percentile.

Tahlia's poor growth was investigated when she was 7.5 years of age. A full blood count and erythrocyte sedimentation ratio (ESR) and a biochemical screen were normal. She was euthyroid and had a negative coeliac screen. A bone age X-ray showed a bone age of 4 years, well below her chronological age. Several weeks later the chromosome result became available, and showed that Tahlia had mosaic Turner syndrome. Tahlia and her parents were referred to a paediatric endocrinologist, who advised them that Tahlia's growth could be improved with growth hormone injections, and that it was very likely that she would need hormonal induction of puberty and would have later infertility due to the presence of gonadal (ovarian) dysgenesis as part of Turner syndrome. They were also informed that Tahlia would need ongoing medical care into adult life to monitor for other possible health problems, including hypertension, dyslipidaemia and type 2 diabetes, all of which occur more commonly in individuals with Turner syndrome.

Endocrine

Endocrine causes of short stature are the least common pathological cause and include hypothyroidism, growth hormone deficiency (possibly associated with other pituitary hormone deficiencies), Cushing syndrome (hypercortisolism) and adrenal insufficiency. In all of these cases the fall-off in linear growth exceeds the fall in weight gain.

Assessment

Issues to determine

Assessment of short stature involves determination of the following issues:

- is s/he short?
- is s/he growing slowly (could this be pathological)?
- what is the underlying cause?
- what is the adult height prognosis?
- how is s/he coping with the short stature?
- is any specific therapy warranted?
- is any supportive therapy indicated?

The approach to the assessment of short stature should include history, examination, investigations if necessary, therapy and follow-up.

History

When taking the history, the following should be sought:

- what is the height compared to peers? How long has the child been short? Who is concerned about the short stature and is there teasing at school? What is the school performance?
- what are the birth details and past medical history? Was there unexplained neonatal hypoglycaemia (suggesting pituitary hormone deficiency) or early illnesses? Determine the dental and milestone development, specific disease symptoms and nutritional status. Has puberty commenced? Are previous growth measurements available (child health record or measurements from local doctor or school)?
- what are the heights and ages of pubertal onset of the parents and siblings? Is there a family history of specific diseases?

Examination

On examination ensure/look for:

- accurate height and weight (using a reliable measuring device, particularly for height); body proportions (span, upper and lower segments)
- assessment of pubertal status. Pubertal stages for boys and girls are summarized in Table 19.1.4. The

---

Table 19.1.4 Stages of puberty

Males: genital (penis) development

- *Stage 1:* Preadolescent, testes, scrotum and penis are of about the same size and proportion as in early childhood
- *Stage 2:* Enlargement of scrotum and testes. Skin of scrotum reddens and changes in texture. Little or no enlargement of penis at this stage
- *Stage 3:* Enlargement of the penis, which occurs at first mainly in length. Further growth of the testes and scrotum
- *Stage 4:* Increased size of penis with growth in breadth and development of glans. Testes and scrotum larger; scrotal skin darkened
- *Stage 5:* Genitalia adult in size and shape

Females: breast development

- *Stage 1:* Preadolescent: elevation of papilla only
- *Stage 2:* Breast bud stage: elevation of breast and papilla as small mound. Enlargement of areola diameter
- *Stage 3:* Further enlargement and elevation of breast and areola, with no separation of their contours
- *Stage 4:* Projection of areola and papilla to form a secondary mound above the level of the breast
- *Stage 5:* Mature stage: projection of papilla only, due to recession of the areola to the general contour of the breast

Both sexes: pubic hair

- *Stage 1:* Preadolescent: the vellus over the pubes is not further developed than that over the abdominal wall, that is, no pubic hair
- *Stage 2:* Sparse growth of long, slightly pigmented downy hair, straight or slightly curled at the base of the penis in boys, or chiefly along labia in girls
- *Stage 3:* Considerably darker, coarser and more curled. The hair spreads sparsely over the junction of the pubes
- *Stage 4:* Hair now adult in type, but area covered is still considerably smaller than in adult. No spread to the medial surface of thighs
- *Stage 5:* Adult in quantity and type with distribution of the horizontal (or classic 'feminine') pattern. Spread to medial surface of thighs but not up linea alba or elsewhere above the base of the inverse triangle (spread up linea alba occurs late and is rated stage 6)

---

characteristic pubertal changes in males and females are illustrated in Figures 19.1.6 and 19.1.7. Further issues regarding puberty will be considered later in this section
- general physical examination including evidence of chronic disease, nutritional state and dysmorphic features suggesting a syndrome
- any sign of goitre or clinical signs of hypothyroidism, including dry hair and skin, bradycardia and delayed reflexes
- evidence of 'midline brain development syndromes' which may result in hypopituitarism. This includes cleft palate, single central incisor and small male

669

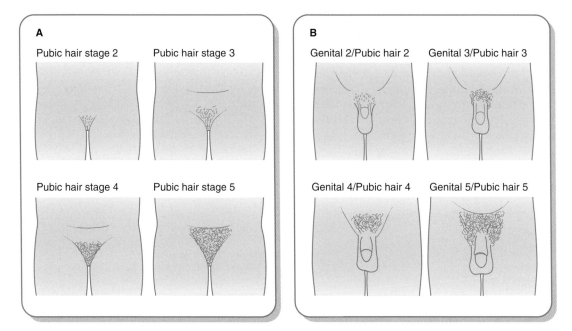

A

Pubic hair stage 2   Pubic hair stage 3

Pubic hair stage 4   Pubic hair stage 5

B

Genital 2/Pubic hair 2   Genital 3/Pubic hair 3

Genital 4/Pubic hair 4   Genital 5/Pubic hair 5

Fig. 19.1.6 **A** Pubertal pubic hair changes in the female. **B** Pubertal genital and pubic hair changes in the male. A more detailed explanation is given in Table 19.1.4.

genitalia (associated with gonadotrophin deficiency in utero). The combination of neonatal hypoglycaemia and small genitalia suggests hypopituitarism
- examination of visual fields and optic fundi to exclude the possibility of a pituitary lesion, in particular craniopharyngioma.

Management

The single most important aspect of the management of short stature is to plot the current and previous heights and weights and parental heights on a percentile chart in order to answer the following questions:

- is the child short and below the 3rd height centile? Is this appropriate for midparental height?
- is the child growing slowly and is there evidence that the height is falling across the percentile lines? This can be further plotted on a height velocity chart (Fig. 19.1.4).

A velocity below the 25th centile for bone age is potentially abnormal in a short child. A reliable height velocity requires at least 6 months of growth data, and preferably 12 months with consistent measurements at 3–4-monthly intervals over that time. Examination of the growth data plus the points obtained in history and examination should allow distinction between a variation of normal or a pathological cause of short stature.

Investigations

Investigations should be performed if there is any evidence of specific chronic disease, if there is a suggestion of chromosomal abnormality or if the growth velocity is subnormal. The following investigations may be performed:

- bone age X-ray
- full blood count and ESR
- urea, creatinine and electrolytes
- urinalysis ± microscopy and culture
- calcium and phosphate
- thyroid function tests
- chromosomes (girls only)
- screening test for coeliac disease (total IgA and endomysial antibodies or tissue transglutaminase antibodies).

It is important to note that all girls with unexplained short stature should have a karyotype performed to exclude the possibility of Turner syndrome.

If puberty is markedly delayed it may be worthwhile measuring gonadotrophins (FSH/LH) and testosterone or estradiol.

These investigations provide a screen for underlying chronic disease, infection or nutritional deficiency as well as hypothyroidism and Turner syndrome. Other investigations may be indicated by specific physical findings. In a child with unexplained combined weight and height fall-off, a malabsorptive disorder should be excluded and consideration should

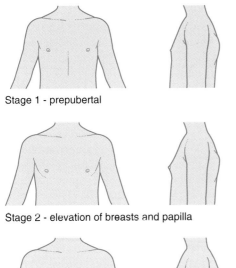

Stage 1 - prepubertal

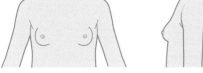

Stage 2 - elevation of breasts and papilla

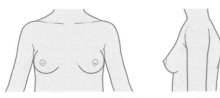

Stage 3 - further enlargement and elevation of breast and areola but no separation of contour

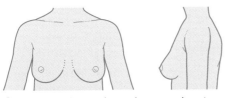

Stage 4 - areola and papilla form a secondary mound above level of the breast

Stage 5 - areola recedes to the general contour of the breast

Fig. 19.1.7 Pubertal breast changes in the female. A more detailed explanation is given in Table 19.1.4.

Clinical example

Ben was a 14-year-old boy whose mother complained that he did not seem to be growing at all. She said to her general practitioner that she had not needed to buy Ben any new clothes for the past 3 years. She remembered that her older son was always growing out of his clothes at this age. She was also concerned because Ben did not seem to have as much stamina as other boys his age, and certainly he ate much less than she would have expected at this age, based on her experience with her older son.

Further history revealed that Ben had always been a very healthy boy in the past, with no significant medical problems. He had become a fussy eater during the past couple of years. He said that many foods he had previously eaten now made him feel sick in the stomach and gave him stomach cramps. When asked if he had diarrhoea, Ben said 'no', but when asked how many times he went to the toilet he admitted that he needed to go at least 6 times per day, and that this pattern had only developed in the last year. Ben said he thought this was normal.

Physical examination confirmed that Ben's height and weight were almost the same as when he was 11 years old. Apart from being a little bit pale, there were no other abnormal physical findings on general examination. Ben was prepubertal.

Baseline investigations included a full blood count and ESR. These showed that Ben had a low haemoglobin and his ESR was 79. All the other baseline tests including electrolytes, liver function tests, renal function, screening tests for coeliac disease and thyroid function tests were normal. Ben's bone age was very delayed. At 14 years of age his bone age was only 10 years.

The history of poor growth and the abdominal symptoms together with the low haemoglobin and raised ESR suggested the possibility of a chronic gastrointestinal problem such as inflammatory bowel disease. Ben was referred to a paediatric gastroenterologist and had an endoscopy and colonoscopy, which demonstrated that he had Crohn disease. Ben was treated with steroids and salazopyrine for his Crohn disease and his symptoms improved. He started to gain weight and over the next 12 months his growth also improved.

be given to measuring endomysial antibodies as a possible indicator of the presence of coeliac disease. If these are elevated, a small bowel biopsy may be necessary.

Investigation for growth hormone deficiency

Growth hormone deficiency may be suggested by association with midline defects or if other pituitary hormone deficiencies, including hypothyroidism or gonadotrophin deficiency, are present. The presence of biochemical growth hormone deficiency suggests a need for magnetic resonance imaging (MRI) of the central nervous system (CNS) and biochemical testing for other pituitary deficits. Specific underlying causes of growth hormone deficiency include idiopathic (most common), pituitary or hypothalamic tumours/structural abnormalities, cranial irradiation and genetic growth hormone deficiency (e.g. gene defects of pituitary transcription factors). Specific tests to determine the presence of growth hormone deficiency include:

- physiological tests of growth hormone sufficiency, including:

- exercise growth hormone (GH) tests: performed in the fasting state on a bicycle ergometer with blood for GH levels taken before and 30 minutes after exercise. This is a screening test with 20% of normal children failing to reach cut off levels
- overnight sleep studies of growth hormone secretion
- measurement of IGF-I and IGFBP-3 levels. This test is used for screening for GH deficiency prior to proceeding to more involved pharmacological tests. As yet the data are not sufficiently reliable to recommend that these tests be performed as a single diagnostic entity in a clinical setting. They may, however, be useful when considered in combination with other clinical information, results of MRI brain scans and growth hormone tests
- pharmacological tests of growth hormone sufficiency, including:
  - glucagon stimulation test
  - arginine–insulin hypoglycaemia test
  - clonidine stimulation test.

Although no one test is superior to another, the glucagon stimulation test is at present the preferred pharmacological test of GH secretion. The glucagon stimulation test also provides information about the adrenocorticotrophin–cortisol axis. The arginine–insulin hypoglycaemia test is used rarely in paediatric practice as hypoglycaemia is an obligate part of this test and is potentially dangerous.

For the purposes of defining GH deficiency and assessing eligibility for hGH as a pharmaceutical benefit in Australia, biochemical growth hormone deficiency is defined as failure to achieve a peak serum GH concentration of more than 10 mU/l in response to two stimulation tests, at least one of which would be a pharmacological test, or in response to one test in the presence of other evidence suggestive of GH deficiency, such as structural CNS abnormalities or low plasma IGF-I and IGFBP-3 levels.

Treatment

Short stature is considered by some children and their families to be a physical and psychosocial disability. Extreme short stature can certainly be considered as a handicap in both a social and medical sense. Many paediatricians and paediatric endocrinologists consider that, if the estimated final height of a female will be less than 152.4 cm (5 ft) or a male less than 162.6 cm (5 ft 4 in), then consideration should be given to the use of a growth promoting agent. The major growth promoting agent used in the treatment of short stature is biosynthetic growth hormone. Biosynthetic growth hormone has been available commercially in Australia since 1985. In 1988, the *Guidelines for the Use of Growth Hormone in Australia* were liberalized, allowing the use of growth hormone in short children who are growing poorly but are not growth-hormone-deficient.

Growth hormone can be administered only by subcutaneous injections, usually given 6–7 days per week. Despite the availability of biosynthetic growth hormone, the annual cost of growth hormone therapy remains very high. Growth hormone should therefore only be used for children who have short stature and who could potentially benefit from the therapy.

The Commonwealth Department of Health and Family Services has provided guidelines for the use of growth hormone in Australia. These can be summarized as follows:

> A child must have abnormally short stature (height less than the 1st percentile) with an abnormally low growth rate, measured over a minimum period of 1 year at intervals of not greater than 6 months. The child should be growing at a height velocity below the 25th centile for skeletal age and sex.

Variations to these guidelines exist for particular groups of patients, such as Turner syndrome, growth hormone deficiency, combined growth hormone deficiency and precocious puberty, chronic renal insufficiency and those patients with growth retardation secondary to an intracranial lesion or cranial irradiation.

Growth hormone treatment has been shown to be of benefit in the following conditions:

- growth hormone deficiency
- Turner syndrome (final height can be improved by up to 8–10 cm)
- growth retardation secondary to renal insufficiency.

In general, results of growth hormone therapy for short stature associated with constitutional delay, intrauterine growth retardation, glucocorticoid-induced growth failure, chromosomal and genetic disorders and skeletal dysplasias have been less promising. Although the definite indications for growth hormone treatment of short stature are limited, any child who is short and growing slowly with a poor ultimate height prognosis should be referred for assessment. After assessment it may be appropriate to offer the child a trial of growth hormone therapy.

Other specific agents used in the treatment of short stature associated with constitutional delay have included oxandrolone (a biosynthetic testosterone analogue) and low dose oral testosterone preparations.

Psychological support and counselling

Psychological support and counselling are undoubtedly the most important part of the management of short stature and can be provided by either health professionals or lay support groups. Often reassurance regarding the normality of the child and the reassurance of a reasonable height prognosis is all that is required. If the height prognosis is poor, then counselling and support should be used in conjunction with growth promoting agents. Families should be advised to encourage self esteem in the child by promoting the child's strengths, for example, sporting, musical or academic, rather than concentrating on the perceived limitations imposed by short stature. Lay support groups associated with growth hormone deficiency or Turner syndrome are now quite common in most large cities, and have active programmes for children and their families. On occasions it may be necessary to seek formal psychological or psychiatric help for a child or family who are very distressed by the problem of short stature.

Tall stature

Tall stature is a relatively infrequent problem compared with the number of children who present because of short stature. In general, very few tall children have an organic disease process as a basis for their disease. The most common reason for tall stature is genetic tall stature. Compared to 20 years ago, relatively few teenagers and their parents are concerned about tall stature, as it is now more socially acceptable for girls to be tall. However, girls may be presented for assessment of their final height if it is thought that they will be in excess of 178 cm (5 ft 10 in). A final height of 183 cm (6 ft) may be acceptable for a girl if her parents and other siblings are also tall. As with short stature, there is no clear demarcation between normal and tall stature. A child whose height is above the 97th percentile for age should be considered tall.

Causes

The following may be causes of tall stature:

- familial or normal variant
- precocious puberty
- syndromes: Marfan, Klinefelter, triple X, homocystinuria, Sotos
- endocrine causes: hyperthyroidism and pituitary gigantism.

Familial/normal variant tall stature

Most tall children are normal in all respects and their height is genetically determined. Some children with early but otherwise normal pubertal development (8–10 years in girls, 10–12 years in boys) will appear tall in relation to their peers and family during adolescence, but will have a predicted final height within the accepted normal range. These early developers have an advanced bone age and are at the opposite end of the spectrum to the short children with delayed maturation, who have delayed puberty but who will also reach a normal adult height commensurate with their midparental height.

Precocious puberty

Precocious puberty is defined as pubertal development at less than 8 years of age in girls and less than 9.5 years in boys. Because of rapid acceleration of bone maturation and early epiphysial closure, many children with precocious puberty are excessively tall in early to mid childhood but finish up as relatively short adults (Fig. 19.1.8). It is important to recognize precocious puberty, as treatment can be provided to switch off the premature activation of the hypothalamic–pituitary–gonadal axis. It is also important to ascertain whether the appearance of precocious puberty may be due to an aberrant source of androgen or oestrogen production, such as an adrenal or ovarian tumour. Occasionally the appearance of precocious puberty may be due to iatrogenic causes, such as oestrogen cream application or excessive administration of anabolic steroids to improve appetite and growth.

Syndromes causing tall stature

Marfan syndrome may present with the classical picture of arachnodactyly, ligamentous laxity, chest deformity, cardiac abnormalities, high arched palate and subluxation of the lenses. Often, however, one sees tall, thin children with some marfanoid features who are difficult to classify. Children with homocystinuria have a marfanoid phenotype but are retarded intellectually. Homocystinuria may be diagnosed by a study of urinary and serum amino acids. Tall girls with intellectual retardation should also be screened for the triple X syndrome, and tall boys with disorders of pubertal maturation, with small testes, gynaecomastia and sometimes behavioural disturbance, should have chromosomal analysis. They may have either XYY syndrome or Klinefelter syndrome (XXY).

Endocrine causes of tall stature

Hyperthyroidism is relatively uncommon in childhood and is an infrequent cause of tall stature. The clinical features of hyperthyroidism are discussed in Chapter 19.2. Pituitary gigantism is extremely rare but should be suspected if the history and

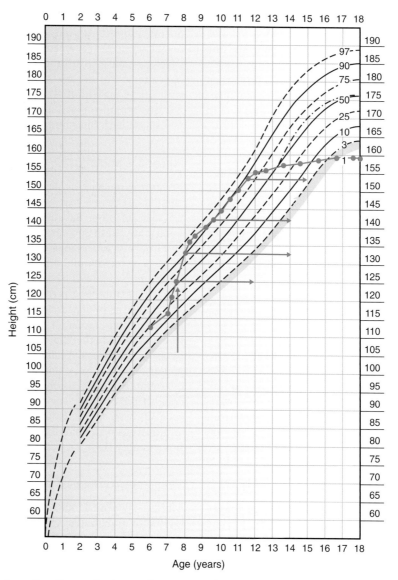

Fig. 19.1.8 The typical growth pattern and outcome of precocious puberty. The vertical arrow indicates commencement of specific therapy to halt/slow down the precocious puberty. The horizontal arrows indicate the degree of bone age at the given chronological ages, advancement (e.g. bone age 12 years at chronological age 7.5 years) ultimately leading to premature fusion of the epiphyses and early cessation of growth.

examination suggest pituitary involvement in association with tall stature. Children with pituitary gigantism will have an abnormally rapid growth rate as well as tall stature, in contrast to genetically tall children who grow above but parallel to the 97th centile but have a normal growth velocity.

Approach to diagnosis and treatment

The approach to diagnosis in a tall child consists of a full history, including a history of family heights and pubertal maturation patterns. In addition, it is important to ascertain whether there are associated

abnormalities or developmental delay which may suggest one of the chromosomal or syndromal disorders causing tall stature.

A full physical examination is essential, with emphasis on accurate height measurement, body build, limb proportions and pubertal status. Neurological assessment should include funduscopy, assessment of visual fields and intellectual function and should determine any evidence of hyperthyroidism.

In most instances a tall child will in fact have a normal growth velocity above but parallel to the 97th centile. An accurate height measurement and bone age assessment by an experienced radiologist or paediatric endocrinologist will enable an adult height prediction to be made. Frequently this is found to be at or below 178 cm (5 ft 10 in) for a girl or 193 cm (6 ft 4 in) for a boy and no further action is necessary.

In the past, sex steroids have been used to reduce the final height in both males and females where the estimate of final height was thought to be excessive. High-dose oestrogen treatment was used in tall girls in the past. However, recent studies have suggested impaired fertility in women treated with high-dose oestrogen for tall stature in adolescence, and this treatment is now rarely advocated. It should only be considered after paediatric endocrinology input and fully informed consent of the both the parent and young person.

Variations of pubertal development

Early normal puberty

In many countries, including Australia, children appear to be going through puberty at an age which is much younger than children in previous generations. This is called the secular trend in growth and development. The earlier age of puberty is probably due to effects of improved nutrition and living circumstances and absence of chronic disease. This seems to be particularly true for girls, with many girls showing early signs of breast development just before 8 years of age and starting to have menstrual periods while still in primary school. In most cases this early puberty is just a variation of normal. After assessment by a specialist, no specific treatment is usually required. The girl and her family need to have the situation explained. Enlisting the help of the teacher is also very helpful.

Delayed puberty

Delayed puberty is very common and occurs in approximately 2% of the adolescent population. Delayed puberty is defined as the absence of pubertal changes over the age of 14 years for girls and over the age of 14–15 years for boys. In general, adolescents have a heightened awareness of body image and are often preoccupied with the normality or otherwise of their pubertal development. Boys in particular may suffer major psychological effects resulting from delayed puberty as they may experience bullying, may be left out of sporting teams and may be less generally able to compete with their peers due to poor muscular development. The most common causes of delayed puberty are familial or constitu-

Clinical example

Sophie Jones was taken to see her general practitioner when she was 10 years old. Mrs Jones was very concerned that Sophie was too young to cope with menstrual periods, and was worried that the periods would commence very soon. Mrs Jones insisted on speaking to the doctor privately, before Sophie came into the consulting room, and she became very upset about Sophie's development when speaking to the doctor. She recalled when she was an adolescent and had 'terrible period pain', which prevented her going to school and being in the netball team. Mrs Jones wanted the doctor to give Sophie medication to 'put puberty on hold' until Sophie was much older. When asked, Mrs Jones did say that Sophie did not seem to be upset about her development and that a few other girls in Sophie's class at school appeared to be at a similar stage of development.

Sophie was a very healthy girl who was in grade 5 at school. She had a group of friends at school, and enjoyed being part of the local Little Athletics Team. She was the eldest child in her family and had two younger brothers aged 6.5 and 4 years. She had no significant medical problems.

Sophie had developed some 'breast budding' when she was 9.5 years old, and in the past 12 months had started using a deodorant. She also reported that she had developed some pubic hair and had a few facial blackheads. Examination showed that Sophie's height was on the 75th percentile and her weight was on the 50th percentile for her age, and confirmed the presence of breast stage 2 and pubic hair stage 2, with some facial seborrhoea. The rest of the physical examination was normal.

The doctor advised Mrs Jones that Sophie's pubertal development was completely normal for her age and that the usual interval from the beginning of breast budding to menarche was usually 18–24 months. She also advised Mrs Jones that it would not be the best option for Sophie to suppress an otherwise normal developmental process. She advised Mrs Jones that Sophie would experience her pubertal growth spurt in the time leading up to menarche, and that Sophie's growth would then slow down over the following 2 years until Sophie was fully grown. Given the current growth pattern, the doctor advised Mrs Jones that Sophie's height would end up being consistent with family expectations. She also advised Mrs Jones that the best thing she could do as a mother was to calmly talk to Sophie about the physical changes of puberty, so that Sophie would understand and be prepared for her menstrual periods when they started.

During the next 2 years, Sophie and Mrs Jones saw their GP every few months. Mrs Jones took her GP's advice and, when Sophie started her periods at the age of 11.5 years, she coped very well.

tional delay in puberty for which there is often a family history, particularly in the father of a teenage boy. Puberty may also be delayed in the presence of any chronic illness of childhood or adolescence. The causes of delayed puberty are usually considered on

Table 19.1.5 Causes of delayed puberty

Associated with normal or low serum gonadotrophins

Constitutional delay	Usually familial: associated with slow growth and a delayed bone age
Chronic illness	Poor nutrition, e.g. cystic fibrosis, juvenile arthritis, inflammatory bowel disease
Endocrine causes	Hypopituitarism, isolated gonadotrophin deficiency, Kallmann syndrome, hypothyroidism, hyperprolactinaemia

Associated with elevated serum gonadotrophins*

Gonadal dysgenesis	Turner syndrome, Klinefelter syndrome, Noonan syndrome
Anorchia	
Gonadal damage, vascular events	Vascular damage, irradiation, infection (mumps), torsion or autoimmune disease

* This usually signifies primary gonadal dysfunction.

the basis of the serum gonadotrophins (LH/FSH) and are outlined in Table 19.1.5.

Diagnosis and management

Assessment of delayed puberty requires a complete history, including a family history of pubertal maturation patterns. Also, it is important to look carefully for the possibility of occult chronic disease, such as inflammatory bowel disease, which may become apparent initially as a delay in the onset of puberty. If the history is suggestive of familial or constitutional delayed puberty, and this is confirmed by physical examination, no further investigation may be necessary. If the diagnosis is not clear, then the following investigations may need to be performed:

- full blood count and ESR
- urea/creatinine and electrolytes
- liver function tests
- screening test for coeliac disease (total IgA and endomysial antibodies or tissue transglutaminase antibodies)
- thyroid function tests
- chromosomes
- bone age X-ray
- serum FSH and LH, testosterone or estradiol
- serum prolactin
- ±growth hormone studies.

Treatment

Indications for treatment of delayed puberty are primarily psychological. Induction of pubertal development in boys through the judicious use of intramuscular or oral testosterone preparations may be very useful in alleviating the psychological stress caused by delayed puberty. Recent research also suggests that treatment of delayed puberty is important, as puberty is the time when peak bone mass is accumulated. Failure to achieve peak bone mass in adolescence may place individuals at risk of osteoporosis in adult life. Treatment of delayed puberty should only be carried out by paediatricians and endocrinologists experienced in this area, as excessive administration of sex steroids can adversely accelerate bony epiphysial maturation and affect long-term height outcome (Fig. 19.1.9).

Psychological support and counselling

Psychological support and counselling are an extremely important part of the management of pubertal delay and in some instances may be all that is required while waiting for the onset of spontaneous pubertal development. It is very important to

Clinical example

Andrew was a 15.5-year-old boy whose father was concerned that Andrew was growing poorly, and that he was underdeveloped for his age. Andrew's father had also been a late developer, and he remembered being bullied at school by some of the other boys and also being left out of the rugby team because of his size. He reported that he was still growing when he left school and became an apprentice mechanic. The mechanics he worked with used to call him 'Shorty'.

Further history revealed that Andrew was a healthy young man who had always grown along the 3rd percentile, but from 14 years of age his height had fallen away from the 3rd percentile line. He was a very keen sportsman and had always been a very fast runner but could no longer compete successfully with boys his age. Because of this he had recently taken up golf, which he and his father played together every Saturday. Andrew's physical examination confirmed that he was completely prepubertal, with an otherwise normal physical examination.

The most likely diagnosis was familial delayed puberty. Andrew was not distressed at all by his delayed puberty, and his father was reassured when the diagnosis was explained. During the next 3 years, Andrew's growth rate increased and he went through a delayed but otherwise normal puberty, eventually being the same height as his father.

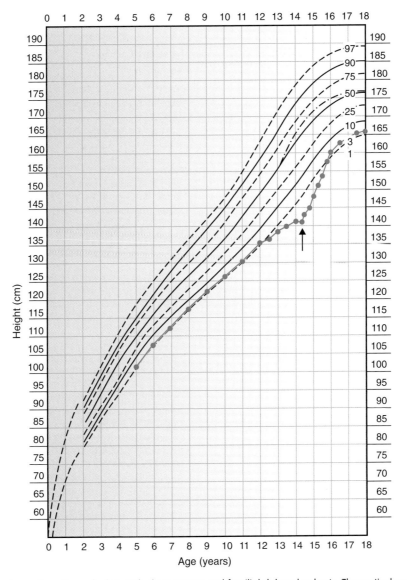

Fig. 19.1.9 The typical growth pattern of a boy with short stature and familial delayed puberty. The vertical arrow indicates the point at which a short course of testosterone therapy was given with a resulting growth spurt, onset of pubertal development and resumption of normal growth and variations in growth.

reassure the adolescent and his/her family that s/he is normal and that appropriate pubertal and sexual development will occur or can be relatively easily assisted with hormonal intervention. Such reassurance and support can profoundly improve an adolescent's self-esteem and can help reverse problems such as truanting from school, oppositional behaviour and bullying.

Precocious puberty

Precocious puberty is a rare problem and occurs much less frequently than delayed puberty. Preco-

cious puberty is defined as pubertal development before age 8 years in girls and 9.5 years in boys. True or central precocious puberty is associated with raised gonadotrophins. True precocious puberty is much more common in girls than boys, and girls are less likely to have an identifiable underlying pathological cause than boys. Girls with this disorder will have accelerated growth and development of both breasts and pubic hair. Boys with true precocious puberty have evidence of enlargement of both testes as well as accelerated linear and genital growth and pubic hair development. The most common cause of central precocious puberty is a hypothalamic hamartoma, but many tumours involving the hypo-thalamic–pituitary area can be associated with an increased prevalence of precocious puberty.

Gonadotrophin-independent (pseudo) precocious puberty may be seen with congenital adrenal hyper-plasia, adrenal, testicular or ovarian neoplasms and tumours that secrete non-pituitary gonadotrophin such as chorionic gonadotrophin. The McCune–Albright syndrome is also a cause of gonadotrophin-independent precocious puberty.

If precocious puberty is suspected, referral should be made to a paediatric endocrinologist who will organize appropriate investigations, which will include measurement of serum FSH and LH, testos-terone or estradiol, dynamic tests of gonadotrophin secretion such as luteinizing hormone releasing hormone (LHRH) testing, bone age assessment and cerebral imaging including computed tomography (CT) and/or MRI head scanning. Treatment of pre-cocious puberty should be managed by a paediatric endocrinologist experienced in this area. Treatment options include LHRH superagonists, medroxypro-gesterone acetate or cyproterone acetate. Indications for treatment for precocious puberty will include factors such as the age of the child and the rate of progression of the pubertal development.

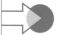

Practical points

Delayed puberty
- Delayed puberty is a very common pubertal problem
- Delayed puberty is defined as absence of pubertal development in girls older than 14 years and boys older than 14–15 years
- Familial delayed puberty and constitutional delayed puberty are the most common causes, particularly in boys, often with a positive family history
- Chronic disease may cause delayed puberty

Conditions resembling precocious puberty

Premature thelarche

Isolated breast development, either unilateral or bilateral, is relatively common in girls older than 2 years of age and may occur at any time throughout childhood. By definition, premature thelarche has no other features of precocious puberty. All cases should be referred for assessment by a paediatrician or endocrinologist; however, in most cases observation and follow-up is all that is required.

Clinical example

Amy was a 12-month-old girl whose parents were very worried that she was going into early puberty. They reported that Amy had bilateral breast development, which had been present from birth.

Amy was the first child of her parents. The pregnancy had been uncomplicated and she born 2 weeks post-term via a normal vaginal delivery. Her birth weight was 3570 g. At birth she was noted to have swollen breasts, which the midwife had said could occur in newborn babies because of the mother's hormones and would go away. However, the breast development had persisted, and now the family were very worried.

Further history revealed that Amy was a very healthy baby who had not had any significant medical problems and had grown and developed normally for her age. At 12 months she was already walking and could say several words. Her weight, height and head circumference were all progressing along the 25th percentile for age. She was not on any medications, health foods or tonics and ate a normal toddler diet.

Physical examination revealed that Amy did have breast enlargement (1.5 cm diameter), but there was no sign of any pubic hair development or other pubertal changes. General examination was normal.

The most likely diagnosis was premature thelarche (isolated premature breast development), which may persist after neonatal breast engorgement has subsided. Premature thelarche may be unilateral or bilateral, and the breast size may wax and wane. There are no associated pubertal changes in this condition and no growth acceleration. The condition may persist through infancy and childhood, and true puberty and menarche occur at a normal time, consistent with familial patterns. Investigations including measurement of LH, FSH and oestradiol, bone age assessment and pelvic ultrasound are normal for age.

Premature adrenarche

The appearance of isolated pubic hair development under the age of 8 years in a girl may occur as a variant of normal but may also be associated with an adrenal disorder such as a non-classical form of congenital adrenal hyperplasia. Careful assessment for any associated signs of virilization, such as clito-ral enlargement, hirsutism or acne, should be per-formed. The appearance of pubic hair in a boy before the age of 9 years rarely occurs as a normal variant and should always be investigated. In all cases of premature pubic hair development, referral should be made to a paediatrician or paediatric endocri-nologist so that appropriate investigation of adrenal androgens can be performed.

Isolated premature menarche

At the beginning of normal puberty in a girl, the small amounts of oestrogen made by the ovary switch 'on and off'. If enough lining of the womb is made with each 'switch on', there may be a small vaginal bleed when the 'switch off' occurs. This may happen several months in a row, then disappears as total oestrogen increases and normal puberty progresses. It is a normal variant and usually needs no treatment. Before the diagnosis of premature menarche is accepted, all other causes of premature oestrogen secretion and/or any local causes of vaginal bleeding must be eliminated by the specialist.

Pubertal gynaecomastia

Gynaecomastia is a very common finding in adolescent boys, occurring in 40–70% of 14-year-olds. In most instances the breast development is minor, transient and regresses. Rare causes of marked pubertal gynaecomastia include Klinefelter syndrome, adrenal and gonadal tumours, and drugs such as cimetidine, digoxin, spironolactone and marijuana use. If significant breast enlargement is causing psychosocial difficulties it may be necessary to refer a teenage boy to a plastic surgeon for consideration for subareolar mastectomy. Hormonal therapy does not influence the natural history of pubertal gynecomastia.

Asymmetrical breast development

Asymmetrical breast development can occur in both males and females. In males, it is clearly a variant of pubertal gynaecomastia. In females, breast development can be asymmetrical at the beginning of breast budding or subsequently through breast development. The degree of asymmetry can be quite marked. Consideration should be given to the possibility of an underlying chest wall or pectoral muscle abnormality and examination should be conducted appropriately. However, in most cases asymmetrical

Clinical example

Adam was a 15-year-old boy with bilateral breast enlargement. The breast enlargement had begun not long after his 14th birthday, and had progressed during the next 12 months. Adam was a healthy adolescent, with no significant medical problems. His parents reported that he was growing rapidly and had developed a large appetite.

Physical examination revealed a male teenager who had stage 3 pubic hair development and 12 ml testes. He had palpable breast tissue bilaterally (2.5 cm diameter), with normal pectoral muscles and underlying chest wall. The breast tissue was uniform and non-tender, and the associated lymph nodes were not enlarged.

Adam had gynaecomastia, which is a very common pubertal problem in teenage males. In the presence of a normal past history and examination, no investigations are usually necessary.

Adam and his family were reassured that the gynaecomastia was a common pubertal condition in males and, over the following 3 years, as Adam completed his growth and pubertal development, the gynaecomastia resolved.

breast development is just a physiological variant of puberty.

In rare cases, an underlying vascular abnormality or lipoma may cause one breast to appear larger than the other. This can usually be readily determined by a physical examination and confirmed by ultrasound. Reassurance and monitoring are all that are usually required. For self-esteem and cosmetic reasons, advice should be given to teenage girls about temporary use of breast prostheses or even shoulder pads to equalize the breast form. Most girls cope with the situation by wearing loose fitting garments and T shirts over swimwear. In most situations, the asymmetry resolves with full pubertal development. On rare occasions, however, referral to a reconstructive surgeon for breast reduction or augmentation may need to be considered.

19.2 Thyroid disorders in childhood and adolescence

F. Cameron, J. Brown

Normal thyroid function throughout infancy, childhood and adolescence is essential for a normal developmental and physiological outcome. Thyroid disease is one of the most common groups of endocrine disorders in childhood and adolescence, with approximately 1–2% of all children having a thyroid disorder at some time. Therefore, knowledge of thyroid disease and its management is fundamental to paediatric medicine.

Thyroid physiology

The thyroid gland removes iodide from the blood stream, combines it with tyrosine and releases iodinated tyrosine to the peripheral tissues. The thyroid gland is able to trap iodide and synthesize iodothyronine from 70 days gestation. Release of thyroxine, however, does not occur until 18–20 weeks gestation. Thyroid gland growth is regulated by thyroid stimulating hormone (TSH), released from the anterior pituitary gland, which is in turn regulated by thyrotropin regulating hormone (TRH), released from the hypothalamus. These regulating hormones are in turn controlled by negative feedback from triiodothyronine (T_3), the active metabolite of the major thyroid hormone thyroxine (or tetraiodothyronine, T_4).

The thyroid gland is extremely effective at trapping serum iodide, with a concentration gradient from thyroid to serum of 30–40. This gradient increases in times of iodide deficiency. Once trapped, iodide is oxidized to iodine and organification occurs. Organification is the iodination of thyroglobulin-bound tyrosyl residues to form monoiodotyrosine (MIT) and diiodotyrosine (DIT).

Organification and iodide oxidation (to iodine) are catalysed by thyroid peroxidase. Thyroid peroxidase couples the iodotyrosines to form iodothyronines within the thyroglobulin molecule, resulting in T_4 and T_3. In the absence of iodine deficiency the T_4 to T_3 synthesis ratio is 10–20:1. In adults, the release rate of T_4 to T_3 is 3:1. Once released, both hormones bind to thyroxine binding globulin (TBG). 80% of circulating T_3 results from deiodinatination of T_4 in peripheral tissues. Thyroid hormones bind to a nuclear receptor. T_3 binds to this receptor with 10 times the affinity of T_4. Once bound, thyroid hormones regulate gene transcription, increasing cytoplasmic proteins, which stimulate mitochondrial activity, thus increasing metabolic rate.

Disorders of thyroid function in childhood can be divided into the following categories:

- hypothyroidism
- hyperthyroidism
- thyroid masses.

Hypothyroidism

Congenital

Screening for congenital hypothyroidism has been performed in most developed countries for the last 15–20 years. In Australia, screening for congenital hypothyroidism, phenylketonuria and cystic fibrosis occurs on day 3–5 of life. Because of such screening the clinical picture of 'cretinism' (the later effects of congenital hypothyroidism, including severe intellectual disability) thankfully is now rarely seen.

Incidence

One in 3000–5000, with some geographical variation.

Aetiology and genetics

Some 75% of cases are due to dysgenesis (agenesis, ectopia), 10% to dyshormonogenesis, 5% to hypothalamic–pituitary deficiency (central hypothyroidism) and 10% to transient hypothyroidism (iodine exposure, maternal antithyroid antibodies, etc.). While thyroid disease appears to be sporadic in the majority of children born with hypothyroidism, evidence for a genetic component is increasing. In up to 2% of cases, hypothyroidism is familial, and children with congenital hypothyroidism have a higher incidence of associated abnormalities (cardiac, renal, hip dysplasia) than the general population.

Studies in mouse models with congenital defects of thyroid development have provided the basis for molecular genetic studies in humans with congenital hypothyroidism. Mutations have been described in a number of genes, resulting in absent, misplaced, hypoplastic or unresponsive glands (Table 19.2.1). In some instances, a specific phenotype can be recognized, and prognosis is affected. For example, in individuals with the *NKX2.1* mutation, neurological outcome is poor despite early thyroxine treatment.

Hypothyroid patients with normally located and normally sized glands have defects in thyroid hormone biosynthesis. Recessive mutations in thyroglobulin, thyroid peroxidase, pendrin (causing Pendred syndrome – sensorineural deafness and hypothyroidism) and sodium/iodide symporter (NIS) genes have been described. Mutations in the TRH receptor gene, TSH beta subunit and transcription factors regulating pituitary development have also been described in some individuals with central hypothyroidism.

Clinical picture

Often the condition is subclinical and is detected on routine screening. Clinical features that should be looked for are jaundice, dry skin, a hoarse cry, puffy face, prominent tongue, listlessness, umbilical hernia, hypothermia, bradycardia and failure to thrive.

Investigation results

An unconjugated hyperbilirubinaemia (due to glucuronyl transferase deficiency) is common. An elevated TSH detected on testing of a heelprick drop of blood collected on filter paper on day 3–5 of life is seen in primary hypothyroidism.

Management

Confirmatory investigations are needed if the screening tests suggest an abnormality: repeat T$_4$ and TSH; thyroid scan (showing absent, lingual or increased uptake of radioisotope), X-ray distal femoral epiphysis (absence implying prolonged/prenatal hypothyroidism), and assessment and imaging of the pituitary gland if indicated. Treatment involves commencement of therapy (thyroxine replacement at 8–10 μg/kg/d). Thyroid imaging results for congenital hypothyroidism of varying causes are shown in Figure 19.2.1.

Prognosis

Normal intellectual and physical development is likely if treatment is commenced promptly and monitored closely. Overtreatment may result in craniosynostosis.

Acquired

Acquired hypothyroidism in the child or adolescent is relatively uncommon. In iodine-sufficient regions of the world the most common cause is autoimmune

Table 19.2.1   Mutations in genes involved in thyroid development resulting in congenital hypothyroidism

Gene	Thyroid gland imaging	Clinical features	Genetics	Comments
PAX-8	Hypoplastic and cystic; ectopic	Mild to moderate congenital hypothyroidism	Familial and sporadic Autosomal dominant heterozygous mutations	
TTF-2	Thyroid agenesis	Developmental delay, cleft palate, choanal atresia, spiky hair	Familial, homozygous mutations	Rare 'Bamforth syndrome'
NKX2.1/ TTF-1	Normal, hypoplastic gland or agenesis	Congenital hypothyroidism, lung disease, hypotonia, developmental delay and choreoathetosis	Sporadic; heterozygous loss of function mutations	Poor neurological outcome despite thyroid replacement
TSH-R	Normal to severely hypoplastic, normally located	Compensated hypothyroidism to severe congenital hypothyroidism	Recessive, inactivating mutations in compound heterozygotes	Heterozygous carrier state may be relatively common in Caucasians Activating mutations cause congenital hyperthyroidism

TTF: thyroid transcription factor; TSH-R: thyroid stimulating hormone receptor.

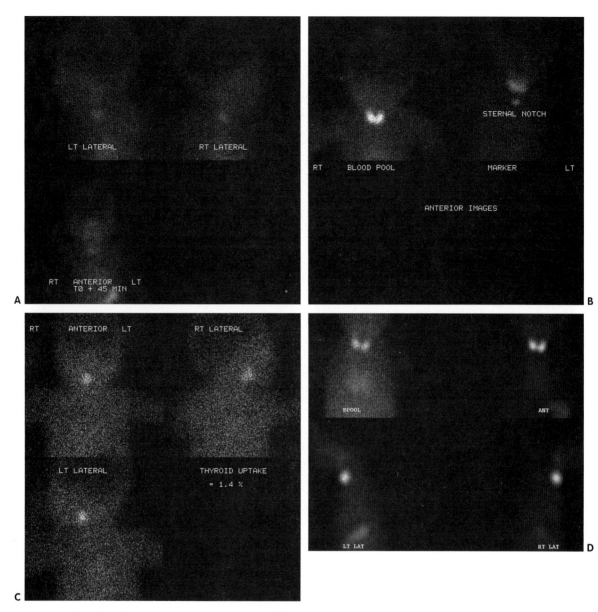

Fig. 19.2.1 Thyroid uptake scan appearances in congenital hypothyroidism. **A** Thyroid agenesis. No functioning thyroid tissue present in the neck or in the usual ectopic sites. **B** Dyshormonogenesis. The radioangiogram reveals increased thyroid perfusion. The uptake of pertechnetate in 20 min is 14% (normal = 2–5%). The thyroid scan reveals a diffuse goitre normally located in the neck. **C** Lingual thyroid. There is no evidence of perfused thyroid tissue in the neck. The thyroid scan reveals a prominent midline lingual thyroid. The uptake of pertechnetate in 20 min is 1% (normal = 2–5%). **D** Normal thyroid. The radioangiogram of the head, neck and upper torso is unremarkable. The uptake of pertechnetate in 20 min is 5% (normal = 2–5%). The thyroid scan reveals a normally located bilobular gland.

thyroiditis. Accordingly, acquired hypothyroidism is seen twice as commonly in females than in males, usually manifesting in early puberty.

Prevalence

Between the ages of 1 and 18 years the prevalence is 1.2%. Acquired hypothyroidism is rare prior to 4 years of age.

Aetiology

The causes in order of frequency are as follows: primary hypothyroidism – chronic lymphocytic, autoimmune (Hashimoto) thyroiditis, late-appearing congenital dyshormonogenesis, exogenous factors (high-dose iodine exposure (Wolff–Chaikoff effect), radiation) and severe iodine deficiency; and central hypothyroidism – congenital and acquired hypopituitarism.

Clinical picture

The most common presentation is growth retardation and goitre. In addition, the triad of short stature, obesity and mental dullness indicates hypothyroidism until proven otherwise. Growth impairment usually mainly affects the limbs so that body proportions predominantly remain infantile. Other features include hypothermia, bradycardia, slow reflex relaxation, constipation, dry hair and skin, pallor, facial puffiness ('myxoedema') and dental delay. The onset is often insidious, with delays of up to 4–5 years being reported between the onset of growth retardation and the diagnosis of hypothyroidism. While delayed puberty usually occurs, some cases of precocious puberty have been reported.

Autoimmune thyroiditis may be associated with other autoimmune diseases (autoimmune polyglandular syndromes) such as type 1 diabetes, autoimmune adrenalitis (Addison disease), vitiligo and pernicious anaemia. Occasionally, autoimmune hypothyroidism can be preceded by a period of transient hyperthyroidism.

Investigation results

Goitre (detected either clinically or sonographically) is common in acquired hypothyroidism. Blood tests show a low circulating T_4 and (usually) a high circulating TSH. Bone age is delayed and there may be positive thyroid autoantibodies (in autoimmune thyroiditis). There is patchy uptake of isotope on thyroid scan (in autoimmune thyroiditis). Hypothalamic or pituitary anomalies may be seen on computed tomography (CT) or magnetic resonance imaging (MRI) (in tertiary or secondary disease).

Management

Replacement thyroxine (usually 50–100 µg/day in a single dose) is required. An appropriate individual dose is determined by measuring serum TSH at 2 or more weeks after commencing therapy.

Prognosis

Severely hypothyroid children often show dramatic clinical changes with treatment. These include: weight loss, rapid growth, loss of primary teeth, some transient hair loss and increased energy/alertness. The long-term neurodevelopmental outcome is good, given that the rapid growth phase of the brain in the first 2 years of life has usually been protected. Despite short-term rapid catch-up growth, restoration of full growth potential often does not occur, because of rapid advancement of bone age in the first 18 months of treatment. Long-term treatment is usually required.

Hyperthyroidism

Congenital

This is always due to maternal thyrotoxicosis and is a rare clinical event. However, if unrecognized and untreated, neonatal hyperthyroidism may be fatal.

Incidence

Maternal thyrotoxicosis is uncommon (1–2 cases per 1000 pregnancies). Neonatal disease occurs in 1 per 70 cases of pregnancies affected by thyrotoxicosis.

Aetiology

Neonatal hyperthyroidism is the result of the transplacental passage of TSH receptor stimulating antibodies from a mother with either active or inactive Graves disease. Measurement of maternal antibody status, rather than thyroxine levels, is predictive of the likelihood of neonatal hyperthyroidism.

Clinical example

Sarah had been struggling at school ever since she started year 7. At the age of 13 years, her parents had become concerned that she was having difficulty settling into her new school as she was always complaining of feeling tired and having 'tummy pains'. Sarah's parents were at a loss to explain why she was behaving this way as she was a good student at primary school and had lots of friends. More recently Sarah's parents had noted that her weight had increased dramatically (they attributed this to her lack of activity, as she didn't seem to eat all that much), so much so that she now had a very 'fat' neck. She was also complaining of feeling cold all the time and was constantly wearing extra clothes even when the weather was warm. Her parents were concerned that she had a body image problem as a consequence of her recent weight gain. The school counsellor felt that Sarah might be depressed and her parents were most concerned.

On examination Sarah was moderately overweight with cool hands and she had a resting pulse rate of 50. She had dry hair and skin. She had a smooth, uniformly enlarged thyroid gland. Her reflexes showed a markedly delayed relaxation phase.

Investigations revealed that Sarah had a serum TSH level of 35 IU/ml (high) associated with a T_4 of 5 nmol/l (low). Her bone age was equivalent to 10 years and a plain X-ray of her abdomen showed faecal loading. Her antithyroid microsomal antibody titre was positive.

Sarah was commenced on 100 µg of thyroxine per day. Within 2 weeks she was reporting much improved energy levels and affect. At 1 month review she had lost 5 kg in weight, her school performance had improved and her goitre was showing some signs of shrinkage.

Clinical picture

Neonates may present with any of the following: irritability, poor weight gain, tachycardia, cardiac arrhythmias, flushing, hypertension, goitre, exomphalos, jaundice and hepatosplenomegaly. While presentation soon after birth is more common, if the mother has been taking antithyroid drugs, presentation may be delayed until day 8–9 after birth, when the antithyroid medication has been eliminated from the neonate's circulation.

Investigation results

High circulating T_4 or T_3 levels and low TSH levels are detected in the neonatal blood sample.

Management

Immediately after diagnosis, sedation and treatment with either beta-blockade or digoxin may be required. Subsequent treatment with antithyroid medication (carbimazole, methimazole or propylthiouracil) is usually required. A therapeutic response should be seen within 24–36 hours after commencing treatment.

Prognosis

Mortality rates of up to 25% have been reported. The half life of thyroid stimulating antibodies in the fetal circulation is approximately 12 days; however, the clinical course may extend for a period of up to 12 weeks.

Acquired

Hyperthyroidism in childhood and adolescence is less common than either euthyroid goitre or hypothyroidism. As with acquired hypothyroidism, it is most commonly due to autoimmune disease and is usually seen in young adolescent females.

Incidence

Females are affected 6–8 times more commonly than males. Some ethnic groups (such as Asian females) have a greater reported incidence of autoimmune hyperthyroidism.

Aetiology

Autoimmune hyperthyroidism (Graves disease) is the most common form of acquired hyperthyroidism in childhood and adolescence. Less frequent causes include the acute toxic phase of autoimmune hypothyroidism (Hashimoto disease; hashitoxicosis) and a toxic thyroid nodule (rare). There is often a family history of autoimmune thyroid disease (either Graves or Hashimoto disease). The primary defect is the presence of stimulating autoantibodies (thyroid receptor antibodies) which mimic the action of TSH. Overstimulation of the TSH receptor leads to thyroid growth and excess thyroxine production. There is often an associated ophthalmopathy due to the deposition of proteoglycans in the extraocular muscles and retro-orbital spaces.

Clinical picture

The clinical features of hyperthyroidism result from sympathetic drive causing a hypermetabolic state. Many of the florid signs of thyrotoxicosis that are seen in adults are less pronounced in children. Symptoms include deteriorating school performance, weakness/fatigue, restlessness/sleeplessness, polyuria, hunger, heat intolerance, excessive sweating, anxiety and diarrhoea and weight loss. Clinical signs include: goitre or localized thyroid mass, tremor, tachycardia and brisk reflexes. Approximately 30% of children will have associated proptosis and other signs of thyroidal ophthalmopathy (lid lag, lid retraction and ophthalmoplegia).

Investigation results

Suppressed serum TSH levels are seen and are associated with elevated T_4 or T_3 levels. There will also be elevated levels of thyroid autoantibodies (TSH-receptor-antibody-positive in Graves disease). The bone age is advanced and there is sonographic evidence of thyromegaly. Generalized and localized increased uptake of isotope is seen in Graves disease and toxic adenoma respectively.

Management

In the setting of autoimmune hyperthyroidism there are three treatment options. The first of these, antithyroid medication, is the most commonly used. Carbimazole and methimazole have traditionally been used most commonly in Australia and Europe, whereas propylthiouracil has been more commonly used in North America. Both types of medication block organification and are similarly efficacious, with comparable side effect profiles. Beta-blockade (with propranolol) may also be used in the first 2–4 weeks of therapy to gain symptom control. This is contraindicated in children who suffer from asthma. Treatment with organification blocking drugs is continued for 2 years in the first instance. Other treatment options include thyroidectomy (subtotal or total) and radioactive iodine. In the setting of toxic adenoma, surgery is usually the preferred treatment option.

Prognosis

After 2 years of medical therapy, approximately 20–50% of patients can be expected to enter spontaneous remission, with resolution of thyroid autoantibody status. Among those patients who do not remit spontaneously, long-term drug therapy is both safe and effective. In the advent of poor compliance with medical therapy, lack of control or increasing thyromegaly, a second treatment option – surgical subtotal or complete thyroidectomy – is considered. This results in 20% of patients becoming euthyroid, 50% of patients becoming hypothyroid and 30% of patients becoming thyrotoxic in the long term. Other paediatric and adult centres use a third treatment option, that of radioactive iodine. This treatment results in total thyroid ablation and requires subsequent lifelong thyroxine replacement therapy.

Clinical example

Tina, aged 15, had noticed increasing anxiety levels recently. She was quite bright academically and had set high standards for herself at school. Her parents were concerned that her anxiety was associated with some recent difficulties in concentrating during classes. Her teachers complained that she 'fidgeted' all the time and was quite restless. Despite a healthy appetite ('she eats more than anyone else in the family') Tina had been losing weight and had frequent loose bowel actions. Her mother also reported that, despite it being winter, Tina refused to wear appropriate cold weather clothing, preferring a T shirt most of the time.

On examination, Tina appeared quite anxious and had very prominent eyes (proptosis). She had difficulty in sitting still on the examination couch and squirmed around quite a lot. Her resting pulse was 110 and she had a fine tremor when her hands were held out. Her palms were very sweaty. She had a firm, smooth goitre with an audible bruit. Her reflexes were very brisk and she had difficulty standing from a squatting position.

A provisional diagnosis of Graves disease was made. This was confirmed by finding that Tina's serum TSH levels were unrecordably low in the face of a T_4 level of 52 nmol/l (high). Her anti-TSH receptor antibody titre was elevated. A thyroid ultrasound demonstrated a uniformly enlarged thyroid with no focal changes.

Tina was commenced initially on both carbimazole and propranolol. Her symptoms had largely abated within 3 weeks and her propranolol was ceased at this time. Ophthalmological review confirmed the presence of proptosis, with no other thyroidal eye signs being present. Over the following year Tina's goitre diminished in size; however, her proptosis remained unchanged. She was initially treated with carbimazole for 2 years. At this time she was still TSH-receptor-antibody-positive and it was decided to continue treatment for a further 2 years.

Thyroid masses

Goitre

The commonest cause of goitre on a worldwide basis remains iodine deficiency. In developed countries this had become rare until recent times, with the iodisation of table salt and some infant milks. Recently, iodine deficiency has been reported again in Australian populations, presumably due to low-salt diets encouraged for cardiovascular health reasons.

Incidence

Goitres or diffuse enlargement of the thyroid gland occur in 4–5% of all children. They are more common in girls during puberty and are often not detected.

Aetiology

In Australia the main causes in order of frequency are: Hashimoto thyroiditis (majority are euthyroid), Graves disease, mild dyshormonogenesis, tumour (benign/malignant), acute/subacute thyroiditis and iodine deficiency. Foods that inhibit thyroxine synthesis and can lead to goitre (goitrogens) include cabbage, soybeans and cassava.

Clinical picture

Most often the goitre is asymptomatic and is frequently detected on routine examination undertaken for other reasons. Thyroid hypofunction or hyperfunction will present with the signs and symptoms described above. Occasionally, pressure symptoms related to the enlarged thyroid (dysphagia, stridor or neck discomfort) may be the presenting feature. Thyroidal tenderness is seen in acute/subacute thyroiditis. Regional lymphadenopathy associated with a goitre or thyroid nodule is suggestive of malignancy and is an ominous sign.

Investigation results

Sonography, serum thyroid function tests and serum thyroid antibody levels will distinguish most causes of goitre. Fasting urinary iodine levels will also help to define iodine status. Thyroid scanning will show increased uptake with mild dyshormonogenesis and patchy distribution in Hashimoto thyroiditis.

Management

Smoothly enlarged goitres with normal thyroid function can be managed simply by observation and iodine supplementation if required. Goitres with functional consequences will require either thyroxine supplementation or suppressive medication.

Prognosis

This depends on the cause of the goitre. As most cases of asymptomatic goitre result in no disturbance of thyroid function, the prognosis is usually good.

Thyroid nodules

Nodules within the thyroid gland are palpable, localized swellings. They may be single or multiple. The Chernobyl nuclear reactor disaster in 1986 led to a markedly increased incidence of benign and malignant thyroid nodules in children from the surrounding iodine-deficient areas.

Incidence

Fewer than 2% of children have thyroid nodules. Of these, approximately 2% are malignant. If the nodule is single the risk of malignancy increases to 30–40%, higher than in adults.

Aetiology

Benign nodules include cysts, cystic adenomas and variations of Hashimoto thyroiditis. Malignant nodules are carcinomas and occur in the following order: papillary/mixed, follicular, medullary and anaplastic. In one series of children with thyroid cancers reported in the 1950s, 80% had a history of having received head/neck radiotherapy. However, head/neck irradiation is now less commonly used and the aetiology of most thyroid cancers remains obscure. Radiation-exposed children need close follow-up, and regular ultrasound surveillance substantially increases the detection of thyroid malignancy. Medullary carcinomas may be sporadic, familial (autosomal dominant mode of inheritance) or part of a multiple endocrine neoplasia (MEN2) complex. Patients with MEN2 have been found to have mutations in the *RET* proto-oncogene.

Clinical picture

The most common presentation is the lobular, irregular thyroid gland seen in Hashimoto thyroiditis. Nodules are usually asymptomatic and are often detected coincidentally upon routine examination. Rarely, nodules may be hyperfunctional ('toxic adenoma'). Medullary carcinomas may be associated with phaeochromocytoma (in later life) and parathyroid hyperplasia (MEN2A), or multiple mucosal neuromas, Marfan-like habitus and phaeo-chromocytoma (MEN2B). It is very rare for a child with MEN2 to present with clinical disease. They are usually detected as part of a kindred subjected to genetic screening.

Investigations

Nodules may be detected both sonographically and by thyroid scanning. The finding of multiple hot nodules associated with positive thyroid antibody titres and/or disturbed thyroid function is against a diagnosis of malignancy. Alternatively, a single cold nodule with or without serum calcitonin levels (associated with medullary carcinomas) is suggestive of malignancy. Fine-needle aspiration is not widely used in the diagnosis of thyroid nodules in children.

Management

If there is any doubt as to the nature of any thyroid nodule it is appropriate to proceed to open biopsy. Solitary benign nodules are usually excised. Papillary thyroid cancers are treated with total thyroid excision, with subsequent radioactive iodine therapy if metastases are thought to be present. Medullary thyroid cancers are unresponsive to radioactive iodine and early total thyroidectomy remains the treatment of choice. In individuals with *RET* proto-oncogene mutations from families with a strong history of medullary carcinomas, prophylactic thyroidectomy is considered.

Prognosis

Most thyroid nodules are benign and have an excellent prognosis. In the case of papillary carcinomas, serial thyroid scans for the first 3 years after surgery

---

Practical points

- Normal thyroid function is essential for normal growth and development
- Thyroid disorders are common and affect up to 2% of children and adolescents
- Neonatal screening for congenital hypothyroidism allows early detection and treatment, resulting in normal development in the majority of affected infants
- Symptoms of acquired hypothyroidism may be subtle in childhood and adolescence. Short stature may be the only presenting feature of hypothyroidism
- Hyperthyroidism is much less common than hypothyroidism and non-specific associated symptoms may result in delay in diagnosis
- Thyroid malignancy in isolated thyroid nodules is much more common in children than in adults

will detect any residual thyroid tissue or tumour recurrence. In patients suffering from medullary carcinomas, serial measures of serum calcitonin levels are the monitoring strategy of choice.

In summary, disorders of the thyroid gland can have many manifestations: hypofunction, hyperfunction, pressure symptoms and incidental tumours.

Given the importance of normal thyroid function for both neurological and physical development, and the potential for malignancy in thyroid nodules, a clinical awareness of potential thyroid problems in paediatrics is essential. Once detected, most thyroid problems can be successfully managed, with excellent clinical outcomes.

The child of uncertain sex

J. Fairchild

The child of uncertain sex has a genital appearance that does not permit gender assignment. This includes infants with bilateral undescended testes, perineal hypospadias with a bifid scrotum, clitoromegaly, posterior labial fusion, a phenotypical female with a palpable gonad and those with discordant genitalia and sex chromosomes.

The birth of a child of uncertain sex presents a psychosocial crisis for the family and may indicate an underlying medical condition such as congenital adrenal hyperplasia, which could be life-threatening if undiagnosed and untreated.

These disorders are rare, often complex and always require urgent expert consultation.

Normal prenatal development

An understanding of normal prenatal development is essential in the evaluation of the child of uncertain sex. Normal sexual development in the embryo consists of three related sequential processes:

1. establishment of chromosomal sex at fertilization, with XY as male and XX as female
2. determination of gonadal sex when the indifferent gonad develops into a testis or an ovary
3. development of phenotypic sex as a result of gonadal differentiation and gonadal hormone production.

Internal genitalia

Up until about 7 weeks, male and female embryos develop in an identical fashion, with bipotential gonads and both wolffian and müllerian internal genital ducts present (Fig. 19.3.1).

In males, the presence of the sex determining region on the Y chromosome (*SRY* gene) directs the bipotential gonad to become a testis. At least four other genes are also required for normal testicular development. By 7–8 weeks the testis has recognizable tubules and starts producing androgens, including testosterone from the Leydig cells and müllerian-inhibiting substance (MIS) from the Sertoli cells. Circulating hormone levels are low and masculinization of the internal genital ducts occurs

by locally acting (exocrine) secretion of these hormones down the wolffian duct.

High levels of testosterone promote the ipsilateral development of the wolffian duct to become the epididymis, vas deferens and seminal vesicle. High levels of MIS lead to ipsilateral müllerian duct regression. This process occurs during a critical period between 8 and 12 weeks. The Leydig cells also produce a relaxin-like factor that, together with MIS and androgens, masculinizes the gubernaculum. The gubernaculum holds the testis near the inguinal ligament during early development and from 25 weeks it begins to elongate, steering the testis towards the scrotum.

Clinical example

A healthy, full-term infant was born with ambiguous genitalia. On examination there was an enlarged clitoris (2 cm in length), posterior fusion of the labia, with a single opening visible, and no gonads were palpable. The genitalia were noted to be hyperpigmented. There was no history of consanguinity but a previous male sibling had died at 2 weeks of age after a vomiting illness.

Initial investigations confirmed that the baby's chromosomes were 46XX and a pelvic ultrasound showed the presence of a normal uterus and ovaries. The 17-hydroxyprogesterone level at 48 hours of age was markedly elevated, confirming the diagnosis of congenital adrenal hyperplasia due to 21-hydroxylase deficiency. Treatment with hydrocortisone was commenced. Daily electrolytes were normal until the 6th day of life, when hyperkalaemia developed, confirming the salt-wasting form of the condition. Fludrocortisone therapy was then added. The child was referred to a paediatric surgeon for corrective genital surgery. She will require lifelong replacement therapy and monitoring.

The hyperpigmentation was due to the adrenocorticotrophic hormone (ACTH) excess and resolved with adequate replacement therapy. It was likely that the previous male sibling also had the condition, as it is inherited as an autosomal recessive trait. The genitalia of affected males are usually normal at birth apart from some hyperpigmentation and affected male infants typically present with a salt-wasting crisis in the first few weeks of life. It is often confused with pyloric stenosis, which also presents at this age with vomiting and dehydration.

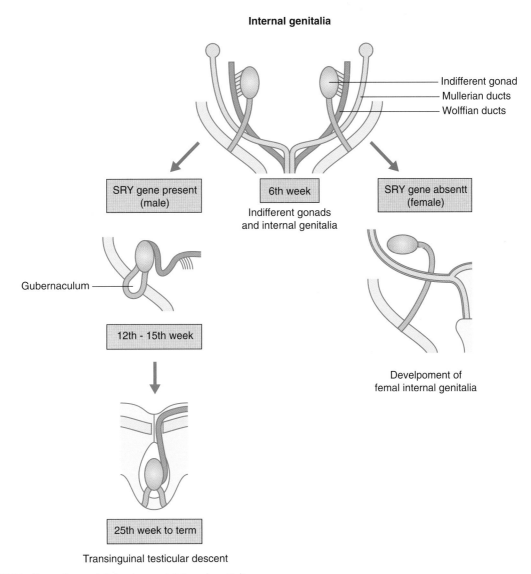

Internal genitalia

Indifferent gonad
Mullerian ducts
Wolffian ducts

SRY gene present
(male)

6th week

Indifferent gonads
and internal genitalia

SRY gene absentt
(female)

Gubernaculum

12th - 15th week

Develpoment of
femal internal genitalia

25th week to term

Transinguinal testicular descent

Fig. 19.3.1   Normal prenatal development: internal genitalia.

In females, the absence of testosterone and MIS leads to wolffian duct regression and müllerian duct preservation. The müllerian ducts develop into the uterus, fallopian tubes and upper vagina.

External genitalia

Up until about 8 weeks, the external genitalia of male and female embryos also have an identical appearance. Both sexes have a genital tubercle, two genital swellings and two genital folds (Fig. 19.3.2).

In males, between 8 and 12 weeks, androgen action on the external genitalia results in the development of normal male genitalia. Circulating levels of testosterone are insufficient for this action but testosterone is converted in the periphery to dihydrotestosterone (DHT) by the enzyme 5α-reductase. Dihydrotestos-

terone binds to the androgen receptors much more strongly than testosterone, thereby amplifying its effect. The genital tubercle develops into the glans penis, the genital swellings fuse to form the scrotum and the genital folds elongate and fuse to become the shaft of the penis and the penile urethra. The prostate forms in the wall of the urogenital sinus. With the exception of the phallus, circulating androgens masculinize the external genitalia only during a critical period between 8 and 12 weeks.

In females, in the absence of androgen, the genital tubercle forms the glans clitoris and the short female urethra. The genital swellings remain unfused and become the labia majora. The genital folds become the labia minora and the vaginal plate, a thickening of the posterior wall of the urogenital sinus, canalizes to form the lower vagina.

External genitalia

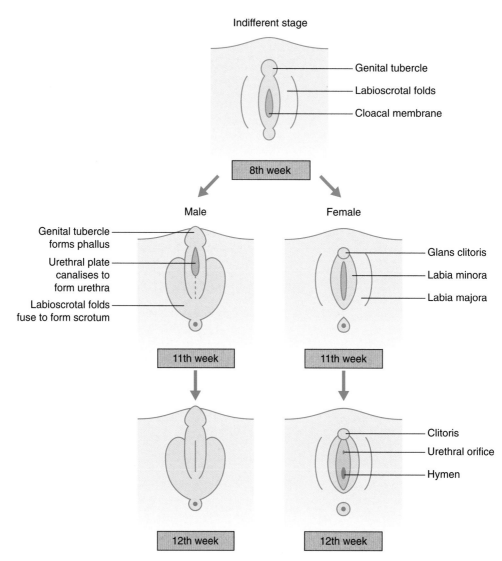

Fig. 19.3.2 Normal prenatal development: external genitalia.

Evaluation of the child of uncertain sex

The initial evaluation of the child of uncertain sex should include a history, clinical examination, assessment of adrenal secretion, sex chromosomes and internal anatomy.

History

A careful history should include:

- any prenatal exposure to androgens
- maternal virilization during pregnancy
- family history of intersex disorders, females who are childless or females who have amenorrhoea

- family history of unexplained infantile deaths
- consanguinity.

Clinical examination

The clinical examination should include:

- inspection of the external genitalia
- palpation to determine the presence, location and symmetry of the gonads:
  - if both gonads are palpable and symmetrical they are almost always testes
  - gonadal asymmetry implies one testis present, suggesting a mixed chromosomal pattern
  - if both gonads are impalpable the gonadal and duct status is unknown
- general examination looking for:

Clinical example

A full-term infant with normal birth weight (3.1 kg) was noted to have a small penis (stretched penile length 1.5 cm, normal >2.5 cm) and undescended testes. The infant had had two episodes of hypoglycaemia treated with intravenous dextrose and on general examination was noted to have a small cleft in the palate.

Hypoglycaemia is unusual in a full-term infant of normal birth weight and in the presence of a midline defect raises the possibility of hypopituitarism.

A diagnostic blood sample taken at the time of the hypoglycaemia revealed low levels of cortisol, growth hormone and free thyroxine, confirming the diagnosis. The baby was commenced on hydrocortisone and thyroxine with resolution of the hypoglycaemia. He was given a short course of testosterone at 6 months of age, which resulted in an increase in his penile length to 2.5 cm. Growth hormone therapy was commenced when his growth rate slowed at 12 months of age.

Micropenis and cryptorchidism can occur with either gonadotrophin deficiency or growth hormone deficiency and is a useful clinical sign of congenital hypopituitarism in male infants.

- dysmorphic features or non-genital abnormalities that may point to the diagnosis of a specific disorder
- hyperpigmentation and/or systemic illness, which may suggest congenital adrenal hyperplasia.

Initial investigations

The initial investigations that should be undertaken are:

- urgent karyotype:
  - permits classification of the infant into one of three diagnostic categories and determines further evaluation
- imaging of internal anatomy:
  - ultrasound to determine the presence of gonads, uterus and vagina
  - urogenital sinogram to visualize the urethral and vaginal anatomy
- exclude congenital adrenal hyperplasia:
  - serum electrolytes and blood glucose series
  - serum 17-hydroxyprogesterone and other adrenal steroids

Further evaluation

This may include:

- serum profile of adrenal steroids, gonadal androgens and their precursors

- human chorionic gonadotrophin (hCG) stimulation test to confirm a normal rise in gonadal hormones with stimulation, with the testosterone/DHT ratio reflecting 5α-reductase activity
- surgical procedures: genital skin biopsies for androgen receptor assay, panendoscopy and/or laparotomy to delineate internal genitalia ± gonadal biopsy.

Practical points

Initial evaluation of the child of uncertain sex
- *History:* androgen exposure, family history of intersex or infant deaths, consanguinity
- *Examination:* determine the presence of palpable gonads, hyperpigmentation, systemic illness, non-genital abnormalities
- *Investigations:* include an urgent karyotype, assessment of adrenal secretion, ultrasound ± urogenital sinogram to assess internal anatomy
- Assignment to one of the three diagnostic categories will determine further evaluation: virilized XX, undervirilized XY or mixed chromosome pattern

Diagnostic categories

The results of the karyotype, in particular the sex chromosomes, will allow the infant to be classified into one of three diagnostic categories which will determine further evaluation:

- virilized XX
- undervirilized XY
- mixed chromosome pattern.

Virilized XX

In the virilized XX child, the gonads are ovaries and the internal genitalia are female, therefore no gonads are palpable (Fig. 19.3.3). The external genitalia are virilized to a variable degree, from mild clitoromegaly to complete labial fusion with urethral tubularization to the tip of the enlarged phallus (Fig. 19.3.4). If the exposure occurred after 12 weeks there will be isolated clitoromegaly without labial fusion.

Causes of the virilized XX state may be:

- androgen excess from the fetal adrenals:
  - congenital adrenal hyperplasia (most common cause)
- androgen excess from the mother:
  - maternal ingestion of androgens
  - androgen-producing tumour
  - placental aromatase deficiency.

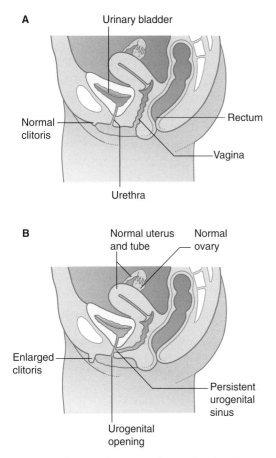

A

- Urinary bladder
- Normal clitoris
- Rectum
- Vagina
- Urethra

B

- Normal uterus and tube
- Normal ovary
- Enlarged clitoris
- Persistent urogenital sinus
- Urogenital opening

Fig. 19.3.3 Schematic illustration of normal and ambiguous female genitalia as in congenital adrenal hyperplasia. Note the urogenital sinus leading to a single opening and the enlarged clitoris induced by androgens (Adapted from Moore and Persaud, 1993).

Undervirilized XY

The undervirilized XY child usually presents with a small phallus, posterior hypospadias, poorly developed, bifid scrotum and testicular maldescent.

The causes of the undervirilized XY state may be:

- inadequate androgen production:
  - hypoplastic testes (luteinizing hormone (LH) deficiency)
  - dysplastic testes
  - testosterone synthesis defects
  - inability to convert testosterone to DHT (5α-reductase deficiency)
- impaired response to androgen:
  - androgen insensitivity syndrome.

Clinical example

A 16-year-old girl presented for investigation of primary amenorrhea. On examination she was found to be a tall girl for her family. She had breast development at stage 5 but sparse pubic hair (stage 2–3) and no axillary hair. She also had an inguinal mass, which was occasionally painful when knocked during sport. Investigations revealed a 46XY karyotype, no uterus on pelvic ultrasound and serum levels of testosterone characteristic of normal men.

A diagnosis of complete androgen insensitivity was made. Gonadectomy was performed as there is a high incidence of germ cell cancer and oestrogen replacement therapy was commenced. Psychological support was important in helping her come to terms with the diagnosis.

Mixed chromosomal pattern

True hermaphroditism

In true hermaphroditism, both testicular and ovarian tissues coexist. The gonads are usually ovary and testis or ovary and ovotestis. The chromosomes are usually 46XX, although 46XY mosaicism can occur. Asymmetry of the gonads, internal and external genitalia is the hallmark of this condition.

Mixed gonadal dysgenesis

In mixed gonadal dysgenesis there is also gonadal asymmetry with a testis on one side and a streak gonad on the other. The testis may be dysgenetic and the streak gonad usually contains ovarian stroma without oocytes. The chromosomes are commonly 45XO/46XY, and these infants may have the phenotypic features of Turner syndrome, but other mosaic

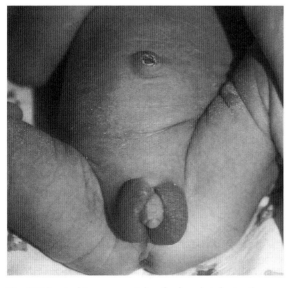

Fig. 19.3.4 Ambiguous genitalia of a female infant with congenital adrenal hyperplasia associated with salt wasting.

patterns can occur. The risk of gonadoblastoma is high in dysgenetic testes and gonadectomy in the first decade of life is recommended.

Intersex disorders with unambiguous genitalia

It is important to note that some patients with intersex disorders will have unambiguous genitalia. These patients have complete sex reversal with a phenotype the reverse of what would be expected from their genotype. Examples of this would be an XY child with complete gonadal dysgenesis or complete androgen insensitivity syndrome.

Intersex abnormalities may be missed if the diagnosis of hypospadias is made without due care. This diagnosis should never be made without full investigations, unless both testes are descended in a fused scrotum.

Management

The birth of a child of uncertain sex presents a unique set of challenging and often difficult management issues. A multidisciplinary team approach involving the paediatrician, paediatric endocrinologist, surgeon, geneticist, psychologist, social worker and adolescent gynaecologist is required for optimal management.

Initial management

The initial management of the child of uncertain sex requires attention to medical and psychosocial issues. Evaluation of the child must be carried out urgently, so that a decision about the sex of rearing can be made as quickly as possible and life-threatening medical conditions can be identified. Urgent expert consultation should always be sought.

The birth of a child of uncertain sex is a psychosocial crisis for the family and must be handled sensitively. The parents should be honestly informed that you do not yet know the sex that their baby is meant to be, but reassured that this will be determined as soon as possible. Instruct all staff to refer to the infant as 'your baby', not he, she or it. The parents will require guidance as to how to deal with family and friends and the support of an experienced social worker or psychologist is invaluable. Every effort should be made to encourage the parents to bond with their baby. The parents should be advised not to name the baby or register the birth until sex assignment is decided.

The urgent medical issue is the exclusion of congenital adrenal hyperplasia and the attendant risk of adrenal crisis. Congenital adrenal hyperplasia is the most common cause of XX virilization and one of the causes of XY undervirilization. Serum electrolytes and blood glucose should be monitored closely and serum sent for urgent measurement of 17-hydroxyprogesterone and other adrenal steroids.

Congenital adrenal hyperplasia refers to a group of autosomal recessive disorders resulting from the deficiency of one of the five enzymes required for the synthesis of cortisol in the adrenal cortex. The most common enzyme deficiency is 21-hydroxylase deficiency, accounting for more than 90% of cases. The deficiency of cortisol results in adrenocorticotrophic hormone (ACTH)-mediated adrenal hypertrophy and excessive production of cortisol precursors, which are diverted to the synthesis of androgens. Concomitant aldosterone deficiency leads to salt wasting in 75% of cases.

Symptoms and signs of a salt-wasting adrenal crisis include vomiting, diarrhoea, hypovolaemia, hyponatraemia with hyperkalaemia, hypoglycaemia and cardiovascular collapse and can occur within the first few days to weeks of life. If symptoms or signs of adrenal crisis are present, stress doses of hydrocortisone and intravenous fluid therapy with normal saline and 5% dextrose should be started immediately. The stress dose of hydrocortisone is 100 mg/m^2/day and is given intravenously.

Practical points

Management goals for the child of uncertain sex
- An accurate and expeditious diagnosis is essential – and requires urgent expert consultation
- Rational sex assignment is important
- Therapy is directed towards achieving successful sex assignment
- Psychological support for the family is required
- Genetic counselling is an integral part of management

Gender issues

The issue of timing and approach to genital reconstruction is controversial and evolving. An evidence-based approach is hampered by the lack of long-term outcome studies involving large numbers of patients. Gender assignment and sex of rearing should be based on the most probable adult gender identity and potential for adult function. It involves consideration of the diagnosis, degree of virilization, capacity to respond to androgen, potential for adult sexual function and fertility as well as the parent's social and cultural background. There are no data demonstrating a link between early genital surgery and psychosexual orientation and, although early surgery may make life easier for the parents and the child, these irrevocable decisions may complicate the lives of adults. Decisions about sex of rearing and genital reconstruction should only be made by an informed family after careful evaluation and counselling by an experienced multidisciplinary team.

Long-term management

Once gender is assigned, every effort should be made to encourage the child's sex of rearing. Both the child and parents will benefit from long-term psychosocial support and many individuals and their families derive benefit from support groups.

Specific management of the gonadal tissue in infants of uncertain sex may be required to reduce the risk of gonadal malignancy, torsion and infertility. Abdominal gonads bearing Y material should be brought into the scrotum or removed surgically. The age of surgery will vary according to the underlying condition.

Sex steroid replacement should be provided consistent with the sex of rearing and age of the child to ensure adequate growth and pubertal development and prevent osteoporosis.

Childhood diabetes 19.4

J. Couper

Diabetes mellitus

Diabetes mellitus is caused by a deficiency in the production or action of insulin. It is the second most common chronic disease of childhood and causes considerable morbidity due to acute metabolic derangements and long-term microvascular and macrovascular complications. In childhood, the majority of diabetes is type 1 diabetes (previously known as insulin-dependent diabetes). However, in parallel with the increasing incidence of type 2 diabetes in childhood in North America, this is also the trend in Australia and New Zealand, especially in Aboriginal and Polynesian populations.

The prevalence of type 1 diabetes mellitus in Australia is approximately 1 in 750 for children under the age of 15 years, with an annual incidence of 12–13 per 100 000 population. Prospective registers show a continuing increase in incidence, especially in the under-5 age group. Similar incidences are reported for New Zealand, USA and the UK. In Asia the incidence is low, whereas in parts of Scandinavia it exceeds 30 per 100 000. The reasons for these variations are presumed to be both genetic and environmental. The sex ratio in diabetes is equal. Diabetes is uncommon in infancy. In childhood the incidence shows two peaks, at ages 4–6 years and 10–14 years.

Pathogenesis of type 1 diabetes

There are two major factors that contribute to the pathogenesis of diabetes:

- genetic predisposition
- environmental triggers or protectors.

Autoimmune destruction of beta cells

Type 1 diabetes is caused by autoimmune destruction of the beta cells (insulin-producing cells) of the islets of Langerhans. T-cell infiltration of the islets and circulating autoantibodies precede the development of diabetes for months to years. Target antigens are insulin, glutamic acid decarboxylase and a tyrosine phosphatase. This preclinical phase, when blood glucose is normal and circulating antibodies are present, provides clues for prevention or postponement of the onset of clinical diabetes. There is an increased frequency of certain HLA types (HLA DR3/DQ2 and DR4/DQ8) in children with diabetes. The HLA genes are located on chromosome 6 and encode HLA molecules on the beta cells.

Environmental factors that are potential candidates in the initiation of autoimmunity or that might act as progression factors are viruses (particularly enteroviruses) and dietary factors (cereals and cow's milk). However, only congenital rubella is a proven environmental trigger and this is a rare cause of type 1 diabetes. The increase in childhood obesity may also account for an earlier presentation of type 1 diabetes due to insulin resistance and beta cell exhaustion but the extent of this contribution to the increasing incidence of type 1 diabetes is unresolved.

Metabolic effects of insulin

Insulin is the hormone of energy storage and anabolism. It allows glucose to enter cells to be stored as glycogen in the liver and muscle and as triglyceride in fat. Insulin deficiency prevents glycogen and triglyceride storage and causes their breakdown as well as that of protein. In addition, insulin deficiency promotes hepatic gluconeogenesis. The combined effects of glycogen breakdown, enhanced gluconeogenesis and failure of glucose entry into cells results in a rise in blood glucose. When the renal threshold is exceeded, glycosuria occurs. The osmotic effect of the glycosuria causes polyuria and dehydration. The breakdown of triglyceride (lipolysis) releases free fatty acids into the circulation. In the liver these are converted to ketoacids (ketogenesis), with eventual development of ketoacidosis.

When the autoimmune process has destroyed approximately 90% of the beta cell mass, persistent hyperglycaemia indicates the onset of clinical diabetes. The diagnosis can be made before symptoms when subjects at risk are followed prospectively in natural history and intervention trials. In routine practice, symptoms are usually present for several weeks before the diagnosis is made; however, a child with a suspected diagnosis of diabetes should be investigated immediately.

As the insulin deficiency proceeds, diabetic ketosis and then ketoacidosis develop and, if not treated, result in death. Ketoacidosis causes vomiting and, later, rapid deep breathing (Kussmaul respiration). The hyperventilation is a compensatory response for the metabolic acidosis by removing carbon dioxide. Chemical breakdown of acetoacetic acid in the body yields acetone, which can be detected on the patient's breath. Breakdown of fat and protein and dehydration lead to weight loss. Abdominal pain mimicking an acute surgical abdomen may occur. Dehydration (shock) occurs with continuing massive urinary losses caused by the osmotic diuresis. The acidosis, dehydration and changes in plasma osmolality cause initial irritability, then confusion, drowsiness and eventually coma. Because immune function becomes compromised, the possibility of serious infection should always be considered, although it is rarely present. A summary of the clinical features and useful investigations at the time of presentation of type 1 diabetes is presented in Table 19.4.1.

Table 19.4.1 Type 1 diabetes: clinical features at presentation and useful investigations at diagnosis

Clinical presentation
- Polyuria and polydipsia
- Enuresis and nocturia
- Weight loss and fatigue
- Thrush
- Vomiting (with increasing ketosis)
- Kussmaul breathing and coma (with increasing acidosis)

Investigations
- Urinalysis for glucose and ketones
- Random blood glucose (postprandial)
- Blood electrolytes and acid–base when unwell
- Blood or other cultures and blood count (if infection suspected)
- Islet antibodies (if type 2 diabetes suspected)

Clinical example

For the previous 2 weeks, a mother had noted her 4-year-old son, Tom, to be irritable, thirsty and wetting the bed at night, having previously been dry. After being generally less well for 24 hours he became lethargic and began vomiting. On presentation at casualty, he was noted to be drowsy, he was dehydrated and he had deep sighing respirations (Kussmaul breathing). The diagnosis of diabetic ketoacidosis was confirmed when he was found to have a blood glucose of 22 mmol/l, blood ketones were 5.2 mmol/l, serum sodium 126 mmol/l, potassium 5.2 mmol/l, bicarbonate 10 mmol/l, pH 7.15 and the base deficit 26. Therapy consisted of intravenous isotonic fluids, intravenous potassium and intravenous insulin.

Tom was discharged 4 days later, on two injections of insulin per day, a diabetes food plan and a programme of home blood glucose testing. During the hospital admission his family received education from the diabetes educator and dietitian, and the education programme was continued as an outpatient. A community diabetes educator visited Tom's kindergarten to educate the staff about hypoglycaemia.

Differential diagnoses

The diagnosis of type 1 diabetes in childhood is not usually difficult, provided that the physician is aware that this condition occurs even in the very young. The most common misdiagnoses are to mistake:

- polyuria for a urinary tract infection
- the overbreathing of metabolic acidosis for a respiratory tract infection or asthma
- vomiting and abdominal pain for gastroenteritis or an acute abdomen.

Children with intercurrent infections, acute asthma or hypernatraemic dehydration may have transient hyperglycaemia and glycosuria that resolves with the intercurrent illness. Only very rarely do these children develop type 1 diabetes. Islet autoantibodies can be tested to determine whether the child is developing type 1 diabetes.

Treatment of diabetic ketoacidosis

The aims of therapy are:

- emergency fluid replacement (10–20 ml/kg/h), using volume expanders, if shock is present so that the circulation is restored
- correction of dehydration slowly over 24–48 hours, using normal (isotonic or 0.9%) saline
- replacement of electrolyte losses and slow correction of acidosis. Supplemental potassium of 40–60 mmol/l in intravenous fluids is required to maintain normal serum potassium levels once insulin therapy has begun. Higher levels of supplementation will require ECG monitoring
- correction of the insulin deficiency, with an infusion of soluble insulin.

Treatment should be undertaken only in a centre equipped with paediatric intensive care facilities; the child may need to be transported there by an expert retrieval team. Frequent biochemical monitoring of the blood glucose, electrolytes and blood gases is required. The initial rate of insulin infusion of 0.1 unit/kg per hour is adjusted to produce a slow fall in the blood glucose. Rapid reductions in the blood glucose level and/or a fall in serum sodium concentration alter the plasma osmolality too quickly and increase the risks of life-threatening cerebral oedema.

When ketones disappear, subcutaneous insulin is begun with regular food intake. Most children are stabilized on two to four daily injections of ultra-short and intermediate-acting insulins. Within days to weeks of the introduction of insulin, some recovery of the remaining viable beta cells may occur. During this period of partial remission (also known as the 'honeymoon' phase), insulin requirements fall. This phase may last for weeks or months but, as the underlying autoimmune destruction of beta cells is still in progress, more complete insulin deficiency occurs, so that blood glucose levels and insulin requirements eventually rise permanently. There is recent evidence that the process of islet destruction and regeneration may continue for years, providing an exciting research avenue to increase viable beta cells.

Management

Aims of management

Type 1 diabetes is a permanent disorder. By definition, insulin treatment is necessary and in childhood at present it can only be given by injection (inhaled insulins can supplement long-acting subcutaneous insulin in adults). The long-term aims are for the child to achieve normal physical and emotional development, to lead a fulfilling life, with as little restriction on lifestyle and occupation as possible, and to minimize the risk of long-term microvascular and macrovascular complications.

Management principles

The attainment of these aims depends largely on maintaining good diabetic (metabolic) control. This is often difficult to achieve and is especially difficult in the under-5-year age group and for the adolescent. The aim is to keep the blood glucose levels as close to normal as possible pre- and postprandially. To measure the blood glucose, a spring-loaded lancet is used to prick a finger, the blood is placed on a reagent strip and the glucose can be measured accurately by a variety of meters designed for home use. Most children measure their blood glucose two to four times a day. The key elements in achieving stability in the blood glucose levels are:

- insulin
- diet
- exercise.

Insulin

Insulin therapy is individualized. Generally, prepubertal children require 0.8–1 unit/kg body weight per day, given as two to four subcutaneous injections daily. This requirement increases with more variability during puberty. Preschool children may be very sensitive to short-acting insulin and therefore receive predominantly intermediate-acting insulin. Regimens using bolus doses of ultra-short-acting insulin before meals and an intermediate or longer-acting insulin before bed, or insulin pump regimens (basal insulin infusion subcutaneously and bolus doses of insulin with meals and snacks) are especially suitable for the adolescent needing more flexibility in the treatment schedule. These regimens may improve metabolic control and reduce hypoglycaemia and, in the case of pump therapy, weight gain, provided compliance is excellent and there is accompanying blood glucose monitoring.

The dose of insulin is adjusted according to blood glucose measurements, anticipated diet and exercise. Glycosylated haemoglobin (HbA_{1C}) levels indicate the level of control during the preceding 6–8 weeks and often provide the most meaningful guide when blood glucose levels are erratic. The target range for HbA_{1C} is less than or equal to 7.5%, and has fallen considerably during the last 5 years. Target blood glucose levels are generally 4–8 mmol/l but may need to be higher in preschool children or children with a history of recurrent severe hypoglycaemia.

> **Practical points**
>
> **Poor metabolic control with high HbA1c**
> - Is the prescribed insulin dose adequate?
> - Is insulin omission a problem?
> - Is food intake excessive or inappropriate?
> - Consider education/dietary/psychological review
> - Consider an eating disorder, especially in girls
> - Consider increasing doses, changing insulin types and intensifying the insulin schedule if insulin omission is not a problem

Diet

Food raises the blood glucose level and this must be balanced by the glucose-lowering effect of insulin and exercise. This balance is usually achieved by having the diabetic diet supply carbohydrate throughout the day with three meals (breakfast, lunch, dinner) and three snacks (morning tea, afternoon tea and supper). However, toddlers will usually have a grazing pattern of food intake and older adolescents may not need three snacks per day. Children receiving insulin pump therapy have more flexibility, with lower carbohydrate intake if desired.

The usual diabetic diet is relatively high in complex carbohydrates, low in simple carbohydrates (sugar) and low in saturated fats. Dietitians frequently use the glycaemic index of foods to guide the child and family to appropriate food choices. The glycaemic index is a classification of foods based on their post-prandial blood glucose response and, as such, is a more predictable guide than merely measuring the carbohydrate content of foods. The diet must be adequate nutritionally for normal growth and must be acceptable and satisfying to the child. Individual and changing food plans are essential if the diet is to be adhered to. It is also necessary to account for pre-existing family and cultural traditions. Frequent review by an experienced dietitian is necessary to cope with changing requirements as the child grows. Extra food may need to be taken with exercise to prevent hypoglycaemia.

Exercise

Exercise increases the uptake of glucose by the exercising muscles and lowers the blood glucose level. This effect is seen only if the diabetes is in good control and adequate serum levels of insulin are present (exercise undertaken during poor control and with low insulin levels may paradoxically raise the blood glucose levels). To combat the hypoglycaemic effect of exercise, the child may need extra carbohydrate food. Regular exercise schedules in the older child may be better managed by a small reduction in the preceding insulin dose. Regular exercise should be encouraged. It does not, per se, improve metabolic control in children but it may do so indi-

rectly in some individuals by modifying appetite and improving wellbeing and self esteem.

Outpatient management

For most children with diabetes, the initial hospitalization or day stay admission at diagnosis for stabilization and education is their only hospital admission. Much or all of the early education programme can be provided by the diabetes educator and dietitian as an outpatient, provided there are adequate resources for this and no contraindications exist, such as severe parental distress or communication difficulties. Follow-up visits are usually every 3 months once the child is stabilized to assess:

- general wellbeing
- history of hypoglycaemic episodes
- home blood glucose monitoring
- insulin schedule
- food plan
- school progress and absenteeism
- height and weight
- injection sites
- size of the thyroid gland
- presence of skin infections.

The blood glucose profile is examined in the logbook kept by the patient, or is downloaded from the patient's blood glucose monitor, and the adequacy of the dietary and insulin regimen is assessed. Continuous blood glucose monitoring (Fig. 19.4.1) is

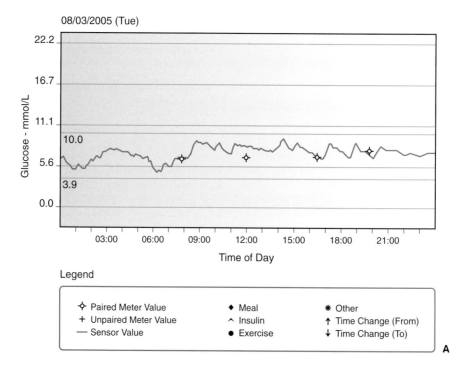

Fig. 19.4.1 Continuous interstitial glucose monitoring obtained from an indwelling subcutaneous sensor in three patients with type 1 diabetes. In **A**, the pattern of results shows that the patient is in the remission phase.

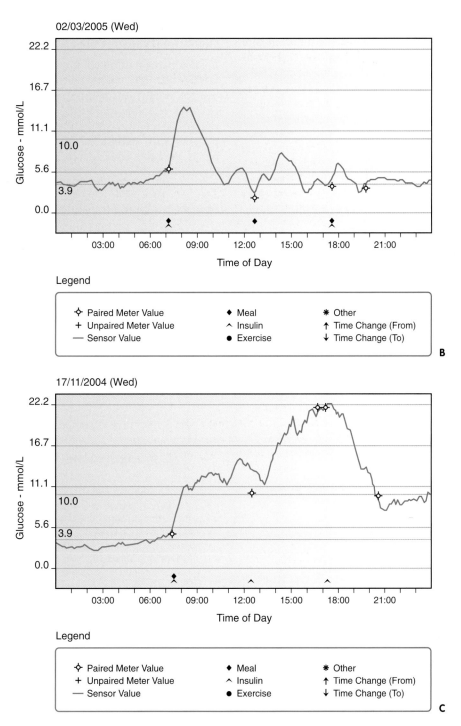

Fig. 19.4.1, cont'd   In **B,** excellent control is seen, but the a.m. rise in glucose concentration requires an increase in a.m. ultra-short insulin. In **C,** the results show asymptomatic nocturnal hypoglycaemia and daytime hyperglycaemia. This requires adjustment of night-time long-acting insulin and daytime ultra-short insulin.

particularly useful when fine tuning of the insulin schedule is required, after a change to a new insulin schedule or insulin pump, or when there are concerns of undetectable nocturnal hypoglycaemia. The glycosylated haemoglobin (also called HbA_{1C}) measures the degree of glycosylation of haemoglobin, while the serum fructosamine measures the extent of non-enzymatic glycosylation of serum proteins. These parameters give an indication of the glycaemic control during the life span of the red cells (120 days) and the serum proteins (3 weeks). HbA_{1C} levels can be measured in capillary blood within minutes in the outpatient clinic setting, which is ideal. With the combined efforts of the parents, the child and the diabetes management team (physician, dietitian, diabetes educator, social worker and psychologist) most children grow and develop normally, achieve their educational potential and have a satisfying childhood and adolescence. However, fewer than 50% of children in Australia achieve target HbA1c levels below 7.5%.

Long-term microvascular and macrovascular complications

Long-term microvascular and macrovascular complications which may occur in children with diabetes are:

- nephropathy
- retinopathy
- neuropathy
- cardiovascular disease
- peripheral vascular disease.

It is extremely rare for children and adolescents to show clinical signs of these complications but subclinical signs can be detected, particularly from adolescence onwards. These form the basis of complication screening programmes. It is recommended that, from 5 years duration of type 1 diabetes, the patient has an annual review including:

- measurement of resting blood pressure
- assessment of urinary albumin excretion, either by an overnight urine collection or an early morning sample
- fundoscopy on dilated pupils by an ophthalmologist.

Serum lipids also are relevant, particularly when there is a family history of a lipid disorder or of premature cardiovascular disease. The major risk factors for the development of complications are:

- degree of metabolic control
- duration of type 1 diabetes
- smoking
- hypertension.
- family history.

It should be reinforced for the patient and their family that any improvement in their glycaemic control, even if it is still not ideal, will reduce their risk of developing complications. The early introduction of angiotensin converting enzyme inhibitors, in patients with persistent microalbuminuria before blood pressure rises, delays the onset of chronic renal failure.

Special problems in management

Hypoglycaemia

For parents, the occurrence of severe hypoglycaemia in their child (loss of consciousness or a convulsion) is one of the most distressing aspects of diabetes management. Usually, no long-term harmful effects result from a severe hypoglycaemic episode. However, the concern remains of possible neurological damage in the very young child, or in the adolescent with a cocktail of other drugs such as alcohol, and the possible development of hypoglycaemic unawareness with recurrent episodes of hypoglycaemia.

> **Practical points**
>
> **Recurrent hypoglycaemia**
> - Is it severe, moderate or mild; is it daytime or nocturnal?
> - Is there hypoglycaemic unawareness?
> - What is the HbA1c level?
> - Consider a change of insulin dose, insulin type (e.g. ultrashort analogues) or insulin schedule
> - Consider continuous glucose monitoring, particularly if nocturnal hypoglycaemia is suspected
> - Consider continuous subcutaneous insulin infusions (insulin pump therapy)

Minor hypoglycaemic episodes are relatively frequent and reflect the difficulties in achieving stable control with current insulin delivery to the systemic circulation, particularly as an improving HbA_{1C} increases the risk of hypoglycaemia. However, the advent of insulin analogues (ultra-short and peakless basal) and insulin pumps has reduced the risk of hypoglycaemia. All patients with type 1 diabetes should carry some rapidly absorbable carbohydrate (e.g. glucose tablets or jelly beans) for immediate treatment of hypoglycaemic symptoms.

Hypoglycaemia may occur if the insulin dose is excessive, if insufficient food is eaten or if extra exercise is undertaken. Severe hypoglycaemia is most common during the night when the glucose threshold for counter-regulatory hormone responses is lower.

The clinical features of hypoglycaemia can be divided into:

- stimulation of the sympathetic nervous system: anxiety, palpitations, tachycardia, pallor, perspiration, headaches and abdominal pain
- effects on the central nervous system: lethargy, dizziness, ataxia, weakness, confusion, personality changes, visual disturbance, unconsciousness, localized and generalized convulsions.

These clinical features appear rapidly in a previously well child and there is no difficulty in differentiating hypoglycaemic coma from the coma of diabetic ketoacidosis.

The emergency treatment for the unconscious hypoglycaemic child is to lie them on their side and check the airway. Oral fluids must not be given. Intramuscular or subcutaneous glucagon (0.5 mg for children under 5 years of age and 1 mg for older children and adults) or intravenous glucose (2.5 ml of 20% dextrose per kilogram of body weight) is administered. All families with a diabetic child should have glucagon at home and should be able to give it subcutaneously. The response to therapy is seen within minutes. For the less severely affected child, so called mild hypoglycaemia can be treated with oral glucose, e.g. half a glass of sugar-containing non-diet lemonade, or jelly beans. On improvement after the emergency treatment, the child should receive some complex carbohydrate.

Management of sick days

Children with well controlled diabetes are no more prone to infections than the non-diabetic child. However, the stress of the infection, especially if associated with fever, causes a temporary insulin resistance and more insulin is required. Blood glucose tends to rise despite a poor oral intake. Ketosis may occur. This is a sign of significant insulin deficiency and, if untreated, diabetic ketoacidosis could develop. Parents are taught to measure blood glucose levels frequently, monitor the presence of ketosis (home measurement of blood ketones is more accurate than for urinary ketones) and give frequent small doses (10–20% of daily requirements) of short-acting insulin every 3–4 hours until the diabetes is stabilized again. Generally regular phone contact with the diabetes consultant or educator will keep the child out of hospital, except when vomiting and persistent ketosis complicates home management. Low doses of glucagon can also help prevent hypoglycaemia in the vomiting child at home, but the parents should be in close contact with a diabetes specialist for advice.

Growth and delayed puberty

Because insulin is the principal hormone of energy storage and anabolism, growth disturbances and pubertal delay can occur if diabetes control is poor. Mauriac syndrome is an extreme example of this, with short stature and hepatic enlargement due to fatty infiltration of the liver. The possibilities of Hashimoto thyroiditis, coeliac disease or, less commonly, adrenal insufficiency should also be considered because of their association with type 1 diabetes: many clinics routinely screen for thyroid function and coeliac disease.

Psychological stresses

Major problems arise with diabetic control in the presence of psychological stresses. Easily identifiable acute stresses such as school examinations do not usually cause significant problems. However, family conflicts, parental separation, teenage rebellion and other emotional problems may cause a more profound instability, and psychological counselling or formal psychotherapy may be required for the child and the whole family.

The relevance of psychological wellbeing to good diabetes control is of such importance that the social worker or psychologist is an integral part of the management team. Most units also have patient and parent support groups. Diabetes camps also nurture self-esteem and confidence.

Adherence

Excellent diabetes control in childhood and adolescence is difficult in the best of circumstances. It becomes impossible when the child or the family become non-compliant with diet, monitoring or injections of insulin. Refusal to perform blood tests and to conform to the prescribed diet are not unusual periodically and represent a normal rebellion against the never ending discipline that characterizes diabetes management.

The commonest cause of recurrent diabetic ketoacidosis and chronic poor metabolic control in adolescence is insulin omission. Patience and counselling are necessary, especially in adolescence, when normal risk-taking behaviour and growing independence do not combine well with diabetes. The adolescent and family should not be made to feel guilty when diabetes control is less than ideal. It is often useful for the frustrated doctor or educator to consider how well s/he would have coped with the tedious diabetes regimen during adolescence.

Clinical example

Jacinta, a 14-year-old girl with a 5-year history of diabetes, had had three episodes of diabetic ketoacidosis in 3 months. Her blood glucose logbook showed the values to be 4–10 mmol/l but a glycosylated haemoglobin level (HbA$_{1C}$) was 10.8% (normal range 4–6%). Her insulin dose was 0.9 units/kg per day and the recorded blood glucose levels appeared spurious.

Admission to hospital for stabilization confirmed elevated blood glucose levels. Management required appropriate increases in insulin dose, education and counselling. The dietitian suspected that Jacinta might also have had an eating disorder complicating her insulin omission, and psychological review was arranged.

Sometimes it is necessary for someone else (e.g. the parents or a community nurse) to temporarily take over responsibility for the insulin injections when there is a serious problem with insulin omission.

Factors limiting management

Factors that are often present when diabetes is proving difficult to manage, and that need to be considered further, are:

- difficulties in family functioning
- hypoglycaemia, which may be unrecognized
- adherence problems and psychological stresses (particularly in adolescence).

Future directions

Families frequently ask about research advances and it is important that they have access to up-to-date information through regular seminars and reliable websites. New synthetic insulin analogues provide a better range of very short, intermediate and peakless long-acting insulins. Inhaled, oral and transdermal insulins are under investigation.

Specific immunotherapy of the autoimmune process is being trialled in subjects with preclinical diabetes in an attempt to prevent diabetes and to prolong life of beta cells after diagnosis.

Novel approaches to preventing vascular complications include targeting the intracellular mechanisms by which glucose is toxic, e.g. inhibitors of protein kinase C and agents that interfere with the accumulation of advanced glycation end-products. Transplantation of isolated islets of Langerhans in adults has shown recent promise with less beta-cell toxic immunosuppressive drugs. Whole pancreas transplants can occur successfully in conjunction with renal transplantation. Prevention of rejection of the transplant requires lifelong immunosuppression and donors of the pancreatic graft are not plentiful. Stem cells and islet regeneration are now major research directions.

Table 19.4.2   Characteristics of type 2 diabetes at diagnosis

- Obesity
- Acanthosis nigricans
- Family history of type 2 diabetes
- Absent or mild ketosis (although ketosis and ketoacidosis can occur)
- Absence of islet antibodies
- Raised C peptide/insulin levels
- Microvascular complications, hypertension and lipid abnormalities may be present
- Hyperandrogenism maybe present
- More common in Aboriginal and Polynesian populations

Type 2 diabetes

The true incidence of type 2 diabetes is not known, as patients are frequently asymptomatic. Characteristics of type 2 diabetes at diagnosis are shown in Table 19.4.2.

The distinction between type 1 and type 2 diabetes in childhood may be difficult to make on clinical grounds alone (for example, many children with type 1 diabetes are overweight and have a family history of type 2 diabetes). Measurement of islet antibodies to show their absence is usually necessary to confirm the diagnosis. The distinction is important, as patients with type 2 diabetes are treated with a weight-reducing diabetes diet and oral hypoglycaemics as first-line measures. Insulin may still be required, especially during intercurrent acute infections, when ketoacidosis can occur. Screening for microvascular and macrovascular complications should begin from the time of diagnosis in type 2 diabetes. There is an association between hyperandrogenism in adolescent females and type 2 diabetes.

Bone mineral disorders

C. Jones

Hypocalcaemia, rickets and hypercalcaemia are the most common manifestations of disorders of calcium, phosphate and vitamin D metabolism. Disorders of magnesium metabolism are rare but share many features of calcium disorders.

Calcium, magnesium and phosphorus (Table 19.5.1)

Calcium and phosphate form the major structural components of bone in the form of hydroxyapatite. The majority of magnesium is also found in bones. A large proportion of each mineral in bone is freely exchangeable with the extracellular fluid (ECF). Calcium and phosphate ions, under normal circumstances, are present in a supersaturated solution. A rise in phosphate will lead to the deposition of more calcium phosphate into bone as hydroxyapatite and cause hypocalcaemia. The distribution of calcium and phosphate between bone and the ECF is determined by hormonal regulation of the concentrations of these minerals. The most important hormones are 1,25-dihydroxyvitamin D_3 (activated vitamin D) and parathyroid hormone (PTH). The actions of these hormones are summarized in Figure 19.5.1.

The ionized ECF forms of calcium and magnesium are responsible for their physiological effects. The ionized form of calcium should be measured to confirm that true abnormalities in concentration are present because the equilibrium between the ionized and protein bound forms can change. For instance, an increase of 0.1 pH unit decreases the ionized calcium by 10%, and hypoalbuminaemia reduces total serum calcium but not the ionized calcium concentration because 90% of bound calcium is bound to albumin.

Hypocalcaemia

In the neonatal period, hypocalcaemia is defined as a total serum calcium concentration below 1.8 mmol/l (ionized calcium 1.0 mmol/l). Beyond this age, a total plasma calcium below 2.1 mmol/l (ionized calcium 1.2 mmol/l) constitutes hypocalcaemia. Clinical signs usually only occur when the total serum calcium is below 2 mmol/l (ionized calcium 0.75 mmol/l), although some patients will tolerate much lower levels and will still remain asymptomatic.

The signs of hypocalcaemia are due to neuromuscular excitability. Jitteriness, apnoea, laryngeal spasm causing stridor and convulsions are frequent in infants. Tetany, carpopedal spasm and the Chvostek (facial twitch on percussion of the facial nerve near the temporomandibular joint) and Trousseau (tetany produced by inflating the sphygmomanometer above systolic blood pressure for up to 2 min) signs are seen mainly in older children. Intracerebral calcification and cataracts are complications. The ECG may show a prolonged QT interval.

The causes of hypocalcaemia are listed in Table 19.5.2.

Early neonatal hypocalcaemia is common in premature infants and in infants of diabetic mothers. In premature infants, it is possibly an exaggerated response to the normal interruption of the maternofetal calcium transfer; the serum calcium falls following delivery to a nadir reached at a few days of age and then increases to normal levels at 1–2 weeks of age. The signs are seen within hours of birth, become most severe about 48 hours after birth and

Clinical example

Kylie, a 6-year-old girl, had nephritis with a metabolic acidosis (pH 7.32, [HCO_3^-] 15 mmol/l, P_{CO_2} 30 mmHg). She had an albumin of 20 g/l, the serum total [Ca^{2+}] was 1.0 mmol/l and the serum [phosphate] was 3.6 mmol/l.

Would it have been safe to correct the acidosis with intravenous $NaHCO_3$? From Table 19.5.1, if the serum albumin was normal, 46% of the total serum Ca^{2+} would be ionized. However, the serum albumin concentration was reduced by 50%, so the amount of calcium bound to albumin would be reduced by 50% (the proportion of total calcium bound to albumin would be reduced to approximately 20%), leaving the ionized proportion of total serum calcium increased from the normal 46% to approximately 66%, equivalent to 0.66 mmol/l. Increasing the pH to 7.4 could reduce the ionized portion and precipitate overt symptoms of hypocalcaemia. Thus, the calcium concentration needed to be corrected before giving $NaHCO_3$.

Table 19.5.1 Distribution, serum concentrations, dietary requirements and sources of calcium, magnesium and phosphate

	Calcium	Magnesium	Phosphorus
Body distribution (%)			
Bone*	99	60	80
Intracellular	–	40	20
Serum status (%)			
Ionized[†]	46	55	85
Complexed	14	25	5
Protein bound	40	20	10
Serum levels (mmol/l)			
Cord blood[‡]	2.4	0.7	1.6
Neonatal	2.1–2.7	0.75–1.1	2.0–3.3
Adult	2.2–2.6	0.75–1.1	1.0–1.3[§]
Dietary intake RDI (mg/d)			
0.6 months	300	40	150
6–12 months	550	60	300
1–10 years	800	100	800
11–18 years	1200	200	1200
Milk content (mg/l)			
Human	300–500	40	100–300
Cow	1500	130	1000
Other food sources	Tinned fish, dairy products	Green vegetables, seeds, nuts	Meats, dairy products

* Ionic exchange occurs readily between extracellular fluid (ECF) and bone, enabling ECF concentrations to be kept fairly constant. [†] The ionized form of phosphorus at pH 7.4 is HPO_4^{2-} (70%) and $H_2PO_4^-$ (20%). [‡] Cord-blood concentrations are higher than maternal blood concentrations, indicating active transport mechanisms are involved in transplacental transfer. Parathyroid-hormone-related peptide (PTHRP) is probably involved in these processes. [§] Levels of phosphate slowly decline during childhood and reach adult levels on completion of bone growth.
RDI, recommended dietary intake.

then improve spontaneously. It may be aggravated by early phosphate-rich formula feeding or hypoxic–ischaemic injury. Treatment of symptomatic infants involves intravenous calcium and commencement of an appropriate diet, following the guidelines provided in Table 19.5.3.

Late neonatal hypocalcaemia usually presents as tetany after the first few days of life. The main cause is transient hypoparathyroidism, as demonstrated by high plasma phosphate and low serum PTH concentrations in the face of hypocalcaemia. A similar clinical picture is seen in infants of mothers with hyperparathyroidism and in infants with congenital heart disease. Treatment may involve calcium infusion, calcitriol, oral calcium supplementation and a low phosphate formula. The infant can often be weaned from this treatment after a few weeks. Persistence of the hypocalcaemia beyond this time should prompt a search for other causes of hypoparathyroidism such as DiGeorge syndrome (aplasia of the parathyroids, thymic aplasia with T cell immu-nodeficiency and cardiovascular abnormalities), hypomagnesaemia or idiopathic congenital hypoparathyroidism. An abnormality of the calcium sensing receptor on the parathyroid cells (an activating mutation decreasing PTH release) is also a cause. Treatment is based on the use of calcitriol, often in combination with phosphate restriction.

Late onset hypoparathyroidism may occur with destructive injury of the parathyroids, e.g. copper deposition in Wilson disease, iron deposition in haemosiderosis or autoimmune type I polyglandular syndrome. In this latter condition, children, usually girls, present with tetany or convulsions and may have candidiasis and adrenal insufficiency, or other autoimmune disorders such as alopecia, malabsorption, thyroiditis and diabetes. Pseudohypoparathyroidism is due to end-organ resistance to PTH and blood levels of PTH are high. Mental deficiency and skeletal abnormalities (particularly a short fourth metacarpal) may be associated. Treatment is the same as for hypoparathyroidism.

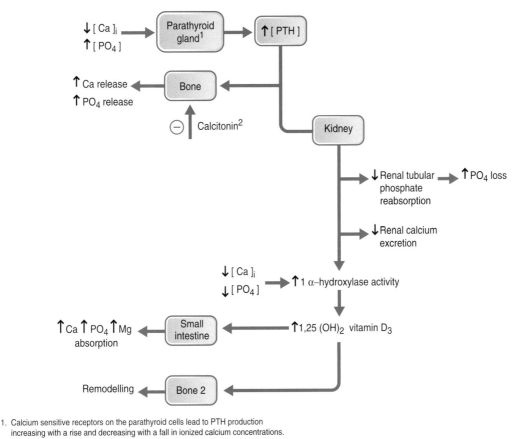

1. Calcium sensitive receptors on the parathyroid cells lead to PTH production increasing with a rise and decreasing with a fall in ionized calcium concentrations.

2. Calcitonin is a hormone produced in the medullary (parafollicular) cells of the thyroid gland in response to an increase in calcium concentrations. It inhibits reabsorption of bone.

Fig. 19.5.1 Hormonal control of calcium, magnesium and phosphate.

Clinical example

Stephanie had received induction treatment for T-cell lymphoma. She developed hypocalcaemia associated with a raised serum phosphate in the days following this treatment. How should the hypocalcaemia have been managed? The administration of intravenous calcium would have resulted in metastatic deposition of calcium phosphate, as the solubility product of calcium phosphate, was exceeded. The calcification would occur in blood vessels and soft tissues. Such an approach might, in fact, have been necessary if Stephanie had symptomatic hypocalcaemia (convulsions) but it would have been preferable to lower the serum phosphate first. This was be achieved by implementing a low phosphate diet, and administering oral phosphate binders (such as calcium carbonate), which bind the phosphate in the gut (calcium complexes phosphate and is not absorbed by the intestine). It would be uncommon to use dialysis or haemofiltration but these treatments would also lower serum phosphate concentrations.

Hyperphosphataemia can cause hypocalcaemia acutely (as seen in tumour lysis syndrome, where cell death following the initiation of chemotherapy for bulky tumours results in the release of phosphate). Acute renal failure with retention of phosphate is associated with hypocalcaemia. The primary treatment in these conditions is to reduce serum phosphate concentrations through dietary restriction of phosphate, the use of phosphate binders (such as calcium carbonate) and dialysis. Rickets due to vitamin D deficiency or disorders of vitamin D metabolism may cause hypocalcaemia (see below.)

Rickets

Rickets is impaired mineralization of osteoid tissue in the growing child. The mineralization defect affects the epiphysial growth plates, where cartilage cells proliferate, and unmineralized osteoid tissue

Table 19.5.2 Causes of hypocalcaemia

• Neonatal
  Early neonatal – prematurity, IDM, IUGR, birth asphyxia
  Late neonatal – di George syndrome
  – Phosphate load
  – Low magnesium
  – IDM
• Pseudohypocalcaemia
  Hypoalbuminaemia
• Vitamin D deficiency
  Nutritional deficiency
  Disorders of vitamin D metabolism
    1α-hydroxylase deficiency
    Vitamin-D-dependent rickets
• Parathyroid-hormone associated
  Hypoparathyroidism
    Idiopathic
    Autoimmune polyglandular disease (with mucocutaneous candidiasis, or Addison disease)
    Calcium-sensing receptor activating mutations or antibodies
    Hypomagnesaemia
    Destructive lesions of the glands
    Hypoplasia
    PTH receptor defect – pseudohypoparathyroidism
• Hyperphosphataemia
  Tumour lysis
  Renal failure
• Pancreatitis
• Medical treatment
  Large blood transfusion/exchange transfusion

PTH, parathyroid hormone; IDM, infant of diabetic mother; IUGR, intrauterine growth retardation.

Table 19.5.3 Treatment of hypocalcaemia
Emergency • Patients with hypocalcaemia and symptoms should be treated with intravenous calcium* • Electrocardiography monitor (bradycardia) • Intravenous calcium chloride 10%, 0.2 ml/kg/dose (max 1 g), repeated at 4–6 h or followed by Infusion of 1 mmol (= 1.5 ml of 10% CaCl$_2$)/kg/d • Correct the concurrent hypomagnesaemia (magnesium chloride, 0.2 mmol/kg over 1 h)
Maintenance • Treat the underlying condition (see text)
* Note: extravasations of intravenous calcium cause skin and subcutaneous tissue necrosis.

Practical points

Hypocalcaemia

- Suspect symptomatic hypocalcaemia when there is tetany, unexplained stridor, irritability or convulsions
- Confirm the diagnosis of hypocalcaemia with total and ionized calcium concentrations and take blood for magnesium, phosphate and parathyroid hormone concentrations
- Treat symptomatic hypocalcaemia with intravenous 10% calcium chloride 0.2 ml/kg/dose, given into a well placed intravenous line slowly, and monitor the ECG during the infusion.

accumulates, resulting in widening metaphyses, weak bones and development of deformities, particularly in the weight-bearing bones. In established bones there is continued bone resorption but failure of mineralization results in soft, rarefied bones (this is osteomalacia, which is the same disease as rickets, in the adult).

Causes of rickets are deficiency of the effect of vitamin D and phosphate depletion. Figure 19.5.2 outlines the causes of vitamin D deficiency and abnormal metabolism of vitamin D in relation to the physiological production of the active product, 1,25-dihydroxyvitamin D$_3$.

The recommended dietary intake of vitamin D is 400 international units (IU) per day. With exposure to a small amount of afternoon sunlight, vitamin D supplementation is unnecessary. Breast milk contains 20–50 IU/l of vitamin D, yet rickets is uncommon in breastfed infants in the first year of life, provided the mother does not have osteomalacia. Most commercial milk formulas have 400 IU/l of vitamin D.

In the last 25 years, the incidence of vitamin D deficiency has increased in Australia. This increase has been seen in the children of migrants from the Middle East, southern Europe and Asia, especially where the mother wears a hejab. Reduced sunlight and darkly pigmented skin combined with a range of social factors, including poor housing, lack of adequate infant welfare services for non-English-speaking migrants and unusual feeding patterns, have combined to make rickets more prevalent.

Malabsorption associated with gastrointestinal, hepatic or pancreatic disease can cause vitamin D deficiency. In approximately 50% of cases hypocalcaemia is present at the time of diagnosis. Severe liver disease and prolonged use of anticonvulsant therapy with diphenylhydantoin or phenobarbital (through an increased hepatic turnover of vitamin D) can cause rickets.

1α-hydroxylase deficiency (type 1 vitamin-D-dependent rickets, characterized by normal or high 25 dihydroxyvitamin D$_3$ levels and low 1,25 dihydroxyvitamin D$_3$ levels) and peripheral resistance to

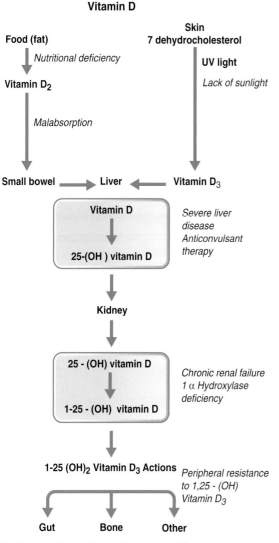

Vitamin D

Food (fat)

Nutritional deficiency

Vitamin D$_2$

Malabsorption

Skin
7 dehydrocholesterol

UV light

Lack of sunlight

Small bowel → Liver ← Vitamin D$_3$

Vitamin D

25-(OH) vitamin D

*Severe liver disease
Anticonvulsant therapy*

Kidney

25 - (OH) vitamin D

1-25 - (OH) vitamin D

*Chronic renal failure
1 α Hydroxylase deficiency*

1-25 (OH)$_2$ Vitamin D$_3$ Actions

*Peripheral resistance
to 1,25 - (OH)
Vitamin D$_3$*

Gut   Bone   Other

Fig. 19.5.2   Vitamin D metabolism and rickets.

1,25 dihydroxyvitamin D$_3$ (type II vitamin-D-dependent rickets, characterized by high concentrations of 1,25 dihydroxyvitamin D$_3$) present as severe hypocalcaemic vitamin D deficiency that fails to respond to treatment with vitamin D.

The clinical features of these forms of rickets are quite variable: young children may present with tetany and convulsions; older children may present incidentally when a chest X-ray is performed for an intercurrent chest infection. Early signs in nutritional rickets include weakness of the outer table of the skull (craniotabes), thickening of the costochondral junctions (the 'rachitic rosary') and widening of the wrists and ankles. Later, asymmetry of the head with delayed closure of the anterior fontanelle, frontal and occipital bossing of the skull, development of a Harrison groove, scoliosis and lumbar lordosis,

delayed dentition and bowing and bending of the legs develop. Muscular weakness, ligament laxity and fractures are common.

The radiology of the ends of long bones is characteristic, showing widening of the space between metaphysis and epiphysis (Fig. 19.5.3). The metaphyseal ends of the long bones are widened and appear cupped and frayed. The biochemical changes are a normal or a low serum calcium, a low serum phosphate, a high serum alkaline phosphatase and a high PTH.

Treatment of nutritional vitamin D deficiency is with oral vitamin D at a dose of 3000–5000 IU/day for 6 weeks. In some cases, treatment precipitates uptake of calcium into bones ('hungry bones') to such an extent that hypocalcaemia is accentuated and large doses of calcium supplement may be required to maintain normocalcaemia for the first week(s). In the longer term, an adequate calcium intake (600–1500 mg/d) needs to be maintained, as does an adequate intake of vitamin D (400 IU/d to age 4 years). In cases where poor compliance may be suspected, 'stoss therapy' using 50 000 IU of vitamin D every 6 weeks may be used.

Radiological improvement is usually apparent within 4 weeks. Some cases are refractory and require longer treatment periods. If there is no response, tests for 1α-hydroxylase deficiency, peripheral resistance to 1,25 dihydroxyvitamin D$_3$ or hypophosphataemic rickets should be undertaken.

Hypophosphataemic rickets

X-linked dominant hypophosphataemic (vitamin-D-resistant) rickets is caused by failure of phosphate reabsorption in the renal tubule and lack of an appropriate increase in 1α-hydroxylase activity (low phosphate concentrations normally increase the activity of this enzyme, which produces 1,25

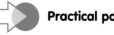

Practical points

Rickets
- Suspect rickets when there is bowing of the long bones, exaggerated lumbar lordosis, splayed wrists and other rachitic changes in an irritable child
- Examine for signs of hypocalcaemia and treat symptomatic hypocalcaemia
- Suspect nutritional vitamin D deficiency in breastfed infants of mothers where covering clothing is worn at all times, children of dark skin colour and children with malabsorption or liver disease
- Suspect another cause if there is failure to respond to vitamin D, low PTH concentrations and very low phosphate concentrations

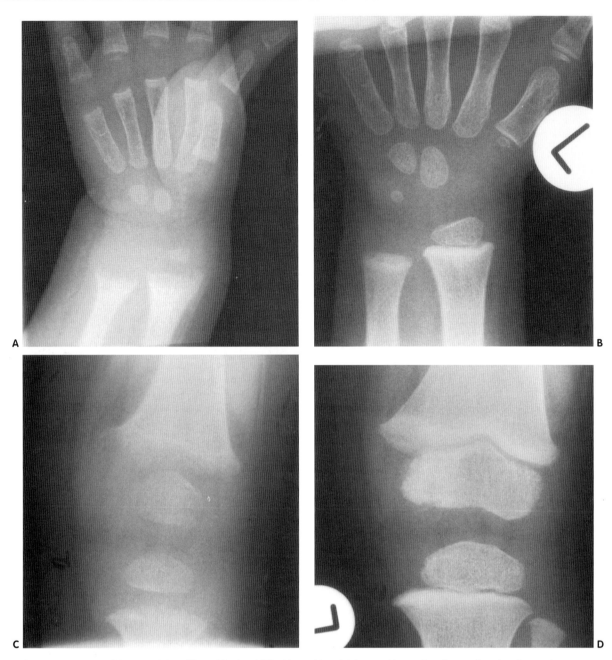

A

B

C

D

Fig. 19.5.3   X-rays of the wrist (A) and knee (C) of a child with nutritional rickets at 18 months of age when the diagnosis was made, and 8 months later (B, D) after treatment was finished.

dihydroxyvitamin D$_3$). In 50% of cases it is familial; the rest of the cases are due to new mutations. Clinically, the rickets affects the lower limbs predominantly, and investigations show that the calcium and PTH concentrations are normal, while the phosphate concentration is quite low. Males are more severely affected than females. Treatment consists of large amounts of dietary phosphate supplementation and large doses of calcitriol.

Chronic phosphate deficiency (e.g. renal Fanconi syndrome, dietary phosphate deficiency) from any cause will result in rickets.

Renal osteodystrophy

This condition predictably occurs when the glomerular filtration rate in chronic renal failure decreases to less than 25% of normal. It occurs as a result of a combination of events, including an increase in plasma phosphate and decreased 1α-hydroxylation of 25 hydroxyvitamin D_3 in the kidney, leading to a fall in 1,25 dihydroxyvitamin D_3 production. This leads to hypocalcaemia and an increase in PTH. The combination of rickets and secondary hyperparathyroidism can result in gross skeletal deformation. Treatment consists of a graded range of measures beginning with dietary phosphate restriction, use of phosphate binders (calcium carbonate) and addition of calcitriol.

Hypercalcaemia

Hypercalcaemia is defined as a total serum calcium above 2.7 mmol/l (ionized calcium >1.3 mmol/l). Symptoms of hypercalcaemia include nausea and vomiting, polyuria and polydipsia, hypertension and failure to thrive. Ensuing hypercalciuria may cause nephrocalcinosis and urinary calculi. The ECG may show a shortened QT interval.

A list of causes of hypercalcaemia is given in Table 19.5.4. Most of these are rare. Primary hyperparathyroidism occurs with some frequency in the second decade of life and is due to hyperplasia or adenoma of the parathyroid glands. It may occur as part of the multiple endocrine neoplasia syndromes (type I hyperparathyroidism associated with prolactinoma or gastrinoma; type II with hyperfunction of the adrenal, parathyroid and medullary cells of the thyroid). Investigations reveal high PTH concentrations, and X-ray appearances include subperiosteal resorption of bone (particularly the phalanges), 'salt and pepper' appearance of the cranium and cyst formation in long bones. Treatment of symptomatic disease usually involves subtotal parathyroidectomy.

Familial hypocalciuric hypercalcaemia is an autosomal dominant disorder and is usually an asymptomatic condition caused by an inactivating mutation of the parathyroid calcium sensing receptor.

Idiopathic hypercalcaemia of infancy is a condition in which there is increased absorption of dietary calcium. The condition usually resolves by the end of the first year of life. Occasionally it is associated with cardiovascular abnormalities (supravalvular aortic stenosis) and dysmorphic facial 'elfin' features (as in Williams syndrome). The genetic defect for Williams syndrome involves the elastin gene and many cases can be diagnosed using fluorescent in situ hybridization (FISH) studies.

Treatment is directed at the cause of the hypercalcaemia. Severe symptoms may necessitate initiation of a diuresis using sodium chloride infusions, dietary phosphate supplements to bind calcium, glucocorticoids to reduce intestinal calcium absorption in vitamin D excess and bisphosphonates to prevent calcium release from bone. A low calcium milk formula is used to treat idiopathic hypercalcaemia of infancy.

Hypercalciuria

The normal upper limit of urinary calcium excretion is 0.15 mmol/kg/d or <0.7 mmol per mmol creatinine. Hypercalcaemia usually causes hypercalciuria (Table 19.5.4), with the notable exception of familial hypocalciuric hypercalcaemia. Normocalcaemic hypercalciuria is caused by furosemide or corticosteroid therapy, immobilization of limb fractures, distal renal tubular acidosis and some rare syndromes.

Idiopathic hypercalciuria is common and appears to be an autosomal dominant condition with incomplete penetrance. On a calcium-rich or calcium-sufficient diet there is intestinal hyperabsorption of calcium and the PTH and 1,25-dihydroxyvitamin D concentrations are normal. On a lower calcium diet, 'renal' loss of calcium occurs and higher levels of PTH and 1,25 dihydroxyvitamin D are found. Excessive bone resorption occurs in some patients and can cause osteoporosis. Thus, the therapeutic safety of a low calcium diet is limited because of the risks of development of osteoporosis. Hypercalciuria can cause nephrocalcinosis (Fig. 19.5.4) and urinary calculi. Where treatment is necessary, thiazide diuretics have proved useful.

Table 19.5.4 Causes of hypercalcaemia

- Neonatal
  Hyperparathyroidism – primary
   – maternal hypoparathyroidism
   – maternal pseudohypoparathyroidism
  Idiopathic infantile hypercalcaemia
  Williams syndrome
  Familial hypocalciuric hypercalcaemia
  Subcutaneous fat necrosis
- Vitamin D excess
  Iatrogenic
  Ectopic production – sarcoidosis, tuberculosis, lymphoma
- Parathyroid hormone excess
  Primary hyperparathyroidism multiple endocrine neoplasia (MEN) syndromes
  Familial hypocalciuric hypercalcaemia
  Abnormalities related to PTH receptor or PTH-related peptide (PTHRP)
- Other
  Bone disease, trauma and immobilization
  Thyrotoxicosis and hypothyroidism
  Neonatal fat necrosis

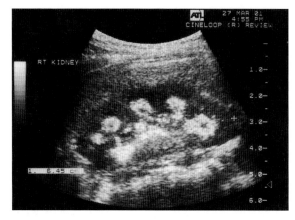

Fig. 19.5.4 Renal ultrasound showing nephrocalcinosis of the medullary pyramids in a 4-year-old child with idiopathic nephrocalcinosis.

Table 19.5.6 Causes of hypomagnesaemia and hypermagnesaemia

Hypomagnesaemia
- Malabsorption, prolonged intravenous therapy
- Diuretic therapy
- Renal tubular acidosis
- Hereditary disorders of renal tubular reabsorption

Hypermagnesaemia
- Neonate of mother given $MgSO_4$ for pre eclampsia
- Medications containing magnesium given to patients with renal failure

---

Table 19.5.5 Causes of osteoporosis

- Calcium deficiency
    Nutritional
    Malabsorption
- Malignancy
    Leukaemia
- Glucocorticoid excess
    Iatrogenic
    Cushing disease
- Homocystinuria
- Osteogenesis imperfecta
- Immobilization
- Idiopathic juvenile osteoporosis

Osteoporosis

Osteoporosis is a condition where there is a decreased mineral content of the skeleton. Measurement of bone mineral density has improved over the last decade with the use of dual energy X-ray absorptiometry (DEXA). However, DEXA must be carefully interpreted with regard to the size of the bone where measurements are taken and the age of the patient, especially with regard to pubertal development of the child. Osteoporosis is only apparent radiologically when approximately half of the bone mineral content has been lost. Causes of osteoporosis are given in Table 19.5.5.

Idiopathic juvenile osteoporosis is a rare condition that occurs in mid childhood with gross demineralization of the skeleton, which can result in extensive fractures (particularly vertebral crush fractures). The disease remits spontaneously with the onset of puberty.

Osteopetrosis

Osteopetrosis is a rare familial disorder of the skeleton in which there is a defect in bone and cartilage resorption and hence a deficiency of bone remodelling. This leads to a dense but brittle type of bone that fractures easily. Infants usually present early in life with a severe leukoerythroblastic anaemia, symptoms of compression of cranial nerves (particularly optic atrophy leading to blindness) and marked hepatosplenomegaly. The bones show a characteristic dense and poorly modelled X-ray appearance.

Magnesium disorders

Causes of hypomagnesaemia are given in Table 19.5.6. The symptoms of hypomagnesaemia resemble those of hypocalcaemia, with increased neuromuscular irritability. Severe hypomagnesaemia interferes with the release of PTH and consequently hypomagnesaemia and hypocalcaemia often coexist.

Hypermagnesaemia occurs rarely in the absence of renal failure. The exception is the neonate born prematurely to a mother given magnesium sulphate for pre-eclampsia.

DISORDERS OF THE GASTROINTESTINAL TRACT AND HEPATIC DISORDERS

Abdominal pain and vomiting in children

20.1

S. W. Beasley

Acute abdominal pain and vomiting are common symptoms in children and a frequent reason for children to be taken to the doctor. Their causes are many and diverse; those that require surgery must be distinguished from those with a medical origin. While there is considerable overlap of age in many disorders (e.g. gastro-oesophageal reflux), other conditions only occur within a specific age range; for example, pyloric stenosis is not seen after the age of 3 months.

Abdominal pain in the first 3 months of life

Abdominal pain without other symptoms is unusual in early infancy. Severe pain may be accompanied by vomiting, abdominal distension, constipation or other features, in which situation it is more likely to have a surgical cause, e.g. malrotation with volvulus.

Infantile colic is an extremely common condition that usually commences in the first few weeks of life. The cause is poorly understood. The term 'colic' is used because of the common assumption that this pattern of behaviour is due to colicky abdominal pain but this explanation is controversial, and there are other hypotheses including an irritable temperament (Ch. 4.1).

The infant:

- has attacks of screaming
- draws up the legs
- is unable to be comforted.

Vomiting is absent, bowel actions are passed normally and the infant is otherwise thriving well. There is no evidence of a strangulated inguinal hernia. The colic almost invariably disappears by the fourth month of age; until then, treatment is supportive. In some infants, apparent colic may be due to oesophagitis from gastro-oesophageal reflux or to hunger in inadequately breastfed babies. Crying babies may cause stress in the family, which in turn may increase the child's irritability. In a vulnerable or unstable family situation this may place the infant at risk of abuse.

Abdominal pain later in the first year

The main surgical cause of abdominal pain between 3 and 12 months of age is intussusception. Vomiting is a frequent accompanying feature, such that, when the colicky abdominal pain is not pronounced, intussusception must be distinguished from other causes of vomiting in this age group (see below).

Intussusception

In intussusception, the distal ileum (the intussusceptum) telescopes into adjoining distal bowel (the intussuscipiens), resulting in intestinal obstruction. It can occur at any age but is most likely in the infant between 3 and 18 months who suddenly develops screaming attacks of pain with vomiting. During each episode of pain the infant becomes pale and may draw up the legs.

The spasms of pain tend to last 2–3 minutes and occur at intervals of about 10–20 minutes, although after a while the pain becomes more persistent. Vomiting is an early symptom. The passage of a few loose stools early on represents evacuation of the bowel distal to the obstruction. The small volume and limited duration of loose stools in intussusception helps differentiate it from acute gastroenteritis. Congestion of the intussusceptum may lead to the passage of bloodstained or 'redcurrant' stools. Many infants with intussusception present with little more than pallor, lethargy and vomiting and may have little evidence of abdominal pain. Should these symptoms be ignored, the infant may progress to develop signs of septicaemia or shock.

The infant with intussusception looks pale, lethargic, anxious and unwell. A vague mass may be felt in the right or left upper quadrants of the abdomen but, once abdominal distension has developed, the mass becomes obscure and difficult to palpate. The apex of the intussusceptum may be palpable on rectal examination in a few, and the examining glove may be bloodstained. A plain X-ray of the abdomen will often be normal but may show an unusual bowel gas distribution or features of bowel obstruction. Ultrasound examination may be helpful in making the diagnosis. Where intussusception is suspected clinically or confirmed on ultrasonography, a gas or barium enema must be performed unless the child has peritonitis. The enema will demonstrate the position of the apex of the intussusception.

Treatment

Intussusception can be reduced non-operatively by gas enema or by hydrostatic reduction under ultrasonographic control; these techniques are successful in 80–90% of patients (Fig. 20.1.1). If gas enema facilities are not available, a barium enema under continuous fluoroscopic control is a less effective but satisfactory alternative. Peritonitis and septicaemia, which suggest the presence of dead bowel, are the only contraindications to attempted enema reduction. A dehydrated child should have intravenous fluid resuscitation and be wrapped in warm blankets before commencing an enema reduction. The success of enema reduction is recognized when there is sudden or rapid flow of gas or barium into the ileum. If partial reduction is achieved, and the child remains in good clinical condition, a further enema should be attempted after several hours (so called 'delayed repeat enema'), and in about half of these patients it will be successful. Recurrence of intussusception occurs in about 9% of children after enema reduction, usually within days. Surgery is reserved for:

- those in whom enema reduction has failed
- those who have clinical evidence of necrotic bowel, such as peritonitis and septicaemia
- those in whom there is evidence of pathological lesions at the lead point.

Differential diagnosis

Gastroenteritis is often confused with intussusception but becomes obvious on clinical grounds by the volume and persistence of the fluid stools. The plain radiological appearance of the abdomen may be similar in both conditions. Where doubt persists, ultrasonography or a gas or barium enema is indicated. Other causes of intestinal obstruction include volvulus secondary to malrotation, a band from a Meckel diverticulum, a duplication cyst or a strangulated inguinal hernia. Examination of the groin will detect the irreducible tender lump of a strangulated hernia.

Acute abdominal pain in older children

Children often present with abdominal pain and in most no specific cause is found. Constipation and mesenteric adenitis are probably the most common non-surgical identifiable causes.

Acute appendicitis

Appendicitis may occur at any age, although it is rare under 5 years of age. Early diagnosis is difficult in the young child (under 5 years) and in the mentally retarded child; the majority of these children have established peritonitis or an appendix abscess at presentation. Delays in the diagnosis of acute appendicitis in childhood is related in part to its variable symptomatology. For example, there may be relatively little abdominal pain, vomiting may be absent and diarrhoea may be a misleading feature.

Nevertheless, the most important and consistent feature is localized abdominal pain. The pain may be intermittent and colicky initially, or situated in the epigastrium or periumbilical region, but soon shifts to the right iliac fossa. Constant pain that is worse with movement is the result of peritoneal irritation ('peritonism'). Vomiting occurs in the majority of children, and some may pass a loose stool. The temperature is usually normal or slightly elevated but occasionally may be in excess of 38°C.

Physical examination of the abdomen should be directed at showing that movement of adjacent peritoneal surfaces exacerbates the pain. The child's cooperation makes assessment easier, and repeated

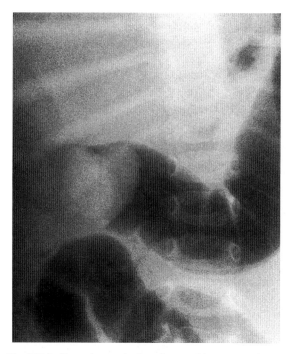

Fig. 20.1.1 X-ray demonstration of apex of intussusception during reduction using a gas enema.

examination of the abdomen may be required to make the diagnosis. A child with appendicitis usually will exhibit tenderness and guarding localized to the right iliac fossa. Gentle palpation and percussion tenderness, performed while observing the child's face, will provide the most reliable evidence of abdominal tenderness and involuntary guarding. Rebound tenderness is an unreliable sign in children, and attempts to elicit the sign may cause unnecessary pain and destroy the child's confidence in the doctor. Rectal examination is required rarely and is primarily indicated if a pelvic appendix or pelvic collection is suspected. It should not be performed if examination of the ventral abdominal wall has already enabled a confident diagnosis of acute appendicitis to be made. Bowel sounds may be normal or reduced and contribute little to the diagnosis.

Peritonitis should be suspected when the child is acutely ill with abdominal pain and fever and is reluctant to move. On examination, there will be generalized abdominal tenderness and guarding.

Laboratory studies and radiology are rarely helpful in making the diagnosis. However, the urine should be checked routinely.

Clinical example

Mark, a 10-year-old boy, had 36 hours of constant lower abdominal pain, which steadily became more severe. He vomited once initially, and was 'off his food'. Movement made the pain worse. On examination, he was afebrile but appeared flushed. He was tender to gentle palpation in the right iliac fossa and had percussion tenderness in the same region. The urine contained a few white and red cells but no bacteria. No other investigation was performed. At laparoscopy an acutely inflamed appendix was removed.

Differential diagnosis

Mesenteric adenitis is the most difficult disorder to distinguish from acute appendicitis. In general, localization of pain and tenderness is variable and less specific, and the temperature may be higher. Guarding is rarely present in mesenteric lymphadenitis.

Other conditions that may mimic acute appendicitis are relatively uncommon. Meckel diverticulitis has symptoms identical to those of appendicitis, such that differentiation is possible only at laparoscopy or laparotomy. Pain in the right iliac fossa may represent radiation from torsion of the right testis or a strangulated inguinal hernia, and highlights the importance of examination of the genitalia in all boys with lower abdominal symptoms (Ch. 9.1). Acute abdominal pain may occur with renal colic, pyelonephritis and, at times, acute glomerulonephri-

tis. Pain and tenderness is usually referred to the loin. Urine analysis and radiology will confirm the diagnosis. In Henoch–Schönlein purpura, the abdominal pain is often severe and colicky, and may be accompanied by vomiting. The characteristic skin lesions over the buttock and legs may be inconspicuous or absent when the child is first examined.

In the appropriate ethnic group, sickle cell anaemia is a prominent cause of acute abdominal pain and should be considered in a pale child with splenomegaly.

Children with cystic fibrosis frequently experience episodes of abdominal pain from faecal impaction (called 'meconium ileus equivalent'), a well known manifestation of this disease. The symptoms resolve following a bowel washout.

It is unusual for constipation in an otherwise normal child to produce sufficient abdominal pain to suggest a surgical emergency. A plain X-ray of the abdomen will demonstrate the extent of faecal accumulation (Fig. 20.1.2). It should be remembered, however, that the diagnosis of constipation is usually made on clinical grounds and that X-ray examination should be reserved for other indications or more complex cases.

Less common causes of abdominal pain include urinary tract infection, haemolytic–uraemic syndrome and diabetes. Acute hepatitis, cholecystitis and pancreatitis, although all rare in childhood, may

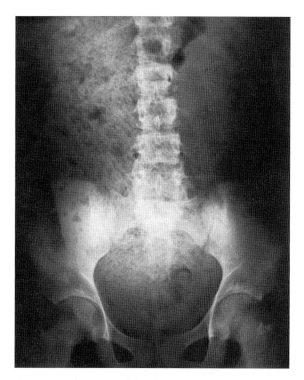

Fig. 20.1.2 Plain X-ray of the abdomen demonstrating gross faecal overload in a child with severe constipation causing abdominal pain. The child also had soiling of his underwear.

also cause abdominal pain. In pancreatitis, vomiting is prominent and epigastric tenderness with guarding may be marked. These children often look ill and obtunded. Pancreatitis may follow a blunt injury to the abdomen, e.g. a handlebar injury, and several weeks later may produce a pancreatic pseudocyst. The diagnosis is suggested by estimation of the plasma or urinary amylase or plasma lipase, and is confirmed with computed tomography (CT) or magnetic resonance imaging (MRI). The management of acute pancreatitis involves correction of shock, intravenous fluid administration, nasogastric suction to keep the stomach empty, and analgesia.

Right lower lobe pneumonia may masquerade as appendicitis. The child is usually febrile, with an increased respiratory rate, and has a cough. Signs of pneumonia may be difficult to elicit clinically, so that a chest X-ray will be required.

A general summary of disorders associated with abdominal pain is listed in Table 20.1.1.

Peptic ulceration

The abdominal pain of peptic ulceration is epigastric and usually is unrelated to meals. Nausea and vomiting may occur. Haematemesis and melaena suggest the diagnosis; alternatively it may be made following investigation of iron deficiency anaemia.

Acute gastritis and acute duodenitis produce abdominal pain with epigastric tenderness. A positive hydrogen breath test is suggestive of *Helicobacter pylori* infection. Culture of biopsy specimens taken during endoscopic examination of the upper gastrointestinal tract will confirm *H. pylori* (Ch. 20.4). Treatment with ampicillin, metronidazole or tripotassium dicitratobismuthate (De-Nol) is usually successful but relapses are common.

Reflux oesophagitis

Gastro-oesophageal reflux is common in infancy but usually resolves with growth. Sometimes it may persist into later childhood, with symptoms of belching, acid eructation and intermittent vomiting. Substernal and epigastric pain ('heartburn') suggests reflux oesophagitis. Oesophageal pH monitoring measures lower oesophageal pH over a period of 24 hours and can establish the relationship of reflux to symptoms (Ch. 20.4). Oesophagoscopy and biopsy may confirm oesophagitis. Initial management may involve the administration of H_2-receptor antagonists but, where non-operative measures fail or if an oesophageal stricture is present, surgical correction of the reflux by laparoscopic fundoplication may be indicated.

Recurrent abdominal pain in children

Recurrent bouts of abdominal pain is a fairly common paediatric presentation and one that may cause great anxiety to parents. The clinical example is illustrative of this syndrome.

Table 20.1.1 Causes of abdominal pain in childhood

Common
- Appendicitis
- Mesenteric adenitis
- Constipation
- Intussusception
- Urinary tract infection
- Torsion of the testis

Uncommon
- Volvulus secondary to malrotation
- Meckel diverticulitis
- Renal colic
- Pyelonephritis
- Acute glomerulonephritis
- Glandular fever
- Drug ingestion, e.g. salicylates, non-steroidal anti-inflammatory drugs, corticosteroids, some antibiotics, imipramine, phenytoin, iron preparations
- Peptic ulceration
- Reflux oesophagitis

Rare
- Sickle cell anaemia
- Henoch–Schönlein purpura
- Pancreatitis
- Cholecystitis
- Acute hepatitis
- Diabetes mellitus
- Haemolytic–uraemic syndrome
- Inflammatory bowel disease, e.g. Crohn disease

Clinical example

Thomas, aged 7 years, was brought in by his mother, who stated that for the last 4 months he had had severe bouts of abdominal pain. The attacks occurred at any time, but were more frequent at breakfast time. He was never awakened at night by them. Vomiting was not a feature, and his bowels had been regular. The pain usually was localized to the periumbilical region and usually lasted less than 1 hour. His parents felt that Thomas was pale and had a poor appetite. He was of normal height and weight. Physical examination was unremarkable. The urine was clear. Further questioning elicited the fact that the bouts of abdominal pain had occurred periodically since the age of 3 years.

Doctors will be impressed by the concern exhibited by parents of these children, who vividly describe the severe pain the child experiences; but there is a disparity between the parents' description and the physical findings on examination of the abdomen. Investigation almost invariably produces negative results. Enquiry into the personality of the child and into the home situation may reveal that the child is anxious or stressed, but often the pain occurs for no apparent reason. Sometimes the episodes of pain appear to be related to stress within the family. A diagnosis of non-organic recurrent abdominal pain can be made only after careful appraisal of the child in relation to the environment, and when the physical examination is normal. Most children need no investigations apart from urine culture. Further investigation is required if the abdominal pain is associated with abdominal tenderness or distension, bile stained vomiting, persistent diarrhoea, fever, weight loss or urinary symptoms. This may include full blood examination, erythrocyte sedimentation ratio (ESR), C reactive protein (CRP), radiological and endoscopic studies of the gastrointestinal tract, and specific investigations for malabsorption and inflammatory bowel disease. The urine should be examined. If the vomitus is bile-stained, malrotation with volvulus should be excluded by an urgent barium meal.

The general status of the patient must be assessed. Retardation of height and growth may occur in chronic inflammatory bowel disease, malabsorption syndromes and tuberculosis. Pallor may be associated with anaemia or conditions such as lead poisoning, sickle cell anaemia and other haemolytic diseases.

Management

Parents will find it helpful to realize that the problem has been taken seriously by the doctor, and the doctor must understand the parents' perception of the abdominal pain. With this knowledge and the negative physical findings, reassurance can be given more positively. Once parents are convinced that there is no significant organic basis to the recurrent abdominal pain they are usually much relieved. The child should be encouraged in all activities and self-esteem improved. Recurrent pain tends to disappear by the age of 12 years but in females may recur at the time of menarche. However, some children with recurrent pain in childhood present in adult life with symptoms of irritable bowel syndrome. In some, as time goes by the child's abdominal pain may become associated with and eventually replaced by migraine headaches.

Vomiting in the neonatal period

Neonates frequently vomit small amounts of mucus and blood swallowed during labour. This vomiting usually clears spontaneously within 24 hours. If not, gastric lavage with normal saline will usually relieve it. In the early weeks of life, many normal newborn babies regurgitate after feeds. The cause of this 'spitting up' or 'possetting' is not clear but is presumably related to gastro-oesophageal reflux.

Systemic infection

Vomiting is one of the many non-specific signs of infection in the neonate. Thus, unexplained vomiting should be an indication to culture the blood, urine and cerebrospinal fluid. Urine will usually be obtained by suprapubic aspiration in this age group.

Bowel obstruction

In duodenal obstruction, vomiting appears early and is bile-stained because the site of the obstruction is almost always at the second part of the duodenum, just distal to the ampulla of Vater. In duodenal atresia, there may be other abnormalities such as Down syndrome and imperforate anus. The bile-stained vomiting commences from birth. The diagnosis is made on plain X-ray of the abdomen (Ch. 11.5). Where there is bowel obstruction beyond the duodenum (e.g. small bowel atresia, Hirschsprung disease and meconium ileus), vomiting commences slightly later and is associated with increasing abdominal distension (Ch. 11.5). A strangulated inguinal hernia may cause a bowel obstruction when a loop of ileum becomes trapped within the hernial sac at the external inguinal ring. The diagnosis becomes evident when a tender irreducible lump is observed in the groin (Ch. 9.1).

Malrotation with volvulus

Volvulus in a neonate or infant with malrotation causes a high bowel obstruction and produces bile-stained vomiting. The volvulus may cut off the blood supply to the midgut and lead to small bowel infarction, septicaemia and death if not treated promptly. Any infant with bile-stained vomiting, otherwise unexplained, should be assumed to have malrotation with volvulus until proven otherwise. A barium meal will confirm the diagnosis. An urgent laparotomy is required to untwist the bowel (Fig. 20.1.3) and to perform a Ladd procedure to broaden the mesentery of the small bowel: this will prevent subsequent volvulus.

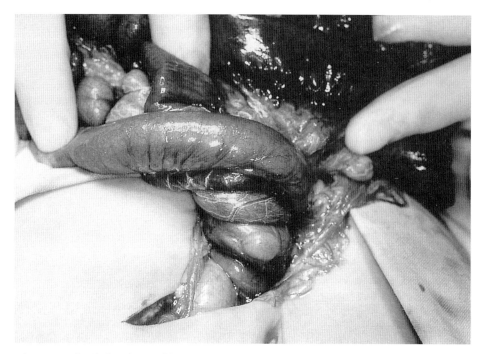

Fig. 20.1.3 Malrotation with volvulus: the small bowel is twisted on its mesentery.

Cerebral hypoxia

There is often a history of fetal distress during labour and asphyxia at birth requiring resuscitation. Following this, some infants remain lethargic and feed poorly, while others may be abnormally wide awake, excessively irritable and cry frequently. The cry may be high-pitched and associated with intermittent twitching and hypertonia; there is head retraction and the thumbs are adducted across the palms with flexion of the fingers. The Moro reflex may be exaggerated but in severe cerebral anoxia it may be lost. The fontanelle tension is not increased initially, unless there has been cerebral haemorrhage, but within 24 hours cerebral oedema occurs and causes a rise in the fontanelle tension. In cerebral anoxia the vomiting occurs before or after feeding, and may be forceful.

Treatment

Cerebral haemorrhage is shown on ultrasonography, which may also demonstrate cerebral oedema. Treatment is symptomatic: sedation with diazepam 0.1–0.3 mg/kg i.v. or phenobarbital 2 mg/kg i.m. may be required. The pulse, temperature, state of consciousness and degree of dehydration should be monitored. Aspiration of vomitus is potentially dangerous. Oral fluids are given in small volume and are offered frequently. An intravenous infusion may be necessary but fluid requirements on the first day of life are only 60 ml/kg. This amount increases gradually each day until the end of the first week, when they reach 150 ml/kg. Frequent blood glucose estimations will detect hypoglycaemia early, before it exacerbates the cerebral disturbance and accentuates the vomiting.

Subdural haematoma

With the current high standard of obstetrics, a subdural haematoma is now rare in the neonatal period. In about 50% of infants, vomiting is the only symptom. In others, vomiting is accompanied by developmental delay, convulsions, an expanding head and retinal haemorrhages. The diagnosis is confirmed on ultrasonography and CT. A subdural haematoma later in childhood must alert the clinician to the possibility of child abuse.

Hypoglycaemia

Vomiting may be the only symptom of hypoglycaemia in the neonatal period. It is more common in 'small for dates' babies and in infants of diabetic mothers but may be seen in any stressful situation in the neonatal period, including low birth weight, neonatal meningitis, septicaemia and severe Rhesus isoimmunization. Symptomatic hypoglycaemia does not usually occur with a blood glucose in excess of 2 mmol/l.

Renal disease

In the neonatal period, urinary infection and renal insufficiency may present with vomiting and poor weight gain, reflecting an underlying urinary tract abnormality. Initial urological investigation will include urine culture, renal ultrasonography, micturating cystourethrography and estimation of electrolytes, urea and creatinine. Renal tubular lesions occasionally present in the neonatal period with vomiting.

Adrenal insufficiency

Congenital adrenal hyperplasia, in which there is deficiency of the enzyme 21-hydroxylase (Ch. 19.3), presents with ambiguous genitalia in the female. If this is not recognized (as in the male), it may lead to unexplained vomiting, dehydration and collapse early in the second week of life. If the adrenal insufficiency is of the salt-losing type, the diagnosis is further suspected by finding low levels of sodium and elevated levels of potassium in the serum, and is confirmed by appropriate hormonal studies.

Inborn metabolic errors

Although individually rare, there are a number of inborn errors involving, separately, amino acid, carbohydrate and organic acid metabolism. Most are inherited recessively, and a number can now be treated. Frequently, the presentation is with unexplained vomiting, lethargy, collapse, seizures and coma (Ch. 10.5).

Vomiting in infancy

Vomiting is a common non-specific symptom in infancy, and disease of almost every system may present with vomiting.

Infection

Vomiting is frequently caused by infections such as tonsillitis, otitis media, pneumonia, meningitis and urinary tract infection. Physical examination will exclude many of these but early signs may be minimal in meningitis and pneumonia, such that a lumbar puncture and chest X-ray will be required if these are suspected. In infants with urinary tract infection, dysuria, frequency of passing urine and loin pain cannot be relied upon for diagnosis, and the urine must always be examined. When infection is controlled, the urinary tract should be imaged to exclude underlying structural abnormalities.

Lesions of the gastrointestinal tract

Conditions that produce vomiting in infancy are different from those seen in the neonatal period, except for duodenal obstruction from volvulus complicating malrotation, and gastro-oesophageal reflux. Failure to recognize malrotation with volvulus may result in infarction of the entire midgut (Ch. 11.5). Bowel trapped in a strangulated inguinal hernia in an infant will also produce vomiting. The diagnosis can be made easily if the inguinal orifices are examined (Ch. 9.1).

Gastro-oesophageal reflux

See Chapter 20.4.

Pyloric stenosis

This is one of the most dramatic causes of vomiting in infancy. Typically, the onset is dramatic, commencing between the second and sixth week of life. Males are affected five times more often than females and there is a definite familial incidence. Before the onset of vomiting, these infants fed well and were thriving. The vomiting is forceful and rapidly becomes projectile. The infant loses weight and becomes dehydrated. Despite vomiting, these infants remain hungry and are keen to feed even immediately after vomiting. The vomitus is not bile-stained but may contain altered blood. The diagnosis is made clinically by feeling the thickened pylorus ('pyloric tumour') in the midline in the epigastrium between the rectus abdominis muscles or in the angle between the right rectus and the liver edge. The pyloric tumour is palpable as a hard mobile mass about the size of a small pebble or olive. Peristaltic waves passing from the left costal margin to the right hypochondrium ('golf ball waves') may be visible long after the last feed. Palpation of the tumour is sufficient to establish the diagnosis. Pyloric stenosis can also be shown on ultrasonography (which reveals a thickened pylorus) and barium meal (which shows delayed gastric emptying and a narrow pyloric canal). These infants develop a hypokalaemic, hypochloraemic metabolic alkalosis which, together with dehydration, must be corrected before surgery. Pyloromyotomy is curative (Fig. 20.1.4).

Gastroenteritis

Vomiting in association with fluid stools is suggestive of gastroenteritis, particularly if the stools contain mucus or blood. However, these features may be seen in a variety of other medical and surgical disorders, which include intussusception and appendicitis. The diagnosis and management of gastroenteritis is discussed in Chapter 20.2.

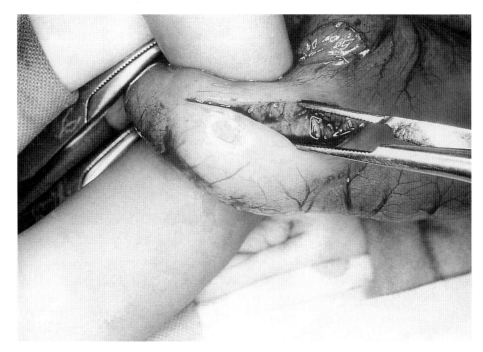

Fig. 20.1.4   Thickened pylorus in pyloric stenosis as seen during pyloromyotomy.

Malabsorption

In the majority of malabsorption syndromes vomiting is not a feature. At times, in the more severe cases of coeliac disease (gluten enteropathy, Ch. 20.3) vomiting may be prominent. A gluten-free diet rapidly reverses the clinical features of this disorder.

Intussusception

Vomiting commences early in intussusception and is the most consistent symptom. The general features, diagnosis and treatment are discussed in more detail on pages 709–710.

Clinical example

Bruce was a healthy 5-month-old baby boy until 24 hours prior to admission, when he commenced vomiting, refused feeds, was lethargic and had marked pallor. His mother had noted that at times he appeared to be in pain. There was an impression of a slightly tender mass in the right upper quadrant. There was no blood rectally. A provisional diagnosis of intussusception was made, and at gas enema an intussusception in the mid-transverse colon was encountered. This was reduced, with rapid relief of symptoms. Bruce was observed overnight before being discharged the next morning.

Strangulated inguinal hernia

Strangulation of an inguinal hernia is common in infants and young children. All irreducible inguinal hernias should be assumed to be strangulated. In practice, the vast majority of so-called irreducible hernias can be reduced manually by skilled hands (Ch. 9.1).

Vomiting in older children

Vomiting in older children is usually associated with infection, particularly viral or bacterial infection of the respiratory and gastrointestinal tracts. Nevertheless, there are some other less frequent but important causes of vomiting.

The possibility of an intracranial neoplasm should always be considered in a child with unexplained vomiting. There may be signs of increased intracranial pressure with midline cerebellar tumours, tumours involving the fourth ventricle and tumours involving the pons or medulla. Initially, vomiting tends to occur in the morning before breakfast. There may be remissions for several days but the vomiting invariably returns.

Migraine

In the older child, the association of severe paroxysmal frontal headache with pallor and vomiting is suggestive of migraine (Ch. 17.5). A positive family history is common. Transient loss of vision, transient hemiparesis, cerebellar ataxia or ophthalmoplegia may be evident. In some children migraine is precipitated by minor trauma. In the younger child, attacks of pallor or vomiting may be the only symptom. The diagnosis of migraine is made on clinical history but, where it is difficult to exclude an intracranial space-occupying lesion clinically, cerebral CT may be required.

Acute appendicitis and peritonitis

In acute appendicitis in childhood, vomiting is a frequent early symptom but is usually preceded by pain. The general features of appendicitis are described on pages 710–712. In the young child (under 5 years), vomiting with or without diarrhoea may be the only obvious symptom. Physical examination in this age group can be difficult and unreliable; the child will prefer to lie still, as movement worsens the pain. This pain and the fear of its exacerbation by palpation may make the child appear uncooperative. It is only by repeated examination of the abdomen and an ongoing high index of suspicion that the diagnosis will be made before widespread peritonitis has developed.

Poisoning

Vomiting and respiratory and circulatory collapse in a previously well child should raise the possibility of poisoning (Ch. 5.3). Non-accidental poisoning is becoming more frequent, and the age incidence of children attempting suicide is decreasing. A history of family discord and emotional problems in the child is not always volunteered.

Psychological causes of vomiting

Psychogenic vomiting may occur in any age group. It can be associated with attempts to force-feed a toddler or a schoolchild, after punishment, and as an attempt to avoid situations perceived as threatening, such as going to preschool or school. Almost any stressful situation may precipitate vomiting in a tense or anxious child. The absence of abnormal physical signs will be a feature.

Cyclical vomiting

Cyclical vomiting is a syndrome of persistent periodic vomiting of childhood. The severity varies, but ketosis and metabolic acidosis may develop rapidly. The aetiology is unknown and attacks usually cease spontaneously. Children with cyclical vomiting are often tense and anxious and may develop migraine or psychosomatic disease later in life. Recurring episodes of volvulus from malrotation, and metabolic disease, should be excluded before labelling these children as having cyclical vomiting.

Diarrhoea is defined as a measured stool volume greater than 10 ml/kg per day. Both the consistency of the stool (loose or watery) and frequency (usually at least three stools in a 24-hour period) are important defining features of diarrhoea. Acute diarrhoea lasts less than 10 days and has a major impact on both fluid and electrolyte status, while chronic diarrhoea suggests that the symptom is present for more than 2–3 weeks and can have a significant effect on the nutritional state of a child. The basic pathological mechanisms causing diarrhoea include osmotic, secretory and inflammatory processes (Table 20.2.1). Often more than one mechanism may operate simultaneously to cause diarrhoea. The commonest cause of acute diarrhoea in children is an enteric infection (acute gastroenteritis).

Acute gastroenteritis

Aetiology

Rotavirus infection (Fig. 20.2.1) is the most common cause of acute gastroenteritis in children under 5 years of age in developed countries, causing 40–50% of cases where hospital admission is required. It accounts for more severe episodes in infants in developing countries than any other single pathogen; it is more likely to cause dehydration, and is associated with a higher mortality than most other agents. The mucosal damage it causes (Fig. 20.2.2), and hence the need for structural repair, has considerable nutritional implications for malnourished children. Asymptomatic reinfection can occur several times and helps maintain immunity.

Enteric adenoviruses (types 40 and 41) cause 5–15% of cases requiring admission to hospital, and several other virus pathogens have been recognized, such as calicivirus, astrovirus and other small viruses, which accounts for a further 15%.

Bacteria cause fewer episodes than viruses in developed countries. *Campylobacter jejuni* is responsible for 5–10% of cases. *Salmonella* spp., *Shigella* spp. and various types of *Escherichia coli* each account for a small percentage. In developing countries, *E. coli* (enterotoxigenic, enteropathogenic and enteroinvasive) and *Shigella* spp. are especially important: *E. coli* because of the huge number of episodes it causes, and *Shigella* because it causes prolonged debilitating illness and antibiotic-resistant strains are emerging.

Giardia lamblia rarely causes acute dehydrating diarrhoea but another parasite, *Cryptosporidium,* is now known to cause 1–4% of cases of acute diarrhoea in infants admitted to hospital.

Clinical features

Symptoms of acute gastroenteritis include vomiting, fever and watery diarrhoea (up to 10–20 stools daily).

Blood, mucus and the passage of small frequent bowel actions accompanied by abdominal pain suggests a diagnosis of bacterial gastroenteritis.

Acute gastroenteritis is a diagnosis of exclusion. A few loose stools and vomiting does not necessarily equate with the diagnosis. There are several systemic disorders and surgical emergencies that can mimic infective gastroenteritis (Table 20.2.2).

Management

Once the diagnosis of acute gastroenteritis is made on thorough clinical history and physical examination, the next step is to assess the degree of dehydration and institute an appropriate plan for rehydration. This should be combined with nutritional support that aids the patient during the recovery phase.

Dehydration

This risk is related to the child's age, with young infants being at greatest risk. This is because infants less than 1 year of age have a high surface area:body volume ratio, resulting in increased insensible fluid loss. They also have a tendency to more severe vomiting and diarrhoea compared with older children and adults.

Fluid loss is usually assessed on the basis of percentage body weight loss. Physical signs of dehydration are not usually apparent until 4% of body weight is lost.

The signs of dehydration traditionally described are outlined in Table 20.2.3. However, three signs

Table 20.2.1 Classification of diarrhoea

	Osmotic	Secretory	Inflammatory
Clinical features	Ceases when enteral feeding is ceased	Continues when enteral feeding is ceased	Presence of blood and mucus in the faeces
Stool volume	<200 ml/day	>200 ml/day	Variable, usually <200 ml/day
Faecal sodium	<60 mosmol/l	90 mosmol/l	Variable

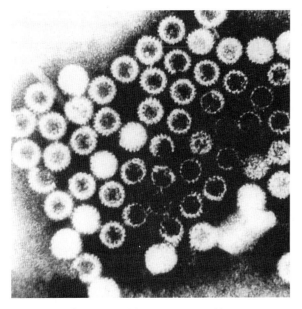

Fig. 20.2.1 The rotavirus (electron micrograph).

Table 20.2.2 Differential diagnosis of acute diarrhoea and vomiting in infants and children

Enteric infection
- Rotavirus
- Other viruses
- Bacterial
  - *Salmonella* spp.
  - *Shigella* spp.
  - *Escherichia coli*
  - *Campylobacter jejuni*
- Protozoa
  - *Cryptosporidium*
  - *Giardia lamblia*
  - *Entamoeba histolytica*
- Food poisoning
- Staphylococcal toxin

Systemic infection
- Urinary tract infection
- Pneumonia
- Septicaemia

Surgical condition
- Appendicitis
- Intussusception
- Partial bowel obstruction
- Hirschsprung disease

Other
- Diabetes mellitus
- Antibiotic diarrhoea
- Haemolytic–uraemic syndrome

discriminate adequately between dehydration and adequate hydration: deep breathing, decreased skin turgor and poor peripheral perfusion.

Electrolyte loss

This is usually isotonic (water and electrolytes being lost in equal amounts). Hypertonic hypernatraemic dehydration (fluid loss > electrolyte loss) occurs in 5–10% of cases of acute gastroenteritis, and hypotonic hyponatraemic dehydration (electrolyte loss > fluid loss) can occur if the colon (a major site of sodium reabsorption) is out of circuit, e.g. short gut syndrome.

If corrected too rapidly, hypernatraemic dehydration will result in convulsions due to rapid shifts of water into cells. Hyponatraemic dehydration can also cause significant neurological morbidity and mortality and, in contrast to the hypernatraemic state, requires vigorous replacement of sodium.

Rehydration guidelines

See also Chapter 6.1

No dehydration

- Nutritional intake and fluids should not be modified but should be offered ad libitum to keep up with ongoing losses

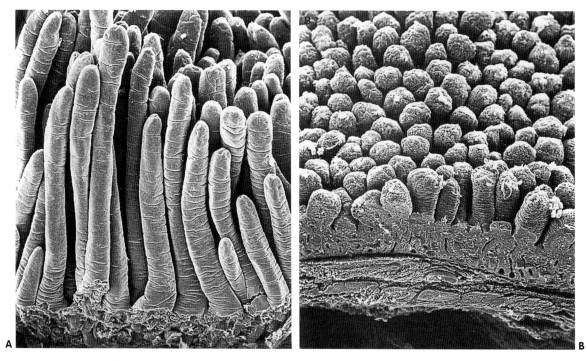

Fig. 20.2.2 Scanning electron microscope appearances of (**A**) normal and (**B**) rotavirus-infected calf jejunum. Villi are short, the epithelium is damaged and crypts are deep. (Courtesy of D. G. A. Hall, Institute for Animal Health, Compton, UK. With permission from Walker et al 1991.)

Table 20.2.3   Assessment of dehydration

Mild (≤5% body weight loss)
- Dry mucous membranes
- Decreased peripheral perfusion*
- Thirsty, alert, restless

Moderate (6–9% body weight loss)
- Exaggeration of the above
- Lethargic but irritable
- Rapid pulse, normal blood pressure
- Sunken eyes, sunken fontanelle
- Oliguria is usually obvious
- Pinched skin retracts slowly (1–2 s)*

Severe (≥10% body weight loss)
- General appearance
  - Infants: drowsy, limp, cold sweaty, cyanotic limbs, comatose
  - Older children: apprehensive, cold, sweaty, cyanotic limbs
- Rapid feeble pulse, low blood pressure
- Sunken eyes and fontanelle
- Pinched skin retracts slowly (>2 s)*
- Deep acidotic breathing*

* These are the only signs proven to discriminate between hydration and dehydration.

Table 20.2.4   Oral rehydration preparations available in Australia

	Na	K	Cl	Citrate	Glucose
WHO	90	20	80	10	90
Hydralyte	45	20	45	30	90
Gastrolyte	60	20	60	10	90
Repalyte	60	20	60	10	90

Concentration expressed as mmol/l.

Mild to moderate dehydration

- Oral rehydration solution (ORS) is the cornerstone of successful rehydration and is recommended globally for the management of acute diarrhoea
- The success of ORS is based on the basic observation that intestinal sodium transport is enhanced by glucose transport in the small intestine and that this sodium-coupled mechanism for glucose transport remains intact during acute gastroenteritis
- To facilitate optimal absorption of sodium, glucose and water, the sodium and glucose must be in the range recommended (Table 20.2.4)

Table 20.2.5 An infant of 10 kg estimated at 8% dehydration has fluid requirements equal to
Maintenance 100 × 10 kg = 1000 ml Deficit 8% of 10 kg = 800 ml Total = 1800 ml Using oral rehydration the deficit can be replaced in 6 hours rather than 24 hours, so in the above example the infant would be offered fluid as follows:
First 6 hours Deficit = 800 ml Maintenance 6/24 of 1000 = 250 ml Total = 1050 ml (175 ml/h)
Next 18 hours Maintenance 18/24 of 1000 = 750 ml (45 ml/h) Another simple method which gives about the right answer is to calculate the fluid deficit, double it, and give that volume over 6–12 hours.

Table 20.2.6 A 10 kg child with 15% dehydration and shock
Total fluid deficit = 15% of 10 kg = 1.5 l = 1500 ml Assume a total of 40 ml/kg (400 ml) normal saline needed to restore circulation Remaining deficit = 1500 – 400 = 1100 ml Maintenance fluid requirement is 100 ml/kg/d = 10 × 100 = 1000 ml Fluid in next 24 h = remaining deficit + maintenance = 1100 + 1000 = 2100 ml = 90 ml/h Therefore, give 400 ml normal saline quickly, then 90 ml/h of 5% dextrose in N/2 saline with KCl 40 mmol/l for the next 24 h

• Rehydration should take place over 4–6 hours and can be given orally or, if either vomiting or fluid refusal is a problem, a nasogastric tube may be used to achieve a steady infusion of fluid
• Volume required for rehydration = estimated deficit and maintenance; maintenance for:
  • 1–3 months of age = 120 ml/kg/24 h
  • 3–12 months of age = 100 ml/kg/24 h
  • 12 months onwards = 80 ml/kg/24 h
  (see Tables 20.2.5 and 20.2.6)

Severe dehydration (10% plus)

• Circulatory insufficiency is present and intravenous therapy is required. The usual requirement is to fill the vascular compartment quickly to restore circulation. This will require rapid rehydration, often using boluses of normal saline by intravenous or intraosseous infusion
• Once dehydration is corrected and normal organ perfusion is restored, ORS can be used in conjunc-

tion with intravenous fluids. The latter is rarely required for longer than 24 hours
• Clinical observations must be highlighted: this allows the physician to reassess the patient's state of hydration and also helps confirm the diagnosis of acute gastroenteritis
• All patients with dehydration require regular checks on pulse, temperature and respiration, and strict fluid balance charts must be kept. The child should be weighed on admission and, in severe cases, after 6 hours and 24 hours, with an increase in weight being a reliable sign of rehydration. However, in some patients weight may not fall even in the presence of severe dehydration, especially if the child has an ileus, so other signs of dehydration must be sought.

Recommendations on nutritional management

Breastfeeding should continue through rehydration and maintenance phases of treatment, and formula feeds need to be restarted after rehydration. Use of special formulas or diluted formulas is unjustified.

Pharmacotherapy

• Infants and children with acute gastroenteritis should not be treated with antidiarrhoeal agents
• Antibiotic treatment may be indicated in *Salmonella* spp. gastroenteritis in the very young (<3 months), those who are immunocompromised or those who are systemically unwell. It may also be indicated in *C. jejuni* infection in compromised hosts and *Yersinia enterocolitica* in children with sickle cell disease
• Pathogens for which antibacterial therapy is always indicated include *Shigella* spp. and *G. lamblia*
• Certain types of probiotic have a modest effect in acute infective gastroenteritis; however, their routine use is not recommended until further large-scale trials have been undertaken.

Complications of acute gastroenteritis

Febrile convulsions

These are generally uncommon, but rotavirus infection can cause fevers as high as 39–40°C.

Sugar malabsorption

This is more common in infants less than 6 months of age and recognized by the persistent nature of the diarrhoea when nutrition is reintroduced.

Stools are often watery, frothy and tend to excoriate the buttocks. If sugar intolerance is suspected, the napkin should be lined with thin plastic material, or a rectal examination should be performed and the fluid stool collected and tested for reducing substances. It is pointless to test solid stool material.

To test for lactose intolerance, mix 5 drops of liquid stool with 10 drops of water and add a Clinitest tablet. A positive test of more than 0.5% indicates lactose or glucose malabsorption, but not sucrose, which is not a reducing sugar.

Diarrhoea due to lactose malabsorption resolves rapidly on a lactose-free diet, which should be continued for approximately 4 weeks. A very small proportion of infants continue to have diarrhoea despite the exclusion of lactose and sucrose. Under these circumstances, a carbohydrate-free feed is given, with glucose and fructose (different transport mechanisms across the enterocyte) added to tolerance.

Prevention of acute gastroenteritis

A simple and effective prevention of transmission of the condition is via handwashing when in contact with an index case, especially in the hospital setting.

Prophylactic passive immunization is provided by oral administration of hyperimmune bovine antirotavirus colostrums. It reduces nosocomial infection in infants in high-risk settings but its effect stops with cessation of administration. Anti-*E.-coli* colostrum tablets are available to help prevent the most common type of traveller's diarrhoea.

Vaccines against typhoid and cholera infection are available and *E. coli* vaccines are under development.

Two live attenuated oral rotavirus vaccines are becoming available, one of which is already licensed in several countries. One is a human strain (Rotarix, GSK), which relies on immunity being stimulated across serotypes. Both vaccines appear to be free from the rare serious side effect of intussusception, which led to the withdrawal of an earlier candidate vaccine based on a Rhesus monkey rotavirus strain. Other candidates are under development in developing countries as a strategy to ensure that rotavirus vaccine becomes widely available to children worldwide.

> ### Practical points
>
> **Acute gastroenteritis**
> - Is commonly caused by viruses and is self-limiting
> - Assess dehydration carefully and correct appropriately, but reassess constantly
> - Not all children with diarrhoea have gastroenteritis; be aware of other conditions that may mimic it
> - Proper handwashing is the best measure to avoid transmission

---

Chronic diarrhoea

This is defined as the presence of diarrhoea for more than 2–3 weeks. It can follow a bout of acute gastroenteritis but usually begins insidiously.

Many causes of chronic diarrhoea are associated with malabsorption of nutrients and are dealt with in detail in Chapter 20.3. Only chronic non-specific diarrhoea, postinfective diarrhoea, sucrase–isomaltase deficiency and inflammatory bowel disease will be discussed in this chapter.

An approach to diagnosis

Answers to a small number of key questions will usually get very close to a definitive diagnosis. Figure 20.2.3 outlines a suggested scheme. Performance of simple stool tests is all that is necessary to guide selection of the appropriate definitive tests. Many of the specific causes are discussed in Chapter 20.3. Others are dealt with here.

Chronic non-specific diarrhoea

- Seen in children between the ages of 12 months and 4 years and current scientific evidence suggests that disturbed intestinal motility is pivotal in the pathogenesis of this condition. It is also commonly referred to as toddlers' diarrhoea
- The history is one of frequent, poorly formed and slightly offensive stools. Food material is often recognized in the stool, suggesting rapid gastrointestinal transit. The condition often resolves spontaneously at about 3–4 years of age

---

Clinical example

Tim, a previously well 22-month-old infant, suddenly became unwell with onset of vomiting and a temperature of 38.5°C. Within 12 hours he started passing frequent, loose motions. Associated with this he appeared to have bouts of abdominal pain. On the second day the vomiting stopped but the diarrhoea persisted at a rate of more than eight stools per day. On presentation to the emergency department, Tim's weight was 13.6 kg compared with 14.5 kg 3 weeks previously. He was clinically assessed to be 5–8% dehydrated and was treated with an oral rehydration solution via a nasogastric tube. A provisional diagnosis of acute gastroenteritis was made. His temperature gradually settled over 24 hours days and oral feeds were introduced once rehydration was complete. His stools returned to their normal pattern after 5 days. Rapid stool testing for rotavirus antigen was positive.

1. EXCLUDE RETENTION WITH OVERFLOW

2. IS THERE FAILURE TO THRIVE?

YES   ALWAYS investigate

NO   Sometimes investigate
             Time is on your side.

3. IS STOOL VOLUME INCREASED?

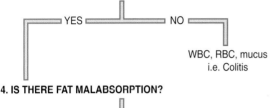

WBC, RBC, mucus
i.e. Colitis

4. IS THERE FAT MALABSORPTION?

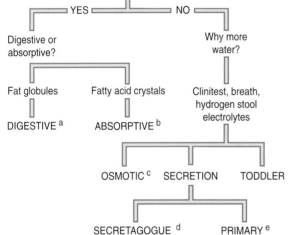

5. IS THERE PROTEIN LOSING ENTEROPATHY?

Raised alpha -1-AT clearance [f]

a. Digestive pancreatic insufficiency (confirmed by low trypsin) liver disease obvious)

b. Absorptive mucosal damage: coeliac disease, giardias, protein hypersensitivity, IBD. lymphatic block: lymphangiectasis.

c. Osmotic disaccharidase deficiency monosaccharide transport: glucose-galatose transport overload: high sugar fluids, fruits, sorbitol

d. Secretagogue bacterial toxin *(C. difficile)* deconjugated bile salts

e. Primary transport defect (rare) chlorideorrhoea

f. Protein losing enteropathy lymphangiectasia, polyposis

Fig. 20.2.3   Investigation of chronic diarrhoea.

• The child is usually active, with unimpaired growth, appetite is normal and there is a history of increased fluid intake. Further questioning about diet often reveals a high intake of fruit juices and cordial

• The cornerstone of successful treatment includes restriction of fruit juice in the diet, normalizing fluid intake and (re-)introduction of wholemeal and other dietary fibres, which add bulk to the stool

• It has also been suggested that many of these children are on a relatively low fat diet, and normalizing fat content acts to slow proximal gastrointestinal transit and improve symptoms.

Postinfective diarrhoea

• This is defined as the persistence of diarrhoea and failure to gain weight for more than 7 days after hospital admission for gastroenteritis

• It is generally due to a sugar intolerance, which can be confirmed on the basis of stool analysis for reducing sugars and will resolve with elimination of the sugar from the diet

• Other causes include cow's milk protein hypersensitivity or a persistent gastrointestinal infection.

Sucrase–isomaltase deficiency

• This is an uncommon inherited disorder (autosomal recessive), with symptoms beginning after sucrose is introduced into the diet

• Symptoms consist of watery diarrhoea and abdominal distension. Growth is usually normal

• Diagnosis is dependent on a positive breath hydrogen test using sucrose as the test sugar. Alternatively, a small bowel biopsy containing very low isomaltase and sucrase levels will establish the diagnosis

• Management is based on dietary restriction of sucrose.

Chronic inflammatory bowel disease

The incidence of Crohn disease has increased annually; that of ulcerative colitis has shown an annual fluctuation without an upward trend. Current opinion regarding the cause of inflammatory bowel disease (IBD) favours the hypothesis that these two conditions result from an interaction between immunological, genetic and environmental factors.

Crohn disease can present in several ways:

• extraintestinal manifestations include growth retardation, anorexia, fatigue, delayed puberty, erythema nodosum, arthritis, clubbing, hepatitis and uveitis

• oropharyngeal involvement include orofacial granulomatosis and recurrent mouth ulcers

• oesophageal, gastric and small bowel Crohn may present as, nausea, vomiting, abdominal pain and diarrhoea

• colonic involvement, presents with passage of blood or mucous per rectum

• perianal involvement include skin tags, fissures, fistulas and abscess.

Children with ulcerative colitis will usually present with lower abdominal pain, urgency, diarrhoea and rectal bleeding; additionally:

- systemic symptoms are less marked
- the child can develop arthritis, which usually correlates with disease activity
- pyoderma gangrenosum occurs more commonly in ulcerative colitis
- the child can develop sclerosing cholangitis.

Children may experience the same symptoms, clinical presentations, complications and response to treatment as adults with IBD. This chapter will highlight some of the features of IBD that have particular importance in the paediatric patient.

Investigation

Several laboratory tests will support the diagnosis of IBD; however, endoscopy is the gold standard. Gastroscopy and colonoscopy (with ileoscopy) is essential, taking biopsies at all levels of the gut, whether or not there is macroscopic disease. Biopsies from a normal-appearing stomach or duodenum may contain granulomas, making the diagnosis clear. Pathological alterations above the ileum exclude the diagnosis of ulcerative colitis. A barium meal and follow-through or a labelled white cell scan can be helpful in assessing the area of the gut that is involved in Crohn disease. Capsule endoscopy is a new and evolving technology that is being used to image the small bowel mucosa.

Treatment

Enteral therapy

- Provides a similar remission rate to corticosteroids in the treatment of childhood Crohn disease (not ulcerative colitis) and improves growth and inflammatory markers
- Probably exerts its beneficial effects by alterations in gut flora, enterocyte nutrition and modulation of endogenous growth factors
- Chronic supplementary enteral therapy reduces relapse rates in Crohn disease but not ulcerative colitis
- Often utilizes polymeric and elemental feeds, which are probably equally effective but are not generally palatable and may require nasogastric infusion. All other oral intake is ceased during this treatment, which usually lasts 6–8 weeks

Corticosteroids

- Used in the dose range of 1–2 mg/kg of prednisolone for moderate to severe ulcerative colitis or Crohn disease, usually for a 2–3-month period with a gradual dose reduction
- Can adversely affect growth and have many unpleasant cosmetic and systemic side effects
- Can have a significant effect on bone mineral density and lead to osteoporosis later in life
- Newer corticosteroids, such as budesonide, have fewer side effects and are particularly useful for ileal and right-sided colonic disease
- Steroid enemas are helpful in the management of lower colonic inflammation in both Crohn disease and ulcerative colitis.

Other pharmacological treatments

- Aminosalicylates can be used in both an oral and topical form to manage colitis in both Crohn disease and ulcerative colitis. This is often used in mild ulcerative colitis to achieve remission and in both ulcerative colitis and Crohn colitis as maintenance therapy
- Azathioprine is often used in children with both ulcerative colitis and Crohn disease if they are steroid-dependent but will take 12–14 weeks to be clinically effective
- Medications such as tacrolimus, ciclosporin and methotrexate may be used in the most severe disease; however, the effectiveness of such agents has only been assessed in open-label studies
- Anti-tumour necrosis factor (TNF)α has shown promising results in the management of adults with severe Crohn disease but has been used sparingly in children. Side effects such as severe allergic reactions and the possible development of lymphoproliferative disorders are a major concern
- Antibiotics, e.g. metronidazole, are useful in perianal and colonic Crohn disease

Surgery

- Usually indicated in children with Crohn disease who have growth failure and have not responded to pharmacological or nutritional therapies. This usually applies to an area of localized disease
- Appropriately timed surgery in children with Crohn disease may accelerate growth and advance puberty
- Colectomy is rarely required in children with ulcerative colitis unless there is uncontrolled bleeding or if toxic megacolon is present

Cancer risk

- Greatest in children with ulcerative colitis, particularly those with pancolitis for more than 10 years who also have coexisting sclerosing cholangitis

• Observed accumulative incidences range from 5 to 10% after 20 years disease duration and 12–20% after 30 years. This implies that a person with ulcerative colitis has a roughly 12% chance of developing colorectal cancer between 10 and 15 years after the onset of the IBD

• To avoid colonic cancer, patients with long-standing extensive colitis face either prophylactic colectomy or regular surveillance colonoscopy. Neither option is perfect; a more reliable, cheaper process of screening needs to be found

• This general approach also applies to children and adults with extensive and long-standing colonic Crohn disease.

Clinical example

Sarah presented at the age of 14 years with a 3-month history of recurrent abdominal pain and diarrhoea. Her stools are described as watery with variable amounts of blood and mucus. Clinical examination revealed mild pallor and, on abdominal examination, there was tenderness in both the left and the right iliac fossa. Blood test revealed a microcytic anaemia (Hb 90 g/dl and an MCV of 69) and an ESR of 25 mm/h. Stool microscopy showed red blood cells and white blood cells. Repeated stool cultures for viruses, bacteria and also *Clostridium difficile* toxin was negative. At colonoscopy, there was a pancolitis and a normal ileum. A provisional diagnosis of ulcerative colitis was made and this was supported by the histology. Sarah was treated initially with high-dose steroids and later was maintained on sulfasalazine, with good clinical response.

Practical points

Inflammatory bowel disease
• Potentially a multisystem chronic relapsing disease
• Assessment of distribution of the disease may require multiple modalities, i.e. endoscopy and biopsy and imaging modalities
• Treatment is individually tailored, based on site and severity of disease
• Be aware of long-term malignant risk, especially in ulcerative colitis, and also side effects of various medication used

Malabsorption is not a clinical entity. It can be defined as the failure to absorb nutrients. A wide range of intestinal, pancreatic and hepatic disorders can be associated with malabsorption. To understand how one approaches the problem of malabsorption in the clinical setting, an understanding of the normal physiology of nutrient digestion and salt, water and macronutrient and micronutrient absorption is essential. This information is available in general physiology texts.

Diagnostic approach

A large number of children have loose stools without having underlying gastrointestinal disease. In young children this is called 'toddlers' diarrhoea'. A major clinical challenge is to differentiate well children with loose stools from children who have gastrointestinal disease. The diagnosis of the majority of children with malabsorption can be established with thorough clinical assessment, stool examination and simple ancillary tests.

Clinical assessment

Initial assessment can reveal whether a child is ill. If so, immediate evaluation will be required. In the well child, a 'wait and see' approach may be more rewarding than immediate investigation.

Malabsorption does not present as malabsorption per se. Rather, individuals with malabsorption can present with a wide array of symptoms and physical signs (Table 20.3.1). Diarrhoea is the most common presentation and may be accompanied by loss of appetite, decreased physical activity, lethargy and growth failure. Children with coeliac disease may have decreased appetite, and are often cranky and irritable. In contrast, children with pancreatic insufficiency often develop a voracious appetite. In children with failure to thrive, a detailed dietary history is required. Occasionally, parents manipulate the child's diet in an attempt to control the diarrhoea, which can lead to significant dietary insufficiency with attendant weight loss. Assessment of the age of introduction of various foods into the diet may give insight to the underlying diagnosis. Onset of symptoms 3–6 months after the introduction of wheat products suggests the possibility of coeliac disease. Onset shortly after introduction of cow's milk suggests cow's milk protein intolerance. History of overseas travel is important, as some unusual infections, such as amoebic dysentery, can cause chronic bloody diarrhoea.

The nature of the loose stool is important to ascertain, as it provides important clues to the pathophysiology and thus aetiology. Diarrhoea can be thought of in terms of fatty stools (steatorrhoea), watery diarrhoea (osmotic because of carbohydrate malabsorption or secretory) and bloody diarrhoea. Table 20.3.2 provides a differential diagnosis of chronic diarrhoea and malabsorption categorized by the nature of the stool.

Assessment of general health is important, as many gastrointestinal disorders exhibit extraintestinal manifestations. Cystic fibrosis (Ch. 14.6), Shwachman syndrome and immunodeficiency disorders (Ch. 13.2) are associated with infections, particularly sinopulmonary infections. Delayed pubertal development can accompany many chronic disorders but is particularly prevalent in Crohn disease (Ch. 20.2).

Family history may be of note. Cystic fibrosis, primary disaccharidase deficiencies and abetalipoproteinaemia are recessively inherited. Coeliac disease and inflammatory bowel disease are more frequently observed in first-degree relatives.

Physical examination includes assessment of growth, nutritional status and pubertal development. Plotting percentile charts is mandatory. A child who is growing normally is unlikely to be suffering from serious gastrointestinal disease. Plotting longitudinal measurements, if available, is very important as it may give clues to the onset of disease and could indicate the diagnosis. Other physical signs of malabsorption and specific nutritional deficiencies include: loss of muscle bulk and subcutaneous fat; peripheral oedema (hypoproteinaemia); bruising (vitamin K deficiency); glossitis and angular stomatitis (iron deficiency); finger clubbing (cystic fibrosis, Crohn disease, coeliac disease); skin rashes in coeliac disease (dermatitis herpetiformis) and inflammatory bowel disease (erythema nodosum, pyoderma gangrenosum); and specific skin disorders associated with zinc, vitamin A and essential fatty acid deficiencies

Table 20.3.1 Some symptoms and signs of nutrient deficiencies

Protein		Growth failure
		Muscle wasting
		Hypoproteinaemic oedema
Fat		Weight loss
		Muscle wasting
		Manifestation of deficiency of vitamins A, D, E, K
Carbohydrate		Weight loss
Salt/water		Electrolyte disturbances
		Growth failure (chronic salt deficiency)
		Dehydration (acute loss)
Vitamins	A	Night blindness
		Skin rash
		Dry eyes (xerophthalmia)
	D	Rickets
		Hypocalcaemia
	K	Bruising (coagulation defects)
	E	Anaemia
		Peripheral neuropathy
	B_{12}	Megaloblastic anaemia
		Irritability
		Hypotonia
		Peripheral neuropathy
	Folate	Megaloblastic anaemia
		Irritability
Minerals	Iron	Microcytic anaemia
		Delayed development
	Calcium	Rickets
		Irritability
		Seizures
	Zinc	Diarrhoea
		Skin rash (mouth, perineum, fingers and toes)
		Poor growth

Table 20.3.2 Differential diagnosis of chronic diarrhoea and malabsorption categorized according to type of stool

Steatorrhoea
Pancreatic insufficiency
- Cystic fibrosis
- Shwachman syndrome
- Chronic pancreatitis
- Malnutrition (developing world)
- Isolated lipase deficiency

Inadequate bile salt concentration
- Biliary atresia
- Cholestatic syndromes
  - Congenital
  - Acquired
- End stage liver disease
- Bacterial overgrowth syndrome
- Bile salt malabsorption (ileal resection)

Inadequate absorptive surface
- Coeliac disease
- Surgical resection (short gut syndrome)
- Milk protein intolerance
- Immunodeficiency

Enterocyte defect
- Abetalipoproteinaemia

Defective lymphatic drainage
- Intestinal lymphangiectasia
- Constrictive pericarditis

Watery diarrhoea
Osmotic
Disaccharidase deficiency
- Lactase
- Sucrase–isomaltase

Glucose–galactose malabsorption
Excessive intake
- Sorbitol
- Fructose

Abnormal water and electrolyte transport
Congenital electrolyte transporter defects
- Congenital chloride diarrhoea
- Congenital sodium diarrhoea

Infection
Mucosal disease
- Coeliac disease
- Milk protein intolerance
- Inflammatory conditions (inflammatory bowel disease)
- Immunodeficiency disorders
- Autoimmune enteropathy

Bile salt malabsorption
- Congenital
- Ileal resection

Bacterial overgrowth syndromes
- Gastrointestinal motility disorders
- Anatomical (blind loop)

Bloody diarrhoea
Infection
- Bacterial
- Parasitic

Inflammatory bowel disease
- Crohn disease
- Ulcerative colitis
- Milk protein intolerance

(Fig. 20.3.1). Rickets (vitamin D deficiency) is very uncommon in sunny climates, even in conditions with severe steatorrhoea. It is important to examine carefully as there are many extraintestinal manifestations of gastrointestinal disease and malnutrition.

Stool examination

Stool examination is very simple and provides very important information. The presence of numerous white and red cells indicates colitis. This is usually due to bacterial or parasitic infection, to chronic inflammatory disorders of the large bowel, or to milk protein intolerance when identified in infants. Leukocytes are not increased in the stool of individuals

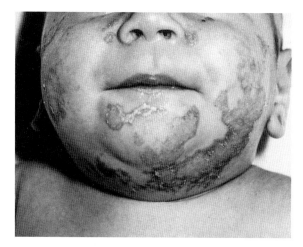

Fig. 20.3.1 Exfoliative rash of zinc deficiency.

with small bowel or pancreatic disease. Cysts of parasites such as *Giardia lamblia* indicate giardiasis.

Oil droplets seen on stool microscopy are always abnormal outside the newborn period and usually indicate fat maldigestion, as occurs with pancreatic insufficiency, e.g. in cystic fibrosis. Mucosal disease, such as coeliac disease, in general does not interfere with fat digestion because pancreatic function is usually normal. Mucosal disease interferes with the absorption of triglyceride products. These products are observed as fatty acid crystals on polarizing microscopy.

The presence of carbohydrate in the stool can be detected with Clinitest tablets. This is a commercially available bedside test in which the reaction between stool sugars such as lactose causes a colour change when added to the tablets. Greater than 500 mg/dl indicates carbohydrate malabsorption. Measurement of stool electrolytes and osmolality in the stool water is also a very useful test. When the sum of the stool electrolytes, i.e. sodium + potassium + chloride + bicarbonate, equals measured osmolality, a secretory diarrhoea is present. If the sum of the electrolytes is substantially less than the measured osmolality (>100 mosmol/l), this indicates an osmotic diarrhoea.

Malabsorption with chronic diarrhoea

Diarrhoea is the most common presentation of malabsorption. Diarrhoea can be defined as increased frequency, fluidity and volume of stool. The following discussion will provide a systematic approach to

the child with malabsorption and diarrhoea based on the type of stool, i.e.:

• fatty
• watery or
• bloody.

Some illustrative cases will be provided.

Fatty diarrhoea (steatorrhoea)

The differential diagnosis of fat malabsorption is quite wide ranging (Table 20.3.2); however, if one understands the normal physiology of fat digestion and absorption, the differential diagnosis is much less daunting. Conditions that cause steatorrhoea can also be associated with protein maldigestion

Clinical example

Mary was 9 months old. She presented with poor weight gain, chronic diarrhoea and a history of recurrent respiratory illnesses, including one admission at age 3 months with 'bronchiolitis'. Loose stools were found each time her nappy was changed. On occasion mother had noted oil drops in the stool. Despite the poor weight gain, Mary had an excellent appetite and was described as a voracious eater. She consumed a mixed diet, including infant formula, appropriate for age. Cereal was introduced at age 6 months. Mother also commented that she tasted salty when she kissed Mary.

On examination, Mary was found to be a thin wasted girl. Her height was on the 50th percentile and her weight was less than the 3rd percentile. She had mild finger clubbing, peripheral oedema, pallor of the tongue and palmar creases but no signs of chronic liver disease. There was no abdominal distension of note, although she had a fine scaling rash over her trunk. Respiratory examination was normal. No other abnormal physical signs were present.

Results of investigations included Hb 85 g/l (normal range, 110–140) with a normocytic normochromic film, normal white cell count and differential; albumin 24 g/l (normal range, 34–44) and normal liver function tests. Stool microscopy revealed copious fat droplets. 3-day faecal fat excretion estimation demonstrated an output of 35% of ingested fat (normal <7% of intake).

Mary's diarrhoea was due to fat malabsorption, as evidenced by her mother's observation of fat droplets in the stool.

Mary's sweat test demonstrated a sweat chloride of 80 mmol/l (a result of >60 mmol/l is diagnostic of cystic fibrosis). Genetic testing indicated that she was homozygous ΔF508 (the commonest mutation), consistent with her relatively severe symptoms. Introduction of pancreatic exocrine replacement therapy, a high fat diet and vitamin supplements alleviated her diarrhoea and eventually corrected her failure to thrive, anaemia and skin rash.

and/or malabsorption, although symptoms most commonly relate to the malabsorption of fat. The presence of fat in the stool is also more readily observed than protein.

Fat and protein digestion and absorption

Ingested fat in the form of triglycerides, cholesterol and phospholipids is, to a large extent, digested in the lumen of the small intestine and absorbed in the jejunum. This requires bile salts, which form micelles and solubilize the fat; pancreatic enzymes, such as lipase and colipase, which digest the fat; and an intact intestinal mucosa, which is required for absorption of the products of digestion. Following digestion in the micelles, breakdown products diffuse across the enterocyte apical membrane and are reconstituted in the cell into chylomicrons. These are small packets of triglyceride, phospholipid and cholesterol which associate with carrier proteins, such as beta lipoprotein, essential for cellular trafficking of the chylomicrons. After the chylomicrons are reconstituted they exit the mucosa into the lymphatic system and subsequently pass into the systemic circulation. Some small chain triglycerides can bypass this system and enter the portal venous system directly.

Protein digestion begins in the stomach by the action of pepsin and acid. However, most protein hydrolysis occurs in the lumen of the jejunum by action of pancreatic proteases. These are secreted as inactive precursors. Chymotrypsin is converted to trypsin by the action of the small intestinal enzyme enterokinase. Activated trypsin further activates chymotrypsin and other proteases, such as carboxypeptidase. The products of protein hydrolysis are amino acids and oligopeptides. The latter are further hydrolysed to mono-, di- and tripeptides by brush border hydrolyases and are absorbed by specific membrane transporters. Di- and tripeptides undergo hydrolysis to amino acids in the cytoplasm of the enterocyte. Isolated protein maldigestion/malabsorption is extremely rare. It usually occurs in association with malabsorption of other macronutrients.

Fat malabsorption

Diseases of the pancreas and the small intestine are the usual causes of steatorrhoea in children. Chronic liver disease may cause steatorrhoea but this is in the setting of severe and obvious liver disease (such as the patient who is cirrhotic and jaundiced) and is not usually a diagnostic problem.

Steatorrhoea causes bulky stools and can lead to other nutritional deficits. Fat is responsible for approximately 40% of caloric intake in the Western diet. Thus, fat malabsorption can lead to failure to thrive due to an energy-deficient diet. Some vitamins are fat-soluble and require normal fat digestion for their absorption. These include A, D, E and K. Thus patients with steatorrhoea may also develop signs of fat-soluble vitamin deficiency, as described above. Essential fatty acids such as arachidonic acid are also malabsorbed in patients with pancreatic malabsorption. A scaling skin rash is one physical manifestation of essential fatty acid deficiency.

Pancreatic and intestinal diseases associated with fat malabsorption can also result in protein and carbohydrate maldigestion/malabsorption. Thus it is not uncommon to find a mixed picture of malabsorption. Protein maldigestion/malabsorption results in hypoproteinaemia. The main physical manifestations are growth failure, peripheral oedema and ascites.

Pancreatic disease

Cystic fibrosis
See also Chapter 14.6.

Cystic fibrosis:

- is the commonest cause of pancreatic malabsorption in the Caucasian population
- has an incidence in the population of approximately 1 per 2000
- is an inborn error in epithelial chloride secretion (cystic fibrosis transmembrane conductance regulator (CFTR)).

Organs affected include:

- gastrointestinal tract and liver
- sinopulmonary tract
- pancreas
- exocrine portion of the sweat glands
- vas deferens
- sweat duct (CFTR absorbs rather than secretes chloride in this organ).

Because of the fluid and salt transport defects, patients with cystic fibrosis produce more viscous secretions in lung, gut, pancreas and vas deferens, leading to:

- chronic suppurative lung disease
- nasal polyps
- pancreatic insufficiency
- intussusception
- meconium ileus and distal intestinal obstruction syndrome
- infertility
- elevated sweat sodium and chloride, which can lead to heat prostration in warmer climates.

Chronic liver disease will develop in 10–15% of children with cystic fibrosis.

Malabsorption in cystic fibrosis frequently results in malnutrition and there may be symptoms and signs of specific nutrient deficits such as hypoalbuminaemic oedema, night blindness due to vitamin A deficiency or skin rash due to essential fatty acid deficiency. Median life expectancy is 30 years, with death usually from respiratory failure or haemorrhage from portal hypertension and oesophageal varices.

Many mutations have been identified in the CFTR. Depending on what part of the channel the mutation affects, the phenotype can vary from mild to severe disease. Individuals with milder mutations have milder lung disease and do not usually have malabsorption, as pancreatic function is normal.

Newborn screening:

- can detect cystic fibrosis in the neonatal period
- involves measurement of immunoreactive trypsinogen and/or CFTR mutations
- is the commonest mode of presentation when it is performed.

In children with the severe phenotype who are missed by screening, or in countries where screening is not performed, presentation is usually in the first year with chronic diarrhoea and failure to thrive, with or without respiratory symptoms. In milder phenotypes, patients may not present until adult life with respiratory disease or infertility.

Diagnostic investigations for cystic fibrosis are:

- elevated sweat sodium and chloride ('sweat test') – simplest and cheapest
- CFTR mutation analysis.

Treatment is usually undertaken in a tertiary referral multidisciplinary clinic and involves:

- physiotherapy, inhalation therapy and antibiotics for chest disease
- pancreatic enzyme supplements and nutritional support
- specific therapy may be required for the other intestinal/liver complications.

Shwachman syndrome

The features of Shwachman syndrome are:

- agenesis of the pancreatic acinus
- short stature
- dysplasia of the metaphysis of the long bones
- cyclical neutropenia.

There is no specific diagnostic test; treatment includes pancreatic exocrine replacement and treatment of infections.

Chronic pancreatitis

Causes of chronic pancreatitis include:

- protein energy malnutrition
- hereditary pancreatitis (rare)
- idiopathic fibrosing pancreatitis (rare).

Small bowel disease

Coeliac disease (gluten enteropathy)

Coeliac disease is a disorder characterized by intestinal injury induced by the cereal protein gluten. Gluten is a glycoprotein found in wheat, barley and rye and, to a lesser extent, oats. In susceptible individuals, the ingestion of gluten induces a cell-mediated injury of the intestinal mucosa resulting in severe villous atrophy, crypt hyperplasia and infiltration of the epithelium with lymphocytes (intraepithelial lymphocytes). In Western countries, the incidence of coeliac disease in the general population may be as high as 1 in 70, although not all affected individuals develop the classical manifestations of coeliac disease.

Modes of presentation include:

- 'Classical' coeliac disease (Fig. 20.3.2)
  - between 9 and 18 months of age
  - anorexia, weight loss, abdominal distension and wasting

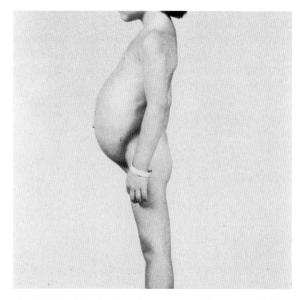

Fig. 20.3.2 Typical physical appearance of a young child with coeliac disease. Note the protuberant abdomen, buttock and shoulder girdle wasting and oedema of the lower limbs. Courtesy of Professor K. Gaskin.

- chronic diarrhoea with or without:
  - iron deficiency anaemia
  - hypoproteinaemic oedema
  - fat-soluble vitamin deficiency
- The older child with:
  - growth failure
  - chronic diarrhoea
  - iron deficiency
- Positive antibody screening (now the commonest form of assessment leading to diagnosis).

Examples of antibodies used to screen when there is suspicion of coeliac disease include:

- antigliadin
- anti endomysial
- antitissue transglutaminase antibodies.

Antiendomysial and antitissue transglutaminase antibodies have sensitivity and specificity of greater than 95%. However, it is important to note that these are screening tests only.

The following are important points in the approach to the diagnosis of coeliac disease in childhood:

- small bowel biopsy is mandatory for the diagnosis (Fig. 20.3.3)
- small bowel biopsy should be performed while the patient is on an unrestricted diet
- there is no place for an empirical trial of a gluten-free diet
- definitive diagnosis is important, as treatment is a lifelong gluten-free diet.

A second biopsy can be undertaken to establish that the intestine has returned to normal on a restricted diet. If there is doubt about the diagnosis, a subsequent gluten challenge with repeat biopsy can be undertaken.

Enterocyte defect
Abetalipoproteinaemia is a recessively inherited defect in chylomicron assembly. Patients develop steatorrhoea early in life with:

- fat-soluble vitamin deficiencies
- low serum cholesterol and triglycerides.

Small bowel biopsy reveals fat laden enterocytes.

Impaired lymphatic drainage
Obstructed lymphatic drainage prevents chylomicrons from migrating from the gut to the systemic circulation. The main cause is intestinal lymphangiectasia. This can lead to:

- fat malabsorption
- low serum cholesterol and triglycerides
- hypoproteinaemia and lymphopenia (loss of lymph into gut lumen)
- abnormal mucosal biopsy.

Other causes of reduced mucosal surface and reduced contact time
Miscellaneous inflammatory and surgical conditions can lead to loss of absorptive surface or reduced contact between chyme and the mucosa. Such conditions include:

- milk protein intolerance (severe)
- infections such as rotavirus infection
- severe immunodeficiency disorders
- autoimmune enteropathy
- short gut syndrome (surgical removal)
- motility disorders causing very rapid intestinal transit.

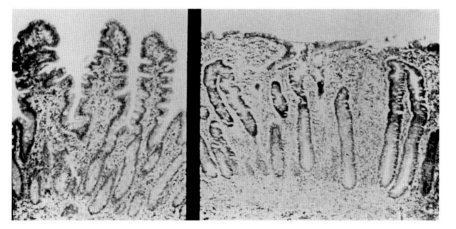

Fig. 20.3.3 Micrographs of normal intestine (left) demonstrating normal crypt villus structure, and coeliac disease (right) with marked crypt hyperplasia and villous atrophy.

Watery diarrhoea

Clinical example

George was 9 years old. He presented with a 6-month history of intermittent bloating, abdominal pain and diarrhoea up to 6–7 times per day. He had lost 1 kg in weight in the past 2 months. He reported that dairy products such as milk and ice-cream made his symptoms worse. He had no past history of significant illness. George was the oldest son of Greek migrants. His mother reported that she could not drink milk, as it made her feel sick.

On examination he was well looking. His weight was on the 50th percentile and his height was on the 10th percentile. There was no abdominal distension, organomegaly, signs of chronic liver disease or evidence of nutritional deficiency such as anaemia or peripheral oedema. Examination of his anus did not reveal any evidence of perianal disease.

Investigations included a normal full blood count, differential white cell count and ESR. C reactive protein was less than 1 g/l. Lactose breath hydrogen measurement following oral ingestion of 50 g of lactose increased 100 parts per million above baseline levels within 60 minutes of ingestion of lactose (normal rise 20 parts per million), indicating lactose intolerance.

George was diagnosed as having lactose intolerance. His history suggested ontogenic lactase deficiency. This was confirmed by small bowel biopsy, which demonstrated normal morphology, and disaccharidase measurement, which revealed very low lactase activity but normal sucrase and maltase activities. Treatment is a low-lactose diet.

Carbohydrate digestion and absorption

Dietary carbohydrates are primarily starch (polysaccharides, amylose and amylopectin), disaccharides (sucrose, in table sugar; lactose, in milk) and some monosaccharides such as fructose.

Starch polymers are large molecules composed of long chains of glucose. These chains are broken down by the action of salivary and pancreatic amylase, which release a disaccharide (amylose), trisaccharide (maltotriose) and a series of branched oligosaccharides (alpha limit dextrins). These molecules are further digested by the brush border enzymes, sucrase–isomaltase and glucoamylase, to the monosaccharide glucose.

The disaccharides sucrose and lactose are metabolized by disaccharidases on the intestinal brush border. Sucrase breaks sucrose down to glucose and fructose and lactase breaks down lactose into glucose and galactose. Glucose and galactose are absorbed by the enterocyte sodium–glucose cotransporter (SGLT), which absorbs the monosaccharides in an energy dependent fashion. Fructose is absorbed by facilitated diffusion (non-energy-dependent) by the transporter termed GLUT-5.

Carbohydrate malabsorption

The presence of non-absorbed osmotically active nutrients in the gut lumen results in osmotic retardation of water absorption, leading to watery diarrhoea. This is referred to as osmotic diarrhoea. Osmotically active compounds are usually low-molecular-weight compounds such as monosaccharides and disaccharides. Osmotic diarrhoea is usually due to maldigestion and/or malabsorption of carbohydrates but can be caused by the ingestion of laxatives such as sorbitol or $MgCl_2$. Unabsorbed carbohydrate present in the lumen of the large bowel is fermented to short chain fatty acids such as butyrate. This results in a highly acidic stool, which can cause perianal excoriation. The colon can absorb the anionic forms of these acids in exchange for bicarbonate, causing a mild hyperchloraemic acidosis.

While stating the obvious, it is important to appreciate that one cannot malabsorb a nutrient that has not been ingested. Thus it is useful to obtain a dietary history in patients suspected of osmotic diarrhoea. One needs to ascertain the nature of the carbohydrates being ingested, and in some instances the age of introduction of the carbohydrate, which can then be compared with the age of onset of symptoms. For example, the onset of osmotic diarrhoea commensurate with the introduction of fruit into the diet suggests the diagnosis of congenital sucrase–isomaltase deficiency.

Disaccharidase deficiencies and monosaccharide malabsorption

Congenital

Ontogenic lactase deficiency:

- occurs in most of the non-Caucasian population of the world
- is dominantly inherited
- is physiological (due to the disappearance of lactase)
- presents in late childhood.

Ingesting lactose causes diarrhoea, bloating, excessive flatus and weight loss. Treatment is a low-lactose diet.

Congenital sucrase–isomaltase deficiency is caused by inactivating mutations in the sucrase–isomaltase gene. These mutations:

- are recessively inherited
- lead to similar symptoms as for lactase deficiency with the ingestion of sucrose

- cause onset of symptoms at the time of weaning when fruit is introduced to the diet.

Treatment is a low-sucrose diet.

Congenital monosaccharide malabsorption refers to defective glucose/galactose malabsorption. Features are:

- mutations in SGLT1
- recessively inherited
- present in the neonatal period.

Treatment is substitution of fructose for glucose–galactose.

Acquired
Except for ontogenic lactase deficiency, acquired disorders are much more common than inherited deficiencies. Lactase is more susceptible to injury than sucrase.

Causes of disaccharidase deficiencies include:

- viral gastroenteritis
- coeliac disease
- chronic giardiasis
- milk protein enteropathy
- small bowel bacterial overgrowth syndrome
- immunodeficiency disorders
- autoimmune enteropathy.

Monosaccharide transporters are less susceptible to injury because, unlike disaccharidase enzymes, they are deeply embedded in the brush border membrane. However, severe enteropathies can occasionally result in monosaccharide malabsorption. Examples include:

- congential villous atrophy (which presents in newborns)
- severe postinfectious enteritis
- milk protein intolerance
- autoimmune enteropathy.

Monosaccharide malabsorption is life-threatening and requires a level of care found only in tertiary paediatric centres. The treatment is to remove t he offending carbohydrate from the diet and substitute an alternative. In acquired disorders, treatment may also be required for the primary mucosal disease.

Disorders of fluid and electrolyte transport

In the normal child approximately 5 litres (depending on size!) of fluid and electrolytes enters the upper gastrointestinal tract per day. One litre is ingested and the remaining volume is from normal secretions into the lumen. The majority of this fluid is absorbed before reaching the colon. Stool weights range from 75 to 150 g per day, of which approximately 75% is water. Small increases in stool water, as little as 30–40 ml/d are enough to produce diarrhoea.

Water is absorbed by osmosis through paracellular pathways in the mucosa. Electrolytes are absorbed by a variety of active transport or passive transport processes. Anions such as chloride and bicarbonate can be absorbed or actively secreted. This varies according to the region of small or large intestine. Regulation of gastrointestinal fluid and electrolyte transport is closely integrated by humoral and neural factors involved in fluid and electrolyte homeostasis. Abnormal fluid and electrolyte transport can be due to inherited defects in specific electrolyte transporters, but more commonly it is due to mucosal damage or inflammation.

Congenital
Congenital sodium diarrhoea and congenital chloride diarrhoea are rare inherited disorders of Na/H exchange and Cl/HCO exchange, respectively. They cause:

- diarrhoea in utero which results in polyhydramnios
- profuse diarrhoea, obvious from birth
- systemic electrolyte disturbances.

Acquired
Isolated water and salt malabsorption is very rare in childhood in the developed world. However, defective salt and water transport can contribute to diarrhoea in:

- disorders which damage or inflame the mucosa of small or large intestine
- bile salt malabsorption (bile acids irritate the colonic mucosa and act as potent stimulants of secretion).

Excessive salt and water loss in the stool may lead to dehydration and electrolyte disturbances. Treatment may require salt and water replacement in addition to treatment of the underlying disease.

Bloody diarrhoea

Chronic bloody diarrhoea is usually caused by inflammatory disorders of the colon such as:

- milk colitis in infants
- infections such as bacteria or parasites
- inflammatory bowel disease in older children.
  The two major forms are:
  - ulcerative colitis
  - Crohn disease.

Blood is not always obvious in the stool. However, the presence of leukocytes on stool microscopy (Fig. 20.3.4) indicates the presence of colitis.

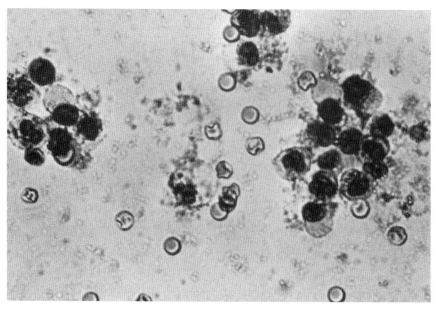

Fig. 20.3.4 Microscopic appearance of leukocytes in a stool smear. The large dark structures are polymorphonuclear leukocytes; the small round objects are red blood cells

Malabsorption of fluid and electrolytes by the inflamed colonic mucosa is a major factor contributing to diarrhoea. Malabsorption of nutrients is uncommon in milk colitis and inflammatory bowel disease. In contrast, excessive blood and protein loss from the inflamed intestinal mucosa can cause iron deficiency anaemia and hypoproteinaemic oedema. This is called protein-losing enteropathy.

Nutrient malabsorption with little or no diarrhoea

Children present with symptoms and signs of nutrient deficiency with little or no accompanying diarrhoea. This is often due to dietary insufficiency, e.g. inadequate iron intake, but sometimes it can be due to malabsorption of the specific nutrient.

Vitamin B$_{12}$

Vitamin B$_{12}$ is ingested in animal protein and is liberated by pepsin in the stomach. In the stomach, the free vitamin B$_{12}$ binds to a binding protein (R protein) which has greater affinity for the vitamin than intrinsic factor (carrier protein). Intrinsic factor is produced by epithelial cells in the gastric mucosa. The vitamin B$_{12}$–R protein complex moves to the duodenum where trypsin cleaves the complex, releasing free vitamin B$_{12}$, which then binds to intrinsic factor. The intrinsic factor–vitamin B$_{12}$ complex moves to

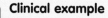

Clinical example

John was 9 months old. He presented with a 6-week history of poor weight gain, irritability and pallor. His mother was also concerned about his development. He was able to sit but could not pull himself to standing. His language had not progressed from babbling, which was in stark contrast to his older sibling, who had several single words at this age. John had a poor appetite but no diarrhoea. He was originally breastfed and his mother ingested a normal diet during pregnancy and lactation.

On examination, John was a pale irritable boy. He had moderate abdominal distension but no organomegaly. He could sit up unsupported but was mildly hypotonic and would not weight bear. There were no focal neurological signs.

Investigation results included: Hb of 65 g/l (normal 120–150) with a megaloblastic blood film, serum B$_{12}$ 50 pmol/l (normal 120–600) and red blood cell folate 350 nmol/l (normal 200–1000). A Shilling test revealed urinary excretion of ingested radioactive vitamin B$_{12}$ (after parenteral administration of a non-radioactive flushing dose of 1 mg vitamin B$_{12}$) of 1% (normal 8%), with no enhancement of urinary excretion with the addition of intrinsic factor.

John's Shilling test suggested a defect in the ileal vitamin B$_{12}$ transporter, as the test was abnormal and did not recover with the addition of intrinsic factor. His age of presentation and lack of prior intestinal surgery suggest a congenital defect. His symptoms and megaloblastic anaemia corrected with administration of parenteral vitamin B$_{12}$.

the ileum where it is absorbed into the enterocytes by carrier mediated transport. On entry into the enterocyte, vitamin B_{12} is separated from intrinsic factor and subsequently exits the enterocyte into the circulation bound to transcobalamin, which carries the vitamin to sites distant from the intestine.

Both congenital and acquired disorders can lead to vitamin B_{12} malabsorption.

Congenital disorders

Congenital defects in:

- ileal vitamin B_{12} transporter
- intrinsic factor
- transcobalamin

can lead to vitamin B_{12} malabsorption and deficiency. This usually presents in the second 6 months of life after the vitamin B_{12} accumulated during intrauterine life is exhausted.

Symptoms are due to megaloblastic anaemia and the central nervous system effects of deficiency. Babies born to vegan mothers (who ingest no animal product and thus can themselves be vitamin-B_{12}-deficient) and weaned on to a vegan diet can present with a similar picture, although usually in the first 6 months, as they are deficient from birth. Dietary history is important to differentiate between dietary deficiency and malabsorption.

Acquired disorders

Acquired disorders that lead to B_{12} malabsorption are:

- surgical resection of the ileum
- atrophic gastritis
- gastric surgery
- autoimmune pernicious anaemia (blocking antibodies to intrinsic factor)
- pancreatic insufficiency (failure to hydrolyse vitamin B_{12}–R protein)
- small bowel bacterial overgrowth (competition for vitamin B_{12} by bacteria).

Iron

Iron absorption occurs in the duodenum and proximal jejunum. An apical enterocyte carrier called the divalent metal cation transporter mediates uptake into the enterocyte. Iron is exported to the circulation via a basolateral process which has not yet been fully defined. In non-breastfed children, only 5–10% of dietary iron is absorbed. The efficiency of iron absorption is greater in breastfed infants because the iron carrier transferrin is present in breast milk. Iron absorption is finely regulated at the level of the enterocyte so that absorption does not exceed requirements. Excessive iron accumulation can lead to multiple organ damage (haemochromatosis).

Iron deficiency is the commonest nutritional deficiency in humans and is usually due to:

- inadequate dietary intake
- excessive gastrointestinal blood loss (bleeding lesions or inflammation).

Inherited defects in iron uptake mechanisms leading to iron deficiency not responsive to oral iron have been described but have not yet been delineated at the molecular or genetic level.

Acquired disorders
Iron deficiency anaemia can occasionally be the primary presenting feature of small intestinal disease such as:

- coeliac disease
- milk protein intolerance
- Crohn disease.

Miscellaneous nutrients

Calcium

Calcium absorption occurs in the duodenum and proximal jejunum and is largely under the regulation of vitamin D:

- hypocalcaemia can be associated with a wide variety of digestive disorders affecting intestinal calcium uptake or the biosynthesis and availability of vitamin D (Ch. 19.5)
- it commonly presents with tetany of the fingers and occasionally seizures.

Zinc

Zinc is absorbed by the small intestine. Zinc deficiency can be due to:

- low breast milk zinc levels in solely breastfed infants
- an inherited defect in zinc absorption (acrodermatitis enteropathica)
- conditions associated with steatorrhoea
- intestinal inflammatory disorders.

Zinc deficiency can cause diarrhoea but the most dramatic manifestation is an erythematous scaly rash on the finger tips and around the perineum and mouth (Fig. 20.3.1).

Magnesium

Magnesium is absorbed in the proximal small intestine. Magnesium malabsorption leading to deficiency can be:

- inherited (primary hypomagnesaemia)
- secondary to other conditions leading to malabsorption.

Hypomagnesaemia causes similar symptoms to calcium deficiency.

Isolated protein malabsorption

Enterokinase deficiency:

- is a very rare disorder
- presents with diarrhoea, growth failure and severe hypoproteinaemia.

Amino acids

Defective amino acid absorption due to mutations in amino acid transporters can occur in:

- Hartnup disease
- cystinuria
- lysinuric protein intolerance.

These defects are rare disorders affecting amino acid transport in gut and kidney and in other organs in the last case. They do not have gastrointestinal symptoms and there are no nutritional consequences because of compensatory absorptive mechanisms for peptide and amino acid absorption.

Summary of the diagnostic approach to suspected malabsorption

Initial clinical assessment and stool examination will suggest the diagnosis in most children. Stool microscopy and measurement of stool-reducing substances can be performed in the clinician's office and are readily available 'bedside' tests. If the diagnosis is not immediately obvious, the clinician will be in a position to investigate a limited differential list with simple and well directed diagnostic tests.

In patients with steatorrhoea the following will be useful but are not necessarily indicated for each patient:

- full blood count and differential white cell count
- serum triglycerides/cholesterol

- sweat test
- small bowel biopsy
- X-ray of long bones.

In patients with carbohydrate maldigestion/malabsorption the following might be indicated:

- breath hydrogen testing: challenge with the carbohydrate of interest (e.g. lactose)
- small bowel biopsy/mucosal disaccharidase activities
- occasionally with monosaccharide malabsorption
- inpatient dietary manipulation with close observation of stool output.

In patients with bloody diarrhoea (if stool cultures negative for pathogens) consider:

- gastroscopy and colonoscopy
- biopsy of small bowel and colon
- sometimes radiology looking for inflammatory bowel disease in jejunum/ileum.

Sometimes highly specialized investigations will be required to establish the diagnosis of some disorders:

- measurement of micronutrients such as iron, zinc and calcium for suspected deficiency
- Schilling test is required for the workup of vitamin B_{12} deficiency. Abnormally low urinary excretion of the ingested radioactive vitamin B_{12} indicates vitamin B_{12} malabsorption
- Schilling test can be used to assess patients with bile salt malabsorption due to ileal resection
- specialized breath tests are used in the workup of bacterial overgrowth syndrome
- immunoglobulins and B- and T-cell subset determination for detection of immunodeficiency disorders.

Practical points

- Diagnosis is not by exclusion
- A thorough history, physical examination and stool examination will suggest the diagnosis in most disorders
- simple well-directed investigations usually confirm the clinical diagnosis
- there is no such thing as a 'malabsorption workup'

Gastro-oesophageal reflux and *Helicobacter pylori* infection

G. Davidson

This chapter discusses gastro-ocsophageal reflux (GOR) a very common clinical problem in infants and children, and *Helicobacter pylori*, an infectious agent that colonizes the stomach in more than 50% of the world's population. *H. pylori* infection is acquired in early childhood but its disease manifestations usually do not occur until adulthood. It is also possible that there may be a relationship between the two, and this will be discussed.

Gastro-oesophageal reflux

Gastro-oesophageal reflux can be defined as the spontaneous or involuntary passage of gastric content into the oesophagus. The origin of the gastric content can vary and includes saliva, ingested food and fluid, gastric secretions and pancreatic or biliary secretions that have first been refluxed into the stomach (duodenogastric reflux). The difference between physiological reflux and gastro-oesophageal reflux disease (GORD) is often blurred by the anxiety engendered in parents, particularly first-time parents, by symptoms such as vomiting and irritability. Physiological reflux manifested by spilling, regurgitation and occasional vomiting occurs in more than 60% of healthy infants by 4 months of age, resolves in the majority by 12 months and rarely leads to GORD. Conservative management is important, particularly in an otherwise healthy infant, so as not to label the condition as a disease state when in fact it is not.

The symptoms of GORD in children aged 3–18 years ranges from 1.8–22% and are more refractory and associated with complications such as pain, vomiting, haematemesis, oesophagitis, stricture, growth failure, swallowing difficulties, respiratory symptoms and apnoea.

Pathophysiology (Table 20.4.1)

The main barrier to GOR is the pressure gradient across the lower oesophageal sphincter (LOS) which is formed by the intrinsic LOS (thickened smooth muscle of the lower oesophagus) and the extrinsic striated muscle of the crural diaphragm. Both components work together to generate LOS pressure, which can be measured by intraluminal manometry. The current understanding of LOS function suggests that a LOS pressure of 5–10 mmHg above intragastric pressure is sufficient to maintain an antireflux barrier. Sphincter incompetence as a pathological mechanism for GORD is extremely unlikely. Transient lower oesophageal sphincter relaxation (TLOSR) is the major mechanism responsible for GOR in infants, children and adults. A TLOSR is defined as an abrupt decrease in LOS pressure unrelated to swallowing or oesophageal body peristalsis. TLOSRs are significantly longer in duration than swallow-related sphincter relaxation and also have a lower nadir pressure. It is unclear at present whether GORD in children is characterized by either a higher rate of TLOSR or a greater incidence of GOR episodes during TLOSRs. Both have been noted in adults.

Abdominal straining

Abdominal straining, which occurs frequently in infants, probably exacerbates GOR only when there is simultaneous TLOSR, because both LOS tone and the crural diaphragm are inhibited. The neuroregulation of TLOSR is controlled via a vagovagal reflex. The afferent arm of the reflex is initiated by mechanoreceptors in the wall of the proximal stomach, and the efferent arm via a brain-stem pattern generator. The presynaptic neurotransmitter is acetylcholine and the postsynaptic neurotransmitter is nitric oxide. Feeding is a potent stimulus for TLOSRs, evidenced by the fact that, in children with GORD, TLOSRs increase from four per hour in the fasting state to eight per hour in the fed state.

Oesophageal body peristalsis

Assessment of oesophageal volume clearance is difficult because of the lack of defined motility criteria. Primary oesophageal body peristalsis following a swallow facilitates clearance. Secondary peristalsis

Table 20.4.1   Pathophysiological mechanisms of gastro-oesophageal reflux in infants, children and adolescents

- Delayed volume clearance
  - Impaired primary or secondary peristalsis
  - Reduced pressure wave amplitude
- Increased occurrence of GOR:
  - Transient LOS relaxation
  - Straining
  - LOS sphincter hypotonia
  - LOS pressure drift
- Delayed gastric emptying

Modified from Davidson GP, Omari TI 2001 Pathophysiological mechanisms of gastroesophageal reflux disease in children. Current Gastroenterology Reports 3: 257–262.

Table 20.4.2   Causes of regurgitation and vomiting in infants and children

Gastrointestinal tract
- Oesophagus
- Achalasia
- GOR
- Foreign body
- Congenital defects
- Stomach
- Pyloric stenosis
- Peptic ulcer disease/gastritis
- Duodenum
- Malrotation
- Duodenal ulcer
- Superior mesenteric artery syndrome
- Small intestine/colon
- Infectious diarrhoea
- Intussusception
- Soy cow's milk protein intolerance
- Meconium ileus
- Inflammatory bowel disease
- Appendicitis
- Other organs
- Hepatitis
- Gallbladder disease
- Pancreatitis

Extraintestinal disorders
- Generalized sepsis
- Rumination
- Intoxications
- Intracranial lesions, e.g. tumour, hydrocephalus
- Adrenal insufficiency
- Metabolic disorders

is initiated by an abrupt sustained increase in intra-oesophageal pressure that accompanies a reflux episode. The frequency of swallowing and type of pressure wave sequence propagated determine the effectiveness of volume clearance. While severe GORD with reflux oesophagitis is associated with a 30–50% decrease in pressure wave amplitude, this in itself may not impair bolus clearance.

Gastric emptying

The role of gastric emptying in the pathophysiology of GORD is not clear. Delayed gastric emptying could exacerbate GOR by prolonging gastric distension and increasing the frequency of TLOSRs. Studies attempting to correlate a delay in gastric emptying with acid GOR have been inconclusive. While the final answer to this question awaits the development of more sophisticated investigative techniques, there are some children at the severe end of the GORD spectrum in whom delayed gastric emptying may be an issue, especially those with neurological or respiratory disease.

Clinical manifestations

There are many causes of regurgitation and vomiting in infants and children, both within the gastrointestinal tract and external to it. The more common causes are outlined in Table 20.4.2.

Regurgitation can be defined as effortless spilling of gastric content that is usually benign. Vomiting, on the other hand, is a forceful emptying of gastric content that should always be explained. The content of the vomitus is important because of the likely cause, as is the age at onset. Bile staining implies small bowel obstruction and should be examined immediately. Blood staining implies ulceration or gastritis.

Table 20.4.3 highlights the symptoms suggestive of GORD in infants and children. Symptoms do vary according to age. Infants more frequently regurgitate but can also have reflux-related behaviours, which include apparent discomfort, yawning, stretching, stridor or mouthing. Irritability and crying as the sole manifestation of GOR should be assessed with caution as it has been shown recently that in children with proven GORD there was no association and no response to proton pump inhibitors. More serious complications include apnoea, acute life-threatening events and recurrent chest disease secondary to aspiration. Chronic cough without associated lung disease is unlikely to be reflux-related.

Older children, usually over the age of 4 years, can describe common symptoms such as heartburn, chest pain and a sick or sour taste in the mouth, implying refluxate. Some younger children may complain of a hot feeling in the chest, abdomen or throat.

Table 20.4.3 Symptoms suggestive of gastro-oesophageal reflux disease in infants and children

	Infants	Children
Vomiting		
Gastrointestinal	Feeding difficulties	Waterbrash
	Failure to thrive	Nausea
	Malnutrition	Dysphagia
	Cow's milk protein intolerance	
Respiratory	Cough, stridor	Chronic cough
	Cyanotic episodes	
	Apnoea	
	Acute life-threatening events	
Acid reflux		
Gastrointestinal	Apnoea, cyanotic episodes	Heartburn
	Colic, irritability	Oesophageal obstruction
	Sleep disturbance	Dysphagia, odynophagia
	Flexion patterns after feeds	Night waking
	Hiccoughs	Haematemesis
	Iron deficiency	
Respiratory	Apnoea, cyanotic episodes	
	Stridor	
Neurobehavioural	Sandifer syndrome	
	Seizure-like events (similar to infantile spasms)	

Table 20.4.4 Potential extraintestinal manifestations of gastro-oesophageal reflux disease

Pulmonary	Ear, nose and throat	Others
Asthma	Chronic cough	Dental erosions
Chronic bronchitis	Laryngitis	Non-cardiac chest pain
Bronchiectasis	Hoarseness	Sleep apnoea
Pulmonary fibrosis	Pharyngitis	
Pneumonia	Sinusitis	
	Vocal cord granuloma	
	Recurrent granuloma	

Adapted from Richter JE 2000 Extraesophageal manifestations of gastroesophageal reflux disease. An overview. American Journal of Gastroenterology 95: 51–53.

GORD is a common problem in neurologically impaired children and, while regurgitation is the most likely symptom, problems such as recurrent chest disease, feeding difficulties and food refusal, anaemia, weight loss and behavioural changes can all be manifestations of GORD.

There are many potential extra-oesophageal manifestations of GORD and these are highlighted in Table 20.4.4, and need to be considered as they may be the only presenting symptom or sign. Ear nose and throat manifestations such as otitis media, sinusitis and dental erosions are now being recognized

Eosinophilic oesophagitis

This condition has only been recognized in the past decade. GORD is distinguished from eosinophilic oesophagitis by the presence of eosinophils in the oesophageal mucosa. Their presence had previously been thought to be due to acid reflux. The density of eosinophils in the mucosa (<20 per high power field) defines the difference between these two conditions.

Dysphagia with solid food, epigastric pain, food impaction, and vomiting. Food allergy is present in more than 60% and at present the only proven effective therapy is strict avoidance of the offending allergen. Topical steroids seem capable of inducing remission if a food is not identified.

Diagnostic tests

Physiological GOR should be diagnosed on clinical grounds and diagnostic tests are not required. There is no single test for the diagnosis of GORD. If there are symptoms or signs of pathological reflux, such as pain, growth failure or respiratory symptoms, then

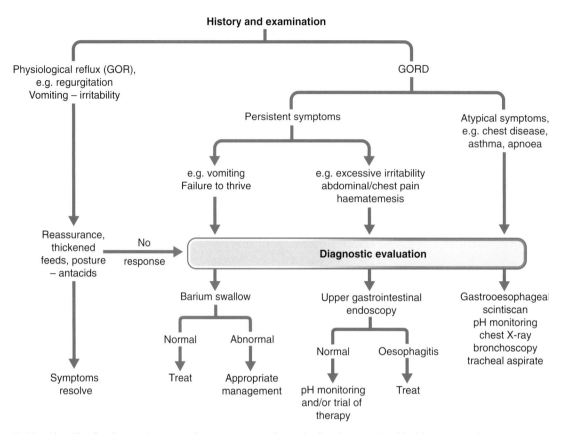

History and examination

Physiological reflux (GOR),
e.g. regurgitation
Vomiting – irritability

GORD

Persistent symptoms

Atypical symptoms,
e.g. chest disease,
asthma, apnoea

e.g. vomiting
Failure to thrive

e.g. excessive irritability
abdominal/chest pain
haematemesis

Reassurance,
thickened
feeds, posture
– antacids

No
response

Diagnostic evaluation

Barium swallow

Upper gastrointestinal
endoscopy

Gastrooesophageal
scintiscan
pH monitoring
chest X-ray
bronchoscopy
tracheal aspirate

Normal   Abnormal

Normal   Oesophagitis

Symptoms
resolve

Treat   Appropriate
management

pH monitoring
and/or trial of
therapy

Treat

Fig. 20.4.1 Algorithm for diagnostic approach to gastro-oesophageal reflux disease. (Modified from Youssef NN, Orenstein SR. Clinical Perspectives in Gastroenterology Jan/Feb 2001: 11–17.)

Table 20.4.5   Commonly used diagnostic tests for gastro-oesophageal reflux disease

- Barium oesophagram
- Radionuclide scintigraphy (milk scan)
- Upper gastrointestinal endoscopy and biopsies
- 24-hour intraoesophageal pH monitoring
- Oesophageal manometry

---

further testing is required (Fig. 20.4.1). The test used will depend on the age of the child, the types of test available and the type and severity of symptoms. The most commonly used tests are outlined in Table 20.4.5.

Barium oesophagram

Most commonly used but least sensitive for the diagnosis of GOR. Useful for detecting structural abnormalities such as pyloric stenosis, malrotation and strictures, and may be useful to assess swallowing function or aspiration. Most useful in children with persistent vomiting.

Radionuclide scintigraphy

Radioactive ^{99}Tc–sulphur colloid is added to an age-appropriate liquid meal and can be used as a direct measure of reflux. It has the benefit of measuring all refluxate. It can also be used to evaluate gastric emptying and to document aspiration due to reflux.

Upper gastrointestinal endoscopy and biopsies

Endoscopic examination of the upper gastrointestinal tract is indicated in GORD with complications such as chest or epigastric pain, heartburn, haematemesis or persistent unexplained iron deficiency.

Unlike in adult medicine, oesophageal biopsies form an important part of the diagnostic strategy in GORD in children. They can support a reflux aetiology and exclude other less common causes of oesophagitis, such as infections (cytomegalovirus, herpes simplex virus, candidiasis), Crohn disease or eosinophilic oesophagitis.

24-hour intraoesophageal pH monitoring

This provides an assessment of oesophageal acid exposure. In the majority of infants with GOR, this test is not required and it should only be carried out if it will alter diagnosis, treatment or outcome. Current indications for its use are outlined in Table 20.4.6.

This is not a simple test and should be carried out only in a specialist centre, as many factors need to be considered, including pretest preparation, insertion and positioning of the catheter medication, symptom assessment and analysis of results.

Oesophageal manometry and multichannel intraluminal impedance

Oesophageal manometry is rarely needed clinically in the diagnosis of GORD in children but may be useful prior to fundoplication in children with a suspected motility disorder. It also has a place in children with swallowing difficulties and in the diagnosis of achalasia.

Multichannel intraluminal impedance measures the flow of liquid or gas in the oesophagus and thus has an advantage over pH monitoring, which only recognizes fluid flow with a pH below 4. It is a relatively new technique and its role in clinical practice is still being evaluated. In young infants and children where regurgitation is often an issue it may have an important role, particularly in delineating an association between reflux and apnoea.

Diagnostic approach to gastro-oesophageal reflux disease

The diagnostic approach depends largely on the severity of symptoms and the presence or absence of complications. In the otherwise healthy infant whose main symptoms are vomiting or regurgitation, parental reassurance is all that is required.

If symptoms persist despite simple therapies such as posture and formula thickening, a barium oesophagram should be carried out to exclude an anatomical abnormality such as stricture, gastric outlet obstruction or malrotation.

Infants presenting with acid-reflux-related symptoms suggestive of oesophagitis require endoscopy and biopsies. In infants with atypical symptoms, the approach is more difficult but initially aspiration needs to be considered. Barium oesophagram, chest X-ray and a gastro-oesophageal scintiscan may provide support for this diagnosis. Referral to a respiratory physician may also be indicated for bronchoscopy and computed tomography (CT) scan. Ambulatory 24-hour pH monitoring may detect evidence of GOR but this does not prove the association. Presence of pepsin in a tracheal aspirate taken at bronchoscopy may be a useful adjunct but as yet remains unproven.

Clinical example

Sophie, the 7-month-old daughter of Greek parents, presented with a history of recurrent haematemesis, with bright and altered blood noted in regurgitated fluid and also dark stains on bibs and pillow. She was generally quite happy and thriving, although clinically a little pale. She did not have any evidence of abdominal tenderness.

In view of the recurrent bleeding and the possibility of oesophagitis or gastritis, an upper gastrointestinal endoscopy was carried out and this showed macroscopically ulcerative oesophagitis but normal stomach and duodenum. Sophie was treated with omeprazole 10 mg b.d. and after 4 weeks the bleeding had stopped clinically and the spilling had also decreased. A repeat endoscopy 8 weeks later showed macroscopic healing but still histological evidence of moderate oesophagitis. Sophie remained on omeprazole for a further 4 months but following a trial off therapy her symptoms recurred and she underwent a Nissen fundoplication. When reviewed at the age of 2 years she was well and asymptomatic.

Treatment approach (Table 20.4.7)

The ideal therapy would include the use of a drug that specifically reduces the frequency of TLOSRs, but this is currently not available.

Table 20.4.6   Current indications for 24-hour intraoesophageal pH monitoring

- Diagnose occult reflux in:
  - Unexplained recurrent pneumonia
  - Patients with bradycardia, apnoea
  - Non-gastrointestinal symptoms caused by reflux, such as stridor, laryngeal symptoms, atypical chest pain, severe irritability
- Assessment of adequacy of medical therapy in cases of severe intractable GORD

Table 20.4.7   Treatment approach to gastro-oesophageal reflux disease

- General
  - Reassurance
  - Positioning
  - Thickened feeds
- Drug therapy
  - Antacids
  - Proton pump inhibitors
- Continuous nasogastric feeds
- Surgery

General measures

These include reassurance, positioning and thickening feeds. The importance of reassurance in relation to the otherwise healthy infant cannot be overstated, It is important to avoid numerous dietary changes, unnecessary investigations and multiple drug therapies, which are often recommended by others or tried by parents.

Previously the only posture proven scientifically to be effective was the prone position, but this is no longer recommended because of the increased risk of sudden infant death syndrome (Ch. 3.10). New evidence suggests that laying children on their left side following a meal significantly reduces regurgitation and the frequency of TLSORs. Feed thickening has also been shown to reduce symptoms of regurgitation and vomiting by reducing the height the reflux-ate comes up the oesophagus. There are now commercially available infant formulas that contain thickening compounds. The risk is that the attenuation of overt symptoms may mask complications of GORD.

Prokinetic drugs

There are no prokinetic agents that have been shown to be beneficial and thus none can be recommended at present.

Acid suppression

This is effective in reduction of symptoms due to acid irritation of the oesophagus. Acid suppressing agents are:

• *antacids.* In infants with mild symptoms suggestive of heartburn such as irritability between feeds, a trial of 0.5–1 ml/kg per dose three to six times a day may be worthwhile. Antacids only have a brief duration of action and a response can be noted within several days; if not then do not persist
• *H_2-receptor antagonists.* Ranitidine has proved the most effective, in doses often higher than used in adults. It does have potentially serious adverse effects such as fulminant hepatic failure. The dose recommended is 3–4 mg/kg per dose three times a day
• *proton pump inhibitors.* These are the most potent acid-suppressing agents and are used if acid-related symptoms fail to respond to other therapies. They are superior to H_2-receptor antagonists in efficacy because of their ability to maintain intragastric pH above 4 for longer periods of time and to inhibit meal-stimulated acid secretion. They are often used as first-line treatment where more complete acid suppression is required, e.g. in chronic respiratory disease, neurologically disabled children and repaired

tracheo-oesophageal fistula. There is also a school of thought that the 'treat then test' principle should be used as the medication is so effective and if there is no response then GORD is less likely. Omeprazole has been most extensively studied in adults but there is very little paediatric data. It is used in doses ranging from 0.7–3.5 mg/kg once daily just before the first meal of the day. Twice-daily dosing may be indicated in certain situations such as severe oesophagitis, peptic stricture, persistent nocturnal reflux symptoms and extraoesophageal GORD.

Continuous feeding

Children with intractable vomiting and growth failure may respond to continuous nasogastric tube or gastrostomy feeding, with catch-up growth, and surgery may be avoided.

Surgery

The Nissen fundoplication is the most common surgical procedure and the indications are shown in Table 20.4.8. It can now be carried out laparoscopically in children. This may work, not by acting as a valve or increasing LOS pressure but by decreasing TLOSRs due to reduction in the fundal surface area. Fundal distension is an important trigger for TLOSRs. There is also evidence that it increases the nadir pressure in the LOS. This option needs very careful consideration in children because of the risk of complications and failure of the effectiveness of surgery.

Summary

It is important to realize that only a small percentage of children with GOR go on to develop GORD. For

---

Table 20.4.8 Indications for anti-reflux surgery in children

Absolute
• Acute life-threatening event or chronic lung disease due to aspiration
• Severely neurologically impaired children
• Continuing severe oesophagitis or oesophageal ulceration despite adequate therapy
• Oesophageal stricture secondary to GOR
• Intractable vomiting with growth failure secondary to GOR

Relative
• Persistent symptoms with oesophagitis or growth failure
• Severe asthma or respiratory disease unresponsive to therapy

most infants, symptoms resolve completely before 12 months of age. Unfortunately, many of these children are overdiagnosed and overtreated. It is equally important that those with continuing symptoms are recognized and treated effectively.

Practical points

- GOR in infants is usually a benign, self-limiting condition
- Reassurance and minor interventions, e.g. posture, feed thickening, often suffice
- GORD always requires further assessment and possibly investigation
- GORD has a number of extra-oesophageal manifestations that need to be considered
- Proton pump inhibitor therapy should be first-line therapy for treatment of GORD

Helicobacter pylori infection in children

Helicobacter pylori is the commonest bacterial pathogen in humans, infecting more than 50% of the world's population. This infection (initially called *Campylobacter pylori*), discovered by Warren and Marshall in Perth, Australia in 1982, ranks as one of the most important medical discoveries of the last century and resulted in them being awarded the Nobel Prize for medicine in 2005. They cultured the organism from the gastric antrum of adults with peptic ulcer disease. It meets Koch's postulates as a human pathogen causing chronic active gastritis. *H. pylori* as a paediatric infection is usually acquired in the first 2 years of life but the disease consequences rarely arise in childhood. A consensus conference sponsored by the Canadian Helicobacter Study Group met in 2005 to develop evidence-based guidelines for the approach to *H. pylori* infection in children.

Epidemiology

Socioeconomic differences are the most important predictor of *H. pylori* infection prevalence in any population group. In developed countries the prevalence in children seems to be declining but there is variability in the burden of infection with higher levels in immigrants and indigenous populations. This is particularly the case in aboriginal children, of whom at least 80% are infected. This is similar to developing countries, where up to 80% of children are infected by the age of 2 years, with a lower preva-

Table 20.4.9   Risk factors for *Helicobacter pylori* infection

- Poor socioeconomic status
- Household crowding
- Ethnicity
- Migration from high prevalence areas
- Infected parent, particularly mother
- Contaminated water

lence in breastfed infants. In developed countries, only 10% of all children are infected by the age of 10 years.

The route of transmission is probably similar to other enteric pathogens, being faecal–oral, oral–oral or gastric–oral. *H. pylori* has been detected in vomitus, saliva, faeces and on children's dummies, and also in contaminated water and food prepared with contaminated water. The housefly has also been implicated as a vector. The spread of infection within families is high, most probably from infected mother to child, although there is good evidence of sibling-to-sibling spread, especially in households with high infection rates in all family groups. Risk factors for *H. pylori* infection in children are shown in Table 20.4.9.

The natural history of *H. pylori* infection in childhood remains obscure. A significant finding has been spontaneous clearing and reacquisition of gastric infections in preschool children, as spontaneous eradication does not appear to occur in adults.

Helicobacter pylori-associated disease

General

In the past, gastric and duodenal ulcers in children have been described as primary or secondary. Secondary ulcers, which are more common in younger children (10 years) are caused by systemic stresses, such as trauma, burns, septic shock, corticosteroids or non-steroidal anti-inflammatory drugs. Primary ulcers, which usually occur in older children, give rise to symptoms similar to those in adults, with epigastric nocturnal abdominal pain and vomiting and often a positive family history of peptic ulceration. It is now clear in this latter group that the disease is due to *H. pylori* infection of gastric mucosa.

All *H. pylori* strains produce urease, which is thought to be important in the inflammatory reaction in the stomach and also in maintaining the ideal submucous environment for the organism. The urease reaction is also exploited in a number of diagnostic tests.

Table 20.4.10   Consequences of *Helicobacter pylori* infection

Gastrointestinal
- Gastritis
- Duodenal ulcer
- Gastric ulcer
- Gastric adenocarcinoma
- Gastric lymphoma and MALT lymphoma

Extragastric
- Gastro-oesophageal reflux
- Iron deficiency anaemia
- Short stature

Genetic analysis of *H. pylori* has demonstrated strains with certain virulence factors, e.g. vacuolating cytotoxin (Vac A), and cytotoxin-associated genes (*cagA, cagE*). In adult ulcer disease there is a correlation between *cagA* positivity and peptic ulcer, but this is less clear in children. A study has shown a strong correlation between disease severity and the *cagE* genotype in children.

Gastrointestinal infection (Table 20.4.10)

Gastritis

H. pylori colonization of gastric mucosa in children is almost always associated with gastritis, which resolves with eradication of the organism. Endoscopy can be negative and biopsy is essential for diagnosis, although on occasions nodular antral hyperplasia can be seen and is diagnostic of infection.

Duodenal ulcer

H. pylori gastritis is found in 90% of children with duodenal ulcers. Ulcers heal faster if anti-*H. pylori* therapy is given, compared with acid suppression alone. Importantly, ulcers do not recur if the infection is successfully eradicated.

Gastric ulcers

H. pylori infection as a cause of gastric ulcers is much less common in children than adults, probably reflecting the fact that the majority are secondary to systemic causes.

Gastric adenocarcinoma

The epidemiological association between *H. pylori* infection and gastric cancer has been judged by the World Health Organization to be sufficiently strong for it to classify *H. pylori* as the first bacterium to be a human carcinogen. *H.-pylori*-induced gastric cancer has not been reported in children.

Gastric lymphoma and MALT lymphoma

Seroepidemiological studies support an association between long-standing *H. pylori* infection and lymphoma and mucosa-associated lymphoid type (MALT) lymphomas. Eradication of *H. pylori* has resulted in regression of MALT lymphoma in some cases. Both these tumours are rare in children.

Recurrent abdominal pain

In adults, a link between non-ulcer dyspepsia (possibly the equivalent of recurrent abdominal pain in childhood) and *H. pylori* has been suggested by a recent meta-analysis of a large number of controlled studies. A comparable study in children with recurrent abdominal pain does not support an association. The major problem with studies in children is the lack of a standardized validated reproducible symptom assessment instrument. It is possible that there is a subset of children in whom *H.-pylori*-induced gastritis is responsible for recurrent abdominal pain, but more information is required. The current consensus is that recurrent abdominal pain of childhood is not an indication to test for *H. pylori* infection.

Extragastric disease

Gastro-oesophageal reflux

It is postulated that certain *H. pylori* strains cause decreased acid production and atrophic gastritis and that, with eradication of *H. pylori,* acid rebound occurs, causing GOR disease. This is still a controversial area in adults and there is very little supporting evidence in children.

Iron deficiency/growth stunting

Iron deficiency has been described in growth-retarded adolescents with *H. pylori* infection. Eradication of *H. pylori* infection corrected the deficiency and led to growth improvement. The current consensus is that testing for *H. pylori* infection should be considered in children with refractory iron deficiency anaemia where no other cause is found.

A large Australian study has shown a relationship between small-for-gestational-age infants and maternal *H. pylori* infection. Growth delay in height and weight has also been shown in *H.-pylori*-infected children but this may be biased by socioeconomic status.

Diagnostic tests (Table 20.4.11)

Endoscopy and biopsy is the only method that can provide evidence of disease activity such as gastritis or an ulcer. Urease testing of biopsy material gives indirect identification of infection

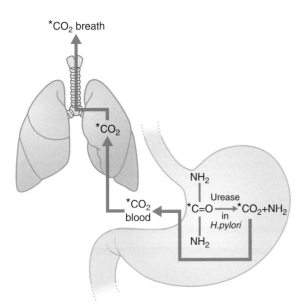

Fig. 20.4.2   The principle of the $^{13/14}$C-urea breath test.

Table 20.4.12   Those who should be tested for *Helicobacter pylori* infection
Yes • Endoscopic/radiologically proven gastric or duodenal ulcers • Confirmation of eradication of *H. pylori* infection
No • Recurrent abdominal pain without ulcer disease • Asymptomatic children • Children in families with history of gastric cancer of ulcer disease

Table 20.4.13   Who should be treated for *Helicobacter pylori* infection
• Histologically proven infection with gastrointestinal symptoms • Duodenal/gastric ulcers • Lymphoma • Atrophic gastritis with intestinal metaplasia

Table 20.4.11   Diagnostic tests for *Helicobacter pylori*
Endoscopic • Biopsy and histology • Rapid urease test • Bacterial culture
Indirect tests • Serum antibody (IgA, IgG) • Stool culture/stool antigen • Urea breath test

but has only a 50% positive predictive value in children.

The ^{13}C-urea breath test is currently the best non-invasive diagnostic test for *H. pylori* infection in children. It has a greater than 95% positive and negative predictive value. The principle of the test is outlined in Figure 20.4.2. Urea can be labelled with either radioactive ^{14}C or stable isotope ^{13}C. In children and women of childbearing age, ^{13}C-urea is recommended.

Serology, while commercially available, is frequently unreliable and cannot distinguish between past and present infection. Of the other non-invasive tests under trial the most promising is the use of a monoclonal antibody to detect *H. pylori* antigen in faeces.

The aim of testing is not to detect the presence of infection but to find the cause of clinical symptoms, and therefore the important question is who should be tested (Table 20.4.12).

Treatment

The discovery of *H. pylori* as the cause of primary peptic ulceration and gastric ulcers has changed their management, as eradication of the organism cures the disease and prevents recurrence. This has meant that peptic ulcer disease is now a curable condition eliminating the need for long-term or destructive surgery.

If endoscopy is indicated to investigate organic disease and *H. pylori* is found, the child should receive treatment (Table 20.4.13); however, if no ulcer is found the patient/parents should be informed that *H. pylori* eradication may not relieve the symptoms.

The traditional treatments do not eradicate *H. pylori* infection and current treatment in children advocates a combined regimen using two antibiotics and a proton pump inhibitor, based on adult treatment regimens. At present there is only one peer-reviewed controlled study of successful use of the triple therapy treatment regimen in children.

The currently recommended first-line treatment is a combination of a proton pump inhibitor, clarithromycin and amoxicillin twice daily for 7 days. Metronidazole can be substituted for either amoxicillin or clarithromycin but there is a high resistance to this drug and its use may lead to treatment failure. Failure of eradication leads to the use of second-line options,

Clinical example

A 10-year-old Vietnamese child, Than, who had resided in Australia since birth, presented with a long history of recurrent epigastric pain that woke him from his sleep at night. His appetite was described as poor. There was a family history of peptic ulcer disease. Examination reveals a thin child on the 3rd percentile for weight and 25th centile for height. Epigastric tenderness was present. The signs and symptoms suggested peptic ulcer disease and at endoscopy antral nodular hyperplastic gastritis was noted, as well as an ulcer in the first part of the duodenum. Histology showed evidence of *H. pylori* infection. Treatment with triple therapy (clarithromycin, amoxicillin and omeprazole) for 1 week led to resolution of symptoms within 4 weeks. 6 weeks after stopping therapy a ^{13}C-urea breath test was carried out and was negative, confirming eradication. At review 12 months later, Than was well and his height and weight were on the 25th percentile.

which usually include bismuth subsalicylate in a triple or quadruple therapy regimen.

The burden of illness and socioeconomic costs of *H.-pylori*-related illness is considerable, making the development of a prophylactic vaccine to prevent infection or a therapeutic vaccine to eliminate existing infection desirable, but to date no vaccine is available.

Liver diseases in childhood

D. Forbes

Compared with many other childhood problems, liver disease is infrequent beyond the newborn period; however, it is important because early recognition and diagnosis can be critical to the outcome of some disorders and because chronic liver disease carries a high burden of disability for children and their families.

The liver has a central role in:

- intermediary metabolism and homeostasis
- synthesis of proteins
- bile acid metabolism
- bilirubin metabolism (uptake, conjugation and excretion)
- detoxification reactions.

Liver disease disturbs these processes, resulting in one or typically more than one of the following problems:

- abnormalities of liver size and consistency (an enlarged or firm liver)
- jaundice
- hepatitis (jaundice and/or elevation of liver transaminases)
- metabolic dysfunction (such as hypoglycaemia)
- liver failure:
  - failure of synthetic function (bleeding or oedema)
  - failure of detoxification and waste elimination (encephalopathy)
- obstruction to blood flow through the portal system (portal hypertension).

Features that help us understand the nature of liver problems include:

- dark urine (excretion of bilirubin and urobilinogen in urine)
- pale stools (with biliary obstruction or severe impairment of hepatic function)
- tender liver (liver capsule stretched)
- hard liver (chronic liver disease with cirrhosis)
- splenic enlargement (in portal hypertension)
- bruising and bleeding (failure of synthesis of coagulant proteins)
- oedema and ascites (failure of albumin synthesis).

Liver size is proportional to body weight (rather than height) and increases during childhood. The physical findings of liver examination and the landmarks of the liver change during childhood. Liver size is best determined by percussing the upper border of the liver, usually at the fifth intercostal space in the midclavicular line anteriorly, gently palpating up from the right lower quadrant to determine the liver edge, and then measuring the 'span' between the upper and lower borders in the midclavicular line.

Overly firm palpation may make it difficult to palpate the liver edge. The normal liver span at different ages is shown in Table 20.5.1. During infancy the normal liver is usually palpable 2–4 cm below the costal margin. Variants in liver shape that make the liver seem enlarged include a prominent Riedel lobe, felt well below the right costal margin, and a prominent left lobe of liver felt in the epigastrium. The normal liver is soft and the surface is smooth and yielding. The consistency of the liver frequently changes when it is abnormal, generally becoming harder. It may also become tender.

The liver enlarges through the accumulation of additional tissue or fluid because of:

- inflammation
- infiltration
- storage
- congestion.

Causes of liver enlargement are shown in Table 20.5.2.

Jaundice

Jaundice occurs because of failure of the liver to excrete the bilirubin load owing to:

- excess bilirubin load due to haemolysis
- deficiency of conjugating enzymes
- obstruction of the biliary tree
- secretory defect
- damage to liver cells with leakage of bilirubin into the circulation.

Jaundice in infancy

Jaundice is very common in newborn infants. Up to 50% of Caucasian babies will become jaundiced and

Table 20.5.1 Liver span (cm) during childhood

Age	Mean	Range
Birth	5.5	4–7
1 year	6	5.5–7
2 years	6.5	6–8
3 years	7	6–9
4 years	7.5	6–9
5 years	8	6–9
12 years	9	7–11

Table 20.5.2 Causes of hepatomegaly

Inflammation
- Infectious hepatitis
- Autoimmune hepatitis
- Drug reactions

Infiltration
- Primary neoplastic liver cancers
- Primary non neoplastic liver cancers
- Secondary liver cancers: leukaemia, lymphoma, neuroblastoma

Storage
- Glycogen storage disorders
- Lipid storage disorders
- Steatohepatitis: obesity, steroids, diabetes mellitus, starvation

Vascular congestion
- Congestive heart failure
- Pericardial disease
- Hepatic vein thrombosis

even higher proportions of Asian babies may be jaundiced in the first weeks of life.

Physiological jaundice usually develops after the first 24 hours of life and by the fourth day of life and resolves by 10–14 days of age. It is discussed in Chapter 11.2. Jaundice requires further investigation when it:

- develops within the first 24 hours of life
- is severe
- is associated with fever or other symptoms of systemic illness
- persists beyond the first 2 weeks of life.

The first step is to differentiate between conjugated and unconjugated hyperbilirubinaemia by measuring the total bilirubin level and the conjugated fraction. Most newborn babies will have unconjugated hyperbilirubinaemia. Non-physiological causes of an elevation of unconjugated bilirubin include:

- breast milk jaundice
- haemolysis
- duodenal atresia
- pyloric stenosis
- hypothyroidism
- conjugating enzyme deficiency syndromes.

Breast milk jaundice

Elevation of the unconjugated bilirubin fraction associated with breastfeeding is common, occurring once in every 50–200 breastfed infants. It is a benign disorder recognized by:

- jaundice persisting beyond 2 weeks of life
- a thriving healthy baby
- no evidence of other disease
- resolution of jaundice with temporary interruption of breastfeeding.

Conjugated hyperbilirubinaemia

Conjugated hyperbilirubinaemia occurs with:

- obstruction to bile flow in intrahepatic or extrahepatic ducts, or with a scretory defect
- liver cell damage (hepatitis).

Conjugated hyperbilirubinaemia is considered to be present if more than 20% of the total bilirubin level is conjugated. It may develop soon after birth but may also manifest later in infancy after dietary change exposes a metabolic defect. This is an uncommon problem (1 in every 2500 infants) but an important syndrome to recognize. Every infant with jaundice persisting beyond the first 2 weeks of life should have the conjugated fraction of their bilirubin determined.

Bile duct obstruction and hepatitis are difficult to differentiate in this age group because of overlap of the disease processes and clinical features. It is useful, however, to attempt to differentiate these clinical syndromes and identify infants who have treatable disease: obstruction of the large ducts, infections and metabolic diseases. Early recognition and treatment is necessary for satisfactory outcome of these diseases. The clinical approach requires recognition of features suggesting neonatal hepatitis or bile duct obstruction (Table 20.5.3) and the application of general and then specific tests leading to a diagnosis.

Table 20.5.3 Clinical features of biliary obstruction and neonatal hepatitis syndromes

	Neonatal hepatitis	Biliary obstruction
Growth	Often impaired	Usually normal
Wellbeing	Often sickly	Usually well
Pale stools	Variable	Usual
Dysmorphic features	Common	May occur
Synthetic function	Often impaired	Preserved until late
Hypoglycaemia	Common	Uncommon

Table 20.5.4 Causes of conjugated hyperbilirubinaemia in infancy

Biliary obstruction syndromes in infancy
Surgical obstruction of large extrahepatic ducts
Choledochal cyst
Extrahepatic biliary atresia
Spontaneous perforation of the common bile duct
Paucity of intrahepatic ducts
• Alagille syndrome
• Non-syndromic paucity of intrahepatic ducts

Neonatal hepatitis syndromes in infancy
Infections
• Bacterial
    • Listeria
    • Escherichia coli
    • Syphilis
• Protozoan
    • Toxoplasmosis
• Viral
    • Cytomegalovirus
    • Rubella
    • Parvovirus
    • Herpesvirus
    • Coxsackie virus
    • Echovirus family
    • Hepatitis B virus

Metabolic disorders
Alpha–1-Antitrypsin deficiency
Cystic fibrosis
Carbohydrate metabolic defects
• Galactosaemia
• Fructosaemia
• Glycogen storage disorder type IV
Amino acid metabolic defects
• Tyrosinaemia
Lipid metabolic defects
• Cholesterol ester storage disease
• Wolman disease
• Gaucher disease
• Niemann–Pick disease
Disorders of bile acid metabolism

Endocrine disorders
Hypopituitarism
Hypothyroidism

Chromosomal disorders

Toxic disorders
Parenteral nutrition

Idiopathic neonatal hepatitis

Tests used to distinguish biliary obstruction from neonatal hepatitis include:

• ultrasound examination of the biliary tree to identify dilatation of extrahepatic ducts
• radioisotope (iminodiacetic acid) scanning to demonstrate bile flow or obstruction
• liver biopsy to identify characteristic features of hepatitis or cholestasis syndromes
• operative cholangiogram to document the patency of extrahepatic biliary structures.

Most of the identifiable causes of neonatal hepatitis syndrome and cholestatic syndromes are rare (Table 20.5.4). The major clinical issue is differentiation of idiopathic neonatal hepatitis from biliary atresia.

The outcome for neonatal hepatitis syndromes varies greatly, depending upon the specific cause. Idiopathic neonatal hepatitis and many infections have a good prognosis for spontaneous and complete recovery. Extrahepatic biliary atresia is potentially fatal and is treated surgically. Infants with biliary atresia who are treated within the first 60 days of life have a much greater potential for establishing bile flow and restoring liver function than infants who are treated after this time. Late treatment frequently results in biliary cirrhosis and progressive liver failure.

The acutely ill, jaundiced infant should be considered differently from infants with biliary duct obstruction or neonatal hepatitis syndromes, as these babies are likely to have a metabolic defect or an infection (Table 20.5.5). They usually have a conjugated hyperbilirubinaemia and often manifest all the features of liver failure: jaundice, bleeding, oedema and encephalopathy (drowsiness, irritability, deteriorating mental function, convulsions). They require urgent assessment and urgent treatment is frequently provided on the basis of a presumed diagnosis, pending confirmation by specific tests.

Table 20.5.5 The acutely ill jaundiced baby	
Infections	Metabolic disorders
E. coli bacteraemia	Mitochondrial disorders
Echovirus	Galactosaemia
Coxsackie virus	Alpha-1-antitrypsin deficiency
Cytomegalovirus	Organic acidaemias
Adenovirus	Tyrosinaemia
Herpes simplex virus	Urea cycle defects
Parvovirus	Fatty acid oxidation defect
	Reye syndrome
	Neonatal iron storage disorder

Table 20.5.6   Hepatitis in older children

Infections
- Hepatitis A
- Hepatitis B
- Hepatitis C
- Hepatitis D (Delta agent: coinfection with hepatitis B)
- Hepatitis E
- Hepatitis G
- Infectious mononucleosis/Epstein–Barr virus
- Cytomegalovirus
- Herpesvirus
- Parvovirus

Autoimmune disease
- Autoimmune hepatitis
- Sclerosing cholangitis

Metabolic disease
- Alpha -1-antitrypsin deficiency
- Hereditary fructose intolerance
- Tyrosinaemia
- Wilson disease
- Cystic fibrosis
- Reye syndrome

Clinical example

Sarah was a healthy, full-term, breastfed infant who was jaundiced at the third day of life but completely recovered by the eighth day of life. She gained weight normally. She again became jaundiced at 4 weeks of age. The jaundice increased and she started passing dark urine and had intermittent but increasingly pale stools. When seen at 7 weeks of age she looked healthy but was deeply jaundiced. Her liver was firm and had a span of 7 cm. Blood tests revealed that her bilirubin was elevated at 240 µmol/l with a conjugated fraction of 190 µmol/l, her alanine aminotransferase was 210 µmol/l, her gamma-glutamyl transpeptidase was 148 µmol/l and albumin 30 g/l. Ultrasound examination failed to visualize the gallbladder or the common bile duct. A liver biopsy demonstrated bilirubin plugs and bile duct proliferation, together with inflammation of the hepatic parenchyma. A radioisotope DESIDA scan showed no excretion.

These findings were suggestive of biliary atresia and so an operative cholangiogram was undertaken, with injection of contrast into the small atretic gallbladder found at laparotomy. This showed some dilatation of intrahepatic biliary ducts but no excretion of contrast via the common bile duct. The surgeon therefore proceeded to a portoenterostomy (Kasai procedure). Within a week of surgery Sarah had some pigmented stools, indicating that some biliary flow had been established.

Jaundice in older children

Jaundice occurs in children because of:

- hepatitis (liver cell damage)
- biliary duct obstruction.

Most older children who develop hepatitis have an infectious illness but drug toxicity, autoimmune and metabolic disorders may also be the cause (Table 20.5.6).

The apparent length of history of jaundice or other symptoms is often not a reliable guide to the duration of liver disease, and children with a short history may in fact have long-standing liver problems. Because of limited opportunities for the effective treatment of some liver disease it is very important to establish a diagnosis for all children who develop hepatitis.

Chronic liver disease should be suspected in any child who has persistent elevation of liver enzymes 3 months or more after a presumed acute infection. Hepatitis in these circumstances is likely to be associated with progressive liver damage.

Chronic liver disease is identified by clinical features in both history and examination:

History

- Recurrent hepatitis
- Prolonged jaundice
- Lethargy
- Anorexia
- Bruising
- Pruritus
- Poor growth.

Examination

- Jaundice
- Muscle wasting
- Poor growth
- Clubbing
- Spider naevi
- Oedema
- Hard liver

- Splenomegaly
- Ascites.

Evidence of liver fibrosis and cirrhosis may be documented on ultrasound and confirmed with liver biopsy and histology.

Infectious hepatitis

The clinical features of infectious hepatitis depend upon the age of the child as well as the specific infectious agent (Table 20.5.6). Younger children may remain asymptomatic despite evidence of significant hepatitis but as children get older they are more likely to have symptoms of nausea, lethargy, fever, vomiting and abdominal pain. A small proportion of children with hepatitis from any cause may develop rapidly progressive, severe hepatitis, known as fulminant hepatitis, which will result in some deaths.

In Australia and New Zealand most children with acute hepatitis will have an acute viral infection. Typically they are jaundiced, have a tender enlarged liver and variable splenic enlargement. They have elevation of their liver transaminase enzymes (alanine aminotransferase, aspartate aminotransferase) and gamma-glutamyl transpeptidase, and elevation of serum bilirubin (usually). The urine contains bilirubin and urobilinogen. The specific viral hepatitis agents are labeled A–G. Hepatitis A, hepatitis B and hepatitis C are numerically the most important agents.

Hepatitis A
The commonest cause of hepatitis, hepatitis A typically:

- is spread by orofaecal transmission
- has an incubation period of around 30 days
- causes an acute illness with malaise, nausea, vomiting and diarrhoea
- is associated with examination findings of jaundice, dark urine and an enlarged, tender liver.

Hepatitis A virus excretion in faeces occurs prior to the onset of jaundice. Complete recovery from infection is usual, although a small proportion of children will develop fulminant hepatitis. Immunity develops following infection, and may be stimulated in unexposed individuals with hepatitis A vaccine, an inactivated virus vaccine. Recent infection can be confirmed by a rise in antihepatitis A virus IgM antibody, and immunity by the presence of specific IgG antibodies.

Hepatitis B
Infection with hepatitis B virus (HBV) is a worldwide problem that is more frequent among socially disadvantaged groups and those Australian and New Zealand children who come from Pacific Island, Asian and African backgrounds. Transmission occurs via body fluids, and vertical transmission from mother to baby readily occurs. Hepatitis B infection can result in an acute hepatitis, but the majority of acute infections are asymptomatic.

HBV is a DNA-containing hepadnavirus with distinct surface and core proteins, which act as antigens. Infection is confirmed by the presence in serum of these antigens. Antibody to these proteins indicates development of immunity. HBV surface antigen (HBsAg) is the first antigen detectable after exposure and persists until recovery occurs. HBV e antigen (HBeAg) also appears in the acute phase of the infection and is indicative of a high viral load and high infectivity (up to 80% of infants of HBeAg-positive mothers will acquire hepatitis B infection). The response of the infected host is initially an anticore antibody (HbcAb), and subsequently HbeAb and HbsAb.

Chronic HBV infection is most likely to occur with perinatal infection. Infection is usually not recognized at the time, and may only be identified when the child is found to have elevated liver enzymes at a later date. It may also present as an arteritis, arthritis or nephritis. It carries increased risks of cirrhosis and hepatocellular carcinoma later in life.

Passive immunization against hepatitis B using immunoglobulin rich in antihepatitis B antibodies should be initiated at the time of exposure (such as at birth). Active immunization should be undertaken in all high-risk groups. HBV immunization is now part of routine immunization programmes in Australasia (Ch. 3.5).

Treatment of chronic HBV infection is indicated in children with persistent elevation of liver enzymes, carriage of HBV antigens and DNA, and who have biopsy evidence of chronic hepatitis. Treatment is undertaken with alpha-interferon or lamivudine for 4–6 months.

Clinical example

Claire was a 4-year-old girl who had been adopted in Korea in infancy. She was well but during a recent febrile illness she had had elevation of her transaminases and was subsequently found to be positive for HBsAg and HbeAg. Physical examination was normal. She was not immunized against hepatitis B in the newborn period. Claire was a chronic, asymptomatic carrier of hepatitis B, almost certainly infected in the perinatal period, and was at risk of chronic hepatitis and hepatocellular carcinoma. Hepatitis B can be transmitted to other children and so immunization of all children in her school group was encouraged.

Hepatitis C

The hepatitis C virus (HCV) is an RNA-containing virus that often causes chronic infection. Children acquire HCV infection via blood transfusions, from their mother at or around birth, and from a number of other as yet unknown sources. Children who have received multiple blood product infusions because of thalassaemia, cancer or haemophilia are at increased risk of HCV infection. Shared needles are an important source of infection in drug-using populations. A high proportion of infected children will develop chronic liver disease. HCV infection should be suspected in high-risk individuals who have elevated transaminases and can be confirmed by detection of HCV antibody or HCV RNA. Children who have progressive liver disease may be treated with alpha-interferon, although the best approach to treatment is still not known.

Infectious hepatitis and day-care and school attendance

Children with hepatitis A should be excluded from school until asymptomatic, or until at least 1 week after the onset of the jaundice, by which time they have typically stopped excreting the virus. Because of the highly infectious nature of hepatitis and the risks to other children, the school should be informed of the reason for the student's absence.

Chronic HBV carriage is associated with some risk of spread to other young children in day-care and kindergarten settings. Biting and scratching behaviour may increase this risk and should be actively discouraged. Despite this it is generally not considered appropriate to exclude children from school. It is important, however, to ensure that all children are immunized against hepatitis B.

Hepatitis C poses similar risks to hepatitis B but to date there is no vaccine to prevent transmission to non-infected individuals. Biting and scratching by young children should be discouraged but exclusion of chronic carriers from day care and school is generally not appropriate.

Drug-induced hepatitis

After infections, drug injury is the commonest cause of hepatitis. The most commonly incriminated agent is paracetamol. Initially the clinical syndrome is often indistinguishable from viral infections, and so drug toxicity should always be considered as a cause of hepatitis. Paracetamol liver toxicity is dose-related. Early recognition, estimation of plasma paracetamol levels to identify those at risk of liver failure and then initiation of treatment with *N*-acetyl cysteine are important in preventing acute liver failure. Chronic anticonvulsant therapy is often associated with abnormalities in transaminases.

These abnormalities do not carry the same risks as acute drug toxicity.

Steatohepatosis and steatohepatitis

A number of children, particularly adolescents, will be found to have abnormal liver enzymes (elevated alananine aminotransferase and aspartate aminotransferase) and sometimes an enlarged liver, but no evidence of other diseases associated with hepatitis, and with additional testing are found to have increased amounts of fat in their liver cells. Biopsy may show the presence of fat globules in liver cells (steatohepatosis) or the presence of intraheptaocyte fat globules and liver inflammation (steatohepatitis) This syndrome is known by several names, including non-alcoholic fatty liver disease (NAFLD) and non-alcoholic steatohepatosis (NASH). Children at especial risk of steatohepatosis and steatohepatitis are those who are obese, who have insulin-dependent diabetes and other metabolic diseases, the undernourished and those on long-term corticosteroid therapy. Steatohepatitis carries risks of progressive liver disease and so needs to be treated seriously. Treament strageies include weight reduction, improved diabetic control and high-dose vitamin E.

Autoimmune hepatitis

This can occur at any age, although it is more likely to occur in the older child and adolescent than in infancy, and can be confined to the liver or be part of a systemic autoimmune illness. It may be triggered by viral infections, or drugs, but commonly has no identifiable antecedents. Girls are affected more commonly than boys. The onset is frequently insidious and often comes to light with vague non-specific symptoms or with elevated liver enzymes. Different types can be identified, based upon the pattern of auto antibodies:

- type 1: antinuclear antibody and antismooth muscle antibody
- type 2: anti-liver–kidney microsomal antibody
- type 3: anti-soluble-liver-antigen antibody.

Treatment involves immunosuppression, usually with steroids and another immunomodulator, such as azathioprine or ciclosporin, often for prolonged periods of time. Liver transplantation is used in children with progressive, chronic liver disease that results in liver failure.

Alpha-1-antitrypsin deficiency

This disorder is commonly identified as a cause of neonatal hepatitis but may present at any stage of life

Clinical example

Elizabeth was an 8-year-old girl who was seen by her general practitioner because of recurrent hives. She was found to have elevated immunoglobulin concentrations and then elevation of her transaminases (alanine aminotransferase 320 U/l and aspartate aminotransferase 250 U/l). Screening for alpha-1-antitrypsin deficiency, Wilson disease, hepatitis B and C was negative, but she had elevated anti-liver–kidney microsomal antibody. A liver biopsy showed evidence of active inflammation with piecemeal necrosis, and fibrosis. A diagnosis of autoimmune hepatitis was made and Elizabeth was commenced on prednisolone, 2 mg/kg per day, which was tapered to a lower dose over 3 months. There was an initial decrease in the levels of transaminases but these rebounded when the steroid dose was decreased. Azathioprine 1 mg/kg per day was added to her therapy, with subsequent normalization of transaminases. A follow-up liver biopsy showed a marked decrease in the inflammatory infiltrate and no progression of fibrosis. Attempts at withdrawing therapy after 2 years resulted in an increase in liver transaminases.

Clinical example

Samuel became jaundiced at about 4 weeks of age. He was otherwise well, was breastfeeding and was gaining weight. His stools were normally pigmented but he had dark urine. His bilirubin was 180 μmol/1 with a conjugated fraction of 120 μmol/1. His alanine aminotransferase was 260 U/l. Because he had a conjugated hyperbilirubinaemia with evidence of hepatitis, Samuel had serological testing for viral infections (negative), urine testing for non-glucose reducing sugars (negative, making galactosaemia unlikely), a urine microscopy and culture, measurement of serum alpha-1-antitrypsin (very low) and Pi type (ZZ). An ultrasound of his biliary tree showed normal gallbladder and no evidence of duct dilatation. A liver biopsy revealed a giant cell hepatitis with accumulation of bilirubin plugs within bile ducts and accumulation of alpha-1-antitrypsin granules within the liver cells. A diagnosis of neonatal hepatitis due to alpha-1-antitrypsin deficiency was established. Samuel was commenced on ursodeoxycholic acid to promote bile flow, plus the fat-soluble vitamins A, E and K. His jaundice gradually cleared and he grew satisfactorily during early childhood, although his transaminases never returned to normal. In middle childhood he developed easy bruising and prolongation of his prothrombin time, hypoalbuminaemia, muscle wasting and oedema. He received a liver transplant when he was aged 8 years, and remains well, although on long-term immunosuppression.

with elevated liver enzymes, jaundice or advanced liver disease. It is due to a gene mutation that results in dysfunctional protease inhibitors in the liver and lung, leading to hepatitis and emphysema. Associated hepatitis eventually leads to cirrhosis.

Wilson disease

This disease arises as a result of failure of copper excretion into the bile, secondary to a defect in a transport protein. The disorder leads to accumulation of copper in the liver, brain, kidneys and bone. Liver disease typically becomes apparent in late childhood as hepatitis, portal hypertension or liver failure. Patients usually have so called Kayser–Fleischer rings of copper accumulation in the peripheral cornea by the time they manifest liver disease. Diagnosis is established by demonstrating low plasma caeruloplasmin (a copper-containing protein), increased urinary copper excretion and increased liver copper. Although this disorder is uncommon, recognition of Wilson disease is important because it is a treatable cause of chronic liver disease and will often present in childhood. Treatment is with a low-copper diet and long-term penicillamine, which increases the urinary excretion of copper.

Hepatitis, or liver inflammation, is typically recognized because of the development of jaundice but asymptomatic children may be found to have elevated liver enzymes and can have any of the disease processes discussed above.

It is important to remember that jaundice in older children may also be due to obstruction of biliary ducts due to:

- a choledochal cyst
- congenital abnormalities of the biliary tree
- gallstones
- parasites.

These children may have features of hepatitis but may also present with pale stools, dark urine and abdominal pain. They need assessment with liver biochemistry to determine whether they have elevation of alkaline phosphatase and gamma-glutamyl transpeptidase out of proportion to elevation of their transamimases. Imaging with ultrasound, computed tomography (CT) or magnetic resonance imaging (MRI) is necessary to define the anatomy of the biliary ducts.

Liver failure

This is the end result of failure of the metabolic and synthetic functions of the liver. The clinical features of liver failure are relatively common for all causes at different ages. Jaundice may not be seen until late in the course of liver failure. The earliest evidence is usually failing production of the vitamin-K-dependent clotting factors, resulting in prolongation of the prothrombin time and, eventually, easy bruising and bleeding. Oedema due to hypoalbuminaemia is generally a late feature of liver disease. Encephalopathy is a late effect of failure of elimination of neurotoxic factors. It may be subtle initially, with drowsiness and then later confusion and tremor.

Portal hypertension

Portal hypertension develops because of increased resistance to blood flow through the portal venous system, resulting in distension of the portal vasculature and oesophageal, gastric or perianal varices, splenic enlargement, neutropenia and thrombocytopenia. Portal hypertension occurs with liver disease with cirrhosis but, in up to one-third of cases, with portal vein obstruction in the absence of liver disease. These cases probably arise after neonatal portal venous thrombosis. Portal hypertension should be suspected in children with splenomegaly, especially if associated with thrombocytopenia, and in any child who has a significant haematemesis. Uncomplicated portal hypertension does not require intervention but children should be kept under surveillance and should avoid aspirin or other factors likely to increase the risk of bleeding. Underlying liver disease should be treated in those children who have cirrhosis.

Variceal haemorrhage is a medical emergency treated with resuscitation and then control of haemorrhage by decreasing portal blood flow with vasopressin or octreotide or with local compression. Endoscopic injection or banding of varices is frequently required to control bleeding and prevent further bleeding. Following variceal bleeding, consideration should be given to lowering portal blood pressure with propranolol or by the surgical creation of a 'shunt'.

Treatment

Treatment of chronic liver disease is aimed at anticipating and treating the complications of malnutrition and deficiency of energy and fat-soluble vitamins, failure of protein synthesis, portal hypertension and encephalopathy for as long as possible. Treatment involves the following components:

- Nutritional support
  - increased dietary energy with food and special supplements
  - supplementation with vitamins A, D, E and K
- Coagulopathy
  - vitamin K, fresh frozen plasma, cryoprecipitate, platelets
- Fluid balance
  - avoid excess sodium
  - diuretics such as spironolactone or furosemide
  - albumen infusions
- Encephalopathy
  - low-protein diet
  - lactulose
- Portal hypertension
  - monitoring of white blood cells and platelets
  - lowering of portal blood pressure with beta-blockers.

Liver transplantation is life-saving in children with acute or chronic, irreversible end-stage liver failure, evidenced by coagulopathy, hypoalbuminaemia, encephalopathy and variceal haemorrhage. The commonest problems leading to paediatric liver transplantation are biliary atresia, alpha-1-antitrypsin deficiency and other rarer metabolic disorders, chronic autoimmune hepatitis and fulminant hepatitis secondary to paracetamol toxicity, or infections. Three-quarters of children undergoing liver transplantation will survive at least 4 years, the majority leading healthy lives. They generally need to take immunosuppressive therapy for life.

> ### Practical points
>
> - It is normal to be able to palpate 2–4 cm of liver below the costal margin in infants
> - Any newborn with jaundice persisting beyond the first 2 weeks of age must have the conjugated bilirubin fraction measured
> - Newborn conjugated hyperbilirubinameia must be assessed as early as possible in life to ensure the best outcome
> - Acutely ill infants who are jaundiced are likely to have serious infections or metabolic disorders
> - It is important never to assume that abnormal liver biochemistry is due to infection; this may be the only chance for diagnosis of potentially treatable but life-threatening liver disease
> - Children with acute hepatitis A should be excluded from school until asymptomatic, while children with chronic carriage of hepatitis B or C rarely need to be excluded

PART 21

SKIN DISORDERS

Skin disorders in infancy and childhood

M. Rogers

Neonatal conditions

Pustular lesions in the neonate

There are many conditions that present in the neonatal period with pustules or pustule-like lesions. Some of these are benign and transient and of no systemic significance; however, many potentially serious infections can present with similar pustular lesions and it is vital to exclude infection in any pustular eruption in a neonate.

Sterile benign transient pustular disorders

Toxic erythema of the newborn
Widespread red macules each surmounted by a papule or pustule; onset in the first 2 days of life and disappear by the end of the first week.

Transient neonatal pustular dermatosis
Onset at birth of flaccid pustules that dry out in 48 hours, leaving postinflammatory hyperpigmentation in dark-skinned infants (Fig. 21.1.1).

Infantile acropustulosis
Crops of spontaneously resolving pustules on the hands and feet during the first few months of life.

Eosinophilic pustular folliculitis of the scalp
Recurrent groups of pustules on a red base on the scalp and later occasionally elsewhere.

Pustular miliaria or sweat duct occlusion rash
Short-lived pustules in among more typical red papules of miliaria, occurring particularly on the face, scalp and upper trunk.

Benign transient lesions simulating pustules

Milia
Firm, white papules especially on the face, which extrude in early weeks of life. These are sebaceous retention cysts.

Sebaceous hyperplasia
Yellow papules on the nose, resolve in early weeks.

Infective disorders presenting with pustules

- Staphylococcal infection
- Folliculitis
- Impetigo
- *Candida*
- Herpes simplex
- Varicella

Rare disorder presenting with pustules

Incontinentia pigmenti
A linear arrangement of pustules and blisters, particularly on the limbs; important associations are seizures and cataracts.

Blistering lesions in the neonate

There is some overlap between pustular and blistering disorders in the neonatal period. Several conditions may present with blisters and then become pustular.

Infections

- Herpes simplex
- Bullous impetigo
- Staphylococcal scalded skin syndrome
- Congenital syphilis

Other

- *Zinc deficiency.* Blistered and crusted lesions around mouth, nose and in napkin area
- *Epidermolysis bullosa.* Blistering in areas of trauma
- *Bullous ichthyosis.* Blisters on the base of a bright red skin; skin thickens in early days
- *Bullous mastocytosis.* Blisters on the background of a leathery skin with a peau d'orange appearance
- *Langerhans cell histiocytosis.* Vesicles and purpuric crusted lesions; a serious disease
- *Incontinentia pigmenti.* A linear arrangement of blisters

The red, scaly neonate or young infant

A number of important conditions can present with diffuse redness and variable scaliness in the neonate; affected infants often have major problems with

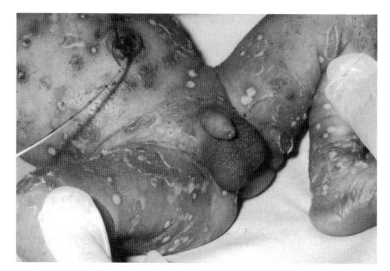

Fig. 21.1.1 Transient neonatal pustulosis.

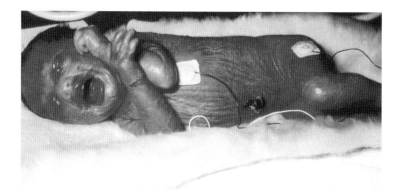

Fig. 21.1.2 Neonate with congenital ichthyosis covered in tight, thick, red membrane.

temperature regulation and fluid balance and may seriously fail to thrive:

• *Seborrhoeic dermatitis.* Dull red erythema with a greasy, yellow scale involving particularly the scalp, centrofacial area and all flexures. The scale may be absent in the flexures and secondary monilia is common. Usually asymptomatic and self-limiting after the early months of life. Responds to weak steroids and antimonilial agents

• *Atopic dermatitis.* Rarely this condition presents in very early infancy with a widespread red scaly and itchy rash. These patients often have food allergies and will go on to develop difficult long-term disease

• *Ichthyoses* (Fig. 21.1.2). Some of these conditions present with the child covered in a shiny, red membrane that peels off in the early weeks of life to leave a red scaly skin. Some commence with a dramatic degree of redness and scale, without the membrane

• *Immunodeficiencies.* Patients with severe combined immunodeficiency and other immunodeficiencies

may present with a widespread, red, scaly rash in the neonatal period or early infancy. In some cases this represents a congenital graft-versus-host disease

• *Staphylococcal scalded skin syndrome.* The child is initially bright red and then blisters appear, initially involving the face and flexures and then widespread; these subsequently dry up into scaly crusts.

Birthmarks and other naevoid conditions

Pigmented birthmarks

Congenital melanocytic naevi (Fig. 21.1.3)
These occur at birth as raised verrucous or lobulated lesions of varying shades of brown to black, sometimes with blue or pink components, with an irregular margin and often growing long dark hairs. They may become increasingly hairy with time. Giant-sized lesions may produce considerable redundancy of skin and often occur in a 'garment' distribution on the trunk and adjacent limbs. In patients with

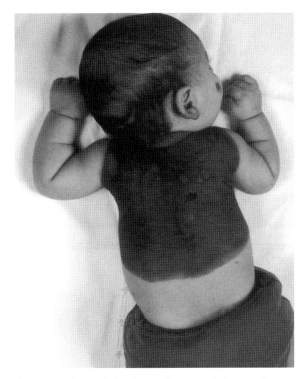

Fig. 21.1.3 Congenital melanocytic naevus in 'garment' distribution on the back.

large naevi an eruption of smaller, but essentially similar lesions may occur during the first few years of life. Malignancy in giant naevi can occur in childhood and the incidence over a lifetime is possibly of the order of 2%. In medium and small lesions the risk is much lower and any development of malignancy is always postpubertal. When large lesions occur over the axial spine, and in particular when multiple satellite lesions are present there is a risk of intracranial lesions, both melanocytic involving the meninges and structural in the posterior cranial fossa.

Naevoid pigmentary disorders
These are flat areas of hyper- or hypopigmented skin, obvious at or very soon after birth. They occur in characteristic patterns – either segmental, or whorled and streaky following the lines of Blaschko. These distributions are now recognized as genetic mosaic patterns. The lesions usually have rather irregular edges. Sometimes the condition is extensive, resembling a marble cake, and both hypo- and hyperpigmented lesions are present in the one individual. These lesions usually occur as isolated phenomena but may be associated, as part of certain mosaic phenotypes, with neurological, skeletal and other abnormalities. An important differential diagnosis is the café au lait spots of neurofibromatosis, which are rarely present at birth and which continue to increase in number.

Mongolian spot
These are flat, blue or slate-grey lesions with poorly defined margins. They may be single or multiple and occur particularly on the lumbosacral area, although the shoulders, upper back and occasionally other areas may be involved. They are found in over 80% of Oriental and black infants and in up to 10% of white infants, particularly those of Mediterranean origin. They usually fade considerably by puberty but may remain unaltered through life.

Naevus of Ota
This is a patchy blue-grey discoloration of the skin of the face, particularly on the cheek, periorbital area and brow. It is usually unilateral and often there is a similar pigmentation of the sclera of the ipsilateral eye. It is most common in Oriental individuals and is present at birth in over 50% of cases. It is a permanent lesion. Associated sensorineural deafness is reported, and very rarely these lesions may be complicated in adult life by development of malignant melanoma.

Epidermal naevi

Epidermal naevi (Fig. 21.1.4) arise from the basal layer of the embryonic epidermis, which gives rise to skin appendages as well as keratinocytes. These naevi have been conventionally classified, according to the tissue of origin, into keratinocytic, sebaceous and follicular types. They can involve any area of skin. They may be present at birth or appear in the first few years of life; they may simply grow with the patient or can extend well beyond their original distribution. On the scalp and face the naevi have a yellowish colour, due to prominent sebaceous glands, and present as a hairless, often linear plaque, usually flat in infancy and childhood and becoming verrucous at puberty.

Lesions elsewhere are usually dark brown but are occasionally paler than the normal skin. They occur as single or multiple warty plaques or lines, often arranged in a linear or swirled pattern. It is now clear that the linear and swirled patterns taken by epidermal naevi follow the lines of Blaschko and that all epidermal naevi can be explained on the basis of genetic mosaicism, with each type of naevus representing the cutaneous manifestation of a different mosaic phenotype. In most patients the naevus is the only detectable manifestation but in some patients there are associated abnormalities in other organ systems, particularly skeletal, neurological and ocular. Skeletal abnormalities occur particularly with naevi of keratinocytic type on the limbs, and

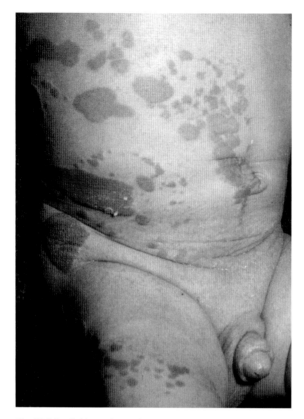

Fig. 21.1.4 Epidermal naevi.

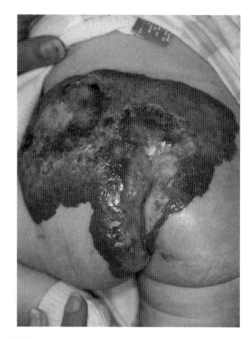

Fig. 21.1.5 Superficial haemangioma.

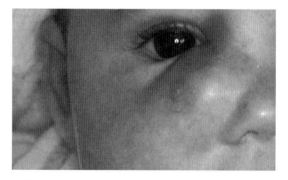

Fig. 21.1.6 Deep haemangioma presenting as bluish tumour.

neurological and ocular abnormalities with naevi of sebaceous type on the head.

Vascular birthmarks

These can be divided into:

- haemangiomas, which are proliferative vascular tumours
- vascular malformations, which represent fixed collections of dilated abnormal vessels.

Haemangiomas

Haemangiomas usually appear just after birth, undergo a fast growth phase and then, over a long period, tend to spontaneous resolution. It is now clear that haemangiomas, whether superficially or deeply located in the skin, have the same structure, being composed in the early stage of proliferating masses of endothelial cells with occasional lumina and later, as they resolve, of large endothelium-lined spaces. The terms capillary, cavernous and capillary–cavernous are misleading and should be abandoned in favour of the simple term haemangioma.

Superficial haemangiomas (Fig. 21.1.5). These usually appear in the first weeks of life as an area of pallor, followed by a telangiectatic patch. They then grow rapidly into a lobulated, well demarcated, bright red tumour. Rapid growth continues over the first 6 months of life; the growth rate then slows and further growth after 10 months is unusual. After a stationary phase, signs of involution begin, with the appearance of grey areas which enlarge and coalesce. The tumour becomes softer and less bulky and then disappears in 90% of cases by 9 years of age.

Deeper haemangiomas (Fig. 21.1.6). These may occur alone or beneath a superficial lesion (Fig. 21.1.7). The overlying skin is normal or bluish in colour. As they resolve, they soften and shrink and complete disappearance occurs in many cases.

Complications.
- Incomplete resolution – redundant tissue, residual telangiectasia, scarring following ulceration

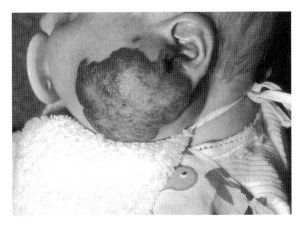

Fig. 21.1.7 Combined superficial and deep haemangioma.

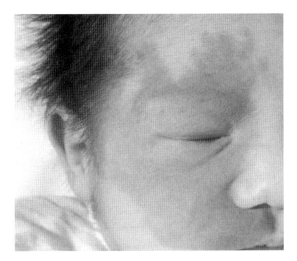

Fig. 21.1.8 Capillary malformation on the face, involving the brow, which suggests the possibility of the Sturge–Weber syndrome.

• Ulceration – full-thickness tissue loss on 'edge structures' (lip, lid, ala), inevitable scarring, cicatricial ectropion from scarring of eyelids, cicatricial alopecia
• Obstruction – of eye, producing amblyopia, of nose, leading to difficulty in breathing during feeding, of lip, leading to problems with sucking, of larynx (a 'beard' distribution haemangioma is a marker for possible laryngeal involvement).

Management. Simple observation and reassurance while awaiting natural resolution is the ideal approach for most haemangiomas. Indications for active intervention are an alarming growth rate, threatening ulceration in areas where serious complications could ensue, interference with vital structures and severe bleeding. Oral corticosteroids will slow the growth of potentially dangerous or cosmetically serious lesions.

Vascular malformations

These are collections of dilated abnormal vessels divided according to the vessels of origin. All vascular malformations are present at birth and grow only in proportion to the growth of the child. They show no tendency to involution.

The most appropriate terminology refers to the component vessels and many outdated terms (in brackets below) can be abandoned:

• *Capillary malformation* (port wine stain, Fig. 21.1.8) – flat purple stain, most commonly on the face but may occur anywhere
• *Venous malformation* (varix) – bluish tumour, empties with pressure and when elevated; fills when dependent; phleboliths may develop within it
• *Lymphatic malformation* (lymphangioma, cystic hygroma) – macrocystic deep lesions present as skin-coloured tumours, often with bruising; superficial microcystic lesions present as groups of haemorrhagic vesicles or warty lesions
• *Arteriovenous malformation* – skin-coloured lump that may expand, become painful and bleed at puberty
• *Other mixed malformations.*

Moles (acquired melanocytic naevi)

These usually first appear after the age of 1 year and increase in number throughout childhood. They

Clinical example

Harriet was born with a blanched area of skin bilaterally on the lower face, extending under the chin. A week later there was a tracery of telangiectases and over the subsequent 4 weeks bright red raised dots appeared in the area, gradually coalescing. When the baby was 5 weeks old her mother, Jane, noticed that Harriet had become very noisy when she was feeding. A general practitioner reassured Jane that this was probably due to 'a floppy larynx'. The child was referred to a dermatologist to discuss the management of the facial haemangioma. An urgent appointment was obtained and the child was 6 weeks old when it came up. By this time breathing was noisy whether or not Harriet was feeding. The dermatologist recognized this as stridor and arranged a lateral airways X-ray, which demonstrated narrowing in the subglottic area. An urgent endoscopy was arranged and this confirmed subglottic haemangioma. The infant was admitted to hospital and observed carefully. High-dose oral steroids were commenced and after 5 days the stridor had almost disappeared. The steroid treatment was continued over a 5-month period, in gradually reducing doses and Harriet remained free of respiratory symptoms.

commence as brown or black macules, some of which become raised and enlarge laterally as they develop. They are usually of uniform colour and well circumscribed. The risk of melanoma arising from acquired melanocytic naevi is very low (less than 0.1%); melanoma almost never occurs in childhood so their prophylactic removal in young patients is not justified.

Halo naevi

A depigmented halo may occur around a melanocytic naevus; the lesion may appear inflamed and often disappears, leaving a white spot, which may eventually repigment. This is a completely benign change.

Dysplastic or atypical naevi

A subtype of acquired melanocytic naevi with characteristic clinicopathological features and a marker for an increased risk of developing malignant melanoma. They differ from more typical moles by being larger (more than 5 mm diameter), having irregular and indistinct margins and irregular tan brown coloration, often with an erythematous component. They are predominantly macular, sometimes with a central elevated portion. They may appear in childhood as small, typical-appearing naevi which after puberty develop the atypical features. Characteristic dysplastic naevi may appear on the scalp in childhood. The final confirmation is based on the finding of some or all of a constellation of histopathological features. Patients with multiple dysplastic naevi should be observed frequently and monitored with serial photography. Any such naevus showing significant alteration should be removed immediately.

Cutaneous infections and infestations

Mollusca contagiosa

This is a poxvirus infection that is rare under 1 year of age and occurs particularly in the 2–5-year age group. The spread of lesions is enhanced in warm water and outbreaks occur among children who swim together or share baths or spas. Further spread of mollusca in the individual is also encouraged by being in warm water.

Clinical features

• Typical lesions are spherical and pearly white with a central umbilication, but they may vary from tiny, 1 mm papules to large nodules over 1 cm in diameter. They occur on any part of the skin surface, with common sites being the axillae and sides of the trunk, the lower abdomen and the anogenital area. Rarely they occur on the eyelids, where they may cause conjunctivitis and punctate keratitis
• A secondary eczema often occurs around lesions, particularly in atopic children
• Secondary bacterial infection may occur, producing crusting, redness and pus formation. However, these same changes may be seen during spontaneous resolution, which occurs in most within several months, leaving normal skin or small, varicella-like scars

Management

Each lesion lasts for only weeks and, if the child is kept out of heated pools and spas and has showers rather than baths at home, the proliferation is curbed and the number of lesions usually decreases quickly. If these measures are rigidly adhered to, treatment is rarely required:

• mollusca are surprisingly resistant to chemical therapies
• the most definitive treatment is deroofing of the lesion with a large cutting-edged needle and wiping out the contents
• with multiple small lesions in a young child, spontaneous resolution should be awaited but, if the lesions are troublesome because of their site, surrounding eczema or frequent secondary infection, removal under nitrous oxide sedation may be considered.

Warts

These are benign tumours caused by infection with a variety of papilloma viruses of the papova group:

• the common wart (verruca vulgaris) occurs particularly on hands, knees and elbows
• plane or flat warts, 1–3 mm, pink or brown, barely raised papules, occur on the face and often spread along scratch marks or cuts
• plantar warts occur particularly over pressure points on the soles and can be differentiated from calluses by a loss of skin markings over the skin surface
• warts at mucocutaneous junctions often have a filiform or fronded appearance
• anogenital warts may be acquired from maternal infection during delivery but their presence should always raise the suspicion of sexual abuse

Management

Various forms of treatment are available; they depend on the area, the type of wart and the age of the patient. Because spontaneous disappearance is common, aggressive treatment is often inappropriate. Treatments include:

- keratolytic wart paints (e.g. salicylic acid, lactic acid and collodion) – for common warts and plantar warts
- retinoic acid preparations – for facial plane warts
- podophyllotoxin and imiquimod – for anogenital warts, used under strict supervision
- a 20% formalin solution – for plantar warts, combined with serial paring
- cautery or diathermy – useful for lesions on the lips or anogenital area but elsewhere recurrence is fairly frequent following their use and there is also a risk of producing a painful scar, particularly over the joints of digits or on the palms or soles
- liquid nitrogen cryotherapy – a successful method of dealing with common warts that is useful for older children.
- oral cimetidine – has recently been demonstrated to be a useful treatment in some cases of multiple refractory warts.

Dermatological presentations of herpes simplex

Herpes simplex virus (HSV) infections are extremely common in children, and serological studies confirm that more than 90% of the population have been infected by the time of reaching adulthood. The commonest type is HSV1, although HSV2 is more important in adulthood, being the cause of genital herpes. Several distinct presentations are recognized in childhood.

Intrauterine herpes simplex

- Cutaneous lesions include blisters and erosions, sometimes in a dermatomal distribution, and irregular, often linear scars
- Other features are microcephaly, short digits, cardiac abnormalities and a variety of ocular abnormalities

Neonatal herpes simplex

- The skin lesions are grouped blisters, localized initially on the presenting part, usually the head, with the onset usually between the fourth and eighth days of life. The eruption may become widespread, with individual lesions a few millimetres across coalescing to produce large erosions
- A rapid immunofluorescence test on material from the blister base enables a diagnosis within a few hours
- Assess immediately for the presence of and extent of other organ involvement, of which the most potentially devastating is neurological
- Immediate treatment with intravenous aciclovir is indicated.

Primary herpetic gingivostomatitis

The child is systemically unwell with a high fever and there is severe swelling, erosion and bleeding of the gums and the anterior part of the buccal mucosa. Spread to the lips and the facial skin often occurs. There may be considerable soft tissue swelling and prominent lymphadenopathy. See also Chapter 14.1.

Primary cutaneous herpes simplex

- Can occur anywhere on the body, depending on the source of infection; painful grouped blisters or pustules on an erythematous base that soon break to produce erosions or crusted lesions
- Often there is local swelling and regional lymphadenopathy and the child may be febrile
- When a primary lesion occurs on the thick skin of a finger, the blisters do not break easily and intact, grouped pustules last for several days
- When primary herpes simplex occurs in the napkin area it presents as a severe erosive napkin rash. This is usually contracted from a herpes lesion on the lip of a carer, directly or via the hands, but occasionally occurs as a result of sexual abuse.

Recurrent cutaneous herpes simplex

- Recurrent herpes simplex of the face, particularly around the lips (herpes labialis), is common in childhood. As in adults, various factors, including fever and sun exposure, may reactivate the virus
- Recurrent herpes on a finger, presenting as long-lasting intact pustules (Fig. 21.1.9), is often mistaken for a recurrent bacterial infection.

Disseminated herpes simplex (eczema herpeticum)

This occurs as a complication of atopic eczema and in immunosuppressed patients (Fig. 21.1.10). It may originate from a primary or recurrent infection or from external reinfection. Spread is both on the surface of the skin and also by haematogenous dissemination. The lesions are vesicles or pustules 2–4 mm across, which may spread with alarming rapidity and have a tendency to coalescence to produce geographical-shaped erosions with scalloped edges. If there are more than very few lesions the patient should be hospitalized. Secondary bacterial infection should be treated with oral antibiotics and saline or tap water packs used to relieve discomfort and dry out the lesions. In severe cases, systemic aciclovir is indicated.

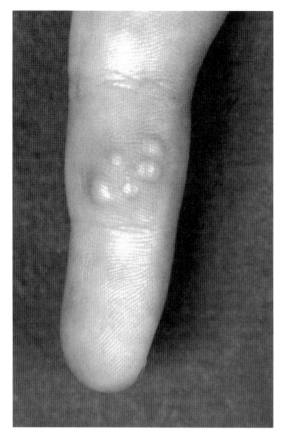

Fig. 21.1.9 Herpes simplex on a finger, presenting as intact pustules.

Indolent ulceration in the immunosuppressed patient

An unusual presentation of herpes simplex in immunosuppressed patients is as a chronic, slowly growing ulcer, often with rather overhanging edges. The outline is usually irregular, reminiscent of the geographical shapes produced by coalescing lesions in the more typical forms of herpes simplex. It requires systemic antiviral therapy.

Impetigo

Impetigo is a bacterial infection caused by *Staphylococcus aureus*, group A streptococcus or a combination of these organisms; it occurs in two forms, bullous and non-bullous (or crusted).

Clinical features

• Bullous impetigo (Fig. 21.1.11) is always due to staphylococci. Blisters arise on previously normal skin and increase rapidly in size and number, soon rupturing to produce superficial erosions with a

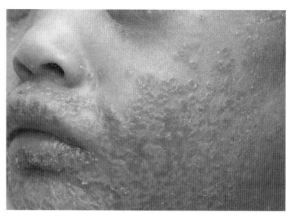

Fig. 21.1.10 Disseminated herpes simplex in a child with atopic dermatitis.

peripheral brown crust. The erosions continue to expand, sometimes clearing centrally to produce annular lesions.

• Non-bullous impetigo may be due to either organism or to a combination. The lesions begin with a small, transient vesicle on an erythematous base. The serum exuding from the ruptured vesicle produces a thick soft yellow crust, below which there is a moist superficial erosion

• Impetigo is often superimposed on other skin diseases such as insect bites, scabies, pediculosis and atopic eczema

• Staphylococcal impetigo does not scar but deep streptococcal lesions may

• Postinflammatory pigmentation can occur, particularly in dark-skinned patients.

Management

• Saline bathing may be used to dry out the lesions
• A swab for culture and sensitivity testing should always be taken
• Topical mupirocin may be successful for localized early disease
• In general, oral antibiotics should be used. Because of the rarity in most areas of pure streptococcal impetigo, a penicillinase-resistant penicillin (e.g. flucloxacillin or Augmentin (amoxicillin plus clavulanic acid)) or erythromycin are the treatments of choice while awaiting culture results
• If a group A streptococcus is isolated the patient should be treated with penicillin and watched for 8 weeks for signs of glomerulonephritis.

Staphylococcal scalded skin syndrome

Staphylococcal scalded skin syndrome (Fig. 21.1.12) is a widespread blistering disease caused by the

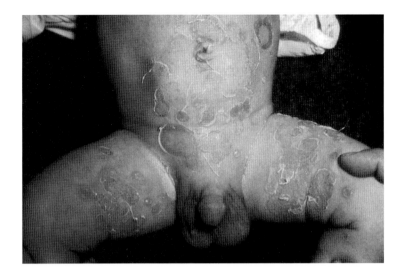

Fig. 21.1.11 Bullous impetigo in a neonate.

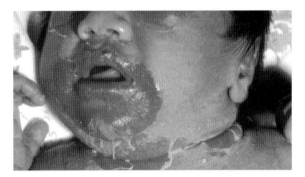

Fig. 21.1.12 Staphylococcal scalded skin syndrome in a neonate.

epidermolytic toxin produced by certain strains of *Staphylococcus aureus*, most often of phage group 2, types 70/71 or 51 but occasionally of phage group 1. This toxin produces a superficial splitting of the skin, with the level of split being high in the epidermis. Clinical disease occurs when there is sufficient toxin load produced from an infection with these organisms.

Clinical features

• The commonest sites of infection are the umbilicus (in neonates), the nose, nasopharynx or throat, the conjunctiva and deep wounds
• The condition commences with a macular erythema, initially on the face and in the major flexures and then becoming generalized. The skin is exquisitely tender and the child draws back from contact. After 2 days flaccid bullae develop and the skin wrinkles and shears off. The exfoliation is most marked

in the groin, neck fold and around the mouth and may involve the entire body surface, but mucosae remain uninvolved
• The child is usually febrile but, because of the superficial level of the split, fluid loss is rarely significant. The erosions crust and dry and heal with desquamation over the next 4–8 days leaving no sequelae

Clinical example

At the age of 13 months Oscar developed conjunctivitis. Oral amoxicillin was prescribed by his GP. 4 days after commencement of this Oscar developed a red, macular rash on his face and in the groin and axillary areas. Oscar was febrile and irritable and screamed when his mother tried to pick him up. The rash was diagnosed as a drug reaction and the antibiotic was ceased. The red rash continued to spread and flaccid blisters appeared in the groin, with the skin lifting off easily. A Gram stain from the blistered groin skin demonstrated no organisms. By this time the result from the conjunctival swab had returned, demonstrating *Staphylococcus aureus* insensitive to penicillin but sensitive to flucloxacillin, which was immediately commenced. The rash worsened over the next 12 hours, with sheeting off of skin all over the body, most marked around mouth and in axilla, groin and neck fold. The child was brought to a paediatric emergency department, where a diagnosis of staphylococcal scalded skin syndrome was made and intravenous flucloxacillin was started. Over the next 4 days the redness settled, the blisters dried out and Oscar became comfortable and cheerful. He was discharged on oral flucloxacillin for a further 4 days.

• Cultures from skin and blister fluid are usually negative. Cultures should be obtained from any area of obvious infection but, if none is apparent, from nasopharynx and throat.

Management

• Nurse the child naked on a non-stick material and handle as little as possible
• Avoid topical agents in the early stages
• A penicillinase-resistant penicillin (e.g. flucloxacillin or Augmentin (amoxicillin plus clavulanic acid)) is the treatment of choice and is usually given intravenously
• Analgesia is often necessary in the early stages
• Emollients are useful once the skin dries and desquamation commences

Boils (furuncles)

Boils are cutaneous abscesses, centred on hair follicles, caused by certain species of coagulase-positive *Staphylococcus aureus*.

Clinical features

• Local predisposing factors are cutaneous injury, friction and sweating
• Episodes are often recurrent and many patients with recurrences are found to carry furuncle producing strains of *Staphylococcus aureus* in nostrils, axilla or groin or to have had close contact with someone who does.

Management

• Early lesions should be treated with warm compresses and oral penicillinase resistant penicillins penicillin (e.g. flucloxacillin or Augmentin (amoxicillin plus clavulanic acid)). Erythromycin may be used in patients allergic to the preferred antibiotics
• For older lesions which have matured and pointed, incision and drainage may occasionally be indicated in conjunction with the use of antibiotics
• Chronic and recurrent furunculosis should be treated with a course of antibiotics of several weeks duration. While the patient is on antibiotics, all clothing, towels and bed linen that have contacted the affected areas should be washed in hot water. Attempts should be made to deal with the carrier state in the patient and/or close contacts. Washing of the groin, axilla and hands with an antiseptic soap can help, as can topical nasal antibiotics such as mupirocin. An oral rifampicin and fusidic acid combination has also been successful in reducing carriage.

Streptococcal perianal disease

This is a distinctive perianal eruption due to group A beta-haemolytic streptococcus (GABHS):

• peak incidence is in children 3–4 years of age but it may occur in infants
• a likely mode of transmission is digital contamination from an infected oropharynx, although symptoms of pharyngitis are rarely present
• the child complains of pain on defecation and often refuses to open the bowels
• bright blood is frequently seen on the stool. A bright pink erythema extends from the anal rim, which is often fissured and macerated, 2–3 cm out from the anus; the skin is tender but not indurated
• lymphangitis and lymphadenopathy are absent
• there may be an associated GABHS balanitis or vulvovaginitis
• diagnosis is established by culture, on blood agar, of GABHS from a swab of the perianal skin
• the treatment of choice is oral penicillin V 50 mg/kg per day in four divided doses, combined with the use of topical mupirocin twice a day. Recurrences are very frequent without this combined therapy, which should be continued for 10 days. Erythromycin is appropriate in penicillin-allergic patients.

Tinea

This is an infection due to dermatophyte fungi; the source of the fungus is an animal (e.g. dog, cat, guinea pig, cattle), the soil or another human. Tinea occurs on any part of the skin surface and can involve hair and nails.

Clinical features and diagnosis

• Classical features of tinea on the general body skin are itch, erythema studded with papules or pustules, annular or geographical lesions with a tendency to central clearing and a superficial scale (Fig. 21.1.13)
• Tinea is often unilateral and always asymmetrical, whereas eczema and psoriasis, which it may resemble, are often symmetrical in distribution
• Between the toes maceration with a thick white scale is the main finding and an annular lesion may extend on to the dorsum of the foot
• Nail tinea produces a white discoloration and crumbling of the nail plate with an accumulation of subungual debris
• On the soles there are deep seated blisters or pustules that dry to produce brown crusts
• On the scalp there is a characteristic combination of alopecia and inflammation with the hair loss being due to breaking of the hair shafts. Depending on the pattern of hair invasion by the fungus, the hairs are

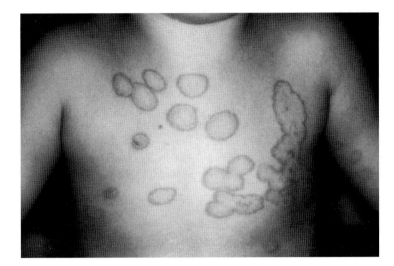

Fig. 21.1.13 Annular lesions of tinea.

either broken off flush with the scalp or at lengths of up to 2–3 mm, but in an individual case all the hairs break at the same length. The inflammation varies from mild erythema and a fine, dandruff-like scale to a pustular carbuncle-like lesion (kerion)
• A Wood light (an ultraviolet lamp) is useful in the diagnosis of some varieties of scalp tinea, with the infected hairs fluorescing bright green. Other varieties of scalp tinea produce no typical fluorescence and the Wood light has no place in the diagnosis of tinea on the skin surface
• The diagnosis of tinea is confirmed by scraping hairs or scales on to a slide, adding 20% potassium hydroxide and examining the specimen microscopically. Septate branching hyphae are seen in skin scales and spores are found in hair. The fungus can be cultured on appropriate media.

Management

• Topical antifungals may be satisfactory for small, localized patches of tinea on the skin
• Oral griseofulvin is the treatment of choice for long-standing or severe cutaneous tinea and hair tinea. This fat-soluble drug is best taken after meals, preferably with a glass of milk. In general a 3-month course is used
• Nail tinea is particularly resistant to treatment and may require other antifungals such as terbinafine.

Tinea versicolor

This is an infection with *Pityrosporum* species, which are part of the normal skin flora. It occurs mainly in tropical and temperate zones and usually affects adolescents and young adults.

Clinical features and diagnosis

• Presents as well demarcated, asymptomatic or slightly itchy macules with a fine, branny scale that is often only obvious on light scratching of the lesions. Primary macules 1–10 mm in diameter coalesce into larger patches
• Lesions occur in two colours – red-brown, especially in the fair-skinned, and hypopigmented in darker-skinned children
• The hypopigmented form must be differentiated from vitiligo, where the depigmentation is total and scale is absent, and pityriasis alba, where lesions are less well demarcated and some erythema may be seen
• In young children it often presents with only facial lesions and almost invariably a parent or older relative will have tinea versicolor in the typical distribution
• Diagnosis is confirmed by microscopic examination of skin scrapings to which 20% potassium hydroxide has been added. Grape-like clusters of spores and short fragments of thick mycelia are seen.

Management

• Untreated, the condition is persistent, although some improvement may occur in winter
• The treatment of choice is with topical imidazole creams
• With the depigmented form, therapy deals with the scale but sun exposure is required for full repigmentation
• Rarely in severe disease in adolescents a short course of oral ketoconazole is required

Scabies

Scabies (Fig. 21.1.14) is due to *Sarcoptes scabei*, an eight-legged, oval-shaped mite less than 0.5 mm in length. The disease is transmitted by close physical contact, with transmission by fomites being exceptional. A small number of mites burrow into the skin in certain sites, particularly between the fingers, the ulnar border of the hand, around the wrists and elbows, the anterior axillary fold, nipples and penis and, in infants, the palms and soles.

Clinical features and diagnosis

- The pathognomonic primary lesion, a typical burrow, is rarely seen. It is a 2–3 mm long curved grey line with a vesicle at the anterior end
- Other lesions that mark the sites of burrows are small blisters or papules, larger blisters on the palms and soles of infants, scratch marks, secondary eczema and secondary bacterial infection
- Eczema or impetigo in the target areas for scabies should always raise suspicion of this disease, as should blisters on the palms and soles of infants

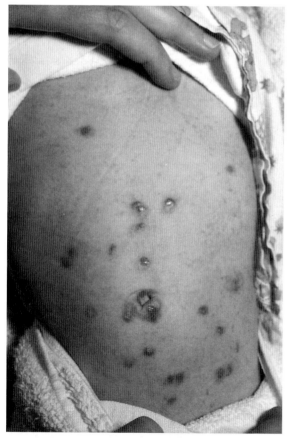

Fig. 21.1.14 Scabies nodules.

- Often more prominent than the evidence of burrows is the so called secondary eruption of scabies. This presents as multiple, very pruritic, urticarial papules, which are soon excoriated. They occur particularly on the abdomen, thighs and buttocks
- Large inflammatory nodules may form part of the secondary eruption, occurring particularly on covered areas, especially on axillae, scrotum, penis and buttocks. They may, however, be very widespread, producing diagnostic difficulties. They may persist for months after effective scabies treatment
- The diagnosis of scabies is usually a clinical one but can be confirmed by demonstration of the mite. A burrow, which may be softened by the application of 20% potassium hydroxide, is scraped and the material is smeared on a slide for microscopic examination. Burrows may be more easily identified by rubbing a thick, black marking pen over suspicious areas and wiping with an alcohol swab, leaving a burrow outlined with ink.

Management

- The patient and all close contacts should be treated simultaneously
- 5% permethrin cream is the treatment of choice and should be applied to all body surfaces from the neck down and left on overnight. A repeat application should be administered after 1 week
- In extremely young infants 6% precipitated sulphur is preferred
- Bedclothes and clothing should be washed in the normal way with no disinfection required
- An irritant dermatitis may follow scabies treatment, particularly in atopic children, and may require emollients and topical steroids once the miticide therapy is fully completed
- Persistent nodules may respond to topical corticosteroids but a coal tar solution painted on is preferable for the very resistant ones.

Pediculosis

Human lice are six-legged insects without wings, grey in colour or brown-red when engorged with blood. The body louse and the head louse have a thin body 2–4 mm long and three similar pairs of legs; the pubic louse is wider and shorter and the second and third pair of legs are larger than the first, producing a crab-like appearance. The ova (nits) appear as oval, grey-white, 0.5 mm specks, attached by a firm chitin ring to hairs or clothes.

Pediculosis capitis (head lice)

This is a common infestation, often occurring in epidemics in schools. The occipital area of the scalp is preferentially involved and may be the only site affected. The condition is itchy, leading to scratching with excoriations and also eczematization and secondary infection, which may mask the underlying infestation. Permethrin shampoos are effective pediculicides but may not destroy ova and a repeat application after a few days is recommended to kill further hatched lice. Removal of nit cases with a fine comb is easier if the chitin is softened by a prior application of vinegar.

Pediculosis corporis (body lice)

This is rare in children except in severely overcrowded conditions with poor hygiene. The organism infests bedding and clothing and the nits are not found on the human host. The lice hatch with body warmth and puncture the skin, producing very itchy, small, red papules with haemorrhagic puncta. Spots of dried blood may be found on the clothing and bed linen. Treatment is directed towards removal of the organisms from materials with hot water laundering and hot ironing or the use of a hot electric dryer.

Pediculosis pubis (pubic lice, crab lice)

This is mainly an adult disease. The pubic louse has as its normal habitat the anogenital area but in children it is particularly seen on the eyelashes. Eyelash infestation in children may occur from innocent close contact with an affected adult but the possibility of sexual abuse must always be considered. Pediculosis of the eyelashes is best treated with petroleum jelly applied thickly twice a day for a week.

Arthropod bites

Patients with arthropod bites present to a dermatologist in two situations: the severe local allergic reaction and the more chronic hypersensitivity condition called 'papular urticaria'. The arthropods most encountered are mosquitos, sand flies, fleas and grass mites. The distribution of the bites helps to suggest the causative agent.

Severe local reactions

- Include blisters, purpura and cellulitis and lymphangitis even in the absence of infection
- As the lesions are extremely itchy, scratching occurs, leading to secondary eczematization and secondary infection.

Papular urticaria

- A very common condition in children, particularly between 10 months and 4 years

- In a child who has been sensitized by previous exposure the bite produces an itchy urticarial (hive-like) weal, which is succeeded by a firm itchy papule that lasts for many days
- The weal and papule usually show a central punctum and the papule may be surmounted by a tiny blister
- The persistence and severity of the condition are explained by the fact that new bites by the same species will often cause a recrudescence of activity in resolving lesions
- Secondary infection and eczematization from scratching also contribute to the chronicity of the condition, which may plague the child through an entire summer
- Management involves avoidance of insect attack, with the use of insect repellents, insecticides, protective clothing and changes in activities, which clearly are difficult in an active child. Wrapping the affected areas in wet dressings overnight as soon as new bites occur is helpful in reducing the itch and preventing scratching, which leads to the secondary eczema and infection. Topical corticosteroids will improve the secondary eczema and have some effect in dampening the severity of the actual bite reaction but must not be used for prolonged periods. Oral antibiotics are required if there is significant secondary infection.

Forms of dermatitis

Atopic dermatitis (atopic eczema)

Atopy is a genetically determined disorder with an increased tendency to form IgE antibody to inhalants and foods and increased susceptibility to asthma, allergic rhinitis and atopic eczema (Ch. 13.1). This eczema may begin at any age but 75% of patients show the first signs by 6 months.

Clinical features

The characteristic clinical features are a generalized dryness and a tendency to lichenification or thickening of the skin, pruritus and excoriations and patches of acute, subacute or chronic eczema. Involvement of the whole cutaneous surface may occur but the predominant areas are the face in infants, extensor aspects of the limbs as the child begins to crawl and the limb flexures in older children. In severe cases the whole skin may be erythematous and in these patients white dermographism is often a prominent feature: this indicates that the condition is likely to be unstable and difficult.

Complications

Patients with atopic eczema may develop secondary bacterial infection that presents either as yellow crusting impetigo or folliculitis, or simply as worsening eczema. Mollusca contagiosa are common and atopic patients are at risk of developing severe widespread herpes simplex infections. The usual childhood immunizations are quite safe.

Management

Explanation and education

The most important aspect of the management of atopic eczema is explanation of the condition to the patient or, more commonly, his/her parents. The family should understand that the child has been born with an inherently dry, irritable skin and that this will be a lifelong tendency. While the skin does become more stable with time, it will always require extra care. It is essential to talk in terms of control rather than cure, otherwise the family search for an endpoint after which care will no longer be required and this is an unrealistic expectation. The condition should be explained as a multifactorial disorder as it must be appreciated that, just as there is no 'cure', there is no single 'cause'.

Avoidance of irritants

Factors that will often irritate the atopic skin should be discussed. Woollen material in direct contact with the skin is a major irritant; apart from the child's own clothing it is important to remember the parent's clothing, carpets, blankets, stroller and car seat covers, furniture and toys. Shiny nylon materials and some acrylics irritate but cotton–polyester mixtures are usually well tolerated. Sand contact is often troublesome, especially with prolonged close contact as in playing in a sandpit. Chlorinated water may aggravate but this is variable. Soap in excess and bubble baths over-dry the skin, and many perfumed and 'medicated' products, disinfectants and strong cleansers cause irritation.

Dealing with dryness

Bath oils and oatmeal-containing products are useful and prevent the defatting of the skin that bathing can induce. It is essential to find a suitable moisturizer that can be applied all over twice a day, whether or not there is active eczema. Glycerine 10% in Sorbolene cream is useful in many cases but more or less greasy preparations are available to suit individual patients and climatic conditions. Urea-containing products sting broken skin and are unsuitable.

Topical corticosteroids

These are an essential part of treatment. In general, ointment bases are preferred because they are more emollient than cream bases. Nothing stronger than 1% hydrocortisone should be used on the face or in the axillae or groin. Medium-strength fluorinated corticosteroids are usually adequate for lesions on the trunk and limbs; the stronger preparations are rarely required. These preparations are best used three times a day and, of course, ceased as soon as the eczema is clear.

Wet dressings

These are useful in severe widespread eczema. A water-based emollient is applied all over; a corticosteroid cream (rather than ointment in this case because cream is more water-miscible) is applied to the areas of active eczema; sheeting soaked in tap water is applied and bandaged on with a crepe bandage and a net material is used to hold the dressings in place. The procedure is repeated three times a day. These dressings cool the skin down, reduce itching, physically prevent scratching, increase the hydration of the skin and enhance the penetration of topical steroids. This treatment is usually effective in clearing the eczema in 3–4 days. If dressings are required for longer periods the corticosteroid should be used only once a day. Particular care should be taken with infants.

Systemic therapy

If significant bacterial infection occurs a swab should be taken and oral antibiotics used. Nocturnal sedation is often valuable during severe episodes but daytime sedation should be avoided; antihistamines are the preferred sedatives. While they may be essential for associated diseases, oral corticosteroids should never be instituted for the eczema itself; a severe rebound can occur on their withdrawal and after several courses the eczema can become very unstable.

Dietary manipulation

No alteration should be made to the patient's diet unless the atopic eczema has failed to respond to conventional therapy properly carried out. There is only a small group of patients with unstable eczema with an associated urticarial element in whom dietary factors are of major significance; skin prick tests are useful in this group to give a guide for dietary manipulation, which should be instituted only by those with a full understanding of the nutritional requirements of young children.

Dust mite allergy

This is important in a selected group of patients. In these children the eczema is usually particularly troublesome on the face and neck. The family should be given details of dust mite reduction strategies.

Discoid eczema

• In children this is often a manifestation of a combined atopic and psoriatic diathesis

- Well-defined patches of acute eczema occur in a strikingly symmetrical distribution. In infants the commonest sites are the upper back and the tops of the shoulders; in older patients the extensor aspects of the limbs are particularly involved. The lesions may be very thick and exudative and they are very itchy
- Discoid eczema should be distinguished from tinea and impetigo, which are less symmetrical, and classical psoriasis, which is rarely moist
- Management involves emollients and topical steroids as for atopic dermatitis, with the continued use of emollient helping to prevent recurrences.

Pityriasis alba

This condition probably represents a very mild eczema, which, however, produces a striking postin-flammatory depigmentation. The condition is more common in atopics, and occasionally some areas will show erythema and more definite eczematous changes:

- appears as poorly defined, slightly scaly, hypopig-mented patches occurring particularly on the face and the upper arms
- the mild irritation and signs of mild eczema respond to emollients and weak topical corticoste-roids but the hypopigmentation may be very per-sistent and require sun exposure over a prolonged period before repigmentation is complete
- the condition should be differentiated from viti-ligo, where there is total depigmentation and no scale, and from tinea versicolor, which is rare on the face, has very well demarcated lesions and has a very fine branny scale.

Clinical example

Harry, aged 4, presented with a swelling and redness around one eye. It was diagnosed by the ophthalmology registrar as preseptal orbital cellulitis, the child was admitted to hospital and intravenous antibiotics were started. It was remarked that a lack of fever and pain was unusual in a child with cellulitis. The next day the area was more swollen and some blistering had occurred. Harry was noted also to have multiple linear blistered red lesions on his arm. Harry's mother told the registrar that Harry's best friend from the preschool had similar lesions on the arms and face, which had been diagnosed by a dermatologist as a plant contact dermatitis. The history obtained was that the preschool garden had been landscaped by parents over the previous weekend and the two children carried Robyn Gordon grevilleas in the car for planting. Harry's antibiotics were ceased and he was discharged from hospital on a 5-day course of oral steroids. The swelling resolved in 2 days and in 6 days all the rash had disappeared. The following weekend the Robyn Gordon grevilleas were removed from the preschool.

Contact allergic dermatitis from plants (Fig. 21.1.15)

- The commonest causative agents in Australia are rhus and a variety of grevilleas, including Robyn Gordon, Ned Kelly and Hookerana
- The dermatitis is usually very severe and blistering often occurs
- It often occurs in a streaky pattern where the plant has brushed against the skin
- Initially there may be much oedema, especially on the face, and cellulitis is often suspected;

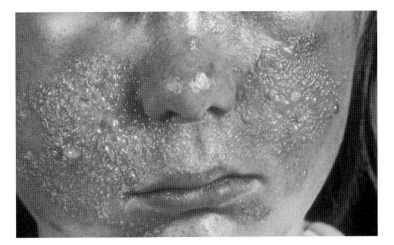

Fig. 21.1.15 Acute vesicular plant contact dermatitis.

however, the child is afebrile and the area is itchy rather than painful
- The condition may be spread beyond areas of initial contact as a result of retention of allergen on clothing and under the nails
- A strong topical steroid may be adequate for localized areas but a short course of oral steroids is usually indicated.

Napkin rashes

Common causes

- *Seborrhoeic dermatitis.* Presents as a dull red rash covering most of the napkin area, sometimes with a greasy yellow scale, although this is characteristically absent in this moist area
- *Monilia.* Manifested as a thick, white material deep in the folds and as small annular lesions with an overhanging white macerated scale at their margin
- *Irritant dermatitis from urine and faeces.* Irritant dermatitis due to urine affects mainly the convex surfaces, with relative sparing of the flexures; irritation due to faeces particularly affects the natal cleft. Napkin dermatitis is rarely caused by irritant or allergic reactions to laundering products
- *Miliaria.* Sweat duct occlusion may occur alone or in combination with other elements. This presents as small red papules, which are very transient so the pattern varies considerably from hour to hour.

Variants of common types

- *Gluteal granulomas.* Occur on top of a pre-existing napkin rash as purplish nodules that tend to be oval in shape, following the lines of the skin folds
- *Erosive napkin rash.* Occurs in the perianal and natal cleft area and usually follows a period of diarrhoea. It is seen in infants with lactose intolerance
- *Ulcerated nodules.* Most often occur in the vulval area in a situation of a constant urinary leak in the presence of major congenital anomalies
- *'Frog plaster' napkin rash.* Due to the accumulation of faeces, and to a lesser extent, urine under the plaster used in cases of developmental dysplasia of the hip, and usually of a mixed erosive and ulcerated nodule type.

Other causes

- *Psoriasis* (Fig. 21.1.16). Produces a bright red, glazed, clearly marginated napkin rash. This may develop into the condition called 'napkin psoriasis'. A few small scaly spots occur on the trunk above the

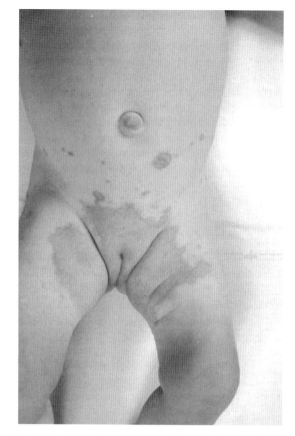

Fig. 21.1.16 Psoriatic napkin rash with early dissemination.

psoriatic napkin rash, followed by a sudden explosion of typical psoriatic lesions on scalp, face and all over the trunk. The infant is well and the condition is usually asymptomatic. The eruption is self-limiting in a few weeks
- *Impetigo.* Presents as small, pus-filled blisters that quickly rupture and expand into large superficial erosions, usually asymptomatic
- *Herpes simplex.* Punched-out 3–8 mm individual erosions that coalesce to form geographical-shaped lesions; considerable swelling is usually seen and there is associated lymphadenopathy and fever
- *Staphylococcal scalded skin syndrome.* May present in the napkin area with a very painful bright red rash with superficial blistering
- *Kawasaki disease.* Often presents in the napkin area with a tender red scaly rash in a febrile child
- *Langerhans cell histiocytosis.* Produces a severe napkin rash with a brownish scale, erosions and purpuric spots
- *Zinc deficiency.* Produces a well marginated shiny rash rather similar to psoriasis, but with a characteristic dark peripheral scale. Similar lesions are present around the mouth and nose.

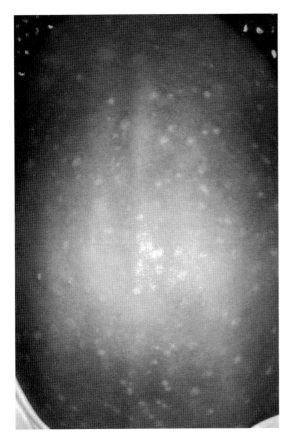

Fig. 21.1.17 Small plaque psoriasis leaving a striking hypopigmentation.

Psoriasis

Psoriasis is a hereditary disease: it is probably an autosomal dominant condition with variable penetrance. It commences by the age of 15 years in 30% of patients. It may present in the typical adult form of large erythematous plaques, with a thick, silvery white scale, predominantly on the knees, elbows, buttocks and scalp, but certain differences are seen in childhood disease:

- plaques are usually smaller and with a finer scale (Fig. 21.1.17)
- a particularly common presentation is acute guttate psoriasis with the eruption of tiny papules in a widespread distribution. The eruption is often preceded by an intercurrent illness, particularly a streptococcal throat infection
- the face and intertriginous sites are commonly affected in children
- children presenting with vulvitis, balanitis and perianal itching may be found to have psoriasis. In these areas the typical scale is absent and the con-dition presents as a glazed erythema, often with fissuring
- nail involvement is usually absent or minimal with minor pitting
- pustular psoriasis and psoriatic arthropathy are extremely rare in children
- there is a particular type of well marginated, bright red napkin rash, described above, that is a marker for psoriasis
- many therapies used in adults are inappropriate in children. In general, psoriasis in children is better treated with tars than topical corticosteroids. No treatment can alter the course of the condition.

Photosensitivity

Photosensitivity may be manifested by exaggerated sunburn or another rash appearing in a light exposed area. There are many causes and some are briefly reviewed here:

- *Phytophotodermatitis* – contact with a phototoxic agent (e.g. lime juice, perfumes) followed by sun exposure causes an exaggerated sunburn reaction
- *Drug reactions* – rare in children
- *Polymorphous light reaction* – may produce recurring erythematous, itchy vesicles and papules on the cheeks, ears, side of the neck and exposed limbs. The onset of the eruption may be delayed 1–2 days after sun exposure, but the distribution of the lesions and history of exacerbation in the summer months are typical
- *Solar urticaria* – a very transient urticarial rash appearing immediately after sun exposure
- *Connective tissue diseases*
  - lupus erythematosus
  - dermatomyositis
- *Porphyrias*
  - erythropoietic protoporphyria
  - congenital erythropoietic porphyria
- Other genetic disorders leading to increased sun sensitivity
  - albinism
  - xeroderma pigmentosum
  - Bloom syndrome
  - Rothmund–Thomson syndrome.

Hair loss in children

There are two major types of hair loss (alopecia): diffuse and patchy. The commonest cause of localized alopecia is telogen effluvium and the main causes of patchy alopecia are tinea, alopecia areata and trichotillomania.

Diffuse alopecia

- *Telogen effluvium* – high fever causes a large number of hairs to enter the resting or telogen stage of the hair cycle prematurely; 2–3 months later these inevitably fall. The hairs have a club-shaped end visible as a white dot with the naked eye. New hairs immediately appear in the empty follicles. The condition may continue for several months but is fully reversible.
- Some other causes are:
  - drugs
  - malnutrition
  - iron deficiency
  - various aminoacidurias
  - hereditary hair shaft abnormality syndromes
  - congenital atrichia
  - alopecia as a part of other genetic syndromes.

Patchy alopecia

- *Tinea* – combination of inflammation of varying degree and broken hairs
- *Alopecia areata* – autoimmune disease with areas of total hair loss and no obvious inflammation; there may be some short, so-called 'exclamation mark hairs' at the edges
- *Trichotillomania* – hair twisting or plucking. Hairs broken at different lengths, usually no inflammation

- Some other causes:
  - hair cutting as a form of artifactual skin disease
  - *traction*: from tight hair styles
  - *infections*: boils, erysipelas, herpes simplex, herpes zoster, tick bites
  - localized scleroderma.

Practical points

- A haemangioma in a beard distribution can be a marker for subglottic haemangioma
- Haemangiomas usually appear after birth, always grow out of proportion to the growth of the child and always undergo resolution
- Vascular malformations are always present at birth, grow only in proportion to the child's growth and never resolve
- Herpes simplex lesions are grouped and tend to coalesce forming geographical-shaped erosions
- Painful defaecation, bright blood on the stool and a bright red rash in the immediate perianal area point to streptococcal perianal infection
- The combination of broken hairs and inflammation suggests tinea capitis
- Scabies nodules can persist for months after effective scabies treatment
- Apparent cellulitis that is itchy, occurs in a well, afebrile child and begins on the second day to blister suggests allergic contact dermatitis to a plant
- A bright red, well marginated napkin rash suggests psoriasis

---

Systemic implications of skin disease in children

R. Phillips

Virtually all systemic diseases lead to skin changes sooner or later. Conversely, many skin conditions have the potential to cause dysfunction in other body systems. This chapter focuses on skin changes in children that require examination and/or investigation for systemic problems. The systemic problem may be the cause of the rash, or it may be caused by the skin disease.

In this chapter, we discuss the significance of different morphological types of rash in turn, namely vesicles and pustules, ulcers, papules, scaly rashes, eczematous rashes, erythematous rashes and purpuric rashes. Vascular and other birthmarks, pigmentary changes, anogenital rashes, skin texture and hair are considered separately.

Practical points

- Many diseases can present with a rash as the first sign
- Widespread chronic eczema is usually associated with systemic complications including psychosocial and growth problems
- Chronic generalized skin disease from any cause is often associated with morbidity in growth and nutrition
- Beware of a common rash presenting in an unusual way, such as early-onset acne
- Drug reactions are common. Most drugs used for systemic disease can cause a rash and most drugs used for skin disease can cause systemic disease
- Purpuric rashes require immediate assessment to exclude life-threatening conditions such as meningococcal disease

---

Vesicular, bullous or pustular rashes

Vesicles and pustules are considered together in this section as there is substantial clinical overlap. Vesicles from any cause usually become pustular in a couple of days if they have not ruptured.

In the neonatal period, pustules may be part of several transient dermatological conditions (Ch. 21.1) but pustules or vesicles may also be a marker of serious underlying illness, even in the absence of fever and lethargy. Consider:

- infection, either congenital or acquired. Herpes simplex virus (Ch. 21.1), varicella, *Listeria*, *Staphylococcus*, *Streptococcus*, *Haemophilus*, *Neisseria* or *Candida* species may be present
- neutropenia from any cause. Superficial bacterial pustules may be the only sign of congenital neutropenia
- incontinentia pigmenti. This disease is X-linked and fatal in male fetuses. Girls present with lesions distributed in linear patterns following the lines of Blaschko (not dermatomal lines; Fig. 21.2.1). Lesions evolve through vesicular and warty phases to eventually leave permanent hyperpigmented streaks. Seizures and developmental, ocular and dental problems may occur (Fig. 21.2.2).

At any age, consider:

- Langerhans cell histiocytosis
- drug reactions. These can manifest as phototoxic or photosensitive reactions (Ch. 21.1) or bullous drug reactions. Stevens–Johnson syndrome presents with mucocutaneous erosions and blistering in association with erythematous or purpuric macules, lethargy, fever, lymphadenopathy and conjunctivitis, occasionally leading to death or blindness. Most cases are secondary to medications, often non-steroidal anti-inflammatory drugs
- dermatitis herpetiformis. This may present in older children as itchy papules or vesicles, often on extensor surfaces. Most patients have gluten enteropathy (coeliac disease) and may have abdominal discomfort, diarrhoea or anaemia.

Acneiform rashes

Some degree of acne is occasionally seen on the face in infancy and is common on the face and upper trunk during puberty. Comedonal acne may be the first sign of puberty. Acne, particularly if severe, can lead to significant depression in adolescents and is a risk factor for suicide. Both the depression and the acne need to be recognized and treated. Acne that is atypical in age of onset, distribution, morphology or severity may be associated with systemic disease. Consider:

- glucocorticoid excess, either exogenous or endogenous. This can give a monomorphic acneiform

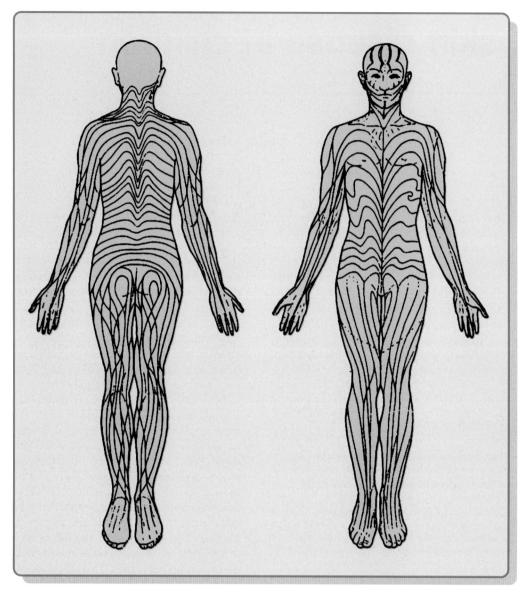

Fig. 21.2.1 Lines of Blaschko.

rash on the face and trunk. Other cushingoid stigmata are usually present
- androgen excess. Look for accelerated growth, body odour, pubic hair, clitoromegaly (but not breast development) and penile (but not testicular) enlargement (Fig. 21.2.3). In teenage females, polycystic ovary syndrome is commonly the cause
- precocious puberty
- medications. In postpubertal children, antiepileptic medications, especially phenytoin and phenobarbital, may induce acne
- tuberosclerosis. Facial angiofibromas may be the first sign of tuberosclerosis and may be misdiagnosed initially as acne or plane warts.

Chronic erosions or ulcers

Any itchy condition such as scabies or papular urticaria can lead to chronic erosions via persistent scratching. Several primary skin conditions can cause chronic erosions or ulcers in children. Consider:

- immunodeficiencies. Recurrent boils can be seen in chronic granulomatous disease and hyper IgE syndrome. Poor wound healing is a feature of leukocyte adhesion defects
- skin fragility syndromes. In junctional and dystrophic forms of epidermolysis bullosa, chronic ulcers

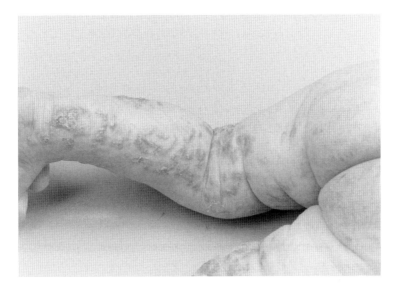

Fig. 21.2.2   Widespread vesicles in a 6-day-old girl. Recognizing the streaky blaschkoid patterns of the vesicles on the back leads to the diagnosis of incontinentia pigmenti.

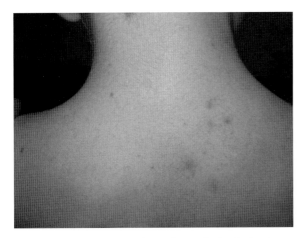

Fig. 21.2.3   Comedones and papules on the back of a 6-year-old boy. He was within normal limits for height but crossing centiles upward. Examination was otherwise normal. He requires investigation for androgen excess.

related to minimal skin trauma may be seen in association with failure to thrive, anaemia and gastrointestinal tract involvement
• porphyria. Several enzyme defects in haem metabolism are associated with chronic erosive lesions, photosensitivity and hyperpigmentation. Episodes of acute pain or neurological dysfunction are rarely seen in childhood porphyrias.

Recurrent mouth ulcers

These are generally due to aphthous stomatitis. Such ulcers are usually small and resolve in a few days. Recurrent mouth ulcers can also be seen in:

• iron, folate or vitamin B₁₂ deficiency
• gastrointestinal disorders. Coeliac disease, Crohn disease and ulcerative colitis are all associated with mouth ulceration. Recurrent abdominal pain, intermittent diarrhoea and failure to thrive may be present
• connective tissue disorders. Patients with Behçet disease usually present in late childhood with ulcers at one site (mouth or genitals) and it may be many years before a second site is involved. Systemic lupus erythematosus and juvenile rheumatoid arthritis may cause recurrent mouth ulcers
• immunodeficiency states, human immunodeficiency virus (HIV) infection
• malignancy. Lymphoma and histiocytosis can present with non-healing mouth ulcers.

Papular rashes

Papules or nodules may occur in a number of disorders, including acute rheumatic fever, juvenile chronic arthritis, systemic lupus erythematosus and neurofibromatosis, but are rarely the presenting feature. Erythematous papules, often itchy, scaly or purpuric, may be widespread in acute Langerhans cell histiocytosis. Severe, recalcitrant 'cradle cap' or weeping intertriginous lesions may also be present, along with single or multiple bone lesions, mucosal ulceration and involvement of other organs. In neonates, Langerhans cell histiocytosis may present as a few nodules, classically with a raised border and

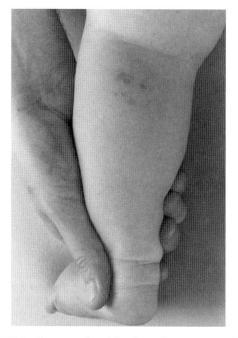

Fig. 21.2.4 These small, rock hard papules were present for several months behind the knee and at two other sites on the trunk of a 1-year-old girl with mild developmental delay. In conjunction with her short fourth metacarpal bones, a diagnosis of pseudohypoparathyroidism was made.

central necrosis. This congenital self-healing form usually shows complete regression within months but visceral involvement may occur. Local or generalized disorders of parathyroid or calcium metabolism can present as calcified or ossified papules (Fig. 21.2.4).

In children, yellow papules are commonly xanthogranulomas. The yellow colour is best seen by pressing over the papule to blanch the overlying capillaries. Xanthogranulomas are often isolated lesions that resolve within a few years. They are not associated with lipid disorders. By contrast, multiple eruptive xanthomas, tuberous xanthomas (usually distributed over the elbows, knuckles, buttocks, knees and heels) and tendinous xanthomas (usually on tendons around the elbow, wrist, hand or ankle) are associated with elevated cholesterol levels. Consider:

- primary hyperlipoproteinaemias. Skin lesions may present between 5 and 15 years of age, sometimes as tendinitis or tenosynovitis. Look for signs of atherosclerotic disease and a family history of high cholesterol, early myocardial infarcts or strokes
- secondary hypercholesterolaemia. This can occur in hypothyroidism, biliary cirrhosis, diabetes mellitus, glycogen storage disease and nephrotic syndrome.

Scaly rashes

Ichthyosis refers to generalized scaly skin. Some ichthyoses only affect the skin but several involve other organs:

- X-linked ichthyosis is quite common but may be undiagnosed. A fine scaling at birth is later replaced by larger, brown scales. Diagnosis is confirmed by leukocyte enzyme analysis. Boys with X-linked ichthyosis need to be monitored for hypogonadism, cryptorchidism, anosmia, short stature and mental retardation. Female carriers may have obstetric difficulties
- in Sjögren–Larsson syndrome, a yellow-brown lichenified appearance is present in infancy. This evolves into a more florid scaling with a symmetric spastic paralysis and mental retardation
- in some trichothiodystrophies, ichthyosis is associated with brittle hair and mental and growth retardation
- several ichthyoses are linked with deafness, cataracts or other eye problems. Mild, generalized scaling may be the first feature in later-onset Refsum disease, before development of multiple visual problems, deafness and neuropathy.

Ectodermal dysplasias are a heterogeneous group of conditions characterized by congenital, non-progressive abnormalities of hair, teeth, nails and sweat glands. The skin is dry and may be hyper-pigmented. Deficient sweating may cause overheating in summer. Teeth are often poorly developed or absent. Cleft lip and palate, limb abnormalities and mucous retention in the upper airway and ear may be present.

Clinical example

A 2-year-old boy attended because he had twice collapsed on hot days over summer. Examination revealed dry skin with sparse hair and deficient dental development. His nails were somewhat hypoplastic. This story is suggestive of ectodermal dysplasia, probably X-linked. History and examination confirmed the near-total absence of sweating. He was at risk of overheating and his family needed to be counselled about strategies to prevent this. Siblings and other family members should be examined and genetic counselling provided.

Eczematous rashes

Atopic eczema is common and in most cases can be readily controlled with minimal sequelae (Ch. 21.1). However, a few children have chronic and severe disease requiring frequent, time-consuming applications of topical medicines and wet dressings. These children may have recurrent infections, particularly with *Staphylococcus aureus* and herpes simplex virus. There may be failure to thrive. Severe psychosocial, behavioural and marital problems are common in these severely affected children, although often hidden from medical staff. These problems need to be identified and addressed.

Eczematous skin lesions can also be associated with:

- immunodeficiency syndromes. Thrombocytopenia, immunodeficiency and eczema are seen in Wiskott–Aldrich syndrome. Failure to thrive, petechiae, recurrent infections, diarrhoea or haematological abnormalities may suggest this or other immunodeficiencies that are variably associated with eczema
- multiple food allergies with consequent dietary restrictions and secondary nutritional and psychosocial problems
- metabolic or nutritional disorders. Phenylketonuria often presents with eczema. Less typical eczematous lesions, more prominent in periorificial areas, are seen in biotin, essential fatty acid and zinc deficiency syndromes. Malnutrition and organoacidaemias, e.g. methylmalonicacidaemia, can result in similar lesions.

Erythematous (red blanching) rashes

Neonatal erythroderma

Erythroderma (inflammation of almost all the skin surface) in the neonatal period requires close monitoring and early investigation to identify the underlying cause. Eczema rarely presents as erythroderma. Exclude staphylococcal-toxin-mediated infections and congenital candidiasis. Metabolic causes include inherited carboxylase deficiencies and essential fatty acid deficiency secondary to any severe malabsorption, and can be associated with severe acidosis and coma. Omenn syndrome (familial reticuloendotheliosis with eosinophilia), maternal graft-versus-host disease and other severe immunodeficiencies can present as erythroderma. Drug reactions are an unlikely cause at this age. Some variants of ichthyosis can present as erythroderma and may be associated with multiple infections, failure to thrive or cataracts.

Annular rashes

Annular lesions are ring-shaped with relatively normal skin centrally. Such lesions are typical of tinea corporis, urticaria and granuloma annulare but may require investigation for neonatal lupus (caused by transfer of maternal antinuclear antibodies across the placenta; look for heart block and maternal antinuclear antibodies), rheumatic fever, syphilis and Lyme disease.

Clinical example

A 4-week-old baby presented with multiple red scaly rings on her face and trunk.

These had been treated as eczema with hydrocortisone, without response. A trial of clotrimazole cream for tinea corporis was also ineffective. Upon questioning, the mother remarked that the 8-year-old brother had also developed a persistent annular rash as an infant. Testing the mother confirmed the presence of antinuclear antibodies, consistent with a diagnosis of neonatal lupus in the two children. Neither sibling had congenital heart block. The mother remains clinically normal.

Erythema nodosum

Erythema nodosum can occur at any age and presents initially as subcutaneous erythematous lesions mainly on the anterior lower legs. They may progress to extensive bruise-like lesions. Erythema nodosum may be idiopathic or associated with chronic streptococcal disease, pulmonary or other tuberculosis, Crohn disease, chronic gastrointestinal infections, sarcoidosis and *Mycoplasma* infection. It may also be secondary to a number of drugs.

Urticaria

Urticaria describes circular erythematous macules or swellings, often with central pallor, that appear, migrate and disappear over minutes or hours. It is common. Usually no cause is found but recurrent or chronic urticaria may be related to underlying inflammatory conditions such as systemic lupus erythematosus, juvenile chronic arthritis, other vasculitic diseases and parasitic infection. In a child who is very unwell, consider Kawasaki disease.

Generalized erythematous rashes

Erythematous rashes with fever are common in children. Many widespread childhood viruses may be accompanied by an erythematous rash. Occasionally the clinical pattern is distinctive and a confident diagnosis can be made. Usually the diagnosis cannot be made clinically. If the diagnosis is not clear, decide if the child is significantly unwell. Any signs of decreased responsiveness, lethargy or shock may require urgent investigation for causes such as septicaemia and Kawasaki disease. In otherwise well children, consider whether the rash may be a drug reaction. If any relatives may be at risk (e.g. immunosuppressed siblings, pregnant women), serological and virological testing to identify a cause may be appropriate. Usually, no investigation is needed:

- the skin lesions of systemic lupus erythematosus include a characteristic butterfly distribution over both cheeks and the base of the nose. Patchy lesions may also present over the ears, neck and less commonly the limbs. In acute systemic lupus erythematosus, erythematous macules are also seen about the nail beds, on the tips of the fingers, the toes, and on the palms of the hands and soles of the feet
- an erythematous maculopapular rash is often seen in the systemic form of juvenile chronic arthritis. This rash usually has a salmon pink colour and tends to come and go, being particularly evident at the time when the fever is at its height. It may be urticarial
- the lesions of Henoch–Schönlein purpura may be erythematous and urticarial rather than purpuric
- an erythematous rash that is distributed over the extensor surfaces of the joints, particularly over the knuckles, elbows and knees, is characteristic of dermatomyositis. In addition, most children with this disorder show a violaceous facial rash and periorbital oedema
- an erythematous rash accompanied by oedema of the palms and soles is often prominent in Kawasaki disease. Other early features include prolonged high fever, conjunctivitis, redness, swelling or ulceration of mucosal surfaces and enlargement of lymph nodes. Desquamation of the hands and feet is a later finding.

Purpuric rashes

Most children presenting with fever and petechiae (pinpoint purpura) but who are otherwise well have an enteroviral infection without other findings. However, purpuric rashes are associated with several life-threatening diseases. They require urgent assessment.

Neonatal purpura

Purpuric rashes in the neonatal period may be an early presentation of any cause of childhood purpura (see below). In addition, consider:

- congenital infection, including rubella, cytomegalovirus, toxoplasmosis, and herpes simplex
- haemolytic disease of the newborn
- malignancy, including neuroblastoma, Langerhans cell histiocytosis and leukaemia
- iatrogenic injury, including birth trauma, extravasation of drugs and arterial injury during catheterization.

Childhood purpura

Purpuric rashes in childhood are usually secondary to vascular dysfunction rather than a low platelet count. Consider:

- septicaemia. An unwell febrile child with purpura should be treated for meningococcal septicaemia without waiting for the results of investigations. Septicaemia from *Haemophilus influenzae*, streptococci, staphylococci and some Gram-negative organisms may cause purpura. Less extensive, but diagnostically useful, are the purpuric lesions of subacute bacterial endocarditis, typhus and typhoid fever. Purpura may also occur in certain viral haemorrhagic fevers
- coagulation disorders. There may be a history of joint pain or swelling, or bleeding from other sites
- Henoch–Schönlein purpura. This is quite common in childhood. Purpuric lesions on the legs and buttocks may be the only finding in Henoch–Schönlein purpura or there may be associated abdominal pain, arthritis or renal involvement. Children with Henoch–Schönlein purpura should be monitored for months for the development of nephritis
- other vasculitic diseases
- Langerhans cell histiocytosis (Fig. 21.2.5)
- glucocorticoid excess
- any cause of abnormal skin elasticity
- scurvy. Irritability, bone pain, gum sponginess and bleeding may be present. Wrist X-rays are diagnostic
- child abuse. Bruises of different ages and at unusual sites may be seen
- trauma.

Childhood purpura with thrombocytopenia

Purpura in association with a low platelet count is often associated with bruising and signs of bleeding elsewhere. Idiopathic thrombocytopenic purpura is the most common cause. Children need to be examined and investigated for leukaemia, pancytopenia, splenomegaly and drug-induced thrombocytopenia

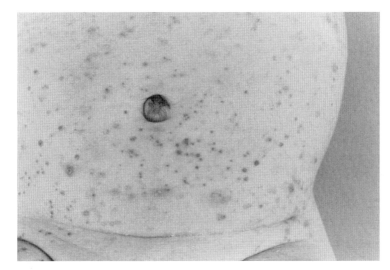

Fig. 21.2.5 This 3-month-old girl was being treated for eczema. However, the distribution and morphology of the chronic rash were unusual. Some lesions were purpuric, suggesting the correct diagnosis of Langerhans cell histiocytosis.

or aplastic anaemia (chloramphenicol, antithyroid medications).

Haemangiomas and vascular malformations

Haemangiomas and vascular malformations are discussed in Chapter 21.1. They are often isolated lesions but may be part of systemic disease. Consider:

- ocular involvement. Children with any vascular lesion around the eye should be screened for glaucoma and other eye abnormalities. Children with haemangiomas adjacent to the eye may develop amblyopia (blindness) secondary to the visual axis being obstructed or secondary to astigmatism caused by pressure of the tumour on the globe
- intracranial involvement. Children with capillary malformations involving the region of the first division of the trigeminal nerve may also have intracranial involvement and develop epilepsy, strokes, hemiplegia or mental retardation (Sturge–Weber syndrome)
- occult spinal abnormalities
- intestinal lesions. Multiple cutaneous and visceral vascular lesions occur in blue rubber bleb syndrome and may cause intestinal bleeding. Telangiectases in hereditary haemorrhagic telangiectasia usually appear on the face, mouth and nose. Nose bleeds become frequent in late childhood and gastrointestinal bleeding occurs in adult life
- overgrowth syndromes. Extensive vascular malformations can be associated with limb overgrowth and other organ involvement in Klippel–Trénauney and Proteus syndromes

- cutis marmorata telangiectatica congenita. Reticulated, vascular lesions on the skin may be associated with asymmetric limb growth (sometimes distant from the skin involvement) and glaucoma
- coagulopathy (Kasabach–Merritt syndrome). This occurs with rare subtypes of haemangioma. Rapid enlargement of the haemangioma accompanies purpura and bleeding, thrombocytopenia and disseminated intravascular coagulation
- Fabry disease. Angiokeratomas (flat or raised, slightly warty, telangiectatic or vascular lesions) appear on the lower trunk, pelvis and thighs. There may be limb pain or paraesthesia, or corneal opacities. Renal, cardiac and central nervous system problems occur later
- fucosidosis. Severely affected children die early. In mild cases, children may present with angiokeratomas and anhidrosis in later childhood. Look for coarse facies, developmental delay and growth retardation
- telangiectasia ataxia. Some degree of ataxia is usually present by the time conjunctival telangiectases are noted.

Lumbosacral birthmarks

Congenital lesions over the lumbosacral area may be associated with occult spinal abnormalities such as a tethered cord. These spinal anomalies may not cause problems until later in childhood when they can present insidiously with irreversible bladder, bowel or limb dysfunction. These problems can be prevented by early magnetic resonance imaging (MRI) screening and surgical correction. Congenital lesions that have been associated with underlying spinal problems include haemangiomas, capillary malformations, lipomas, dimples, sinuses and hairy patches.

Hypopigmented lesions

Generalized hypopigmentation

Generalized hypopigmentation, blonde hair and grey-blue eyes are seen in several genodermatoses involving chromosomes 11 or 15. The clinical presentations vary from mild to complete loss of pigmentation and individuals may go undiagnosed unless compared to their siblings and parents. Early diagnosis and investigation is important to ensure early ophthalmological intervention and rigorous sun protection. Look for:

- poor vision, photophobia and nystagmus. Type 1 oculocutaneous albinism usually results in more severe disease than type 2
- bleeding diathesis, due to a platelet defect in Hermansky–Pudlak syndrome
- recurrent infections in Chédiak–Higashi syndrome
- mental retardation, obesity. Both Angelman and Prader–Willi syndromes can present with albinism.

Localized hypopigmentation

Localized patches of hypopigmented skin or hair may be due to piebaldism, pityriasis versicolor (usually in adolescence), pityriasis alba (usually in mid-childhood), previous inflammation and vitiligo. Also consider:

- endocrinopathies. Vitiligo in children is weakly associated with other endocrine conditions. Children with vitiligo should be reviewed for features of diabetes and thyroid dysfunction
- tuberosclerosis. Hypopigmented patches may be the first sign of tuberosclerosis. These patches can be regular or irregular in shape. An isolated hypopigmented patch in a young child is far more likely to be a simple achromic naevus than to be part of tuberosclerosis, but multiple hypopigmented patches increase the likelihood of tuberosclerosis. Look also for forehead plaques (pink, initially flat but later slightly raised) and shagreen patches (rough, slightly thickened skin, usually over the back). Other skin findings such as periungual fibromas and facial angiofibromas usually appear in older children. The diagnosis of tuberosclerosis may require imaging of eyes, brain, heart and kidneys and investigation of relatives

- streaks, lines and whorls of hyper- or hypopigmentation that may be present from birth. These patterns reflect mosaicism. Usually these children are otherwise normal but a wide range of associated abnormalities in other systems have been reported. Apart from audiological and ophthalmological examination, investigations are not required unless suggested by clinical findings, but these children should be reviewed until settled in school to assess whether any developmental difficulties are present
- leprosy. Focal pale patches may be the only marker of leprosy in an individual from an endemic area.

Hyperpigmented lesions

Generalized hyperpigmentation or skin colour

Generalized darkening of the skin is often most obvious on the palmar creases, linea alba and areola. It is uncommon in childhood. Consider:

- endocrine disease. Addison disease, Cushing syndrome of pituitary origin, exogenous adrenocorticotrophic hormone (ACTH) administration and acromegaly can all cause hyperpigmentation
- renal failure may cause greying of the skin
- haemochromatosis. In children, this is usually secondary to transfusions
- photosensitivity
- lipoidoses. A yellow-brown darkening of skin, most prominent in sun exposed areas, can occur in the Niemann–Pick diseases. Look for waxy indurated skin, purpura, hepatosplenomegaly and neurological deterioration. Although a similar colour can be seen in adult-onset Gaucher disease, it is not a feature of the earlier-onset forms.

Localized hyperpigmentation

Many normal children have one or two well-defined pigmented macules, generally not present at birth but appearing in the early years. In a child with pigmented macular lesions, consider:

- neurofibromatosis. Five or more café au lait spots greater than 0.5 cm in diameter are strong evidence for neurofibromatosis. Examine for other features (axillary 'freckling', pigmented or thickened skin over plexiform neurofibromas, iris pigmentation, optic tumours, skeletal abnormalities, short stature, skin neurofibromas, macrocephaly and learning difficulties). The diagnosis may be uncertain early in life. Regular follow-up is needed, including assessment of intellectual progress. Apart from audiologicalandophthalmologicalexamination,investigations are not required unless suggested by clinical findings

- McCune–Albright syndrome. Macules are often large and may stop at the midline. Look for fibrous dysplasia, sexual precocity and mental retardation
- incontinentia pigmenti. Hyperpigmented streaks may be the presenting feature if the early vesicular/warty phases occurred in utero or were undiagnosed in infancy and then forgotten
- Peutz–Jeghers syndrome. Small pigmented macules present on the lips and mucosa from birth are associated with intestinal polyposis. Care must be taken when assessing any episodes of abdominal pain in these children as they are at higher risk of intussusception and collapse
- naevoid hyperpigmentation (see Localized hypopigmentation, above)
- pellagra. Hyperpigmentation and erythema on sun-exposed areas, cheilitis, perineal inflammation and diarrhoea may be seen.

If areas of hyperpigmentation are roughened, raised, depressed or warty, consider:

- congenital pigmented naevi. Depending on their site and size, infants with congenital pigmented naevi over the posterior scalp or spine may require imaging to look for meningeal involvement, obstructive hydrocephalus, cerebellar malformation or tethered cord
- genodermatoses such as dyskeratosis congenita. Congenital nail dystrophy, pancytopenia, skeletal and eye anomalies may be present
- necrobiosis lipoidica. Atrophic pigmented patches on the lower legs may be the first sign of diabetes in childhood
- acanthosis nigricans. Rough 'dirty' skin on the neck or axillary folds is usually associated with obesity and/or the polycystic ovary syndrome but consider other insulin-resistance syndromes and hypothyroidism. Look for menstrual irregularities and obstructive sleep apnoea. Consider investigation, including liver enzymes and a fasting insulin level to assess for incipient diabetes. If abnormal, perform a formal glucose tolerance test and consider weight-loss strategies and, especially if menstrual irregularities are present, metformin.

Skin texture

Lax, hyperextensible skin is seen in Ehlers–Danlos syndrome. There may be bruising, scarring at sites of minor trauma, joint hyperextensibility and arthritis, and recurrent urinary infections.

Unusually firm skin is an early feature of systemic sclerosis. In children, there is usually widespread skin involvement. Raynaud's phenomenon may be present, and involvement of lungs, heart, kidneys and gastrointestinal tract usually occurs within a few years.

Waxy indurated skin may accompany neurological degeneration and hepatosplenomegaly in type A Niemann–Pick disease.

Anogenital rashes

Common causes of anogenital rashes include irritant napkin dermatitis, seborrhoeic dermatitis and yeast infection. These usually settle rapidly with treatment. More resistant rashes may be due to psoriasis or perianal streptococcal infection, but also consider:

- Langerhans cell histiocytosis. This may present in infancy as a chronic inguinal rash, often erosive and unresponsive to treatment. A scaly, papular eruption on the scalp or trunk may appear (Fig. 21.2.5). Petechiae, purpura, fever, diarrhoea or hepatosplenomegaly may be present
- nutritional deficiencies. Anogenital lesions are an early and prominent manifestation of zinc deficiency. Look for perioral and acral rashes, alopecia, diarrhoea and failure to thrive. Serum zinc levels do not correlate well with body zinc status. Biotin and essential fatty acid deficiency syndromes can give a similar picture
- malabsorption. Both an intractable irritant napkin dermatitis and secondary nutritional deficiencies may contribute to anogenital rashes in malabsorptive conditions
- congenital syphilis. Perianal erosions and moist warty lesions may be seen in early infancy, with erythema on the palms and soles, fever, failure to thrive and hepatosplenomegaly
- HIV can present as severe, erosive napkin dermatitis, which may be secondarily infected
- family factors. Irritant or traumatic anogenital rashes may be seen in circumstances of suboptimal care, emotional abuse or physical abuse.

Hair problems

Hair loss

See Chapter 21.1.

Hypertrichosis

Generalized hypertrichosis (increased hair in all areas) may be an isolated finding or may be related to:

- inherited syndromes, including Hurler and De Lange syndromes
- medications, especially minoxidil, phenytoin and ciclosporin

- gastrointestinal disease, including coeliac disease
- hypothyroidism
- porphyria; look for photosensitivity and blisters.

Hirsutism

Increased pubic or axillary hair in young children may be due to adrenal, gonadal or central nervous system disease and requires investigation. Hirsutism in adolescent females may be an isolated finding or may be seen with obesity and amenorrhea in polycystic ovary syndrome. Cushing syndrome, mild congenital adrenal hyperplasia, virilizing adrenal and ovarian tumours and thyroid dysfunction may cause hirsutism.

PART 22

ENT, EYE AND DENTAL DISORDERS

Ear, nose and throat, and head and neck surgery problems

B. Benjamin

Paediatric ear, nose and throat (ENT) disorders cover a wide field of congenital and acquired diseases of the ear, nose and paranasal sinuses, oral cavity, tongue, pharynx, larynx, tracheobronchial tree and oesophagus. They include craniofacial abnormalities, tumours and cysts of the head and neck, deafness and speech, language and communication problems. This section covers the common disorders.

The ear

The external auditory canal and the tympanic membrane are usually inspected (if necessary and if possible after removal of wax) using a handheld, battery-operated otoscope or a Seigle magnifying pneumatic speculum. An ENT specialist uses a slim, short telescope or a microscope for more detailed examination.

The external ear

Congenital abnormalities

Differences in the shape of the pinna are common – small ears, large ears, accessory skin tags and unusual configuration of the helix and antihelix – but usually no treatment is needed except for unsightly protruding ears, which can be corrected surgically. Major abnormalities of the external canal such as stenosis or atresia are sometimes associated with small, malformed pinnae, abnormalities of the ossicles and possibly hypoplastic inner ear abnormalities with consequent major hearing problems. When these anomalies affect both ears, hearing aids or reconstructive surgical procedures may be necessary.

Otitis externa

Swimming in contaminated or heavily chlorinated water predisposes the delicate skin lining the ear canal to infection with bacteria or fungi. Otitis externa causes itch, soreness, discharge and partial deafness. Treatment includes removal of debris by swabbing and/or syringing followed by careful drying and regular administration of appropriate antibiotic/steroid drops. Water in the ear should be avoided.

Severe pain and exquisite tenderness indicate acute localized or acute diffuse infection requiring systemic antibiotics, especially when there is surrounding cellulitis, lymphadenitis or generalized toxicity. ENT referral and hospitalization may be required in severe or intractable cases.

Wax

Black, brown, yellow or pale wax is a mixture of sebaceous material and ceruminous gland secretion combined with desquamated epithelium. Although normally removed by the self-cleaning chewing movement of the temporomandibular joint and evaporation, wax occasionally accumulates to occlude the canal, causing a hearing loss and a sensation of blockage. Obsessive parental attempts to 'clean' normal wax with cotton buds or a matchstick or repeated daily insertion of a hearing aid mould may cause impaction of the wax, requiring removal by syringing or use of special blunt probes and suction by an ENT specialist. Sometimes, in obstinate cases, wax must be removed under general anaesthesia with the aid of an operating microscope.

Foreign bodies

Foreign bodies such as beads, pips, pieces of paper, insects, etc. sometimes become lodged in the external auditory canal where they cause discomfort, pain and partial deafness. Occasionally they are discovered by chance. If attempts at careful extraction using a syringe or small grasping forceps are unsuccessful in a young or fractious child, referral to a specialist is indicated for removal, if necessary under general anaesthesia. Rough or ill-judged attempts at removal may cause damage to the tympanic membrane or the middle ear ossicles.

Injury of the tympanic membrane

Indirect trauma such as a slap or blow to the ear, a blast injury or impact with water can compress the column of air in the ear canal and rupture the tympanic membrane. Direct trauma may be caused by a cotton bud, hairpin or an incorrect syringing technique. There is pain, bleeding, deafness and some initial unsteadiness. On inspection, bleeding or a tear may be visible. The ear should not be cleaned and no drops should be given. Antibiotics are usually given to prevent infection. Almost all traumatic injuries will heal within a month or two: if not, a graft may eventually be necessary.

The middle ear

This air-containing, irregularly shaped, bony cavity is lined by mucous membrane and includes the mastoid air cells posteriorly and the eustachian tube anteromedially. The latter opens and closes on swallowing, yawning and blowing the nose and has an active mucociliary lining to cleanse, ventilate and maintain air pressure in the middle ear. Motion of the tympanic membrane and the lever action of the three small, articulated ossicles create an efficient transducer mechanism to transfer sound energy at the air–water interface. As the footplate of the stapes moves rapidly in the oval window, vibrations in air become wave motion in the perilymph fluid of the inner ear.

Acute suppurative otitis media

Acute suppurative otitis media (ASOM) is due to infection of part or all of the mucoperiosteum that lines the spaces of the middle ear. The diagnosis can be verified only by examination of the tympanic membrane.

It is much more common in infants and children than in adults, with a peak incidence under 2 years of age and again between 5 and 7 years. It is more common in winter and where there is overcrowding and malnutrition. About 50% of children will have experienced an attack before the age of 2 years and about 75% by the age of 3 years. This high incidence is apparently due to an immature immune response and increased frequency of upper respiratory tract infections in this age group. The overall incidence is also much higher in Aboriginal children in Australia.

Many factors predispose to middle ear infection:

- pre-existing middle ear effusion or 'glue ear'
- infants and small children have a short, wide, straight eustachian tube, the dynamic protective function of which is less effective in minimizing middle ear contamination from the nasopharynx than the mature adult eustachian tube
- nasopharyngeal disease, such as seen with acute or chronic upper respiratory tract infection, enlarged

infected adenoids and (to a lesser extent) tonsils or rhinosinusitis can act as a focus of infection
- coexistent chronic middle ear disease such as chronic otitis media or a pre-existing tympanic membrane perforation
- cleft palate or repaired cleft palate or other rarer craniofacial structural abnormality affects the normal opening by the palate muscles and the normal closure by the spring action of the cartilaginous portion of the eustachian tube
- contamination of the nasopharynx in babies being bottlefed in the recumbent position or in infants who are vomiting
- attendance at preschool or kindergarten with exposure to pathogens
- parental cigarette smoking
- deficiency of surface-tension-lowering substance, surfactant, in the tube
- abnormality of mucociliary action affecting the normal cleansing mechanism
- immunodeficiency syndromes.

In ASOM, the pathological sequence of events in the air spaces and mucosa of the middle ear proceeds rapidly with oedema, hyperaemia and exudate into the middle ear, more often than not following a head cold or upper respiratory tract infection. Inflammatory swelling occludes the eustachian tube. The serous fluid becomes purulent after secondary bacterial infection and causes bulging of the pain-sensitive tympanic membrane. The body's natural defences, with or without assistance from antibiotics, usually achieve resolution. If not, the tympanic membrane continues to bulge, forming an area of ischaemic necrosis that ultimately ruptures.

The microbiology of ASOM primarily involves bacteria but in 5–10% viruses may play a role, usually paving the way for secondary bacterial invasion. Common organisms include *Streptococcus pneumoniae*, *Streptococcus pyogenes*, *Branhamella catarrhalis*, *Haemophilus influenzae* (especially in younger children), *Staphylococcus aureus* and some Gram-negative or mixed infections. About 30–40% of aspirates will yield no pathogen.

The clinical features of ASOM vary with the age of the child, the efficiency of the host defence and the effectiveness of treatment. Severe, throbbing pain in one or both ears is the commonest feature. There may be minor earache for an hour or two or a fulminating febrile illness with acute pain. These symptoms are often worse in the evening or at night when the child is lying down. Infants may present with fever, attempts to pull at the affected ear, irritability, vomiting and abdominal pain. Rupture of the tympanic membrane, with bloodstained then purulent discharge, relieves the pain and allows a culture and sensitivity to be obtained. If perforation occurs it usually heals within a few weeks.

The diagnosis is confirmed by the appearance of the tympanic membrane. However, many sick, irritable infants and smaller children are difficult, if not impossible, to examine, so in some cases a clinical diagnosis is made and treatment is commenced without visualization of the tympanic membrane.

The progression of ASOM can be divided into four stages:

1. Eustachian tube obstruction with a stuffy, blocked feeling of discomfort in the ear and a slightly retracted, pink tympanic membrane
2. Early infection with increasing earache, fever, and redness due to some mucoid or purulent material behind the tympanic membrane
3. Suppurative stage with severe local pain, constitutional symptoms and purulent exudate under pressure, leading to bulging of the tympanic membrane, which develops a yellowish colour with ischaemic necrosis prior to rupture
4. Resolution stage with dramatic lessening of pain and improvement of the tympanic membrane.

Treatment usually requires bed rest, adequate fluid intake, antipyretics and sufficient analgesic medication. Sometimes local warmth is helpful.

Although there is discussion about whether antibiotics are given too freely, many experienced physicians believe that antibiotics limit the disease, control pain and minimize possible complications. Others suggest that antibiotics should be withheld in nonsevere cases pending further observation and given to those not recovering in 24–48 hours. It is generally agreed that children under 2 years of age should be treated with antibiotics rather than adopting a wait and see policy.

As a first-line treatment amoxicillin for 5–10 days is the drug of choice and is generally well tolerated. Erythromycin, sulfamethoxazole–trimethoprim or cefaclor are alternatives. Very occasionally a resistant or complicated infection requires myringotomy. Severe, otherwise uncontrolled infections require intravenous treatment in hospital.

There are no data to support the use of decongestants or antihistamines: in fact there is some evidence that they may be harmful. Topical antibiotic drops have no place in the treatment of acute suppurative otitis media.

The untoward sequelae of otitis media include:

• incomplete resolution with persistence of effusion ('glue ear')
• rarely, a ruptured tympanic membrane that will not heal. The chronic perforation will require grafting

• acute mastoiditis or its complications, which are still seen despite the use of antibiotics and usually present as a subperiosteal abscess behind the ear
• labyrinthitis with severe vertigo and vomiting
• intracranial complications, including lateral venous sinus thrombosis, extradural or subdural abscess, meningitis, cortical thrombophlebitis and intracerebral or intracerebellar abscess.

Remember that otitis media has not been 'cured' until both the appearance of the tympanic membrane and the hearing have returned to normal. The recently introduced universal pneumococcal immunization programme in Australia may be helpful in preventing recurrent ASOM, particularly for children attending day school.

Clinical example

Emma, aged 3 years 8 months, complained of a 'sore' ear late in the afternoon, refused her dinner and later developed distressing pain and a fever of 39.4°C. The family doctor found a crying, upset, vomiting child and an agitated mother. Otoscopy showed a red, bulging tympanic membrane on the left and a thickened, pink membrane on the right. The advice was bed rest, fluids as tolerated, paracetamol, amoxicillin and a progress examination next day.

Note that acute suppurative otitis media causes severe pain, often worse in the evening. Both ears and the upper respiratory tract must be examined.

Glue ear or otitis media with effusion

A confusion of names have been applied to 'glue ear' but otitis media with effusion (OME) or secretory otitis media are those used most often. It is a common cause of repeated earaches, fluctuating mild to moderate conduction deafness and educational impairment.

The aetiology is uncertain but the ventilation, drainage and clearing mechanism of the eustachian tube is abnormal. Organisms similar to those found in ASOM can be cultured in 30–50% of cases – the effusion apparently follows incomplete resolution of ASOM. A mucoid, non-purulent effusion, containing leukocytes, dead or live bacteria, serum protein and mucus, accumulates in the middle ear. The effusion may be thin, thick, gelatinous or, in advanced cases, even 'rubbery'.

The middle ear mucosa becomes oedematous and granular in appearance. Microscopically, the goblet cells and mucous glands increase dramatically in number and small cysts filled with watery or inspissated mucus can be seen in the thickened sub-epithelial layer, which is infiltrated by chronic inflammatory cells. It is now believed that biofilm (a blanket of bacteria in a very low metabolic state and enclosed in a polymeric matrix) in the middle ear may be a contributing factor in otitis media with effusion.

The clinical features of OME are common up to 8–10 years of age, are usually seen first in winter and are sometimes variable and unpredictable. Symptoms often follow a viral upper respiratory tract infection or incompletely resolved ASOM. Because at first there may be no symptoms the condition may remain unrecognized. Earache and deafness are the two important features.

Earache presents in two ways. Firstly, as a flare-up during an acute respiratory infection there may be typical ASOM with severe pain. Secondly, repeated 'small' earaches, lasting for minutes rather than hours, may wake the child at night or occur at school and settle quickly.

Deafness is often suspected by the parents or teacher or may be discovered at a routine screening hearing test. School performance is often affected: 'doesn't pay attention', 'can do better' or 'not concentrating' are frequent remarks. Non-specific symptoms include poor school achievement, decreased learning skills, interference with language development, an adverse affect on emotional growth, irritability and personality changes. The child may be at an educational disadvantage. A few children become clumsy if their balance is mildly affected. Infants may be irritable, crying or constantly unsettled at night.

Recognition of physical signs in the tympanic membrane is often difficult for the inexperienced: a good pneumatic otoscope with magnification is invaluable. The common physical signs include:

- yellow or amber appearance of the tympanic membrane
- vascular dilatation, which is easier to see with magnification
- thickening and dullness of the tympanic membrane
- indrawing of the tympanic membrane, giving a concave appearance so that the handle of the malleus appears short
- in advanced cases there may be atelectasis in the middle ear with atrophy and thinning of the tympanic membrane.

Sluggish or poor movement of the tympanic membrane detected using a pneumatic otoscope is a most important physical sign. The thicker the fluid, the less the 'bounce'. In children old enough to perform a pure tone audiogram (Fig. 22.1.1) a mild to moderate conduction deafness will be detected. Impedance

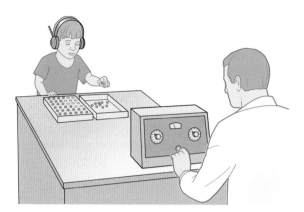

Fig. 22.1.1 Pure tone audiometry at 3–4 years of age. The child drops a coloured bead into the box when a sound is heard. A reasonably reliable pure tone audiogram can be obtained.

tympanometry tests the bounce of the tympanic membrane and typically shows a 'flat' curve.

In many children OME will resolve without treatment over weeks or months. However, referral for specialist assessment is indicated:

- when infants and toddlers are persistently irritable, sleep poorly at night and rub or pull at their ears
- when older children have repeated earaches and/ or persistent hearing loss.

There is no evidence that antibiotics, antihistamines, decongestants, mucolytics or antiallergy treatment have any significant beneficial effect.

In some cases, after adequate observation indicates that the effusion has been present for 3 months or more, myringotomy, suction removal of the fluid and insertion of tympanostomy tubes for middle ear ventilation/drainage is indicated. The tube remains in the tympanic membrane, functioning as a 'temporary' artificial eustachian tube providing sustained middle ear ventilation, discouraging recurrent effusions and promoting recovery, usually without any complications. The tube is extruded through natural mechanisms after 6–12 months but the effusion can recur. Insertion of the tubes may need to be repeated if the symptoms warrant it. In some children, predisposing causes such as infection and hypertrophy of the adenoids or upper respiratory tract mucosal disease or rhinosinusitis need treatment.

If untreated, the long-term irreversible complications of OME include atrophic thinning of the tympanic membrane, atelectasis of the middle ear space, damage to the middle ear mucosa, adhesive otitis media, retraction pockets, avascular necrosis of the incus and stapes, tympanosclerosis, cholesteatoma and cholesterol granuloma.

Clinical example

John's mother was called to his school because he complained of earache and the teacher observed that he was not hearing well. She stated that her 6-year-old son had suffered four attacks of 'ear abscess' in the last 10 months. On examination, both tympanic membranes were dull and dilated vessels were seen to be running in a radial fashion. The tympanogram was 'flat'. Referral to an ENT surgeon for treatment of glue ears was arranged. In fact, John had probably had otitis media with effusions (OME) for 10 months. Parents may be unaware of the hearing loss in OME. Variable deafness and ear infections almost always indicate OME.

Practical points

Possible sequelae of acute suppurative otitis media are:
- Complete resolution
- Residual 'glue ear' and minor deafness
- Acute mastoiditis or a complication of mastoiditis
- 'Masked mastoiditis'
- Open chronic perforation

Chronic suppurative otitis media

In this condition the tympanic membrane is perforated. The patient complains of partial deafness and painless, recurrent or persistent discharge.

There are two types of chronic suppurative otitis media (CSOM):

- mucoperiosteal disease with a central perforation from pinhole size up to complete destruction of the tympanic membrane. The basic middle ear disease is chronic, persistent or intermittent infection with a purulent, sometimes profuse, discharge due to infection of the mucoperiosteum of the middle ear space. For this reason it is often called tubotympanic disease. Because complications are rare this is known as a 'safe' ear. A clean, dry, chronic, central perforation, whether large or small, is suitable for tympanoplasty, using fascia or perichondrium, usually waiting until the child is 7–8 years old. Grafting is successful in about 95%, prevents recurrent infections causing further damage, restores hearing and allows swimming without the risk of infection
- bony disease with a small marginal perforation at the superior bony edge of the tympanic membrane is usually associated with cholesteatoma and chronic, often smelly discharge. Complications are likely; hence this is an 'unsafe' ear.

A cholesteatoma is not a tumour but is a very slowly enlarging, pearl-like pocket of misplaced squamous epithelium accompanied by enzymatic destruction of the surrounding bone and ossicles. It is sometimes called atticoantral disease because of its position high in the middle ear.

Mucoperiosteal infection is usually controlled by repeated dry mopping or suction cleaning of the ear and use of appropriate topical antibiotic drops. Water must not get into the ear. The common organisms are *Pseudomonas aeruginosa*, *Bacillus proteus* and *Escherichia coli*. Therefore a chronic or intermittently discharging ear must not be neglected. Cholesteatoma and bony disease usually requires surgical mastoidectomy to remove the disease, combined with tympanoplasty to repair the tympanic membrane and reconstruct the ossicular chain to preserve hearing.

The complications of cholesteatoma include erosion and destruction of the ossicles, osteitis, petrositis, mastoiditis, labyrinthitis, facial nerve paralysis, thrombosis of the sigmoid venous sinus, meningitis, extradural, subdural or cerebral abscess and septicaemia. Some of these complications are life threatening.

Deafness

The accurate assessment of the type, degree and cause of deafness is essential for optimum treatment.

The type of hearing loss is usually described according to the site of pathology:

- '*Conductive*' deafness. Sound vibrations are not conducted normally via the ear canal (for example, obstructing wax), the tympanic membrane (for example, perforation) or the ossicles (e.g. congenital malformation). Conduction deafness is usually treatable
- '*Sensorineural*' deafness. There is malfunction of the sensory (cochlear) components (for example, rubella deafness) or the neural (retrocochlear) components (e.g. acoustic neuroma). Sensorineural deafness is often congenital, may be acquired and cannot be cured. If severe enough, sensorineural deafness requires a hearing aid for amplification, or consideration for cochlear implant.

Universal newborn screening for deafness. Language and communication will ultimately be better when deafness is identified early so that a hearing aid and a support programme can be provided. However, it has been difficult to assess the hearing of small children with the traditional informal and special testing techniques (described below) which require a child to be old enough for some cooperation. It is now hoped that universal hearing screening tests which are being introduced for the newborn in Australia will detect most congenital deafness.

When a sound is heard by the ear a tiny corresponding 'echo' can be measured by a computer using a small probe placed in a baby's ear canal – the basis for a non-invasive screening technique called oto-acoustic emissions (OAE) testing. Because the test takes only a few minutes and does not rely on the participation of the baby it is suitable for newborn hearing screening. If the initial result is unreliable, for example if the baby is restless or irritable, further evaluation is necessary. A small number of babies will need referral for auditory brainstem response tests (see below), which can give more reliable information about the hearing

Certain 'at risk' criteria can be used to select babies, all of whom should have hearing screening tests soon after birth, usually before leaving hospital, including those with a family history of deafness, craniofacial abnormalities, exposure to ototoxic drugs and those who needed more than 48 hours in a neonatal intensive care unit.

In infants with deafness not detected by screening tests or those developing deafness after the newborn period hearing loss is commonly suspected by the child's mother (Fig. 22.1.2). The degree of loss is assessed by informal and special audiological methods according to age:

- in infants days or weeks old, the normal but non-quantitative response to a sudden loud sound is the 'blink' or 'startle' reaction (Fig. 22.1.3). This test is best done with the infant lightly asleep. However, the universal screening programmes using OAE above will, when fully introduced, be a better form of testing
- in special units, computerized electrophysiological tests are available to record small electrical changes evoked in the inner ear during transmission of acoustic signals. An accurate measure of function in the brainstem and the ear can be provided by electrocochleography and auditory brainstem tests in infants and children, including those with behavioural problems or multiple handicaps
- in babies from 4 months of age, normal head turning responses (Fig. 22.1.4) are elicited towards the side of a sound stimulus, which can be varied from a soft whisper to the jingle of keys or the crumple of paper. An approximate, clinical quantitative estimate of hearing can be obtained
- older toddlers can be assessed in specialized paediatric units by behavioural methods, observing the child's reaction to ambient sounds or by conditioning them to respond to a puppet or peep show – known as condition-oriented response (COR) audiometry

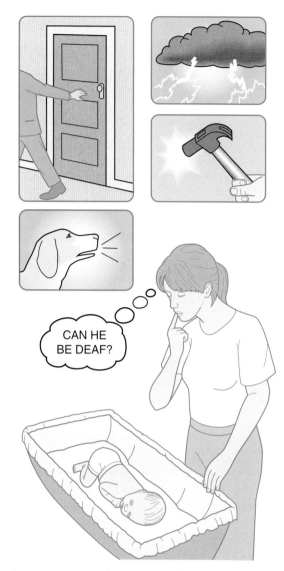

Fig. 22.1.2 Parents often suspect deafness if the baby consistently fails to respond to loud sounds and 'sleeps peacefully'. Their suspicion of deafness should be investigated.

- children of 3 or 4 years of age or older can usually cooperate so that a quantitative pure tone threshold audiogram (Fig. 22.1.1) can be obtained for different frequencies for both air conduction and bone conduction.

The cause of deafness determines the need for treatment. The many causes of conduction deafness each need specific attention, e.g.:

- removal of wax
- operation for congenital external ear canal atresia
- myringoplasty for tympanic membrane perforation
- ventilating tube for persistent otitis media with effusion

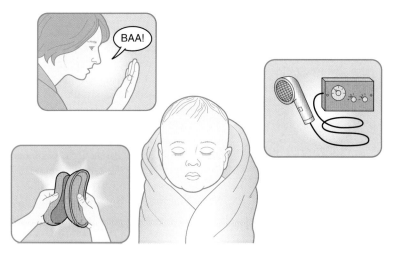

Fig. 22.1.3 There are a number of tests for screening the hearing of newborn babies. The normal response to a sudden loud sound (80–90 dB) is a 'blink' or 'startle' reaction. This test is best done with the infant lightly asleep.

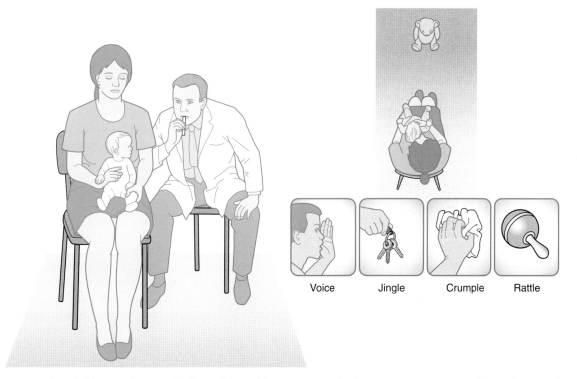

| Voice | Jingle | Crumple | Rattle |

Fig. 22.1.4 Most babies over the age of 4–5 months are able to turn to a noise from an unseen source, so that each ear can be tested. The intensity of the sound may be varied to estimate the level at which response occurs.

- reconstruction of congenital ossicular chain abnormality.

Approximately 1 baby in 1000 is born with severe deafness, and approximately 1 in 1000 infants become deaf before they have developed speech. In many cases the cause of sensorineural deafness is difficult to determine. The known causes can be considered in four groups, as below.

Prenatal hereditary deafness

This is transmitted by a dominant gene in 10%. If one parent carries the gene, up to 50% of children will be affected. There is a recessive gene in 90%, and in this situation both parents must carry the gene and 25% of children will be affected. Consanguinity increases recessive transmission. There is, therefore, sometimes a positive family history of deafness.

There are many hereditary syndromes with hearing loss as a feature. Some examples include:

- Waardenburg syndrome – epicanthic folds, different-coloured irises, white forelock
- Usher syndrome – retinitis pigmentosa, epilepsy
- Pendred syndrome – sporadic thyroid disease
- Alport syndrome – progressive renal disease
- Hurler syndrome – gargoylism
- Fanconi syndrome – anaemia, skin pigmentation, skeletal deformities, mental retardation.

Prenatal acquired deafness

Damage in the first trimester can affect the developing cochlea. Detailed radiological imaging will define the Michel deformity, which is total absence, and the Mondini deformity, which is partial maldevelopment of the bony cochlea. The Scheibe deformity has a normal bony cochlea but damaged hair cells in the organ of Corti. Causes of prenatal acquired deafness include maternal infection such as rubella, cytomegalovirus, toxoplasmosis, herpes and congenital syphilis. Drugs that are ototoxic to the embryo include aminoglycosides, loop diuretics, quinine and thalidomide.

Perinatal acquired deafness

Causes include prematurity, prolonged or difficult labour, hypoxia, Rhesus incompatibility, kernicterus, ototoxins, infectious diseases and others.

Deafness in infancy and childhood

The common causes of acquired deafness at this age are mumps, measles, meningitis, traumatic fracture of the petrous bone through the inner ear or acoustic nerve, and patent cochlear aqueduct. Fortunately in these cases, if only one ear is affected, the handicap is not as devastating as with bilateral deafness.

Treatment of sensorineural deafness

Most deaf children have normal intellectual capacity and some usable residual inner ear function. The diagnosis must be made early and the child fitted with hearing aids or be considered for a cochlear implant. He or she should receive early and continued auditory training. Many such deaf children learn to understand the spoken word, to develop intelligible speech and play an active role in society. However, the hearing of speech sounds does not guarantee normal understanding, as amplification may be accompanied by distortion and decreased intelligibility. Thus general practitioners, paediatricians and otologists have an enormous responsibility to take the mother's suspicion of deafness seriously and arrange prompt investigation and assessment. Early diagnosis is the key to optimal outcome.

A geneticist should give advice to parents who have had a deaf child and who want to know the chances of having another – is the problem dominant deafness or recessive? The ability to identify previously undiagnosed cases of hereditary deafness on the basis of specific genetic testing has improved. DNA-based testing is available for the diagnosis of mutations that cause deafness, often those in the *GJB2* gene which encodes the protein connexin 26. Up to 50% of those with non-syndromic deafness have mutations in the gap junction protein beta-2 gene.

The nose

Congenital conditions

Many congenital anomalies affect the nasal structures:

- craniofacial and external nasal malformations
- cleft lip, palate and face clefts
- haemangioma and vascular malformations
- dermoid, encephalocele, nasolacrimal duct cyst and other rare masses
- bilateral congenital choanal atresia poses the greatest threat to life because neonates, being obligate nose breathers, develop increasing cyanosis and even fatal asphyxia when their nasal airways are completely obstructed. However, if the baby cries and takes a breath through the mouth the obstruction is momentarily relieved until the mouth closes. Choanal atresia can be confirmed by failure to pass a 3 mm diameter plastic catheter through the nose into the oropharynx. The airway can be maintained using a Guedel oral airway or an endotracheal tube pending computed tomography (CT) assessment and surgical correction
- unilateral choanal atresia presents as persistent glairy discharge later in life.

Acute rhinosinusitis

Acute infective rhinosinusitis presents with purulent nasal discharge, nasal obstruction, pain and tenderness over the involved sinuses, and general malaise. The acute episode often follows an upper respiratory tract infection, swimming or diving and usually affects the maxillary sinuses, and in older children the ethmoid sinuses. Plain X-rays and CT are required only in difficult cases. Treatment is symptomatic, using decongestant nasal drops or oral decongestants and paracetamol. Antibiotics are given in severe, persistent, recurrent or complicated cases. Amoxicillin for 7–10 days to cover the common upper respiratory tract pathogens is the drug of first choice. In penicillin-hypersensitive patients use cefaclor, erythromycin or doxycycline (not in children under 8 years).

Infective rhinosinusitis in infants and children usually responds to medical treatment. Surgical drainage may be necessary for chronic disease or for acute complications such as subperiosteal abscess, periorbital cellulitis, osteomyelitis or intracranial spread.

Chronic rhinosinusitis

Chronic rhinitis often has an allergic basis, with secondary bacterial infection being common. In younger children it is aggravated by, or inseparable from, hypertrophy and infection of the adenoids. Swollen turbinates cause intermittent or persistent nasal stuffiness and catarrhal discharge. Therapy with antihistamines and pseudoephedrine may be helpful but symptoms are more often controlled with regular use of intranasal metered aerosol steroid spray. Nasal allergy, often with hay fever or asthma, may be traced to specific allergens, which should be avoided where possible. Desensitization can be considered in older children. In severe, persistent cases cautery, laser or surgical reduction of the inferior turbinates may provide substantial relief. Nasal polyps in children strongly suggest cystic fibrosis.

Nasopharyngeal tumours and cysts

Antrochoanal polyp, dermoid cyst, meningoencephalocele, glioma and chordoma are rare benign conditions. Nasopharyngeal angiofibroma is an uncommon locally destructive, non-metastasizing very vascular tumour occurring mostly in adolescent boys. It usually presents as frequent, often severe, epistaxes and nasal obstruction. Treatment is surgical removal after embolization of the feeding vessels, although some advocate radical radiotherapy. Rhabdomyosarcoma or lymphosarcoma are rare malignant nasopharyngeal tumours.

Trauma

Fracture or dislocation deformity of the external nose and nasal septum sometimes occurs during a difficult birth or after forceps delivery. The degree of displacement and nasal obstruction are occasionally severe enough to require correction in the neonatal period. Injuries of the nose, nasal bones and nasal septum occur commonly when toddlers fall during vigorous play and in older children during contact sports. Depressed, displaced nasal bones require correction within 10 days. Haematomas of the nasal septum should be drained and treated with antibiotics to minimize development of a septal abscess, which destroys cartilage and can lead to a saddle nose deformity.

Foreign bodies

Unilateral purulent, sometimes bloodstained nasal discharge in a young child suggests the presence of a foreign body, such as a bead, eraser, piece of vegetable or other material, until proven otherwise. Unreactive inorganic objects may remain undetected for months or years. The most dangerous foreign body is an alkaline battery, which emits a small current and leaks its caustic contents, rapidly causing local tissue necrosis; it must be treated as an emergency. Removal may require general anaesthesia.

Epistaxis

Bleeding from a prominent vessel on the anterior nasal septum (Little's area) is common and is sometimes frightening for parents. It may be aggravated by accidental trauma, nose picking, nose blowing and infection. Occasionally epistaxis may be the presentation of a blood dyscrasia or a nasopharyngeal angiofibroma. First aid is to apply constant pressure to the side of the nose with a cold face cloth for at least 5 minutes. Packing with ribbon gauze controls many persistent cases. If the bleeding continues and the vessel can be identified, it can be thermally or chemically cauterized using topical anaesthesia in older cooperative children or under general anaesthesia in others.

Clinical example

Benjamin, aged 9, was struck on the nose by the seat of a swing while he was playing in the park. His nose bled, appeared 'crooked' and became swollen. He was taken to the casualty department, where the ENT registrar confirmed traumatic fracture of the nasal bones by clinical examination. Corrective surgery was arranged for later in the week.

Bruising and swelling will rapidly hide the deformity. Careful palpation usually confirms the displacement without the need for X-ray.

The oropharynx

Acute sore throat (AST) in children is a common problem. The illness can be due to viral, bacterial, fungal or other infectious microorganisms or of unknown aetiology. Most children have a cold and nothing more and are better in less than a week. A number of questions arise. Is the infection due to a respiratory virus or to a bacterial infection? Is a throat swab useful? Are antibiotics justified? Is the sore throat a manifestation of a more serious systemic disease? Is admission to hospital necessary?

Arbitrary division of the acute infectious process into the descriptive 'diagnostic' categories rhinitis, nasopharyngitis, stomatitis, pharyngitis and tonsillitis is somewhat unsatisfactory because the inflammation often extends to overlap nearby areas. Nevertheless, the majority of patients with an acute sore throat can be described as having either acute 'pharyngitis' or 'tonsillitis'.

Inflammation is widespread in the mucous membrane in 'pharyngitis' which can be caused by one of many viruses, whereas in more localized 'tonsillitis' the pathogen is usually either group A beta-haemolytic streptococcus (*S. pyogenes*) or a virus – adenovirus, Epstein–Barr virus (EBV) or Coxsackie A virus. The differentiation of bacterial from viral infection on clinical grounds is far from easy – often no more than an educated guess – because, for the most part, the symptoms and local signs accompanying AST correlate poorly with the presumed (or later proven) aetiological microorganism. Most acute upper respiratory tract infections that cause sore throat, fever and swallowing discomfort last 3–6 days, are viral and are mild in severity. They seldom warrant antibiotic treatment.

In approximately 50% of patients with acute sore throat beta-haemolytic streptococci can be isolated by surface throat culture; it seems reasonable to assume a cause and effect relationship. In fact this organism is more likely to be pathogenic when there are also local clinical findings of intense cellulitis of the uvula and soft palate and haemorrhagic palatal petechiae. Remember that 10–20% of otherwise normal children may be carriers of beta-haemolytic streptococci.

What, then, is acute tonsillitis? Acute tonsillitis has been defined clinically as a condition in which not only is inflammation mostly confined to the tonsils but the clinical features also include acute sore throat, fever, difficulty in swallowing, enlarged tender regional cervical lymph nodes, halitosis and constitutional symptoms such as lethargy, nausea and vomiting. Sometimes there is abdominal pain.

Examination can show various appearances in tonsillitis:

- red mucosa over the tonsils and oedematous, generalized inflammation (parenchymatous tonsillitis)
- yellowish-white exudate in the crypts of the tonsils (follicular tonsillitis)
- the crypts become filled with 'debris', an exudate of desquamated epithelium and pus
- coalescence of these follicles can form a thin, white, non-confluent, patchy membrane that peels away without bleeding (membranous tonsillitis)
- the typical redness, oedema and purulent secretion (exudative tonsillitis). Note that this appearance is not necessarily diagnostic of streptococcal infection.

Acute sore throat is one of the commonest complaints seen in general practice. It is occasionally a manifestation of a serious systemic disease. A useful classification of causes includes:

- acute viral pharyngitis. Examples are coryza, influenza, parainfluenza, the viral exanthemas and infections with Coxsackie viruses (herpangina), the ECHO virus group and many others. Coryza (common cold, viral nasopharyngitis, viral catarrh) is usually caused by rhinoviruses and coronaviruses in winter and spring and by enteroviruses in summer and autumn and at other times by other viruses. Coryza is highly infectious. There is an initial burning sensation above the palate, then sore throat, which is generally not severe, minimal fever, stuffy nose, rhinorrhoea and conjunctivitis. It usually resolves in 4–5 days. Complications include acute sinusitis, otitis media and lower respiratory tract infections
- acute bacterial tonsillitis, often due to beta-haemolytic streptococci but occasionally to other bacterial organisms in immunocompromised patients. It seems also that adenoviruses and Epstein–Barr viruses may lie dormant in tonsils for years and can be activated by non-specific environmental factors such as fever, chilling and stress
- infectious mononucleosis (glandular fever), caused by the Epstein–Barr virus, has many manifestations. Acute sore throat is consistently a prominent feature
- thrush, due to *Candida albicans* and predisposed to by diabetes, general debility, immunosuppression, nutritional deficiency and disturbances in the normal flora due to prolonged administration of antimicrobial agents. There is a wide range of appearances but characteristically there are white, curd-like, adherent patches overlying inflamed mucosa on the gingival surfaces

- Vincent angina (also known as ulceromembranous gingivostomatitis), caused by a combination of the normal spirochaetes of the mouth and mixed anaerobic bacteria often in injured necrotic tissue of the gums, which provides the necessary anaerobic environment
- diphtheria is now uncommon yet it remains a potentially lethal acute infection, caused by *Corynebacterium diphtheriae*, which produces a powerful exotoxin. A sore throat is part of the much more serious systemic toxic illness
- aphthous stomatitis. The cause is unknown. These recurrent, non-infective, well demarcated, painful ulcers have an erythematous border and are usually in the anterior part of the oral cavity on the mucosa of the lips, mouth and gingivae and the borders of the tongue, but when they occur in the soft palate or the fauces the patient complains of sore throat
- patients with acute leukaemia, agranulocytosis, aplastic anaemia or HIV infection may present with an acute sore throat.

Approximately 50% of cases of acute sore throat are eventually proved to be bacterial. Pending the result of culture it would seem prudent to immediately treat with an antibiotic those children who are extremely ill or toxic, and to await the result of culture in other children.

Examination of the mouth and throat

Older children are examined sitting up in a chair or on a bed and younger children sitting on mother's lap or lying on the bed. It may be helpful to have an assistant steady the head. A torch with a bright light and a wooden tongue depressor is usually used but, where available, a headlight and an angled metal tongue depressor will provide a better view of the oropharynx. The lips, buccal mucosa, teeth and gums, floor of the mouth and the tongue are examined and then the palate, tonsils and posterior pharyngeal wall.

In severely ill children, brief examination of the oropharynx will eliminate grossly enlarged tonsils, peritonsillar abscess, retropharyngeal abscess and the rare case of diphtheria. In suspected acute epiglottitis care must be taken not to worsen airway obstruction, and the oropharynx should only be examined under expert controlled conditions if epiglottitis is a significant possibility.

Throat swab and rapid antigen testing

Pharyngitis caused by adenoviruses or herpes simplex is generally indistinguishable from that caused by *S. pyogenes*. Viral studies are rarely helpful. The only way to confirm a bacterial infection and justify treatment is to identify the streptococcal organism using a rapid antigen test or to take a throat swab, if facilities for culture and laboratory identification are available. Although not diagnostic, at times a Gram stain for tentative identification would be a reasonable basis for the commencement of antibiotic therapy. Identification of *S. pyogenes* allows logical use of an antibiotic for those few who are judged to be unduly ill or those 'at risk' (see below under Antibiotics) and as a valuable reference in a patient who may later be suspected of having rheumatic fever.

Although seldom used, rapid immunological tests employ antiserum against group A streptococcal antigen. Streptococci obtained from a throat swab by chemical or enzymatic extraction are tested for agglutination using antibodies to group A *Streptococcus*. Such tests are reasonably accurate but the false-negative rate can be up to 30% – then a throat swab may be necessary.

A throat swab should preferably be taken before any antibiotics are given. Technique is important – with adequate exposure and illumination, sterile cotton wool swabs are rubbed vigorously on the areas of inflammation or exudate on the tonsils and posterior pharyngeal wall and put directly into a sterile container. Because the throat is normally colonized by many organisms, laboratory tests taking 24–48 hours are done to single out and identify the group A beta-haemolytic streptococcus. Remember, if diphtheria is a possibility the laboratory should be contacted as special tests are necessary.

Antibiotics

The difficult dilemma is that, although it might often seem reasonable to give antibiotics to a sick child with a sore throat, available evidence does not support their administration whether the infection is streptococcal or viral. When laboratory confirmation of a bacterial cause is available it is rational to give antibiotics to those at risk of remote complications such as post-streptococcal rheumatic fever or, less likely, acute glomerulonephritis. In others, the risk of these complications is not increased by delay in giving antibiotics for 24–48 hours: in fact treatment begun within 7–9 days of the onset is effective. Bear in mind that 10–20% of otherwise normal children may be carriers of *S. pyogenes* and that considerably fewer than 50% of cases of AST are eventually proved to be bacterial. In many cases no pathogen is isolated.

Antibiotics confer minimal worthwhile benefit (symptoms may last for 1 day less) over purely symptomatic treatment (rest, paracetamol and fluids) and are seldom effective in preventing suppurative complications except in high-risk groups. Nevertheless, pending the result of a throat swab, it might be prudent to immediately treat those who are unduly ill or toxic or those at risk, including diabetics, immunocompromised individuals and Aboriginal, Torres Strait and Pacific Islander children.

There are many proprietary 'remedies' available for upper respiratory infections and sore throat but none can be recommended. Throat lozenges, including those containing antibiotic, are of no use and antihistamine/decongestant preparations can lead to troublesome side effects.

Practical points

Features associated with an acute sore throat which should alert a perceptive medical attendant to a possible serious condition:
- Undue toxicity – the child appears sicker than might be expected
- Signs of respiratory distress, stridor or restlessness
- Difficulty swallowing or drooling
- Dehydration
- Marked or generalized lymphadenopathy
- Unilateral swelling in the pharynx
- Bruising or bleeding
- An adherent or obstructive membrane

Clinical example

The family doctor saw Andrew, a 7-year-old boy who had had a sore throat, difficulty in swallowing and fever for 2 days. The appearance in the throat was described as 'tonsillitis'. An antibiotic was prescribed but when he was no better 3 days later it was changed to a different antibiotic. Again, Andrew was no better and in addition was complaining of feeling weak, with aching in the muscles and headache. Careful examination 8 days after the illness had commenced revealed tender, enlarged lymph nodes in the neck, axilla and inguinal region. His spleen was enlarged and tender. Blood tests were diagnostic of infectious mononucleosis.

An atypical sore throat needs caution about the diagnosis. Infectious mononucleosis is a systemic illness whose principal features are sore throat, fever, cervical (often generalized) lymphadenopathy and a feeling of malaise. Many organs in the body can be affected with protean manifestations. Antibiotics have no therapeutic value.

Indications for tonsillectomy and adenoidectomy

There is now reliable information to prove that the frequency of throat infections is reduced in selected patients undergoing these procedures. Operation is clearly indicated in a small number of children. There may be disagreement about the operation in individual cases and at times a second opinion may be in the best interests of the patient.

Indications for tonsillectomy

The indications for tonsillectomy are:

- repeated attacks of acute tonsillitis: at least three documented attacks a year for 2 years or more, making a minimum of 6 attacks in 2 years
- acute or chronic upper airway obstruction caused by enlarged lymphoid tissue. There may be an obstructive sleep pattern, even apnoea. Some cases with severe obstruction develop cardiac changes and cor pulmonale
- chronic tonsillitis. This usually applies to older children and adults
- peritonsillar abscess (quinsy). Two or more attacks are a definite indication for tonsillectomy
- biopsy excision for suspected new growth.

Indications for adenoidectomy

The indications for adenoidectomy are:

- enlargement causing severe nasal obstruction and breathing discomfort
- persistent discharge of infected mucopurulent material caused by large and infected adenoids
- possible benefit in repeated acute or chronic ear disease.

The tonsils and adenoids are often removed in a single, combined operation but there are clear indications for tonsillectomy alone or adenoidectomy alone. There is now greater awareness of the incidence and severity of obstructive sleep problems, which occur in an age range from 6 months to 10 years of age.

Contraindications to tonsillectomy and adenoidectomy

Tonsillectomy and/or adenoidectomy should not be performed if there is:

- a lack of staff or facilities to recognize and manage the potential complications
- recent respiratory tract infection, within the previous 2 weeks

- a systemic disorder, such as poorly controlled diabetes
- a bleeding disorder
- pharyngeal insufficiency, such as repaired cleft palate, submucous cleft palate or paralysis or paresis of the palate and so called 'short' palate. Adenoidectomy may cause or worsen escape of air through the nose (hypernasality), making speech difficult to understand.

Injuries of the tongue and oropharynx

Children with, for example, a pencil in the mouth may fall and injure the soft palate, tonsils or pharyngeal wall. At other times it is not uncommon for the teeth to lacerate the tongue and cause considerable bleeding. It is usually necessary to suture only the most severe of these injuries.

The larynx and trachea

Features of upper airway disease include:

- stridor: a prominent, audible manifestation of upper airway obstruction caused by turbulent airflow through a narrowed airway, usually the larynx or sometimes the trachea. It is most often inspiratory, sometimes expiratory and occasionally both
- other signs of partial or severe airway obstruction: tachypnoea, chest retraction
- cyanotic or apnoeic attacks
- husky, weak or absent cry
- repeated aspiration
- recurrent or atypical croup
- features of weakness, compression or stenosis of the trachea and/or bronchi.

Laryngomalacia

This is a common cause of stridor in infants. It is also appropriately called 'floppy larynx', both names implying collapse of the supraglottic tissues during inspiration. The cause is unknown. The features are intermittent inspiratory stridor, signs of upper airway obstruction, a normal cry and general health that is usually (but not always) normal. The features are often alarming to parents. As the condition is usually self-limiting there is seldom any need for treatment once a certain diagnosis has been established to differentiate laryngomalacia from the many other causes of stridor in infants. Occasionally, severe cases warrant laser removal of part of the redundant, floppy, supraglottic tissues.

Clinical example

Suzanna, a 7-week-old baby with intermittent 'noisy breathing' for 3–4 weeks, was brought to the family doctor because the noise was getting worse and had become more worrying for her parents. There had been no cyanotic or apnoeic episodes, her cry was normal, she was otherwise progressing well and she was gaining weight normally. Chest X-ray was normal. She was seen by a paediatrician who found no abnormality other than the stridor and referred her to a paediatric ENT surgeon. At laryngobronchoscopy under general anaesthesia the characteristic supraglottic changes of laryngomalacia were seen but there was no other abnormality of the upper aerodigestive tract. Suzanna's parents were reassured that there was no serious disease, there was no relationship to 'cot death' and that, with time, the stridor would resolve without treatment.

The descriptive terms 'congenital laryngeal stridor' and 'infantile stridor' are not diagnoses. This baby could have had a serious problem, such as an enlarging cyst, subglottic stenosis, subglottic haemangioma, vascular compression of the trachea, mediastinal tumour or developmental cyst or other rare conditions. Imaging and endoscopy will lead to a definitive diagnosis.

Congenital and acquired subglottic stenosis

The reported incidence of subglottic stenosis has increased, partly because of the improved survival of premature babies who have been treated by prolonged intubation and partly because of more accurate diagnosis. Severe cases require tracheotomy and later repair by rib graft laryngotracheoplasty or even cricotracheal resection.

Vocal cord paralysis

Unilateral paralysis causes few symptoms in infants and children. Bilateral vocal cord paralysis is the cause of stridor in about 10% of infants with airway obstruction and is associated with a central nervous system anomaly (e.g. Arnold–Chiari malformation) in many cases. Tracheotomy is usually, but not always, required for bilateral paralysis.

Other causes of stridor

Laryngeal web, laryngeal atresia and laryngeal cleft are uncommon anomalies. Cysts causing clinical features include retention cysts, congenital cysts and cystic hygroma. Subglottic haemangioma is the commonest laryngeal tumour in infants and presents with inspiratory stridor in the first 6–8 weeks. The clinical features of tracheal obstruction are caused by tracheomalacia, tracheal compression by a vascular ring or other anomalies or congenital tracheal stenosis.

Investigations include X-rays, CT, contrast oesophagogram and ultrasound of the neck or mediastinum. Flexible laryngoscopy and direct laryngoscopy, bronchoscopy and possibly oesophagoscopy under general anaesthesia ultimately establish a firm diagnosis.

Acute inflammatory airway obstruction

Acute infectious diseases of the upper respiratory tract that cause airway obstruction fall into two groups:

- *Oropharynx.* Acute bacterial or viral infection with obstructive hypertrophy of the tonsils and adenoids; infectious mononucleosis causing obstructive enlargement of the tonsils and adenoids; peritonsillar abscess; retropharyngeal or parapharyngeal abscess and Ludwig's angina
- *Larynx and trachea.* Acute laryngotracheobronchitis or croup; spasmodic croup; bacterial tracheitis; acute supraglottitis or epiglottitis (with a frighteningly rapid onset) and diphtheria. Some cases (especially patients with acute supraglottitis, epiglottitis or diphtheria) have critical, life-threatening airway obstruction, a situation that requires immediate recognition and transfer to a paediatric hospital for relief of airway obstruction, if necessary by endotracheal intubation or tracheotomy, and intensive care management.

Important advances in treatment of these diseases include more effective antibiotics, diphtheria immunization, diphtheria antitoxin, the use of racemic adrenaline (epinephrine) for croup, steroids for croup, Hib vaccine, which has dramatically reduced the incidence of *H. influenzae* supraglottitis and epiglottitis, and the use of intubation in place of tracheotomy.

Multiple respiratory papillomas

Papillomas are the most common benign growths in the larynx. Human papillomavirus (HPV) type 6, type 11 and occasionally type 16 cause papillomas in the respiratory tract, most often in the mucosa of the larynx. About two-thirds of patients are younger than 15 years and one-third older than 15 years, with the highest incidence before the age of 5 years. There is a tendency for recurrence after removal, although sometimes unexpected spontaneous improvement can occur. In infants, large obstructing masses may threaten life. There is a strong association between recurrent respiratory papillomas in infants and children and maternal condylomata acuminata or genital warts but transmission of HPV during passage through the birth canal is unlikely, as some infants have papillomas already in their larynx at birth.

Growth may be slow and persistent or irregular and unpredictable. The commonest presentation is a change in the cry or voice, sometimes with increasing airway obstruction, and often an erroneous diagnosis of asthma, laryngitis, bronchitis or croup has been made. Therefore, persistent or progressive huskiness in an infant or child should suggest the possibility of papillomas. The mainstay of treatment is repeated removal at microlaryngeal surgery under general anaesthesia, using forceps or the carbon dioxide laser, which is a precise modality attended by minimal bleeding, causing little pain and limited local scarring. Many adjunctive treatments have been tried because of frustration and recurrence of the tumour but none of these have proved beneficial over the long term. There is no tendency for regression or disappearance at puberty, as was formerly thought.

Ingested and inhaled foreign bodies

Foreign bodies in the pharynx and oesophagus

Children often swallow foreign bodies. Sharp objects such as fishbones can impact in the tonsils, base of the tongue or the pyriform fossa. More often objects such as coins, buttons, lumps of meat or vegetable, plastic or pins lodge somewhere in the oesophagus, usually at the upper end but occasionally at a site of pathological narrowing (stenosis). Some show on X-ray but, ultimately, if an impacted foreign body is

Clinical example

Simon, aged 2 years and 6 months, ran to his mother in great distress, gasping for breath, coughing and crying. She rushed him to the nearby emergency department. The respiratory distress had lessened but pulse oximetry showed only 90% saturation. There was a wheeze and decreased air entry on the right side. An expiratory chest X-ray showed air trapping on the same side with shift of the mediastinum to the left. Simon was observed in the high-dependency ward until an impacted peanut was removed from the right main bronchus under general anaesthesia 90 minutes later. He made an uneventful recovery thereafter.

With inhalation of foreign bodies into major airways, if death does not occur in the first few minutes after inhalation, the situation usually improves but the implications remain serious. In this case the peanut, acting as a ball valve in the right main bronchus, let air into that side, but as the bronchus narrowed during expiration air was trapped in the lung.

suspected, oesophagoscopy is necessary. Remember most small smooth objects will pass through the oesophagus and the gastrointestinal tract and be recovered in the stools; however, ingestion of a small alkaline button battery is extremely destructive of surrounding tissue and must be treated as an acute emergency to prevent perforation of the oesophagus and mediastinitis.

Foreign bodies in the larynx and tracheobronchial tree

The highest incidence of inhaled foreign bodies is in the second and third years of life and about 60% of deaths occur in children less than 4 years of age. Occasionally they lodge in the larynx or subglottic region but more often in one or other main bronchus. Diagnosis is made by awareness of the possibility and from a history of inhalation of a foreign body (a history of possible inhalation is present in about 65% of cases).

The clinical presentation may be:

- immediate, with sudden coughing, choking, gasping, spasm and cyanosis. Fortunately, few deaths occur in this stage

- delayed, with wheeze, chronic cough, atypical pneumonia, and chest X-ray changes (but about 20% show no abnormality). The foreign body may be found days, weeks or even months later
- symptomless. Although most foreign bodies will ultimately cause symptoms, occasionally some are found by chance on a chest X-ray or at endoscopy.

Only 5–10% of ingested foreign bodies impact in the larynx or subglottic region and then stridor, laryngospasm, dyspnoea, a husky voice, inspiratory wheeze or repeated atypical croup dominate the clinical picture. If death does not occur in the first few minutes after the foreign body is inhaled, the prognosis is good if the patient is promptly transported by road or air ambulance to a major paediatric unit where experienced personnel and adequate instruments are available. Ill-advised attempts at bronchoscopic diagnosis or removal by inexperienced surgeons or anaesthetists often worsen the situation.

Two-thirds of inhaled foreign bodies are nuts. Parents should be made aware that children under 4 years of age should be denied access to nuts, especially peanuts, in the hope that aspiration accidents will be minimized.

22.2 Eye disorders in childhood

J. E. Elder

A systematic approach to children's eye disease allows rapid determination of the correct diagnosis or initiation of appropriate further investigation.

Visual development

A rapid sequence of anatomical and functional changes in the visual apparatus enables vision to develop from a very low level after birth to near adult levels by 12–18 months of age. At birth an infant has visual acuity of approximately 6/120 and by 12 months this has improved to about 6/12. This rapid development is the result of retinal maturation, myelination of the visual pathways, the ability to accommodate (change the focal length of the eye) and maturation within the visual cortex. The first three of these processes (retinal maturation, myelination and accommodation) are complete by 4–6 months of age. The maturation of the visual cortex occurs more gradually, over a 6–8-year period, with the most rapid phase being in the first 2 years. Anything that interferes with this gradual cortical maturation may result in the development of amblyopia, which is one of the commonest ophthalmic abnormalities of childhood (see Amblyopia, below).

Measurement of vision in children

Measurement of visual acuity in preverbal children presents a challenge. Asking the parent 'Does your child see well?' or 'How well do you think your child sees?' often gives useful information about an infant's visual function. If a parent expresses concern about an infant's vision, take note, as this concern is often well founded.

An understanding of normal visual behaviour is vital to estimating visual function in infancy. At birth, when alert, an infant should be able to fix on a face briefly. By 6 weeks of age most infants smile in a visually responsive fashion to a face. At this age the infant will also be able to follow a face or light through an arc of 90°. By 6 months of age an infant can reach for a small object and can actively follow objects in the visual environment. At 12 months of age a child should be able to reach and pick up tiny objects such as hundreds-and-thousands ('sprinkles').

More formal assessment of visual acuity becomes possible with the development of language. Children with specific language delay or more general intellectual delay will have difficulty with these tests of visual acuity. Picture-naming tests can be done by children between 2 and 3 years of age. Single letter-matching tests are within the abilities of most 3–4-year-olds. The standard Snellen chart test is often not performed well until the child is between 5 and 6 years of age. The vision should be tested for each eye individually. As with all testing in children, patience and an encouraging manner are vital to obtain the best results. Repeat the test on another occasion if the test results seem inaccurate.

The notation for documenting visual acuity is the Snellen fraction, e.g. 6/6. Most visual acuity tests use standard distances of 3 or 6 m between subject and chart. The numerator of the Snellen fraction is the distance from the chart while the denominator indicates which line on the chart was the smallest to be seen. If the vision is poor the subject should be brought closer to the chart. The vision then may be recorded as 2/18 or 1/60, etc., depending on how close the subject is to the chart and which line is read.

What level of vision is abnormal? (or, when to refer!)

This depends on the age of the child. An infant who is not fixing and following by 3–4 months, or reaching for small objects and tracking objects in the visual environment by 8–12 months, deserves further examination and investigation.

If the child is able to do a more formal test of acuity, a difference between the two eyes of two or more lines (that is 6/6 and 6/12) indicates the need for further assessment. In children less than 3 years of age vision of 6/18 or less in either eye should prompt referral and in children older than 3 years 6/12 is an acceptable cut-off for referral.

Assessment of a child with a possible eye problem

History

Prematurity, perinatal difficulties (e.g. birth asphyxia), significant syndromes (e.g. Down syndrome) and other sensory impairment (e.g. deafness) are associated with an increased risk of eye disease. Developmental delay often interferes with assessment of visual acuity, especially if language or intellect is affected. Common childhood eye problems such as strabismus and refractive errors have a clearly identified familial tendency, although the precise genetics are not well understood. Finally, the parents' perception of a child's visual function is important, particularly if there is concern that the vision is poor.

Examination

In keeping with paediatrics in general, observation without approaching or touching a child often supplies a great deal of information. By observation it is possible to rapidly determine an infant's use of vision. Does the child smile at a face? Is the child looking around the room? If something moves, does the child look to it? If there is a noise, does the child look to the source of the noise? A blind child will become still and will often drop the head down while using hearing to further localize the source of the sound, but will not look towards this source.

Most eyelid, eyelash and ocular surface abnormalities can be detected readily by simple observation. Many intraocular abnormalities can be detected by examination of the 'red reflex'. This is the red to orange colour seen within the pupil when the line of illumination and observation are approximately coaxial (that is, the same). This situation is most easily obtained by observing the child's eye with a direct ophthalmoscope from a distance of about 1 m. It is then easy to compare the reflexes for the two eyes and the child is not threatened by the examiner getting too close. A dull or absent red reflex indicates an opacity, such as a cataract, in the normally clear media of the eye. A white reflex results from an abnormally pale reflecting surface within the eye, such as a white retinal tumour (retinoblastoma). While these intraocular disorders are rare, they are important in terms of the severe effect on vision or threat to life.

Misalignment of the eyes

Strabismus or squint is common in childhood and accurate assessment to confirm or refute the presence of misalignment is an important skill for anyone who deals with children.

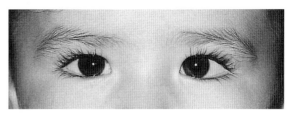

Fig. 22.2.1 This infant has prominent epicanthic folds, giving rise to the appearance of misaligned eyes. This is pseudostrabismus. Note that the corneal light reflections are symmetrical. Cover testing failed to reveal misalignment of either eye.

Observation will confirm the presence of large-angle strabismus. However, a broad nasal bridge or prominent epicanthic folds will mimic milder degrees of strabismus, especially in younger infants. This situation is known as pseudostrabismus (Fig. 22.2.1). The epicanthic folds cover the sclera on the medial aspect of the globe while the lateral sclera is easily visible. This creates the appearance of misalignment, particularly when the child looks laterally. Examining the symmetry of corneal light reflections will help to avoid being misled by pseudostrabismus.

The cover test is by far the most reliable method of detecting strabismus. The cover test is done by first getting the child to fix on an object while the observer determines which eye appears to be misaligned. The eye that appears to be fixing on the object (and not misaligned) is then covered while the apparently misaligned eye is observed. If strabismus is present a corrective movement of the misaligned eye will be seen as this eye takes up fixation on the object of regard (Fig. 22.2.2). If no movement is seen then the eye is uncovered.

The cover test is then repeated but the other eye is covered this time and the eye that is not covered is again observed for a corrective movement and, if present, strabismus is confirmed. The test can be repeated as many times as necessary. If no movement is seen following repeated covering of either eye, then no strabismus is present. Care must be taken to let the child fix with both eyes open before covering either eye, otherwise normal binocular control may be prevented and a small latent squint (phoria) may be detected. Latent squints are normal variants and are of no significance.

Common eye problems in childhood

Amblyopia

Amblyopia is the cortical response to abnormal input from the eyes and is manifest as reduced visual

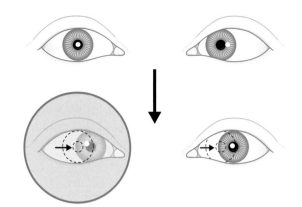

Fig. 22.2.2 Cover test. First the child's attention is attracted with a toy (top). Then the eye that appears to be looking directly at the toy is covered and the other eye is observed for a refixation movement (bottom). If there is a convergent squint there will be an outward movement of the uncovered eye (pictured) and if there is a divergent squint there will be an inward movement of the eye. If no movement is detected, the test should be repeated but covering the other eye first.

acuity in one or both eyes. This abnormal input may result from a refractive (spectacle) error, a structural abnormality of the eye (e.g. cataract) or strabismus. Provided it is detected early enough, while the developing visual cortex is immature, amblyopia is treatable. Conversely, if the amblyopia is not treated before visual cortex maturation (about 7 years of age), it may not be reversible later in life. Detection of amblyopia is one of the major reasons for routine visual screening in childhood.

Common causes of amblyopia are strabismus and refractive errors. Refractive errors cause a poorly focused image to form on the retina and thus a poor-quality image to be transmitted to the cortex. Such input does not stimulate normal cortical development and amblyopia results. Strabismic (misaligned) eyes are not necessarily out of focus; however, if the cortex 'paid attention' to the image from each eye diplopia would result, as each eye is sending a different view of the world. In children, the immature visual cortex is capable of ignoring the image from one eye. If this situation is allowed to persist the cortex may completely ignore or suppress the input from a deviating eye and amblyopia will result.

Treatment of amblyopia involves correcting any focusing errors with appropriate spectacles and forcing the brain to use the amblyopic eye by depriving the brain of clear input from the better-seeing eye, most commonly with a patch. Unfortunately, simply realigning strabismic eyes is not enough to overcome amblyopia secondary to strabismus.

Strabismus

A squint or misaligned eye is important to detect as it is frequently associated with amblyopia. Most childhood strabismus is the result of failure of binocular control at a cortical level within the central nervous system (CNS). Less commonly it is the result of cranial nerve lesions or extraocular muscle disease. In most children this CNS abnormality in eye movement control is an isolated abnormality with no other associated neurological or intellectual problems. However, children with widespread CNS abnormalities have an increased risk of developing strabismus. Down syndrome is a good example of this, with an approximately tenfold increase in the risk of developing strabismus.

The diagnosis of strabismus is outlined above and detailed consideration of the therapy of strabismus is beyond the scope of this chapter. The following is a brief description of the commoner patterns of strabismus seen in childhood and an outline of management.

Infantile esotropia

This is a large-angle convergent squint seen before 6 months of age. Strabismic amblyopia is common in infantile esotropia but refractive errors are rare. Patching followed by surgery is the most common initial treatment. Children with infantile esotropia need to be followed up throughout childhood, as about one-third need more than one operation and amblyopia can occur following apparently successful initial treatment.

Intermittent divergent strabismus

This occurs from 18 months of age onwards. It is often more noticeable on distance fixation and may be associated with closure of the deviating eye, especially in bright light. Amblyopia is uncommon, as the deviation is intermittent and presumably when the eyes are straight normal visual development proceeds. In some cases the divergence becomes more constant and in such situations surgery may be undertaken to improve alignment.

Accommodative esotropia

This occurs in children who are excessively longsighted (hypermetropic). To overcome hypermetropia and focus a clear image on the retina, accommodative effort is used. Accommodation consists of the combination of changing focal length of the lens and converging the eyes (so that both are directed at the nearer object of regard). Thus in children with excessive hypermetropia there is increased focusing and at times excessive convergence; that is, a convergent squint (esotropia) appears as a result of the increased accommodative effort used by these children. Accommodative esotropia can be completely or partially corrected by prescribing glasses that compensate for the appropriate amount of hypermetropia. Amblyopia is often seen in association with accommodative esotropia and requires treatment. If glasses only partly correct the esotropia, surgery may be indicated to obtain optimal alignment.

Clinical example

A 3-year-old girl presented with a history of a worsening inward turn of her left eye over four months. The cover test confirmed a left convergent squint and the red reflex was normal in each eye. Subsequent assessment by an ophthalmologist confirmed the findings and her visual acuities were 3/3 in the right eye and 3/9 in the left with refraction showing she was long-sighted. When next seen 6 months later she was wearing glasses and had been patching her right eye 2 hours a day. Her eyes were straight to cover test and her parents reported that her left vision was slowly improving and that surgery was not going to be required in her case.

Refractive problems

Refractive problems are the result of defects in the focusing components of the eye. These defects include abnormality of corneal curvature (a frequent cause of astigmatism) and abnormalities of lens power and axial length of the eye (which may result in hypermetropia or myopia – short-sightedness). Children will rarely complain of poor vision related to refractive error. Rather, they readily accept the vision they have and get on with life. Children with high myopia will often manifest myopic behaviour (they will go very close to objects to look at them). Different refraction in either eye will often result in amblyopia because one eye will generally have a clearer image than the other and thus enable better cortical development for that eye.

Routine screening of visual acuity is the only reliable way of detecting the majority of refractive errors in children. In many countries there are both preschool and school entry tests of visual acuity for this reason. Such screening testing needs to be reliable, available to all of the target population and followed up with appropriate intervention when defects are identified. As cortical maturation of vision occurs at about 7 years of age, screening should ideally

commence in 3–4-year-olds, before any amblyopia becomes difficult to reverse.

If a refractive error is suspected in a young child because of strabismus or poor visual acuity, then accurate and objective testing with cycloplegic retinoscopy is required. If a child is prescribed glasses, these should be worn the majority of the time.

Practical points

Vision assessment and strabismus
- The parents' assessment of their infant child's vision is often very accurate; if they are concerned their child is not seeing you should be concerned also
- Always try to gain as much information as possible by observation before actively engaging a child in an examination. Red reflexes can be observed from a distance. Urgent referral is required if an abnormal red reflex is found
- Children under 7 years of age will rarely complain of visual difficulty relating to refractive errors (reduced visual acuity). A vision screening programme is the most reliable method of detecting reduced visual acuity in children of this age
- Strabismus is a common cause of amblyopia. All suspected or confirmed strabismus should be referred to an ophthalmologist for further assessment and management
- Cover testing is the most accurate clinical method of diagnosing strabismus. When doing a cover test always make sure that the child is looking at a interesting fixation target – a small toy is useful for near fixation and a picture or larger toy for distance fixation
- Amblyopia is generally reversible if it is detected early and appropriate management is initiated

Watery and sticky eyes

This occurs commonly in infancy as the result of congenital nasolacrimal duct obstruction. About 10% of newborn infants have obstructed nasolacrimal ducts. This will present as a watery and sticky eye in the first few weeks of life. Despite the persistent discharge the eye is generally not red or inflamed. An inflamed eye suggests an alternative diagnosis such as infective conjunctivitis. If the obstruction persists, the lower lid will often become red and sometimes slightly scaly as a result of the skin being constantly moist.

The differential diagnosis includes trauma, conjunctivitis and infantile glaucoma. These conditions are all described below.

Most congenital nasolacrimal duct obstructions resolve spontaneously. Approximately 95% of cases have resolved by the time of the first birthday, with most doing so in the first 6 months. In persistent cases, probing under a general anaesthetic is recommended after 1 year of age.

Trauma

Trauma to the eye can take many forms. Physical trauma to the eye and surrounding structures may be blunt or sharp. Trauma can also result from radiation (thermal and electromagnetic) and chemical agents.

Direct blunt trauma to the eye may disrupt iris blood vessels, causing bleeding in the anterior chamber of the eye (hyphema), tear the iris, dislocate the lens, rupture the choroid and rarely rupture the eye wall (sclera) if the force is sufficient. Simple inspection of the eye will reveal most of these injuries and choroid and globe rupture may be suspected on the basis of the nature of the injury and associated poor vision. Referral to an ophthalmologist is necessary in these cases for confirmation of the injury and further management.

Sharp trauma may be due to a range of causes, from tiny objects such as a subtarsal foreign body causing a corneal abrasion, to fingernail scratches through to penetration of the eye by sharp objects such as a scissors blade or dart. Surface trauma can be diagnosed easily with the help of fluorescein staining and a cobalt blue light. Areas of epithelial abrasion will fluoresce green. If a round ulcer and/or vertical linear abrasions are seen, suspect a subtarsal foreign body and the upper lid should be everted. If identified, most subtarsal foreign bodies can be removed with a moistened cotton bud. Superficial trauma is treated with antibiotic ointment and a patch and daily review until any epithelial defect (ulcer or abrasion) is healed.

If the wall of the eye (cornea or sclera) has been penetrated, intraocular contents may prolapse out through the wound, the iris and pupil may appear distorted or the anterior chamber may be shallower than normal. Any suspected penetration of the eye must be referred to an ophthalmologist for further investigation and management. The eye should be protected with a cone that does not exert any pressure on the eye. If vomiting is likely or occurs an anti-emetic should be given to prevent further prolapse of intraocular tissue.

Thermal injuries to the eye itself are rare, as in most burn situations the eyelids are firmly closed and thus protect the eye. Facial burns may cause scarring that interferes with lid function, leading to exposure and drying of the eye's surface. If a primary thermal injury to the eye is suspected, fluorescein dye should be used to detect any ulceration. If ulceration is found, treatment is with antibiotic ointment and a patch.

Radiation injuries to the eye are rare in childhood and most are the result of intentional irradiation as part of medical therapy for facial and ocular neoplasia. Typical injuries are cataract, dry eye syndrome, radiation retinopathy and optic neuropathy. These changes are seen some considerable time after the irradiation.

Chemical burns to the eye are unusual in childhood but potentially are very serious, especially if the chemical is alkaline. Many domestic cleaning agents are alkaline. Strong alkali will denature and dissolve protein and penetrate deeply into the surface of the eye. Acids tend to coagulate surface structures and this often prevents deeper penetration of the acidic chemical into the eye. Immediate first aid should consist of copious irrigation with water at the site of the accident and this should be continued for at least 10 minutes. Following adequate irrigation all chemical burns of the eye should be referred to an ophthalmologist.

Practical points

Blocked tear ducts and eye injury

- Most blocked tear ducts resolve spontaneously by 1 year of age
- Simple inspection with the addition of fluorescein staining will enable the diagnosis of most physical trauma to the eye
- All chemical injuries to the eye should be regarded as serious. Copious irrigation is the cornerstone of immediate management of all chemical injuries to the eye

---

Conjunctivitis

Conjunctivitis may result from infective, allergic or chemical agents interacting with the conjunctiva. Symptoms are itch, pain and irritation or a gritty sensation. Signs are epiphora (watering), discharge and erythema of conjunctiva and lids. The relative prominence of different symptoms and signs varies with the cause of the conjunctivitis (Table 22.2.1).

Conjunctivitis occurring in the first few weeks of life is generally bacterial and frequently acquired from the birth canal. *Neisseria gonorrhoeae* and *Chlamydia trachomatis* both cause a conjunctivitis with copious discharge and marked erythema in the neonatal period, termed ophthalmia neonatorum. Gonococcal conjunctivitis is serious because of the risk of spontaneous perforation of the cornea and resultant loss of vision and also the risk of more generalized sepsis. Chlamydial conjunctivitis is significant because of the risk of more generalized

Table 22.2.1 Signs and symptoms of conjunctivitis		
Cause of conjunctivitis	Symptoms	Signs
Viral	Moderate discomfort	Moderate epiphora Mild discharge Mild to moderate erythema
Bacterial	Moderate to severe discomfort	Moderate epiphora Copious discharge Moderate to severe erythema
Allergic	Itch often prominent	Mild to moderate epiphora Stringy discharge Mild erythema
Chemical	Pain intense	Severe epiphora Mild discharge Moderate to severe erythema
The descriptions in this table are intended to be a guide; there may be considerable variation and overlap in the signs and symptoms of conjunctivitis due to different causes.		

chlamydial sepsis. For accurate and prompt diagnosis of these infections, microbiological diagnosis and systemic as well as topical antibiotic therapy is needed. For culture, conjunctival swabs should be directly inoculated onto culture medium plates and conjunctival scrapings for Gram staining and immunofluorescent staining should be taken.

Bacterial conjunctivitis occurring outside the first few weeks of life in children is usually the result of relatively innocuous organisms (e.g. *Staphylococcus* spp. and *Haemophilus* spp.) Microbiological investigation is not usually indicated and a broad-spectrum topical antibiotic should be prescribed (such as neomycin/polymyxin or chloramphenicol). Concern has been raised about topical chloramphenicol preparations because of a perceived risk of secondary agranulocytosis. It is the author's belief that this risk is extremely low but does exist and should not stop short-term use of topical chloramphenicol.

Viral conjunctivitis is relatively common at all ages and clinically may be very difficult to differentiate from bacterial conjunctivitis. The discharge may be somewhat less with viral conjunctivitis. Viral conjunctivitis is frequently associated with upper respiratory tract infection symptoms. If the aetiology is uncertain, topical antibiotics as for bacterial conjunctivitis should be used.

Allergic conjunctivitis is common in children of all age groups and has itch as its most prominent symptom. House dust mite, grass and other plant pollens are common allergens that precipitate allergic conjunctivitis. Therapy depends on the severity of the symptoms. If mild, cold compresses may be all

that is needed. For more severe symptoms soothing topical astringent agents that include a topical antihistamine are helpful. In more persistent and severe cases topical sodium cromoglycate and steroid preparations may be indicated. Topical steroid should be used with the supervision of an ophthalmologist because of the risk of significant side effects, including cataract and glaucoma.

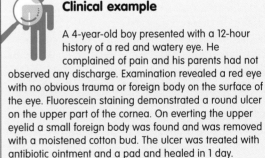

Clinical example

A 4-year-old boy presented with a 12-hour history of a red and watery eye. He complained of pain and his parents had not observed any discharge. Examination revealed a red eye with no obvious trauma or foreign body on the surface of the eye. Fluorescein staining demonstrated a round ulcer on the upper part of the cornea. On everting the upper eyelid a small foreign body was found and was removed with a moistened cotton bud. The ulcer was treated with antibiotic ointment and a pad and healed in 1 day.

Lid infections

These are common in children and most arise in the skin appendages of the eyelids (lash follicles and meibomian glands). Infection of a lash follicle is called a stye (or hordeolum externum) and acute infection of a meibomian gland is known as hordeolum internum. Unless there is significant secondary erythema of the surrounding lid, topical and systemic antibiotics are not indicated. Occasionally, severe preseptal cellulitis will follow a focal lid infection and systemic (often intravenous) antibiotics will then be needed for treatment.

More chronic inflammation of a meibomian gland is known as a chalazion. This is generally the result of sterile chemical inflammation rather than infection and occurs when the contents of a meibomian gland escape into the lid following blockage of the opening of the gland at the lid margin. A chalazion will appear as a lump in the substance of the lid and is often not particularly inflamed in appearance. Topical antibiotics seldom hasten resolution. Warm compresses may give symptomatic relief and help drainage. Chalazia may persist for many months. Some will discharge through the conjunctiva or the skin. On occasions surgical drainage is indicated for a persistently inflamed and large chalazion.

Practical points

Conjunctivitis and chalazion
- Neonatal conjunctivitis may be sight-threatening and a threat to the newborn infant's health. Immediate investigation with appropriate treatment is needed
- If a child does not have itch as a major symptom then allergic conjunctivitis is unlikely. Think of other causes of conjunctivitis in this situation
- Most chalazia are not infected and redness and swelling is the result of sterile inflammation. Consequently topical and oral antibiotics are of little use in treatment. Most chalazia resolve spontaneously

Ptosis

Ptosis, also called blepharoptosis, is a droopy upper eyelid and results from innervational or muscular defects of the levator superioris or Muller muscles. Innervational defects include third cranial nerve palsy, Horner syndrome (sympathetic nervous system) and myasthenia gravis. Congenital ptosis is the commonest muscle defect causing ptosis in children. Ptosis will cause visual defects when the lid is so low that it occludes the visual axis or if it induces astigmatism by altering the corneal curvature. Ptosis is also a cosmetic concern in that it may make an affected child look sleepy or dull. Surgical correction is possible in most cases.

Learning difficulties

Learning difficulties are common in school-age children and are the result of a neurobiological disorder, i.e. brain dysfunction. The majority of reading difficulties are the result of defects in phonological awareness. It is commonly assumed that there may be a visual abnormality that contributes to or even causes the learning difficulty. This assumption is ill founded and arises because vision is so obviously involved with activities such as reading and writing. Children with learning difficulties are no more or less likely to have visual problems than children without evidence of learning problems. Rather than expending effort on therapies for perceived ocular abnormalities, parents should be encouraged to take an educational approach to their child's learning difficulties.

Visual handicap

Visual handicap in childhood may be the result of ocular and/or cortical visual abnormalities and may be associated with other abnormalities, e.g. deafness, motor defects and intellectual defects. Intervention and support for a particular child needs to be planned after a thorough assessment of the child's visual and associated handicaps. From a purely visual point of view, interventions may include mobility training, low vision aids, such as magnifiers and closed circuit television, and training in alternative means of communication, such as 'reading' braille and using a computer to write.

The presence of additional handicap such as deafness or an intellectual deficit compounds the situation and necessitates skilled intervention over many years to achieve optimal outcomes.

Rare but important eye problems in childhood

These are mentioned briefly because prompt recognition enables early treatment and optimal outcomes.

Poor vision in infancy

This first comes to attention when a child fails to achieve normal milestones of visual development (see Measurement of vision in children, above). If the cause of severe visual impairment is within the eye, sensory nystagmus will develop at about 3–4 months of age. This nystagmus is often slow and somewhat pendular rather than jerky in appearance. Severe visual loss secondary to CNS abnormality does not cause nystagmus. Causes of poor vision in infancy include:

- cataracts
- albinism
- retinal colobomas
- infantile glaucoma

- congenital retinal dystrophy
- retinoblastoma
- delayed visual maturation
- cortical visual impairment.

Prompt recognition is vital as there may be a treatable cause (e.g. cataracts) and, even if no treatment is possible, early and appropriate intervention minimizes the negative effects of severe visual impairment on general development.

Cataract

A cataract is any opacity within the lens. Bilateral congenital cataracts will often cause poor vision in infancy, while unilateral congenital cataract may go unrecognized, as one eye has normal vision. Both bilateral and unilateral congenital cataracts are treatable if diagnosed early. Cataracts are detected readily by inspection of the red reflex with the direct ophthalmoscope.

There are numerous causes of congenital cataracts, including: hereditary (dominant, recessive and X linked); metabolic (e.g. galactosaemia); association with systemic syndromes (e.g. Down syndrome), and congenital infection (e.g. rubella embryopathy). Many, especially unilateral cataracts, are idiopathic.

Retinoblastoma

This is a rare childhood cancer arising within the retina. Sporadic and hereditary forms are recognized. The sporadic form is the result of two separate mutations that negate the action of the retinoblastoma (Rb) gene within a single retinoblast cell, and thus is always unilateral. The hereditary form arises when the first of these two mutations occurs in one Rb gene within a germ cell (most often a sperm). The second mutation occurs within the retinoblast. As all retinoblasts descended from an affected germ cell have the first mutation, by chance more than one retinoblastoma will usually develop and hence the hereditary form is often, but not always, bilateral.

Retinoblastoma most often presents with leukocoria (white pupillary reflection: the white tumour is seen immediately behind the lens), strabismus, poor vision, or a known family history of retinoblastoma. Prompt recognition is vital as early treatment will increase the possibility of preserving vision and life. With current treatments the 5-year survival of this childhood cancer is about 98%.

Glaucoma

Glaucoma in infancy presents with a cloudy and enlarged cornea with associated epiphora (watery eye) and photophobia. It may be unilateral or bilateral and is usually an isolated ocular abnormality. If unrecognized it will result in severe and untreatable visual loss over weeks to months. Prompt diagnosis allows surgical treatment, which controls the glaucoma in the majority of cases.

Colobomas

These defects result from failure of complete fusion of the embryonic fissure of the developing eye between the fourth and sixth week of gestation. If the optic nerve or macular area of the retina is involved then vision will be significantly affected. An iris coloboma may or may not be present in association with a visually more important posterior pole colobomas. Colobomas are not treatable.

Practical points

Further important considerations
- Learning difficulties are seldom the result of simple eye problems
- Examine the red reflexes of all infants suspected of having poor vision and all infants with strabismus. An abnormal red reflex in this situation may be due to retinoblastoma and urgent referral is mandatory
- Think glaucoma if a child has one eye that bigger than the other. Then look for co-existing clouding of the cornea and seek history of watery eye and photophobia

---

The eye in paediatric systemic disease

The following is a brief account of the common ocular features of some paediatric systemic diseases.

Extreme prematurity

Marked prematurity gives rise to eye problems by interfering with the orderly development of retinal blood vessels. This disorder is known as retinopathy of prematurity (ROP). Mild ROP is seen in 30–50% of infants weighing less than 1250 g at birth and then regresses without ill effect on vision. In some infants the ROP progresses and a fibrovascular proliferation develops within the eye that detaches the retina, with resultant loss of vision.

Excess oxygen administration to premature infants has been known to be a potent cause of severe ROP since the 1950s. Curtailment of oxygen use to amounts sufficient to limit respiratory and neurological sequelae has greatly reduced the incidence of blinding ROP but has not completely prevented it. In general it is the sicker and smaller infants that are still at risk of severe ROP.

Screening of at-risk infants (birth weight <1250 g) by an ophthalmologist enables detection of significant ROP before retinal detachment occurs. Retinal ablation with laser will then greatly reduce the risk of the development of retinal detachment.

Juvenile chronic arthritis

Childhood chronic arthritis gives rise to inflammation of the iris (iritis or anterior uveitis) in some affected children. Those at particular risk are young girls with oligoarticular juvenile chronic arthritis who are antinuclear antibody positive, although it also occurs in other presentations of juvenile arthritis also. The iritis that occurs in these children is painless and chronic and will, if untreated, often cause cataract and glaucoma. Periodic assessment by an ophthalmologist will detect early iritis and permit treatment to minimize the risk of visual loss.

Down syndrome

Down syndrome is associated with an approximately tenfold increase in the risk of developing eye problems during childhood when compared with the normal incidence. The eye problems are the same as for any child. An increased index of suspicion for eye problems should be maintained for individuals with Down syndrome.

Physical child abuse

Non-accidental injury may involve the eye. Direct trauma to the eye or eyelids will generally be obvious on inspection. Violent shaking of a small child is often associated with the development of retinal haemorrhages and a severe closed brain injury. Although not pathognomonic for child abuse, the presence of retinal haemorrhage is highly suggestive of abuse in cases of unexplained severe brain injury in a young child.

Diabetes mellitus

Diabetes mellitus is common in childhood. However, the duration of diabetes in children is often insufficient for there to be much risk of the development of eye complications during childhood itself. Screening for eye complications should begin at about puberty and occur 2-yearly thereafter if the examination is normal. Significant retinal abnormalities are seen in a small number of diabetic children in mid to late adolescence, particularly if the disease was of early onset and control has been poor.

Disorders of teeth and the oral cavity

N. Kilpatrick

The oral cavity can be considered the gateway to the body. It is the start of the alimentary tract and is integrally involved in the initial phases of digestion. The oral cavity consists of teeth sitting in sockets in the alveolar processes of the maxillary and mandibular bones supported by a fibrous sling known as the periodontal ligament. The oral cavity is lined by a combination of attached gingival tissue (gums) and more generalized mucous membranes. As with the rest of the body, the oral cavity is susceptible to both developmental and acquired disorders that can occur in isolation or as part of more general medical conditions or genetic syndromes.

It is becoming increasingly well recognized that oral health plays a significant role in maintaining good general health and wellbeing. This chapter will, therefore, summarize the key features of normal oral development and highlight the common disorders that affect both the teeth and their supporting structures. It will also identify the oral manifestations of some of the more common paediatric diseases.

Development

Teeth start to form from the 5th week in utero and may continue until the late teens or early 20s with the eruption of the third permanent molars (or wisdom teeth) (Table 22.3.1). The first tooth to erupt is usually the lower central incisor at around 7 months of age. By the age of 2.5 years most children will have a complete primary dentition. consisting of 20 teeth; 8 incisors, 4 canines, 8 molars. At around the age of 6, the primary incisors become mobile and fall out. Most people have 32 permanent teeth, the first of which to erupt is usually the lower first permanent molars at around 6 years of age. The period that follows, referred to as the mixed dentition phase, is highly variable.

Permanent upper incisors are usually more proclined than their predecessors, which allows the mandible to grow forward and encourages the development of what is described as a normal occlusion. This is known as a class I occlusion and while described as 'normal' is actually relatively uncommon, and the development of the permanent dentition is frequently neither well organized nor ideal.

Variations of the norm are common, particularly in the anteroposterior dimension, which causes changes to the relationship between the upper and lower incisors. Cases where the maxilla is forward relative to the mandible and the upper incisors protrude creating an increase in 'overjet' are known as a class II malocclusion. Conversely those cases in which the mandible is relatively prognathic and the upper front teeth develop behind the lower ones the result is a class III malocclusion, or reverse overjet. These malocclusions may result from growth anomalies in either or both jaws and may be further complicated by the pattern of eruption of the dentition, the size of the teeth and other external influences such as thumb sucking. Recognizing malocclusions is not only important in determining the need for and nature of treatment but can also be important in diagnosing growth disorders and in syndrome identification, as jaw discrepancies are common in such conditions.

> **Practical points**
>
> - Eruption times vary widely
> - Providing the sequence of eruption of the teeth is in order (central incisors before lateral incisors, etc.) delays per se are not a cause for concern
> - Asymmetrical eruption, particularly of the permanent incisors, should be reviewed by a dentist in order to check that there is no obstruction (such as an extra tooth) to the eruption of the appropriate tooth
> - The simultaneous presence of primary and permanent teeth during the mixed dentition phase is generally not a problem
> - Premature loss of primary teeth can be a sign of underlying systemic disease and should be reviewed by a paediatric dentist

Developmental anomalies of the soft tissues

There are only a limited number of developmental anomalies that occur in the newborn or very young child. As it is unusual for infants to be seen by a dental health professional, it is important that the medical practitioner examine the oral cavity periodically and refer to a paediatric dentist as appropriate.

Table 22.3.1 A summary of the eruption times for primary and permanent teeth							
Primary dentition (months after birth)							
Central incisors 6–12		Lateral incisors 9–16		Canines 16–23	First molars 13–19		Second molars 23–33
Permanent dentition (years of age)							
Central incisors 6–8	Lateral incisors 6.5–8.5	Canines 9–13	First premolars 9.5–11.5	Second premolars 10–13	First molars 5.5–7.0	Second molars 11–13	Third molars 17+

Congenital epulis

- a benign pedunculated soft tissue tumour on the alveolar ridge, present at birth
- composed of sheets of granular cells
- management is by careful surgical excision
- does not recur.

Oral alveolar developmental cysts (Bohn's nodules)

- multiple 1–5 mm creamy nodules on the outer surface of the alveolar ridges (normally shed in utero)
- composed of epithelial remnants
- sometimes mistaken for prematurely erupting teeth
- similar nodules, found along the palatal midline, are known as Epstein's pearls
- no treatment indicated as the contents discharge spontaneously by 3rd month.

Palatal odontogenic hamartoma

- unilateral or bilateral 3–5 mm dome like swellings adjacent to the midline of the palate behind the incisive papilla
- contain odontogenic epithelium or a developing tooth (demonstrated on occlusal radiograph)
- appear from 8–12 months of age
- managed by elective surgical excision (can be deferred to 12 months of age).

Eruption cyst

- a blue or clear swelling overlying the crown of an erupting tooth, most frequently in the incisor region of the maxilla
- eruption is slightly delayed and discomfort or pain may occur
- management is symptomatic only. Surgical intervention is contraindicated.

Melanotic neuroectodermal tumour of infancy (MNTI)

- very rare solid benign but locally invasive blue-black pigmented tumour
- cells of neural crest origin (two cell types: neuroblasts and black pigment cells)
- tumour cells associated with each primary tooth in one jaw quadrant
- commences in utero and always presents before 3 months age
- management by careful surgical excision, and removal of associated teeth; does not recur if completely removed
- computed tomography essential to locate all individual tumour deposits.

This tumour should not be confused with an eruption cyst or haematoma. It is the only oral lesion that can appear blue-black in this region at this age.

Natal and neonatal teeth

- present at 1 in 3000 births, or erupt in the neonatal period – usually in the mandibular incisor region
- in infants with cleft lip and palate commonly occur high in the cleft
- most are prematurely erupted normal primary teeth, but some may be 'supernumerary' or extra teeth
- can interfere with breast feeding (nipple trauma)
- removal is commonly indicated to alleviate parental anxiety and is simple (using topical local anaesthesia and a haemostat). Parents should be reminded that it is likely that there will be teeth missing in this region until the permanent dentition begins to erupt at around 6 years of age.

Teething

Teething is a normal process by which an infant begins to cut their first teeth (primary dentition). A variety of symptoms can accompany teething, including sensitive and painful gums, mouth ulceration, drooling, feeding difficulties, lack of sleep, fevers, diarrhoea and crying. The scientific evidence that any of these symptoms are directly related to tooth eruption is controversial. Nevertheless, they are commonly reported and can cause significant distress to the child and anxious parent. Similarly there is no evidence base to support any particular management strategy. The use of chilled teething rings, hard, sugar-free rusk biscuits and finger pressure appears to help. Over-the-counter teething preparations are of limited use. Not only do many contain choline salicylate and significant amounts of ethanol and are contra-indicated in very young infants but also repeated use can cause ulceration of the gums. Some lidocaine (lignocaine)-based gels are thought to be slightly more effective and may be mildly antiseptic. Mild elevations in temperature can be managed with systemic oral medication but temperatures of 38°C and higher or other serious symptoms (e.g. convulsions) should not be ascribed to teething and should be assessed independently.

Developmental anomalies of the teeth

Teeth start forming from the 5th week in utero. Any disturbance in metabolism can cause damage to or even the death of the sensitive enamel-forming cells (the ameloblasts). Such a disturbance will leave a permanent developmental defect on the tooth surface that will appear as a loss of tooth substance (hypoplasia) or a deficiency in the quality of the enamel (hypomineralization) once the tooth erupts. By using published tables (or diagrams) of normal tooth development, enamel defects can frequently be related chronologically to:

- prenatal events (usually occurring between the 3rd and 7th month in utero), such as maternal rubella virus or cytomegalovirus (CMV) infection, maternal syphilis and pregnancy toxaemia
- perinatal events: may be prematurity, hypoxia and hyperbilirubinaemia
- postnatal events: measles virus infection, gastrointestinal disease, hypoparathyroidism and administration of tetracycline are some of the over 100 possible aetiological factors capable of inducing developmental defects of tooth enamel.

These defects will be found symmetrically and developmentally chronologically distributed on areas of the tooth crown that were at that particular developmental stage at the time of insult (Fig. 22.3.1). First permanent molars (the so called 6-year-old molars) are particularly susceptible to enamel defects as they are developing at the time of birth. Children with other health issues such as congenital heart disease or cerebral palsy are more likely to have developmental defects of their teeth as a result of systemic illness, fevers, periods of hypoxia, etc., in infancy and early childhood. When isolated defects occur in just one or two permanent teeth they may also be due to infection or trauma of the primary

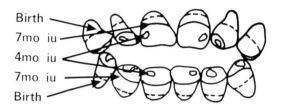

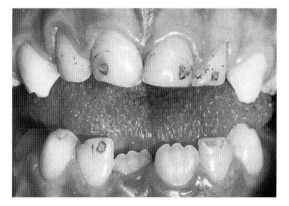

Fig. 22.3.1 Developmental defects of primary tooth enamel at 4 months in utero (iu), 7 months in utero, and birth stages of tooth development.

precursor tooth. Early identification of these defects is important, as the quality of the tooth enamel is compromised and the teeth may be sensitive, particularly to oral hygiene measures, and more likely to develop decay.

Clinical example

Miranda, aged 2 years, had been born normally at term with a normal birth weight. Since then she had demonstrated slow developmental milestones and mild hemiplegia with no obvious cause. Dental examination revealed a caries-free primary dentition, which, however, had chronologically distributed enamel hypoplastic (developmental) defects, affecting the teeth at the 4–7 months in utero stage of development. On questioning, her mother could not recall any major abnormal event during pregnancy; however, the grandmother had recorded in her diary the dates when her daughter had a severe viral infection and was in bed for several days (and she had gone to look after her).

Antibodies to CMV were detected on testing. CMV was the presumptive cause of the enamel defects and possibly also of the mild neurological defect and hemiplegia. This diagnosis helped early planning for future assessment and care. These enamel defects can increase the risk of developing dental caries, as the surface of the teeth are often more porous and retain plaque, and they can be quite sensitive. Such teeth can be protected with a tooth-coloured adhesive material and the parents should be encouraged to assist Miranda with her oral hygiene and to maintain regular dental visits.

Acquired disorders of the teeth

Dental caries

Despite a decline in prevalence worldwide, dental caries (decay) remains one of the most common chronic diseases in childhood. As with many diseases there are considerable inequalities in terms of caries experience throughout the population. In Australia just over 60% of 5-year-old children are caries-free but, of those who do have caries, a mean of three teeth per child are affected. Furthermore 10% of the 4-year-old children who do have caries have more than nine affected teeth. In fact, 80% of all decay is experienced by just 20% of children. It is therefore important to identify children at high risk of developing decay and target them for proactive prevention. Given that very few pre-school-age children get taken to a dental health professional, the responsibility lies with medical and nursing health professionals to identify infants at risk of developing decay and to provide appropriate anticipatory preventive advice.

Dental caries (or decay) is an infectious disease caused by the presence of certain bacteria (predominantly mutans streptococci) in the oral cavity. The mutans streptococci (MS) metabolize sugars and starches to produced acids, which lower the pH of the oral cavity and promote loss of minerals from the tooth surface. Minerals in the oral cavity, including fluoride, are redeposited on the tooth surface once the neutral pH is restored (normally after about 20 minutes). This process is dynamic and as long as minerals are replaced the tooth surface remains sound and intact. If, however, the drop in pH is prolonged and/or frequent there will be a net loss of minerals, leading to a weakening and eventual breakdown (cavitation) of the tooth surface. The early sign of mineral loss is characterized by precavitated or 'white spot' lesions, usually around the necks of the teeth where the MS tend to accumulate in a biofilm (known as dental plaque) on the teeth. Early identification of these precavitated lesions is important as they signal the need for proactive preventive measures to encourage remineralization. Failure to change the oral environment to one that encourages remineralization will result in cavities. If this occurs, then restorations (fillings) are necessary.

Early childhood caries (ECC; historically also referred to as nursing bottle caries, baby bottle decay and many other terms) is a distinct form of dental caries affecting pre-school-age children. ECC is particularly virulent, causing massive destruction to the primary dentition in children as young as 18 months of age. At birth MS do not inhabit the oral cavity; however, the earlier colonization occurs the greater the risk of ECC. The most common source for transmission of MS has been shown to be the primary care giver, usually the mother. Poor maternal oral health coupled with inappropriate feeding behaviours such as prolonged on-demand feeding, particularly through the night, places an infant at high risk of developing ECC. Medical practitioners, paediatricians and maternal child health nurses are all in a strategically good position to identify individuals at risk of developing ECC (Table 22.3.2).

Prevention of dental caries

Strategies to prevent dental caries should start as soon as the first primary teeth erupt (Table 22.3.3).

Fluoride
Fluoride is the single most effective way to protect teeth from decay. It acts in two ways; it can enhance the ability of teeth to resist demineralization caused by intraoral acids and it can also inhibit oral bacterial enzymes to reduce the conversion of sugars in to acids. However, the latter effect is relatively small in comparison to its biochemical modification of the structure of tooth enamel.

Fluoride can be delivered both systemically and topically. Fluoridation of the water supplies allows for both effects. Water ingested during development of the teeth allows fluoride to be incorporated into the developing dental enamel. However, it is as a topical agent that water has its most beneficial effect, as low-dose fluoride comes in to frequent contact with the teeth before being ingested. As such, water fluoridation is considered a very cost-effective public health intervention. However, many homes in rural and remote areas do not enjoy 'town water' and so miss out on the advantages of water fluoridation.

The other common source of fluoride comes in the form of toothpaste. In Australia and New Zealand (and most parts of Europe) there are two common strengths of fluoride toothpaste; most adult toothpastes contain around 1000 ppm (parts per million) fluoride whilst junior toothpastes contain lower concentrations of fluoride, around 400 ppm. The early exposure of primary teeth to fluoridated toothpaste is very effective in preventing caries, as the newly erupted immature tooth surface is highly susceptible to the beneficial maturation effect of fluoride. For most infants a junior toothpaste will be appropriate; however, for those infants at high risk (see Table 23.3.2) exposure to an adult strength toothpaste may be more appropriate. Advice from a paediatric dentist should be sought. The use of additional topical fluoride supplements (tablets or drops) can be of benefit on an individual basis; however, the universal prescription of fluoride supplements is no

Table 22.3.2	The common risk factors for dental caries
Risk factor	Influence
Fluoride exposure	Exposure to fluoridated water source and the regular use of fluoridated toothpaste are two key factors that reduce caries risk
Sugar exposure	Infant feeding habits are very important with frequency of exposure being most relevant. High risk associated with prolonged on-demand night-time feeds
Family oral health history	Poor parental oral health places child at risk of decay as cariogenic bacteria can be transmitted to infants from their primary care giver (usually the mother)
Social and family practices	Poor, indigenous, ethnic and migrant groups have higher levels of dental disease
Medical history	Medically compromised children are more at risk of dental decay the impact of which, on their general health, can be considerable. They are also less likely to receive appropriate treatment
Saliva flow	Children with reduced salivary flow are at significant risk of developing caries as the acids in the oral cavity cannot be diluted, buffered and cleared effectively. Examples of such children are those on certain medications (e.g. anti-depressants, anticholinergics), exposed to radiotherapy or with certain conditions, e.g. Prader Willi and Velocardiofacial Syndrome.

Table 22.3.3	A summary of caries preventive strategies
Fluoride	A smear of toothpaste should be applied regularly to an infant's teeth within 6 months of their eruption For most individuals a junior toothpaste (400 ppm fluoride) will be adequate until about the age of 5–6. However, for children with additional risk factors, an adult toothpaste may be more appropriate Teeth should be brushed twice a day with nothing to eat or drink after the night-time brushing Parents should supervise toothbrushing until around 8 years of age The use of additional topical fluoride supplements (tablets or drops) can be of benefit to a few individuals but should be prescribed by an appropriate dental professional
Diet	Reduce the total amount and frequency of intake of sugary foods and drinks Avoid on-demand feeding through the night Limit sugary snacks to meal times, when salivary flow is optimal Avoid sugary snacks close to bedtime Increase water intake
Dental attendance	Parents should be encouraged to take their infant to a dental professional within 6 months of the eruption of their first teeth Regular monitoring by a dental professional should continue in to adulthood
Remineralizing products	Products containing calcium phosphopeptides, e.g. Tooth Mousse (GC Corporation, Itabashi-ku, Tokyo, Japan), are available through dental practitioners. These promote remineralization of early carious lesions

longer recommended and advice should be sought from an appropriate dental professional.

Diet
In addition to encouraging optimal exposure to fluoride, providing advice on healthy dietary practices that reduce the length of time that the oral cavity spends with an acidic demineralizing pH will also reduce the risk of caries. At all ages, trying to reduce both the total amount and frequency of intake of sugary foods and drinks is important. For infants only milk, formula or water should be put in the nursing bottle and on-demand nocturnal feeding should be discouraged. In particular, children put to

bed and allowed to sleep with a nursing bottle are likely to develop decay. As children get older, encouraging water drinking and limiting sugary snacks/drinks to meal times when salivary flow is optimal will optimize the buffering capacity of the oral cavity.

Remineralization products

Recently new products have been developed that contain casein phosphopeptide–amorphous calcium phosphate (CPP-ACP). These products, either as a chewing gum (Recaldent, Cadbury Japan Limited, Adams Division) or as topical cream (Tooth Mousse, GC Corporation, Itabashi-ku, Tokyo, Japan) act as a reservoir for calcium phosphate, maintaining a state of supersaturation around the tooth with respect to calcium and phosphate thereby depressing the demineralization of tooth tissue and promoting its remineralization. These products can be used in conjunction with fluoride products such as toothpaste as they act synergistically to promote remineralization in the oral cavity. With the exception of being contraindicated in individuals with milk protein allergy, they are safe and effective. These products are currently only available through dental surgery outlets but are being increasingly used, particularly in individuals who continue to develop caries despite optimal fluoride exposure.

Fluorosis

High serum levels of fluoride can produce a developmental abnormality of enamel maturation known as fluorosis. Mild cases usually appear clinically, as a white flecking or linear opacity of the enamel. Mild fluorosis is sometimes difficult to distinguish from developmental defects of enamel arising from other causes. The use of low-fluoride (440 ppm fluoride) junior toothpastes and the very cautious use of systemic supplementation reduce the risks of fluorosis. When recommending fluoride strategies, the risks of developing fluorosis (which can potentially create relatively minor aesthetic challenges in the permanent dentition) need to be weighed against the risk of developing dental caries and all its potential sequelae. Discussion between a paediatric dentist and the family is important in order to optimize prevention but reduce unwanted side effects.

Dental abscesses

If dental caries is undiagnosed, untreated or treated inappropriately it can cause pain, systemic infection and abscesses. Once the bacterial acids have caused breakdown of the tooth surface, the cavity becomes colonized with a range of microorganisms. If left,

these will penetrate through the tooth to the pulp (or nerve), prompting a characteristic inflammatory reaction, a component of which is pain. Initially, the inflammation is reversible, the pain is sporadic and occurs only in response to stimuli such as changes in temperature. However, as the process continues the inflammation becomes irreversible, the pulp necroses and becomes colonized by bacteria and an abscess forms.

In the primary dentition an abscess can be superficial, pointing beneath the gum usually on the cheek side of the tooth and is often relatively painless. Alternatively and more seriously, an infection from a necrosed tooth can spread in to the deeper soft tissue planes and lymph nodes. Cellulitis is accompanied by systemic illness, high fever, facial swelling and often limited mouth opening. In the upper jaw this can cause closure of the eye while in the lower jaw can compromise the airway as the submandibular and sublingual spaces become involved. This is more common with an abscessed permanent molar tooth as the roots are located deep in the alveolar process of the mandible. In most cases a simple clinical examination will identify the affected tooth; however, a panoral radiograph is useful to confirm the diagnosis. Once antibiotic control has been established the involved tooth should be extracted as soon as possible (often under general anaesthesia).

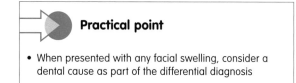

Practical point

- When presented with any facial swelling, consider a dental cause as part of the differential diagnosis

Trauma

Up to one-third of children will experience some sort of injury to either their primary or permanent teeth. The peak ages are between 18 months and 3 years when infants are learning to walk and prone to falling and again in early teens when boys in particular are participating in more adventurous games and sports. Most injuries in children are accidental in nature, as opposed to adults, where fights and traffic accidents are not uncommon.

Dental injuries can affect the teeth, bone and soft tissues or any combination of the three, with injuries to the teeth and lacerations of the tongue and lips being the most common. Jaw fractures are relatively uncommon in children and are not covered further here.

Clinical example

Jimmy, aged 3 years and 6 months, presented with his mother because he had been crying when he ate or drank at the day-care centre. Recently his mother had noticed that he sometimes woke up at night crying because of the pain in his mouth. On being asked about his health his mother reported that he had seen a heart doctor at the children's hospital because he had a 'hole in the heart' and she had been told that he would need an antibiotic if he 'had to have his teeth out'. She also acknowledged that Jimmy still took a bottle of milk to bed at night and that she sometimes put a little of his favourite chocolate powder in the milk to help him sleep.

Oral examination confirmed the presence of early childhood dental caries, with extensive decay involving the incisor teeth in both upper and lower jaws as well as the upper first primary molars and some white areas of early enamel demineralization on the recently erupted second molars. In addition, Jimmy's gums were slightly inflamed and there were widespread deposits of white, furry plaque over this teeth and gums.

From the history of spontaneous pain particularly at night it was apparent that the decay was well advanced and involved the nerve (pulp) of at least some of the teeth. The presence of generalized plaque deposits around the teeth and gums suggested that toothbrushing did not happen regularly, if at all. In addition to posing a risk of bacteraemia (and hence for endocarditis in Jimmy, who has a pre-existing cardiac history) the presence of gingivitis also suggested that Jimmy was not receiving the optimum benefits to be gained from regular topical fluoride (toothpaste) exposure.

Management was in two stages. First, the immediate relief of pain and elimination of infection was achieved through the removal of all pulpally involved teeth and restoration of non-pulpally involved teeth. This was completed under general anaesthesia (because of Jimmy's age and the extent of the treatment to be carried out) with an appropriate antibiotic cover of amoxicillin given at the time of anaesthetic induction. Second, proactive preventive advice was provided at the follow-up outpatient appointment. This advice included recommending (and demonstrating) toothbrushing using a fluoridated junior toothpaste, to be done by Jimmy's mother twice a day, at the same time ceasing immediately the night time use of the infant feeding bottle. Finally, information was provided to Jimmy's mother on the particular importance of good oral health for people with congenital heart disease.

Oral health for children who have other healthcare needs is often not high on the list of parental priorities. Close cooperation is necessary between doctors, paediatricians and paediatric dentists to assist parents of such children in appreciating the importance of oral health for their child and providing advice on how to minimize potential future problems. It is never too early to start to talk about teeth.

Primary dentition

Injuries to the primary dentition most commonly involve displacement of the upper primary incisors from their sockets with or without some soft tissue lacerations. In general infants are very resilient and parents are often more stressed than the affected child.

Injury to the primary teeth can, in some instances, affect the development of the underlying permanent successor. Primary teeth are never reimplanted as this too can have a detrimental affect on the permanent successor, however, parents can be reassured that early loss of primary incisors has no lasting effecting on speech, function or appearance.

Practical points

- Check that there are no other signs of injury such as limb fractures or head injury
- Refer to an appropriate dental professional
- If the displacement is mild and not affecting function (i.e. the child can bring their teeth together) regular monitoring may be appropriate
- If the tooth is more severely displaced, it should be removed, either under local or general anaesthesia depending on the age of the child and nature of the injury
- An avulsed primary is never repositioned

Permanent dentition

Injuries to the permanent dentition range from a small tooth fracture, to complete loss (avulsion) of multiple teeth and significant soft tissue lacerations. Injuries to the permanent dentition are often missed or incorrectly diagnosed. Appropriate emergency management of traumatized teeth impacts significantly on the ultimate outcome of the injury.

Unless replaced immediately the long-term prognosis for an avulsed permanent tooth is guarded. Given that this rarely occurs, the avulsed tooth should be handled as little as possible and stored in milk. The child should be referred immediately by telephone to an appropriate dental provider. Direct contact with the dentist will ensure that s/he is prepared to accept the child for treatment, thus avoiding further delays. In many instances this will be a paediatric dentist or hospital-based dental unit. Dental management of displaced teeth usually involves repositioning accompanied by placement of a thin wire splint bonded to the affected and some unaffected teeth to stabilize the injury for several days. In some cases further endodontic (root canal) therapy may be required and treatment can continue for many years after the initial injury. In many cases the prognosis for retaining traumatized teeth in the long term is very good. However, avulsion and severe intrusion injuries, particularly those with additional bony fractures, do not have a good prognosis in the long term. The aim of treatment in these cases is to retain a child's natural teeth through adolescence so that once growth is complete a permanent prosthetic replacement of the compromised teeth can be considered.

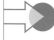

Practical points

- All injuries should be carefully examined intraorally
- Ideally, an avulsed permanent tooth should be repositioned immediately
- Irrespective of the degree of seriousness of the injury, trauma to the permanent dentition should be referred promptly (by telephone) to a willing dental professional

---

Non-accidental injury

Orofacial trauma is present in 50% of reported cases of child abuse. Bruising and laceration of lips and alveolar mucosa, damage to teeth, alveolar bone fractures, finger and bite marks on face and neck are all frequent signs of child abuse. These result from slapping, punching, hand over mouth, forcible feeding with spoon or fork and forcible intrusion or removal of a feeding bottle, dummy or toy from the mouth. Tears to the upper midline frenum in pre-ambulatory infants are highly suspicious and oral bruising and palatal contusion can be seen in cases of sexual abuse. Oral signs should not be neglected when considering the possibility of child abuse and an intraoral examination should form part of routine surveillance. (See also Ch. 3.9.)

Riga–Fédé ulceration

A Riga–Fédé ulcer is an ulcer that develops on the underside of the tongue. It is most common in infants with significant intellectual impairment or those with sensory deficits such as Riley–Day syndrome who continually rub the tongue backward and forward over the sharp edges of the lower incisor teeth. In some cases these ulcers interfere with feeding and become infected. Conservative management, covering the lower incisors with a small bonded splint, can be successful in allowing healing. If not then removal of the appropriate teeth is required.

Dental erosion

Dental erosion is defined as a chronic localized loss of dental hard tissue chemically etched away from the tooth surface without bacterial involvement (which differentiates it from caries, which is bacterial in aetiology). Many young children show wear of their primary incisors but more worrying is the fact that up to one-third of adolescents have significant wear of their permanent teeth as well. The appearance of erosive tooth wear is quite characteristic but possibly a little difficult for most non-dental professionals to diagnose. There is a general loss of lustre from the surface enamel, thinning and chipping of the upper incisors and there may be smooth exposed dentine, pulpal exposure and sensitivity.

As with dental caries the aetiology is multifactorial but is associated with an increase exposure of the teeth to acid (Table 22.3.4). These non-bacterial acids may be extrinsic (essentially dietary) or intrinsic (from the gastric tract).

Given the high prevalence of asthma, particularly in Australia and New Zealand, a suggested association between it and dental erosion is of note. This association appears to be more of a problem in adults than children, and one large study in children showed no such association. There are theoretical reasons

Table 22.3.4 The potential sources of acid responsible for dental erosion

Extrinsic	Intrinsic
Dietary Citrus fruits and juice Carbonated drinks (including 'diet' products) Sports drinks Wine	**Gastric reflux** Cerebral palsy Dysphagia Gastro-oesophageal reflux
Environmental/occupational Swimming (poorly regulated pool water) Nutrition regimes for elite athletes	**Eating disorders** Bulimia nervosa
Lifestyle Recreational drugs	**Rumination**
Medications Topical effect – aspirin, vitamin C, phenylketonuria supplements, nebulized asthma medications (although this is controversial, and probably a minor problem more likely to affect adults) Systemic effect on saliva – antidepressants, anticholinergics Some mouthwashes	

Table 22.3.5	Strategies to prevent dental erosion
Reducing acid exposure	Inform patients of types of foods and drinks that have greatest erosive potential Consumption of still/non-carbonated drinks as an alternative Limiting the intake of acidic foods/drinks to meal times Advocate consumption of a neutral food, e.g. cheese, immediately after a meal Rinsing mouth out after acid exposure, i.e. after an episode of vomiting, but delaying brushing teeth immediately after the exposure as this increases wear of tooth tissue.
Optimizing salivary function	Increased water intake Use of water bottles in school bags Advise use of sugar-free chewing gum to enhance salivary flow.
Enhancing resistance to erosion	Suitable products include: neutral fluoride mouthwashes, Recaldent chewing gum and Tooth Mousse (Cadbury Japan Limited)
Adams Division; GC Corporation Itabashi.ku, Tokyo, Japan	

that this might occur, e.g. chronic mouth breathing from associated allergic rhinitis leading to mouth dryness; higher incidence of gastro-oesophageal reflux, which may result in more acid in the oral cavity; an acidic base to some nebulizer solutions.

Children with dysphagia and other conditions associated with abnormal muscle tone tend to have more gastric reflux and are more likely to have dental erosion. In addition, those children with muscle spasticity tend to grind their teeth, which, superimposed upon the softening caused by acidic erosion, can lead to rapid tooth tissue loss.

The role of the medical practitioner in managing dental erosion is to be aware of the risk factors, to provide generic preventive advice (Table 22.3.5) and refer the child to a dentist for ongoing monitoring. If caught early enough, little active dental treatment will be required; however, if significant tooth tissue loss occurs in the young permanent dentition then pain and aesthetic considerations may mean that restorative treatment is required.

Practical point

- Any child with a history of gastric reflux should be counselled as to the potential for erosive tooth tissue loss and advised to seek dental review

Acquired disorders of the soft tissues

Bleeding gums

Gingivitis is the most common cause of bleeding gums. Gingivitis is a non-specific inflammation of the gingival tissues (gums) that reflects the bacterial challenge to the host when dental plaque accumulates. Dental plaque is a complex biofilm that starts to accumulate around the teeth immediately after toothbrushing. It consists of 70% microorganisms and 30% food debris and if brushing is ineffective the gums mount a subclinical inflammatory response within 2 days that will become clinically apparent by 10 days. The characteristic signs of chronic gingivitis include red inflamed gums that bleed when brushed and that can deteriorate to a point where there is bleeding on eating and, in some cases, even spontaneous bleeding. Gingivitis is relatively easily reversed with appropriate oral hygiene practices to remove the plaque.

If left untreated, gingivitis may progress to periodontitis, in which the inflammatory response becomes more destructive within the underlying supporting tissues. This can lead to significant bone loss around the teeth, which become mobile and may ultimately be lost. There is a high degree of individual susceptibility to periodontal disease, with certain subgroups, e.g. individuals with Down syndrome, being particularly prone to destructive periodontal disease. Fortunately, with the exception of some specific conditions, e.g. Ehlers–Danlos syndrome, and individuals with cyclic neutropenia children and adolescents do not experience significant periodontal disease.

Non-plaque-related causes of bleeding gums include; local trauma, exfoliating teeth, hormonal changes, e.g. puberty, underlying haematological conditions, e.g. leukaemia, and some drugs, e.g. cytotoxics and anticoagulants.

Oral ulceration

Ulceration of the oral cavity is often a sign of underlying systemic disease and if so treatment of the oral lesions will be essentially symptomatic whilst the underlying disorder should obviously be attended to appropriately.

A careful history and examination should be completed in order to assist with the diagnosis.

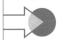

Practical points

In a child with oral ulcers take a good history of:
- general health status, including appetite, weight loss, fever
- the ulcers, including frequency, position, duration, stimuli

Complete a thorough examination of:
- general health, including appearance, weight, psychological state, signs of inflammatory bowel disease
- oral cavity, including location, size, appearance, obvious traumatic aetiology

Useful special tests:
- full blood screen, full blood count, erythrocyte sedimentation ratio, iron, serum B_{12}, folate, antibody screen for coeliac disease

Infections

The most common oral infection seen in children is primary herpetic gingivostomatitis. The signs are of a systemic viral infection with fever, lassitude, lack of appetite and very sore oral cavity with characteristic painful ulcerated gingival tissues as well as occasional ulcers on the tongue and buccal mucosa. Other viral infections can involve the oral cavity including hand, foot and mouth disease and chicken pox.

Treatment
Treatment is symptomatic, involving fluids and analgesia and encouraging the parents to maintain oral hygiene although this can be difficult when the mouth is very sore (Ch. 14.1).

Trauma

Single ulcers located in specific sites around the oral cavity can be caused by both physical or chemical trauma. Use of a toothpick to relieve food packing between teeth can cause ulceration interdentally while the placement of an aspirin tablet directly on to the buccal gum in order to relieve toothache has been known to produce a nasty chemical ulcer. In most cases of a traumatic ulcer, the aetiology will be relatively clear; however, it is important to bear in mind the possibility of self-inflicted injury. Particularly in instances of apparently random and repeated episodes of traumatic ulceration, there may be an associated condition involving insensitivity to pain, such as Riley–Day syndrome.

Treatment
The elimination of the irritant, e.g. a fractured filling, poorly contoured orthodontic appliance, or cessation of the injurious behaviour.

Aphthous ulcers

In many situations an obvious aetiology is not forthcoming. These are referred to as aphthous ulcers. Fortunately, they are relatively uncommon in children, as they are difficult to treat. They are noninfective, extremely painful ulcers occurring most commonly on the labial and buccal mucosa and tongue borders. A prodromal burning sensation precedes breakdown of an initially white papule to form an ulcer with a crateriform base that heals slowly over 8–10 days. Aphthous ulcers may be of minor or major type and are often associated with stress; however, they may also be associated with an underlying iron or folate deficiency. They may be recurrent and associated with menstruation in adolescent girls.

Treatment
Aphthous ulcers are difficult to manage and treatment is rarely totally successful. Chlorhexidine gluconate or a tetracycline/nystatin combination mouthrinse along with diligent toothbrushing helps to relieve pain and control secondary infection. Other strategies for aphthae include topical anaesthetics, systemic analgesics and topical antiinflammatories, including steroids. However, these medications will at best reduce the duration of the ulcer experience rather than cure it.

Haematological

Children suffering from an underlying haematological disorder, including neutropenia and leukaemia, can experience oral ulceration. Children with leukaemia may present initially with bleeding gums in the absence of poor oral hygiene. Ulceration accompanied by mucositis and secondary infection is also common as a sequel to chemotherapy. Those with cyclic neutropenia in particular experience cyclical bouts of severe gingivitis accompanied by significant periodontal bone loss resulting in premature loss of both primary and later permanent teeth. Children with this condition need regular review and management by a paediatric dentist or periodontist in order to try and retard the process.

Gastrointestinal

As the oral cavity is the start of the gastrointestinal tract it is unsurprising that disorders affecting the rest of the tract can affect the mouth. Individuals with inflammatory bowel diseases, Crohn disease and ulcerative colitis (Chs 20.2 and 20.3) may experience oral ulceration. In addition, those with Crohn disease can have other significant oral manifestations, often described as orofacial granulomatosis, including:

- marked lip enlargement, together with enlargement of the buccal mucosa
- mucosal erythematous granulomatosis in the anterior regions of the maxilla
- large, linear ulceration in the buccal sulci posteriorly.

These oral findings can occur on their own or together with anal fissuring, genital swelling and gastrointestinal changes.

In patients with coeliac disease, a higher incidence of recurrent aphthous ulceration has been suggested but not proved. Such patients may also have dental enamel defects in the permanent teeth.

Treatment
If there are any concerns about gastric symptoms, e.g. weight loss, blood in the stools, the child should be referred to a paediatric gastroenterologist and paediatric dentist for a combined evaluation.

Dermatological

Oral ulcers occur in many of the rarer dermatological conditions such as epidermolysis bullosa, pemphigus and pemphigoid. However, these conditions are usually diagnosed from their more general manifestations rather than from their oral symptoms.

Malignancy

Oral malignancy is rare in children; however, single persistent, large ulcers that have no obvious traumatic aetiology nor are associated with acute systemic illness should be viewed with suspicion and referred for investigation to a paediatric dentist/maxillofacial surgeon.

Gingival swelling

Swelling of the gingival tissues can be congenital or acquired; however, the former are relatively rare. Individuals with any of the mucopolysaccharidosis disorders may have very enlarged gums, often to the extent that teeth fail to erupt or are ectopically displaced. Similar disruption to the developing dentition can occur in individuals with vascular anomalies such as a lymphangioma, which may affect both soft and hard tissues of the jaws.

Of the acquired causes of gum enlargement, drugs are most commonly implicated, specifically the anti-seizure medication phenytoin and the immunosuppressant cyclosporin A. The latter has been widely used in organ transplant protocols and in children has caused significant aesthetic and psychological problems as the gums enlarge in an unsightly fashion and teeth fail to erupt or are covered in excess gum

tissue. The advent of tacrolimus as an alternative to cyclosporin A has improved the quality of life for these children significantly by reducing not only the gum overgrowth but also the hirsutism. Most of the enlargement resolves once the causative drug, be it phenytoin or cyclosporin A, is ceased. Other more localized swellings of the gingival tissues include giant cell granuloma, histiocytosis and lymphoma and, while rare, such swellings are of obvious clinical significance and should be reviewed by a paediatric dentist.

Children with special healthcare needs

Children with significant medical conditions, developmental disabilities and craniofacial disorders face multiple health issues, among which is often an increased risk of dental disease coupled with barriers in accessing appropriate dental services. Given that many dental problems are relatively simple to prevent and manage if diagnosed early, close collaboration between the general health-care professional (medical practitioner, paediatrician or nurse) and the dental profession is essential. Identifying an appropriate 'dental home' for children with special health-care needs is important so that these complex children have access to timely and appropriate oral health-care. Many general dentists are not comfortable managing children with special health-care needs, whereas paediatric dentists are trained specifically in this area. Establishing a close collaboration between medical and dental clinicians not only optimizes the child's oral health but significantly improves their general health and wellbeing as well as reducing the need for extensive, costly and burdensome dental treatment.

Medications

Many children with special healthcare needs are on multiple medications for prolonged periods of time. With the exceptions of the anticonvulsant phenytoin, the immunosuppressant cyclosporin and nifedipine, all of which cause gingival overgrowth, very few drugs directly affect the oral tissues. However, there is an increased risk of developing caries associated with the long term use of sugar-based liquid medications. As many of the common liquid medications are over-the-counter formulations, parents should be warned to check that, where possible, they purchase a sugar-free brand of medication such as cough linctus or analgesic.

While the evidence regarding the impact of asthma, and its treatment, on oral health is weak (see Dental erosion, above), nevertheless, ensuring that all children are registered with a dentist who is familiar with their general health issues will optimize their general wellbeing.

Congenital heart disease

Parents of infants diagnosed with a congenital heart anomaly should be provided with clear information regarding the implications of oral health on the general health of their child. Parental information sheets exist in most paediatric units to provide information and advice (http://www.rch.org.au/emplibrary/cardiology/dentalheart.pdf). Despite a lack of convincing evidence that dental disease and/or its treatment actually does cause bacterial endocarditis, proactive prevention (to minimize disease experience) and prophylactic antibiotic cover for any dental procedure that is likely to cause bleeding is still considered best practice (Ch. 15.2). Many parents are confused as to whether their child has a significant structural heart anomaly and whether they really do need antibiotic cover. When taking their child to a dental professional, parents should be provided with written confirmation of their cardiac status together with a clear indication of the risk of endocarditis and the need for prophylaxis endorsed by their cardiologist. This will facilitate the smooth provision of appropriate dental care and minimize the unnecessary prescription of antibiotics.

> ### Practical points
>
> - Every child with a special health-care need should have a regular dentist familiar with the implications of their medical history
> - Good communication between paediatricians and paediatric dentists will optimize health outcomes for individuals and their families
> - The specific prescription for sugar-free alternatives should be part of routine clinical practice
> - Parents of children with a congenital heart defect should be provided with written confirmation of their child's cardiac status with respect to endocarditis
> - Standard protocols for prophylactic antibiotic cover should be followed when a child with a significant congenital heart defect requires any invasive dental procedures. The protocols can be accessed at: http://www.rch.org.au/cardiology/health-info.cfm

Index